Bailey & Scott's **Diagnostic Microbiology**

Bailey & Scott's

Diagnostic Microbiology

Ellen Jo Baron

Ph.D., Diplomate (ABMM)

Adjunct Assistant Professor of Medicine
University of California School of Medicine
Los Angeles, California

Sydney M. Finegold

MD., SM(AAM), Diplomate (ABMM)

Associate Chief of Staff for Research and Development
Wadsworth V.A. Medical Center
Professor of Medicine and of Microbiology and Immunology
University of California School of Medicine
Los Angeles, California

EIGHTH EDITION

with 313 color illustrations

The C. V. Mosby Company

ST. LOUIS • BALTIMORE • PHILADELPHIA • TORONTO   1990

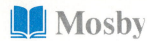

Editor: Stephanie Manning
Assistant Editor: Anne Gunter
Design: Rey Umali
Editing and Production: CRACOM Corporation

EIGHTH EDITION

The C. V. Mosby Company
11830 Westline Industrial Drive, St. Louis, Missouri 63146

Library of Congress Cataloging-in-Publication Data

Baron, Ellen Jo.
 Bailey and Scott's diagnostic microbiology. —8th ed./Ellen Jo
Baron, Sydney M. Finegold.
  p. cm.
 Rev. ed. of: Baily and Scott's diagnostic microbiology. 7th ed./
Sydney M. Finegold, Ellen Jo Baron. 1986.
 Includes bibliographical references.
 ISBN 0-8016-0344-7
 1. Diagnostic microbiology. I. Bailey, W. Robert (William
Robert), 1917- Diagnostic microbiology. II. Finegold, Sydney, M.,
1921-   III. Title. IV. Title: Diagnostic microbiology.
 [DNLM: 1. Microbiological Technics. QW 25 B265b]
QR67.B37 1990
616'.01'028—dc20
DNLM/DLC
for Library of Congress   89-13698
               CIP

GW/VH/VH 9 8 7 6 5 4 3 2 1

To
James C. Taylor,
Alma and Lee Baron,
and **Mary L. Finegold**
with loving appreciation for
their constant guidance
and continued understanding
again

Contributors

CHAPTER AUTHORS

O. George W. Berlin, Ph.D., M.A., MT(ASCP)
Clinical Microbiology Laboratory, Medical Center, University of California—Los Angeles

W. Lawrence Drew, M.D., Ph.D.
Department of Microbiology and Infectious Diseases, Mount Zion Hospital and Medical Center, San Francisco, California; University of California—San Francisco

Martha A.C. Edelstein, B.A., MT(ASCP)
Clinical Microbiology Laboratory, Hospital of the University of Pennsylvania, Philadelphia

Lynne Shore Garcia, M.S., CLS(NCA), MT(ASCP)
Clinical Microbiology Laboratory, Medical Center, University of California—Los Angeles

Glenn D. Roberts, Ph.D.
Department of Laboratory Medicine, Section of Clinical Microbiology, Mayo Medical School, Mayo Clinic and Mayo Foundation, Rochester, Minnesota

CHAPTER CONSULTANTS

Richard R. Facklam, Ph.D.
Respiratory and Special Pathogens Laboratory Branch, Centers for Disease Control, Atlanta, Georgia

Gerald L. Gilardi, Ph.D.

Department of Microbiology,
North General Hospital, New York, New York

Janet A. Hindler, M.S., MT(ASCP)

Clinical Microbiology Laboratory, Medical Center,
University of California—Los Angeles

J. Michael Janda, Ph.D.

Microbiology Diseases Laboratory,
California Department of Health Services,
Berkeley, California

Michael Pfaller, M.D.

Veterans Administration Medical Center;
Department of Pathology, University of Iowa
College of Medicine, Iowa City, Iowa

Ella M. Swierkosz, Ph.D.

Department of Diagnostic Microbiology and
Virology, Cardinal Glennon Children's Hospital;
St. Louis University School of Medicine,
St. Louis, Missouri.

Preface

Diagnostic Microbiology presents a comprehensive view of medical microbiology from the standpoints of the organization and function of a clinical microbiology laboratory (Part One), likely agents associated with infectious syndromes (Part Three), and procedures for identification and susceptibility testing of infecting agents (Parts Two and Four). Reviews of the previous edition suggested that *Diagnostic Microbiology* is valuable as a textbook for students of medical technology, medical microbiology, pathology, infectious diseases, and infection control and as a laboratory reference manual and procedure book. We have strived to maintain that focus.

We welcome the continued participation of W. Lawrence Drew (virology), Martha A. C. Edelstein (anaerobes), Lynne Shore Garcia (parasitology), and Glenn D. Roberts (mycology), whose authoritative chapters add so much to the book. We have also received able assistance from several new contributors, George Berlin (mycobacteriology), Michael Pfaller (non-spore-forming, gram-positive bacilli), and Ella Swierkosz (chlamydiae), who helped to provide the updated information presented in this edition.

Certain chapters were evaluated extensively by Gerald Gilardi, Janet Hindler, J. Michael Janda, Richard Facklam, and Maurice White. Henry Isenberg's suggestions are always valuable. Several of the new photographs were taken by Peter Rose. We are grateful for their expert contributions. Stephanie Manning at Mosby and Mary Espenschied at CRACOM have been able editors, and we appreciate their support and expertise. As always, we welcome input from our readers, many of whom helped us to correct errors and modify topics that were presented in the seventh edition.

The eighth edition continues the format introduced in the seventh edition, with chapter outlines listed at the beginning of each chapter. The major format change is the introduction of full color throughout, which allows all illustrations to be placed adjacent to their corresponding text. Procedures, still presented in boxes on one page or facing pages, now include a statement of the principle of the test, quality control guidelines, expected results, and performance schedule recommendations, in addition to the method itself. Chapter 4 has been retitled to reflect its current content, which has been expanded to include material on laboratory manage-

ment and test selection. Of course, the entire book has been updated, and new identification tables have been added in certain areas. We urge readers to peruse How to Use This Book, p. xi, which explains the organization of the text and outlines the content.

The importance of microbiology continues to expand in this era of new infectious agents and difficult-to-manage infections. Although there is a definite trend toward automation and newer techniques, such as DNA probes, there will always be a place for conventional microbiology and for competent microbiologists.

Ellen Jo Baron
Sydney M. Finegold

How To Use
This Book

The organization of the seventh edition of this book has been retained. Part One contains material of general importance to the practice of diagnostic clinical microbiology, including laboratory safety, quality assurance, and laboratory management, as well as the role of the microbiology laboratory in infection control and epidemiologic studies. Part Two encompasses methods for specimen handling, initial observations, and procedures used to detect agents of infectious diseases. New technologies, automation, and immunologic methods are included in this section, as are methods for susceptibility testing. The pathogenesis of infectious diseases in relation to the site of infection or the organ system involved is covered in Part Three, which highlights the agents likely to be recovered from each body site or syndrome. Part Four details methods for detection and identification of specific infectious agents.

Each chapter begins with an outline of the sections within to facilitate finding a particular area and to provide a quick overview of the contents. Reference material has been reorganized into three appendixes and the glossary. Appendix A contains formulas for media and reagents, Appendix B contains formulas for commonly used stains, and Appendix C lists the names and addresses of commercial product suppliers, whose names are simply mentioned in parentheses in the text when they are cited. Even companies not cited specifically in the book are listed; Appendix C should be a valuable resource for laboratory managers. The Glossary has been expanded to include numerous new terms and the abbreviations used throughout the text are incorporated alphabetically into the Glossary. The use of boldface type in the text identifies all terms that have been defined in the Glossary.

Contents

Bailey & Scott's Diagnostic
Microbiology

Part One

Organization and Function
of the Clinical Microbiology
Laboratory

1 Diagnostic Microbiology: Purpose and Philosophy

Clinical microbiologists are part of the health team and serve an important role in the diagnosis, management, and prevention of infections in patients. Microbiologists should take pride in this role and should feel responsibility commensurate with it.

1.1. Purpose of Diagnostic Microbiology

The purpose of clinical microbiology is to work closely with clinicians and other health team members to provide diagnosis and optimum management of infectious disease in patients and to prevent the spread of infection to other individuals. In general, it is important to document the presence of infection, to determine its specific nature, and to provide appropriate therapy early in the course of the illness. Early diagnosis and treatment are usually more urgent with infectious diseases than with any other type of disease process. In many infections, speedy treatment is crucial. Both mortality and morbidity may be reduced significantly if proper treatment is provided early. In others, hospitalization may be avoided or shortened and surgery may be avoided if specific antimicrobial therapy is provided early. While the responsibility is large, the satisfaction that may be achieved in successfully diagnosing and treating patients with infectious diseases can be great. It is very gratifying to see rapid improvement in a critically ill patient; all members of the health team share in this gratification.

1.2. Responsibility to the Clinician and to the Patient

Microbiology laboratory service must be available at all times. This means that microbiologists must be

3

on call if it is not reasonable to have the laboratory staffed at all times. Others may be able to set up certain types of specimens in the absence of the microbiologist, but the expertise of the microbiologist may be required to properly interpret a Gram stain or colonial morphology late at night. In assessing early findings, one should provide as much detail as possible and one should not hesitate to indicate the various possibilities as to the microbiological diagnosis. The clinician sets up his or her own differential diagnosis based on the clinical picture, roentgenograms, blood studies, and so on. The diagnostic possibilities, as seen by a competent microbiologist, are of paramount importance to the clinician in further narrowing down or substantiating a diagnosis. The microbiologist must be alert to unusual findings. As suggested earlier, speed is critical in serious illness caused by infectious agents. Good microbiologists can usually find one or more ways to expedite presumptive identification of microorganisms in clinical specimens. If the health team is to function with maximum efficiency, the members of that team must communicate freely and frequently, particularly when dealing with seriously ill patients. The physician should lead in this respect, but if he or she does not, the others on the team should initiate communication when it may be helpful. Our primary concern always must be the patient. The clinician should supply the microbiologist with pertinent historical and other data regarding the patient's illness; the microbiologist should be able to utilize this information.

The microbiologist can also be of service to the clinician by instructing him or her concerning the importance of proper specimen collection and transport and regarding specific techniques to be used. An interested physician can be taught how to judge the quality of a sputum specimen and how to interpret a Gram stain properly.

Microbiologists also have a responsibility to notify infection control personnel or epidemiologists and public health authorities. Urgent matters should be communicated by telephone.

The microbiologist also has an obligation to the patient aside from considerations of rapid, accurate diagnosis. Professionalism demands that microbiologists, as well as other members of the health team, not hesitate to deal with certain specimens or patients and that they respect the patient's rights and feelings with regard to sensitive information. At times the microbiologist may be pressured to release

information on a patient to the patient, his or her family, or others; such pressure must be resisted. Demands of this nature should be referred to the physician.

1.3. Specimen Collection and Transport

Specimen collection and transportation are urgent considerations because the quality of a laboratory's work may be limited by the nature of a specimen and its condition on arrival in the laboratory. Chapter 6 includes a detailed discussion of correct collection and transportation methods.

Specimens should be obtained so as to preclude or minimize the possibility of introducing extraneous microorganisms that are not involved in the infectious process. The problem is greatest when the specimen may become contaminated with elements of the normal (or colonizing) flora that may serve as pathogens in the entity being studied (e.g., *Klebsiella* as an oral cavity colonizer in a patient with pneumonia). Even normally sterile body fluids may be contaminated during specimen collection in such a way as to cause significant difficulty in interpretation. For example, a patient suspected of having bacterial endocarditis, although he does not really have the disease, has one or more blood cultures that have become contaminated with coagulase-negative staphylococci during venipuncture. Since this organism can cause endocarditis in numerous clinical settings, this patient's contaminated cultures may lead to additional testing, administration of unnecessary antibiotics, and a prolonged hospital stay for the patient. Careful skin preparation before procedures such as blood cultures and spinal taps and techniques for bypassing areas of normal flora when this is important and feasible (e.g., percutaneous transtracheal aspiration in critically ill patients with pneumonia) will prevent many problems. Personnel must be instructed to label all specimens submitted to the laboratory with data such as the patient's name, hospital number, date and time, and exact nature and source of the specimen, as discussed in Chapter 3.

1.4. Noncultural Methods of Diagnosis

As noted previously, the physician depends on data from many sources in arriving at tentative and definitive diagnoses. In addition to the usual medical history and physical examination, the competent clinician explores epidemiologic information (travel history; exposure to animals, ticks, or other vectors;

illness in the family or neighborhood; previous illness in the patient that might have relapsed). He or she also obtains a number of laboratory tests (e.g., complete blood count, blood chemistry tests, liver function tests, spinal fluid examination) and special tests such as a chest roentgenogram, computed tomography or magnetic resonance imaging, radionuclide scans, and ultrasound studies. In the case of suspected infection, examination of direct preparations such as wet mounts, Gram stains, and darkfield examinations may provide information quickly. The use of monoclonal antibodies or genetic probes may provide remarkable specificity in direct examination of clinical specimens (Chapter 10). Certain skin tests may be useful diagnostically. Rapid examination for products of microorganisms (e.g., gas-liquid chromatography for demonstration of volatile metabolic end products) may be helpful on occasion. Finally, the physician looks for an immunologic response to a given microorganism, usually in the patient's serum (see Chapter 12). This, of course, requires that an infection has been present sufficiently long that such a response could have taken place.

1.5. Rejection of Specimens

It is important that criteria be set up for specimen rejection; such criteria are indicated in appropriate places in this book. However, it is an important rule always to talk to the requesting physicians *before* rejecting specimens, since they are primarily responsible for the patients' welfare. They may need support and advice. They may know or think they know that an unorthodox specimen may provide useful information. If this is not the case, the microbiologist must explain why it is not and must work with physicians to resolve the disagreement.

Frequently it is necessary and important to do the best possible job on a less than optimal specimen. It may be necessary to educate the clinician, and the best way to do this is to review individual specimens in a friendly and cooperative manner.

1.6. Extent of Identification Required

We lean heavily toward *definitive* identification. For example, identification to species within the *Bacteroides* genus may be useful. Merely identifying an organism as "*Bacteroides ureolyticus* group" is inadequate. *B. gracilis* is more pathogenic and more resistant to antimicrobial agents than *B. ureolyticus* and other members of the group.

An outbreak of infantile diarrhea of serious pro-

portion persisted for many months in a large general hospital in the southwestern United States because stool cultures did not reveal any pathogens. Until the *Escherichia coli* isolates were tested for enterotoxin production and found to be positive, all therapeutic and control measures attempted proved futile. Definitive identification of the unusual blood culture isolates from a number of outbreaks—and these were not really recognized initially as outbreaks—finally permitted determination that commercial intravenous fluid bottles were contaminated; this led to definitive control measures.[3] Many cases of bacteremia and many outbreaks across the country were attributable to this source.

Identification of a clostridial blood culture isolate as *Clostridium septicum* will alert the clinician to the possibility of malignancy or other disease, usually in the colon, because of the strong association between these two events.[1] Identification of an organism thought to be *Bacteroides fragilis* group in a patient with bacteremia of unknown source as actually being a *Bacteroides splanchnicus* could indicate that the source is probably in the gastrointestinal tract, whereas *B. fragilis* might also be in the genital tract or even another site.

Precise information of organisms from a patient with two distinct episodes of infection at an interval of some months might permit establishing that the second infection represents a recurrence rather than a new infection, or it might permit excluding that possibility. Recurrent infection may suggest a foreign body or an abscess from prior surgery; in the absence of prior surgery, it suggests the possibility of malignancy or other underlying process. Definitive identification of an atypical mycobacterium may permit more accurate assessment as to whether the organism is truly involved in the disease, what the source might be, its drug susceptibility pattern, and the likelihood of its responding to the therapeutic regimen chosen.

In the case of certain organisms, especially the anaerobes, incomplete identification may lead to very serious errors in identification. Things that we learn in our first course of microbiology—that certain organisms produce spores, that some are gram-positive and some are gram-negative, and so on—do not necessarily help with the anaerobes. It may be very difficult to demonstrate spores in sporulating anaerobes. Gram-positive anaerobes are very commonly decolorized and may appear gram-negative, even early in the course of growth. Cocci may be mistaken for bacilli, or, more commonly, bacilli may be mistaken for cocci. It may even be difficult to define what an anaerobe actually is, considering that certain organisms, such as some clostridia (aerotolerant), are capable of relatively good growth under aerobic conditions. There are several outstanding examples in the literature of serious errors of this type in identification. For example, *B. melaninogenicus* has been incorrectly reported as being an anaerobic gram-positive streptococcus, and even such a great anaerobist as Prévot mistakenly classified as a *Fusobacterium (F. biacutum)* an organism subsequently shown to be gram-positive and a sporeformer *(Clostridium)*. Determination of the specific species of a group D *Streptococcus* (e.g., *S. bovis* as opposed to *Enterococcus faecalis*)[2] may permit the use of less toxic and less expensive therapeutic remedies. It may also have implications with regard to serious underlying disease. Organisms as diverse as *Listeria monocytogenes* and *Actinomyces viscosus* have been incorrectly identified as diphtheroids (even in reports in the literature) when shortcuts were taken.

Careful bacteriologic studies permit us to define the role of various organisms in different infectious processes, the prognosis associated with these, and so forth. Finally, definitive identification is important in educating clinicians as to the role of various organisms in infectious processes and, perhaps most importantly, prevents deterioration of the skills and interest of the microbiologist.

At the same time, some shortcuts and use of limited identification procedures in certain cases are necessary in most clinical laboratories. Careful application of knowledge of the significance of various organisms in specific situations and thoughtful use of limited approaches will keep expenses in line and keep the laboratory's workload manageable, while providing for optimum patient care.

1.7. Quantitation of Results

The concept of quantitation has not been adequately stressed in microbiology except in the case of urine cultures. Quantitation is useful in other situations as well. It may help to distinguish between an organism present as a "contaminant" and an organism actively involved in infection. It is often useful in determining the relative importance of different organisms recovered from mixed infections. Ordinarily, formal quantitation by dilution procedure or even by means of a quantitative loop is not necessary or desirable. Numbers of organisms present can be graded as "many" ("heavy growth"), "moderate numbers," or "few" ("light growth") on the basis of Gram stain appearance and the amount of growth on a plate. For example, does a given colony type extend to the secondary streak, tertiary streak, and so on? The Gram stain is important because differences in amount of growth or rate of growth of different organisms may be related to the fastidiousness of the organism.

1.8. Expediting Results

The need for speed in identification and susceptibility testing is another crucial area that has been neglected, as noted earlier. Few diseases are as dynamic and rapid acting as the infectious diseases. In certain serious infections, such as bacteremia, endocarditis, meningitis, and certain pneumonias, delay of a few hours (or even less in more critical cases) in providing proper therapy may lead to death. It is not always feasible or safe to try to "cover" all possible types of infecting organisms with antimicrobial therapy. Clearly, the clinician must use this type of empirical approach initially, but the microbiologist must be prepared to assist in choosing a rational approach through knowledge of the role of various organisms in different disease processes and through interpretation of direct smears. In such cases the microbiologist should offer something more than routine daily inspection and subculture so that any necessary or desirable modification of therapy can be made as soon as possible; of course, the clinician must communicate with the laboratory about problem cases. Cultures can be examined at 6- to 12-hour intervals, and the processing can be speeded up considerably for selected cases (Chapter 4). Aside from lowering mortality and morbidity, rapid provision of data may shorten hospitalization and thus save money for the patient or the hospital. It may help avoid a surgical procedure.

A limited number of organisms are responsible for the majority of infections. Simple procedures (e.g., Gram stain, colony morphology, catalase, coagulase, bile solubility, oxidase, spot indole, and rapid susceptibility tests) often may provide accurate presumptive identification quickly. Automated rapid procedures can be very helpful.

1.9. Interaction with the Clinician

In communicating with the physician, the microbiologist can avoid confusion and misunderstanding by not using jargon or abbreviations and by providing reports with clear-cut conclusions. Do not assume that the clinician is fully familiar with laboratory procedures or the latest taxonomic schemes. When feasible, provide interpretation on the written report, along with the specific results. However, *never provide only your interpretation* without the actual bacteriologic data (e.g., "Only normal flora isolated").

Monthly newsletters may be used to supplement laboratory manuals in order to provide physicians with material such as details of your procedures, new nomenclature, and changes in usual susceptibility patterns of given organisms in your hospital's setting.

REFERENCES

1. Alpern, R.J., and Dowell, V.R. Jr. 1969. *Clostridium septicum* infections and malignancy. J.A.M.A. 209:385.
2. Facklam, R.R., and Carey, R.B. 1985. Streptococci and aerococci. p. 154-175. In Lennette, E.H., Balows, A., Hausler, W.J. Jr., and Shadomy, H.J., editors. Manual of clinical microbiology, ed. 4. American Society for Microbiology, Washington, D.C.
3. Maki, D.G., Rhame, F.S., Goldmann, D.A., and Mandell, G.L. 1973. The infection hazard posed by contaminated intravenous infusion fluid. In Sonnenwirth, A.C., editor. Bacteremia: laboratory and clinical aspects. Charles C Thomas, Publisher, Springfield, Ill.

BIBLIOGRAPHY

Neu, H.C. 1978. What should the clinician expect from the microbiology laboratory? Ann. Intern. Med. 89(Part 2):781.

2 Laboratory Safety

Microbiology laboratories are unique environments in relation to the safety of those who work within them. Clinical specimens received from patients pose a hazard to personnel because of infectious agents they may contain. Spurred on by the spread of **acquired immunodeficiency syndrome (AIDS)**, the United States Centers for Disease Control has recommended new safety precautions concerning the handling of patient materials by health-care workers.[5] These recommendations, known as Universal Precautions (or universal blood and body-fluid precautions), stress that since not all patients carrying blood-borne pathogens can be reliably identified, all persons whose activities involve contact with patients or with blood or other body fluids from patients in a health-care setting should exercise the same consistent precautions.[4] These precautions are detailed below.

Cultures of infectious agents also pose a threat. Education of employees who routinely handle the potentially infectious agents and education (by means of biohazard notices as well as written and verbal instruction) for those people who have only limited exposure to the environment, such as custodial personnel, delivery personnel, and visitors, are the most important measures available for preventing laboratory-acquired infection. Risks from a microbiology laboratory may extend to adjacent laboratories and to families of those who work in the microbiology laboratory. For example, Blaser and Feldman[1] noted that 5 of 31 individuals who contracted typhoid fever from proficiency testing specimens did not work in a microbiology laboratory. Two patients were family members of a microbiologist who had worked with *Salmonella typhi*, two were students whose afternoon class was in a laboratory where the organism had been cultured that morning, and one worked in an adjacent chemistry laboratory. The last several documented cases of smallpox in the world were acquired by employees working in a different area in the building where a smallpox research laboratory was located. The principal investigator was so dismayed that his possibly deficient safety practices led to these smallpox cases that he committed suicide. It is the ultimate responsibility of the laboratory director or supervisor to ensure that proper safety guidelines are followed.

2.1. General Safety Considerations

In addition to the threat of infection, microbiology laboratories also contain the safety risks associated with any laboratory or institutional environment, those of fire, electrical hazards, chemical hazards, hazardous environmental situations (slippery floors, faulty air-handling systems), radioactive materials, equipment malfunction, and dangers imposed by natural disasters. Each section of the microbiology laboratory should have a safety manual containing information about procedures to follow in case of fire, flood, earthquake, or other natural disaster; location of all safety equipment; and practices to follow in the event of a situation posing a safety hazard. These considerations are universal to all laboratories and are addressed in references on general laboratory safety. Guidelines for the storage of flammable materials and caustic chemicals have been delineated by the College of American Pathologists and should be strictly enforced. A good way to assure that all laboratory personnel are familiar with current safety practices is to hold periodic unannounced safety drills. By varying the hypothetical hazardous situation, the safety director allows all personnel the opportunity to become aware of their knowledge of proper action in an emergency and to improve their performance before a real disaster strikes.

2.2. Biohazards and Practices Specific to Microbiology in General

The biohazards present in a clinical microbiology laboratory are a more specific concern of this text. Certain aspects of the organization, design, and functioning of such a laboratory should be accepted generally as good safety practices throughout all specialty areas of the laboratory.

2.2.a. **Laboratory environment.** The microbiology laboratory poses many hazards to unsuspecting and untrained people; therefore, access should be lim-

ited to those who have been informed of which actions they can perform safely. Visitors, especially small children, should be discouraged. Certain areas of high risk, such as the mycobacteriology and virology laboratories, should be closed to visitors. Custodial personnel should be trained to discriminate among the waste containers, dealing only with those that contain noninfectious material.

Care should be taken to prevent insects from infesting any laboratory areas. Mites, for example, have been known to crawl over the surface of media, carrying bacteria from colonies on a plate to other areas. Houseplants can serve as a source of such potential hazards and should be carefully observed for infestation if they are not excluded altogether from the laboratory environment.

The air-handling system of a microbiology laboratory should move air from low to higher risk areas, never the reverse. Ideally, the microbiology laboratory should be under negative pressure and air should not be recirculated after it passes through microbiology. The selected use of biological safety cabinets for those procedures that generate infectious aerosols is critical to laboratory safety. Many infectious diseases, such as plague, tularemia, brucellosis, Q fever, histoplasmosis, tuberculosis, and Legionnaires' disease, may be contracted by inhalation of the infectious particles, often present in a small droplet of liquid. If the droplets are between 2 and 5 μm in diameter, they may easily reach the alveolar spaces of the lung, where they may cause disease. Several common procedures used to process specimens for culture, notably mincing, grinding, vortexing, and preparing direct smears, are known to produce aerosol droplets. These procedures must be performed in a biological safety cabinet.

2.2.b. **Biological safety cabinet.** A biological safety cabinet is a device that encloses a workspace in such a way as to protect workers from aerosol exposure to infectious disease agents. Air that contains the infectious material is sterilized, either by heat, ultraviolet light, or, most commonly, by passage through a **high-efficiency particulate air (HEPA)** filter that removes most particles larger than 0.3 μm in diameter. These cabinets are designated by class according to the degree of biological containment they afford. Class I cabinets allow room (unsterilized) air to pass into the cabinet and around the material within, sterilizing only the air to be exhausted (Fig-

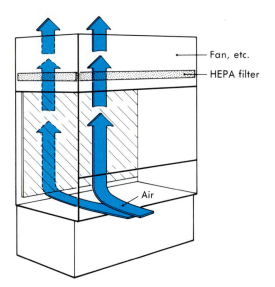

Figure 2.1
Class I biological safety cabinet.

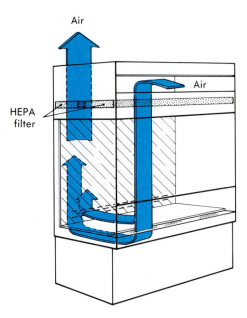

Figure 2.2
Class II biological safety cabinet.

ure 2.1). Class II cabinets sterilize air that flows over the infectious material, as well as air to be exhausted. The air flows in "sheets," which serve as barriers to particles from outside the cabinet, and which direct the flow of contaminated air into the filters (Figure 2.2). Such cabinets are called **laminar flow** biological safety cabinets. Type IIA cabinets have a fixed opening, and Type IIB cabinets have a variable sash opening through which the operator gains access to the work surface. Class III cabinets afford the most protection to the worker since they are completely enclosed, with negative pressure. Air coming into and going out of the cabinet is filter sterilized, and the infectious material within is handled with rubber gloves that are attached and sealed to the cabinet (Figure 2.3).

Most hospital clinical microbiology laboratory technologists use Class II cabinets routinely. The use of biological safety cabinets for certain procedures will be discussed further below. The routine inspection and documentation of adequate function of these cabinets is a critical factor in an ongoing quality assurance program. Important to proper operation of laminar flow cabinets is maintenance of an open area for 3 feet (90 cm) from the cabinet during operation of the air-circulating system (Figure 2.4) to ensure that infectious material is directed through the HEPA filter.

2.2.c. Protective clothing. Microbiologists should wear laboratory coats over their street clothes, and these coats should be removed before leaving the laboratory. If the laboratory protective clothing becomes contaminated with a pathogen, it should be sterilized in an autoclave immediately and cleaned before reusing. Obviously, laboratory workers who plan to enter an area of the hospital in which patients at special risk of acquiring infection are present, such as intensive care units, the nursery, operating rooms, or areas in which immunosuppressive therapy is being administered, should take every precaution to cover their street clothes with clean or sterile protective clothing appropriate to the area being visited. Special protective clothing may be advisable for certain activities, such as working with radioactive substances or caustic chemicals.

2.2.d. Decontamination. All materials contaminated with potentially infectious agents must be decontaminated before disposal. These include unused portions of patient specimens as well as media that have been inoculated, whether pathogens have grown or not. Infectious material to be disposed of should be placed into containers that are labeled as to their biohazard risk. Certain instruments, such as scissors, forceps, and scalpel blade holders, should be placed into a closed metal container until they can be sterilized in an autoclave. Sharp objects, nee-

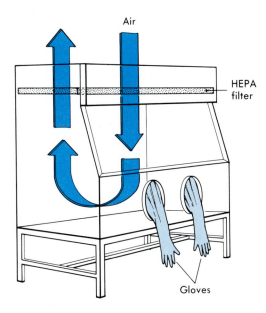

Figure 2.3
Class III biological safety cabinet.

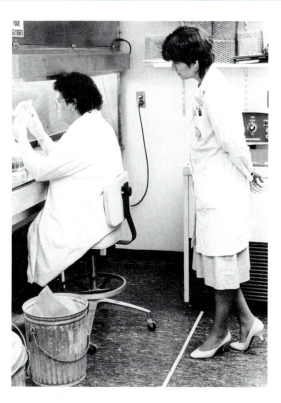

Figure 2.4
An area of at least 3 feet from the front of a Class II biological safety cabinet must be kept clear of people during operation.

dles and scalpel blades, should be inserted into a hard-sided puncture-proof container *without resheathing*. Such containers are commercially available. The container should be clearly labeled as to contents, sterilized in an autoclave, and discarded. Only needles that lock onto syringes or one-piece units should be used. Specially designed holders for resheathing needles without posing a hazard to the worker are now available commercially; simply recapping of needles with their original protective sheaths after use has led to numerous accidental needle-puncture wounds in hospital and laboratory personnel.

Decontamination of potentially infectious material to be discarded from the microbiology laboratory is most often accomplished by steam sterilization in an **autoclave,** an instrument that uses moist heat at greater than atmospheric pressure to kill infectious agents. The pressure allows the steam to be heated above the boiling point, thus decreasing the time needed to sterilize. Material to be sterilized should be packed loosely so that the steam can circulate freely around it. Material of potentially greater hazard, such as cultures and specimens from the mycobacteriology laboratory, is often sterilized for 1 hour instead of the usual 30 to 45 minutes (at 121°C and 15 pounds per square inch [psi] pressure). It is best to locate the autoclave within the laboratory; if

infectious material must be transported for sterilization, however, it should be double-bagged and carried in leakproof, sterilizable containers.

Autoclaves should be monitored regularly for adequate sterilization performance as part of regular quality control practice (discussed in Chapter 3). The proper loading and placement of material in the autoclave does, however, help to determine whether material has been adequately sterilized. An important safety precaution for those operating an autoclave is to open the door slowly after completion of a cycle. Several workers have been severely burned by the rush of steam that escapes through the crack in the autoclave door as it is first being opened. The use of a protective face mask for this procedure will prevent such burn incidents.

Workbenches and other horizontal surfaces should be decontaminated at least after every shift and immediately after every spill by washing with a liquid antiseptic agent, such as a phenolic compound, 70% ethanol, or a 0.5% solution of sodium hypochlorite (10% solution of household bleach in water). Diluted bleach is the most effective agent against viral contaminants such as hepatitis B virus and human immunodeficiency virus (HIV). For those laboratories in which viral contamination is a significant hazard, diluted bleach is recommended as the antiseptic of choice. Bleach can also inactivate the infectious proteins called **prions** (discussed in Chapter 40) that may be the etiologic agents of Creutzfeldt-Jakob disease. Suppliers of commercially available disinfectants are listed in the Appendix. The longer the surface is allowed to remain wet with the agent, the more effective will be the antiseptic action. A minimum of 10 minutes is recommended. Germicides are not active unless they are in solution. Most disinfectants do not destroy bacterial spores, but these forms of pathogens with the exception of anthrax spores, do not usually pose a hazard to personnel. At least one commercially available disinfectant (Alcide) is moderately effective as a sporicidal agent. It is good practice to wipe down the outside surfaces of other laboratory equipment, such as centrifuges, vortex mixers, telephones, and even fluorescent lamps above work surfaces, with disinfectant on a regular basis.

2.2.e. Personnel practices. Careful handling of infectious materials to prevent aerosol formation is an important aspect of microbiological laboratory technique. If open flame burners are used, care must be taken to prevent spattering of material from inoculating needles and loops. The burner should be in a protective container to prevent accidental burns. Incinerator burners offer a less hazardous alternative to an open flame, although as they age and the insulation wears thin, they can pose an electrical hazard. Incinerator burners should be inspected every 6 months for signs of wear in the ceramic core, which must be replaced as necessary. CDC's Universal Precautions for personnel handling blood and body fluids (which in microbiology would include all secretions and excretions containing visible blood in addition to blood, serum, semen, and vaginal secretions[6]) are summarized in the box above.

Universal Precautions do not apply to feces, nasal secretions, saliva, sputum, sweat, tears, urine, or vomitus unless they are grossly bloody.[6] If the risk of aerosol infection during specimen handling is great, such as for tuberculosis, the use of a molded surgical mask is recommended. Additional safety

---

Essentials of Universal Precautions

1. Use of appropriate barrier precautions to prevent skin and mucous membrane exposure, including wearing gloves at all times and masks, goggles, gowns, or aprons if there is a risk of splashes or droplet formation
2. Thorough washing of hands and other skin surfaces after gloves are removed and immediately after any contamination
3. Taking special care to avoid injuries with sharp objects such as needles and scalpels
4. Use of mouthpieces or other ventilation devices with one-way valves for performing any resuscitation measures
5. Refraining from handling patient care equipment or patients if health-care workers have exudative lesions or weeping dermatitis
6. Very stringent adherence to precautions by pregnant workers

---

recommendations for laboratory workers are shown in the box on p. 13.

Mouth pipetting is strictly prohibited; mechanical devices (Figure 2.5) are used for drawing all liquids into pipettes. Eating, drinking, smoking, and applying cosmetics are strictly forbidden in work areas. Food and drink are stored in refrigerators in areas separate from the work area. All personnel should wash their hands with soap and water after handling infectious material and before leaving the laboratory area.

The risk of laboratory-acquired infection with the agent of AIDS (HIV) is extremely low (0.9% of 351 health care workers [laboratory workers would typically have less risk] with percutaneous exposures seroconverted[4]), although the potential consequences are grave. The consistent practice of Universal Precautions by health-care workers handling all patient material will lessen the risks associated with such specimens. However, it is good practice to store sera collected periodically from all health-care workers so that a seroconversion can be documented. Serum should be drawn immediately in the event of a percutaneous contamination accident, whether it

---

Safety Practices for Laboratory Workers

1. Placement of specimens in leakproof, sealed containers for transport and avoiding contamination of specimen container surfaces
2. Changing gloves and washing hands after specimen processing
3. Limiting the use of needles and syringes to those situations in which there are no alternatives
4. Thorough decontamination of any equipment that has been contaminated with any blood or body fluid before it is repaired or transported.

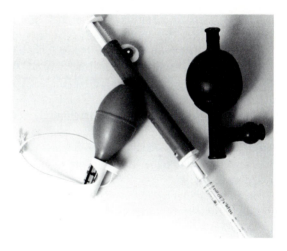

Figure 2.5
Several devices used for drawing liquids into pipettes as alternatives to mouth pipetting.

is examined at the time of the accident or later. More detailed measures are described in the CDC guidelines.[5,6]

An alert and responsible physician will warn the microbiology laboratory personnel about specimens that may contain the agents of highly contagious, dangerous disease such as tularemia or Lassa fever. Again, however, microbiologists should exert caution in working with *all* specimens because the physician may not suspect a special problem.

2.3. Classification of Biological Agents on the Basis of Hazard

The Centers for Disease Control publishes a booklet entitled *Classification of Etiologic Agents on the Basis of Hazard*,[2] which has served as a reference for assessing the relative risks of working with biological agents since 1969. Although many unusual agents will not be mentioned here, we will list a few of the more common agents likely to be encountered in clinical microbiology practice in the United States. An excellent source of more detailed information on handling of biohazardous material can be found in the 1984 booklet *Biosafety in Microbiological and Biomedical Laboratories*.[3] In general, patient specimens pose a greater risk to laboratory workers than do microorganisms in culture because the nature of etiologic agents in patient specimens is unknown.

2.3.a. Specific agents. Biosafety Level 1 agents include those that have no known pathogenic potential for immunocompetent persons. These agents are useful in laboratory teaching exercises for beginning level students of microbiology. Level 1 agents include *Bacillus subtilis* and *Mycobacterium gordonae*. Precautions for working with Level 1 agents include standard good laboratory technique as described in Section 2.2.

Biosafety Level 2 agents are those most commonly being sought in clinical specimens. They include all of the common agents of infectious disease, as well as HIV and several more unusual pathogens.[5] The most common causes of laboratory-acquired infection are: hepatitis B virus, *Coxiella burnetti*, *Brucella* species, *Francisella tularensis*, *Mycobacterium tuberculosis*, *Salmonella* and *Shigella* species, and arboviruses. Many other agents have been documented to cause laboratory-acquired infections. For handling clinical specimens suspected of harboring any of these pathogens, Biosafety Level 2 precautions are sufficient. This level of safety includes the principles outlined in Section 2.2 above and the added measures of limited access to the laboratory during working procedures, training in the handling of pathogenic agents by laboratory personnel, direction by competent supervisors, and the performance of aerosol-generating procedures in a biological safety cabinet.

Biosafety Level 3 procedures have been recommended for the handling of material suspected of harboring certain viruses, including certain arboviruses and arenaviruses, unlikely to be encountered in a routine clinical laboratory. These precautions, in addition to those undertaken for Level 2, include design and engineering features that increase the containment of potentially dangerous material by careful control of air movement and the requirement that personnel wear protective clothing and devices. Persons working with Biosafety Level 3 agents should have baseline sera stored for comparison with acute sera that should be drawn in the event of an unexplained illness.

Biosafety Level 4 agents, which include only certain viruses of the arbovirus, arenavirus, or filovirus groups, none of which are commonly found in the United States, require the use of maximum containment facilities; personnel and all materials are decontaminated before leaving the facility and all procedures are performed under maximum containment (special protective clothing, cabinets). Most of these facilities are research laboratories.

2.4. Special Precautions for Specific Areas of Clinical Microbiology

2.4.a. Bacteriology and general accessioning. Guidelines for the laboratory should require that all respiratory tract specimens must be inoculated to media in a biological safety cabinet. All tissues, whether ground, minced, or touch-cultured, are handled in the cabinet. Inoculating material from Isolator tubes (described in Chapter 14) is also performed under laminar flow air-handling conditions in the cabinet. As recommended by CDC's Universal Precautions, laboratorians should wear gloves when handling patient specimens. Specimen containers should be opened inside the biological safety cabinet. Safety caps should be used when centrifuging materials such as blood (Isolator tubes), sputum, and feces. Always keep in mind that the outer surface of specimen containers may have been contaminated inadvertently with specimen. Work with patient material should be performed slowly and carefully to prevent accidental inoculation or production of aerosols.

Certain bacteria, when present on laboratory media after incubation, should be processed only within a Class II or higher biological safety cabinet. These include situations or colonies suspicious for *Yersinia pestis*, *Brucella* species, *Francisella tularensis*, *Rickettsia* and *Coxiella* species, *Bacillus anthracis*, and

Pseudomonas pseudomallei. If production of aerosols is possible, *Neisseria gonorrhoeae*, *N. meningitidis*, and *Legionella* species should be manipulated in a cabinet.

2.4.b. Mycobacteriology. Processing of all specimens for mycobacteria should take place within a biological safety cabinet. Personnel may choose to wear face-molding masks as an added protective measure. All centrifugations should take place in sealed centrifuge safety cups. The placement of centrifuges under an exhaust system or within a biological safety cabinet will further decrease the hazards associated with centrifugation. Further information can be found in Chapter 41.

2.4.c. Mycology. After inoculation, all plated media should be *taped shut* to prevent accidental opening. Masking tape, certain cellophane tapes, and colored labeling tape have been found satisfactory (the tape must not lose its stickiness in a moist incubator). Complete sealing of edges is not necessary.

All moldlike fungi (those with aerial mycelia, as described in Chapter 43) must be manipulated within a biological safety cabinet. Many laboratories have been plagued by contaminating molds spread throughout all areas by spores from a single culture. When a mold appears on any medium within the laboratory, even if fungi are not being sought, the plate should be sealed immediately and opened thereafter only in the cabinet.

Any white, fuzzy fungus that appears on culture plates should be regarded with extreme suspicion as a possible dimorphic pathogen. Manipulations should be kept to a minimum and performed only by trained technologists with impeccable technique. Slide cultures should not be attempted for identification of fungi that grossly resemble the systemic pathogens *Coccidioides*, *Blastomyces*, and *Histoplasma*. Further discussion of handling such cultures can be found in Chapter 43.

2.4.d. Parasitology. The eggs of certain cestodes, if ingested during the infective stage, can cause disease. Microbiologists should exercise caution when handling suspected infected fecal material, and gloves should be worn if contact with infective material is possible. The use of a biological safety cabinet for handling most parasitic specimens is not necessary. However, for respiratory secretions that may harbor pathogens other than *Pneumocystic carinii* or flukes, manipulation within a safety cabinet is recommended. Cultures of the protozoan agents of primary meningoencephalitis (e.g., *Naegleria fowleri*) should be handled in a safety cabinet. Chapter 44 includes more discussion of handling of these agents.

2.4.e. **Virology.** All virology procedures performed in a routine clinical virology laboratory should be carried out within a biological safety cabinet. All specimens should be handled with gloves. Technologists should hold a 4- by 4-inch square gauze pad soaked in 10% bleach solution so as to completely cover the rubber stopper of serum tubes or other containers as the stopper is pulled off to help to absorb droplets formed during removal of the tops of such containers. Barrier devices, including plastic decapping devices and antiseptic-impregnated material squares, are available for this purpose. Special virology procedures, such as dissection of the heads of animals suspected of rabies infection, require stringent safety precautions. The precautions necessary for laboratories performing routine virology will be discussed further in Chapter 42.

2.4.f. **Serology.** Sera can contain agents that potentially may lead to laboratory-acquired infection. Gloves should be worn during manipulations that might allow skin contact with sera. The production of aerosols during the removal of tube tops or during other manipulations should be avoided. If possible, procedures that generate aerosols, such as vortexing, pouring, shaking incubations, and washing steps for microtiter assays, should be performed in a biological safety cabinet. The careful technique of laboratory workers is the best single safety measure available.

The availability of a proved effective and safe vaccine against hepatitis B should serve to significantly reduce the rate of laboratory-acquired hepatitis. We recommend that all individuals who are required by their duties in the laboratory to have even moderate contact with sera receive the vaccine. *As described above, universal precautions require that all sera and other body fluids should be handled as if they were infectious.*

2.5. Mailing Biologicals

Potentially infectious material must often be sent to distant laboratories for further studies. Etiologic agents, specimens, and biological materials may be shipped following the requirements of the Interstate Shipment of Etiologic Agents code. Cultures should be grown on solid media in a tube, preferably plastic, but most often glass. The cap must be sealed with waterproof tape. This primary container is packed in enough absorbent material to absorb the entire volume of the culture if it should leak or break; it is inserted into a second container, often a metal tube. The second container is capped and is inserted into a shipping container, such as a cardboard mailing tube. Any labeling should be affixed to the outside of the secondary container. The mailing label is affixed to the shipping container along with an official Etiologic Agents label, available from CDC (Figures 2.6 and 2.7). Shipments are limited to 50 ml volume each.

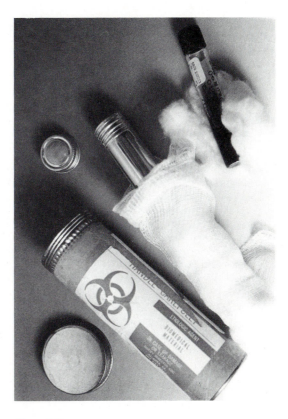

Figure 2.6
Proper containers for mailing etiologic agents.

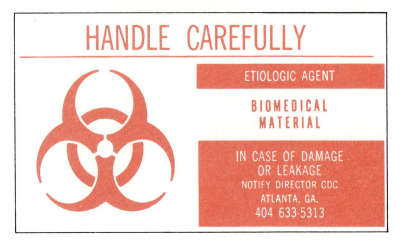

*Figure 2.*7
Label for etiologic agents and biomedical material.

REFERENCES

1. Blaser, M.J., and Feldman, R.A. 1980. Acquisition of typhoid fever from proficiency-testing specimens. N. Engl. J. Med. 303:1481.

2. Centers for Disease Control and National Institutes of Health. 1974. Classification of etiologic agents on the basis of hazard, ed. 4. U.S. Department of Health, Education, and Welfare, Public Health Service, Washington, D.C.

3. Centers for Disease Control and National Institutes of Health. 1984. Biosafety in microbiological and biomedical laboratories. H.H.S. Publication No. (CDC) 84-8395. U.S. Department of Health and Human Services, Public Health Service, Washington, D.C.

4. Centers for Disease Control. 1987. Recommendations for prevention of HIV transmission in health-care setting. M.M.W.R. 36(Suppl.):3s.

5. Centers for Disease Control. 1988. 1988 Agent summary statement for human immunodeficiency virus and report on laboratory-acquired infection with human immunodeficiency virus. M.M.W.R. 37(Suppl.):1.

6. Centers for Disease Control. 1988. Update: Universal precautions for prevention of transmission of human immunodeficiency virus, hepatitis B virus, and other bloodborne pathogens in health-care settings. M.M.W.R. 37:377.

BIBLIOGRAPHY

College of American Pathologists. 1977. Safety inspection checklist. The College, Skokie, Ill.

Inderlied, C.B. 1985. The laboratory environment. In Wagner, K.P., and Kelley, S.G., editors: Clinical microbiology: listen, look, and learn series. Health and Education Resources, Inc., American Society for Microbiology, Washington, D.C.

Miller, B.M., editor. 1986. Laboratory safety: principles and practices. American Society for Microbiology, Washington, D.C.

Richardson, J.N., and Barkley, W.E. 1985. Biological safety in the clinical laboratory. In Lennette, E.H., Balows, A., Hausler, W.J. Jr., and Shadomy, H.J., editors. Manual of clinical microbiology, ed. 4. American Society for Microbiology, Washington, D.C., p. 138.

3 Laboratory Organization and Quality Assurance

With the present and continuing reexamination of health care delivery by the medical, allied health, and governmental communities (see Chapter 4), it is incumbent on the microbiologist to ensure that the laboratory contributes to the highest quality of patient care by its expertise, its accuracy, its relevance, and the prompt reporting of its findings to the clinician. As stated in the revised *Accreditation Manual for Hospitals* published by the Joint Commission on Accreditation of Hospitals (1985), the standard which all hospitals must meet, a hospital must have "an ongoing quality assurance program designed to objectively and systematically monitor and evaluate the quality and appropriateness of patient care. . ." It is only by constant self-evaluation of the laboratory's performance through a comprehensive quality assurance program that such a level of excellence can be developed and maintained. Quality control, the process-oriented monitoring of activities within the laboratory, is only one facet of such a program.[1] The ease with which technologists can perform to the best of their abilities and the extent to which they can work together as a team to accomplish the goal of high quality patient care are determined, in part, by the organization of both the physical environment and the workflow within the laboratory. This chapter discusses general considerations for specimen handling and reporting results that contribute to the overall *quality assurance* that technologists and physicians expect of the laboratory and addresses some actual components of an active quality control/quality assurance program.

3.1. Specimen Procurement and Laboratory Accessioning

The quality of results from the microbiology laboratory and their contribution to good patient care are directly dependent on the freshness, quality, and appropriateness of specimens. Education of nurses and physicians in the proper collection and transport of specimens and in appropriate utilization of the diagnostic capabilities of the laboratory are the first steps in a quality assurance program. An easily accessible handbook containing all information needed for obtaining appropriate specimens, ordering tests correctly, and transporting specimens to the laboratory should be available at every patient care unit. A bulletin or newsletter can inform nurses and physicians of changes in procedures and other important information.

Laboratories should try to provide a central area to which all specimens are brought. This simplifies the delivery process and allows the laboratory to monitor and record all incoming specimens. The ability to determine whether a specimen has been received and at what point in the processing system a given specimen may be found is an important part of the overall organization of the laboratory. This may be called an "audit trail." It is at this point that specimens with requests for testing in more than one area of the laboratory can be divided, if necessary, or their proper routing can be arranged. Monitoring to be certain that specimens are being transported to the laboratory within an acceptable period of time is a worthwhile quality assurance activity.

3.2. Specimen Identification

Proper identification of each specimen includes the patient's name and identification number. The specimen should be tightly capped and in the proper container. Practice of the Universal Precautions (Chapter 2) assures that all incoming specimens are treated as though they may contain a hazardous agent. At the accessioning point, specific criteria for rejection of specimens should be enforced. Table 3.1 contains some suggested reasons for refusal to process a specimen. Other reasons for specimen rejection may be appropriate for individual laboratories. Under certain circumstances, such as receipt of an unlabeled specimen from a site that would be difficult or impossible to collect from again (e.g., cerebrospinal fluid), there should be policies that would permit overriding the original rejection. One such policy might be the acceptance of an unlabeled specimen after the attending physician has personally come to the laboratory to identify and label the specimen and has signed a statement assuming responsibility for the proper identification.

3.3. Laboratory Requisition Form

The request slip accompanying the specimen must contain the patient's identification parameters, the patient's location, the date and time that the specimen was collected, the exact source and type of specimen, the requested studies, and other pertinent information (such as the antimicrobials the patient is receiving), as well as the physician responsible. It is very useful to include the time at which the specimen was received in the laboratory; many laboratories use a time-stamp machine for this purpose. A clean and legible request form is essential to optimal processing. The format of the request form can often influence the way in which physicians order tests. As mentioned in Chapter 4, listing a limited number of possible tests on the request form will contribute to limiting the test requests to those listed. The use of screening procedures and test panels dealing with a series of tests that might aid in identification of a particular infectious agent or type of infection (such as "strep throat screen" or "respiratory virus panel") may simplify the ordering process for physicians and clarify the request for the technologists. If the patient's diagnosis is included on the request, the laboratory can more easily determine which tests to perform to give the most useful information to the physician.

3.4. Reporting Results

Part of the organization of the microbiology laboratory must include a system for delivering results of test procedures to the physician (or patient-care unit). Assuring minimal turnaround time from test receipt to reporting results and ascertaining that accurately relayed results actually reach the healthcare provider are important aspects of ongoing quality assurance. Certain information is important enough to warrant a telephone call. Suggested reports that ought to be relayed immediately include Gram stain results; positive direct visual preparations of any sort; positive antigen detection results from sterile body fluids; growth in blood cultures, cerebrospinal fluid, or from any sterile body fluid or tissue; positive acid fast smears; presence of organ-

Table 3.1
Criteria for Rejection of Requests for Microbiological Tests*

CATEGORY	CRITERION FOR REJECTION	ACTION
Identification	Container not identified	Write "container not identified" and call ordering unit to send someone to verify the ID if the request form is attached to the specimen. Otherwise, do not process. (See text.)
	Container and request form have different ID's	Document on report form. Call ordering unit to send correct request forms or resolve the problem.
Request form	Insufficient information marked on form	Call ordering unit for additional necessary information
Specimen	Specimen grossly contaminated	Call ordering unit to send repeat specimen. If they are unable to re-collect, ask them to come down to clean it in the laboratory. Final resort: clean it with germicide, wear gloves, work in biohazard chamber.
	Specimen submitted in improper container	Notify ordering unit of problem. If unable to re-collect, perform test if possible and make note on report form that improper container was used. If unable to perform test, document reason on report form and discard specimen.
	Excessive delay between specimen collection and arrival in laboratory	If specimen was not stored properly, notify ordering unit and request repeat specimen. Do not process unless patient care is likely to be compromised by delay. Note on report that delay may result in less accurate results.
	Inadequate specimen for number of tests requested	Call physician for priority of requests and to request additional material. Note on report that specimen had inadequate volume as reason for lack of performance of certain tests.
	Some factor renders specimen inadequate for request *Examples:* sputum on a swab or in tissue paper, stool for ova and parasites with gross barium visible, specimen placed into formalin, container broke or leaked during transport	Call ordering unit or physician to inform them of problem. Note problem on report form and do not process specimen.
	Pooled 24-hour urine or sputum received for culture	Call ordering unit to inform them that 24-hour specimens are unacceptable for microbiology. Do not process and send report out with note indicating reason for not performing test.
	Dry swab received for culture	Notify ordering unit that dry swabs are not suitable for culture. Do not process. Send report out with note indicating reason for not performing test.
	Improper specimen for test *Examples:* blood in serum tube with clot for malaria smear, slide with material smeared on for culture, pleural fluid for serologic test	Call ordering unit to verify test request. Do not process, and send documented reason for not performing test on report.
	Foley catheter tip	Call ordering unit to inform them that clinically relevant results cannot be obtained from this specimen. Request a urine for culture. Send out report noting the reason for not processing the specimen.
	Duplicate specimen received (other than blood)	Send notice that only one of the duplicate specimens will be processed unless the laboratory is notified and reasons are given for processing duplicate(s).
	Anaerobic culture requested on improper specimen *Examples:* expectorated sputum, voided urine (not suprapubic tap), vaginal discharge, prostatic secretions, gastrointestinal tract (except in blind loop syndrome), oral material, respiratory secretions not collected by needle aspiration or by special plugged double-lumen catheter device, lochia, environmental material, any specimen exposed to air for extended time	Notify ordering unit that the specimen is unacceptable for such a request. Process aerobically only.

*All specimens not processed should be refrigerated for 3 days before they are discarded as a safeguard against erroneous discarding of an irretrievable specimen. Always discuss with clinician before discarding.

isms that would require the patient to be isolated, such as intestinal pathogens of *Staphylococcus aureus;* and growth of mycobacteria. It is equally important for the technologist to document what information was relayed by telephone, when this was done, and to whom. Other results are usually delivered in written form, either directly from the laboratory or via a computerized system of information processing. The work of the laboratory will only be worthwhile if it is useful in directing care for the patient. One aspect of the more careful scrutiny of hospital practices by government and other third-party payers (Chapter 4) has been a close examination of result reporting from laboratories to the patient care areas. Most administrative policies now require an interim or preliminary written report within 24 or at the most 48 hours after specimen receipt. Those laboratories that have hospital-wide on-line computer capability have a system that facilitates such reporting. Other laboratories must rely on multiple-copy report forms to accomplish this purpose.

Certain results are important to people other than physicians directly responsible for patients. Infection control practitioners monitor the incidence and spread of various infections throughout the hospital and must be given access to relevant information, both on a daily basis and in cumulative fashion. Policies that govern which culture results must be telephoned directly to infection control practitioners should be clearly delineated. The laboratory also has an obligation to report certain infections, such as preventable venereal diseases, tuberculosis, agents of transmissible gastroenteritis, and diseases of grave concern such as botulism and plague, to the local public health authorities. All technologists should be informed as to which results require additional reporting, and standardized procedures should be established for this function.

3.5. Procedure Manual

Every laboratory must provide procedure manuals detailing all aspects of performance of procedures within that laboratory. Such manuals should be easily accessible at all times to the technologists who may wish to consult them. Manuals should discuss safety aspects of working within the laboratory, administrative and technical policies that must be followed by laboratory workers, specimen collection information, specimen acceptability criteria, as well as

criteria for performance of all tests and reporting results. The manual should detail the steps to take in the event of a failure to meet quality control standards established for each procedure. The procedure manual should be the *working reference standard* for the entire staff. The manuals are reviewed regularly, at least annually, by supervisory staff and the procedures are updated as they are modified or replaced. Documenting laboratory procedures, as is done by means of a manual, is as important as documenting the results of quality control procedures outlined below. The National Committee for Clinical Laboratory Standards has established guidelines for writing laboratory procedure manuals.[2]

3.6. Quality Assurance

Quality technologist performance determines the quality of laboratory results, thus establishing and maintaining the high levels of performance that are crucial to quality assurance. The laboratory's physical layout and environment should be adequate for the number of employees and conducive to good performance. New employees should be given thorough orientation to policies and procedures. Maintenance and upgrading of the technical skills of all personnel should be pursued through laboratory rounds, in-service education, opportunities to attend continuing education programs, and by encouraging self-directed learning. Personnel performance should be monitored. Periodic comparisons of ongoing work to work cards and results reports, daily checking by a supervisor of all reports produced during all shifts for errors and omissions, and an occasional evaluation of each technologist's performance by complete investigation of their current culture workups may point out hidden sources of error.

Quality control activities are both internal and external.[4] Internal activities involve monitoring the performance of media, reagents, instruments, products, and equipment. Documentation of performance of quality control measures is as important as the performance itself. The written record for each laboratory procedure or function that is monitored should also contain a section that details any deviation from expected results, problems, or failures and the corrective actions taken in response to such problems. Incidents that occur in the laboratory that are not directly related to performance of tests, such as spills of infectious materials, personal injuries, abusive interactions between technologists and physi-

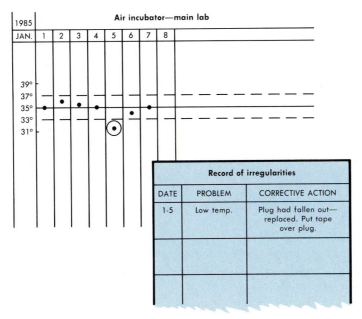

Figure 3.1
Example of incubator quality control performance record.

cians, or any unusual occurrence, should also be documented. A special logbook for corrective actions is very helpful in documenting an ongoing quality control program's effectiveness. Quality control records must be held for a minimum of 2 years; instrument records must be held for the life of the instrument.

Instrument quality control monitoring should include preventive maintenance, temperature charts if applicable, and other records of performance. An example of a quality control log for an incubator is shown in Figure 3.1. Volumetric instruments must be validated at least annually. All perishable products and all solutions must be labeled with the date of receipt or preparation, strength, safety warnings or additional information, when they were first used, and the expiration date. All products prepared in the laboratory should be checked for proper performance. In the case of microbiological media, tests should include sterility and growth of microorganisms with both positive and negative outcomes. Selective media should be monitored for their ability to inhibit the expected organisms as well as for the growth of the sought-for organisms. The National Committee for Clinical Laboratory Standards has recently established guidelines for the testing of microbiological media, including the names of organisms to be tested, expected results, and frequency of testing.[3] These guidelines are further discussed in Chapter 8.

Organisms for use in monitoring media and reagent performance are available commercially in lyophilized form from several suppliers (listed in Appendix C under Quality Control Organisms and Supplies). Test organisms not available commercially should be obtained from a reference laboratory. Organisms can be kept frozen indefinitely at $-70°$ C in skim milk (diluted 1:1 in distilled water and sterilized in an autoclave at 121° C for 10 minutes) in small plastic freezer vials, or they may be maintained for quite some time on nutrient or blood agar slants under a layer of sterile mineral oil. Viability is prolonged when the media are prepared without added sodium chloride or carbohydrate. Yeasts and mycobacteria retain viability for several months stored in suspension in sterile distilled water

Test organisms appropriate for performance monitoring will be mentioned in relationship to tests as they are described throughout this text. The bibliographic references cited at the end of this chapter contain more detailed lists of those media and reagents that should be evaluated and suggestions for organization of quality control programs. Susceptibility testing procedures require particularly stringent quality control, as detailed in Chapter 13. The amount of quality control performed by a laboratory is dictated by the agency under which the laboratory is accredited, such as the Joint Commission on Hospital Accreditation, Health Care Financing Administration, or the state in which the laboratory functions. A laboratory must adjust its practices to satisfy the most stringent regulating agency. The documented recorded history of results within established limits can help to determine how often quality control procedures must be performed by any particular laboratory.

Laboratories can also monitor their overall performance by utilizing a system of internal proficiency testing of outcomes. This is accomplished by occasionally submitting the same sample, divided into two specimens, as a second specimen, unknown to the technologists. Lapses in consistency are often spotted in this way.

External quality control activities include periodic inspection by agents of the regulatory agencies responsible for accreditation of the laboratory and performance of routine procedures on check samples and unknowns provided by an outside resource (proficiency testing). These programs are valuable for comparing one's results with those of many other laboratories, spotting errors in technique, and learning to recognize unusual agents or rare results. It can be argued that outcome measurements as determined by proficiency testing only assess a laboratory's best performance. Nevertheless, they are a valuable and necessary component of an ongoing quality assurance program.

The laboratory is often responsible for helping maintain quality control for other areas of the hospital. Monitoring the effectiveness of autoclaves in surgery, laundry, and other sections may be a function of the microbiology laboratory. Often the laboratory provides sterility checks for the pharmacy, blood bank, milk bank, dialysis service, and other areas. Unless there has been a documented nosocomial infection outbreak, it is not recommended that cultures of environmental surfaces be performed. Such cultures are not necessarily indicated then, either.

3.7. Statistics

Maintaining adequate records of specimens received, procedures performed, and results will be extremely helpful for determining staffing needs and organization of workload. Use of some method for assessing work accomplished, such as the College of American Pathologists workload unit recording system, will enable a laboratory to determine productivity, trends in test requests, and proper pricing structures. Other statistics that are helpful include cumulative susceptibility testing results. An updated compilation of these data, provided to physicians on a regular basis, preferably in a reduced format that allows physicians to carry the information in their white jacket or coat pockets, will aid them in selecting the most efficacious antimicrobial agents, as well as alert them to new trends in susceptibility patterns among isolates from their institution. By comparing a particular organism's susceptibility pattern to the established norm, a technologist may find an error in identification or an unusual isolate that requires further study.

3.8. Information Processing

The number and diversity of the records and statistics that must be generated, evaluated, and stored by the microbiology laboratory have increased just as technological advances have blossomed. Luckily, the development of information-processing systems suitable for use by the laboratory has also been occurring. It is hoped that microbiology laboratories can make use of some of the new technology to aid in the giant task of record-keeping. The use of computers for many tasks within the clinical microbiology laboratory is discussed in Chapter 4.

REFERENCES

1. Barros, A. 1987. Is quality control quality assurance? Med. Laboratory Observer 19:21.
2. NCCLS. 1980. Tentative guidelines for clinical laboratory procedure manuals. National Committee for Clinical Laboratory Standards, Villanova, Penn.
3. NCCLS. 1987. Quality assurance standards for commercially prepared microbiological culture media. Tentative Standard, M22-T. National Committee for Clinical Laboratory Standards, Villanova, Penn.
4. Sommers, H.M. 1985. Towards more effective quality control. In Smith, J.W., editor. The role of clinical microbiology in cost-effective health care. College of American Pathologists, Skokie, Ill.

BIBLIOGRAPHY

Bartlett, R.C. 1974. Medical microbiology: quality, cost, and clinical relevance. John Wiley & Sons, New York.
Bartlett, R.C. 1985. Quality control in clinical microbiology. In Lennette, E.H., Balows, A., Hausler, W.J. Jr., and Shadomy,

H.J., editors. Manual of clinical microbiology, ed. 4. American Society for Microbiology, Washington, D.C.

Blazevic, D.J., Hall, C.T., and Wilson, M.E. 1976. Cumitech 3, Practical quality control procedures for the clinical microbiology laboratory. In Balows, A., coordinating editor. American Society for Microbiology, Washington, D.C.

Environmental Protection Agency. 1986. EPA guide for infectious waste management. (Publication No. PB86.199130.) National Technical Information Service, Port Royal Road, Springfield, VA 22161. Telephone (703) 487-4650.

Miller, J.M. 1983. Quality control in the microbiology laboratory. Centers for Disease Control, U.S. Department of Health and Human Services, Public Health Service, Atlanta.

Miller, J.M., and Wentworth, B.B., editors. 1985. Methods for quality control in diagnostic microbiology. American Public Health Association, Washington, D.C.

Sewell, D.L. 1987. Quality control in the new environment: microbiology. Med. Lab. Observer 19:45.

Weissfeld, A.S., and Bartlett, R.C. 1987. Quality control. In Howard, B., Weissfeld, A.S., and Tilton, R.C. Clinical and pathogenic microbiology. The C.V. Mosby Co., St. Louis.

4

Managing the Clinical Microbiology Laboratory: Maximizing Patient Care in a Cost-Conscious Environment

The federally-mandated system in which hospitals receive reimbursement for costs based primarily on the admission and discharge diagnosis given to a patient, rather than on the cost of medical care generated by that patient (diagnosis related groups [**DRGs**]), has been practiced since 1983. Although numerous factors influence the amount of reimbursement (Medicare or Medicaid) allowed to each hospital, it is immediately obvious that it is to a hospital's financial advantage to keep costs as low as possible. Suddenly the laboratory, which previously had received reimbursement for all charged services and therefore served as a revenue-producing center for the hospital, became a potential drain on the hospital's resources, becoming a cost center. Many third-party payers (insurance companies) found it to their advantage to work out contracts similar to DRGs, such that hospitals without large numbers of Medicare patients still face prospective payment reimbursement in some form.

The challenge that faces hospital-based microbiologists, as well as those working in referral laboratories that rely on reimbursement from health care providers, is to continue to deliver quality results under increasing budgetary constraints. Most laboratories have responded to this challenge, finding new (and sometimes better) ways to deliver quality results rapidly in a cost-efficient manner. Industry has also responded by becoming more involved in developing rapid testing methods and pioneering ways to use new technology to the benefit of microbiology. The ultimate beneficiary of laboratory efforts is the patient; physicians and health care workers try to ensure that he or she receives timely and appropriate treatment, the overall goal is quality patient care. Since the negative impact of slow or incorrect diagnosis of infectious disease is an increased hospital stay (at the attendant increased expenditure), changes made in microbiology to better serve the clinician and patient have a positive impact that is multiplied in terms of cost benefits and quality health care.

Some strategies that can be employed to achieve these goals are presented in this chapter, which is intended as a sampler of ideas to serve as a basis upon which microbiologists can build, not an exhaustive catalogue of the available choices for altering test procedures to achieve maximum cost containment. Microbiologists, in choosing strategies that will work in their unique situations, are helping to shape the future of health care.

4.1. General Approaches to Cost Savings

Knowledge about the true costs of microbiology laboratory procedures and information about the budget allocated to operations are essential in order for administrators of the laboratory to be able to monitor its costs and performance. It is important that laboratory administrators receive timely copies of the appropriate budget, broken down into divisions representing personnel costs, supplies, services, and overhead (if charged to the laboratory). Almost all direct costs in microbiology laboratories are included within salaries (and benefits) and supplies; it is these two areas in which cost containment should be pursued most aggressively. Good measurement practices will allow the results of cost-cutting strategies to be monitored for their effectiveness.

It is also essential to know the actual costs incurred in performance of each procedure. Bartlett and others[2] and Garcia and Bruckner[10] have discussed procedures for gathering this information. An ongoing record of workload units (testing time, usually recorded in minutes) performed by technologists in each area of the microbiology laboratory is also important for assessing trends in the workload, rearranging staffing patterns to fit changing needs, and forecasting future developments, as well as for determining the technologist time expended on each procedure performed. The College of American Pa-

thologists' workload recording units (CAP units) are widely used for this purpose.[4]

Savings in supplies can be realized by substituting clean, nonsterile containers for certain specimens such as stool, urine, and sputum, the microbiological results from which will not be compromised.[14] Throat swabs for isolation of group A β-streptococci can be transported in glassine envelopes, rather than transport media, without losing viability. Forming consortia with other laboratories for buying common supplies in bulk and for negotiating lower supply costs is an effective cost-saving measure; sharing or splitting the performance of tests between neighboring laboratories to maximize utilization of resources can also pay off. A careful evaluation of supply costs coupled with some creative thinking should allow microbiologists to modify existing methods to save resources in many ways.

4.1.a Education. The physician has the ultimate responsibility for patient care; all cost-generating procedures originate with a physician's orders. The first challenge that microbiologists face is that of educating physicians as to proper utilization of the services of the microbiology laboratory. Incoming physicians, those attending and those in training, should be presented with an orientation session detailing the functions and capabilities of the microbiology laboratory. Physicians should be aware of the hours during which microbiologists are available, the extent of diagnostic services provided, and the expected turnaround time for test results. Clinicians should be introduced to microbiologists with whom they may interact, so that communication can be open and often. A general orientation session presented to the house staff by the microbiologist should include suggestions for proper media, timing, and special requests for blood cultures, as well as other specimens that require advance notice or special handling.

Microbiologists must also seek to learn from clinicians. Decisions such as elimination of tests, minimizing identification, and hours that the laboratory should be open should be made jointly by knowledgeable physicians, such as infectious disease clinicians, and microbiologists so as to achieve cost containment without undue risk or discomfort to patients. Elimination of unnecessary tests has been shown to save money.[24] Continuous dialogue between microbiologists and clinicians concerning proper utilization and interpretation of the labora-

---

Suggested Characteristics of Good Microbiological Result Reports

1. Inclusion of interpretive statements
2. Notification of improper specimen collection or handling
3. Reporting of relevant susceptibility results only
4. Clear and unambiguous terminology
5. Explanation of unusual organism names
6. Inclusion of normal values with numerical data

7. Reporting negative results from special tests, for example, "no *Campylobacter* isolated"
8. Reporting normal flora from contaminated sites, for example, "normal skin flora"
9. Reporting of results in semiquantitative form
10. Reporting of all isolates from normally sterile sites
11. Naming a source for further information

Modified from Lee, A., and Gooden, H. 1982. Improving communication of microbiology test results. Am. J. Clin. Pathol. 77:443.

---

tory's services should help to decrease excessive or inappropriate test requests. Guidelines for reporting microbiological data to facilitate physician understanding have been suggested (see box above).

It is necessary to discuss proper laboratory utilization with the nursing staff as well. One strategy that pays off in terms of helping nurses and physicians to submit specimens properly for microbiological analysis is the availability of a small, printed manual containing detailed instructions on proper submission of specimens, including containers, request forms, special handling requirements, timing and numbers of specimens to submit, and other information. Updated at least annually with procedural changes, such a book rapidly becomes an essential reference manual for nurses and clinicians, and the laboratory benefits both in decreased numbers of phone calls and in better quality of specimens. Some of the information to include in such a reference manual is found in Chapter 6.

A quarterly or semiannual publication originating in the microbiology laboratory that seems to impact positively on patient care and minimizing costs is the cumulative antimicrobial susceptibility statistics for the hospital. Information to include in this publication, which is best reduced to a pocket-sized folded card, could include maximum serum, urine, and cerebrospinal fluid levels achievable for appropriate antimicrobial agents, as well as some representative costs. By being aware of susceptibility patterns within the institution, clinicians can prescribe antimicrobial agents that are likely to be the most ef-

fective at the least cost. Although microbiology laboratories don't always have full say in the matter, the antimicrobial susceptibility results for third-generation cephalosporins, broad-spectrum penicillins, and more expensive aminoglycosides should be reported only for those bacteria that exhibit resistance to a predetermined group of first-choice antimicrobial agents, thus shaping the treatment patterns of physicians who consider in vitro susceptibility results in such decisions. Additionally, microbiologists should participate on those committees, usually consisting of representatives from the infectious disease service, medical and surgical services, and pharmacy, that choose which antimicrobial agents are routinely tested in the microbiology laboratory. By educating physicians as to appropriate use of antimicrobial agents, often in such subtle ways as reporting patterns, microbiologists are contributing to cost savings.

4.1.b. Limitations on testing. Laboratories can limit tests in several ways without harming patient care quality. As suggested by Ellner,[6,7] limits on the numbers of specimens in several categories (Table 4.1) that are accepted by the laboratory will contribute to more rational patient management. By offering test panels that automatically offer increasingly specialized tests based on the results of screening tests, laboratories can decrease the number of nonproductive tests run. A number of specimens are inappropriate for culture and may even yield misleading information. Foley catheter tip cultures; surface cultures of decubiti; anaerobic cultures from the

Table 4.1

Suggested Limits for Specimens Accepted for Microbiological Studies

SPECIMEN	LIMIT
Urine, stool, genital, sputum, wounds, upper respiratory area	One daily, maximum three weekly
Blood	Three daily, maximum six per patient admission
Stool for ova and parasites	Three per patient admission
Specimens for fungus culture and serology	Three per patient admission
Virus cultures	One of each type per patient admission
Sputum and gastric aspirate for mycobacteria	Three of each per patient admission
Urine or cerebrospinal fluid for mycobacteria	Infectious disease section approval required

Adapted from Ellner, P.D. 1985. A dozen ways to achieve more cost-effective microbiology. Med. Lab. Observer 17:40.

vagina or cervix, bowel contents, or oral sources; and cultures of periodontal material (except for specialized laboratories) do not contribute to good patient management and should be avoided. The laboratory should limit the testing of *routine* throat cultures to detection of β-hemolytic streptococci and respiratory viruses. Pooling the three formalin-preserved stool specimens received from outpatients for detection of ova and parasites has been shown to yield the same results as examination of the specimens separately.[20] This procedure saves both technologist time and resources.

Cultures of material should be avoided if Gram stains or other direct visual examinations will yield sufficient diagnostic information. For example, a 10% potassium hydroxide (KOH) or calcofluor white wet preparation of scrapings from clinically compatible lesions on the tongue of a child suspected of having thrush or on the vaginal wall of a woman suspected of candidal vaginitis, if positive, provides the diagnosis without culture. The presence of clue cells, lack of lactobacilli, increased pH, and disagreeable odor of vaginal discharge are indicative of bacterial vaginosis (nonspecific vaginitis), and cultures are unnecessary. The presence of multinucleated giant cells in a Tzanck preparation or direct fluorescent antibody stain from a suspected herpetic vesicle precludes the necessity for culture.

Limitations that may be practiced within the laboratory should be undertaken only after careful study and discussions with clinicians to determine that no negative effect on patient care will result. The number of primary plates that are routinely inoculated with clinical material may be decreased. Stool cultures can be plated to two selective and differential media instead of three or four, in addition to blood and *Campylobacter* and MacConkey agars (Chapter 17). It may be possible to eliminate inoculation of stool into enrichment broth for subsequent subculture if it can be shown that no significant additional isolates are recovered by this procedure. The number of media set up for cultivation of mycobacteria and fungi can be limited to support the growth of all etiologic agents in a more general sense. For example, instead of incubating separate sets of fungal media at 37° and 30° C, incubate one set of plates at 30° C, a temperature at which all fungi can grow. Biplates, such as anaerobic *Bacteroides* bile esculin and laked sheep blood with kanamycin and vancomycin, can be inoculated instead of two separate plates. Limitations on all anaerobic bacteriology procedures should be implemented, based on patient-care needs.[8] Blood cultures and stool cultures from hospitalized patients should be limited based on clinical usefulness.[1,11,13] Other cost-saving measures can be undertaken, depending on the individual situation present in each laboratory. Of course, the physicians must be kept well informed of laboratory policy so that special circumstances will be accommodated and patient care will not suffer.

In some circumstances, what appears to be a costly procedure may, in fact, prove cost-effective in the overall achievement of better patient care. Virus culture of cerebrospinal fluids, a seemingly low-yield procedure, was found to shorten hospitalization and prevent unnecessary antibiotic use in a significant number of patients from whom viruses were isolated. The overall cost savings and patient-care improvements more than offset the initial cost of the laboratory test.[3] In other circumstances, such as direct antigen detection in cerebrospinal fluid, the rapid results cannot compensate for lack of sensitivity in serious infections such as meningitis; and test results are unlikely to alter patient management.[12] Usefulness of such tests in each laboratory environment should be evaluated very carefully, with input from clinicians, before they are implemented.

4.1.c. **Screening procedures**. Tremendous cost savings can be achieved if specimens unlikely to yield diagnostic information are not processed beyond initial evaluation. The screening of expectorated sputum for the numbers of polymorphonuclear neutrophils and squamous epithelial cells per low-power field is an effective way to improve the quality of sputum specimens received in the laboratory and to prevent unnecessary work. Sputum can be screened unstained for even greater time and cost savings.[23]

Screening should be extended to wound cultures received on swabs. Even when only one swab is received in the laboratory, both cultures and a Gram-stained smear may be prepared using the following method. The microbiologist vortexes the swab for at least 30 seconds in 0.5 ml of the appropriate diluent (tryptic soy broth or brucella broth) to suspend the material on the swab, places the swab into enrichment broth (thioglycolate), and, with a sterile capillary pipette, inoculates several drops of the remaining suspension to the appropriate media and onto the surface of a slide. The presence of polymorphonuclear neutrophils indicates an infectious process; the presence of squamous epithelial cells indicates surface skin contamination. The appearance of the Gram stain can further be used by technologists to determine the extent of definitive identification and susceptibility testing to be performed on the organisms recovered. The immediate information conveyed to physicians by the results of the Gram stain and the subsequent decrease in unnecessary studies performed on specimens of dubious value should far outweigh the inconvenience and time initially invested in the staining procedure.

A number of recent technical advances, including the use of bioluminescent analysis and colorimetric methods, have been directed toward screening urine (Chapter 18). Since the largest numbers of specimens received by many laboratories are urines, of which over half are culture-negative or not diagnostically significant, a urine screening system can reduce unnecessary work. Physicians will benefit by receiving negative results one day sooner than by conventional culture, which should aid in preventing antibiotic overusage. A urine screen that has been evaluated for its applicability to the specific clinical milieu in which the laboratory functions should be considered.[21]

New technologies are being applied to development of screening procedures for many other clinical specimens. Tests are available for rapid testing of stool filtrates for the presence of *Clostridium difficile* toxin, screening of enrichment broths from stool specimens for presence of *Salmonella* or *Shigella*, and presence of antigens of several infectious agents in urine and other body fluids. Some tests on clinical specimens will have the greatest value as predictors of negative results, thus limiting the number of specimens that must be assessed by more cumbersome methods. Gas chromatography has long been studied as a means to quickly evaluate body fluids for the presence of bacterial metabolic products, although it has not gained widespread usage.

4.1.d. **Strategies for choosing methods.** Microbiology laboratories should make available to physicians all tests necessary for diagnosis and management of the patient population served. Not all tests can be performed reliably or economically by the laboratory. A laboratory must decide which tests to perform in-house and which methods to use; as well as which tests to send to an outside reference laboratory and which reference laboratory to use. The needs of the patients will dictate the numbers and variety of methods that a laboratory should offer.

Based on historical and predicted numbers of test requests, laboratories can remove low-volume tests from their menu to realize cost savings. Cost-accounting information can help determine which tests should be sent out based on direct costs alone. Additional cost factors to be considered include the cost of quality control testing that must be performed with each in-house patient test, the supplies that must be discarded due to outdating if test requests do not exceed supply shelf-life, cost of proficiency-testing surveys to cover the test, clerical time for record keeping and preparing additional forms, and mailing or transport costs to the reference laboratory. Noncost considerations include the ability of an outside laboratory to provide results in time to be useful clinically, the loss of expertise among staff who perform a test infrequently, the quality of available reference laboratories, and the enhanced prestige of the in-house laboratory that offers special tests among clinician-users and the hospital administration (which uses such information in public relations campaigns to attract more patients).

Once it has been decided to perform a test in-house, a method must be chosen. Patient population demographics again influence this decision, as tests vary in their efficiency of detection of a positive result (particular organism or disease state, for example) in relation to the prevalence of that result in the population.

Commonly used measurements of a test's performance include **sensitivity, specificity,** predictive value of a positive test result (**PVP**), and predictive value of a negative test result (**PVN**) (Table 4.2).[9] Inherent in determining the sensitivity and specificity of a test is the concept of a "gold standard" against which the test's performance is measured. This may not always be feasible. For example, new tests for detection of respiratory syncytial virus antigen by fluorescent antibody stain or enzyme-linked immunosorbent assay (ELISA) may be more sensitive than, and as specific as, conventional culture. In such a case, the performance of one of these new test systems should not be judged against standard methods to determine sensitivity. Given a suitable standard of comparison, the sensitivity and specificity of a test method are independent of the patient population tested. Therefore, laboratories need not always conduct extensive studies to evaluate new tests; they should make use of such evaluations carried out by respected and competent microbiologists and published in scientific literature. The choice of a test for in-house evaluation should be based on published performance and perceived utility within the laboratory based on prevalence of the organism or syndrome among the patient population served. The predictive value of a positive test decreases as the prevalence of the disease in the population decreases. Prevalence can thus be used to make initial decisions on types of tests to perform. Only hands-on experience, however, can ultimately determine the appropriateness of a given test for each laboratory setting. An algorithm for choosing a diagnostic test method has been published.[22]

A similar approach to that outlined should be applied to the decision as to whether to automate a given procedure, which instrument to use, and whether to purchase or lease the instrument. Initial equipment costs, ongoing reagent costs, and labor-saving costs (less technologist hand-on time or less skilled workers required to perform the test) must be taken into account when comparing overall economics of instrumentation. The skills and numbers of the available workforce, turnaround time, specimen preparation requirements, record-keeping and report-generating capabilities, and space requirements are nonecomonic considerations. Microbiology, perhaps the least automated of the clinical lab-

Table 4.2

Diagram of Test Reliability Parameters

	TRUE STATE	
TEST RESULT	**CONDITION EXISTS**	**CONDITION DOES NOT EXIST**
Positive test result	TP (true-positives)	FP (false-positives)
Negative test result	FN (false-negatives)	TN (true-negatives)

DEFINITIONS:

Sensitivity $\left(\begin{array}{l}\text{percent true-positives among all positive}\\\text{situations}\end{array}\right)$

$$= \frac{TP}{TP + FN} \times 100$$

Specificity $\left(\begin{array}{l}\text{percent true-negatives among all negative}\\\text{situations}\end{array}\right)$

$$= \frac{TN}{FP + TN} \times 100$$

PVP $\left(\begin{array}{l}\text{predictive value}\\\text{of positive test}\end{array}\right) = \left(\begin{array}{l}\text{percent true-positives}\\\text{among all positive test results}\end{array}\right)$

$$= \frac{TP}{TP + FP} \times 100$$

PVN $\left(\begin{array}{l}\text{predictive value}\\\text{of negative test}\end{array}\right) = \left(\begin{array}{l}\text{percent true-negatives}\\\text{among all negative test results}\end{array}\right)$

$$= \frac{TN}{TN + FN} \times 100$$

Efficiency (percent of correct results, both positive and negative)

$$= \frac{TP + TN}{TP + FP + FN + TN} \times 100$$

oratory disciplines, has adopted such methods slowly. The variety and proved abilities of instruments available today, however, have weakened the objections of most microbiologists. Automation in microbiology has found a place in today's cost-conscious environment.

4.2. Rapid Detection of Etiologic Agents of Infection

4.2.a. Visual tests. As discussed throughout the book, there are numerous methods for rapidly detecting the presence of infectious agents or their products. The easiest to perform are direct wet preparations and simple stains. The Gram stain is probably the single most cost-effective test used in clinical microbiology. Some specific visual methods employ immunological reagents coupled to marker substances. Examples include the rapid detection of *Chlamydia* elementary bodies by a monoclonal antibody conjugated with a fluorescein marker. Horseradish peroxidase, alkaline phosphatase, and other enzymatic markers have been used, particularly for detection of viral subunits, either nucleic acid sequences or surface proteins. Fluorescent reagents are available for specific staining of *Legionella* species, *Neisseria gonorrhoeae*, *Bordetella pertussis*, *Yersinia pestis*, *Francisella tularensis*, *Treponema pallidum*, *Bacteroides fragilis*, some pigmented anaerobic gram-negative bacilli, other bacteria, and a number of fungal and parasitic agents of infectious disease. For specimens that are suspected of harboring these agents, the use of rapid detection methods can save days and directly influence patient care.

4.2.b. **Particle agglutination methods.** Latex agglutination and staphylococcal coagglutination reagents coated with antibodies are available for rapid detection of many antigens. Group A β-hemolytic streptococci can be detected in throat swabbings within 15 minutes of collection of the specimen. Commercial kits are available for rapid detection of the antigens of the most common causes of meningitis, *Haemophilus influenzae* type b, *Neisseria meningitidis*, *Streptococcus pneumoniae*, and *Streptococcus agalactiae*. These tests may detect antigens in urine or serum as well. Cryptococcal antigen can be detected with more sensitivity using latex reagents than by India ink direct preparations. Latex tests for detection of rotavirus in stool filtrates have been compared favorably with electron microscopy and ELISA methods. Latex reagents are also being evaluated for diagnosis of invasive staphylococcal disease (by quantitation of circulating teichoic acid antigens) and invasive *Candida* infections (by quantitation of circulating cell wall mannan). Latex agglutination procedures for detection of herpes-virus in lesion scrapings, *Legionella* antigen in urine, *C. difficile* protein in stool, and so forth are available. Because of limitations of sensitivity, such tests are usually better predictors of positive results than of negative results, although false-positive results also occur.

4.2.c. **Automation.** The plethora of automated microbiology instruments allows rapid detection of the presence or absence of infectious agents and often yields identifications as well (Chapter 11). The use of such instruments can greatly increase microbiology laboratory productivity. Instruments developed to detect the presence of certain etiologic agents, particularly in urine, or to identify isolates are the Vitek AMS, the Abbott MS-2, the new Hewlett-Packard MIS instrument, and the General Diagnostics Autobac. Urines with numbers of microorganisms greater than 10^5/ml are identified within hours, all with greater than 95% sensitivity.

Radiometric and spectrophotometric detection of microbial metabolism, as used by the Johnston Laboratories Bactec system, can significantly decrease the time to detection of mycobacteria in sterile body fluids and concentrated contaminated specimens and in some cases in blood. Other automated blood screening devices are being developed, utilizing colorimetric, electrical impedance, and other technological tools. The *Limulus* lysate test (Chapter 10), although somewhat labor intensive at this time, may be automated for detection of endotoxin. The Abbott Quantum makes use of ELISA technology to detect antigens of gonococci and chlamydia in genital swab specimens. An ELISA test is commonly used to detect the presence of rotavirus antigen in feces. Radioimmunoassay and ELISA methods can be used for rapid diagnose of hepatitis A and B.

4.2.d. **Other strategies.** Additional labor at the receiving end of a specimen may save time and effort later. Two such approaches are used for blood cultures, lysis centrifugation (DuPont Isolator) and antimicrobial removal (Becton Dickinson Antimicrobial Removal Device and Bactec resin bottles). Both systems entail additional initial processing of blood cultures (Bactec simply requires a separate culture collection bottle), but both systems decrease the time to detection of positive results. Rapid initiation of appropriate treatment based on blood culture results should save hospitals money and, more importantly, lead to more successful therapy of patients. Blood cultures not handled by an automated system or by direct plating may reveal positive results more rapidly if an early detection system is employed. These include internal subculture to agar that is enclosed within the system (Gibco biphasic bottle; Roche Septi-Check) and early external subculture or acridine orange stain. Almost 80% of all positive blood cultures will be detected within 24 hours of collection if the vented or aerobic bottle is agitated during initial incubation and examined microscopically by acridine orange or subcultured within 6 to 12 hours after receipt.

4.3. Speeding Up Identification Results

4.3.a. Noncommercial methods. Once microbial growth has occurred, several methods can be used to decrease the time required to ascertain identification and susceptibility results. Spot biochemical tests can reliably identify presumptively several bacteria. The most cost-effective measure available to microbiologists is to identify bacteria presumptively based on colony morphology and simple spot biochemical tests. Several organisms lend themselves to such methods. The indole and oxidase tests are two of the most useful and rapid tests available. Indole-positive, oxidase-negative, lactose-positive, nonmucoid, flat colonies on MacConkey agar can be reported presumptively as *Escherichia coli*. These organisms comprise a substantial percentage of the gram-negative bacilli isolated in most laboratories. Swarming *Proteus* species seen on blood agar may also be identified presumptively with spot indole. Indole-positive *Proteus* is likely to be *P. vulgaris*. Indole-negative *Proteus* is likely to be *P. mirabilis*. Colonies that morphologically resemble *Pseudomonas aeruginosa* may be identified presumptively based on β-hemolysis, blue-green pigment, characteristic odor, and positive oxidase spot test results. When assessing the results of cultures of genital specimens taken from sexually active adults, technologists may presumptively identify colonies of gram-negative diplococci growing on Thayer-Martin media that are oxidase-positive as *Neisseria gonorrhoeae* or *N. meningitidis*. The PYR test can be used for rapid identification of *Streptococcus pyogenes* and *Enterococcus* species from morphologically characteristic colonies.

From cerebrospinal fluid and blood cultures, slightly β-hemolytic colonies of catalase-positive gram-positive short bacilli or coccobacilli can be presumptively identified as *Listeria monocytogenes* if they exhibit characteristic tumbling motility on wet preparation. A positive slide coagulase result on a colony of catalase-positive gram-positive cocci in clusters identifies the isolate as *Staphylococcus aureus*. Yeast cells from certain sources can be presumptively identified as *Candida albicans* if they form germ tubes within 3 hours at 37° C in fetal bovine serum. The Quellung rapid serologic slide test can also be used to identify *S. pneumoniae* and *H. influenzae* type b.

Suspicious colonies on primary stool media can be subcultured to blood agar plates or to Kliger's iron or triple sugar iron agar slants immediately upon discovery. Rapid urease or phenylalanine tests can be set up at the same time to rule out certain nonpathogens. After 4 to 5 hours incubation, enough of a film of growth will have occurred on the blood agar or the slant surface to allow the technologist to perform slide agglutination serologic typing tests.

Carbohydrate fermentation reactions of a number of non-Enterobacteriaceae can be determined within 4 hours using a broth containing 20% carbohydrate, peptone, meat extract, and buffers, described in Chapter 9 (Procedure 9.9). Fastidious bacteria, including *Kingella* species, *Actinobacillus*, *Cardiobacterium*, DF-2, and *Neisseria*, can be rapidly identified biochemically using this medium. Other approaches have been suggested.[16]

Microbiologists should all have additional ideas about the implementation of rapid methods for identification that will fit into the workflow, capabilities, and needs of their individual situations. Many clinical situations exist in which rapid, presumptive information is more important than delayed, definitive information. It is important that the microbiologist ascertain from the infectious disease specialists and other physicians who utilize laboratory results which definitive results can be delayed or even deleted in exchange for early, presumptive information. Sources cited in the bibliography and references should be consulted for other ideas.

4.3.b. Commercial methods. More commercial systems for rapid identification of microorganisms exist than can be mentioned here. Many of them are discussed in Chapter 9. By using enzymatic substrates that yield a colored end product, the presence of enzymes can be used to identify bacteria even in the absence of growth. Rapid enzymatic or biochemical tests systems, made by Key Scientific, General Diagnostics, API, Innovative Diagnostics, Flow Laboratories, BBL Microbiology Systems, Remel Laboratories, Austin Biologicals, and many others, are available for preliminary screening and identification of most gram-negative bacilli, gram-negative cocci, anaerobic bacteria, and some gram-positive cocci. Immunological reagents for identification of organisms by particle agglutination are also available. Such systems (as discussed in Chapter 25) for identification of β-hemolytic streptococci yield results within minutes or a few hours.

An important source of inoculum for direct application to commercial systems is blood culture broth. Broth from a positive blood culture medium may be inoculated directly to identification systems, such as rapid enzymatic test kits, or to coagulase plasma, depending on the Gram stain morphology. Even the particle agglutination identification systems have been shown to accurately identify organisms found in blood culture media when they are performed on properly prepared samples. One technique for preparing a sample suitable for biochemical inoculation is to remove 10 ml of the supernatant from a blood culture bottle shown to contain only one morphological type of organism. The culture medium is centrifuged at $1500 \times g$ for 10 minutes to concentrate the bacteria, the supernatant is discarded, and the pellet is resuspended in distilled water (which serves to lyse blood cells). If desired, a second centrifugation can be performed to wash the bacteria free of blood cell components, but this has not usually been found to be necessary. This suspension is then inoculated to the rapid identification system of choice. Just as for suspicious colonies from stool cultures, blood culture broth may be plated to a blood agar plate and incubated for 3 to 4 hours to allow a sufficient film of growth to develop. This film is removed with a cotton swab, emulsified in water or saline, and used to inoculate rapid systems.

The strategies and products mentioned here and in other sources that address cost containment should be evaluated for their utility in each laboratory, and their use should be considered where appropriate. It is possible that microbiology laboratories may have to respond to the DRG challenge by rearranging the workflow, expanding the hours of operation, hiring more laboratory assistants, utilizing more automated methods, and otherwise changing to conform to the times and the needs of the patient population.

4.4. Speeding Up Susceptibility Results

The susceptibility of a microorganism to antimicrobial agents is even more important than the definitive identification in many cases. Several strategies have been developed to yield faster results in that

area. Exhaustively reviewed by Isenberg and D'Amato,[15] rapid susceptibility testing methods range from reading disk diffusion agar plates after only 5 or 6 hours incubation to direct inoculation of susceptibility testing media with specimen material. The most effective method for rapid susceptibility testing of isolated bacteria appeared to be that of Lorian,[19] in which isolated colonies were suspended in trypticase soy broth to a density equal to a McFarland 1.0 turbidity standard and the suspension was inoculated to Mueller-Hinton agar without preincubation. The standard zone sizes were used for interpretation of results, but Mueller-Hinton with 5% sheep blood was used for all gram-positive cocci. *Qualitative* results obtained after 5 hours incubation agreed with conventional Bauer-Kirby disk diffusion determinations over 97% of the time for all organisms. Rapid methods have not been so standardized for quantitative susceptibility results. New technologies exploiting the ability of growing organisms to produce fluorescent marker metabolic end products or the technological advances that allow laser imaging of tiny amounts of bacterial mass are being actively pursued as possible candidates for rapid susceptibility testing use.

Direct susceptibility testing with urine has not yielded results that correlate well with conventional methods. Positive blood cultures, however, since they are almost universally monomicrobic, can be adapted for direct testing. Methods cited above for preparation of inocula for identification systems can also be used to prepare inocula for direct susceptibility testing. Greater than 95% agreement with interpretative results of conventional testing procedures can be achieved by dropping two to three drops of the well-agitated blood culture broth (Gram-stained to ascertain the presence of only one morphological type) directly to the surface of Mueller-Hinton agar. This inoculum is spread and further handled in the same manner as for standard disk diffusion.[5] Results are thus available 1 day sooner than with conventional methods, which should always be performed to confirm rapid test findings.

Even quantitative susceptibility testing can be speeded up, as reported by Kiehn et al.[17] A 1-ml suspension made of equal amounts of turbid blood culture broth and brain-heart infusion broth, incubated for 3 to 6 hours and diluted 1:500, can be used as the inoculum for a microbroth dilution susceptibility test with results that have greater than 98%

agreement with conventional methods (within two dilutions). Of course, all of these strategies work only with rapidly growing organisms, and results must be confirmed with conventional methods on the following day.

The equivalent of direct susceptibility testing of at least two selected bacterial species can be accomplished extremely rapidly by using chromogenic substrates, as discussed in Chapter 13. The chromogenic cephalosporin *nitrocefin* can be used with pure culture material as well as with pelleted specimen material from cerebrospinal fluids, for example, for detection of β-lactamases. Such information should be generated for isolates of gonococci and *H. influenzae*. Detection of β-lactamases produced by *S. aureus* cocci or *Bacteroides* may require increased reaction time, but the chromogenic substrate is still valuable for rapid detection of antimicrobial resistance. Other chromogenic substrates have been employed in other commercially produced rapid systems, usually impregnated on filter paper. β-lactamases can be detected using other systems, such as acidometric or iodometric, but these methods are slightly more cumbersome than the single filter paper required for the chromogenic substrate tests. A rapid test for detection of the acetyltransferase enzyme that renders an organism resistant to chloramphenicol should be used to test isolates of *H. influenzae* from cerebrospinal fluid in areas where chloramphenicol resistance has been reported and where that agent is used in the initial treatment of meningitis. This test is also available as a filter paper–impregnated disk (Remel Laboratories). It is hoped that new detection systems for resistance to other agents will soon be available.

Automation has made a tremendous impact on susceptibility testing in microbiology. A number of systems are available, as detailed in Chapter 11, that yield qualitative and quantitative results within 4 to 6 hours after the test is inoculated. Although certain types of resistance will not be detected with these systems as they are currently produced (such as inducible cephalosporinases and small numbers of methicillin-resistant staphylococci in a population of bacteria), the information generated by such systems is extremely valuable. Special susceptibility tests that previously required hours of labor, such as synergism studies, can be performed easily with those automated systems that generate curves of bacterial growth as detected nephelometrically (Abbot MS-2, Autobac).

Use of the radiometric system (Bactec) for detection of metabolic activity has revolutionized susceptibility testing of *M. tuberculosis*. Results that used to require up to 3 weeks are now available in several days. The effect of combinations of antimycobacterial agents on growth of isolates can be assessed in this system as well.

4.5. Computerization

The final product of the labors of microbiologists is information and the thrust of this discussion has been toward strategies for decreasing the time until the information is available. The speed with which this information is generated will have no impact on patient care, however, if it is not quickly relayed to the physician with responsibility for patient care. It is in the rapid dissemination of information that the modern laboratory differs from those of the past. A computer system is essential for information storage, sorting, and retrieval.

Cost containment measures that can be aided by computerization include logging in of new specimens. A computer can flag a second specimen from the same patient on a single day to alert the laboratory to (probably) unnecessary test requests. Without an automated system, duplicate specimens are rarely recognized until the next day, after they have been inoculated, if they are discovered at all. A microbiology computer can be used to maintain inventory and avoid costly delays due to lack of products as well as loss of operating costs due to outdating or overstocking. The use of computers for direct test requesting and reporting will save technologist and clerical time. In addition, the information critical to patient care will reach the intended physician directly, without the possible misunderstandings that occur when messages are relayed by telephone or the costly delay while the proper party is being located.

The computer can also be used to assess workload units of procedures, to effect direct billing and thus monitor laboratory usage, and to maintain quality control records. Of course, computers are valuable for preparing cumulative susceptibility data reports and for epidemiologic evaluation. Direct communication between microbiology instruments and laboratory computers can allow data to be transmitted easily after verification. Even if there is no computer access from the laboratory to the nursing stations, answers to telephone queries can be obtained much more quickly by finding the information on a laboratory computer than by leafing through a logbook for a patient's name or number.

Ultimately, it is computers that will help to effect the change in microbiology practices mandated by the need to control rising costs without adversely affecting patient care. The change from slow methods that require time for bacterial growth to more rapid methods for detection of pathogens and prediction of susceptibility patterns has begun late for microbiology in comparison to other laboratory specialities, such as chemistry and hematology. Clinicians, however, realize the value of rapid availability of results and will utilize the information for better patient care; they will demand more and better systems. Once hospital administrators also realize the cost benefit of rapid methods in microbiology, they will support more instrument acquisitions, which will spur the manufacturers to develop new and better systems. The revolution in microbiology, boosted by DRGs, has only begun.

REFERENCES

1. Aronson, M.D., and Bor, D.H. 1987. Blood cultures. Ann. Intern. Med. 106:246.
2. Bartlett, R.C., Kohan, T.S., and Rutz, C. 1979. Comparative costs of microbial identification employing conventional and prepackaged commercial systems. Am. J. Clin. Pathol. 71:194.
3. Chonmaitree, T., Menegus, M.A., and Powell, K.R. 1982. The clinical relevance of 'CSF viral culture.' J.A.M.A. 247:1843.
4. College of American Pathologists. 1988. Manual for laboratory workload recording method. The College, Skokie, Ill.
5. Coyle, M.B., McGonagle, L.A., Plorde, J.J., et al. 1984. Rapid antimicrobial susceptibility testing of isolates from blood cultures by direct inoculation and early reading of disk diffusion tests. J. Clin. Microbiol. 20:473.
6. Ellner, P.D. 1987. Cost-containment strategies for the diagnostic microbiology laboratory. Clin. Microbiol. Newsletter 9:117.
7. Ellner, P.D. 1985. A dozen ways to achieve more cost-effective microbiology. Med. Lab. Observer 17:40.
8. Finegold, S.M., and Edelstein, M.A.C. 1988. Coping with anaerobes in the 80s. pp. 1-10. In Hardie, J.M., and Borriello, S.P., editors. Anaerobes today. John Wiley & Sons, New York.
9. Galen, R.S., and Gambino, S. R. 1975. Beyond normality: the predictive value and efficiency of medical diagnosis. John Wiley & Sons, New York.
10. Garcia, L.S., and Bruckner, D.A. 1985. Microbiology's economics: dissecting procedures and costs. Med. Lab. Observer 17:51.
11. Gilligan, P.H. 1986. Diarrheal disease in the hospitalized patient. Infect. Control 7:607.
12. Granoff, D.M., Murphy, T.V., Ingram, D.L., and Cates, K.L. 1986. Use of rapidly generated results in patient management. Diagn. Microbiol. Infect. Dis 4(Suppl.):157S.
13. Gross, P.A., VanAntwerpen, C.L., Hess, W.A., and Reilly, K.A. 1988. Use and abuse of blood cultures: program to limit use. Am. J. Infect. Control 16:114.
14. Harris, P.C., and Sealey, L.B. 1986. Practical cost savings in microbiology. Med. Lab. Observer 18:32.
15. Isenberg, H.D., and D'Amato, R.F. 1984. Rapid methods for antimicrobic susceptibility testing. In Cunha, B.A., and Ristuccia, A.M., editors. Antimicrobial therapy. Raven Press, New York.
16. Kelly, M.T. 1986. Making organism identification cost-effective. Med. Lab. Observer 18:55.
17. Kiehn, T.E., Capitolo, C., and Armstrong, D. 1982. Comparison of direct and standard microtiter broth dilution susceptibility testing of blood culture isolates. J. Clin. Microbiol. 16:96.
18. Lee, A., and Gooden, H. 1982. Improving communication of microbiology test results. Am J. Clin. Pathol. 77:443.
19. Lorian, V. 1977. A five hour disc antibiotic susceptibility test. In Lorian, V., editor. Significance of medical microbiology in the care of patients. Williams & Wilkins, Baltimore.
20. Peters, C.S., Hernandez, L., Sheffield, et al. 1988. Cost containment of formalin-preserved stool specimens for ova and parasites from outpatients. J. Clin. Microbiol. 26:1584.
21. Pezzlo, M. 1988. Detection of urinary tract infections by rapid methods. Clin. Microbiol. Rev. 1:268.
22. Radetsky, M., and Todd, J.K. 1984. Criteria for the evaluation of new diagnostic tests. Ped. Infect. Dis. 3:461.
23. Wetterau, L.M., Zeimis, R.T., and Hollick, G.E. 1986. Direct examination of unstained smears for the evaluation of sputum specimens. J. Clin. Microbiol. 24:143.
24. Winkel, P., and Statland, B.E. 1984. Assessing cost savings when unnecessary utilization of laboratory tests can be abolished. Am. J. Clin. Pathol. 82:418.

BIBLIOGRAPHY

Bartlett, R.C. 1974. Medical microbiology: quality, cost and clinical relevance. John Wiley & Sons, New York.
Becker, B.L. 1985. Test menus and profiles: signs of change under DRG's. Med. Lab. Observer 17:26.
Doern, G.V., Scott, D.R., and Rashad, A.L. 1982. Clinical impact of rapid antimicrobial susceptibility testing of blood culture isolates. Antimicrob. Agents Chemother. 21:1023.
Everett, G.D., de Blois, S., Chang, P.F., and Holets, T. 1983. Effect of cost education, cost audits, and faculty chart review on the use of laboratory services. Arch. Intern. Med. 143:942.
Garcia, L.S. 1985. A cost containment checklist. Med. Lab. Observer 17:67.
Jorgenson, J.H., editor. 1987. Automation in clinical microbiology. CRC Press, Boca Raton, Fla.
Laboratory Medicine. 1988. Symposium: the practice of real-time diagnostic microbiology. Lab. Med. 19:336 pp. (Entire issue devoted to rapid testing in microbiology.)
Matsen, J.M. 1982. How rapid should rapid methods be? Clin. Microbiol. Newsletter 4:164.

Matsen, J.M., and Kelly, M.T. 1985. Practical clinical microbiology—laboratory perspectives for the era of prospective payment and DRG's. American Society for Clinical Pathology Commission on Continuing Education, Council on Microbiology, Chicago. (Workshop manual.)

McPherson, K.A., and Needham, C.A. 1987. Method evaluation and test selection. pp. 27-33. In Wentworth, B.B., Baselski, V.S., Doern, G.V., et al., editors. Diagnostic procedures for bacterial infections, ed. 7. American Public Health Association, Washington, D.C.

Miller, J.M. 1984. The impact of DRG's on hospital laboratories. Clin. Microbiol. Newsletter 6:57.

Sanders, C.B., and Aldridge, K.E. 1983. The microbiology laboratory: garbage in, garbage out. Clin. Microbiol. Newsletter 5:123.

Tilton, R.C., editor. 1982. Rapid methods and automation in microbiology. American Society for Microbiology, Washington, D.C.

5 Hospital Epidemiology

In addition to its important role in assisting in the diagnosis and guiding treatment of patients, the microbiology laboratory has the opportunity and responsibility to recognize infections of public health importance. The laboratory may identify infections that are capable of being spread from one individual to another, including tuberculosis, venereal disease, and certain diarrheal diseases, among others. Data from clinical microbiology laboratories may suggest or document an epidemic outbreak in the community.

Of particular importance to the microbiology laboratories in hospitals is their role in identifying and investigating nosocomial infection. The balance of this chapter will be devoted to nosocomial infections.

5.1. Nosocomial Infections

Nosocomial infections are those that are acquired in the hospital setting (Chapter 23). These may, of course, first appear after a patient has been discharged from the hospital, depending on the incubation period of the infection in question. Thus, it may be difficult to distinguish between community-acquired and nosocomial infections. Identification by the laboratory of an unusual number of isolates of an uncommon pathogen, of a number of strains of the same organism with an unusual antimicrobial susceptibility pattern or unique biochemical feature (e.g., H_2S-positive *Escherichia coli*), genetic pattern, or clustering of isolates of a given type from an intensive care unit or other discrete area within the hospital suggests the likelihood of an outbreak of nosocomial infection. The laboratory works closely with the infection control team to investigate the epidemiology of such outbreaks and to seek corrective measures. The laboratory assists in preventing infection of other patients and of hospital personnel by indicating which patients are likely to require isolation and by providing guidance in the use of disinfectants and sterilizing procedures.

5.1.a. **Incidence.** The National Nosocomial Infections Study (NNIS) carried out by the Centers for Disease Control indicates that 5% to 6% of hospitalized patients develop nosocomial infection. It is estimated that the average nosocomial infection prolongs hospital stay by about 3.2 days and results in added direct charges of about $1800 (based on 1986 figures). Thus, for the United States as a whole, nosocomial infections cost over $4 billion per year in direct costs alone. This does not take into account charges of physicians, loss of productivity, and costs of death. It appears that at least 1% of nosocomially infected patients die as a direct result of such infection and that nosocomial infection contributes to the deaths of an additional 2% to 3% of infected patients.

Attack rates vary according to the type of hospital, with large referral hospitals having higher rates of nosocomial infection than small community hospitals. Large teaching hospitals have higher infection rates than small teaching hospitals. The difference in risk of infection is probably related to several factors—severity of the illness occasioning hospitalization, frequency of invasive diagnostic and therapeutic procedures, and variation in the effectiveness of infection control programs. Within hospitals, surgical and medical services have the highest rates of infection, and pediatric and nursery units the lowest. Convalescent care facilities and nursing homes also contribute to the number of nosocomial infections. Although not documented as comprehensively as in hospitals, rates in such institutions are estimated to be significant.

5.1.b. **Epidemiology.** Three principal factors determine the likelihood that a given patient will acquire a nosocomial infection: (1) susceptibility of the patient to the infection, (2) the inoculum and virulence of the infecting organism, and (3) the nature of the patient's exposure to the infecting organism. In general, of course, hospitalized persons do have an increased susceptibility to infection, and it is not yet possible to immunize patients against nosocomial infections. Corticosteroids, cancer chemotherapeutic agents, and antimicrobial agents all contribute to the likelihood of nosocomial infection but are nonetheless important agents that are generally much more beneficial than harmful. It is also not possible

to exert influence over the virulence of the infecting organisms. Patients with serious community-acquired infections are admitted to hospitals frequently. It is advisable in the case of an influenza epidemic to avoid hospitalizing patients without serious complications and who are not in real need of hospital care. Nonetheless, it is necessary to admit a number of patients and the disease may spread in this manner. Our best hope to minimize nosocomial infections is to eliminate sources of exposure and to interrupt means of spread of these organisms in the hospital environment.

The most important means of transmission of nosocomial infections is by contact, usually direct but sometimes indirect, as in the case of spread of infection by means of secretions. Infected patients are the primary source of organisms in nosocomial infections, although asymptomatic carriers may transmit such infection. *Handwashing* by personnel before and after contact with each patient is the most important way to prevent direct contact transmission of nosocomial infection. Appropriate isolation of infected patients is also important. The second most common means of spread of hospital-acquired infection is by contaminated vehicles as in so-called common source outbreaks. Included here are contaminated food, water, medications, or medical devices. Other types of materials in the hospital may serve as sources of nosocomial infection or as fomites. A recently described example was wet mattresses, which served as environmental reservoirs of *Acinetobacter* that was involved in an outbreak of infection in a burn center. For the most part airborne spread of infection is less significant in the hospital setting, although it can be implicated in situations such as influenza or pulmonary tuberculosis.

5.1.c. **Types of nosocomial infection.** Urinary tract infection, the most common type of hospital-acquired infection, accounts for some 40% of nosocomial infections. Surgical wound infections account for an additional 20%, lower respiratory tract infections (primarily pneumonia) account for 15%, and nosocomial bacteremia accounts for an additional 5%. Thus, these four categories together account for about 80% of nosocomial infections. Cutaneous infections account for an additional 5% of hospital-acquired infections. *E. coli* is the most common pathogen isolated from urinary tract infections and is usually, but not always, of endogenous origin. However, it is less important in nosocomial infection than *Klebsiella, Enterobacter, Pseudomonas,* and other antimicrobial-resistant organisms. Important factors in nosocomial urinary tract infection are manipulation of indwelling urinary catheters and other types of urologic manipulations carried out for diagnostic or therapeutic purposes. Surgical wound infections often involve indigenous flora, but *Staphylococcus aureus* and a number of different types of gram-negative aerobic or facultative bacilli are more important pathogens in nosocomial infection. Lower respiratory tract infection acquired in the hospital setting often is related to aspiration and thus involves normal oral flora; however, patients in the hospital setting commonly acquire nosocomial pathogens such as *S. aureus* and various gram-negative bacilli in their oropharyngeal flora. If such patients should then aspirate, these organisms, in addition to anaerobes and streptococci from the indigenous flora, may play a role in a subsequent aspiration pneumonia. Respiratory therapy procedures, such as endotracheal suctioning or inhalation therapy, may introduce nosocomial pathogens into the patient's respiratory tract. Contaminated vehicles such as medications or water used for inhalation therapy may also be responsible. Nosocomial bacteremia is most often related to the use of intravascular devices. These catheters or cannulas may be contaminated by direct contact spread via health care personnel or from the patient's own skin flora. Contaminated vehicles such as intravenous fluids or arterial pressure transducers are also important sources of nosocomial infections. About two thirds of nosocomial infections involve a single pathogen and about 20% involve multiple pathogens. Thus, pathogens are identified in 85% of nosocomial infections. Of these, about 85% are aerobic or facultative bacteria, and 7% fungi. The most frequently reported pathogens have been *E. coli, S. aureus,* enterococci, and *P. aeruginosa.* Additional pathogens, in order of frequency of isolation from nosocomial infections, are *Klebsiella* sp., coagulase-negative staphylococci, *Enterobacter* sp., *Proteus* sp., *Candida* sp., and *Serratia* sp. The frequency of isolation of different pathogens varies, of course, according to the service on which the patient is hospitalized and the site of infection. Various *Legionella* sp. have been implicated in outbreaks in hospitals, with the source of the organisms being the water system, air-conditioning system, or cooling tower in most cases. Major enteric pathogens such as *Salmonella* and *Shigella* may cause hospital outbreaks on occasion.

Many or most of the nosocomial bacterial pathogens are resistant to a number of antimicrobial agents. Methicillin-resistant *S. aureus* infections, which initially were encountered primarily at large teaching hospitals, are increasing in frequency in small teaching hospitals and in nonteaching hospitals as well. Various gram-negative bacilli, such as *K. pneumoniae, S. marcescens,* and *P. aeruginosa,* are manifesting increased resistance to aminoglycosides, including amikacin and other agents. The incidence of nosocomial viral infections, including those involving rotavirus, respiratory syncytial virus, and influenza, is beginning to be appreciated with the increase of virus identification capabilities in hospital laboratories. It has been suggested that more than 75,000 nosocomial viral infections occur in the United States annually.[6]

5.1.d. Control programs and role of microbiology laboratory. Hospital infection control programs are designed to detect and monitor hospital-acquired infections and to prevent them where possible. Hospitals have multidisciplinary infection control committees, which should include a representative from the microbiology laboratory. Most hospitals have one or more infection control nurses who collect and analyze surveillance data, monitor patient care practices, and participate in epidemiologic investigations of problems. Some hospitals have physicians or sanitarians as hospital epidemiologists. Infection control personnel are responsible for systematic surveillance of patient disease in order to recognize problems of hospital-acquired infection and to detect epidemics as early as possible. The microbiology laboratory provides important data for this surveillance effort. Obviously, there must be good communication between laboratory personnel and the infection control team. It is desirable for infection control personnel to review the results of cultures in the laboratory on a daily basis. This provides a good opportunity for such people and laboratory microbiologists to exchange information and to learn to work together.

In the past it was common for microbiology laboratories to culture the inanimate environment of the hospital as well as certain fomites routinely. It is now recognized that such activities done on a routine basis provide little or no useful information and are very time-consuming and expensive. However, investigation of a specific problem of nosocomial infection may well be facilitated by cultures of the environment and personnel.

The prompt and accurate performance of routine

microbiology procedures may be very helpful in infection control work. The importance of full identification of isolates is underlined by a recent report of an outbreak of bacteremia and meningitis due to *Streptococcus faecium* in a neonatal intensive care unit.[2] Such outbreaks may not be recognized as outbreaks without full characterization of organisms. Beyond this, the microbiology laboratory must be able to adapt quickly to unexpected infection control problems. The laboratory may be asked to characterize organisms in detail, to perform additional susceptibility tests, and to screen a large number of specimens of various types for a particular pathogen. Infection control problems tend to occur suddenly and unexpectedly, and the microbiology laboratory must be prepared to react promptly and effectively in such situations. The laboratory director must assist the infection control team in planning strategies that are consistent with the nature of the outbreak and the resources of the laboratory. A laboratory should be prepared to ask for help from county or state health departments or other resources, when necessary. It is highly desirable for the laboratory to have contingency plans available for emergencies that might be anticipated. Obviously, laboratory budgets should be adequate to cover routine infection control testing as well as special tests and emergency procedures. More extensive coverage of microbiology procedures as they relate to a comprehensive infection control program can be found in works by McGowan and coworkers.[4,5]

5.1.e. Reporting of results. As noted above, good infection control personnel review microbiology laboratory results on a daily basis, and this should include direct discussions between the two groups. Certain types of results should cause the microbiologist to initiate a phone call to the infection control team or infectious disease physicians, in addition to the attending physician. For example, all positive blood cultures, all positive spinal fluid cultures, all positive acid fast smears, isolations of enteric pathogens such as *Shigella*, and isolation of resistant organisms such as methicillin-resistant *S. aureus* should be reported by phone. Isolation of a new or unusual pathogen should result in prompt relay of information to the infection control team.

Laboratory results should be kept in a readily accessible format such as a logbook if the laboratory is not computerized, and laboratory records, including microbiology work cards, should be kept on file for at least 2 years. If the laboratory changes any of its technical practices that might influence the surveillance data, such as culturing urines with a 0.01-ml calibrated loop instead of the previously used 0.001-ml loop, all affected parties should be notified of the change and a record of the date of institution of the new practice should be kept with the infection control data files. Isolations of unusual organisms or organisms with unique susceptibility patterns are spotted readily. However, it may be much more difficult to recognize a cluster of cases of infection involving a common organism. Computers may be very useful for this purpose. Infection control personnel should be supplied with periodic summaries of selective results. Tables indicating the frequency with which particular organisms have been isolated from various sites on specific wards or units and on specific services are very helpful. This type of data should be expressed in percentages. The antimicrobial susceptibility of various isolates to the more commonly used antimicrobial agents should also be provided on a regular basis in tabular form. For this type of data to be useful, it is important to exclude repeat cultures of the same organism from the same patient.

5.1.f. Characterizing epidemic strains. A good system for typing microbial strains involved in outbreaks is standardized, reproducible, sensitive, stable, readily available, inexpensive, applicable to a wide range of microorganisms, and field tested in conjunction with epidemiologic investigation. No such ideal typing system is available, but it is important for us to appreciate the strengths and weaknesses of the systems that we use. Useful typing methods include biological or biochemical typing (biotype), antimicrobial susceptibility patterns (antibiogram), serologic typing (serotype), bacteriocin typing (including both susceptibility to bacteriocin and production of bacteriocin), bacteriophage typing (phage type), plasmid analysis, and restriction enzyme analysis of plasmid or chromosomal nucleic acids. Biotyping and antibiograms are clearly suitable for all hospital clinical microbiology laboratories. Limited serologic typing may also be performed in clinical laboratories. For the most part, the other typing methods listed above are available only through reference or research laboratories.

Routine identification procedures, if organisms are identified to at least the species level, are very useful in permitting recognition of hospital-acquired infection outbreaks. Failure to fully identify *Pseudomonas* species might lead to overlooking less commonly encountered species such as *P. cepacia* or *P. maltophilia* as causes of an outbreak. Identification of an unusual Enterobacteriaceae strain, such as *Klebsiella oxytoca*, in sputum from several patients with pneumonia may facilitate the discovery of faulty cleaning techniques for respiratory therapy equipment.

Commercially available biochemical test panels, such as the API 20E, Vitek AutoMicrobic System, and Enterotube II (Chapter 9), permit identification to species of the vast majority of fermentative gram-negative rods and, with the addition of a few other tests, also identify many nonfermenters. Such systems provide a computer data base into which biochemical profiles of large numbers of cultures have been entered (Chapter 9). Some of these computerized systems employ "octal numbers," which have been used in epidemiologic investigations. Unfortunately, there is some problem with reproducibility of octal or biotype numbers. Some of the reasons for the lack of reproducibility are inexact descriptions of many of the taxonomic groups, variations in inoculum size, differences in temperatures and times of incubation, and differences in media. Some of these factors apply more to interlaboratory discrepancies, but even within one laboratory there may be significant variation. Rigorous standardization of the test procedure, especially the inoculum, will provide better reproducibility with these systems. It must also be appreciated that certain of the reactions in these panels may be plasmid-mediated and therefore may be either acquired or lost by a strain during an outbreak of nosocomial infection. One should not assign too much significance to variations of just one or two tests in a biotype unless careful studies have been done to define the normal variation that can be expected in these cultures with the test being used. It is hoped that manufacturers of these commercial systems will ultimately provide us with standardized chemically defined media and reagents and carry out studies to examine the reproducibility of individual tests within and between laboratories.

Accurate reproducible susceptibility testing is important to the epidemiologist just as it is to the clinician. Recognition of outbreaks of infection due to gentamicin-resistant Enterobacteriaceae, methicillin-resistant *S. aureus*, and amikacin-resistant *P. aeruginosa*, for example, is very important. In addition, antimicrobial susceptibility patterns may be useful as epidemiologic markers in the same manner as biotyping. It is desirable to include, in the standard set of antimicrobial agents for testing, certain drugs such as nalidixic acid and streptomycin, which are of proved epidemiologic value. It must be remembered, however, that resistance to antimicrobial agents is often plasmid-mediated and therefore may be either lost or acquired by a strain during the course of an outbreak. The type of susceptibility test used and the method of reporting influence the degree to which antibiograms may be used successfully for epidemiologic purposes. Many laboratories use the Bauer-Kirby disk diffusion method (Chapter 13) for susceptibility testing. This method is standardized, reproducible, readily available, and relatively inexpensive. However, it can be used only for rapidly growing bacteria. Reporting of results of such tests as resistant, susceptible, or intermediate is much less useful to the infection control team than reporting of actual zone size measurements. With the Bauer-Kirby technique, however, degrees of resistance may not be appreciated. Absence of any zone of inhibition might be seen for a strain with a minimum inhibitory concentration (MIC) of 16 µg/ml and with another for which the MIC was greater than 1024 µg/ml. Such striking differences in degree of resistance may well indicate entirely different strains for epidemiologic purposes, even though the species was identical. The mechanisms of resistance might well be different also. Broth dilution susceptibility testing is being used more widely now as a result of mechanization and commmercialization. While differences in degrees of resistance, as in the example cited previously, can readily be determined by this type of test, there are other problems. For example, an MIC of 8 µg/ml might actually be anywhere between 4 and 16 µg/ml, given the inherent variability of a twofold serial dilution test. In this situation, an actual zone size measurement would provide less error.

When neither the antibiogram nor the biotype alone adequately characterizes a particular nosocomial strain, it may be useful to expand both typing systems by adding additional antimicrobial agents (or other substances with antimicrobial activity such as heavy metals) or additional biochemicals. One may also combine the results of biochemical and susceptibility testing to produce an "antibiotype."

Serologic typing is also potentially useful in hospital clinical microbiology laboratories and could be applicable to a broad range of microorganisms. How-

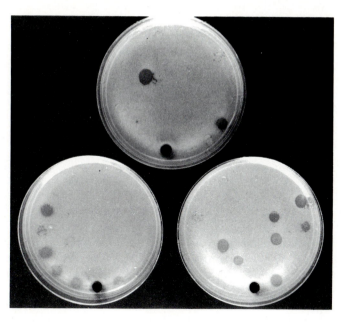

Figure 5.1

Figure 5.1
Example of three *S. aureus* isolates with different phage typing patterns. The organisms are swabbed on agar plates to achieve confluent growth, and suspensions of several different bacteriophages are spotted on the agar surface in a standard pattern. The ability of particular phages to infect and lyse the staphylococci is detected by the presence of a lysed circle, or "plaque." The staphylococci are assigned phage types according to which phages can cause lysis. (Plates courtesy Henry Isenberg.)

ever, its development as an epidemiologic tool is limited because of difficulties with mass production of antisera and with standardization of methods.

5.1.g. Special biotyping procedures. As indicated previously, there are a number of other procedures aside from biotyping, antibiograms, and serologic typing for characterization of epidemic strains. Such procedures are primarily useful in reference laboratory or research settings. Bacteriophage typing, by definition, is limited to bacteria. It has been especially useful with *S. aureus*, *P. aeruginosa* and *Salmonella* species. Phage typing consists of spotting a series of bacteriophages on a "lawn" of the organism to be typed on an agar plate culture. Bacteriophages have a very specific host range, each one attacking only a particular type of a given organism such as *S. aureus*. Thus there are a number of phages active against *S. aureus*, but each one lyses only particular types of *S. aureus*. From the pattern of lysis of the bacterium on the agar plate (see Figure 5.1), one can specify the phage type of a particular strain of *S. aureus*. If only phages numbered 52A and 80 among the whole set of phages used produce zones

of lysis with a given strain of *S. aureus*, that strain is designated phage type 52A, 80. Bacteriocin typing is also limited to bacteria. **Bacteriocins** are a group of heterologous substances produced by bacteria that inhibit the growth of closely related species; they are usually proteins. There are two systems of bacteriocin typing: bacteriocin production, which involves determination of the inhibitory spectrum of bacteriocins produced by a strain to be typed, and bacteriocin susceptibility, in which the susceptibility of the strain to be typed to bacteriocins produced by a set of standard producer strains is determined.

Plasmids are extrachromosomal bits of genetic material that are able to self-replicate. Plasmids may be transferred from one bacterial cell to another by conjugation or transduction. Plasmid analysis has been used primarily to explain the occurrence of unusual or linked antibiotic resistance patterns. It has been shown that plasmid or R factor (resistance genes carried on plasmids) epidemics occur in which a specific plasmid is transmitted from one genus of bacteria to another. Plasmid profiles, patterns created when plasmids are separated on agarose gel by

Table 5.1

Epidemiologic Typing Systems Most Useful for Nosocomial Pathogens

TYPING SYSTEM	MICROORGANISMS
Biotype	*Salmonella, Shigella*, other species of Enterobacteriaceae, *Pseudomonas*, fungi
Antibiogram	Enterobacteriaceae, *Pseudomonas* and other nonfermentative bacteria, *Staphylococcus*
Serotype	Viruses, Enterobacteriaeae, *Pseudomonas*, streptococci, *Legionella, Chlamydia*
Bacteriocin type	*Shigella, Pseudomonas, Serratia*
Bacteriophage type	*Staphylococcus, Pseudomonas, Salmonella, Mycobacterium*
Plasmid profiles	All bacteria, resistant strains
Restriction enzyme analysis	Herpes simplex virus, adenovirus, bacterial plasmid S, bacterial DNA

Modified from Aber, R.C., and Mackel, D.C. 1981. Epidemiologic typing of nosocomial microorganisms. Am. J. Med. 70:899.

electrophoresis, can also be used to characterize the similarity of bacterial strains that carry the plasmids. Relatedness of strains is based on the number and size of plasmids, with strains from identical sources showing identical plasmid profiles. Plasmids themselves or whole chromosomal DNA may be typed by means of restriction endonuclease digestion patterns. Restriction enzymes recognize specific nucleotide sequences in DNA and produce double-stranded cleavages that break the DNA into smaller fragments. There are at least 36 of these enzymes for which the specific recognition sequence and cleavage site have been defined. Figure 5.2 briefly outlines two methods used epidemiologically for nucleic acid analysis of bacterial strains. Restriction enzyme analysis may also be used for characterizing strains of viruses. It has been used particularly for herpes simplex virus. Table 5.1 summarizes the various typing systems that have been found most useful for selected nosocomial pathogens.

5.1.h. **Screening populations.** When a hospital infection outbreak occurs, it may be necessary to determine the extent to which the infecting strain has spread among the patients. Thus, the laboratory may be required to screen a large number of patients in a short period of time. It is important to choose culture sites and culture media so as to avoid unnecessary effort. Sites known to be colonized by a particular pathogen should be selected for culture. In the case of a group B streptococcal outbreak, for example, good sources of cultures would be the umbilicus, throat, and perhaps stool. In the case of a staphylococcal outbreak in a nursery setting, cultures of the umbilicus and nose would be appropriate. For enteric gram-negative bacilli, throat and stool are the major reservoirs.

Selective or differential media, or both, should be used to facilitate recovery of the organism being sought. In the case of an outbreak with an antibiotic-resistant organism, the microbiologist may incorporate an appropriate concentration of the drug or drugs in question in appropriate plate media. With this approach, it is important to test each batch to be certain that it supports the growth of the epidemic strain that is being sought.

Occasionally it is desirable to culture hospital personnel who may be involved in spreading an epidemic strain. It is important to culture only those individuals who are epidemiologically incriminated. Culturing large numbers of the medical staff indiscriminately is expensive, may yield misleading information, and causes anxiety or hostility.

Demonstration of bacteria on the hands of personnel may not only confirm the mechanism of cross-infection but also may serve as an important educational device to impress personnel with the importance of handwashing. A simple hand-culturing procedure is to have personnel press their fingertips, including nail tips, onto the surface of an appropriate agar medium. Unfortunately, this technique is not very sensitive. Detection of hand colonization is much more likely if personnel vigorously wash their hands with 10 to 20 ml of a nutrient broth in an ethylene oxide sterilized plastic bag or plastic glove containing the broth. The broth is then cultured onto agar by a semiquantitative method.

5.1.i. **Storage of strains.** It is important for microbiology laboratories to save unique isolates from patients so that they may be retrieved for further study if an epidemic is recognized later. Such organisms should be retained for at least a month in order to give the infection control team adequate time to re-

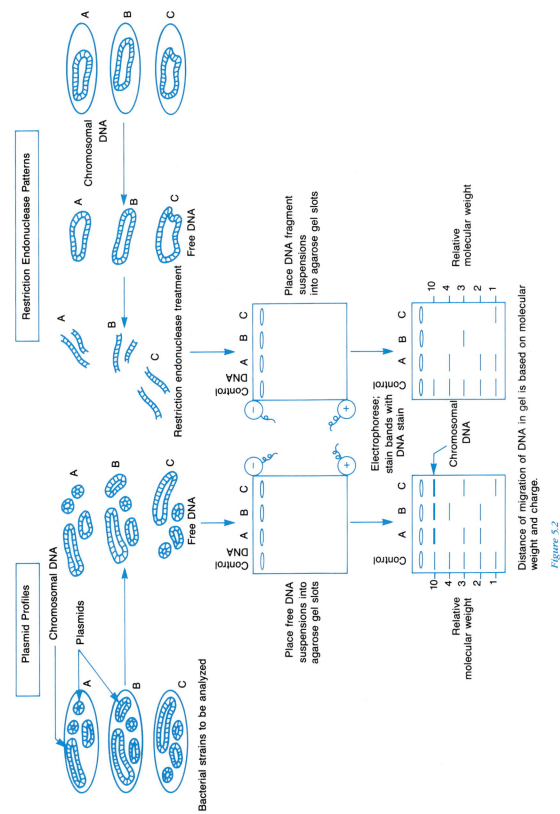

Figure 5.2
Two methods used to type bacteria based on genetic patterns.

view the situation to determine whether further analysis is indicated. Such storage, of course, is also valuable to clinicians who may wish to have additional identification procedures or susceptibility testing performed. Organisms that are documented as being involved in nosocomial infections and organisms with unique susceptibility patterns for the institution should be saved for extended periods of time.

5.2. Monitoring

Bacteriologic monitoring of personnel and of certain medical products or solutions is indicated on occasion, as noted above.

5.2.a. **Personnel monitoring**. Some institutions require preemployment stool cultures on food handlers. This is of limited value. It is much more important to stress that food handlers submit cultures if they develop diarrhea. There should be no routine screening of personnel for nasal carriage of S. *aureus*. A significant percentage of hospital personnel do carry this organism, but such individuals rarely shed enough organisms to pose a hazard and there is no simple way to predict which nasal carriers disseminate staphylococci. Culture of skin or other infections in members of the hospital staff is clearly an important function of the microbiology laboratory. The employee health service should be notified promptly of recovery of significant pathogens from such infections and of isolation of other organisms such as *Shigella* from stool cultures.

5.2.b. **Monitoring of hospital supplies and environment**. Because there have been a few outbreaks of nosocomial infection related to contaminated intravenous fluids and other commercial products, some hospitals have considered routine sampling of products before use. This is not practical and is not recommended. This type of contamination has typically involved only a small fraction of production lots, and the level of contamination is quite low. The quality control provided by the manufacturer is usually much more extensive than would be practical in the hospital microbiology laboratory. The better approach is for the infection control team to monitor patients for the development of nosocomial infections that might be related to the use of contaminated commercial products. In the event of an outbreak or an incident related to suspected contamination of commercial products, an appropriate microbiological study is indicated. Most often, such infections are actually caused by in-use contamination of the system, rather than contamination during the manufacturing process. Suspect lots of fluid and catheter trays should be saved and the Food and Drug Administration notified if contamination is suspected.

Some hospitals prepare their own parenteral solutions, especially hyperalimentation fluids. Microbiological testing is indicated as part of the quality control procedure. Since contamination of such fluids is generally rare and sporadic, it is not practical for most institutions to perform rigorous quality control to guarantee sterility of each lot that is produced. When culture is indicated, approximately 20 ml of fluid should be collected aseptically. A calibrated loop of 0.01 ml capacity may be used to inoculate the surface of a nutrient agar plate. The remaining fluid should be inoculated into a suitable nutrient broth in dilutions as low as 1:2, if necessary. Vacuum-assisted filtration of the fluid through sterile nitro-cellulose filters and subsequent incubation of the filter on suitable agar media is an alternative technique for detecting contamination in large volumes of fluids (>100 ml). Hospitals that prepare infant formula and those that bank human milk should perform microbiological studies to detect possible contamination. Several bottles of formula from each lot produced should be cultured by preparing a nutrient agar pour plate with 1 ml of milk. It has been suggested that no more than 25 colonies should be present after 48 hours of incubation, and none of these should be potential pathogens such as S. *aureus* or group A *Streptococcus*. Further guidelines for culture of milk are being developed.

In the event of a *Legionella* outbreak, environmental sampling should be done. In particular, the potable water supply, the air-conditioning cooling towers, and other elements of the air-conditioning system should be cultured. Details of suitable procedures may be found in the laboratory manual by Edelstein.[3]

REFERENCES

1. Aber, R.C., and Mackel, D.C. 1981. Epidemiologic typing of nosocomial microorganisms. Am. J. Med. 70:899.
2. Coudron, P.E., Mayhall, C.G., Facklam, R.R., Spadora, A.C., Lamb, V.A., Lybrand, M.R., and Dalton, H.P. 1984. *Streptococcus faecium* outbreak in a neonatal intensive care unit. J. Clin. Microbiol. 20:1044.
3. Edelstein, P.H. 1984. Legionnaires' disease laboratory manual. Document PB 84 156 827. National Technical Information Service, Springfield, Va.

4. McGowan, J.E. 1985. Role of the microbiology laboratory in prevention and control of nosocomial infections. In Lennette, E.H., Balows, A., Hausler, W.J. Jr., and Shadomy, H.J., editors. Manual of clinical microbiology, ed. 4. American Society for Microbiology, Washington, D.C.

5. McGowan, J.E. Jr., Weinstein, R.A., and Mallison, G.F. 1986. The role of the laboratory in control of nosocomial infections. In Bennett, J.V., and Brachman, P.S., editors. Hospital infections, ed. 2. Little, Brown & Co., Boston.

6. Valenti, W.M., et al. 1980. Nosocomial viral infection. I. Epidemiology and significance. Infect. Control 1:33.

BIBLIOGRAPHY

Archer, G.L., Dietrick, D.R., and Johnston, J.L. 1985. Molecular epidemiology of transmissible gentamicin resistance among coagulase-negative staphylococci in a cardiac surgery unit. J. Infect. Dis. 151:243.

Centers for Disease Control. 1986 (published annually). National nosocomial infection study report. U.S. Department of Health and Human Services, Public Health Service, Atlanta.

Coyle, M.B., and Schoenknecht, F.D. 1986. The clinical laboratory. In Bennett, J.V., and Brachman, P.S., editors. Hospital infections, ed. 2. Little, Brown & Co., Boston.

Favero, M.S. 1985. Sterilization, disinfection, and antisepsis in the hospital. In Lennette, E.H., Balows, A., Hausler, W.J. Jr., and Shadomy, H.J., editors. Manual of clinical microbiology, ed. 4. American Society for Microbiology, Washington, D.C.

Garner, J.S., and Emori, T.G. 1985. Nosocomial infection surveillance and control programs. In Lennette, E.H., Balows, A., Hausler, W.J. Jr., and Shadomy, H.J., editors. Manual of clinical microbiology, ed. 4. American Society for Microbiology, Washington, D.C.

Gilchrist, M.J.R., and Brooks, L.H. 1989. Nosocomial infections. In Davis, B.G., Bishop, M.L., Mass, D. editors. Clinical laboratory science: strategies for practice. J.B. Lippincott, Philadelphia.

Hayes, J.S., Soule, B.M., and LaRocco, M.T. 1987. Nosocomial infections: an overview. In Howard, B.J., Klaas, J. II, Rubin, S.J., Weissfeld, A.S., and Tilton, R.C. Clinical and pathogenic microbiology. C.V. Mosby Co., St. Louis.

Jarvis, W.R., White, J.W., Munn, V.P., Mosser, J.L., Emori, T.G., Culver, D.H., Thornsberry, C., and Hughes, J.M. 1983. Nosocomial infection surveillance, 1983. M.M.W.R. 33:9SS.

Mayer, L.W. 1988. Use of plasmid profiles in epidemiologic surveillance of disease outbreaks and in tracing the transmission of antibiotic resistance. Clin. Microbiol. Rev. 1:228.

Shands, K.N., Ho, J.L., Meyer, R.D., Gorman, G.W., Edelstein, P.H., Mallison, G.F., Finegold, S.M., and Fraser, D.W. 1985. Potable water as a source of Legionnaires' disease. J.A.M.A. 253:1412.

Smith, P.B. 1983. Biotyping—its value as an epidemiologic tool. Clin. Microbiol. Newsletter 5:165.

Part Two Handling Clinical Specimens for Microbiological Studies

6

Selection, Collection, and Transport of Specimens for Microbiological Examination

6.1. Specimen Selection

The primary considerations here are that the specimen obtained be representative of the disease process and that sufficient material be collected to assure a complete and accurate examination. For example, a small amount of serous drainage from the surface of a diabetic foot ulcer with underlying osteomyelitis may well not yield organisms of the type found in the infected bone; indeed, it may yield no organisms at all. In the example cited, the ideal specimen would be a bone biopsy (to be studied histologically as well as bacteriologically). Although it may often not be feasible to obtain infected tissue, tissue is clearly the ideal specimen. Frankly purulent drainage is next in terms of desirability and is entirely satisfactory. In the case of a spreading lesion of the skin and subcutaneous tissue (such as progressive synergistic bacterial gangrene), material from the active margin of the lesion, rather than from the central portion of the lesion, is most likely to accurately reflect the true bacteriology of the process. Material obtained on a swab from a sinus tract opening often does not yield the true infecting organisms. A deep biopsy of the sinus tract would be much more reliable. Expectorated sputum, particularly if it is not a good purulent specimen (*Legionella pneumophila* is one exception) with minimal salivary contamination, presents major problems, particularly since pneumonia is often a serious infection. Ways around this problem include obtaining blood cultures, examining pleural fluid when present, screening the sputum specimen under $100\times$ magnification to determine its quality (Chapters 4 and 7), and transtracheal aspiration or other invasive procedure. Material from normally sterile sites in the body always provides an excellent specimen if care is taken to avoid contamination with skin flora.

Since anaerobic bacteria may be involved in infections of any type anywhere in the body, one should always culture anaerobically specimens of any variety that are free of contamination with normal flora. Certain specimens are essentially always contaminated with normal flora and therefore should not ordinarily be cultured anaerobically: throat swabs, nasopharyngeal swabs, gingival swabs, expectorated sputum, sputum obtained by nasotracheal or orotracheal suction, specimens obtained via a bronchoscope, gastric contents, small bowel contents (the latter two types of specimens may yield valuable information on culture in the case of "blind loop" and similar syndromes and gastric biopsy in the case of *Campylobacter pylori* infection), large bowel contents or feces (except for *Clostridium difficile* and *Clostridium botulinum*), ileostomy and colostomy effluents, voided or catheterized urine, and vaginal or cervical swabs (except as discussed under specimen collection from patients with endometritis).

6.2. Collection Procedures

Generally a report from the bacteriologic laboratory can indicate only what has been found by microscopic and cultural examination. An etiologic diagnosis is thus confirmed or denied. Failure to isolate the causative organism, however, is not necessarily the fault of inadequate cultural methods; it is frequently the result of faulty collecting or transport technique. In a busy hospital the collection of specimens is too often relegated to persons who do not understand the requirements and consequences of such procedures. The microbiologist may also deserve criticism on occasion for neglecting to provide adequate supplies or proper instructions, which may result in poorly collected samples. The following are *general considerations* regarding the collection of material for culture. Specific instructions for the handling of a variety of specimens are given in subsequent chapters.

Whenever possible, specimens should be obtained *before antimicrobial agents have been administered*. Often cerebrospinal fluid (CSF) from a patient with bacterial meningitis reveals no bacterial pathogens on smear or culture when an antibiotic

has been given within the previous 24 hours. A patient with salmonellosis may have a negative stool culture if the specimen has been collected while he or she was receiving antibacterial therapy that was only suppressive, only to reveal a positive culture several days after therapy has been terminated. If the culture has been taken after initiation of antibacterial therapy, the laboratory should be informed so that specific counteractive measures, such as adding penicillinase or merely diluting the specimen, may be carried out.

It is axiomatic that material should be collected where the suspected organism is *most likely to be found, with as little external contamination as possible*. The skin and all mucosal surfaces are populated with an indigenous flora and may often also acquire a transient flora or even become colonized for extended periods with potential pathogens from the hospital environment. The latter is particularly true of individuals who are quite ill, especially if they are receiving antimicrobial therapy (resistant organisms colonize as normal flora is suppressed). Accordingly, special procedures must be employed to help distinguish between organisms involved in an infectious process and those representing normal flora or "abnormal" colonizers that are not actually causing infection. Four major approaches are utilized to resolve this problem:

1. Cleanse skin surface with germicide using enough friction for mechanical cleansing as well. Start centrally and go out in ever enlarging circles. Repeat this several times, using a new swab each time. Alcohol (70%) is satisfactory for skin, but a full 2 minutes of wet contact time is needed. Iodine (2%) and povidone-iodine work more quickly (1 minute) and are effective against spore-forming organisms. Collection of normally sterile body fluids (such as joint, pleural, or cerebrospinal fluid) by percutaneous needle aspiration should always be preceded by thorough skin decontamination as described here.

2. Bypass areas of normal flora entirely (e.g., percutaneous transtracheal aspiration rather than coughed sputum).

3. Culture only for a specific pathogen (e.g., group A streptococci in the throat).

4. Quantitate culture results as a means of determining the likelihood of organisms being involved in infection (e.g., quantitative urine culture). Less formal quantitation may also be satisfactory

and should *routinely* be used; this may involve grading on a scale of 1+ to 4+, or simply heavy growth, moderate growth, light growth, four colonies, and so forth.

Another factor contributing to the successful isolation of the causative agent is the *stage of the disease* at which the specimen is collected for culture. Enteric pathogens are present in much greater numbers during the *acute*, or diarrheal, stage of intestinal infections and are more likely to be isolated at that time. Viruses responsible for causing meningoencephalitis are isolated from CSF with greater frequency when the fluid is obtained soon after the *onset* of the disease rather than when the symptoms of acute illness have subsided. Subsequent chapters discuss the type of specimen most likely to contain the etiologic agent during different stages of disease.

There are occasions when patients must participate actively in the collection of a specimen, such as a sputum sample. They should be given full instructions (Chapter 16), and cooperation should be encouraged by the ward attendant. Too often a container is placed on the patient's bedside table, with the only instructions being to "spit in this cup."

Another specimen for which proper collection procedures are essential for reliable culture results is the clean-catch, midstream urine specimen. These specimens, usually collected by the patient without the assistance of a trained medical care worker, often comprise a large portion of the specimens received by a clinical microbiology laboratory. Microbiologists may be asked to help prepare guidelines for proper specimen collection. The use of a printed card (bilingual, if necessary) with the procedure clearly described and preferably illustrated (see box on p. 52) can help to ensure patient compliance. Separate cards should be given to males and females. Careful patient education should improve the quality of such urine specimens received by the laboratory.

Specimens should be of a *sufficient quantity* to permit complete examination and should be placed in sterile containers that avoid hazard to the patient, nurse, or ward messenger. A serious danger to the laboratory worker, as well as to all others involved, is the soiled outer surface of a sputum container, a leaking stool sample, or possible contact with blood-containing exudates. The hazard of spreading disease by inadequately trained nonprofessional workers is frequently overlooked. Its control requires contin-

ued education and constant vigilance by those in responsible and supervisory positions.

Provision must be made for the *prompt delivery* of specimens to the laboratory if the results of analysis are to be valid. It is difficult, for example, to isolate *Shigella* from a fecal specimen that has remained on the hospital ward too long, permitting overgrowth by commensal organisms and an increasing death rate of the shigellae. In some instances it may be necessary to take culture (room temperature) media and other equipment to the patient's bedside to ensure prompt inoculation of the specimen. This is an unusual circumstance and requires prior arrangements with the laboratory.

Although most pathogenic microorganisms are not greatly affected by small changes in temperature, they are generally susceptible to drying out, particularly when on cotton applicator sticks. However, some bacteria, such as the meningococcus in CSF, are quite sensitive to low temperatures and require immediate culturing.

Specimens for gonococci can be inoculated directly onto selective media such as modified Thayer-Martin medium with carbon dioxide provided in a device (Transgrow) or by placing a generating tablet in a chamber (Figure 6.1) (Jembec; Chapters 8 and 19). Alternate methods include placing inoculated Thayer-Martin plates immediately into a candle jar (Figure 6.2).

Clinical material likely to contain abundant microbial flora may in most instances be held at 5° C in a refrigerator for several hours before culturing if it cannot be processed right away. This is particularly true with specimens such as urine, feces, and material on swabs taken from a variety of sources, with the exception of wound cultures, which may contain oxygen-sensitive anaerobes. These should be inoculated promptly. Not only will refrigeration preserve the viability of most pathogens, but it will also minimize overgrowth of commensal organisms, increased numbers of which could make the isolation of a significant microbe more difficult. However, the sooner an organism leaving the sheltered environment of its host is transferred to an appropriate artificial culture medium, the better are the chances of its survival and subsequent multiplication.

Although not a function of specimen collection, it is an essential prerequisite that the *laboratory be given sufficient clinical information* to guide the microbiologist in selection of suitable media and ap-

---

Patient Guidelines for Collection of a Urine Specimen

READ ENTIRE DIRECTIONS BEFORE STARTING PROCEDURE

Note: *Proper collection will help us to give useful results to your physician.*

Females

1. Prepare a sterile gauze pad (found on the shelf above the sink) for washing your vagina by wetting the pad in the sink and placing a small amount of soap on the surface so that it is sudsy. Prepare two more sterile gauze pads for rinsing by moistening them with warm water. Last, open the package of a fourth sterile gauze pad and leave it to dry. Take the top off the plastic urine container and set it on the edge of the sink. Set the pads and the container in a row on the edge of the sink so that you can reach them while sitting on the toilet.

2. Pull your panties below your knees so that they will not interfere with your urine collection. With two fingers of one hand, hold the outer folds of your vagina apart. With the other hand, gently wash the vaginal area from the front to the back, using the soapy gauze pad. Discard the gauze in the wastebasket; do not throw it into the toilet.

3. Still holding the outer vaginal skin away from the opening through which you urinate, rinse the area from the front to the back, using first one moistened pad and then the second moistened pad. Last of all, dry the area from the front to the back with the dry gauze pad. Discard all gauze pads in the wastebasket.

4. Continue holding your outer vaginal folds apart and begin to urinate into the toilet. Lean slightly forward so that the urine flows directly down without running along the skin. After the first few teaspoons, place the sterile container under the stream of urine and collect the rest of your urine in the container. Even one-fourth cup is an adequate sample for the test.

5. After you have finished, tighten the cap on the container securely and wash any spilled urine from the outside of the container. Make certain that your name is correctly written on the container.

6. Hand the filled and tightly capped container to the attendant in the outpatient laboratory area.

Males

1. Prepare a sterile gauze pad (found on the shelf above the sink) for washing your penis by wetting it in the sink and placing a small amount of soap on the surface so that it is sudsy. Prepare two more sterile gauze pads for rinsing by moistening them with warm water. Last, open the package of a fourth sterile gauze pad and let it dry. Take the top off the plastic urine container and set it on the edge of the sink. Set the pads and the container in a row on the edge of the sink so that you can reach them while urinating.

2. Holding back your foreskin with one hand, if necessary, use the sudsy gauze pad to gently wash the end of your penis. Discard the gauze pad in the wastebasket; do not throw gauze pads into the toilet.

3. Continue holding back the foreskin and gently rinse the end of your penis, using first one moistened gauze pad and then the other, discarding them in the wastebasket when finished. Use the dry gauze pad to dry the end of your penis.

4. Continue holding back the foreskin and begin to urinate into the toilet. After the first few teaspoons, place the sterile container under the stream of urine and collect the rest of your urine in the container. Even one-fourth cup is an adequate sample for the test.

5. After you have finished, tighten the cap on the container securely and wash any spilled urine from the outside of the container. Make certain that your name is correctly written on the container.

6. Hand the filled and tightly capped container to the attendant in the outpatient laboratory area.

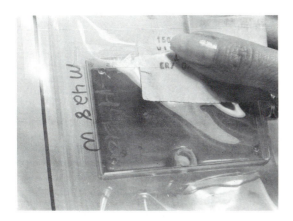

Figure 6.1

Modified Thayer-Martin medium in a square, plastic culture plate for transport and cultivation of *N. gonorrhoeae* (Neigon-Jembec, Flow Laboratories). A white tablet of bicarbonate is placed in a special well within the plate, the top is snapped shut, and the plate is sealed into a ziploc plastic bag to maintain the increased CO_2 atmosphere during transport and incubation.

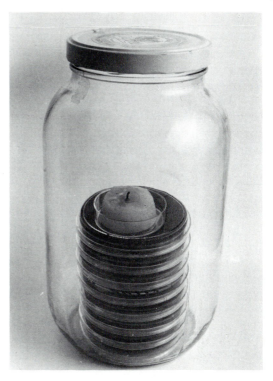

Figure 6.2

Thayer-Martin plates in a candle jar.

propriate techniques. Likewise, it is important for the clinician to appreciate the *limitations and potentials* of the bacteriology laboratory and to realize that a negative report does not necessarily invalidate the diagnosis. It is essential that close cooperation and frequent consultation among the clinician, nurse, and microbiologist be the rule rather than the exception.

Laboratory personnel should reject specimens not obtained in a proper manner and should be supported in this position by infectious disease clinicians or pathologists. In rejecting specimens, of course, the reasons should be explained to the requesting physician. Specimens should never be discarded before discussion with the requesting clinician. Some specimens, such as those taken at the time of surgery, are difficult or impossible to replace. Those specimens that cannot be replaced should be Gram stained and interpreted as carefully as possible. Guidelines for specimen rejection are discussed in Chapter 3 (Table 3.1).

6.2.a. **Anaerobic collection procedures.** Proper collection, or taking care to avoid inclusion of normal flora, cannot be overemphasized because indigenous anaerobes are often present in such large numbers that even minimal contamination of a specimen with normal flora can give very misleading results and cause much wasted effort.

Coughed sputum is unsuitable, because it becomes contaminated with normal flora anaerobes on its passage through the mouth and pharynx. For the same reason, bronchoscopic specimens are those obtained by nasotracheal tube suctioning also should not be cultured anaerobically. The sampling tube always contacts normal flora on its downward path. The efficacy of a double-lumen plugged catheter in preventing such contamination is such that it is possible to obtain reliable results by careful attention to detail in carrying out these procedures and by doing quantitative cultures. Adequate pleuropulmonary specimens for anaerobic culture can be obtained by transtracheal aspiration (TTA), thoracentesis, or direct percutaneous needle puncture and aspiration of lung. Tracheostomy tube specimens may provide useful material when the tube is first placed; when it has been in place for a while there is inevitable contamination with oropharyngeal secretions, whether or not there is an inflated cuff.

Voided urine specimens are unsuitable for anaerobic culture because the distal portion of the urethra and the meatus are colonized with a normal flora containing anaerobes, which will contaminate urine passing through these areas. If a suprapubic bladder catheter or cystostomy or nephrostomy tube is in place, reliable urine specimens may be collected from these sites. Percutaneous aspiration of urines from a full bladder provides a reliable specimen.

Endometritis presents a very difficult problem. Anaerobes are clearly very important in this infection. However, most cases of endometritis follow childbirth, and it has been demonstrated that in the postpartum period, *whether or not there is endometrial infection*, significant numbers of anaerobes and other organisms from the cervical and vaginal flora may be found in the uterine cavity. There may not even be quantitative differences between infected and uninfected patients. This situation may apply also in postabortal endometritis. Thus, one should obtain blood cultures and culture any better sources of material that may be available. Culture for the *Bacteroides fragilis* group may be useful. Since the presence of the *B. fragilis* group in this type of specimen indicates a poorer prognosis and since this organism is more resistant to antimicrobials than other anaerobes, it makes sense to determine whether it is present. Biopsy of endometrial tissue obtained with an endometrial suction curette (Pipelle, Unimar, Inc.) will provide a satisfactory specimen.[4]

Infections of decubitus ulcers commonly involve anaerobic organisms, particularly when the decubitus is in the vicinity of the anus (sacral decubiti and decubiti of the hips and buttocks). Since these areas are subject to fecal contamination (this is how they become infected), the area must be thoroughly cleansed with an antiseptic agent before cultures are taken. Whenever possible, one should aspirate collections of pus from under skin flaps or from deep pockets, using a syringe and a needle. The same considerations apply to other lesions in these areas (e.g., perirectal abscess).

Specimens that are normally sterile (such as spinal fluid and blood and joint fluid) may be collected in the usual fashion after thorough skin decontamination.

In general, material for anaerobic culture is best obtained by tissue biopsy or by using a needle and syringe. All air must be expelled from the syringe and needle (Figure 6.3). Use of swabs is a poor alternative because of excessive exposure of the specimen to the deleterious effects of oxygen and drying.

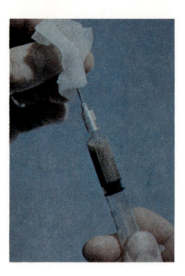

Figure 6.3
Eliminating air bubbles from syringe and needle to protect anaerobes in specimen from exposure to oxygen.

6.3. Specimen Transport

It is essential that the container bearing a specimen does not contribute its own microbial flora. Furthermore, the original flora should neither multiply nor decrease because of prolonged standing on the ward or prolonged refrigeration in the laboratory. In other words, *a sterile container should be used and the specimen should be plated as soon as possible*. Although these are not hard-and-fast rules, any deviation should be the responsibility of the microbiologist.

A variety of containers has been devised for collecting bacteriologic specimens. Many of these can be used repeatedly after proper sterilization and cleaning, whereas others must be incinerated after use. Apart from the sterile Pyrex Petri dish and its modern counterpart, the presterilized and disposable plastic dish, the most used (but not necessarily the most desirable) piece of collecting equipment is the cotton-, calcium alginate–, or Dacron (polyester)–tipped wooden applicator stick. These swabs are best prepared by autoclaving the wooden applicator sticks in Sörensen buffer, pH 7.2, for 5 minutes, drying them, and then tipping them with polyester batting,* calcium alginate (Colab Laboratories), or long-fibered medicinal cotton. One approach uses a sterile disposable culture unit (Culturette, Becton-Dickinson Microbiology Systems)

*Dacron polyester filling, ½-pound bags, Sears, Roebuck and Co.

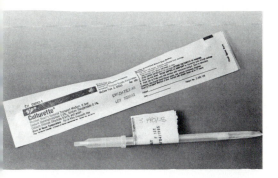

gure 6.4

erile specimen collection unit consisting of a polyester swab
th a plastic shaft inserted into a tight-fitting cap within a
erile tube (Culturette, Becton-Dickinson Microbiology
stems). After the specimen is collected, the glass ampule
ntaining transport medium is broken to moisten and protect
e specimen on the swab.

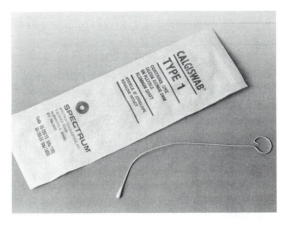

Figure 6.5
Calcium alginate nasopharyngeal swabs on a flexible wire that
can be bent to conform to the shape of the nasal passage
(Spectrum Diagnostics).

'igure 6.4) consisting of a plastic tube containing a
erile polyester-tipped swab and a small glass am-
ule of modified Stuart's holding medium. The unit
removed from its sterile envelope, and the swab
used to collect the specimen. It is then returned
the tube, the ampule is crushed, and the swab is
rced into the released holding medium. This will
rovide sufficient moisture for storage up to 72 hours
room temperature.

Some cotton used for applicators may contain
tty acids that may be detrimental to microbial
owth.[6] An excellent substitute is calcium alginate
ool, derived from alginic acid, a natural plant prod-
ct. This silky-fibered material dissolves in certain
olutions that are compatible with bacterial preser-
ation (such as dilute Ringer's solution with sodium
exametaphosphate) to form a soluble sodium algi-
ate. Calcium anginate–tipped wooden applicators
r flexible aluminum nasopharyngeal swabs (Figure
.5), as well as the citrate or hexametaphosphate
iluents, are available commercially. Calcium algi-
ate should not be used where herpesvirus is antic-
oated, as it may inhibit replication of this virus, or
hen swabs will be used for subsequent direct an-
gen detection, as the calcium alginate will interfere
ith the extraction reagents.

A modification of the cotton applicator uses 28-
auge Nichrome or thin aluminum wire in place of
he wooden stick. Because of its flexibility, the wire
pplicator is recommended for collecting specimens
om the nasopharynx or the urethra. To ensure that
he small amount of cotton adheres to the wire dur-

ing passage through the nasal tract, the end of the
wire must be bent over and some collodion applied
before the wrapping with cotton; otherwise the outfit
remains the same as that previously described. Commercially prepared sterile wire swabs also are available (see Appendix C).

A variety of transport media have been devised
for prolonging the survival of microorganisms when
a significant delay occurs between collection and culturing. Stuart and others[1,7] advocated a medium that
has proved effective in preserving the viability of
pathogenic agents in clinical material. The medium
consists of buffered semisolid agar devoid of nutrients and containing sodium thioglycollate as a reducing agent and is used in conjunction with cotton
swabs. Stuart's medium (available commercially)
maintains a favorable pH and prevents both dehydration of secretions during transport and oxidation
and enzymatic self-destruction of the pathogen present. However, the glycerophosphate present permits multiplication of certain organisms.

A report on a transport medium (available commercially) by Cary and Blair[3] (Figure 6.6) indicates
that salmonellae and shigellae can be recovered from
fecal specimens for as long as 49 days and Vibrio
cholerae for 22 days; Yersinia pestis survives for at
least 75 days. The medium itself remains good after
storage at room temperature for longer than 1½
years.

Polyester-tipped swabs may be used for delayed
recovery of group A streptococci from throat cultures. A report by Hosty and coworkers[5] indicates

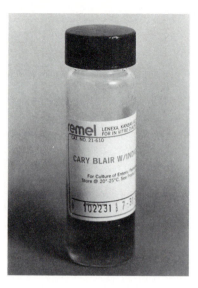

Figure 6.6
Small vial containing Cary-Blair medium for transport and
maintenance of fecal specimens (Remel Laboratories).

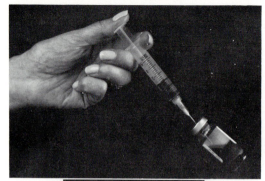

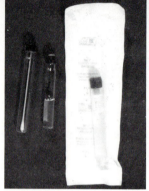

Figure 6.7
A, Anaerobic transport vial containing agar with oxygen tension
indicator. (Becton-Dickinson Microbiology Systems). Liquid
specimen is injected into vial through the rubber septum. **B,**
Examples of additional transport methods for anaerobic
specimens. Tube on left contains swab in oxygen-free
atmosphere (prepared in-house). Sterile pack on right contains
screwcap tube with agar deep suitable for inserting swab
(Becton-Dickinson Microbiology Systems). Tube in middle
incorporates both agar deep and screwcap with a rubber
septum (Anaerobe Systems), suitable for either swab or
injected liquid specimen. (Photographs by Pete Rose.)

that the incorporation of a small amount of silica gel
in the glass tube containing the polyester swab will
further maintain the viability of group A streptococci
in throat swabs for as long as 3 days before plating.

6.3.a. **Anaerobic specimen transport.** The collection of specimens for anaerobic culturing poses a
special problem in that the conventional methods
previously described will not lead to optimal recovery of these air-intolerant microorganisms. A crucial
factor in the final success of anaerobic culturing is
the transport of clinical specimens; the lethal effect
of atmospheric oxygen must be nullified until the
specimen has been processed anaerobically in the
laboratory. We recommend using a double-stop-
pered collection tube or vial, gassed out with oxygen-
free CO_2 or nitrogen and containing an agar or broth
indicator system (Figure 6.7). One injects the specimen (pus, body fluid, or other liquid material)
through the rubber stopper after first expelling all
air from the syringe and the needle. In the laboratory, the material is aspirated from the transport
container by needle and syringe, inoculated to media, and incubated under anaerobic conditions. If
only a swab specimen can be obtained, it may be
collected on a swab that has been maintained in an
anaerobic tube (Figure 6.8) and can then be transferred to a rubber-stoppered tube with a deep column of prereduced and anaerobically sterilized
transport medium (see Appendix C).

An Anaerobic Culturette (Becton-Dickinson Microbiology Systems) generates its own anaerobic atmosphere and contains a small amount of transport
medium to prevent drying. The Bio-Bag (Becton-
Dickinson Microbiology Systems), Anaerobic Pouch
(Difco Laboratories), or GasPak Pouch (BBL Microbiology Systems) (Figure 6.9) offers remarkable flexibility. It is not only suitable for swabs (for short
periods; no specific means are incorporated to maintain a moist environment, nor is there a holding
medium), but it can also be used to transport specimens in rubber-stoppered plastic syringes. It can
be used for tissue (placed first in a loosely capped
sterile tube or vial).

The materials recommended for anaerobic trans-

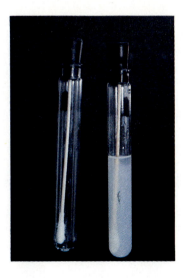

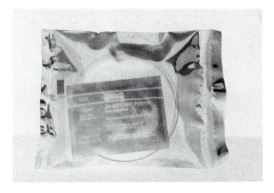

Figure 6.9
Anaerobic pouch with catalyst-free system (Difco Laboratories).
(Photograph by Pete Rose.)

Figure 6.8
Swab in anaerobic atmosphere. Companion tube on right
(shown with specimen on swab in place) contains prereduced
nonnutritive semisolid transport medium.

port actually constitute ideal *universal transport set-ups*, since *all* types of microorganisms should survive well in them. It should be stressed that although the swab is the most widely used transport vehicle, it is preferable to submit a larger specimen whenever possible (e.g., aspirated pus or tissue). When organisms may be scarce (as in some forms of tuberculosis), the larger the specimen the better. Throughout this text, specimen collection and handling methods are discussed in relation to the disease process or the etiologic agent. Procedures should be chosen based on the needs of the patients served by the laboratory.

6.4. Shipping Specimens

On occasion it is necessary to submit specimens to a *reference laboratory* in a distant city, thus requiring transportation by mail or express. If, for example, there is no viral diagnostic service available in the immediate area, it may be necessary to ship specimens at a low temperature to preserve their viability. This is especially true of virus-containing material, such as CSF, throat and rectal swabs, stools, and tissue, which should be refrigerated immediately and shipped in a Styrofoam box with commercial refrigerant packs (e.g., 3M Cryogel). Specimens should not be frozen. Whole blood is *not* shipped. Rather, the serum is separated and sent in a sterile tube.

If a culture of an isolated organism is to be sent to a reference laboratory (state or public health laboratory), it is not necessary to send it in the frozen state.

In most instances microbiological specimens can be satisfactorily shipped through the mails, provided that *special precautions* are taken against breakage and subsequent contamination of the mailing container. According to the Code of Federal Regulations,* a viable organism or its toxin or a diagnostic specimen of a volume less than 50 ml shall be placed in a securely closed, watertight specimen container, which is enclosed in a second durable watertight container, further described in Chapter 2.

Double mailing containers and standardized biohazard labels (Figure 2.7) must be used when the microbiologist considers the specimen to be of a hazardous nature or thinks it may constitute a definite danger to the person handling the container. This includes clinical specimens, cultures for identification, and so forth. Postal regulations may change soon, requiring shippers of etiologic agents to use the more expensive commercial carriers. This change has been suggested but not implemented.

For the shipment of fecal specimens containing salmonellae or shigellae over long distances, the filter paper method may also be employed. In collecting the specimen by this technique, fresh fecal material must be spread fairly thinly over a strip of filter paper or clean blotting paper and allowed to dry at room temperature. Using forceps, the smeared strip is then folded inward from the ends

_____
*Section 72.25 of Part 72, Title 42, amended.

in such a way that the fecal material is covered. The folded specimen may then be inserted in a plastic envelope (polyethylene is recommended) and placed in a container to conform with postal regulations. It is possible to ship a large number of such specimens in one container through the mail. The pathogens are unaffected by this treatment, whereas the normal intestinal flora dies. On receipt at the laboratory the paper specimen may be cut into three pieces. One piece is placed in physiologic saline for suspension and direct plating, and the remaining pieces are placed in selenite and tetrathionate broths, respectively, for enrichment and subsequent plating.[2]

When it is necessary to ship fecal specimens or when such specimens must be held for some time before culturing, it is recommended that they be placed in a preservative solution. Cary-Blair medium has proved satisfactory. It should be discarded if it becomes acid. Approximately 1 g of feces is emulsified in not more than 10 ml of preservative, and the preserved specimen is shipped in a heavy glass container (universal type) with a screw cap in the regular double mailing container just described.

6.5. Handling of Specimens in the Laboratory

In previous sections of this book the importance of a properly collected specimen was stressed and the responsibility of personnel in its collection was indicated. In the following section the subsequent handling of the specimen in the laboratory is considered. In addition, the responsibility of the laboratory worker is pointed out.

Since it is not always practical for many specimens to be inoculated as soon as they arrive in the laboratory, refrigeration at 4° to 6° C offers a safe and dependable method of storing many clinical samples until they can be conveniently handled. However, some may require immediate plating (such as specimens that might contain gonococci or *Bordetella pertussis*), whereas others must be immediately frozen (e.g., serum for subsequent antimicrobial agent assay).

The length of time of refrigeration varies with the type of specimen: swabs from wounds (except for anaerobic cultures), the urogenital tract, throat, and rectum and samples of feces or sputum can be refrigerated for 2 to 3 hours without appreciable loss

of pathogens. Urine specimens for culture may be refrigerated at least 24 hours without affecting the bacterial flora (except the tubercle bacillus, which may be adversely affected by the urine); on the other hand, CSF from a patient with suspected meningitis should be examined *at once*.

Specimens submitted for the isolation of virus should be refrigerated immediately; even for storage up to 5 days, they should be refrigerated and *never frozen*. Specimens of clotted blood for virus serology may also be refrigerated but never frozen, as discussed in Chapter 42.

Gastric washings and resected lung tissue submitted for culture of *Mycobacterium tuberculosis* should be processed soon after delivery, since tubercle bacilli may die rapidly in either type of specimen. Alternatively, gastric specimens and urine may be adjusted to neutral pH if some storage is necessary before processing. Further discussion of handling material for mycobacterial culture is found in Chapter 41.

Pieces of hair or scrapings from the skin and nails submitted for the isolation of fungi may be kept at room temperature (protected from dust) for several days before inoculation. On the other hand, sputum, bronchial secretions, bone marrow, and purulent material from patients suspected of having systemic fungal infection should be inoculated to appropriate media as soon as possible, especially when the diagnosis of histoplasmosis is considered. Further guidelines for collection of specimens for fungal isolation are given in Chapter 43.

6.6. Inoculation of Primary Culture Media

Depending on the etiologic agents suspected, specimens are plated and inoculated to several growth media. Special media for unusual agents (e.g., Bordet-Gengou agar for *B. pertussis*) are inoculated by request. Laboratories in some geographic areas may choose to inoculate routinely media that other laboratories could not justify economically (e.g., selective agar for *Yersinia enterocolitica*). Table 6.1 suggests one approach to the inoculation of specimens for routine bacteriological studies. As discussed in Chapters 14 through 23, etiologic agents other than bacteria (fungi, viruses, parasites) must often be considered and sought in clinical specimens.

Table 6.1
Selection of Primary Plating Media for Bacteriology Specimens

SPECIMEN	DIRECT SMEAR	ROUTINE MEDIA	SUGGESTED ADDITIONAL MEDIA	SPECIAL SITUATIONS	COMMENTS
• Abscess/pus* (closed wound)	+	B, M, An, Thio	As smear indicates; CNA		Wash any granules and "emulsify" in saline.
• Autopsy Blood, tissue			Follow procedure for "living" material		
Blood Peripheral blood		Choc, An	As smear indicates	Brucellosis, tularemia, cell wall-deficient bacteria, leptospirosis, mycobacteria	Smear when evidence of growth
• Bone marrow		B, M, Choc			
Body fluids (except blood, CSF, urine)		Centrifuge fluids for 15 min at 2,500 rpm except when grossly purulent. Stain and culture sediment. Incubate supernatant for 24 h at 37 °C. Filtration is also useful if the filter can be cultured directly.			
Bile	+	B, M, An, Thio	CNA, HE, XLD, GN		Do not use An if collected perorally.
Hematoma	+	Treat as abscess	CNA	PRAS if anaerobes suspected	
Joint	+	B, Choc, Thio		Brucellosis	
Pericardial, peritoneal	+	B, M, An, Choc, Thio	CNA		
Pleural empyema	+	B, M, An, Choc, Thio	CNA	*Legionella, Chlamydia* in infants, *Nocardia, Actinomyces,* mycobacteria	
Catheters Foley		Do not culture			
• Central venous pressure lines, umbilical or intravenous catheters		B	Thio		Roll segment back and forth across agar with sterile forceps 4 times; ≥15 colonies are associated with clinical significance. (See Chapter 14).
• Central nervous system Brain tissue	+	Treat as abscess			

B = blood agar, M = MacConkey agar, An = anaerobic blood agar, Choc = chocolate agar, Thio = thioglycollate broth, TM = Thayer-Martin agar, CNA = Columbia agar with colistin and nalidixic acid, HE = Hektoen enteric agar, XLD = xylose lysine deoxycholate agar, GN = gram-negative broth, HBT = human blood–Tween bilayer agar, Campy = *Campylobacter* agar.

*Bullets before entry indicate specimens that require immediate attention.

Modified from Isenberg, H.D., Schoenknecht, F.D., von Graevenitz, A., and Rubin, S.J. 1979. Collection and processing of bacteriological specimens. Cumitech 9. American Society for Microbiology, Washington, D.C.

Continued.

Table 6.1
Selection of Primary Plating Media for Bacteriology Specimens—cont'd

SPECIMEN	DIRECT SMEAR	ROUTINE MEDIA	SUGGESTED ADDITIONAL MEDIA	SPECIAL SITUATIONS	COMMENTS
CSF, shunt, meningomyelocele, and ventricular fluid	+	If large enough volume, centrifuge for 15 min at 2,500 rpm, and smear, and culture sediment. Incubate supernatant for 48 h at 37° C. B, Choc, Thio	As smear indicates; M, CNA, An	Leptospirosis, mycobacteria	*Haemophilus influenzae* may not sediment at 2,500 rpm and may require 10,000 × g for 10 min. Alternatively, culture entire specimen.
Ear					
Internal	+	B, M, Choc, Thio	CNA	An if aspiration or biopsy material	
External	+	B, M, Choc	CNA		
Eye					
Conjunctiva	+	B, M, Choc, Thio	TM, CNA		
Other	+	B, M, Choc, An, Thio	CNA		
Genital tract—female					
• Amniotic fluid	+	B, M, TM, Choc, An, Thio	CNA		Should be collected without contamination by normal flora
Cervix	±	TM	Choc with 1% IsoVitaleX, HBT		A small number of *Neisseria gonorrhoeae* are susceptible to vancomycin. Choc with 1% IsoVitaleX, especially when there is clinical evidence of gonorrhea and negative cultures (see Chapter 19).
• Cul de sac	+	B, M, Choc, TM, An, Thio	CNA, HBT		
• Uterine material (endometrium, products of conception; fetus, placenta, lochia), tubes, ovaries	+	B, M, Choc, TM, An, Thio	CNA, HBT		Anaerobic culture is done on material collected without contamination by vaginal flora.

Specimen	Presence of cells	Transport/media	Media	Organisms	Comments
Intrauterine device	±	Thio			
Urethra	±	TM	Choc with 1% IsoVitaleX	*Mycoplasma, Chlamydia* (nongonococcal urethritis)	Smears of urethral exudate that are positive for intracellular gram-negative diplococci from females are presumptively diagnostic and must be confirmed by culture.
Vagina (except cuff)	±	TM	HBT, Choc with 1% IsoVitaleX	Selective group B streptococcal media in pregnancy	
• Vulva (Bartholin abscess)	+	B, M, TM, An, Thio	CNS, Choc with 1% IsoVitaleX, HBT		Vaginal cuff infections are treated as abscess/pus
Genital tract—male					
Prostate fluid	+	B, M, TM, Thio	CNA		
Testes and epididymis (aspirate)	+	B, CNA, TM, M			
Urethra	+	TM	TM	*Chlamydia* (nongonococcal urethritis), *Mycoplasma*	
Intestinal tract					
Colostomy, ileostomy, feces, rectal swab	Presence of cells only (polymorphonuclear leukocytes)	B, M, HE, XLD, GN, Campy (42° C)		*Yersinia enterocolitica, Vibrio cholerae, V. parahaemolyticus, Neisseria gonorrhoeae* (rectal swab), *Mycobacterium avium* complex	
Gastric aspirate	+	B, M, Choc	CNA	Mycobacteria	In young child, may be submitted in place of sputum.
Plastic prostheses	−	Thio			
Pus—closed wound		See Abscess/pus			
Respiratory tract					
Throat/pharynx	−	Streptococcal Selective Agar		Vincent's angina, *N. gonorrhoeae, N. meningitidis, Corynebacterium diphtheriae*	Routine culture for group A streptococci only. Incubate ANO₂ or use pour plate. If fluorescent antibody studies are done for group A streptococci, incubate swab for 2 h in Todd-Hewitt broth. May be submitted instead of sputum in cystic fibrosis.

Continued.

Table 6.1
Selection of Primary Plating Media for Bacteriology Specimens—cont'd

SPECIMEN	DIRECT SMEAR	ROUTINE MEDIA	SUGGESTED ADDITIONAL MEDIA	SPECIAL SITUATIONS	COMMENTS
Epiglottis	−	B, Choc			
Nasal sinus	+	B, M, Choc, An, Thio	CNA		
Nasopharynx	−	B, Choc	CNA	*Bordetella pertussis*	
Nose	+	B, CNA	Mannitol salt		
Oral cavity		See Body fluids			
Pleural fluid		See Body fluids			
Sputum	+	B, M, Choc	CNA	*Mycoplasma, Nocardia,* mycobacteria	See Chapter 16.
Bronchial secretions	+	B, M, Choc	CNA	Mycobacteria	
Tracheal aspirate	+	B, M, Choc	CNA		
• Transtracheal aspirate	+	B, M, Choc, An, Thio	CNA	*Mycoplasma,* mycobacteria	
Dental abscess	+	B, M, An, Thio	As smear indicates		
Skin					
• Deep wound (open)	+	B, M, An, Thio	CNA		
Superficial wound	+	B, M	CNA, Choc	Petechiae/pustules (*Neisseria*)	
Traumatized areas (burns, bites, decubitus ulcers)	+	B, M, Thio	As smear indicates; CNA, An	Foul-smelling or gas-containing lesions; culture anaerobically	Quantitative culture of burn tissue may be useful (see Chapter 21).
Rash, nonpurulent lesions	+	B, M, Choc, Thio	CNA		Smear may be diagnostic, especially in meningococcemia.
Tissue		Grind with sterile Alundum (aluminum oxide) with a sterile mortar and pestle or sterile glass tissue grinder or homogenize (Chapter 21). Use enough broth to give a 10%-20% suspension.			
Surgical/biopsy	+	B, M, An, Thio	CNA	Other media on the basis of history, body site, and smear (i.e., tularemia or brucellosis)	
Urine					
Clean-voided, catheterized, or ileal loop urine	±	B, M (See Chapter 18)	CNA	Leptospirosis, mycobacteria	Gram stain on unspun urine may be useful in selected patients. It is not recommended as a routine procedure. (See Chapter 18.)
Suprapubic bladder tap; cystoscopy or ureterostomy urine	+	B, M, An, Thio (0.1 ml per plate)	CNA		

REFERENCES

1. Amies, C.R. 1967. A modified formula for the preparation of Stuart's transport medium. Can. J. Public Health 58:296.
2. Bailey, W.R., and Bynoe, E.T. 1953. The "filter paper" method for collecting and transporting stools to the laboratory for enteric bacteriological examination. Can. J. Public Health 44:468.
3. Cary, S.G., and Blair, E.B. 1964. New transport medium for shipment of clinical specimens. J. Bacteriol. 88:96.
4. Eschenbach, D.A., Rosene, K., Tompkins, L.S., et al. 1986. Endometrial cultures obtained by a triple-lumen method from afebrile and febrile postpartum women. J. Infect. Dis. 153:1038.
5. Hosty, T.S., Johnson, M.B., Freear, M.A., Gaddy, R.E., and Hunter, F.R. 1964. Evaluation of the efficiency of four different types of swabs in the recovery of group A streptococci. Health Lab. Sci. 1:163.
6. Pollock, M.R. 1948. Unsaturated fatty acids in cotton plugs. Nature 161:853.
7. Stuart, R.D., Tosach, S.R., and Patsula, T.M. 1954. The problem of transport of specimens for culture of gonococci. Can. J. Public Health 45:73.

BIBLIOGRAPHY

Forney, J.E., editor. 1968. Collection, handling, and shipment of microbiological specimens. Public Health Serv. Pub. No. 976, Nov. 1968. U.S. Government Printing Office, Washington, D.C.

Higgins, M. 1950. A comparison of the recovery rate of organisms from cotton-wool and calcium alginate wool swabs. Ministry Health Public Lab. Serv. Bull. 43.

Isenberg, H.D., Schoenknecht, F.D., von Graevenitz, A., and Rubin, S.J. 1979. Collection and processing of bacteriological specimens. Cumitech 9. American Society for Microbiology, Washington, D.C.

Rubin, S.J. 1987. Specimen collection and processing. In Howard, B.J., Klass, J. II, Rubin, S.J., Weissfeld, A.S., and Tilton, R.C. Clinical and pathogenic microbiology. The C.V. Mosby Co., St. Louis, Mo.

Sutter, V.L., Citron, D.M., Edelstein, M.A.C., and Finegold, S.M. 1985. Wadsworth anaerobic bacteriology manual, ed. 4. Star Publishing Co., Belmont, Calif.

Washington, J.A. II. 1985. Bacteria, fungi and parasites. In Mandell, G.L., Douglas, R.G. Jr., and Bennett, J.E., editors. Principles and practice of infectious diseases, ed. 2. John Wiley & Sons, New York.

7

Optical Methods for Laboratory Diagnosis of Infectious Diseases

Until the observations of van Leeuwenhoek during the late seventeenth century, the presence of infectious agents smaller than the human eye could see was only speculated upon. Since that time, however, the light microscope has become a most important tool for the diagnosis of infection. Even today, with the emphasis on rapid methods for diagnosis, many of which require complicated instruments or immunological reagents, simple visual inspection of clinical specimens obtained from patients is still the fastest and most specific way to immediately augment a physician's clinical diagnosis.[1] Many infectious agents can be reliably identified with only a few simple stains and a basic microscope. The Gram stain is still the single most efficient and cost-effective test for rapid early diagnosis of bacterial infection. Methods discussed in this chapter include many common visual techniques that have been employed by microbiologists for decades as well as a few relatively recent innovations in microscopy.

Examination of Fresh Material

Most microscopic examinations of material are carried out with *brightfield microscopy*, in which the object to be viewed is illuminated with light from below the field of focus, usually provided by a coiled filament tungsten lamp. The glowing filaments are prevented from causing glare by focusing their light on the substage condenser, rather than on the object. This is known as *Köhler illumination*, after the inventor of the method. Since most pathogens visible with the microscope are of a refractive index similar to that of aqueous suspending liquids, they are in-

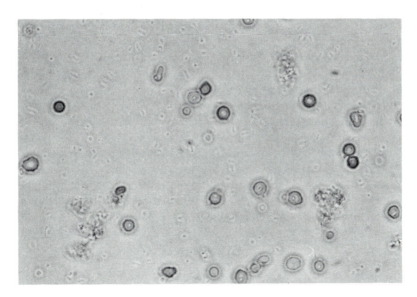

Figure 7.1
Blood culture broth positive for gram-negative bacilli; seen under phase contrast at 1000×.

visible unless they or the technique is modified. Closing the aperture of the condenser slightly may aid in detection of certain organisms, particularly protozoans and fungi, as the light will be hitting the edges of the object at a sharper angle, increasing contrast. For Köhler illumination, which assures the best brightfield viewing of unstained clinical material, the condenser should be properly focused. This is achieved by placing a slide on the stage and viewing it through the 10× objective. After the radiant field diaphragm (the control in the base of the microscope where the light source is) is stopped down, the condenser is moved up or down until the leaves around the edge of the diaphragm are in sharp focus and the condenser is centered so that the circle of light is in the center of the field of view. At this point, the leaves of the radiant field diaphragm are opened until they just disappear from the field of view. The condenser aperture diaphragm must now be adjusted. For best viewing, the aperture should be closed slowly until the sharpest image is obtained. Since the human eye is most sensitive to green light, a green filter over the light source may enhance visualization.

For direct observaton of unstained material, *phase-contrast microscopy* may be helpful. In this lighting method, beams of light pass through the object and are partially deflected by different densities or thicknesses (refractive indices) of the object.

These light beams are deflected again when they impinge on a special objective lens, increasing in light wave amplitude (and brightness) when aligning in phase, as when passing though material of uniform refractive index, and decreasing in amplitude (visualized as darkness) when out of phase, as when passing though areas of differing refractive index. Resolution for phase-contrast microscopy is also heightened with the use of a green filter. Some laboratories routinely perform phase microscopic examination of bacterial colonies emulsified in water or saline or the supernatant of broth cultures (such as blood cultures) and covered by a coverslip and examined under an oil immersion lens (1,000×) (Figure 7.1). With practice, microbiologists can learn to recognize morphologies, motility, and various other characteristics helpful in aiding early presumptive identification. In *oil immersion microscopy* the oil, which fills the space between the objective and the coverglass, helps to keep light rays from dispersing and, since the oil is of the same refractive index as glass, prevents changes in wavelength due to changes in refractivity of the medium through which the light passes. Immersion oil is necessary to achieve enough resolution for the visualization of most bacteria; the 100× objective is usually used for this purpose together with 10× oculars (total magnification = 1,000×).

7.2.a. Direct examination of clinical specimens.
Many clinical specimens may be examined in their native state, under brightfield or phase-contrast microscopy, preferably as soon as they are collected from the patient. Specimens that can be applied directly to the surface of a slide for this purpose include sputum, exudate from lesions, aspirated fluid, stool, vaginal discharge, and urine sediment. Material too thick to easily differentiate suspended material in can be diluted with equal parts of physiologic sterile saline. It is best to prepare all slides made from fresh clinical material within a biohazard hood, since emulsifying material on the surface of a slide often creates aerosols. A coverslip is then gently laid over the surface of the material, and excess liquid is blotted from around the edges with a paper towel or tissue, which is discarded as contaminated material. The technologist should wear gloves if contact with any patient material is anticipated. This sort of preparation, known as a *direct wet mount*, can be preserved for longer viewing time by ringing the edge of the coverslip with nail polish or histological mounting medium. Wet preparations are often used to detect motile trophozoites of fecal parasites such as *Giardia lamblia*, *Entamoeba histolytica*, and *Dientamoeba fragilis*. The eggs and cysts of other parasites, larvae, and adult worms are also often seen in wet mounts made from freshly passed stool. *Trichomonas vaginalis* can be seen moving in wet mounts prepared from vaginal discharge material or spun sediment from fresh urine specimens. Parasites can also be found in direct wet mounts made from material aspirated from the duodenum, lung, or abscess contents.

Stool may be examined directly by phase contrast microscopy for evidence of certain bacterial diseases as well as parasites. Experienced microbiologists can recognize the characteristic darting motility and short, curved morphology of *Campylobacter jejuni*. In areas of endemic cholera, the presence of *Vibrio cholerae* in stool can be established presumptively by microscopy.

Examination of blood, often diluted in saline, can establish the diagnosis of relapsing fever or leptospirosis, as discussed in Chapter 31. Microfilariae, including trypanosomes and hemoflagellates, may also be seen in direct preparations of blood.

7.1.b. Slightly modified direct preparations of clinical material. The use of *10% potassium hydroxide (KOH preparation)* will help to distinguish fungal elements in a direct wet preparation of clinical material. Proteinaceous components, such as host cells, are partially digested by the alkali, leaving intact the polysaccharide-containing fungal cell walls. The material to be examined, whether fluid or skin or nail scrapings, is added to a drop of 10% aqueous KOH on a glass slide (see also Appendix B). The KOH may be preserved with 0.1% thimerosal (Sigma Chemical Co.), or its digestive capabilities may be enhanced by 40% dimethyl sulfoxide (DMSO), as suggested by McGinnis.[6] A coverslip is laid over the preparation, and excess fluid is removed from the edges by gently pressing the slide, coverslip side down, onto several thicknesses of paper towels. If this procedure is followed, the slide may be examined several minutes later for the presence of fungal elements. Gentle heating may speed the activity of the KOH, but it is unnecessary and may be harmful to the specimen if overdone. A small amount of lactophenol cotton blue (available commercially) can be added to the 10% KOH for enhanced visibility of fungal elements, or lactophenol cotton blue may be used alone for wet mount preparations of fungi. One of the most exciting new stains for visualizing fungi and other microorganisms whose cell walls contain cellulose or chitin is calcofluor white, described below in Section 7.3.c.

The presence of encapsulated yeast, suspicious for *Cryptococcus neoformans*, particularly in cerebrospinal fluid specimens, can be determined by adding equal parts of India ink (Pelikan brand) or nigrosin stain to the spun sediment of the spinal fluid. The polysaccharide capsules will exclude the particles of ink and the capsule will appear as a clear halo around the organisms. Direct visualization of fungi in clinical specimens will be discussed further in Chapter 43. Capsules of bacteria may also be demonstrated with India ink or nigrosin stains (Appendix B), although these preparations are rarely used in laboratories today.

Lugol's iodine is often added to direct wet mounts of fecal material to aid the microscopist in differentiating parasitic cysts from host white blood cells. Many cysts will take up the iodine, appearing light brown in color. Other objects remain clear. The glycogen vacuole of cysts of *Iodamoeba bütschlii* is particularly visible after it absorbs the iodine. The use of iodine is delineated in Chapter 44.

Another simple stain, Loeffler's methylene blue, described in Appendix B, may be added to wet

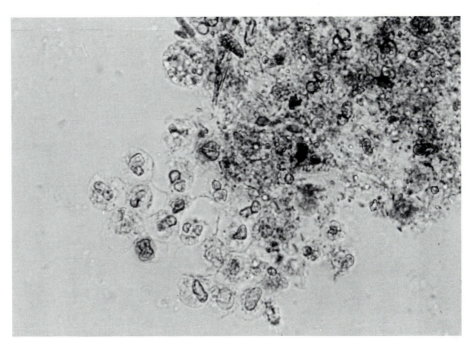

Figure 7.2
Loeffler's methylene blue–stained preparation of feces from a patient with invasive bowel disease, characterized by the presence of many leukocytes.

mounts of feces (equal amounts of stain and feces) for determination of the presence of leukocytes (Figure 7.2). The presence of many polymorphonuclear leukocytes is indicative of invasive disease such as bacterial dysentery or campylobacteriosis, as opposed to the noninflammatory nature of the diarrhea of most parasitic diseases or certain food poisonings.

By adding specific antiserum to a wet preparation of selected clinical material, certain organisms may be identified by a visible antigen-antibody reaction, the *Quellung reaction*. Organisms with capsules, such as *Haemophilus influenzae* type b and *Streptococcus pneumoniae*, exhibit apparent capsular swelling in the presence of homologous antibody. Pathogens in cerebrospinal fluid and sputum can be identified rapidly by this method, although it is less commonly used today than it has been in the past, perhaps because of the recently developed antigen-detection reagents that utilize macroscopically visible endpoints (particle agglutination) instead of microscopically determined endpoints (discussed in Chapter 10).

7.1.c. **Darkfield microscopy.** Certain bacteria are so thin that they cannot be resolved in direct prep-

arations, even with phase contrast microscopy. However, their characteristic motility is an important feature of presumptive identification. These bacteria, primarily spirochetes such as *Borrelia* and treponemes, are best visualized by *darkfield microscopy*, a method of allowing light to be reflected or refracted off the surface of the object, which appears brightly lit against a black background (Figure 7.3). Light from below the object is blocked in a central circle so that only light from the outer ring reaches the object at a sharp angle. The object reflects and scatters this light around the object's edges and the scattered light is viewed through the objective. Large, flat objects such as host cells and clear liquid will not refract much light and will appear very dark. To control the path of light, a drop of immersion oil is placed on the top lens of the darkfield condenser, which is then slowly raised until the oil comes into contact with the bottom of the slide containing the specimen. The condenser height is adjusted until the brightest light is visible reflecting off the numerous small particles in the specimen. The light coming into the condenser from below should be the brightest possible. It may be helpful for the micro-

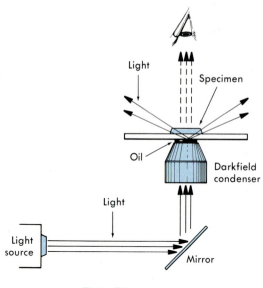

Figure 7.3
Darkfield microscopy.

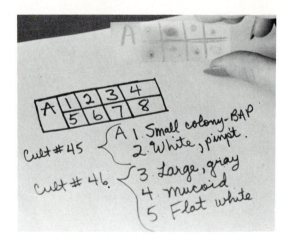

Figure 7.4
Preparation of a slide map for staining several colonies on one slide.

biologist to set the darkfield lighting with a sample slide of a scraping made from the inside of one's cheek emulsified in saline before the actual sample is obtained. In that way, the delicate clinical material can be examined without delay. This method is used most often for the demonstration of motile treponemes in exudate expressed from a primary chancre of syphilis. To best identify these treponemes in darkfield preparations, oil is used on the top of the coverslip to allow viewing with the oil immersion lens at 1,000×. Specimen collection and preparation are discussed in Chapter 19. Motile campylobacters in stool may also be seen under darkfield microscopy.

7.2. Examination of Fixed, Stained Material

Examination of stained material, either direct clinical specimens or samples of growth from cultures, is the most useful method of presumptive identification of bacteria and the presence of certain viruses and for definitive identification of most parasites and many fungi. Individual stains used for special purposes will be mentioned in this chapter and in Appendix B, but specific procedures will usually be found in the section of the book that detail techniques for handling specific specimens or identifying specific pathogens.

Stains are either (1) *simple*, consisting of the addition of one dye that serves to delineate morphology but renders all structures the same hue, or (2) *dif-*

ferential. Differential stains consist of more than one dye added in several steps, and the stained structures are differentiated by color as well as by shape. Certain classical stains are commonly used in clinical microbiology and selected procedures for these stains will be discussed below. Formulas for all reagents not shown here are listed in Appendix B, and procedures not listed here are found in the section of the book describing specific uses for certain staining methods.

7.2.a. **Preparation of a "smear."** Material to be stained is dropped (if liquid) or rolled (if present on a swab) onto the surface of a clean, dry glass slide. Once a swab has touched the surface of a nonsterile slide, it cannot be used for inoculating culture media. A sterile needle may be used to transfer a small amount of the bacterial growth from solid media to the surface of the slide. This material is emulsified in a drop of sterile water or saline on the slide. For very tiny colonies that might become lost in even a small drop of saline, a sterile wooden applicator stick can be used to touch the colony and obtain a bit of growth. This material is then rubbed directly onto the slide, where it can be easily seen. Bacterial morphology is well preserved with this technique. If more than one specimen is to be stained on the same slide, a wax pencil may be used to indicate divisions. It is helpful to draw a "map" of the slide so that different Gram stain results can be recorded in an organized fashion (Figure 7.4). In the case of certain critical specimens, such as cerebrospinal fluid, the use of alcohol-cleaned, sterilized slides is recommended. The material placed on the slide to be stained is allowed to dry or may be heated on a slide warmer to 60° C for at least 10 minutes to kill any pathogens that may be present. If the material is not heated, formalinized, or sterilized in an autoclave, organisms may survive the staining procedure. Therefore, all stained slides should be treated as though they were potentially infectious, and should be discarded with other contaminated material after use. Flaming a slide by passing the slide through the blue flame of a Bunsen burner several times, until the slide it too hot to touch comfortably, will affix the material to the glass but may not be bactericidal. Slides fixed in this way must be allowed to cool before they can be stained.

7.2.b. **Gram stain.** First devised by Hans Christian Gram during the late nineteenth century, the Gram stain can be used to divide most bacterial species effectively into two large groups: those that take up the basic dye, crystal violet (gram-positive) and those that allow the crystal violet dye to wash out easily with the decolorizer alcohol or acetone (gram-negative). The classic Gram stain procedure (Procedure 7.1) entails fixing the material to be stained, either by flaming as described above or by fixing in alcohol. Methanol fixation preserves the morphology of red blood cells as well as bacteria and is especially useful for examining bloody specimen material and blood culture supernatant fluid.[4] Slides are overlaid with 95% methanol for 1 minute, the methanol is allowed to run off, and the slides are air dried before staining.

After fixation, the first step in the Gram stain is the application of the crystal violet. After the crystal violet, a mordant, Gram's iodine, is applied to chemically bond the alkaline dye to the cell wall. The decolorization step distinguishes gram-positive from gram-negative cells. It has recently been shown that the difference in composition between gram-positive cell walls, which contain thick peptidoglycan with numerous teichoic acid crosslinkages, and gram-negative cell walls, consisting of a thin layer of peptidoglycan and a thick external coat of lipopolysaccharides and protein islands, accounts for the differing Gram stain characteristics of these two major groups of organisms.[1,2] Presumably their extensive teichoic acid crosslinks contribute to gram-positive organisms' ability to resist alcohol decolorization. Gram-positive organisms that have lost cell wall integrity due to antibiotic treatment, old age, or action

of autolytic enzymes will also allow the crystal violet to wash out with the decolorizer step. Animal cells, such as red and white blood cells, allow the stain to wash out with the decolorizer as well. At this stage, those organisms that stain gram-positive still retain the crystal violet and those that stain gram-negative are clear. Addition of the counterstain, safranin (or carbol fuchsin, Appendix B) will stain these clear organisms and cells pink or red. Although the counterstain may be taken up by the gram-positive organisms as well, their purple color will not be altered. Yeast cells also stain gram-positive, although fungal mycelia take up the Gram stain variably. Modifications of the classic Gram stain, which include changes in reagents and timing, may be found in Appendix B.

In addition to determining the Gram reaction and morphology of isolated colonies of bacteria, the Gram stain should be used to examine clinical material directly. Sputum can be assessed for suitability for culture by determining the numbers of squamous epithelial cells and polymorphonuclear leukocytes present in the specimen (Chapter 16). If more than 10 epithelial cells are found in an average low-power field ($100 \times$), a sputum sample can be assumed to be contaminated with normal oral flora and unsuitable for culture. The presence of few or no epithelial cells and more than 25 polymorphonuclear leukocytes represents a very good specimen. Obviously, patients with profound granulocytopenia will show few or no polymorphonuclear leukocytes; in sputum specimens from such patients the number of epithelial cells is used to judge the quality of the specimen. The numbers and morphology of bacteria seen in direct smears of clinical material are very valuable as early clues to the cause of disease, as well as for comparison to the growth resulting after incubation. The presence of anaerobic organisms may be signaled, for example, by a culture showing many bacteria on Gram stain that yields light or no growth after aerobic incubation on standard media. Comparing Gram stain results to culture results is an excellent internal method for monitoring quality assurance. Several grading systems for reporting Gram stain results have been published.

Unspun urine can also be Gram-stained to determine the presence of significant bacteriuria. A μl drop of well-mixed unspun urine is allowed to dry on the surface of a slide without being spread out. The presence of one or more bacteria in most oil

PROCEDURE 7.1

Conventional Gram Stain

Principle

Prokaryotes will differentially retain crystal violet depending on cell wall characteristics. Bacteria can be grouped initially based on their Gram stain reactions.

Method

1. Prepare reagents as follows:

    a. Crystal violet
       Crystal violet, 90% dye content   10 g
       Absolute methyl alcohol   500 ml
    b. Iodine
       Iodine crystals   6 g
       Potassium iodide   12 g
       Distilled water   800 ml
    c. Decolorizer
       Acetone   400 ml
       Ethyl alcohol (95%)   200 ml
    d. Counterstain
       Safranin, 99% dye content   10 g
       Distilled water   1000 ml

2. Fix material on slide with methanol or heat fix as detailed in text. If slide is heat fixed, allow it to cool to the touch before applying stain.
3. Flood slide with crystal violet and allow it to remain on the surface without drying for 10 to 30 seconds.
4. Rinse the slide with tap water, shaking off all excess.
5. Flood the slide with iodine and allow it to remain on the surface without drying for twice as long as the crystal violet was in contact with the slide surface (20 seconds of iodine for 10 seconds of crystal violet, for example).
6. Rinse with tap water, shaking off all excess.
7. Flood the slide with decolorizer for 10 seconds and rinse it off immediately with tap water. Repeat this procedure until the blue dye no longer runs off the slide with the decolorizer. Thicker smears require more prolonged decolorizing. Rinse with tap water and shake off excess.
8. Flood the slide with counterstain and allow it to remain on the surface without drying for 30 seconds. Rinse with tap water and gently blot the slide dry with paper towels or bibulous paper or air dry. For delicate smears, such as thin body fluids, air drying is the best method.
9. Examine microscopically under an oil immersion lens at 1000 × for white cells, bacteria, and other structures.

Quality control

Prepare a suspension of mixed *Streptococcus pyogenes* ATCC 19615 and *Escherichia coli* ATCC 25922 in saline. Place a thin drop on the surface of a slide and allow it to air dry. (These can be prepared in advance and stored indefinitely at room temperature in a covered box.) Fix and stain the smear in the same manner as the test slides. Examine it microscopically under oil immersion.

Expected results

One should see purple cocci in chains (the streptococci) and pink rods (the *E. coli*).

Performance schedule

Test each new batch of stains used and test at weekly intervals.

---

immersion fields $(1,000\times)$ is indicative of over 100,000 organisms per milliliter of urine. White blood cells may also be noted. Screening procedures for urine are discussed further in Chapter 18.

    7.2.c. Acid-fast stains. The cell walls of certain parasites and bacteria contain long-chain (50 to 90 carbon atoms) fatty acids (mycolic acids), lending them the property of resistance to destaining of basic dyes by acid alcohol. Thus, they are called "**acid-fast.**" Mycobacteria such as *Mycobacterium tuberculosis* and *Mycobacterium marinum* (Figure 7.5) and coccidian parasites such as *Cryptosporidium* species (Figure 7.6) are characterized by their acid-fast staining properties. The classic acid-fast stain,

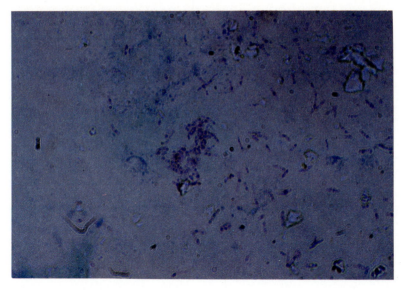

Figure 7.5
Acid-fast stain of *M. marinum* from skin lesion.

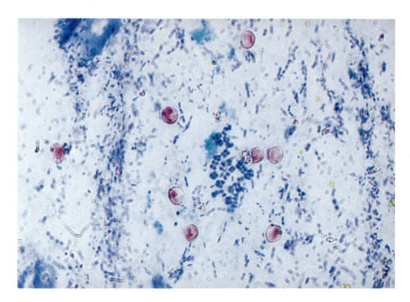

Figure 7.6
Acid-fast stain of *Cryptosporidium* in unconcentrated stool.

Ziehl–Neelsen (Procedure 7.2), requires the addition of heat to allow the stain to enter the wax-containing cell wall. The cold Kinyoun acid-fast stain modification is detailed in Chapter 41. Formulas are listed in Appendix B. A modified acid-fast stain has been developed for differentiating *Nocardia* species, filamentous, branching bacteria that contain fatty acid chains in their cell walls of approximately 50 carbon atoms, from similar non-acid-fast actinomycetes, *Actinomyces* and *Propionibacterium* sp. The *Nocardia* are decolorized by the standard acid-alcohol step, but not by a milder decolorizer, 0.5% to 1% sulfuric acid. These organisms are known as partially or weakly acid-fast bacteria. A procedure for

PROCEDURE 7.2

Ziehl-Neelsen Acid-Fast Stain

Principle

Certain bacteria, parasitic cysts, and rare fungal forms, because of mycolic acids in their cell walls, retain the basic dye carbolfuchsin despite acid-alcohol rinsing. This characteristic differentiates them from other bacteria and is an initial step in their identification.

Note: *Smears should be prepared in a biohazard hood.*

Method

1. Prepare reagents as follows:

    a. Carbolfuchsin
    Basic fuchsin   0.3 g
    Ethanol (95%)   10 ml

    All ingredients are available from Sigma Chemical Co. or other chemical supply houses. Add together and mix. Add the fuchsin solution to 100 ml of 5% phenol solution in distilled water. This solution should then be placed on a stirring platform with a stir-bar in a 37° C incubator overnight; let the stain stand for several days, to allow all components to go into solution, before using the stain.

    b. Decolorizer
    Ethanol (95%)   97 ml
    Concentrated HC1   3 ml

    Add the hydrochloric acid to the ethanol slowly, working in a chemical fume hood.

    c. Counterstain
    Methylene blue   0.3 g
    Distilled water   100 ml

2. Use only new slides. Fix smears on heated surface (60° C for at least 10 minutes). Flood smears with carbolfuchsin and heat to almost boiling by performing the procedure on an electrically heated platform or by passing the flame of a Bunsen burner underneath the slides on a metal rack. The stain on the slides should steam.

3. Allow slides to sit for 5 minutes after heating; do not allow them to dry out.
4. Wash the slides in distilled water (tap water may contain acid-fast bacilli). Shake off excess liquid.
5. Flood slides with decolorizer for approximately 1 minute. Check to see that no more red color runs off the surface when the slide is tipped. Add a bit more decolorizer for very thick slides or those that continue to "bleed" red dye.
6. Wash thoroughly with water and remove the excess.
7. Flood slides with counterstain and allow to remain on surface of slides for 1 minute.
8. Wash with distilled water and stand slides upright on paper towels to air dry. Do not blot dry.
9. Examine microscopically, screening at high power ($400\times$) and confirming all suspicious organisms at $1000\times$ with an oil-immersion lens.

Quality control

Prepare separate suspensions of *M. tuberculosis* H37Ra (suggest ATCC 25177) and *Nocardia asteroides* (suggest ATCC 3308) in Dubos 7H9 broth (use glass beads to disperse the organisms) and place a separate drop of each suspension onto opposite ends of a slide. Allow to dry on a heated slide warmer. (These can be prepared in advance in a biohazard hood and stored indefinitely at room temperature in a covered box.) Fix and stain the slide along with the test slides.

Expected results

The mycobacteria will stain dark red and the nocardia will stain blue.

Performance schedule

Perform each time new stain reagents are used and each time any acid-fast stains are performed.

performing this weak acid-fast stain is given in Chapter 33. Another modification of the acid-fast stain for cryptosporidia is described in Chapter 44.

7.2.d. Methylene blue stain. A simple methylene blue stain of growth from Loeffler's agar slant cultures of possible diphtheria specimens may reveal bacilli with characteristic metachromatic granules of *Corynebacterium diphtheriae*. This same stain will reveal the morphology of fusiform bacteria and of spirochetes in oral specimens.

7.2.e. Differential stains for parasites. Several differential stains are used to highlight the visibility and internal structures of cysts, trophozoites, or other forms of parasites, particularly those found in stool specimens. These stains, further described in Chapter 44, include Wheatley-trichrome and iron hematoxylin. Toluidine O stain, used for rapid examination of respiratory tract material for the presence of *Pneumocystis carinii*, is described in Chapter 44. Silver stains, which stain bacterial and fungal cells, are also used to visualize parasites. Although such stains are usually performed by pathologists, microbiologists may be required to add these procedures to their protocols.

7.2.f. Differential stains for blood smears and tissue sections. Parasites that circulate in the bloodstream may be found within erythrocytes or free in the plasma. Several stains have been developed to help differentiate these parasites from human host cell components. The two stains most commonly used are Wright's and Giemsa (Appendix B). Thin films of blood are fixed with methanol to preserve the red cell morphology so that the relationship of the parasites to the red cells can be seen clearly. The slides are then stained, revealing the nuclei and cytoplasmic features of the parasites. To search a larger quantity of blood for the presence of parasites, a thick film may be prepared by placing a large drop of blood (the size of a nickel) in one area of a slide and defibrinating it by making circles of ever-increasing size from the center outward, using the edge of another glass slide. To visualize the parasites in such a thick smear, the red cells must be lysed with water. Preparation of stains of blood films is discussed in Chapter 44. The Giemsa stain is also used to visualize inclusions in virally or other infected cells, either directly from clinical material, such as the base of a suspected herpetic vesicle or a corneal scraping from a suspected case of *Chlamydia trachomatis* conjunctivitis, or for staining a

monolayer of infected cell cultures, such as the McCoy cells of an in vitro *Chlamydia* culture (discussed further in Chapter 38). The presence of other parasitic infections, such as toxoplasmosis in brain tissue, may be detected using the Giemsa stain. Neither the Wright's nor the Giemsa stain will reliably stain fungal or bacterial elements, so they must be used in conjunction with other stains if the etiology of a suspected infection is totally unknown.

Other stains are used for special purposes, such as the iodine stain for the inclusions of chlamydia-infected monolayer cells, Seller's stain for the Negri bodies in rabies-infected tissues, and the Giménez stain for *Chlamydia* and *Legionella*. These stains are outlined in the chapter in which their use is described or in Appendix B.

7.2.g. Fungal stains. Fungal elements can be seen in fixed material with several stains. The periodic acid–Schiff (PAS) is probably one of the best general stains since most fungal elements in clinical material (such as sputum and tissue) will take up the stain. Methenamine silver, in addition to staining certain parasites, will also stain fungal cell walls a dark blackish brown. This stain, however, usually takes increased time to perform. The polysaccharide capsular material of certain fungi, notably *Cryptococcus neoformans*, stains bright pink with mucicarmine stain, which may prove useful for differentiating this fungus in tissue.

7.3. Fluorescence Microscopy

Certain dyes, called fluors or *fluorochromes*, have the property of becoming excited (raised to a higher energy level) after absorbing ultraviolet (UV) light (light of short wavelength). As the excited molecules return to their normal state, they release the excess energy in the form of visible light of longer wavelength than that which first excited them. This property of becoming self-luminous is called *fluorescence*. Modern microscopic methods have been developed to exploit the enhanced detection possible with this system. Figure 7.7 diagrams a modern fluorescence microscope, in which the light is emitted from above (epifluorescence). An excitation filter passes light of the desired wavelength to excite the fluorochrome, and a barrier filter in the objective prevents the exciting wavelengths from damaging the eyes of the observer. Fluorescing objects appear brightly lit against a dark background, with the color

Figure 7.7
Fluorescence microscope.

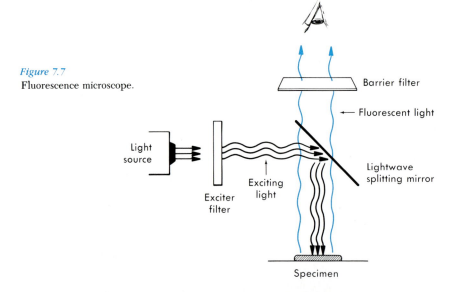

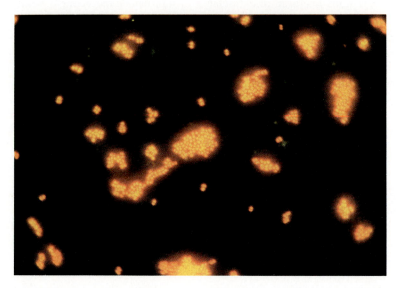

Figure 7.8
Acridine orange–stained staphylococci from blood.

dependent on the dye being used. Many agents will absorb fluorescent dyes directly, as outlined below.

7.3.a. **Acridine orange**. The fluorochrome acridine orange binds to nucleic acid, either in the native or the denatured state. In some formulations of acridine orange, depending on the pH and concentration, the color of the fluorescence will vary (Figure 7.8) Acridine orange has been used as a vital dye, fluorescing green if the organism is alive and red if it is dead. Since the dye intercalates with nucleic acid, however, viable organism will not remain alive for very long after staining. The use of acridine orange for highlighting bacteria in blood culture media (Procedure 7.3) has become widely accepted. Studies have shown the staining of blood cultures with acridine orange to be as sensitive as blind subculture for initial detection of positive cultures.[5] This stain has also been used for detection of cell wall–deficient

PROCEDURE 7.3

Acridine Orange Stain

Principle

Acridine orange, a vital stain, will intercalate with nucleic acid, changing the dye's optical reflecting characteristics so that it will fluoresce bright orange under UV light. Any nucleic acid–containing object will fluoresce.

Method

1. Fix slide, either in methanol or with heat, as described previously.
2. Flood slide with acridine orange stain (Appendix B; also available from BBL Microbiology Products, Difco Laboratories, Remel Laboratories, and other suppliers). Allow stain to remain on surface of slide for 2 minutes without drying.
3. Rinse with tap water and allow the slide to air dry by leaning it upright to drain on paper towels.
4. Examine the slide microscopically under UV light with the same light source as that used for fluorescein. Bacteria will fluoresce bright orange against a green-fluorescing or dark background. The nuclei of blood cells may also fluoresce.

Quality control

Save a culture-positive blood culture broth and prepare a smear at the same time as the unknown sample smear is prepared. Fix and stain both smears simultaneously and examine microscopically under oil immersion.

Expected results

The known positive should show bright orange–fluorescing organisms of the morphology of the organism isolated previously.

Performance schedule

Perform with new reagents and each time the stain is used.

bacteria, such as mycoplasmas, in broth cultures.

7.3.b. **Rhodamine-auramine**. The mycolic acid in the cell walls of mycobacteria has an affinity for the fluorochromes auramine and rhodamine. These dyes will bind to mycobacteria, which appear bright yellow or orange against a greenish background. The counterstain, potassium permanganate, helps to prevent nonspecific fluorescence. All acid-fast objects, including the sporozoan parasites, will stain with auramine or rhodamine as well. One widely used staining procedure, that of Truant and others,[7] is shown in Procedure 7.4.

An important aspect of the rhodamine-auramine stain is that slides may be restained with Ziehl-Neelsen or Kinyoun stain directly over the fluorochrome stain, as long as the oil has been removed. In this way, positive slides can be confirmed with the traditional stain, which will also aid in differentiating morphology.

7.3.c. **Calcofluor white**. The cell walls of fungi will bind the stain calcofluor white, greatly enhancing their visibility in tissue and other specimens. As described by Hageage and Harrington,[3] this stain is used in place of 10% KOH for initial examination of clinical material. It is also used to enhance visualization of morphologic elements of pure cultures of fungi. For many applications, it has supplanted the lactophenol cotton blue stain in some laboratories. Organisms fluoresce blue-white or apple green, depending on the light source (Figure 7.9). The modification of the stain that we suggest is outlined in Procedure 7.5. The fluorescent stain and the KOH are added separately, since they tend to precipitate if combined and stored as a single solution. The stain is also available commercially.

7.4. Antibody-Conjugated Stains

The most specific detectors are antibodies that bind tightly to antigens against which they are directed (Chapter 12). Antibodies can be produced against entire classes of agents that share common antigens or against specific determinants, such as the carbohydrate that is common to the cell walls of *Streptococcus pyogenes*. If antibodies are conjugated to a dye that allows their reactive sites to interact with the homologous antigens, they serve as visible flags for the presence of that antigen. Several of the dyes that are commonly bound to antibodies are described on pages 78 and 79.

PROCEDURE 7.4

Rhodamine-Auramine Acid-Fast Stain

Principle

The nonspecific chromophores rhodamine and auramine bind to mycolic acids in the cell walls of acid-fast organisms and are refractory to rinsing by acid-alcohol. These stains thus exhibit the same characteristics as fuchsin-based, acid-fast stains although they are visualized under UV light. Organisms fluorescing orange-yellow or red are more easily detected than traditionally stained organisms.

Method

1. Prepare reagents as follows:

   a. Rhodamine-auramine

Auramine O (C.I. 41000)	1.5 g
Rhodamine B (C.I. 45170)	0.75 g
Glycerol	75 ml
Melted phenol crystals	10 ml
Distilled water	50 ml

   Reagents are available from Sigma Chemical Co. and other chemical supply companies. Add the phenol and water together; then add the other ingredients. Place on a magnetic stirrer with a stir bar in the incubator. Allow to stir at 37° C overnight, or until all particulates are dissolved. Filter through glass wool and store in a brown glass bottle with a glass stopper. The stain is stable for at least 6 months in the refrigerator.

   b. Decolorizer

Hydrochloric acid (concentrated)	0.5 ml
Ethanol (70%)	100 ml

   c. Counterstain

Potassium permanganate	0.5 g
Distilled water	100 ml

   Mix together, filter through coarse filter paper or glass wool, and store in a brown glass bottle.

Modified from Truant, J.P., Brett, W.A., and Thomas, W. Jr. 1962. Henry Ford Hosp. Med Bull. 10:287.

The solution is stable at room temperature for 6 months.

2. Heat-fix slides as described above.
3. Flood slides with rhodamine-auramine. Allow the stain to remain on the slide for 15 minutes. Do not allow the surface to dry.
4. Rinse the slides with distilled water and shake off excess liquid.
5. Flood slides with decolorizer for 2 to 3 minutes. Slide will still appear pink.
6. Rinse thoroughly with distilled water, shake off excess.
7. Flood slides with counterstain for 3 to 4 minutes. Do not allow slides to dry.
8. Rinse thoroughly with distilled water and allow to air dry as described above for other acid-fast stains.
9. Examine microscopically under the same UV light source as used for fluorescein or other light source dictated by the instrument. Acid-fast bacilli will be visible as bright yellow-orange organisms against a green background. Slides can be screened with high power $(400\times)$ and verified under oil immersion.

Quality control

Same procedure as for Ziehl-Neelsen stain discussed previously.

Expected results

Acid-fast organisms will exhibit bright orange-yellow to red fluorescence, depending on the filter system used. Non-acid-fast organisms will not be visible.

Performance schedule

As for Ziehl-Neelsen stain.

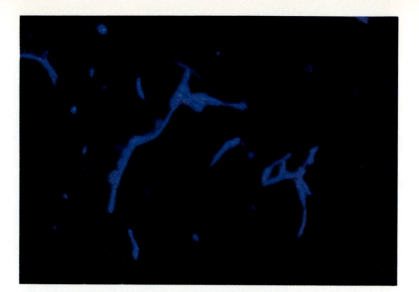

Figure 7.9
Fungal elements stained with calcofluor white.

PROCEDURE 7.5

Examining Clinical Material for the Presence of Fungal Elements

Principle

Cellulose in the cell walls of certain prokaryotes and eukaryotic fungi will bind the nonspecific fluorochrome calcofluor white, allowing detection of fungal elements in wet preparations more easily and rapidly than with conventional KOH preparations and more rapid screening with lower magnification. The dye concentrates in fungal cell walls and fluoresces blue-white or green under UV light, depending on the filter system used.

Method

1. Prepare calcofluor white stain as follows:

Calcofluor white M2R (Polysciences or Sigma Chemical Co.)	0.1 g
Evans blue (Sigma)	0.05 g
Distilled water	100 ml

Mix thoroughly and store in a brown bottle at room temperature. The solution is stable for 1 year.

2. Add one drop of the calcofluor white solution and one drop of 10% KOH (described previously) to the specimen to be examined on a clean glass slide. Place a coverslip over the material and turn the slide face down on several thicknesses of paper toweling, pushing gently to flatten the coverslip down and express excess fluid out from the edges of the coverslip and into the paper towels.

3. Examine the slide under UV light, using a K530 excitation filter and a BG 12 barrier filter, as for fluorescein. Other filter combinations that produce light of blue-white wavelength, such as a G-365 excitation filter and an LP 420 barrier filter, can be used.

4. Fungal elements will appear apple green (or blue-white, depending on the filter combination used), with a much dimmer reddish tinted fluorescing background.

Quality control

Prepare a dilute saline suspension of *Candida albicans* ATCC 10231 and *E. coli* ATCC 25922. Add the calcofluor reagents as described and examine this material on the other end of the test slide or on a separate slide.

Expected results

The large yeast cells will fluoresce brightly and the small rod-shaped *E. coli* will be barely visible as pale outlines.

Performance schedule

Test a quality control suspension when new reagents are prepared and each time the stain is performed.

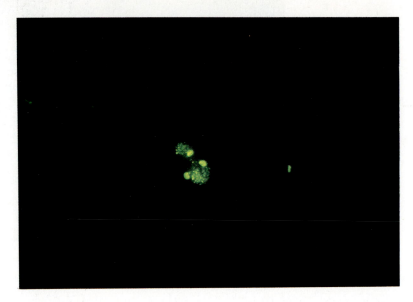

Fluorescent antibody–stained *S. pyogenes* from pure culture.

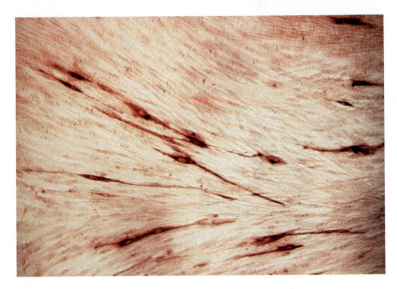

Immunoperoxidase–stained cell culture monolayer infected with herpes simplex virus.

7.4.a. **Fluorescein-conjugated stains.** Antibodies bound to the fluorochrome fluorescein isothiocyanate (FITC) are used to visualize many bacteria in direct specimens. Fluorescein fluoresces an intense apple green when excited. Examples include *Bordetella pertussis* in nasopharyngeal smears from children suspected of having whooping cough, and *Legionella* species in respiratory specimens or tissue of patients with Legionnaires' disease. Monoclonal an-

tibodies (described in Chapter 10) have been successfully conjugated to fluorescein for detection of chlamydiae; herpes, respiratory syncytial, rabies, and other viruses; treponemes and other pathogens in directly stained clinical material. Other fluorescein-conjugated antibodies are used to identify pure cultures of organisms, such as certain *Actinomyces* species, *S. pyogenes* (Figure 7.10), *Neisseria gonorrhoeae*, and others. As more monoclonal antibod-

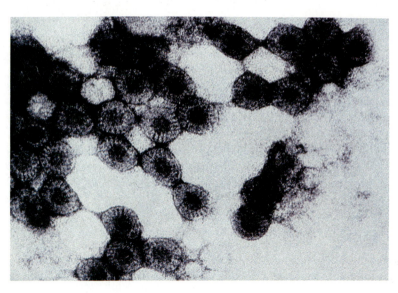

Figure 7.12
Rotavirus particles stained by immunoelectron microscopy.

7.4.a. Fluorescein-conjugated stains. Antibodies bound to the fluorochrome fluorescein isothiocyanate (FITC) are used to visualize many bacteria in direct specimens. Fluorescein fluoresces an intense apple green when excited. Examples include *Bordetella pertussis* in nasopharyngeal smears from children suspected of having whooping cough, and *Legionella* species in respiratory specimens or tissue of patients with Legionnaires' disease. Monoclonal antibodies (described in Chapter 10) have been successfully conjugated to fluorescein for detection of chlamydiae; herpes, respiratory syncytial, rabies, and other viruses; treponemes and other pathogens in directly stained clinical material. Other fluorescein-conjugated antibodies are used to identify pure cultures of organisms, such as certain *Actinomyces* species, *S. pyogenes* (Figure 7.10), *Neisseria gonorrhoeae*, and others. As more monoclonal antibodies are developed, more conjugated stains will be produced for the rapid, direct detection of pathogens in clinical material.

7.4.b. Enzyme-conjugated stains. For those laboratories that do not have access to a fluorescent microscope, enzymes that catalyze the production of a colored precipitin product are an excellent alternative conjugate for specific antibody detector reagents. Horseradish peroxidase is a small enzyme that produces an orange-brown precipitate as its eas-

ily visible endpoint. Conjugated to antibodies, it is known as *immunoperoxidase stain*, and it is used to detect cytomegalovirus and other virus proteins or nucleic acids in cells (Figure 7.11). Although primarily used to detect viral antigens, other antigens could easily be detected with this system. Other enzymes have been conjugated to antibodies. Alkaline phosphatase produces a blue precipitate as its end product, and it, too, has been used as a detector for viral antigens, as well as inclusions of chlamydiae.

7.4.c. Biotin-avidin-enzyme-conjugated stains. Single-stranded nucleic acid probes (described in Chapter 10), antimicrobial antibodies, or antibiotin antibodies can be bound to the small molecule, biotin. This molecule has a strong affinity for the protein avidin, which has four binding sites. Thus, biotin bound to avidin or antibody can be complexed to fluorescent dyes or to color-producing enzymes to form specific detector systems. Products are available for the detection of nucleic acids of cytomegalovirus, herpes I and II viruses, hepatitis B virus, adenovirus 2, Epstein-Barr virus, *Chlamydia*, and other etiologic agents.

7.5. Electron Microscopy

The electron microscope uses electrons instead of light to visualize small objects; thus the resolution is increased relative to the shortness of the wavelength of the electron beams. Instead of lenses, the electrons are focused by electromagnetic fields and form an image on a fluorescent screen, like a television screen. Many new morphologic features of bacteria, bacterial components, fungi, and parasites have been discovered using electron microscopy. For routine microbiological diagnosis, however, the greatest use of electron microscopy has been for detection of viral causes of gastroenteritis. All enteric viruses can be identified in either direct electron microscopic preparations of fecal material or by immunoelectron microscopy, in which fecal samples are mixed with specific antiviral antibody before staining (Figure 7.12). Since an electron microscope is a major capital investment, few laboratories have the capability to use these techniques on a routine basis.

REFERENCES

1. Bottone, E.J. 1988. The gram stain: the century-old quintessential rapid diagnostic test. Lab. Med. 19:288.
2. Davies, J.A., Anderson, G.K., Beveridge, T.J., et al. 1983. Chemical mechanism of the Gram stain and synthesis of a new electron-opaque marker for electron microscopy which replaces the iodine mordant of the stain. J. Bacteriol. 156:837.
3. Hageage, G.J. Jr., and Harrington, B.J. 1984. Use of calcofluor white in clinical mycology. Lab. Med. 15:109.
4. Mangels, J.I., Cox, M.E., and Lindberg, L.H. 1984. Methanol fixation: an alternative to heat fixation of smears before staining. Diagn. Microbiol. Infect. Dis. 2:129.
5. McCarthy, L.R., and Senne, J.E. 1980. Evaluation of acridine orange stain for detection of microorganisms in blood cultures. J. Clin. Microbiol. 11:281.
6. McGinnis, M.R. 1980. Laboratory handbook of medical mycology. Academic Press, New York.
7. Truant, J.P., Brett, W.A., and Thomas, W. Jr. 1962. Fluorescence microscopy of tubercle bacillus stained with auramine and rhodamine. Henry Ford Hosp. Med. Bull. 10:287.

BIBLIOGRAPHY

Clarridge, J.E., and Mullins, J.M. 1987. In Howard, B.J., Klass, J. II, Rubin, S.J., et al. Clinical and pathogenic microbiology. The C.V. Mosby Co., St. Louis.
Douglas, S.D. 1980. Microscopy. In Lennette, E.H., Balows, A., Hausler, W.J. Jr., and Truant, J.P., editors. Manual for clinical microbiology, ed. 3. American Society for Microbiology, Washington, D.C.
Goodman, N.L. 1985. Direct microscopy in diagnosing fungal disease. Diagn. Med. 8:14.
Smith, R.F. 1982. Microscopy and photomicrography: a practical guide. Appleton-Century-Crofts, Norwalk, Conn.
Yong, D.C.T., and Peter, J.B. 1984. Using DEM to detect pediatric viral gastroenteritis. Diagn. Med. 7:45.

8 Cultivation and Isolation of Viable Pathogens

Although future trends in clinical microbiology are clearly pointing in the direction of developing rapid, non-growth-dependent methods for detecting the presence of infectious agents, the isolation and identification of viable pathogens is still the "gold standard" for diagnosis of infectious diseases today and will always remain important. A pure culture of a clone of identical cells has been necessary for performing biochemical differentiation tests and susceptibility studies, since single cells are impossible to work with easily, and mixed cultures yield no useful or even misleading information. In the late nineteenth century, the invention in Robert Koch's laboratory by Frau Hesse of solid agar aided the development of the newly burgeoning science of clinical microbiology. Before solid media plates were available, microbiologists had to rely on the method developed by Lister, employing the principle of limiting dilutions from cultures in broth media for obtaining pure isolates with which to work. General concepts applicable to the in vitro cultivation of pathogens are outlined below.

Methods used to create optimal conditions for the cultivation of pathogens have been developed over years of experimentation. At this time, commercially produced environmental systems, artificial media, cell culture lines, and all other items necessary for the practice of clinical microbiology are readily available to microbiologists in the industrialized world. Laboratorians in less well-developed parts of the world may still need to bleed their own sheep (or other animals) and perform other basic tasks necessary to practice diagnostic microbiology, but most microbiologists now purchase the majority of the materials needed for cultivation, identification, and susceptibility testing of pathogenic microorganisms.

Clinical microbiologists used to rely heavily on inoculation of experimental animals for the isolation and identification of infectious agents. Today, such activities are usually confined to research facilities or public health laboratories. For this reason, animal inoculation techniques will not be mentioned extensively in the rest of this book, unless their application is particularly important for clinical diagnosis.

8.1. Artificial Media

8.1.a. General concepts of artificial media. Over the years varied strategies have been developed for the cultivation of pathogens. Ingredients necessary for the growth of pathogens can be supplied by a living system, as in the human or animal host or in cell culture, or by mixing together the required nutrients in an artificial system. During the nineteenth century, media were prepared in glass containers, from which the phrase *in vitro* (which means "in glass") originated. To encourage the growth of particular organisms from a milieu containing only a few of the desired organisms among large numbers of normal flora, various kinds of laboratory-prepared nutrient-containing solutions were concocted and called **enrichment media.** An example of such a medium is selenite broth, which encourages the growth of small numbers of stool pathogens and suppresses the growth of the much larger numbers of normal stool organisms. A second class of artificial media is called **supportive.** These media contain nutrients that allow most nonfastidious organisms to grow at their natural rates, without affording any particular organism a growth advantage (except for the organism's own metabolism) on the medium. Examples of supportive media are nutrient agar and brain heart infusion agar. Media containing one or more agents inhibitory to all organisms except the organism being sought were developed, first using dyes that exhib-

ited antibacterial characteristics, later using antibiotics, and still later incorporating components that take into consideration certain metabolic activities of the organisms sought. Such media are known as **selective media,** since they select for certain organisms to the disadvantage of others. An example of a selective medium is phenylethyl alcohol agar, which inhibits the growth of aerobic and facultatively anaerobic gram-negative rods and allows gram-positive cocci to grow. The fourth type of medium, **differential,** employs some factor or factors that allows colonies of organisms that possess certain metabolic or cultural characteristics to be morphologically distinguished from those organisms that have different characteristics. The most supportive differential medium is sheep blood agar, which allows many organisms to grow and additionally allows different organisms to be distinguished on the basis of their hemolytic reactions against the sheep red blood cells, production of pigment, and so forth. Table 8.1 lists a number of media that are commonly used in clinical microbiology, along with the ingredients that allow for differential or selective ability.

8.1.b. Preparation of dehydrated artificial media that are to be sterilized in autoclave. Dehydrated media powders should be kept in their original bottles with the caps tightly closed. The date received and the date first opened for use should be recorded on the bottle itself. Media makers should always *read the label* before preparing any medium. Media should be prepared in clean glassware that has been rinsed in distilled or deionized water. To avoid boiling over during heating, a vessel holding a liquid solution to be sterilized in an autoclave should never be filled more than two-thirds full. The proper amount of powder is weighed onto nonabsorbent paper and poured into the container in which it is to be prepared. Distilled water is added next with vigorous swirling to achieve an even suspension. If other liquid ingredients are to be added, they should be incorporated at this point. If the solution is clear, as most broths usually are, it requires no further manipulation before autoclaving; however, most agar solutions require heating almost to the boiling point, with constant agitation, to achieve an even solution. The use of a stirrer–hot plate and a magnetic stirbar will greatly increase the efficiency of this stage of media making. The hot solution must be watched extremely carefully as soon as tiny bubbles begin to appear, as these media tend to boil over very easily.

Table 8.1
Primary Plating Media

MEDIUM	COMPONENTS/COMMENTS	PRIMARY PURPOSE
Bacteroides bile esculin agar (BBE)	Trypticase soy agar base with ferric ammonium citrate, enriched with hemin (5 mg/ml). Bile salts and gentamicin act as inhibitors.	Selective and differential for *Bacteroides fragilis* group. Good for presumptive identification.
Bile esculin agar (BEA)	Nutrient agar base with ferric citrate. Hydrolysis of esculin by group D streptococci imparts a brown color to medium; sodium desoxycholate inhibits many bacteria.	Differential isolation and presumptive identification of group D streptococci
Bismuth sulfite agar (BS)	Peptone agar with dextrose and ferrous sulfate. Gram-positive organisms and other Enterobacteriaceae inhibited by bismuth sulfite and brilliant green.	Selective for isolation of *Salmonella* from stool
Blood agar	Trypticase soy agar, *Brucella* agar, or beef heart infusion base with 5% sheep blood.	Cultivation of fastidious microorganisms, determination of hemolytic reactions
Bordet-Gengou agar	Potato-glycerol-based medium enriched with 15%-20% defibrinated blood. Contaminants inhibited by methicillin (final concentration of 2.5 µg/ml).	Isolation of *Bordetella pertussis*
Buffered charcoal yeast extract agar (BCYE)	Yeast extract, agar, charcoal and salts supplemented with L-cysteine HCl, ferric pyrophosphate, ACES buffer, and α-ketoglutarate.	Selective for *Legionella* sp.
Campy-blood agar	Contains vancomycin (10 mg/L), trimethoprim (5 mg/L), polymixin B (2500 U/L), amphotericin B (2 mg/L), and cephalothin (15 mg/L) in a *Brucella* agar base with sheep blood	Selective for *Campylobacter* sp.
CDC anaerobic blood agar	Trypticase soy agar with 5% sheep blood enriched with hemin, L-cystine, and vitamin K_1.	Isolation of anaerobic and other organisms
Cefsulodin-irgasan-novo-biocin (CIN) agar	Peptone base with yeast extract, mannitol, and bile salts. Supplemented with cefsulodin, irgasan, and novobiocin; neutral red and crystal violet indicators.	Selective for *Yersinia* sp.
Chocolate agar	Peptone base, enriched with solution of 2% hemoglobin or IsoVitaleX (BBL).	Cultivation of *Haemophilus* and *Neisseria* sp.
Columbia colistin-nalidixic acid (CNA) agar	Columbia agar base with 10 mg colistin per liter, 15 mg nalidixic acid per liter, and 5% sheep blood.	Selective isolation of gram-positive cocci
Cooked meat (CM; also called chopped meat)	Solid meat particles initiate growth of bacteria, reducing substances lower oxidation-reduction potential (Eh).	Cultivation of anaerobic organisms
Cycloserine-cefoxitin fructose agar (CCFA)	Egg yolk base with fructose, cycloserine (500 mg/L), and cefoxitin (16 mg/L) added to inhibit stool flora. Neutral red indicator.	Selective for *Clostridium difficile*
Cystine-lactose-electrolyte-deficient (CLED) agar	Peptone base agar with lactose and L-cystine; bromthymol blue indicator inhibits swarming of *Proteus* sp.	Isolation and enumeration of bacteria in urine
Cystine-tellurite blood agar	Infusion agar base with 5% sheep blood. Reduction of potassium tellurite by *Corynebacterium diphtheriae* produces black colonies.	Isolation of *C. diphtheriae*
Dermatophyte test medium (DTM) agar	Nutrient base with glucose and phenol red indicator. Contaminants inhibited by cycloheximide, gentamicin, and tetracycline.	Isolation and identification of dermatophytes
Eosin methylene blue (EMB) agar (Levine)	Peptone base with lactose and sucrose. Eosin and methylene blue as indicators.	Isolation and differentiation of lactose-fermenting and non-lactose-fermenting enteric bacilli
Gram-negative broth (GN)	Peptone base broth with glucose and mannitol. Sodium citrate and sodium desoxycholate act as inhibitory agents.	Selective (enrichment) liquid medium for enteric pathogens

Continued.

Table 8.1

Primary Plating Media—cont'd

MEDIUM	COMPONENTS/COMMENTS	PRIMARY PURPOSE
Hektoen enteric (HE) agar	Peptone base agar with bile salts, lactose, sucrose, salicin, and ferric ammonium citrate. Indicators include bromthymol blue and acid fuchsin.	Differential, selective medium for the isolation and differentiation of *Salmonella* and *Shigella* from other gram-negative enteric bacilli
Kanamycin-vancomycin laked blood agar (KVLB)	*Brucella* agar base with kanamycin (75 µg/ml), vancomycin (7.5 µg/ml), vitamin K_1 (10 µg/ml), and 5% laked blood.	Selective isolation of *Bacteroides* sp.
Lombard-Dowell agar	Casein digest agar enriched with hemin (10 mg/L), vitamin K_1 (10 mg/L), L-cystine (0.4 g/L), and yeast extract.	Isolation and initial testing of anaerobic organisms
Löwenstein-Jensen (L-J) agar	Egg-based medium; contaminants inhibited by malachite green.	Isolation of mycobacteria
MacConkey agar	Peptone base with lactose. Gram-positive organisms inhibited by crystal violet and bile salts. Neutral red as indicator.	Isolation and differentiation of lactose fermenting and non-lactose-fermenting enteric bacilli
Mannitol salt agar	Peptone base, mannitol, and phenol red indicator. Salt concentration of 7.5% inhibits most bacteria.	Selective isolation of coagulase-positive staphylococci
Middlebrook 7H10 agar	Complex base with albumin, salts, enzymatic digest of casein enrichment, and malachite green inhibitor.	Isolation of and antimicrobial susceptibility testing of mycobacteria
Mycosel or mycobiotic agar	Peptone base with glucose; contaminants inhibited by chloramphenicol and cycloheximide.	Isolation of dermatophytes
New York City (NYC) agar	Peptone agar base with cornstarch, supplemented with yeast dialysate, 3% hemoglobin, and horse plasma. Antibiotic supplement includes vancomycin (2 µg/ml), colistin (5.5 µg/ml), amphotericin B (1.2 µg/ml), and trimethoprim (3 µg/ml).	Selective for *Neisseria gonorrhoeae*
Petragnani agar	Coagulated-egg medium with malachite green to inhibit commensals.	Isolation of mycobacteria
Phenylethyl alcohol (PEA) agar	Nutrient agar base. Phenylethanol inhibits growth of gram-negative organisms.	Selective isolation of gram-positive cocci and anaerobic gram-negative bacilli
Sabouraud dextrose agar	Peptone base agar. Final pH of medium (5.6) favors growth of fungi over bacteria.	Isolation of dermatophytes

Some media are ready to be dispensed at this point.

If the medium is to be sterilized in an autoclave, it is capped with either a plastic screw cap or a plug. A good plug can be made from a large wad of non-absorbable cotton wrapped in a square of gauze one layer thick. For sterilization of flasks of agar that are to be poured into plates by hand, we have found a large square of aluminum foil molded to the shape of the flask to be an excellent cover that can be removed and replaced many times and that allows the neck of the flask to remain sterile until the foil is lifted off (Figure 8.1). The solutions are placed in the autoclave and sterilized; the timing of the sterilization should start from the moment the temperature reaches 121° C. Very large quantities of media

may require a longer sterilization time than is recommended on the package label. Once the sterilization cycle is completed, the autoclave chamber is slowly returned to atmospheric pressure, to prevent the liquid from bubbling over. Sterilized media should not be kept in the autoclave once the pressure has equalized, since prolonged heat may alter some of the ingredients.

Sterilization in an autoclave can be dangerous; all the safety precautions outlined in Chapter 2 and the quality control practices outlined in Chapter 3 should be carefully adhered to by operators. Autoclave performance should be monitored for microbial killing ability regularly and for achievement of proper temperature during every use (with autoclave

Table 8.1

Primary Plating Media—cont'd

MEDIUM	COMPONENTS/COMMENTS	PRIMARY PURPOSE
Salmonella-Shigella (SS) agar	Peptone base with lactose, ferric citrate, and sodium citrate. Neutral red as indicator; inhibition of coliforms by brillant green, bile salts.	Selective for *Salmonella* and *Shigella* sp.
Schaedler agar	Peptone and soy protein base agar with yeast extract, dextrose, and buffers. Addition of hemin, L-cystine, and 5% blood enriches for anaerobes.	Nonselective medium for the recovery of anaerobes and aerobes
Selenite broth	Peptone base broth. Sodium selenite toxic for most Enterobacteriaceae.	Enrichment of isloation of *Salmonella*
Skirrow agar	Peptone and soy protein base agar with lysed horse blood. Vancomycin inhibits gram-positive organisms; polymyxin B and trimethoprim inhibit most gram-negative organisms.	Selective for *Campylobacter*, particularly recommended for "*C. pylori*."
Streptococcal selective agar (SSA)	Contains crystal violet, colistin, and trimethoprim-sulfamethoxazole in 5% sheep blood agar base.	Selective for *Streptococcus pyogenes* and *Streptococcus agalactiae*
Tetrathionate broth	Peptone base broth. Bile salts and sodium thiosulfate inhibit gram-positive organisms and Enterobacteriaceae.	Selctive for *Salmonella* and *Shigella*
Thayer-Martin agar	Blood agar base enriched with hemoglobin and supplement B; contaminating organisms inhibited by colistin, nystatin, vancomycin, and trimethoprim.	Selective for *N. gonorrhoeae* and *N. meningitidis*
Thioglycolate broth	Pancreatic digest of casein, soy broth, and glucose enrich growth of most microorganisms. Thioglycolate and agar reduce Eh.	Supports growth of anaerobes, aerobes, microaerophilic, and fastidious microorganisms
Thiosulfate citrate–bile salts (TCBS) agar	Peptone base agar with yeast extract, bile salts, citrate, sucrose, ferric citrate, and sodium thiosulfate. Bromthymol blue acts as indicator.	Selective and differential for vibrios
Vaginalis (V) agar	Columbia agar base supplemented with 5% human blood.	Selective and differential for *Gardnerella vaginalis*
Xylose lysine desoxycholate (XLD) agar	Yeast extract agar with lysine, xylose, lactose, sucrose, and ferric ammonium citrate. Sodium desoxycholate inhibits gram-positive organisms; phenol red as indicator.	Isolation and differentiation of *Salmonella* and *Shigella* from other gram-negative enteric bacilli

tape, for example). Media removed from the autoclave should be placed into a 55° C water bath to cool before any supplements are added or before plates are poured. Liquid media or media that are not to be dispensed may be allowed to cool on the bench top. Agar will tend to settle to the bottom of a flask during sterilization, so all flasks should be swirled in a large circle on the bench top (to avoid making bubbles) before pouring. If a few bubbles appear on the surface of a freshly poured plate, they can be removed by quickly passing the flame from a Bunsen burner over the surface. We have found that leaving the covers of Petri dishes slightly ajar allows contaminants to reach the agar surfaces. Our recommendation is to leave tops closed and incubate plates overnight after they have set, to remove surface moisture and detect contamination.

8.1.c. **Methods of sterilization other than autoclave.** Media that contain serum or certain proteins are often sterilized by **inspissation.** In this intermittent sterilization method, the media are placed in a chamber through which steam continuously flows for approximately 30 minutes each day for several successive days. Loeffler agar and Löwenstein-Jensen agar are prepared by this method.

Delicate media may also be sterilized by allowing the flasks or tubes to remain in a chamber through which steam actively flows. Such a chamber, the Arnold steam sterilizer, is also often used to remelt media that have been prepared in advance and al-

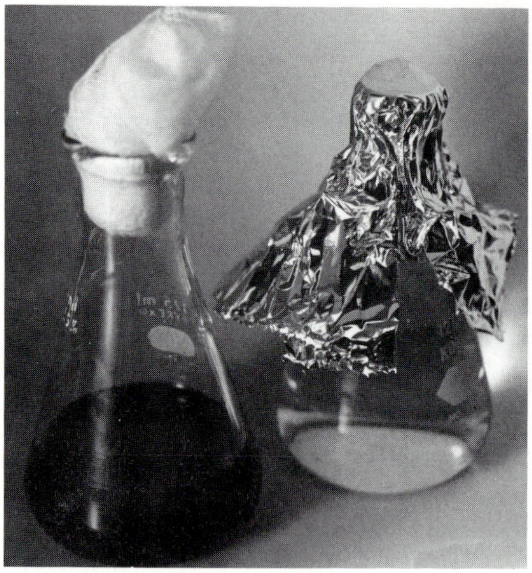

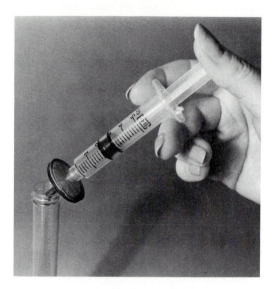

Figure 8.1
Gauze-covered nonabsorbable cotton plug and aluminum foil cover for flasks used in media preparation.

Figure 8.2
Use of a membrane filter system to sterilize solutions nonsterilizable in autoclave.

lowed to harden. This method is particularly useful for pouring fresh agar plates made from previously prepared agar deep tubes, to which a sterile additive not suitable for autoclave sterilization (such as blood) is added immediately before pouring. Plates seldom used but that require fresh enrichments (egg yolk agar, Bordet-Gengou, etc.) can be prepared as needed from agar deep tubes, which have a much longer shelf life than poured plates. Carbohydrate solutions and other liquids that may be denatured by heat can be **filter sterilized** by injecting the liquid through a syringe attached to a membrane filter with pores no larger than 0.2 or 0.45 μm in diameter (Figure 8.2). Disposable closed membrane filtration systems are available commercially (Appendix C).

Most hospitals use **gas sterilization** for instruments and equipment. This method uses ethylene oxide to destroy bacteria and spores. Microbiologists may make use of the gas sterilizer to process reusable plastic ware and instruments. Gas sterilization takes much longer than the other methods described, usually requiring an overnight cycle and aeration time for the ethylene oxide to diffuse away.

8.2. Conditions Necessary for Growth of Pathogens

In order for bacteria or fungi to multiply on or in artificial media, they must have available the re-

quired nutrients, a permissive temperature, enough moisture in the medium and in the atmosphere, the proper gaseous atmosphere, proper salt concentration, an appropriate pH, and there must be no growth-inhibiting factors (such as other bacteria or fungi or artificial compounds that antagonize growth).

8.2.a. Establishing atmospheric conditions required for growth of pathogens other than anaerobes. Pathogenic organisms are either **aerobic,** utilizing oxygen as a terminal electron acceptor and showing good growth in an atmosphere of room air, **anaerobic,** relatively intolerant to the presence of oxygen, or **microaerophilic,** growing best in atmospheres of reduced oxygen tension. Aerobic organisms can be incubated in room air without much difficulty. Most clinically significant "aerobic" organisms are actually **facultatively anaerobic;** they grow under either aerobic or anaerobic conditions. True aerobic organisms include *Pseudomonas* species, members of the Neisseriaceae family, *Brucella* species, *Bordetella* species, and *Francisella* species, as well as mycobacteria, filamentous fungi, and others.

To achieve an atmosphere of incubation other than room air, several strategies have been developed. Organisms that grow best with greater CO_2 concentrations than are found in room air, called **capnophilic,** may be incubated in an atmosphere of

5% to 10% CO_2 in a special incubator with sealed doors. Gas of the proper mixture is fed into the incubator automatically from nearby cylinders. The CO_2 concentration should be checked on a routine basis.

By placing inoculated cultures into a sealable container, evacuating the room air down to a negative pressure of 25 pounds of mercury, and replacing it with a commercially produced artificial mixture of gases placed under pressure in a gas cylinder, microbiologists can produce any desired atmosphere. Three evacuation-replacement cycles are usually necessary to remove all residual normal atmosphere. Sealable plastic bags into which fit the components of a CO_2 and hydrogen generating system or oxygen-binding components and an indicator of the proper atmosphere are also available commercially for the production of specialized atmospheres of incubation (see Appendix C). Bags have been designed for creating either anaerobic or capnophilic atmospheres. These bags are especially convenient for incubating primary plates from important cultures or in other circumstances where few plates are used. The bags accommodate only one or a few culture plates each, but all plates can be examined through the plastic without opening the bag. Some organisms that appear to be microaerophilic or capnophilic are actually **humidophilic;** they require increased moisture in the atmosphere.

Pathogenic campylobacters (except *C. pylori*) require a high CO_2 content (5% to 10%) and no more than 6% oxygen. This atmosphere can be achieved safely by using a premixed gas for evacuation-replacement or by creating the atmosphere in a sealed jar or plastic bag with a commercially available self-contained generator system. These generator systems, which are similar to those available for creating an anaerobic atmosphere in a closed container, consist of an envelope that contains the components of a small hydrogen (and sometimes a CO_2) generating system. Chemical components required to catalyze the reaction between hydrogen and oxygen, forming water, removing oxygen, and thus creating the anaerobic atmosphere in such a system (alumina-coated palladium pellets), may be incorporated into the generator or supplied separately. Other methods for creating the atmosphere required by campylobacters are discussed in Chapter 30.

The proper atmosphere for microaerophilic organisms requires an oxygen tension lower than that of room air. A CO_2 concentration of approximately 3% can be achieved in a **candle jar.** A small white wax candle is lit in a jar with a sealable lid, such as a commercial mayonnaise jar (Figure 6.2 in Chapter 6). The candle uses up just enough oxygen before it goes out (from lack of oxygen) to lower the oxygen tension. The products of combustion are CO_2 and water, both growth factors for the organisms. The candle jar is often used to cultivate *Neisseria gonorrhoeae*. A self-contained culture medium and increased CO_2-producing system has been developed for culturing gonococci. A tablet of sodium bicarbonate (such as Alka-Seltzer) dissolves in the moisture created by sealing the medium in a Ziploc plastic bag and produces enough CO_2 to allow growth of the pathogen (Figure 6.1). Microaerophilic conditions can also be created by adding a small concentration of agar to a liquid medium. By preventing oxygen at the surface from being dispersed throughout the liquid by inhibiting circulating convection currents, the agar serves to create a minimicroaerophilic environment about 1 to 2 cm below the surface of the medium. *Leptospira* species are cultivated in this way.

8.2.b. Methods for establishing anaerobic atmospheric conditions for incubation of primary culture plates.

8.2.b.(1). Conventional method. The most commonly used system for creating specialized anaerobic and capnophilic atmospheres is the anaerobic jar. Available anaerobic jars include the GasPak (BBL Microbiology Systems) and those made by Scott Laboratories and Oxoid U.S.A. These systems utilize a clear, heavy plastic jar with a lid that is clamped down to make it airtight (Figure 8.3).

Anaerobic jars are used primarily with plated media. The introduction of a gas mixture containing hydrogen into a jar is followed by catalytic conversion of the oxygen in the jar with hydrogen to water, thus establishing anaerobiosis. A catalyst composed of palladium-coated alumina pellets held in a wire mesh is preferred, since there is no explosion hazard with this "cold" catalyst and it is more convenient to use. However, the pellets can be inactivated by excess moisture and H_2S. Therefore, they should be reactivated *after each use* by heating the basket or sachet of pellets to 160° C in a drying oven for 1½ to 2 hours. It is convenient to have a few extra baskets or sachets of catalysts for this purpose. Reactivated catalysts should be stored in a dry area until used. We do not recommend the use of jars without catalysts.

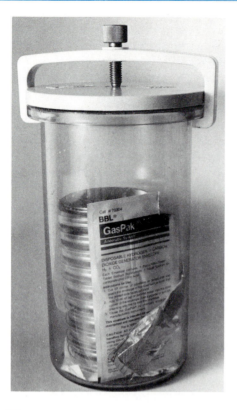

Figure 8.3
GasPak anaerobic jar (BBL Microbiology Systems) containing inoculated plates, gas-generating envelope, catalysts, and indicator strip.

Anaerobic jars can be set up by two different methods. The easiest method utilizes a commercially available hydrogen and CO_2 generator envelope, which is activated by simply adding 10 ml of water. The open envelope is placed in the jar with the inoculated plates, water is added, and the jar is sealed. Production of heat within a few minutes (detected by touching the top of the jar) and subsequent development of moisture on the walls of the jar are indications that the catalyst and generator envelope are functioning properly. Reduced conditions are achieved in 1 to 2 hours, although the methylene blue or resazurin indicators take longer to decolorize. Alternatively, the "evacuation-replacement" system may be used. Air is removed from the sealed jar by drawing a vacuum of 25 inches (62.5 cm) of mercury. This process is repeated two times, filling the jar with an oxygen-free gas such as nitrogen between evacuations. The final fill of the jar is made with a gas mixture containing 80% to 90% nitrogen,

5% to 10% hydrogen, and 5% to 10% CO_2. CO_2 is included since many anaerobes require it for maximal growth. The atmosphere in the jars should be monitored by including an indicator to check anaerobiosis. Anaerobiosis is achieved more quickly by the evacuation-replacement method. However, both methods give comparable yields of anaerobes from clinical specimens if the specimen is properly transported and set up in jars immediately after plates are streaked.

Stringent anaerobic conditions required by some organisms are attainable in an enclosed system, called a **glove box** or an anaerobic chamber. Made of molded or flexible clear plastic, these chambers allow materials to enter through an air lock. The operator uses gloves or sleeves that form airtight seals around his or her arms to handle items inside the chamber (Figure 8.4). Media stored in the chamber are kept oxygen-free and thus able to support the growth of even oxygen-sensitive anaerobic organisms. For practical purposes, most pathogenic anaerobes can tolerate a minimal exposure to oxygen. Methods that make use of fresh media and that allow inoculated cultures to be brought under anaerobic conditions quickly (oxygen-reduction potential less than -10 mV), such as the anaerobic jars or plastic pouches discussed previously, should be adequate for isolation of most clinically significant anaerobes.

8.2.b.(2). Prereduced anaerobically sterilized (PRAS) and roll-tube techniques. Media produced under anaerobic conditions are called **prereduced, anaerobically sterilized (PRAS)** media. PRAS tubes are made by combining the constituents of the medium, boiling the liquid to remove dissolved air, and then gassing-out with an oxygen-free gas. During the remainder of the media-making process (sterilization, inoculation, and subculture), air is prevented from gaining entrance into the containers by a gassing procedure or by keeping the container stoppered or sealed. To lower the oxidation-reduction potential (Eh) of the medium, a reducing agent may be added before sterilization. Details of PRAS media preparation and inoculation are given in the VPI *Anaerobe Laboratory Manual* by Holdeman et al.[1] PRAS media, both tubed and plates, are available from commercial sources (see Appendix C).

PRAS tubes can be inoculated by either the closed or the open method. In the closed method, also known as the Hungate method, a (preferably

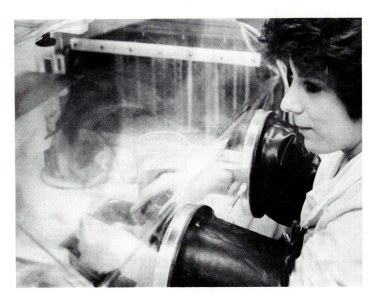

Figure 8.4
Anaerobic chamber (Anaerobe Systems). The rubber sleeves form airtight seals around the operator's
arms, allowing the operator to work without gloves.

"degassed" if working with fastidious anaerobes) syringe and needle are used to inoculate through the rubber seal. Biochemical testing for speciation may be done by this technique.

PRAS tubes can also be inoculated by the open method, which consists of removing the rubber stopper and inserting a cannula that has oxygen-free gas flowing from the tip. While the tube is open and gas flowing, inoculation can be accomplished by loop or Pasteur pipette. Special equipment can be purchased for the inoculating procedure (Bellco Glass and Kontes), or a simple inoculating device can be made using a bent needle attached to tubing and connected to a ring stand. The PRAS tube is held by an adjustable laboratory clamp containing an aluminum test tube cap within which the tube is placed. Some batches of tungsten wire may oxidize PRAS media. It is therefore advisable to use platinum wires and loops for PRAS techniques.

Organisms can be grown in or on a thin layer of PRAS agar that covers the inside walls of tubes. This is called the roll-tube technique because the tubes are rolled and cooled until the melted agar forms the thin layer referred to. Colonies are difficult to subculture and differentiate by this method, and it is our belief that roll-tube techniques are not as practical for clinical work as the other methods discussed

here. Cultivation of anaerobes will be discussed further in Chapter 34.

8.2.c. **Temperatures of incubation.** Human pathogens generally multiply best at temperatures similar to those in the host. Isolation of most pathogens, therefore, can be carried out using incubators of only two temperatures: 35° C, close to the normal internal human body temperature, and 30° C, the temperature of the surface of the body. With the few exceptions noted later, all bacteria and viruses of pathogenic importance may be isolated from cultures incubated at 35° C. Material from lesions suspected of being infected with *Mycobacterium marinum*, blood and urine being tested for leptospires, and all cultures from which fungi are being sought should be incubated at 30° C. Recovery of certain organisms can be enhanced by incubation at unusual temperatures; *Campylobacter jejuni* grows at 42° C, although most other fecal pathogens cannot. Incubation at this temperature, therefore, acts as an enrichment procedure. Certain viruses, such as respiratory syncytial virus, multiply best in tubes incubated in roller drums at 33° to 36° C. Cold enrichment for *Listeria* and *Yersinia enterocolitica* utilizes the same principle.

The temperature of incubators should be monitored by checking each area of the incubator where cultures will be placed, since temperature variations do occur within incubators. The humidity can be controlled automatically by feeding water from an external source into the system as needed, or manually by placing a large pan filled with water on the bottom shelf of the incubator. A little detergent in the water will discourage contaminants.

8.2.d. pH of artificial media. Although commercially produced dehydrated powders are so consistent that even the ultimate pH is usually correct, the hydrogen ion concentration should be checked using a pH meter. Especially after altering the pH of a medium with additives or for special uses, the pH should be reestablished. It is important to remember that pH electrodes are calibrated according to temperature; thus the pH reading of a hot solution will be different than that taken at room temperature. If the calibration temperature for the electrode cannot be adjusted, the pH must be measured at approximately 28° C, or room temperature. Solid media pose an additional problem, since the pH is best adjusted while the media are still in liquid form and thus hotter than 50° C. A surface electrode may be used to measure the pH of agar, but these electrodes are very expensive and the agar must be set, which makes it difficult to alter the pH later if needed. A workable strategy is to allow a small quantity of the molten agar to solidify in a tiny beaker or plastic cup. The pH of this material can be easily determined with a regular pH electrode thrust into the agar after it has been vigorously broken up with a tongue depressor. The moisture in the medium will be enough to allow proper operation of the pH meter.

8.3. Characteristics of Certain Commonly Used Artificial Media

Only a few of the hundreds of available media will be mentioned here, as a sample of the types of media available. The choices of which media should be used to culture clinical specimens will be discussed in the chapters in Part Three that detail laboratory handling of specimens and in chapters in Part Four that deal with individual isolates. Complete descriptions of the composition and use of these and other media are found in the *Difco Manual* (Difco Laboratories), the *Scott Manual* (Scott Laboratories), the *Oxoid Manual* (Oxoid U.S.A.), and the *BBL Manual* (Becton-Dickinson).

8.3.a. *Bacteroides* bile esculin agar (BBE). BBE agar is useful for the rapid isolation and presumptive identification of the *Bacteroides fragilis* group. It contains 100 μg/ml of gentamicin, which inhibits most aerobic organisms; 20% bile, which inhibits most anaerobes except for the *B. fragilis* group and a few other species; and esculin, which aids in detecting the *B. fragilis* group which are usually esculin positive. Other non–*B. fragilis* group organisms that may rarely grow on this medium are *Fusobacterium mortiferum*, *Klebsiella pneumoniae*, *Enterococcus*, and yeast. However, unlike the *B. fragilis* group, their colony size is less than 1 mm in diameter.

8.3.b. Blood agar. Most specimens received in a clinical microbiology laboratory are plated onto blood agar, since it supports all but the most fastidious clinically significant isolates and since most microbiologists have become adept at making decisions about the identification of bacteria from their colonial morphologies on blood agar. These media consist of a base containing a protein source, such as tryptones, soybean protein digest (containing a slight amount of natural carbohydrate), sodium chloride, agar, and 5% blood. In the United States, the blood source is usually sheep, whereas horse blood is often used in Europe. Certain bacteria produce extracellular enzymes that act on the red cells to lyse them completely (beta hemolysis) or to produce a greenish discoloration around the colony (alpha or incomplete hemolysis), while others have no effect (sometimes called gamma hemolysis); this is determined on blood agar (Figure 8.5). Production of hemolysins by bacteria is dependent on many environmental factors, such as pH and atmosphere of incubation. Microbiologists often use colony morphology and hemolysin production as initial screening tests to assist in the decision as to what further steps may be necessary for identification of an isolate. To accurately read the hemolytic reaction on a blood agar plate, the technologist must hold the plate up to the light and observe the plate with the light coming from behind. If the loop used to streak the culture on the blood agar has been stabbed into the medium to cause organisms to grow below the surface, production of oxygen-sensitive beta hemolysin may be enhanced with certain organisms. Alternatively, plates may be incubated anaerobically to demonstrate oxygen-sensitive hemolysis.

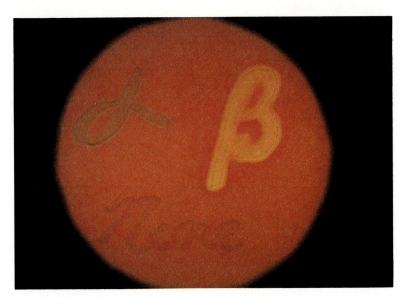

Figure 8.5
Sheep blood agar plate exhibiting all three types of hemolysis.

8.3.c. Brain-heart infusion media. Another nutritionally rich formula, brain heart infusion (BHI), can be used to grow a variety of microorganisms, either as a broth or hardened with agar, with or without added blood. Key ingredients include infusion from several animal tissue sources, added peptone, phosphate buffer, and a small concentration of dextrose. The carbohydrate provides a readily accessible source of energy for the organisms. Brain heart infusion broths are often used as blood culture media and as basal media for many metabolic tests, particularly for identification of streptococci. The usual base for blood agar plates is heart infusion agar, but BHI, trypticase soy agar, or *Brucella* agar is preferred by many workers.

Brain heart infusion agar with 5% to 10% sheep blood and the antimicrobial agents chloramphenicol (16 µg/ml) and gentamicin (5 µg/ml) will inhibit the growth of bacteria while allowing the growth of even the most fastidious dimorphic fungi. This agar should be used as a primary plating medium for the growth of fungi, since it has been shown to yield better recovery than the previously recommended Sabouraud dextrose.

8.3.d. Chocolate agar. This medium uses the same base as blood agar. Originally, red blood was added to the molten base and the temperature raised enough to partially lyse the red blood cells (around 85° C), causing the medium to turn a chocolate-brown color. Now, hemoglobin and the other nutrients present in the lysed red cells, hemin (also known as "X" factor), and the coenzyme nicotine adenine dinucleotide (called "V" factor) are added as supplements to a nutritionally rich agar base. *Neisseria gonorrhoeae* and *Haemophilus* species, among other fastidious organisms, will grow best in the presence of the nutrients supplied by chocolate agar.

8.3.e. Chopped meat broth. With or without added glucose, this medium is used to enrich and preserve the growth of anaerobic organisms. The pieces of meat provide substrates for proteolytic enzymes, serve as reducing substances to maintain the low oxidation-reduction potential, and somehow prevent rapidly growing bacteria from overgrowing slower forms. A mineral oil or vaspar overlay on a chopped meat culture of an anaerobic bacterium will allow many anaerobes to remain viable at room temperature for several months. Chopped meat need not be incubated anaerobically to support the growth of anaerobes.

8.3.f. Columbia CNA agar with blood. Columbia agar base is a nutritionally rich formula containing three peptone sources. Five percent defibrinated blood provides more nutrients and the capability of displaying hemolytic reactions. The antibacterial agents colistin (10 μg/ml) and nalidixic acid (15 μg/ml) completely suppress the growth of Enterobacteriaceae and *Pseudomonas* species while allowing staphylococci, streptococci, and enterococci to grow. Certain gram-negative organisms such as *Gardnerella vaginalis* and some *Bacteroides* species can grow very well on Columbia CNA agar with blood.

8.3.g. GN broth. Used as a selective broth for the cultivation of salmonella and shigella from stool specimens and rectal swabs, GN (which stands for gram negative) broth contains several active ingredients. Sodium citrate and sodium desoxycholate (a bile salt) destroy gram-positive organisms and inhibit the early multiplication of coliforms. The addition of more mannitol than dextrose serves to encourage the growth of mannitol-fermenting pathogens and discourage the growth of *Proteus* species. The medium is buffered to remain at neutral pH, even after production of acid metabolites by bacterial growth. To obtain the optimal benefit of the selective nature of GN broth, it should be subcultured 6 to 8 hours after initial inoculation and incubation. After this time, the coliforms begin to overgrow the pathogens.

8.3.h. Hektoen enteric agar. This medium is included as an example of a selective, differential agar that is not autoclave sterilized. The concentrations of bile salts and the dyes bromthymol blue and acid fuchsin are high enough to inhibit the growth of most normal fecal flora, while inhibiting the growth of *Salmonella* and *Shigella* species only slightly. Because so few organisms can grow on the medium, it is unnecessary to sterilize it prior to dispensing plates. Lactose fermenting organisms, by lowering the pH of the medium in the area of colonies, turn the colonies yellow. The addition of ferric ammonium citrate, a source of iron common to many media formulas, allows the production of H_2S from sodium thiosulfate to be visualized by formation of a black precipitate around colonies.

8.3.i. Kanamycin-vancomycin laked rabbit blood agar (KVLB). KVLB agar is useful for the selective isolation of *Bacteroides* sp. The medium contains 75 μg/ml kanamycin, which inhibits most aerobic, facultative, and anaerobic gram-negative rods except for *Bacteroides*, and 7.5 μg/ml vancomycin, which inhibits most gram-positive organisms. The laked blood allows earlier pigmentation of the pigmented anaerobic gram-negative rods. However, many strains of *B. asaccharolyticus* and *B. gingivalis* will

not grow on this medium because of their susceptibility to vancomycin. Yeast and other kanamycin-resistant organisms sometimes grow on this medium; therefore, one should Gram stain and check the aerotolerance of all isolates.

8.3.j. Löwenstein-Jensen agar. This medium was developed as a selective enrichment agar for mycobacteria. Malachite green dye inhibits the growth of contaminants that are able to survive the initial specimen processing. Löwenstein-based media are the only commonly used formulas that require the addition of homogenized eggs, which necessitates sterilization by inspissation. The utilization of egg protein by some mycobacteria results in production of niacin, an important differentiating characteristic. Many modifications of the basic medium are used, including those of Gruft (added antibiotics and ribonucleic acid growth factor) and Wallenstein (added glycerol).

8.3.k. MacConkey agar. The most commonly used primary selective and differential agar, MacConkey agar, contains crystal violet dye to inhibit the growth of gram-positive cocci and the pH indicator neutral red to impart differential characteristics. Gram-negative bacilli grow readily; lactose fermenters produce acid products of metabolism that cause the pH of the medium close to the colony to fall. The neutral red then turns red at the acid pH (Figure 8.6). Nonlactose fermenters remain colorless and translucent. MacConkey is the most supportive of the selective and differential media used for isolation of *Shigella* species.

8.3.l. Middlebrook agars and broths. These media, made of more defined components than egg base media, are also used for cultivation of mycobacteria. The malachite green and low pH serve to inhibit contaminants and the clear nature of the agar allows technologists to observe colony morphology easily. Middlebrook formulas are also used for antimicrobial susceptibility testing of mycobacteria, since the antimicrobial agents would be damaged by the repeated heating used to prepare inspissated egg base media. The enrichment supplements of oleic acid, albumin, dextrose, and catalase must be added to support the growth of most mycobacteria.

8.3.m. Phenylethyl alcohol agar. By adding phenylethyl alcohol to a peptone and beef extract base, an agar is created that inhibits the growth of gram-negative bacteria. Five percent sheep blood provides nutrients for streptococci and staphylococci.

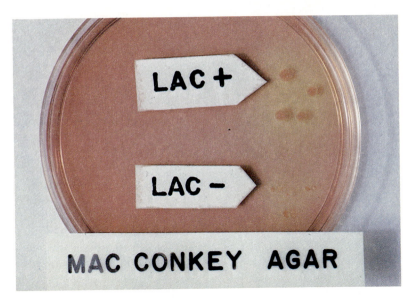

Figure 8.6
Appearance of lactose-fermenting and nonlactose-fermenting colonies on MacConkey agar.

This medium is also used to cultivate anaerobic gram-negative organisms, which are not inhibited by the alcohol. After preparation, phenylethyl alcohol plates smell like roses.

8.3.n. **PPLO agar.** An enrichment medium for mycoplasma (formerly called **pleuropneumonia-like organisms, PPLO**), this formula contains slightly less agar than most bacteriological media and is prepared at a slightly higher pH. Beef heart infusion, peptones, and the added nutrients of serum or ascitic fluid allow the mycoplasma to grow as small colonies with dense centers. Agents such as penicillin and crystal violet can be added to inhibit contaminants.

8.3.o. **Sabouraud dextrose agar.** Developed for the cultivation of pathogenic fungi, particularly the agents of superficial mycoses, this medium contains peptones, dextrose, and agar. It is recommended only for primary isolation of dermatophytes at this time, with the addition of the antimicrobial agents cycloheximide (0.5 µg/ml) and chloramphenicol (16 µg/ml). Subcultures of fungi originally isolated on BHI may exhibit more standard morphology on Sabouraud dextrose; thus it is still useful for identification of molds once they have been isolated. The final pH, around 5.6, is much lower than that of most media and tends to inhibit the growth of bacteria.

8.3.p. **Streptococcal selective agar.** Recently improved, streptococcal selective agar (SSA) is available commercially. A modification of sheep blood agar, this medium contains crystal violet, trimethoprim-sulfamethoxazole, and colistin in concentrations adequate to inhibit most streptococci except for *Streptococcus pyogenes* and *S. agalactiae*. Beta hemolysis is readily observed. The medium is effective for primary plating of throat swabs for detection of group A streptococci.

8.3.q. **Thayer-Martin agar.** Chocolate agar has been modified to be selective for pathogenic Neisseria by the addition of antibiotics, including colistin (to inhibit other gram-negative bacteria), vancomycin (to inhibit gram-positive bacteria), and nystatin or anisomycin (to inhibit yeast). The most widely used formula is that of Thayer and Martin. Thayer-Martin agar incorporates nystatin to inhibit yeasts. Modified Thayer-Martin (MTM) includes trimethoprim to inhibit *Proteus*. While several modifications are available, the most common is Martin-Lewis agar, which substitutes anisomycin (characterized by a longer shelf life and greater activity against yeast) for nystatin.

8.3.r. **Thioglycollate broth.** The most commonly used enrichment broth in clinical microbiology, thioglycollate, uses 0.075% agar to prevent convection currents from carrying atmospheric oxygen throughout the broth. Thioglycolic acid also acts as a reducing agent, lowering the oxidation-reduction potential of the medium. With the addition of many

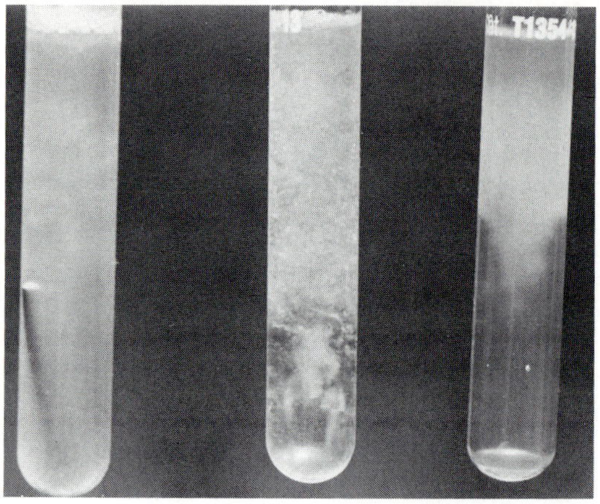

Figure 8.7
Growth of gram-negative bacilli (left tube), gram-positive cocci (center tube), and yeast (right tube) in thioglycollate broth.

nutrient factors, such as casein, yeast and beef extracts, vitamins, and others, this medium enhances the growth of most pathogenic bacteria. Other nutrient supplements, an oxidation-reduction indicator (resazurin), dextrose, vitamin K_1, and hemin, have been added in various modified formulas. Technologists can visualize the difference between the diffuse, even growth of gram-negative, facultative bacilli and the discrete, puffball-type growth of gram-positive cocci. Strict aerobes, such as pseudomonads and yeast, tend to grow in a thin layer on the surface of the broth (Figure 8.7). For cultivation of anaerobes, thioglycollate supplemented with hemin (5 μg/ml), vitamin K_1 (0.1 μg/ml), and sodium bicarbonate (1 mg/ml) is best.

8.3.s. *Trichomonas* **medium.** Developed for isolation of human protozoa, this medium contains antibiotics such as chloramphenicol to inhibit growth of contaminating bacteria. The pH, around 6.0, favors the growth of trichomonads. Nutrients are provided by peptones, maltose, and cysteine.

8.3.t. **Xylose-lysine-desoxycholate agar.** Like Hektoen agar, xylose-lysine-desoxycholate (XLD) agar is selective for *Shigella* and *Salmonella* and is not autoclave sterilized. The salts inhibit many Enterobacteriaceae and gram-positive organisms. The phenol red indicator accounts for the differentiation of nonlactose-fermenters *(Shigella* and *Salmonella)* as colorless (pale pink) colonies. Ferric ammonium citrate allows the visualization of H_2S producing organisms as colonies with black centers. Organisms

that ferment the carbohydrates in the medium (xylose, lactose, and sucrose) produce yellow colonies.

•   •   •

There are many other media available that can be used to cultivate pathogens. We have mentioned examples of supportive, enrichment, selective, and differential media. Our basic recommendations for handling specimens are covered in Part Three. However, for an individual laboratory, the ultimate choice of which primary and secondary media to use for inoculating clinical specimens will depend on the patient population served by the laboratory, the extent of services offered by the laboratory, and the cost-benefit ratio of each additional medium. The laboratory director often needs to make difficult decisions concerning limiting the numbers of media used to obtain the most generally beneficial results. Some of these issues are addressed in Chapter 4.

8.4. Using Streak Plates to Isolate and Enumerate Growth of Pathogens

Inocula are usually spread over the surface of agar plates in a standard pattern, so that the quantity of bacterial growth can be determined, either semi-quantitatively or relatively. A useful streaking pattern is illustrated in Figure 8.8. The relative numbers of organisms in the original specimen can be estimated based on the extent of growth of colonies past the original area of inoculation. For some viscous specimens, such as sputum, and for some highly selective media, such as stool agars, better isolation of all colony types can be achieved if the technologist returns the loop to the original inoculum area on the plate several times during the initial streaking pattern. We have found that flaming the loop between streaking areas is not necessary for most specimens, although turning the loop to access a previously unused edge will enhance isolation. It may be beneficial, however, to flame the inoculating loop between streaking areas when the original inoculum is material from an already growing bacterial colony.

Streaking plates with a measured amount of inoculum, such as that found in a standard calibrated loop (used to quantify colony-forming units [CFU] in fluid specimens like urine), should be done to facilitate counting colonies. For this purpose, the inoculum should be spread out more evenly over the entire plate (Figure 8.9).

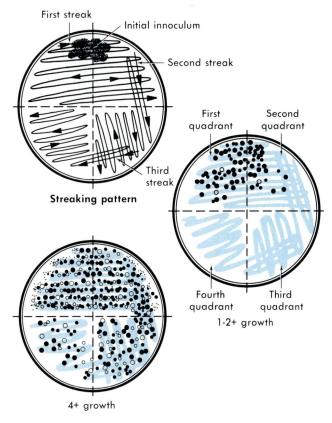

Figure 8.8

Streaking pattern for primary inoculation of plates to achieve isolated colonies. Growth in the initial half of the plate only is semiquantitated as $1+$ or $2+$ (sparse); growth into the third quadrant is reported as $3+$ (moderate); and growth into the fourth quadrant is reported as $4+$ (heavy). If numbers of colonies can be counted, this number should be reported.

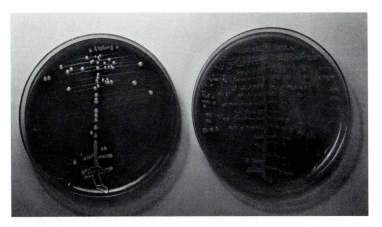

Figure 8.9

Inoculation of plates streaked with a calibrated loop.

8.5. Quality Control of Microbiological Primary Culture Media

Until recently, laboratories were required by regulatory agencies to perform in-house quality control tests on all media prepared or purchased by the laboratory. Such tests were designed to verify that the media were sterile and that they performed as expected. The time and expense of in-house testing placed a strain on already overworked microbiologists and its value, particularly for commercial media, was questioned by a number of critics of the system. The National Committee for Clinical Laboratory Standards studied the issue and subsequently developed recommendations for abbreviated quality control testing procedures for commercially prepared media that would be more relevant.[2] When manufacturers follow the testing methods recommended, the performance of their media has been shown to be adequate and consistent. This standard has since been accepted by most state and national regulatory agencies, including the College of American Pathologists and the Joint Commission on Hospital Accreditation.

In addition to listing those purchased media that microbiologists need not test in-house (see box), the NCCLS guidelines include methods for testing the performance of media that are applicable to all primary growth media that require testing, either by the manufacturer or within the laboratory (Procedure 8.1). For quality control organisms and expected results used for commercially prepared media, the reader is referred to the NCCLS publication M22-T. Organisms and results expected for several of the major purchased media that must still be tested within each laboratory are listed in Table 8.2. Guidelines did not include commercial identification kit media, susceptibility testing media, or media used for isolation of parasites, viruses, chlamydiae, or mycoplasmas. Throughout this text, quality control suggestions will accompany procedures presented. Of course, all media prepared in the laboratory must be fully tested before placing into use. In the absence of standardized guidelines, testing should be performed with clones of stock strains of organisms for which the medium is intended to show expected characteristics, both positive and negative. Quality control organisms are available commercially (see Appendix C).

Commercially Prepared Media for Which User Laboratories Need Not Perform Quality Control Checks*

Nonselective blood agars
Selective blood agars: Columbia CNA agar, phenylethyl alcohol agar
Chocolate agar (This medium has a relatively high failure rate in the NCCLS analysis: users may want to monitor it when it is used for primary isolation.)
MacConkey agar
Eosin methylene blue agars: Levine EMB agar, EMB agar, modified
Media for *Salmonella/Shigella:* Hektoen enteric agar, XLD agar, S-S agar
Mannitol salt agar
Selective media for group D *Streptococci*
Sabouraud dextrose agar
Selective mycology agars
Media for mycobacteria: L-J medium, Middlebrook media
Anaerobic blood agars
Anaerobic broth: thioglycollate media
Enrichment broth for enterics: GN broth, Selenite broth
Media for blood cultures: BHI, Thiol, TSB

*For sterility, growth, selectivity, enrichment, or biochemical response if the manufacturer follows NCCLS guidelines for quality control.
From NCCLS. 1987. Quality assurance for commercially prepared microbiological culture media; Tentative standard. NCCLS, Villanova, PA.

8.6. Cell Cultures for Cultivation of Pathogens

Although fungi and most bacteria grow readily on artificial media, certain pathogens require factors provided only by living cells. Often these organisms are obligate intracellular parasites, but occasionally they are not, although scientists have been unable to isolate the critical growth factors needed to support growth on wholly artificial media. An example of a pathogen of the latter type is *Legionella pneumophila*, which was isolated in chicken embryo culture before the necessary growth factors were dis-

PROCEDURE 8.1

Quality Control Testing for Primary Culture Media

Principle

Certain media, particularly those with blood product additives, must be monitored for sterility, support of growth of desired microorganisms, and performance characteristics within the expected parameters of the media. Organisms of known growth characteristics can be used to verify media performance standards.

Method

1. User must inspect plate media for cracks in the agar or in the plastic Petri dish, unequal filling of plates, hemolysis of blood additives, the mushy appearance that signifies that the plates had been frozen during transport, excessive bubbles, and contamination.
2. User should incubate selected plates before use to ensure that they are sterile.
3. User should test the growth supportive characteristics by inoculating the appropriate quality control organism(s) as follows:
   a. Prepare a fresh subculture of the test organism(s). Organisms can be stored frozen at −70° C in soybean casein digest broth with a final concentration of 10% glycerol, frozen in skim milk or purchased lyophilized (Appendix C). After incubation sufficient to produce isolated colonies, the organism can be used for testing.
   b. Prepare a suspension of several colonies in sterile saline to match a McFarland 0.5 turbidity standard (Procedure 13.1), approximately 5×10^8 colony forming units (CFU) per milliliter. This is the stock suspension.
   c. Dilute this suspension 1:100 in sterile saline and inoculate each plate to be tested with 0.01 ml (use a 10-µL calibrated loop) of the diluted suspension. Spread the inoculum evenly on the plate so that colonies can be counted.
4. User should test the inhibitory characteristics of a selective medium as follows:
   a. Dilute the stock suspension 1:10 in sterile saline and inoculate each plate to be tested with 0.01 ml of the diluted suspension as above.
5. User should test tubed media by inoculating 0.01 ml of the stock suspension into the tube.
6. Incubate all media under the conditions required for normal use.

Expected results

Media are within acceptable limits if they are sterile, if test organisms grow well and display typical colony morphology and if appropriate test organisms are inhibited. Tubed media should display proper positive and negative reactions with appropriate test microorganisms.

Performance schedule

Media prepared in-house should be tested with each batch. Purchased media should be tested with each lot number and with each shipment received at a separate time.

---

covered and incorporated into artificial media by scientists at the Centers for Disease Control in Atlanta. All viruses and chlamydiae are obligate intracellular parasites, growing outside of the host only in tissue cultures or cell cultures. These media are made up of layers of living cells growing on the surface of a solid matrix such as the inside of a glass tube or the bottom of a plastic flask (Figure 8.10). Pathogenic viruses are cultivated in clinical microbiology laboratories on cell cultures of two types, **primary cell lines** and **continuous cell lines.** Primary cell lines are produced by cutting up fresh tissue, often kidney, into tiny pieces. When treated with the proteolytic agent trypsin, the tissue pieces break up into indi-

Table 8.2

Abbreviated List of Quality Control Procedures for Media that Require In-house Testing

MEDIUM	CONTROL ORGANISM (SUGGESTED ATCC NO.)*	EXPECTED RESULTS
Campylobacter agar	*Campylobacter jejuni* (33290)	Growth
	Escherichia coli (25922)	Inhibition (partial)
Agar for isolation of pathogenic *Neisseria* (not modified Thayer-Martin)	*Neisseria gonorrhoeae* (43070)	Growth
	Neisseria meningitidis (13090)	Growth
	Neisseria sicca (9913)	Inhibition (complete)
	Candida albicans (60193)	Inhibition (partial)
	Proteus mirabilis (43071)	Inhibition (partial)
	Staphylococcus epidermidis (12228)	Inhibition (partial)
Rabbit or horse blood agar	*Haemophilus influenzae* (10211)	Growth, no hemolysis
	Haemophilus haemolyticus (33390)	Growth, beta hemolysis
Bordet-Gengou agar	*Bordetella pertussis* (9340)	Growth
Charcoal yeast and buffered charcoal yeast extract agar	*Legionella pneumophila* (33152)	Growth
Thiosulfate–citrate–bile salts–sucrose agar	*Vibrio parahaemolyticus* (17802)	Blue-green colonies
	Vibrio alginolyticus (17749)	Yellow colonies
	E. coli (25922)	Inhibition
Cycloserine–cefoxitin–fructose agar	*Clostridium difficile* (9689)	Yellow colonies
	E. coli (25922)	Inhibition
KVLB agar (anaerobic)	*Bacteroides intermedius* (25261)	Brown colonies
	Bacteroides fragilis (25285)	Growth
	E. coli (25922)	Inhibition

*American Type Culture Collection available from ATCC, Rockville, Md.

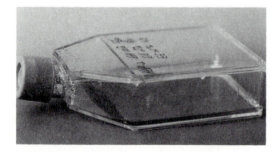

Figure 8.10
Tissue culture flask used for maintaining cell lines.

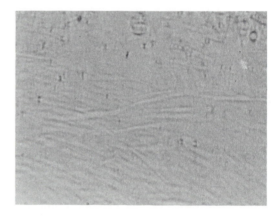

Figure 8.11
Monolayer of uninoculated human fibroblasts, visualized at 400×.

vidual cells, which are seeded into a flask or tube containing growth-supportive media (formulas are given in Appendix A). The cells attach to the inside bottom of the container and multiply until they reach a single layer, a **monolayer,** of confluent growth. Normal cells are inhibited from growing on top of each other. Fibroblast cells, such as human foreskin primary cell line, are spindle shaped (Figure 8.11). Cells from other tissue sources, such as kidney cells, may be shaped more irregularly, like polygons (Fig-

ure 8.12). Primary cell lines usually carry the same number of chromosomes as the natural cells from which they were derived, the diploid number of normal somatic cells, and they will multiply for approximately only 50 generations before they begin to die off. If cells are obtained from a malignant tissue

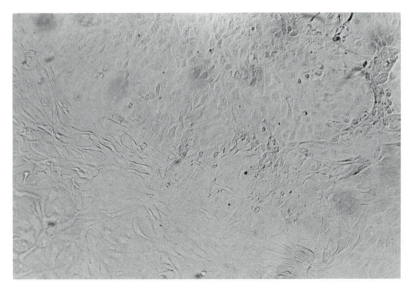

Figure 8.12
Monolayer of African green monkey kidney cells, visualized at 400×.

source, such as a human epithelial cell cancer, they will multiply indefinitely in cell culture and they often contain aberrations in the number of chromosomes they possess (aneuploid). Such cell cultures are called continuous cell lines.

In addition to their use for cultivation of viruses, tissue cultures may be used for other purposes in clinical microbiology. Several cell lines, including Hep-2, HeLa, and Vero, have been used for detection of the cytotoxin of *Clostridium difficile*. Chlamydiae are cultivated on a special cell line, McCoy cells, the monolayer of which is treated with cycloheximide to prevent multiplication before the specimen is inoculated. Maintenance and inoculation of the tissue culture lines used for routine clinical virology are reviewed in Chapter 42.

REFERENCES

1. Holdeman, L.V., Cato, E.P., and Moore, W.E.C. 1977. Anaerobe laboratory manual, ed. 4. Anaerobe Laboratory, Virginia Polytechnic Institute and State University, Blacksburg, Va.
2. National Committee for Clinical Laboratory Standards. 1987. Quality assurance standards for commercially prepared microbiological culture media, Tentative Standard M22-T. Order No. M22-T, available from NCCLS, Villanova, PA 19085. (Enclose check for $20 with your order, plus $5 for overseas postage.)

BIBLIOGRAPHY

Difco manual, ed. 10. 1984. Difco Laboratories, Detroit.
Emmons, C.W., Binford, C.H., Utz, J.P., and Kwon-Chung, K.J. 1977. Medical mycology, ed. 3. Lea & Febiger, Philadelphia.
Estevez, E.G. 1984. Bacteriologic plate media: review of mechanisms of action. Lab. Med. 15:258.
Isenberg, H.D., Washington, J.A. II., Balows, A., and Sonnenwirth, A.C. 1985. Collection, handling, and processing of specimens. In Lennette, E.H., Balows, A., Hausler, W.J. Jr., and Shadomy, H.J., editors. Manual of clinical microbiology, ed. 4. American Society for Microbiology, Washington, D.C.
Joklik, W.K. 1980. The nature, isolation, and measurement of animal viruses. In Joklik, W.K., Wilda, H.P., and Amos, D.B., editors. Zinsser's microbiology, ed. 17. Appleton-Century-Crofts, Norwalk, Conn.
MacFaddin, J.F. 1985. Media for isolation-cultivation-identification-maintenance of medical bacteria, vol 1. Williams & Wilkins, Baltimore.
Oxoid manual, ed. 5. 1982. Oxoid Ltd., Basingstoke, U.K.
Phillips, E., and Nash, P. 1985. Culture media. In Lennette, E.H., Balows, A., Hausler, W.J. Jr., and Shadomy, H.J., editors. Manual of clinical microbiology, ed. 4. American Society for Microbiology, Washington, D.C.
Sutter, V.L., Citron, D.M., Edelstein, M.A.C., and Finegold, S.M. 1985. Wadsworth anaerobic bacteriology manual, ed. 4. Star Publishing Co., Belmont, Calif.
Washington, J.A. II. 1985. Laboratory procedures in clinical microbiology, ed. 2. Springer-Verlag, New York.

9

Conventional and Rapid Microbiological Methods for Identification of Bacteria and Fungi

Cultivation and identification of specific pathogens from material collected from patients suspected of having infection is still the most reliable diagnostic tool, even though it is not the fastest. In some cases (such as with *Rickettsia* species) recovery of the infecting organisms is difficult or impossible (as with *Treponema pallidum*). In those cases, reliance must be placed on serologic or other methods for diagnosis. However, until molecular biological techniques have advanced to the point that the microorganisms contributing to infectious diseases can be pinpointed by totally individual genetic markers, definitive diagnosis of most infections continues to require isolation of an etiologic agent. Chapter 8 discussed various growth media and strategies for encouraging the growth of cultivatable microorganisms. This chapter will discuss basic morphological clues and enzymatic and biochemical tests that are used to identify such pathogens once they have been isolated. In addition, we will mention some of the rapid methods and basic concepts of the commercial systems that are currently available for performing biochemical and enzymatic tests. Certain of the biochemical tests used to identify bacteria are also used for identification of some fungi.

Identification of viruses does not depend primarily on biochemical or enzymatic means. Virus identification relies more heavily on the visual detection of specific damage inflicted on tissue culture cells by invasion and proliferation of viruses. Immunological assays for viral antigens in tissue or tissue culture are also used. Fungi and eukaryotic parasites are identified primarily by visualizing characteristic morphological features of the parasites themselves. Techniques for identification of these agents will be discussed in Chapters 42 to 44. In addition, there are many new methods based on antigenic detection and molecular manipulations that are not covered in this chapter, several of which are discussed in Chapter 10.

9.1. Basic Approaches to Identification of Pathogens

General strategies for determining the category of pathogen isolated and for deciding which further tests are needed for identification will be discussed in this section.

9.1.a. Preliminary identification of colonies growing on solid media. Since most clinical specimens are inoculated onto and into several media, including some selective or differential agars (Chapter 8), the first clue to identification of an isolated colony is the nature of the medium on which the organism is growing. For example, with rare exceptions such as enterococci, only gram-negative bacteria grow well on MacConkey agar or other selective or differential agars for gram-negative bacteria. Plates that contain substances inhibitory to gram-negative bacteria, such as Columbia agar with colistin and nalidixic acid, support growth of gram-positive organisms. Most bacteria and fungi will proliferate on nutrient or supplemented media, such as 5% sheep blood agar, chocolate agar, and brain heart infusion agar.

Moldlike fungi, of course, produce fuzzy or fluffy growth due to their aerial hyphae. If a fuzzy colony is noted on agar plates (Figure 9.1), the plate should be placed into a biological safety cabinet before the plate is opened for further examination. All bacterial colonies should be subcultured to other media. The fungus can then be studied by methods outlined in Chapter 43. Before the plate is removed from the

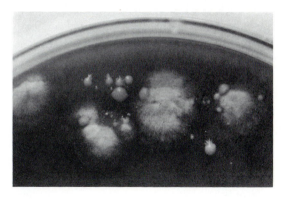

Figure 9.1
A moldlike fungus is growing among the bacterial colonies on this primary blood agar plate inoculated with sputum. The plate must be examined in a biohazard hood to avoid dissemination of the fungus.

cabinet, it should be sealed on two sides with tape to prevent dissemination of spores. Such precautions decrease the chances of laboratory acquisition of systemic fungal infection and prevent contamination of other media during subsequent plate handling or incubation.

It is unwise to place total confidence on colonial morphology for preliminary identification of isolates on primary media, since a microorganism may produce a colony that is not different from colonies of many other species. Yeast colonies often resemble those of staphylococci, for example. Unless colony morphology is distinctive (such as that of typical *Pseudomonas aeruginosa*) or growth appears on selective media, the cellular morphology of the microorganism must be determined. Even colonies on selective media usually require some additional verification (for example, some *Escherichia coli* colonies are indistinguishable from those of *Shigella* species on Hektoen agar). Examination of a wet preparation of bacterial colonies under oil immersion ($1,000\times$) magnification, with or without phase microscopy, can rapidly provide many clues as to possible identity. For example, a wet preparation prepared from a translucent, alpha hemolytic colony on blood agar may yield cocci in chains, a strong indication that the bacteria are probably streptococci; or long, thin, uniform, chaining rods, suspicious for lactobacilli. Motility can often be detected by this initial examination; the presence of yeast cells, mimicking bacterial colonies, can also be discovered.

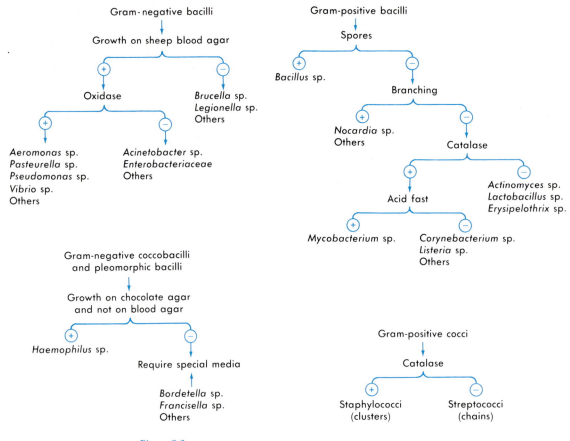

Figure 9.2
Flow chart illustrating basic identification parameters for bacteria.

9.1.b. Gram stain morphology for initial identification of bacteria: classical and nontraditional methods. The microbiologist should perform a Gram stain of material from isolated colonies to gain the most valuable cellular morphological information. Most bacteria can be divided into four distinct groups: gram-positive cocci, gram-negative cocci, gram-positive bacilli, and gram-negative bacilli. Some species are morphologically indistinct and are described by combining the preceding terms, such as "gram-negative coccobacilli" or "gram-variable bacilli." Other morphological shapes encountered include curved rods and spirals. Identification procedures are based on the cellular morphology of bacteria. Once this basic information is known, definitive identification can proceed (Figure 9.2). Gram stain results are not always indicative of the cell wall structure of the organism. For example, certain gram-positive bacteria (and fungi) lose some of their cell wall integrity with age or under adverse conditions (such as exposure to antimicrobial agents) and appear to stain gram-negative. Many *Bacillus* and *Clostridium* species appear gram-negative on stains, resulting in incorrect additional tests for speciation (and much confusion). To try to capture the proper stain reaction of an organism suspected of being gram-positive, it may be useful to stain a very young broth subculture. If this fails, there are at least two nonstain systems available to aid in determination of true Gram stain reaction. The reagent L-alanine-4-nitroanilide (LANA) has been shown by Carlone et al.[2] to differentiate Gram reactivity of aerobic and facultatively anaerobic organisms. This reagent is commercially available (see Rapid Tests in Appendix C) impregnated in cotton swabs, which turn yellow when touched to the colony of a gram-negative bacterium. The potassium hydroxide (KOH) test has also been used successfully for problem organisms.[4] A

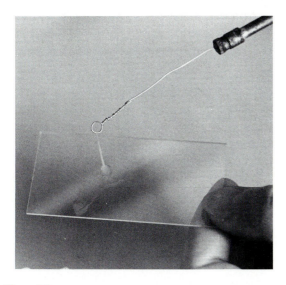

Figure 9.3
The KOH test. Addition of 3% KOH to a gram-negative bacillus causes release of viscous nuclear material.

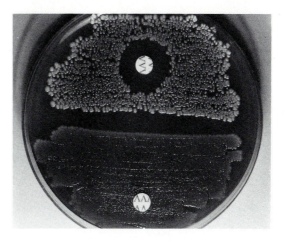

Figure 9.4
Susceptibility to vancomycin (impregnated in a filter paper disk) can differentiate gram-positive bacilli (upper half of plate) from gram-negative bacilli (no zone of inhibition, lower half of plate).

loop of growth from a colony of the organism is emulsified on the surface of a glass slide in a suspension of 3% KOH. The suspension is stirred continuously for 60 seconds, after which the loop is gently pulled from the suspension. Gram-negative cell walls are broken down, releasing viscid chromosomal material, which causes the suspension to become thick and stringy (Figure 9.3). Although useful, neither of these tests is foolproof, as reviewed by von Graevenitz and Bucher.[7] Many gram-positive bacteria (with a few exceptions, such as certain lactobacilli) are susceptible to vancomycin, an antimicrobial agent that acts on the gram-positive cell wall. Inhibition of growth by vancomycin at concentrations as low as 3 μg/ml can often presumptively identify a gram-negative-staining organism as gram-positive. Certain gram-negative organisms, notably *Moraxella* and *Acinetobacter* species, may be vancomycin susceptible. The vancomycin screening test can be easily performed by heavily inoculating the organism onto a portion of the surface of a sheep blood agar plate and placing a 5-μg vancomycin disk (available from Anaerobe Systems, Scott Laboratories, and other disk manufacturers, commonly used for assisting in Gram reaction determination with anaerobic bacteria) on the inoculated agar surface. Any zone of inhibition after overnight incubation is usually indicative of a gram-positive bacterium (Figure 9.4). Conversely, with a few exceptions, most truly

gram-negative organisms are resistant to vancomycin and susceptible to colistin or polymyxin at 10 μg/ml.

9.2. Extremely Rapid Biochemical or Enzymatic Tests That Can Be Performed on Single Colonies Growing on Primary Media

All of the tests described here can be performed directly with colonies seen on primary isolation plates. They all can produce positive reactions in less than an hour and most of them take only a minute or two, although incubation for up to 4 hours may be required. Such tests can help the technologist place an isolate of known morphology into a further subdivision, thus directing the additional procedures needed for identification (Figure 9.2) and providing valuable tentative or preliminary identification in cases of serious infection. In addition to those tests mentioned here, there are others in use in laboratories around the world; still others are constantly being developed.

    9.2.a. Catalase test. The enzyme catalase catalyzes the liberation of water and oxygen from hydrogen peroxide, a metabolic end product toxic to bacteria. All members of the staphylococci are catalase-positive, whereas members of the genus *Streptococcus* are negative. Catalase reactions can also differentiate *Listeria monocytogenes* (catalase-positive) from beta hemolytic streptococci. Most *Neisseria* species are

PROCEDURE 9.1

Catalase Test

Principle

The breakdown of hydrogen peroxide into oxygen and water is mediated by the enzyme catalase. When a small amount of an organism that produces catalase is introduced into hydrogen peroxide, rapid elaboration of bubbles of oxygen, the gaseous product of the enzyme's activity, will be produced.

Method

1. With a loop or sterile wooden stick, transfer a small amount of pure growth from the agar onto the surface of a clean, dry glass slide.
2. Immediately place a drop of 3% hydrogen peroxide (H_2O_2) onto a portion of a colony on the slide.
3. Observe for the evolution of bubbles of gas, indicating a positive test (Figure 9.5).

Quality control

Colonies of *Staphylococcus aureus* ATCC 25923 and *Streptococcus pyogenes* ATCC 19615 are tested.

Expected results

The staphylococci are catalase-positive and produce copious bubbles; streptococci are catalase-negative and do not yield any visible bubbling of the hydrogen peroxide.

Performance schedule

Test quality control organisms with each new batch of reagents placed into usage and each day that tests are performed.

Comments

It has been recommended that the test be performed only on isolates grown on non-blood-containing media. Although red blood cells contain some catalase, a technologist can distinguish the very weak reaction of contaminating red blood cells by performing a control slide catalase test with a small loopful of the blood-containing agar on the same slide with the organism. If the catalase reaction from the colony is much stronger than that from the agar alone, the test can be considered positive.

catalase-positive. Catalase can also help distinguish *Bacillus* species (catalase-positive) from *Clostridium* species (mostly catalase-negative). The test can be performed with a very small amount of growth removed from an agar surface (Procedure 9.1).

  9.2.b. **Clumping factor test ("slide coagulase test").** Gram-positive cocci that are catalase positive belong to the family Micrococcaceae, which includes the staphylococci. The clumping factor test (Procedure 9.2) is used to screen quickly for isolates of *S. aureus*, which are almost always coagulase-positive. Although other species of staphylococci may be coagulase-positive (e.g., *S. intermedius* and *S. hyicus* ss. *hyicus*), they are not important agents of human disease. Clumping factor is a cell-associated substance that binds plasma fibrinogen, causing agglu-

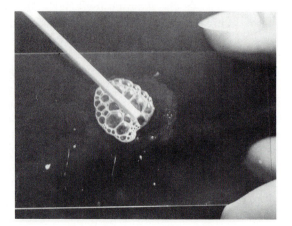

Figure 9.5
Catalase test. Bubbles of gas are released when a catalase-positive organism is emulsified in a drop of hydrogen peroxide on a slide.

PROCEDURE 9.2

Clumping Factor ("Slide Coagulase") Test

Principle

The presence of a cell surface–associated substance that binds fibrinogen and thus allows aggregation of organisms in plasma-containing fibrinogen is detected by observation of clumping of cells.

Method

1. Place a drop of coagulase plasma (rabbit plasma with EDTA or citrate, available commercially from BBL Microbiology Systems, Difco Laboratories, and others) on a clean, dry glass slide.
2. Place a drop of distilled water or saline next to the drop of plasma as a control.
3. With a loop, straight wire, or wooden stick, emulsify an amount of the isolated colony being tested in each drop, inoculating the water or saline first. Try to create a smooth suspension.
4. Observe for clumping in the coagulase plasma drop and a smooth, homogeneous suspension in the control. Clumping in both drops indicates that the organism autoagglutinates and is unsuitable for the slide coagulase test.

Quality control

Colonies of *S. aureus* ATCC 25923 and *S. epidermidis* ATCC 12228 should be tested.

Expected results

Positive organisms such as *S. aureus* exhibit immediate aggregation visible to the naked eye, usually resulting in complete clearing of the background of the suspension. Negative organisms such as *S. epidermidis* will retain the smooth, milky appearance of the original suspension.

Performance schedule

Quality control organisms should be tested with each new batch of coagulase plasma prepared and each day that tests are performed.

tination of the organisms by binding them together with aggregated fibrinogen. With the exception of a newly recognized species, *Staphylococcus lugdunensis*, which is clumping–factor positive but not coagulase-positive, those organisms that produce clumping factor also elaborate the coagulase enzyme and can be identified presumptively as *S. aureus*. Not all *S. aureus* strains produce clumping factor. The reaction must be read within 10 seconds, and the inclusion of an autoagglutination control will decrease the number of false positive results. Rabbit coagulase plasma with ethylenediaminetetraacetic acid (EDTA) or citrate is preferable to human plasma, which may contain substances inhibitory to the reaction. The clumping factor test for presumptive identification of *S. aureus* has been supplanted in many laboratories by specific immunological reagent particle agglutination tests that detect cell surface antigens such as protein A and clumping factor, providing a rapid and definitive identification without the need to perform further tests on clumping factor–negative isolates (discussed in Chapter 10).

9.2.c. Oxidase test. Performed to presumptively identify *Neisseria* species and to initially characterize gram-negative bacilli, the oxidase test indicates the presence of the enzyme cytochrome oxidase. This iron-containing porphyrin enzyme participates in the electron transport mechanism and in the nitrate metabolic pathways of some bacteria. Although the test can be performed by flooding the agar surface of an inoculated plate with the reagent after incubation, it is most easily interpreted when carried out by the Kovac's method (Procedure 9.3). If an iron-containing wire is used to transfer growth, a false positive reaction may result; therefore, platinum wire or wooden sticks are recommended. Certain organisms may show slight positive reactions after the initial 10 seconds have passed; such results are not considered definitive. Passing a culture several times on artificial media and testing a very fresh subculture may sometimes induce an organism that shows a questionable or negative reaction to display its true oxidase positivity. Several manufacturers, including Becton-Dickinson Microbiology Systems, Difco Laboratories, General Diagnostics, Austin Biological Laboratories, and others, produce oxidase test systems consisting of reagent-impregnated filter-paper strips or disposable glass ampules containing small amounts of reagent. Such systems yield results comparable to the conventional test and save preparation time.

PROCEDURE 9.3

Spot Oxidase Test (Kovac's Method)

Principle

The cytochrome oxidase enzyme is able to oxidize the substrate tetramethyl-*p*-phenylenediamine dihydrochloride, forming a colored end product, indophenol. The dark purple end product will be visible if a small amount of growth from a strain that produces the enzyme is rubbed on substrate-impregnated filter paper.

Method

1. Prepare a solution of 1% tetramethyl-*p*-phenylenediamine dihydrochloride (available from Kodak Chemicals, Sigma Chemical Co., and other suppliers) in sterile distilled water each day. To eliminate some work, 50 mg reagent powder can be weighed into each of a large number of plastic, snap-top tubes at one sitting. Each day of use, 5 ml of water is added to one tube (to a predrawn line, for example), which is discarded after that day's use. The reagent is also commercially produced in individually sealed glass ampules for daily use.
2. Place a filter paper circle into a sterile plastic disposable Petri dish and moisten the filter paper with several drops of the fresh reagent.
3. Remove a small portion of the colony to be tested (preferably not more than 24 h old) with a platinum wire or wooden stick and rub the growth on the moistened filter paper.
4. Observe for a color change to blue or purple (Figure 9.6) within 10 s (timing is critical).

Quality control

Test *E. coli* ATCC 25922 and *Neisseria gonorrhoeae* ATCC 43069.

Expected results

Positive organisms such as *Neisseria* species will turn the filter paper dark purple within 10 s; negative organism material such as that from *E. coli* will remain colorless or the color of the colony within 10 s.

Performance schedule

Perform when a new lot number of reagent is received and each day that tests are performed.

Figure 9.6
Kovac's oxidase test. A purple color results when a small portion from a colony of an oxidase-positive organism is rubbed onto filter paper saturated with the oxidase reagent. (From Baron, E. J. 1985. Clinical microbiology, vol. 3: Listen, look, and learn. Health and Education Resources, Bethesda, Md.)

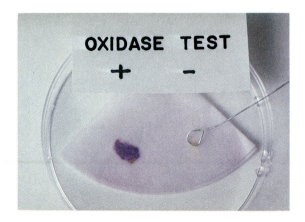

PROCEDURE 9.4

Spot Indole Test

Principle

The indole end product of the action of tryptophanase on tryptophan can be detected by its ability to combine with certain aldehydes to form a colored compound. The blue-green compound formed by indole and cinnamaldehyde is visualized by rubbing bacteria that produce tryptophanase on filter paper impregnated with the substrate.

Method

1. Prepare indole reagent (1% paradimethylaminocinnamaldehyde, available from Sigma Chemical Co. and other chemical supply houses, dissolved in 10% [vol/vol] concentrated hydrochloric acid). Store in a dark bottle in the refrigerator.
2. Saturate a qualitative filter paper (Whatman No. 1 is fine) in the bottom of a Petri dish with the reagent.

3. Using a wooden stick or loop, rub a portion of the colony on the filter paper. Rapid development of a blue color indicates a positive test. Most indole positive organisms will turn blue within 30 s.

Quality control

Test a fresh subculture of *E. coli* ATCC 25922 and *Enterobacter cloacae* ATCC 23355.

Expected results

Positive organisms such as *E. coli* will display a blue-green color on the filter paper; negative organisms such as *E. cloacae* will remain colorless.

Performance schedule

Perform when a new lot number of reagent is received and each day that tests are performed.

9.2.d. Spot indole test. Organisms that produce the enzyme tryptophanase are able to degrade the amino acid tryptophan into pyruvic acid, ammonia, and the product indole. Indole is detected by its combination with the indicator aldehyde (available commercially) to form a colored end product (Procedure 9.4 and Figure 9.7). This test can be used to differentiate swarming *Proteus* species from one another and to begin to presumptively characterize *E. coli*. It has also been found useful for examining anaerobic organisms.

9.2.e. Bile solubility test. *Streptococcus pneumoniae* possesses an active autocatalytic enzyme that lyses the organism's own cell wall during cell division. Under the influence of a bile salt (sodium deoxycholate), the organisms rapidly autolyze. Procedure 9.5 outlines the performance of this test. Other alpha hemolytic streptococci do not possess such an active enzyme and will not dissolve in bile. The bile solubility test may not always work, since old colonies may have lost their active enzyme. Therefore, non-bile-soluble streptococci that resemble pneu-

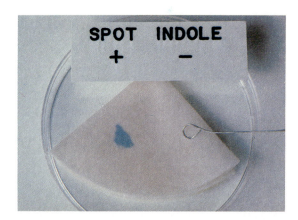

Figure 9.7

Spot indole test. A blue-green color results when a small portion from a colony of an indole-positive organism is rubbed onto filter paper saturated with the indole reagent. (From Baron, E. J. 1985. Clinical microbiology, vol. 3: Listen, look, and learn. Health and Education Resources, Bethesda, Md.)

PROCEDURE 9.5

Bile Solubility Test

Principle

S. pneumoniae will rapidly autocatalyze in the presence of the surfactant sodium deoxycholate (one of the major components of bile). The "melting" or dissolution of a colony within 30 min after exposure to the detergent is indicative of this species.

Method

1. Make a solution of bile salt (10% sodium deoxycholate, available from Difco Laboratories, Sigma Chemical Co., and other sources, in distilled water) and store it at room temperature. The reagent is good for 6 months as long as it remains sterile.
2. Select a well-isolated suspicious colony from a blood agar or chocolate agar plate and place 1 drop of the reagent directly upon the colony.
3. Keeping the plate very level, to prevent the reagent from running and washing a nonpneumococcal colony away, producing a false-positive result, allow the reagent to dry. Placing the plate in an aerobic incubator will speed up this process.

4. When the reagent has dried (in approximately 15 min), examine the area for the absence or flattening of the original colony (Figure 9.8), indicators of bile solubility. Ascertain that an alpha hemolytic streptococcal colony has not merely been washed to another portion of the plate by making certain that the bile drop has remained where it was placed (the blood under the drop becomes slightly hemolyzed).

Quality control

Test a fresh subculture of *S. pneumoniae* ATCC 27336 and *S. mitis* ATCC 15909.

Expected results

Species of *S. pneumoniae* will disappear under the drop and the area will appear flat. Other streptococci will not be affected and the colony elevation will be obvious once the reagent has dried.

Performance schedule

Perform when a new lot number of reagent is received and monthly.

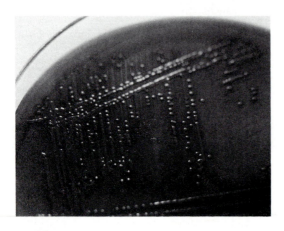

Figure 9.8
Bile solubility test. Within 15 minutes after placing a drop of bile reagent on a colony of *S. pneumoniae*, the colony dissolves.

mococci should be further identified by another method.

9.2.f. PYR (L-pyrrolidonyl-β-naphthylamide hydrolysis) test. *S. pyogenes*, *Enterococcus* species, and some staphylococci are able to hydrolyze the substrate PYR via the enzyme L-pyroglutamyl aminopeptidase. This test is as specific as the more labor-intensive and slower bile esculin agar and salt broth tests used classically to identify enterococci and more specific than the overnight bacitracin test used classically to presumptively identify group A streptococci. Several configurations of the test are available commercially (Figure 9.9). One method is given in Procedure 9.6. Colonies should be catalase negative and morphologically consistent with these two groups of organisms, since certain Micrococcaceae and rare viridans streptococci may also produce the enzyme. *Lactococcus garviae*, a recently recognized

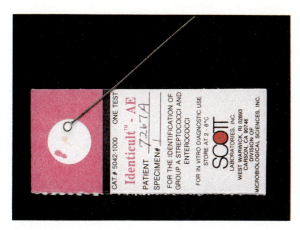

Figure 9.9
PYR test. The presence of the aminopeptidase enzyme results in a pink color change when the indicator is added (organism smeared on left side of paper circle). PYR-negative organisms show no color change (organisms on right side of filter paper circle). The system pictured (Scott Laboratories) is one of several available commercially. (Photograph by Pete Rose.)

streptococcus-like species, can hydrolyze the substrate slowly, resulting in late development of color (10 minutes).

9.2.g. Rapid urease test. *Proteus* species, *Klebsiella* species, some *Citrobacter* species, some *Haemophilus* species, the yeast *Cryptococcus neoformans,* and several other bacteria and fungi produce the enzyme urease, which hydrolyzes urea into ammonia, water, and carbon dioxide. The alkaline end products cause the indicator phenol red to change from yellow to pink or red. This test can be used to screen lactose negative colonies on differential media plated with material from stool specimens, helping to differentiate *Salmonella* and *Shigella* species, which are urease negative, from the urease positive nonpathogens. (Note that *Yersinia enterocolitica,* a stool pathogen, is also urease positive.) Commercial reagents are available for performance of rapid urease tests, including reagent impregnated on a cotton swab that is rubbed across a colony to be tested. A broth method is outlined in Procedure 9.7. Other methods specific for *Cryptococcus* species are discussed in the mycology section of the text.

9.2.h. Rapid thermonuclease test. Another way to distinguish between *S. aureus* and coagulase negative staphylococci (particularly useful for supernatants of blood culture broths growing gram-positive cocci in clusters, for which rapid presumptive identification is essential) is the demonstration of the production of a thermostable deoxyribonuclease by

---

PROCEDURE 9.6

PYR Test

Principle

S. pyogenes and *Enterococcus* species possess the enzyme L-pyroglutamyl aminopeptidase which hydrolyzes an amide substrate with formation of the free β-naphthylamine, which combines with a cinnamaldehyde reagent to form a bright red end product.

Method

1. Rub a small amount of a colony to be tested on the surface of a filter paper impregnated with PYR (available commercially).
2. Add a drop of freshly reconstituted detector reagent, *N*,*N*-dimethylaminocinnamaldehyde with detergent (available commercially) and observe for a red color within 5 min.

Quality control

Test a fresh subculture of *S. pyogenes* ATCC 19615 and *S. agalactiae* ATCC 13813.

Expected results

Positive organisms such as *S. pyogenes* will yield a bright red color change within 5 min; negative organisms, including *S. agalactiae,* will yield either an orange color or no change.

Performance schedule

Test each new batch of reagents received and each day that the test is performed.

S. aureus (Procedure 9.8). Only plates from the manufacturers mentioned have been found to perform satisfactorily in this particular procedure.[3]

9.2.i. Rapid hippurate hydrolysis test. Several species, including group B β-hemolytic streptococci, *Gardnerella vaginalis*, *Listeria* species, and others, are able to hydrolyze hippurate. The presence of the constitutive enzyme, hippuricase, is detected by seeing a colored end product that is formed when ninhydrin oxidizes the amino acids produced during hippurate hydrolysis (Procedure 9.9)

PROCEDURE 9.7

Rapid Urease Test

Principle

Hydrolysis of urea by the enzyme urease releases the end product ammonia, the alkalinity of which causes the indicator phenol red to change from yellow to red. The broth method employs buffers that control the pH change and speed the reaction.

Method

1. Prepare urea broth as follows:

Yeast extract	0.1 g
Monopotassium phosphate	0.091 g
Disodium phosphate	0.095 g
Urea	20 g
Phenol red	0.01 g
Distilled water	1000 ml

Mix ingredients together and store in refrigerator in small plastic snap-top or borosilicate glass screw capped tubes in aliquots of 0.5 ml. The reagent should be stable for 6 months. Do not use if the color is other than pale straw. The rapid urea broth is available commercially.

2. Inoculate a tube of broth with a heavy suspension of the organism to be tested.
3. Incubate the tube at 35° C and observe at 15, 30, and 60 min and up to 4 h for a change in color to pink or red.

Quality control

Test a fresh subculture of *E. coli* ATCC 25922 and *Proteus mirabilis* ATCC 12453.

Expected results

Urease positive organisms such as *Proteus* species will yield a bright pink or red color to the broth; negative organisms such as *E. coli* will not cause a change in the color of the broth.

Performance schedule

Test each new batch of broth and monthly.

9.2.j. Miscellaneous rapidly determined information. Colonial morphology, fluorescence under ultraviolet light (pigmenting *Bacteroides* or *Porphyromonas*), pigment production (e.g., *Pseudomonas* and *Chromobacterium*), spreading (e.g., *Capnocytophaga* and *Proteus*), pitting of agar (e.g., *Eikenella corrodens*), hemolytic reaction on blood agar, odor, and many other characteristics mentioned throughout the text are very helpful in narrowing down identification possibilities.

9.3. Conventional Metabolic Biochemical Tests

A relatively small proportion of the total genetic makeup of bacteria is involved in production of the enzymes that metabolize various substrates. These enzymes have traditionally been used as markers for separating species groups. If an organism possessed a given enzyme and was able to utilize a substrate, an end product would be formed that changed the pH of the medium, causing a visual color change in a pH indicator substance. In some cases, the organism's ability to grow in a medium could be detected by increased turbidity or the presence of colonies on the surface. This approach has been modified in many ways in recent years, but it is still used for identification of unusual pathogens, difficult-to-speciate pathogens, and as the standard against which all other metabolic test methods are compared. There are many conventional tests other than those described in this chapter; some of them will be mentioned in later sections of the book. Detailed explanations of the principles of metabolic reactions can be found in other references, such as *Manual of Clinical Microbiology*, edited by Lennette et al., *Zinsser's Microbiology*, edited by Joklik et al., *Microbiology, Including Immunology and Molecular Genetics*, edited by Davis et al., and other sources.

9.3.a. Oxidation and fermentation tests. The metabolic pathways used by a microorganism during utilization of a substrate for production of cell building material and for energy (usually with the concomitant production of acid by-products) can be either **oxidative** or **fermentative.** Oxidation occurs when the organism uses oxygen as a terminal electron acceptor. This reaction can be observed on the surface of agar slants or in the surface layer of liquid media loosely capped to allow diffusion of air. Fermentation occurs in the absence of oxygen. During fermentation, the organism often produces large amounts of organic acids. Fermentation can be demonstrated by

PROCEDURE 9.8

Rapid Thermonuclease Test

Principle

S. aureus can be reliably identified by production of a heat-stable deoxyribonuclease enzyme. Organisms are heated to destroy non-heat-stable nucleases and are allowed to interact with media containing DNA intercalated with a dye, toluidine blue, that looks blue when bound to DNA and changes color when its conformation is altered. Breakdown of the DNA by the nuclease changes the dye's structure and causes it to reflect a different wavelength of light, appearing red or pink instead of blue.

Method

1. For isolated colonies, inoculate several colonies into 1 ml of brain heart infusion broth and incubate for 2 h at 35° C; then follow the procedure outlined below.
2. Boil approximately 2 ml of blood culture broth (can be mixed or unmixed) or brain heart infusion broth suspension of organisms (as above) in a water bath or microwave oven for 15 min. The red cells will clot in the bottom of the tube. Allow the tube to cool to room temperature.
3. Punch a well in DNAse test agar (Thermal agar, Edge Diagnostics or Thermonuclease agar, Remel) with the large end of a Pasteur pipette or a plastic drinking straw, remove the agar plug, and fill the well with the heated and cooled supernatant above the red cell clot (approximately 2 drops) or broth suspension.
4. Incubate the plate at 37° C in an upright position and inspect the plate after 1 h and again after 2 h.
5. The plate may be refrigerated and reused several times.

Quality control

A portion of a positive control, a negative blood culture seeded with *S. aureus* and passed to a new negative blood culture weekly, should be boiled and tested as above.

Expected results

Positive results, as for *S. aureus*, are indicated by a pink or red halo around the well. No change will be observed around wells filled with supernatants from negative organisms. A small, clear zone around a well is not indicative of a positive test, as some coagulase negative staphylococci can degrade the dye without denaturing the DNA.

Performance schedule

The test should be performed with each new batch or lot number of agar media and each time the test is performed.

Modified from Madison, B.M., and Baselski, V.S. 1983. J. Clin. Microbiol. 18:722; and Ratner, H.B., and Stratton, C.W. 1985. J. Clin. Microbiol. 21:995.

---

overlaying substrate-containing media with mineral oil or a petroleum jelly (Vaseline) and paraffin combination (Vaspar) to exclude oxygen. A special medium containing low concentrations of peptone (oxidative-fermentative [O-F] medium, described in Chapter 28) has been developed for testing this aspect of the metabolism of bacteria. In either case, the final end products are detected by noting a change in the color of the pH indicator incorporated into the medium. It is clear that the pH at which the indicator changes color will substantially affect the outcome of the test. For that reason, the indicator given for a particular medium formula must not be modified. Many substrate utilization tests rely on either bromcresol purple, which changes from purple to yellow at pH 6.3, Andrade's acid fuchsin

PROCEDURE 9.9

Rapid Hippurate Hydrolysis

Principle

The end products of hydrolysis of hippuric acid include glycine and benzoic acid. Glycine is deaminated by the oxidizing agent, ninhydrin, which becomes reduced during the process. The end products of the ninhydrin oxidation react to form a purple colored dye. The test medium must contain only hippurate, since ninhydrin might react with any free amino acids present in growth media or other broths.

Method

1. Prepare 1% sodium hippurate substrate as follows:

Sodium hippurate (Sigma Chemical Co.)	1 g
Distilled water	100 ml

   Mix together and dispense into small (12 × 75 mm) plastic disposable test tubes with snap top caps, 0.4 ml per tube. Store frozen for a maximum of 6 months.

2. Prepare ninhydrin reagent as follows:

Ninhydrin (Sigma)	3.5 g
Acetone	50 ml
Butanol	50 ml

   Mix the acetone and butanol together and then add the ninhydrin. Store at room temperature

Modified from Hwang M. and Ederer G.M. 1975. Rapid hippurate hydrolysis method for presumptive identification of group B streptococci. J. Clin. Microbiol. 1:114.

in a brown bottle with a tight seal for a maximum of 6 months.

3. Defrost the sodium hippurate substrate and heavily inoculate a tube with a pure culture of the organism to be tested. The suspension should be milky.

4. Incubate the capped tubes for 2 h in a 35° C water bath.

5. Add 0.2 ml ninhydrin reagent and reincubate for an additional 15 min. Observe for a change to deep purple, indicating that the hippurate has been hydrolyzed. This test can also be used to identify other organisms, as mentioned throughout the book.

Quality control

Test *S. agalactiae* ATCC 27956 and *Enterococcus faecalis* ATCC 19433.

Expected results

The *S. agalactiae* should turn deep purple (positive), and the enterococcus should remain colorless or slightly yellow-pink (negative) after addition of the ninhydrin reagent.

Performance schedule

Test the quality control organisms each time a new batch of reagents is prepared and occasionally thereafter.

---

indicator, which changes from pale yellow to pink at pH 5.5, or phenol red, which changes from red to yellow at pH 7.9. Formulas for the preparation of media containing certain of these indicators are found in Appendix A.

9.3.b. **Hydrolysis tests.** An enzyme that breaks down a substrate by adding the components of water to key bonds within the substrate molecule is called a **hydrolyzing** enzyme. The products are measured

by some visual reaction. Substrates for such enzymes that are commonly used in differentiating species include sodium hippurate, which can be broken down by *Listeria*, *Streptococcus uberis*, *G. vaginalis*, and group B streptococci *(S. agalactiae)*; deoxyribonucleic acid (DNA), which can be hydrolyzed by certain Enterobacteriaceae, certain species of staphylococci (mentioned previously), and other microorganisms; urea (mentioned previously); and es-

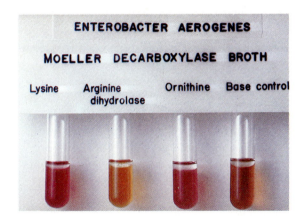

Figure 9.10
Moeller's decarboxylase broth media. (From Baron, E. J. 1985. Clinical microbiology, vol. 3: Listen, look, and learn. Health and Education Resources, Bethesda, Md.)

culin, which is hydrolyzed by *L. monocytogenes*, group D streptococci, some viridans streptococci, and some anaerobes, among others. Hydrolysis of starch, casein, and lecithin is also used for differentiation of species. Certain mycobacteria can be identified by their ability to hydrolyze the detergent, polysorbate-80 (Tween-80). Media for all these reactions can be purchased, either fully prepared or in dry powder form. Use of hydrolysis tests for identification is described throughout the book.

9.3.c. **Amino acid degradation.** Enzymes formed by some organisms either *deaminate, dihydrolyze,* or *decarboxylate* amino acids, breaking them down into smaller components. The amino acid substrates tested often include lysine, arginine, ornithine, tryptophan (described previously for the indole test), and phenylalanine. Certain mycobacteria can be differentiated by their ability to deaminate pyrazinamide. Some of these amino acid–degrading enzymes are active in the absence of oxygen; therefore, such tests are often carried out in the deep butts of agar tubes or in liquid media with vaspar overlay to prevent the products of more active oxidative enzymes from obscuring the results. One such commonly used system is that of Moeller (Figure 10). Amino acids (lysine, arginine, and ornithine) are incorporated into broth media containing 0.05% glucose, to allow the organisms to begin growth, and bromcresol purple indicator. Along with each amino acid being tested, a control tube of the glucose-containing broth base without amino acid is inoculated to serve as a stan-

dard against which to compare the color of the indicator. In the case of most of the amino acid degradation reactions, the end products (such as ammonia) are alkaline and the color indicator changes to its original color: bromcresol purple turns to purple and phenol red changes to red. Phenylalanine deamination, on the other hand, occurs in air and is measured by the production of a green reactant after the addition of 10% ferric chloride. The media for performing all of the tests mentioned here are commercially available (Appendix C).

9.3.d. **Single substrate utilization.** Many organisms can be recognized by their ability to grow in the presence of only a single compound that supplies enough of the organism's nutrient needs. Substrates that can fulfill this function and are helpful in differentiating microorganisms include citrate, malonate, and acetate. Growth on a substrate-containing agar slant, with or without a pH indicator, is used as the end point of this test. Another variant of this test, used to determine whether a yeast is able to grow with only a single carbohydrate or nitrate, is called an **assimilation** test. Filter paper disks impregnated with the substrate are placed on the surface of a Petri dish of agar without nutrients that has been streaked with a suspension of the yeast being tested so as to obtain confluent growth. The yeast grows around the disks that contain substrates that it can utilize, or assimilate.

9.3.e. **Nitrate reactions.** Nitrate serves as the source of nitrogen for many bacteria and fungi, but it must be broken down. The first step in nitrate utilization is reduction to nitrite by removal of one oxygen molecule. The Enterobacteriaceae and many other gram-negative bacilli, mycobacteria, and fungi reduce nitrate to nitrite. Certain microorganisms are able to further reduce nitrite to nitrogen by replacing the remaining oxygens with hydrogens. Some *Pseudomonas* species and other nonfermentative gram-negative bacilli possess this capability, as do other species. The classic nitrate reduction test is described in Procedure 9.10. Spot tests using filter paper disks impregnated with nitrate are used for presumptive testing of anaerobes, although that method is less sensitive than broth methods. The ability of yeasts to utilize nitrate can be determined by the same method used for assimilation tests or by a rapid test that uses a swab, described in the Mycology section.

PROCEDURE 9.10

Conventional Nitrate Reduction Test

Principle

Organisms that possess nitrate reductase can reduce nitrate to nitrite. Nitrite combines with an acidified naphythylamine substrate to form a red-colored end product. If the organism has further reduced nitrite to nitrogen gas, the test for nitrite will yield a negative (colorless) result. An additional test for the presence of unreacted nitrate must be performed to validate such a colorless result. Metallic zinc catalyzes the reduction of nitrate to nitrite; thus, with the addition of zinc a negative test will yield a red color, indicating the presence of unreacted nitrate.

Method

1. Grow the organism in 5 ml of nitrate broth (commercially available) for 24 to 48 h or longer for poorly growing organisms. A small inverted tube, called a Durham tube, may be placed into the broth to trap bubbles of nitrogen gas that may be formed by nitrite-reducing organisms.
2. Prepare the reagents that combine with the nitrite to form colored end products:

Reagent A

Sulfanilic acid	4 g
Acetic acid (5 M)	500 ml

Reagent B

N,N-dimethyl-1-naphthylamine	3 ml
Acetic acid (5 M)	500 ml

3. Add 3 drops of reagent A and then 3 drops of reagent B to the suspension of organisms in broth.
4. Wait 30 min for the production of a red color, indicating the presence of the nitrate reduction product, nitrite.
5. The presence of unreduced nitrate can be detected by adding a pinch of commercially available zinc powder to the broth if the red color did not develop after the initial reagents were added.

Quality control

Inoculate suspensions of *E. coli* ATCC 25922 and *Acinetobacter calcoaceticus* ATCC 19606 into broth and test.

Expected results

Nitrate positive organisms such as all Enterobacteriaceae will either yield a red color after addition of reagents A and B or will yield no color even after the addition of zinc. Negative organisms such as *Acinetobacter* species will show no color after addition of reagents A and B but will turn red with zinc. This red color after the addition of zinc indicates that nitrate was still present in the broth and that the organism could not reduce it.

Performance schedule

Perform with each new batch of nitrate broth, reagents A or B, and monthly.

9.3.f. **Triple sugar iron agar and Kligler's iron agar reactions.** Reactions of bacteria in Kligler's iron agar (**KIA**) or triple sugar iron agar (**TSIA**) can be used to direct the initial identification of gram-negative bacilli, particularly members of the Enterobacteriaceae. KIA and TSIA can detect three primary characteristics of a bacterium: the ability to produce gas from the fermentation of sugars, the production of large amounts of hydrogen sulfide gas (as visualized

by the formation of a black iron-containing precipitate), and the ability to ferment lactose in KIA or lactose and sucrose in TSIA. A small amount of growth from a pure colony is picked onto a straight wire and inoculated to these media by streaking the surface of the slant and stabbing the butt of the tube all the way to the bottom. Only the tops of colonies growing on selective agar should be touched, since inhibited flora may still be present and viable. For the same reason, the needle or loop should not be cooled in the agar of any selective medium. Gas formation is usually visualized as bubbles and cracks in the medium, caused by the pressure of the gas formed in the agar. Therefore, the inoculating wire must be stabbed down the center of the agar butt of the tube; careless inoculation may allow the wire to form a channel in the agar along the inside glass wall of the tube through which the newly formed gas may escape, preventing its detection. The presence of oxygen in the atmosphere is necessary for the proper reaction to occur on the slant; therefore caps must be very loose if screw-capped tubes are used.

Both TSIA and KIA contain a limiting amount of glucose and a tenfold greater lactose concentration. Enterobacteriaceae and other glucose fermenters first begin to metabolize glucose, as glucose utilizing enzymes are present constitutively and the bacteria can gain the most energy from using the simplest sugar. All other sugars must be converted to glucose before they enter the Embden-Meyerhof pathway. Glucose utilization occurs both aerobically on the slant where oxygen is available as a terminal electron acceptor, and in the butt where conditions are anaerobic. Once a glucose fermenting bacterium has reduced all of the available glucose to pyruvate, it will further metabolize pyruvate via the aerobic Krebs cycle (on the slant) to produce acid end products. The acid in the medium causes the pH indicator, phenol red, to assume a yellow color. Thus, after 6 hours of incubation, both the slant and the butt of a TSIA or a KIA that has been inoculated with a glucose fermenter will appear yellow. If the organism cannot ferment glucose, the **butt** will remain red (indicating no change in pH) or become alkaline (may be indicated by a red color slightly deeper than that of the original medium), demonstrating that the organism is not a member of the Enterobacteriaceae.

After depletion of the limited glucose, an organism that is able to do so will begin to utilize lactose or sucrose. Since there is 10 times as much lactose (and sucrose in TSIA) as glucose in the agar, the organism will have enough substrate to continue making acid end products. The slant and butt of the TSIA or KIA will remain yellow after 18 to 24 hours incubation. This reaction is called acid over acid (A/A) and the organism is identified as a lactose fermenter. The production of gas will cause the medium

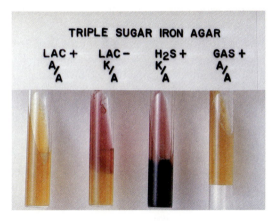

Figure 9.11
Examples of inoculated triple sugar iron agar slants. (From Baron, E. J. 1985. Clinical microbiology, vol. 3: Listen, look, and learn. Health and Education Resources, Bethesda, Md.)

to break up or to be pushed up the tube, so that a gas-producing lactose fermenter will give an A/A plus gas reaction.

If the organism being tested cannot use the lactose in the medium, it must produce energy in a less efficient way by using the proteins and amino acids in the medium as nutrient sources. Protein metabolism occurs primarily on the surface of the slant where oxygen is plentiful. The byproducts of peptone breakdown (such as ammonia) are alkaline and cause the phenol red indicator to revert back to its original red color. After 18 to 24 hours' incubation of a nonlactose fermenter, the TSIA or KIA will thus show a red slant; the butt remains yellow because of the early anaerobic glucose metabolism. This reaction is called alkaline over acid (Alk/A or K/A).

Glucose nonfermenters may also produce alkaline products from peptone utilization on the slant. Such reactions will be alkaline over alkaline (Alk/Alk or K/K) or alkaline over no change (Alk/NC). Figure 9.11 shows several different possible reactions in TSIA.

Either lactose fermenters or nonlactose fermenters can produce hydrogen sulfide, and the black precipitate may mask the true color of the butt. In this case, the ability to ferment or oxidize glucose can be tested by inoculating the organism into **oxidative-fermentative** media. These media are prepared with a low peptone concentration so that the pH change that occurs after metabolism of glucose will not be affected by the alkaline products formed from peptone utilization.

The initial reaction of an inoculum from a pure culture of a bacterial strain in TSIA or KIA gives a microbiologist a great deal of information about what the genus might be, and further tests are often chosen based on this reaction. Although these media are used primarily for gram-negative bacilli, the ability of one species of gram-positive bacilli, *Erysipelothrix rhusiopathiae*, to produce hydrogen sulfide is often detected in TSIA. *Bacillus* species that are inoculated to TSIA or KIA because they are initially thought to be gram-negative bacilli will usually yield an acid slant over a slightly orange (or no change in color) butt. Subtle patterns and colors of reactions, such as a cherry-red slant and very little gas (suggestive of *Serratia* species) or a very dark red slant (suggestive of *Proteus*, *Providencia*, or *Morganella* species) can be recognized by experienced technologists and serve to guide the choice of further tests.

9.4. Modifications of Conventional Biochemical Tests

A number of modifications of conventional biochemicals have been used in recent years to facilitate inoculation of media, to decrease the incubation time, to automate the procedure, or to systematize the determination of species based on reaction patterns. Three types of these systems are briefly described.

9.4.a. **Modified conventional biochemical test systems that utilize small volumes.** A number of conventional methods can be made to yield more rapid results by heavily inoculating a very small volume of substrate. Used successfully for rapid identification of *Neisseria* species, the method of Kellogg[6] uses this principle. A modification of the Kellogg broths (Procedure 9.11) has been used for rapid determination of carbohydrate reactions of fastidious gram-negative bacilli.[5] The reagents can be used to test most bacteria, including *Neisseria* species.[1]

Many tests, including hippurate hydrolysis, nitrate reduction, urease production, decarboxylations, and deaminations, have been modified for rapid results. For these tests, small volumes of media are inoculated with heavy suspensions of the organism to be tested. Media manufacturers produce many such reagents (Appendix C). In several cases commercial suppliers (including Remel Laboratories, Austin Biological Laboratories, and others) produce reagent-impregnated paper disks or filter paper

strips to be eluted in a small volume of water saline to form the test substrate. Key Scientific Products was one of the first commercial suppliers single substrates for elution. In the Key system compressed tablets that could be stored at room temperature are added to small volumes of water needed to produce the substrates for specific reactions. All of these systems obviate the need for the technologist to prepare these media in the usual way. The test organism can then be suspended direct in the substrate. Such small volume, singly performed tests are extremely useful for differentiating two similar species that differ in only one characteristic or for ruling out an organism that is characterized by a single parameter. One example is the use of a rapid urease test that can help eliminate certain nonpathogens from further biochemical testing as possible stool pathogens, many of which (except for *Y. enterocolitica*) are urease negative. The nitrate and niacin tests for mycobacteria have been adapted to this format. Other tests have also been adapted for rapid determination with filter paper reagents.

9.4.b. **Multitest systems.** The simplest multitest system consists of a conventional-type format that can be inoculated once to yield more than one result. By combining reactants, for example, one substrate can be used to determine indole and nitrate results; indole and motility results; motility, indole, and ornithine decarboxylase; or other combinations. The systems are commercially available (powder or prepared media). The R/B system (Flow Laboratories) incorporates several media within one uniquely designed tube (Figure 9.12).

In a widely used type of identification system, conventional biochemicals have been put up smaller volumes and packaged so that they can inoculated easily with one manipulation instead several. When used in conjunction with a computer generated data base (described later), the biochemical patterns generated can be used to predict species identification with much more precision than obtainable using conventional methods with fewer parameters. Several manufacturers produce conventional biochemicals in microdilution trays (Figure 9.13) that are shipped to the user in a frozen state and maintained frozen until they are thawed, inoculated, and used. These systems require overnight incubation, as do conventional biochemicals. The addition of reagents for the demonstration of end products

PROCEDURE 9.11

Rapid Carbohydrate Fermentation Reaction Test

Principle

When carbohydrates are metabolized by organisms with subsequent change in pH, the phenol red indicator changes from red to yellow. The presence of buffers controls the pH change and the heavy inoculum of organisms allows rapid detection of constitutive enzymes.

Method

1. Prepare buffered indicator solution as follows:

KH_2PO_4	0.01 g
K_2HPO_4	0.04 g
KCl	0.80 g
Phenol red	0.004 g (or 0.4 ml of a 1% aqueous solution)
Distilled water	100 ml

   Adjust the pH to 7.0; sterilize by passing the solution through a 0.2 μm diameter pore size membrane filter, and store in a tightly capped brown bottle in the refrigerator (4° C).

2. Prepare 20% stock carbohydrate solutions as follows:

Peptone	10 g
Meat extract	3 g
NaCl	5 g
Distilled water	1000 ml

   Add 20 g of the appropriate carbohydrate (e.g., glucose, sucrose, available from Difco Laboratories) to 100 ml of the peptone broth solution, adjust to pH 7.0, and filter sterilize as above. One portion of the peptone broth should be retained without carbohydrate to serve as a control. These solutions may be stored frozen in small aliquots.

3. Place 0.1 ml of the indicator buffer solution in a plastic or glass disposable culture tube (10 × 75 mm diameter) for each carbohydrate to be tested and for one control. Make an extremely heavy suspension of a pure culture of the organism to be tested in each of the indicator buffer tubes (should be milky).

4. Add 1 drop (approximately 0.04 ml) of the appropriate carbohydrate stock solution to each suspension. Add 1 drop of peptone broth without carbohydrate to one suspension to serve as a negative control.

5. Cap the tubes and incubate them in a water bath or heating block at 35° C for up to 4 h, observing periodically.

Quality control

Test a fresh subculture of an organism that is positive for all carbohydrates prepared, for example, use *Neisseria sicca* ATCC 9913 as a positive control for glucose, maltose, fructose, and sucrose.

Expected results

Positive organisms show a change in indicator from red to yellow. Many reactions will be positive within 30 min; questionable reactions may require up to 24 h for full development. The peptone broth control tube should remain red and serves as an internal negative control for each test.

Performance schedule

Perform with each new batch or reagents prepared.

Modified from Brown, 1974, and Hollis et al., 1980.

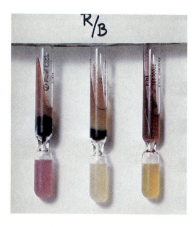

Figure 9.12
Multitest media (R/B System, Flow Laboratories) that allows aerobic reactions on the slant and anaerobic reactions in the pinched-off base of the tube. (From Baron, E. J. 1985. Clinical microbiology, vol. 3: Listen, look, and learn. Health and Education Resources, Bethesda, Md.)

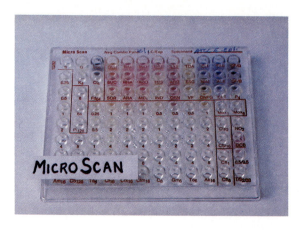

Figure 9.13
Example of a microdilution tray identification/susceptibility system format (American MicroScan). (From Baron, E. J. 1985. Clinical microbiology, vol. 3: Listen, look, and learn. Health and Education Resources, Bethesda, Md.)

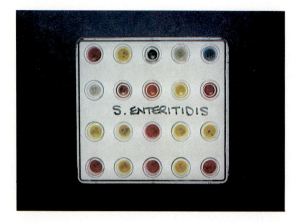

Figure 9.14
The Minitek system (BBL Microbiology Systems), which employs filter paper disks impregnated with substrates.

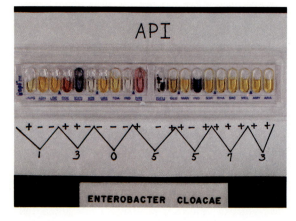

Figure 9.15
The API (Analytab Products, Inc.) miniaturized identification system. (From Baron, E. J. 1985. Clinical microbiology, vol. 3: Listen, look, and learn. Health and Education Resources, Bethesda, Md.)

ucts of reactions is necessary. The Sceptor system (BBL Microbiology Systems) is also based on a microdilution array, but the substrates are dried in the trays, which are rehydrated with a suspension of the organism during inoculation. The Minitek system (also BBL Microbiology Systems) incorporates a microbroth format and allows the user to determine which reactions are to be tested by arbitrarily adding substrate-impregnated filter paper disks to wells in a plastic tray (Figure 9.14). Many different groups of bacteria, including Enterobacteriaceae, anaer-

obes, and *Neisseria* species, can be tested in the versatile Minitek system. If heavy inocula are used to inoculate the Minitek wells, results may be available within 4 hours.

The API 20E for identification of gram-negative bacilli, API 20S for identification of streptococci, API 20C for yeast identification, and API 20A for identification of anaerobes (Analytab Products) incorporate dried reagents in plastic cupules into which a

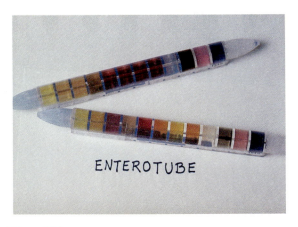

Figure 9.16
The Enterotube II (Roche Diagnostics) miniaturized identification system. (From Baron, E. J. 1985. Clinical microbiology, vol. 3: Listen, look, and learn. Health and Education Resources, Bethesda, Md.)

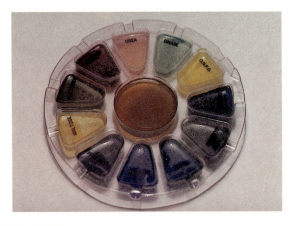

Figure 9.17
The Uni-N/F-Tek plate, an example of the Flow (Flow Laboratories) miniaturized identification system.

suspension of the test organism is placed (Figure 9.15). With a heavy inoculum, results may be read after 4 to 6 hours' incubation in some cases. The API Rapid E for Enterobacteriaceae, Rapid NFT for non-fermentative gram-negative bacilli, and Rapid Strep for streptococcal identification systems (also Analy-tab Products) use the same format, although a number of chromogenic substrates (described later) are incorporated as differential reactants to allow more rapid results (4 hours). The API systems have been adopted by large numbers of laboratories since their introduction in the late 1970s. Because of an extensive computer-generated data base incorporating the results of 21 test results (including the oxidase reaction that is performed separately), use of the API system for identification of Enterobacteriaceae has facilitated the recognition of several of the new species of Enterobacteriaceae and has allowed laboratories to designate species to a more precise level (based on biotype) than was previously possible in a cost-effective manner.

Innovative formats for conventional biochemicals are found in several other systems. The Enterotube II (for lactose fermenters) and Oxi-Ferm (for non-fermenters), produced by Roche Diagnostics, are contained within a large tube. A colony is picked onto the end of a long inoculating needle that is drawn through a series of substrate-containing agar compartments in the plastic tube (Figure 9.16). The Enteric-Tek for Enterobacteriaceae, Uni-Yeast-Tek

for yeast, Anaerobe-Tek for identification of anaerobes, and Uni-N/F-Tek for nonfermentative gram-negative bacilli (Flow Laboratories) employ substrate-containing media in pie-shaped wedges in a circular plastic tray (Figure 9.17). Substrates incorporated into agar plates allow many bacteria to be tested at one time in a cost-effective manner (Cathra Repliscan II System, MCT Diagnostics).

In recent years several of the multitest systems have been adapted to yield results more rapidly, often without requiring overnight incubation. The Micro-ID system (General Diagnostics) was one of the first to exploit the principle that bacterial enzymes can act in the absence of actual viable growth or multiplication. The detection of **preformed enzymes** relies on the inoculation of substrate-containing solutions with an extremely heavy suspension of the organism, resembling the turbidity of skim milk (bacteria $\sim 1 \times 10^9$/ml). Enough of the enzyme will be present in this volume of organisms to cause the substrate reaction to occur, even if the organisms are no longer alive. The Micro-ID system uses a number of substrates that detect preformed enzymes in addition to conventional tests for identification of Enterobacteriaceae. The test organism suspension is inoculated to plastic wells, the tray is incubated, and the entire tray is tipped to allow reactants in a separate chamber to mix with the suspension (Figure 9.18). Results are available after 4 hours' incubation. Tests of this sort (several have been mentioned) yield

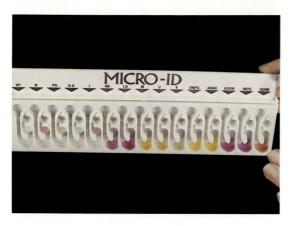

Figure 9.18
The Micro-ID (General Diagnostics) miniaturized identification system. (From Baron, E. J. 1985. Clinical microbiology, vol. 3: Listen, look, and learn. Health and Education Resources, Bethesda, Md.)

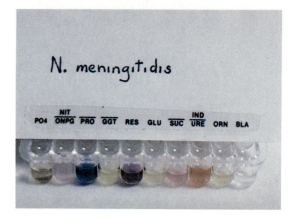

Figure 9.19
The RapID N/H (Innovative Diagnostics) miniaturized identification system.

results after several hours of incubation instead of the overnight incubation required by many conventional methods.

Newer biochemical test systems may also utilize chromogenic substrates. Chromogenic substrates are acted upon by enzymes to form colored products; a separate visual indicator system is unnecessary. Because most of the enzymes being detected by their activity on chromogenic substrates are preformed, results are available within 4 hours for most systems using these substrates. Identification systems that utilize a large number of chromogenic substrates include the RapID ANA anaerobic identification panel and the RapID N/H panel for identification of *Neisseria* and *Haemophilus* species, produced by Innovative Diagnostics (Figure 9.19). Rapid Strep, An-Ident, and Staph-Ident systems by Analytab Products and several other *Neisseria* and *Haemophilus* identification systems also utilize chromogenic substrates.

Most systems that include susceptibility testing as well as identification parameters on the same tray must be incubated overnight to allow enough growth of the organism for accurate test results. Changes in the technology of microbiology are being contemplated, however, that will shorten incubation time by relying on parameters other than growth for measurement of an organism's reaction to an antimicrobial substrate, as further discussed in Chapter 13. Sensititre gram negative identification system microdilution trays employ fluorogenic substrates that

change wavelength and fluoresce when they are acted on by bacterial enzymes. These fluorescent markers of growth can be detected by a fluorometer with greater sensitivity than classical determinants of growth, such as color change due to pH change or turbidity, and thus can identify metabolic activity faster than conventional growth-dependent methods.

9.4.c. **Automated microbial identification systems.** Although they are discussed in more detail in Chapter 11, the most widely used automated identification systems are mentioned briefly here. Systems that utilize a microdilution tray format have been automated to allow hands-off or partially manual reading of results. The MicroScan (Baxter-American MicroScan), Pasco (Difco Laboratories), Sensititre (Radiometer, Inc.), MicroMedia Systems (Beckman Instruments), and Sceptor systems (BBL Microbiology Systems) employ readers that interface with the data base for computer-assisted identification. The Sceptor system includes an automated filling device for rehydrating the wells with a suspension of the test organism. API-compatible systems (UniScept Plus and Aladin, Analytab Products) also incorporate an automated reader that interfaces with their extensive data base. The Aladin instrument adds reagents, reads results, and discards trays without operator assistance.

The Autobac IDX (General Diagnostics) was one of the first automated susceptibility systems. It has been modified to provide bacterial identification.

ble 9.1

eneration and Utilization of Genus-Identification Data Base Probability: Percent Positive Reactions for
0 Known Strains

ORGANISM	BIOCHEMICAL PARAMETER			
	LACTOSE	SUCROSE	INDOLE	ORNITHINE
Escherichia	91	49	99	63
Shigella	1	1	38	20

ble 9.2

eneration and Utilization of Genus-Identification Data Base Probability: Probability that Unknown Strain
is a Member of the Known Genus Based on Results of Each Individual Parameter Tested

ORGANISM	BIOCHEMICAL PARAMETER			
	LACTOSE	SUCROSE	INDOLE	ORNITHINE
X	% +	% +	% −	% +
Escherichia	.91	.49	.01	.63
Shigella	.01	.01	.62	.20

obability that X is *Escherichia* = .91 × .49 × .01 × .63 = .002809
obability that X is *Shigella* = .01 × .01 × .62 × .20 = .000012

rganisms are inoculated into plastic cuvettes con-
ining various inhibitory substances. After 3 to 6
urs' incubation, the identification of a test organ-
m is determined by its growth pattern in the pres-
ice of the different antibacterial agents, as mea-
red by light-scatter photometry. The Auto-
icrobic System (Vitek Systems) determines the
owth of the test strain within tiny substrate-con-
ining wells on a plastic card by measuring turbid-
y. Once the card has been inoculated, the instru-
ent performs all readings without operator assis-
nce; results are available within 4 to 6 hours'
cubation. Cards are available for identification of
am-negative fermenters and nonfermenters, yeast,
aphylococci, and streptococci, some of which re-
iire longer incubation periods for final results. The
vantage system (Abbott Laboratories) utilizes a
astic cartridge with a number of wells containing
ophilized substrates that is manually inoculated in
ie step. The instrument monitors turbidity over
me, yielding results based on kinetic patterns of
owth and metabolism. Separate reagent cartridges
e available for identification of yeasts, nonfer-
enting gram-negative bacilli, and Enterobacteria-
eae.

9.5. Computer-Assisted Data Base Systems

The principles upon which computer-assisted data
base systems for identification of species are based
are simple. The first step in developing a data base
is to accumulate a large number of organisms of
known species. Each strain is subjected to an identical battery of biochemical and enzymatic tests. The
reactions are recorded as positive (+) or negative
(−) and the cumulative results of each test are expressed as a percentage of each genus or species that
possesses that characteristic. For example, suppose
that 100 different known *Escherichia* strains and 100
known *Shigella* strains are tested in four biochemicals, yielding the results illustrated in Table 9.1.
Now an unknown organism, *X*, is tested in the same
four biochemicals, yielding results as follows: lactose
(+), sucrose (+), indole (−), and ornithine (+). The
results of testing the known strains are now converted to the percentage probability that the unknown strain *X* is a member of one of the known
genera based on each separate test result (Table 9.2).
If *Escherichia* sp. are 91% lactose positive, then the
probability that *X* is an *Escherichia* based on lactose
alone is .91. If *Shigella* sp. are 38% indole positive,
then the probability that *X* is a *Shigella* based on
indole alone is .62 (1.00 [all *Shigella*] − 0.38 [per-

Table 9.3

Commercially Available Kits for the Identification of *Enterobacteriaceae*

PRODUCT NAME	DESCRIPTION	SUBSTRATE/TEST	OPERATION	COMMENTS

API 20E (Analytab Products; Plate 2, A)	Twenty miniature cupules containing dehydrated substrates are in plasticized strip. After addition of standardized inoculum (McFarland 0.5) and incubation, color changes are read visually. Reagents must be added to some cupules before reading.	Hydrolysis of o-nitrophenyl-β-galactopyranoside (ONPG)
		Arginine dihydrolase
		Lysine decarboxylase
		Ornithine decarboxylase
		Citrate utilization
		Production of hydrogen sulfide (H_2S)
		Urea hydrolysis
		Tryptophan deaminase
		Formation of indole
		Production of acetoin (Voges-Proskauer test)
		Liquefaction of gelatin
		Fermentation of:
		    Glucose
		    Mannitol
		    Inositol
		    Sorbitol
		    Rhamnose
		    Sucrose
		    Melibiose
		    Amygdalin
		    Arabinose
			Each cupule is manually inoculated with Pasteur pipette. Some cupules are overlaid with oil to provide conditions of reduced oxygen tension. Strip is placed in humid chamber and incubated either 5 h for rapid test or 18-24 h for overnight result. Seven-digit number is derived from scoring the seven sets of three reactions each. Number is then found in code book that reveals identification of bacterium, probability of its being correct, and aberrant test results.	This is largest commercially available microbiologic data base in world. Many reports indicate >90% agreement with conventional methods for both 18-h and 5-h system.

API Rapid E (API Systems, S.A.)	This system is essentially identical to API 20E except that substrates are not buffered and microtubes are smaller.	Hydrolysis of ONPG
		Lysine decarboxylase
		Ornithine decarboxylase
		Urea hydrolysis
		Phenylalanine deaminase
		Esculin
		Citrate utilization
		Malonate utilization
		Indole production
		Voges-Proskauer test
		Fermentation of:
		    Arabinose
		    Xylose
		    Adonitol
		    Rhamnose
		    Cellobiose
		    Melibiose
		    Sucrose
		    Trehalose
		    Raffinose
		    Glucose
			Operation is identical to API 20E except initial incubation period is 4 h.	Results are available in 4 or 18 h. This test is acceptable alternative to API 20E.

cent of positive *Shigella]* = 0.62 [percent of *Shigella* that are indole negative]). The probabilities are then multiplied to achieve a calculated likelihood that *X* is one or the other of the two genera. Ultimately, *X* is more likely to be an *Escherichia*, with a probability of 357:1 (1 divided by 0.0028). This is still a very

unlikely probability, but we have tested only four parameters, and the indole, a very important one, was atypical. As more parameters are added to the formula, the importance of just one test decreases and the overall pattern prevails. It is obvious that with typical organisms being tested for 20 or more

Table 9.3

Commercially Available Kits for the Identification of *Enterobacteriaceae—cont'd*

PRODUCT NAME	DESCRIPTION	SUBSTRATE/TEST	OPERATION	COMMENTS
R/B Enteric (Roche Diagnostics)	Fourteen determinations are available through use of four constricted Beckford tubes containing slanted agar media. Two tubes provide presumptive identification of *Enterobacteriaceae* based on eight tests. Remaining two tubes, called "Expanders," provide additional tests.	R/B 1 Phenylalanine deaminase Lactose fermentation H₂S production Glucose fermentation Lysine decarboxylase R/B 2 Indole production Ornithine decarboxylase R/B Expander (1) Citrate utilization Rhamnose fermentation R/B Expander (2) DNAse production Raffinose fermentation Sorbitol fermentation Arabinose fermentation	Agar tube is stabbed with long needle, and then agar surface is streaked with same needle. Tubes are loosely capped and incubated overnight at 35° C. Color changes and read visually and compared to chart provided in kit.	Results of collaborative study indicate >90% agreement with conventional methods.

Entero-Set (Fisher Scientific Co.)	System is similar in appearance to API. Two cards have 10 miniature plastic cupules each. Cards are used as presumptive and confirmatory test series. Each cupule is inoculated with capillary pipette. Hourglass cupule shape provides anaerobic conditions in bottom sector.	*Entero-Set (1)*
		Resazurin (growth control)
		Malonate utilization
		Phenylalanine deaminase
		H₂S production
		Sucrose fermentation
		Hydrolysis of ONPG
		Lysine decarboxylase
		Ornithine decarboxylase
		Urea hydrolysis
		Indole production
		Entero-Set (2)
		Arginine dihydrolase
		Citrate utilization
		Fermentation of:
		  Salicin
		  Adonitol
		  Inositol
		  Sorbitol
		  Arabinose
		  Maltose
		  Trehalose
		  Xylose
			Single colony is transferred to 5 ml of BHI and incubated for 3 to 4 h. Growth is resuspended in 1.8 ml of H₂O, and strips are inoculated. If chambers are overfilled, significant biosafety hazard may result.	>90% agreement with conventional tests. Test results are available 3 to 4 h after incubation at 35° C.

Continued.

reactions, a computer must be used to generate the probabilities. The more organisms in the data base, the more precise will be the genus or species designations derived. All commercial suppliers of multicomponent biochemical test systems (Table 9.3) provide their customers with a computer, a computer-derived code book, or access to a telephone inquiry center for matching profile numbers to species. By adding large numbers of organisms to the data base, unusual patterns can be recognized. In some cases, new species or unusual species involved in an unsuspected epidemic have been discovered in this way.

Table 9-3

Commercially Available Kits for the Identification of *Enterobacteriaceae*—cont'd

PRODUCT NAME	DESCRIPTION	SUBSTRATE/TEST	OPERATION	COMMENTS
Micro-ID (Organon Teknika) (Plate 2, *C*)	Kit consists of 15 tests in plastic tray. Reaction chamber has inoculation part at top. Five of the chambers have both substrate and detection disk; other five have combination substrate-detection disk. Strip is sealed during incubation.	Voges-Proskauer (production of acetoin) Nitrate reduction Phenylalanine deaminase H₂S production Indole production Ornithine decarboxylase Lysine decarboxylase Malonate utilization Urea hydrolysis Esculin hydrolysis Hydrolysis of ONPG Fermentation of: Arabinose Adonitol Inositol Sorbitol	A heavy suspension (McFarland no. 1 standard) is prepared from the colony to be identified. Each chamber is inoculated with 0.2 ml, and strip is then incubated in upright position. Care must be taken so the substrate strips are moistened but the five separate detection strips remain dry. After 5 h of incubation, strip is rotated 90 degrees to moisten detection strips. Color reactions are read visually.	One of first "rapid" identification systems. Identification is based on constitutive enzyme activity and is not growth dependent. Numerous studies indicate >90% agreement with traditional methods.
Minitek (BBL Systems, Inc.)	This kit contains multiwelled plastic tray, 30 reagent disks, and assorted reagents and accessories.	Thirty substrate disks are included. Manufacturer suggests following for *Enterobacteriaceae:* Arginine Citrate Esculin H₂S Indole Lysine Malonate ONPG PDA Urea Voges-Proskauer test	Operator selects substrates to be tested and adds one disk to each of the 12 wells. Inoculum is prepared to density of McFarland no. 0.5 standard, and 50 μl is added to each well. Disks are overlaid with oil, and results are read using color comparison chart after 18 to 24 h of incubation.	>90% agreement with conventional systems. System can be used for nonfermenters and anaerobes, as well as *Enterobacteriaceae.*
Microdilution identification systems	All microdilution products have capability for identification of *Enterobacteriaceae*, as well as other organisms. Substrates are included in trays either dried or frozen. Panels for identification only or combination identification-antimicrobial susceptibility panels are available.	Most microdilution products include 20 tests similar to those in API 20E strip. There are minor differences.	Standardized inoculum is added either in very small quantity (3 to 5 μl) with disposable multipronged inoculator or as 50 to 100 μl aliquot with semiautomated inoculation device.	>90% agreement with traditional methods. One advantage is combination with antimicrobial susceptibility test.

Table 9.3

Commercially Available Kits for the Identification of *Enterobacteriaceae*—cont'd

PRODUCT NAME	DESCRIPTION	SUBSTRATE/TEST	OPERATION	COMMENTS

Enteric-Tek (Flow Laboratories)	Unlike most kits described, Enteric-Tek is a compartmented wheel with central well and 11 surrounding wedgeshaped chambers containing agar media. Fourteen tests can be performed with one wheel.	Indole production
		Tryptophan-deaminase
		H_2S production
		Citrate utilization
		Malonate utilization
		Lysine decarboxylase
		Ornithine decarboxylase
		Urea hydrolysis
		Fermentation of:
		  Glucose
		  Lactose
		  Rhamnose
		  Adonitol
		  Sorbitol
		  Arabinose
			One drop of inoculum is added to each chamber with Pasteur pipette. To provide anaerobic conditions, medium in central well and lysine and ornithine wells should be stabbed. Wheel is incubated right side up for 18 h at 35° C. Color changes are noted. Spot indole test can be performed from center well.	Agreement is >90% with conventional methods.

Quantum II (Abbott Labs)	This is multipurpose instrumental system using plastic cartridge containing 20 chambers and dual wavelength photometer.	Lysine decarboxylase
		Ornithine decarboxylase
		Urea hydrolysis
		Citrate utilization
		Malonate utilization
		Arginine dihydrolase
		Indole production
		Growth in acetamide
		Polymixin B susceptibility
		Fermentation of:
		  Lactose
		  Arabinose
		  Xylose
		  Adonitol
		  Rhamnose
		  Sucrose
		  Glucose
		  Inositol
		  Mannitol
		  Sorbitol
			Four or five isolated colonies are suspended in sterile H_2O and adjusted to McFarland no. 0.5 standard; 200 µl of inoculum is added to each chamber. Chamber is sealed and incubated for 4 to 5 h before reading.	Enterobacteriaceae identification are more accurate than those of oxidase-positive gram-negative bacilli.

From Howard, B.J., Klaas, J. II, Rubin, S.J., et al. 1987. Clinical and pathogenic microbiology, The C. V. Mosby Co., St. Louis.

REFERENCES

1. Brown, W. J. 1974. Modification of the rapid fermentation test for *Neisseria gonorrhoeae*. Appl. Microbiol. 27:1027.
2. Carlone, G.M., Valadez, M.J. and Pickett, M.J. 1983. Methods for distinguishing gram-positive from gram-negative bacteria. J. Clin. Microbiol. 16:1157.
3. Faruki, H. and Murray, P. 1986. Medium dependence for rapid detection of thermonuclease activity in blood culture broths. J. Clin. Microbiol. 24:482.
4. Halebian, S., Harris, B., Finegold, S.M., et al. 1981. Rapid method that aids in distinguishing gram-positive from gram-negative anaerobic bacteria. J. Clin. Microbiol. 13:444.
5. Hollis, D.G., Sottnek, F.O., Brown, W.J., et al. 1980. Use of the rapid fermentation test in determining carbohydrate reactions of fastidious bacteria in clinical laboratories. J. Clin. Microbiol. 12:620.

6. Kellogg, D.S. , Jr., Holmes, K.K. and Hill, G.A. 1976. Cumitech 4. Laboratory diagnosis of gonorrhea, American Society for Microbiology, Washington, D.C..
7. von Graevenitz, A. and Bucher, C. 1983. Accuracy of the KOH and vancomycin tests in determining the Gram reaction of nonenterobacterial rods. J. Clin. Microbiol. 18:983.

BIBLIOGRAPHY

Blazevic, D.N. and Ederer, G.M. 1975. Biochemical tests in diagnostic microbiology, John Wiley & Sons, New York.

D'Amato, R.F., McLaughlin, J.C., and Ferraro, M.J. 1985. Rapid manual and mechanized/automated methods for the detection and identification of bacteria and yeasts. p. 52-65. In Lennette, E.H., Balows, A., Hausler, W.J., Jr., and Shadomy, H.J., editors. Manual of clinical microbiology, ed. 4. American Society for Microbiology, Washington, D.C.

Davis, B.D., Dulbecco, R., Eizen, H.N., et al. 1980. Microbiology, Including Inmunology and Molecular Genetics, ed. 3. Harper and Row, New York.

Difco manual, ed. 10. 1984. Difco Laboratories, Detroit.

Emmons, C.W., Binnford, C.H., Utz, J.P., et al. 1977. Medical Mycology, ed. 3. Lea & Febiger, Philadelphia.

Estevez, E.G. 1984. Bacteriologic plate media: review of mechanisms in action. Lab. Med. 15:258.

Hanna, B.A. 1988. Clinical microbiology in real time: the high noon of a new era. Lab. Med. 19:292. (Entire issue devoted to automation in clinical microbiology.)

Isenberg, H.D., Washington, J.A. II, Balows, A., et al. 1985. Collection, handling, and processing of specimens. p. 73-98. In Lennette, E.H., Balows, A., Hausler, W.J., Jr., and Shadomy, H.J., editors. Manual of clinical microbiology, ed. 4. American Society for Microbiology, Washington, D.C.

Joklik, W.K. 1980. The nature, isolation, and measurement of animal viruses. In Joklik, W.K., Wilda, H.P. and Amos, D.B., editors. Zinsser's Microbiology, ed. 17. Appleton-Century-Crofts, Norwalk, Conn.

Jorgensen, J.H., editor 1987. Automation in clinical microbiology. CRC Press, Inc. Boca Raton, Fla. (Entire book devoted to automation in clinical microbiology.)

LeBeau, L.J. 1983. Roots of automation in microbiology: an introduction. Am. J. Med. Technol. 49:299.

Lennette, E.H., Balows, A., Hausler, W.J., Jr., and Shadomy, H.J., editors. 1985. Manual of clinical microbiology, ed. 4. American Society for Microbiology, Washington, D.C.

MacFaddin, J. F. 1985. Media for isolation-cultivation-identification-maintenance of medical bacteria, Williams & Wilkins, Baltimore.

Oxoid manual, ed. 5. 1982. Oxoid Ltd., Basingstoke, U.K.

Paik, G. 1980. Reagants, stains, and miscellaneous test procedures. Lennette, E.H., Balows A., Housler W.J., Jr., and Shadomy, H.J., editors. Manual of clinical microbiology, ed. 3. American Society for Microbiology, Washington, D.C..

Phillips, E. and Nash, P. 1985. Culture media. In Lennette, E.H., Balows, A., Hausler, W.J., Jr., and Shadomy, H.J., editors. Manual of clinical microbiology, ed. 4. American Society for Microbiology, Washington, D.C.

Pincus, D.H., Salkin, I.F., and McGinnis, M.R. 1988. Rapid methods in medical mycology. Lab. Med. 19:296. (Entire issue devoted to automation in clinical microbiology.)

Smith, T.F. 1981. Viruses. In Washington, J.A. II, editor. Laboratory procedures in clinical microbiology, Springer-Verlag, New York.

Sutter, V.L., Citron, D.M., Edelstein, M.A.C., et al. 1985. Wadsworth anaerobic bacteriology manual, ed. 4. Star Publishing Co., Belmont, Calif.

Washington, J.A. II, 2. editor. 1985. Laboratory procedures in clinical microbiology, ed. 2. Springer-Verlag, New York.

10 Nontraditional Methods for Identification and Detection of Pathogens or Their Products

The microbiologist has traditionally sought to isolate pathogenic organisms in pure culture in an artificial environment outside the human host. In this way, the morphology, biochemical activity, and antimicrobial susceptibility pattern of each organism could be examined and evaluated. In the case of viral diseases, identification of the pathogen required recognition of a particular cytopathic effect in a predefined cell culture medium, a criterion that demanded a high degree of sophistication in the laboratory and often a fairly long incubation period. Only by definitive identification could the cause of an infection or disease be ascertained. A second and less satisfactory method for diagnosis of disease has been the demonstration (by showing a significant rise in titer) of a specific humoral antibody response to the organism in question. For efficient serologic diagnosis, therefore, the clinician must be able to narrow down the possible causes of disease so that the appropriate antigens can be chosen to test against the patient's serum specimens, since testing sera against all possible antigens would be prohibitive. It often takes 2 weeks (or sometimes considerably longer) for antibodies to appear. As more patients survive with compromised immune systems such that their antibody production is severely curtailed or absent, the use of rising serologic titers for diagnosis has become less universally applicable. In addition, it has been shown that patients may exhibit a nonspecific rise in antibodies in response to certain antigenic stimuli, confounding the interpretation of serologic tests.

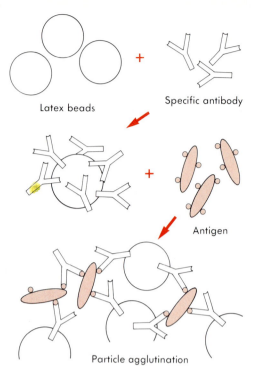

Latex beads

Specific antibody

Antigen

Particle agglutination

Figure 10.1

Alignment of antibody molecules bound to the surface of a latex particle and latex agglutination reaction.

Modern science has developed many new techniques, unthought of in the days of Pasteur, to aid laboratorians in this time of need. The needs are for more rapid specific diagnostic tests, obviating the classic waiting period for growth of microorganisms, and for tests that detect antigens of pathogens without waiting for an antibody response. This chapter briefly describes several of these new methods in a general sense. Only those methods that lend themselves to visual interpretation will be mentioned here; diagnostic microbiological methods that require an automated system or instrument for interpretation of results are discussed in Chapter 11.

10.1. Particle Agglutination

10.1.a. Latex agglutination. Antibody molecules can be bound in a random alignment to the surface of latex (polystyrene) beads (Figure 10.1). Since the number of antibody molecules bound to each latex particle is large, the potential number of antigen binding sites exposed is also large. Antigen present in a solution being tested will bind to the combining sites of the antibody exposed on the surfaces of the

latex beads, forming cross-linked aggregates of latex beads and antigen. The large size of the latex bead (0.8 μm or larger) enhances the ease with which the agglutination reaction is recognized. Levels of bacterial polysaccharides detected by latex agglutination have been shown to be as low as 0.1 ng/ml.[12] The pH, osmolarity, and ionic concentration of the solution will influence the amount of binding that occurs, so that conditions under which latex agglutination procedures are carried out must be carefully standardized. Additionally, some constituents of body fluids have been found to cause false-positive agglutination in the latex agglutination systems available. To counteract this problem, it is recommended that all specimens be pretreated by boiling or with ethylene diamine tetraacetic acid (EDTA) to extract the antigen before testing, as suggested for cerebrospinal fluid and outlined in Chapter 15. A similar pretreatment protocol is included as a standard step in the procedure in some of the commercial systems. Commercial systems should be used intact, following the manufacturer's recommendations, to ensure accurate results. Either a solid, particulate antigen, such as whole bacteria, or soluble antigen, such as capsular polysaccharide, can cause particle agglutination. Microorganisms or their antigenic determinants for which commercial latex agglutination reagents are available are shown in the box on p. 129. As a measure of the widespread adaptation of this technology is the fact that at least a dozen products are available for identification of *Staphylococcus aureus* by particle agglutination (latex agglutination or coagglutination, next section). Some of the more widely used individual products are discussed in those chapters that deal with the organisms being sought. Latex tests for the detection of several bacterial toxins, including enterotoxins of *Vibrio cholerae*, *S. aureus*, *Clostridium perfringens*, and *Escherichia coli*; the staphylococcal toxic shock syndrome toxin, and a *Clostridium difficile*–related protein in stool supernatant are available commercially.

10.1.b. Coagglutination. Similar to latex agglutination, coagglutination utilizes antibody bound to a particle to enhance visibility of the agglutination reaction between antigen and antibody. In this case, the particles are killed and treated *S. aureus* organisms (Cowan I strain), which contain a large amount of an antibody-binding protein, **protein A,** in their cell walls. In contrast to latex particles, these staphylococci bind only the base of the heavy chain portion

---

Infectious Agents for Which Latex Particle Agglutination Tests are Available Commercially

Bacteria

Campylobacter species (*coli, fetus, jejuni, laridis*)
E. coli
Haemophilus influenzae type b
Mycoplasma pneumoniae
Neisseria meningitidis
Neiserria gonorrhoeae
Proteus species
Rickettsia species
Salmonella species
Shigella species
Staphylococcus aureus
Streptococcus pneumoniae
Streptococcus pyogenes
Streptococcus agalactiae
Other beta hemolytic streptococci

Fungi

Candida albicans
Coccidioides immitis
Cryptococcus neoformans
Histoplasma capsulatum
Sporothrix schenckii

Parasites

Toxoplasma gondii
Trichinella spiralis

Viruses

Adenovirus
Cytomegalovirus
Herpes simplex virus
Human immunodeficiency virus (HIV)
Rotavirus

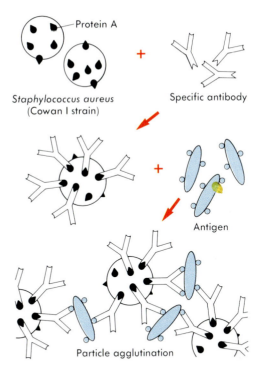

Figure 10.2
Coagglutination.

orrhoeae, and *Haemophilus influenzae* types a to f. The coagglutination reaction is highly specific but may not be as sensitive for detecting small quantities of antigen as is latex agglutination.

10.1.c. Liposome-enhanced latex agglutination. Phospholipid molecules form small closed vesicles under certain controlled conditions. These vesicles, consisting of a single lipid bilayer, are called **liposomes.** Molecules bound to the surface of liposomes act as agglutinating particles in a reaction. By combining liposomes containing reactive molecules on their surfaces and latex particles that harbor antibody-binding sites on their surfaces, reagents are created that have the potential to transform a rather weak antigen-antibody particle agglutination reaction into a stronger, more easily visualized reaction (Figure 10.3). Liposomes have yet to reach their full potential as diagnostic reagents in clinical microbiology.

10.1.d. Lectin assays. Certain proteins or glycoproteins produced as natural biological structural components by various plants and animals, called **lectins,** have the capability of binding sugars and carbohydrates to form stable complexes.[4] Lectins,

of the antibody, leaving both antigen-binding ends free to form complexes with specific antigen (Figure 10.2). Several commercial suppliers have prepared coagglutination reagents for identification of streptococci, including Lancefield groups A, B, C, D, F, G, and N, *S. pneumoniae*, *N. meningitidis*, *N. gon-*

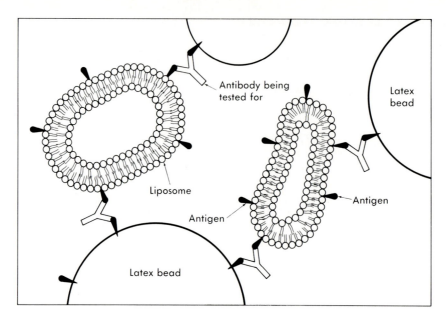

Figure 10.3
Diagram of liposome-latex agglutination reaction.

then, can bind to surface components of bacterial and fungal cells that contain these receptors. Although the exact nature of the binding reaction is unknown, various lectins have been found to bind specifically to species of bacteria and fungi (Table 10-1). Lectins can be conjugated to fluorescent and enzymatic markers to create stable diagnostic reagents. Lectin reagents are not widely available at this time but they are potentially useful.

10.2. Enzyme-Linked Immunosorbent Assay (ELISA)

ELISA systems were first developed during the 1960s by investigators searching for a substitute for radioimmunoassay procedures. The basic ELISA detection system consists of antibodies bonded to enzymes that remain able to catalyze a reaction that yields a visually discernible end product while attached to the antibody. Furthermore, the antibody-binding sites remain free to react with their specific antigen.[3] The use of enzymes as labels has several advantages. The enzyme itself is not changed during activity; it can catalyze the reaction of a large number of substrate molecules, greatly expanding the reaction and thus enhancing the possibility of detection. Enzyme-conjugated substrates are quite stable, unlike radioactive substrates, and can be stored for

Table 10.1

Examples of Lectins Known to Bind to Specific Microbes

LECTIN	MICROBE
Wheat germ agglutinin (*Triticum vulgaris*)	*N. gonorrhoeae*
Soybean agglutinin (*Glycine max*)	*Bacillus anthracis*
Hairy vetch lectin (*Vicia villosa*)	*Trypanosoma rangeli*
Concanavalin A	*Leishmania donovani* promastigotes
Snail agglutinin (*Cepaea hortensis*)	*Streptococcus agalactiae*

relatively long time periods. Additionally, the formation of a colored end product allows direct observation of the reaction or measurement with a simple instrument. There are many aspects of ELISA testing to consider. Excellent discussions of methodology and possible future developments are presented by Yolken[14] and by Meier and Hill.[10] The use of monoclonal antibodies (see section 10.6) has helped increase the specificity of currently available ELISA assays. New ELISA tests are being developed rapidly for detection of etiologic agents, their products, or antibodies. In some instances, such as detection of respiratory syncytial virus, HIV, and certain adenoviruses, ELISA assays are thought to be more sensitive than current culture methods.[7,13] Although several ELISA tests have been developed for visual reading of results, most systems rely on automated spectrophotometric reading of end points. The instruments used for such readings are discussed in Chapter 11. ELISA methodology is arguably the fastest growing new technology in diagnostic microbiology. Individual test systems will be discussed as they relate to specific etiologic agents.

10.2.a. **Solid phase immunoassay (SPIA).** Most ELISA systems developed for detection of infectious agents consist of antibody directed against the agent in question firmly fixed to a solid matrix, either the inside of the wells of a microdilution tray or the outside of a spherical plastic or metal bead, or some other solid matrix. Such systems are called **solid-phase immunosorbent assays (SPIA).** If antigen is present in the fluid to be tested, stable antigen-antibody complexes form when the fluid is added to the matrix. Washing steps to remove nonspecifically adsorbed molecules are very important in ELISA tests. A second antibody against the antigen being sought is then added to the system. This antibody has been complexed to an enzyme, such as alkaline phosphatase or horseradish peroxidase, that catalyzes a reaction that yields a colored end point. If the antigen is present on the solid matrix, it will now bind the second antibody, forming a sandwich with antigen in the middle. After washing has removed unbound labeled antibody, the addition of the substrates for the enzyme completes the reaction, and the visually detectable end point will appear wherever the enzyme is present (Figure 10.4). Because of the expanding nature of the reaction, even minute amounts of antigen (<1 ng/ml) can be detected. The system just described requires a specific enzyme-labeled antibody for each antigen tested. It is simpler to use an indirect assay that uses a second unlabeled antibody to bind to the antigen-antibody complex on the matrix. A third antibody, labeled with enzyme and directed against the nonvariable Fc portion of the unlabeled second antibody, can then be used as the detection marker for a number of different antigen-antibody complexes.

10.2.b. **Membrane-bound SPIA.** The flowthrough and large surface area characteristics of nitrocellulose, nylon, or other membranes can be exploited to enhance the speed and sensitivity of ELISA reactions.[6] The presence of absorbent material below the membrane can serve to pull the liquid reactants through the membrane and help to separate non-reacted components from the antigen-antibody complexes bound to the membrane and simplify the washing steps. Membrane-bound SPIA assays are available for detection of group A beta hemolytic streptococci antigen directly from throat swabs (Figure 10.5), as well as for detection of several antibodies in serum. They are expected to become more prevalent for physicians' office laboratory and home testing systems, in addition to clinical laboratories.

10.3. Fluorogenic Substrates

A fluorophore is a compound that absorbs light of a short, excitatory wavelength and emits light of a longer wavelength. The emitted, fluorescent light can be seen visually and can be measured quantitatively by special photometers called fluorometers.[5] Fluorophores are used in biological reactions by binding them to a substrate, which effectively inhibits their fluorescence. When the substrate is acted on, such as by the metabolic enzymes of microorganisms, the fluorophore is released and fluoresces under ultraviolet or other shortwave light. Substrate-fluorophore combinations are stable and allow the detection of tiny amounts of reactants. The first practical test utilizing this technology was the MUG test (4-methylumbelliferyl-β-D-glucuronide) for rapid identification of *E. coli*. The enzyme β-glucuronidase, produced by *E. coli* and a few species of *Salmonella* and *Shigella*, breaks the bond holding MUG together and releases the potent fluorophore 4-methylumbelliferone. By observing the fluorescence, microbiologists can identify the organism, often within 30 minutes. Commercially available MUG tests have been found to be specific and convenient. Other fluorophores, including luminol, 7-methyl-coumarin amide, and naphthylamine, are being investigated as diagnostic reagents. Quantitative measurements of fluorescence inhibition by bacteria in the presence of antimicrobial agents is available as a rapid alternative method for susceptibility testing.[8] At least for Enterobacteriaceae, this method has correlated well with standard methods. Fluorophores can be coupled to most nucleic acid probes and immunoassay reagents in the same way as enzymes are coupled. The potential exists for developing more sensitive detection systems with such fluorescent markers.

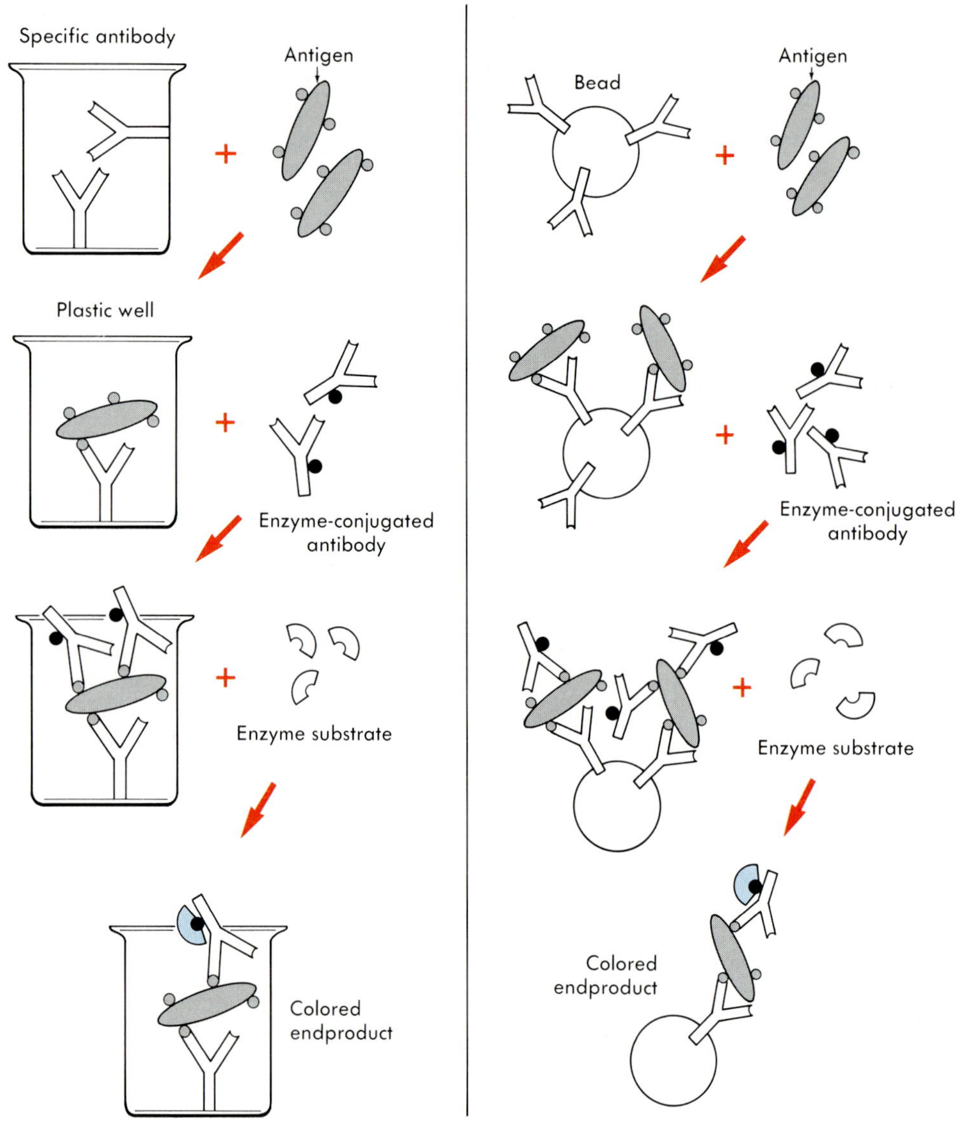

Figure 10.4
Principle of solid-phase enzyme immunosorbent assay.

10.4. Countercurrent Immunoelectrophoresis (CIE)

With some exceptions (e.g., *S. pneumoniae* serotypes 7 and 14), most bacterial antigens are negatively charged in a slightly alkaline environment, while antibodies are neutral. This principle is exploited by CIE assays, in which solutions of antibody and body fluid to be tested are placed in small wells cut into a slab of agarose (a gelatinlike matrix through which molecules can diffuse readily) on a glass sur-

face (Figure 10.6). A paper or fiber wick is used to connect the two opposite sides of the agarose to troughs of buffer, formulated for each antibody-antigen system. When an electric current is applied through the buffer, the negatively charged antigen molecules migrate toward the positive electrode and thus toward the wells filled with antibody. The neutrally charged antibodies are carried toward the negative electrode by the flow of the slightly alkaline buffer. At some point between the wells a zone of

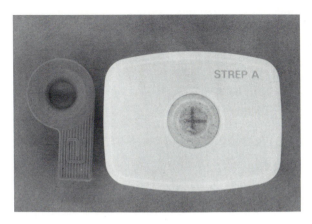

Figure 10.5
Membrane-bound SPIA assay for detection of group A streptococcal cell wall antigen. (Courtesy Abbott Diagnostics.)

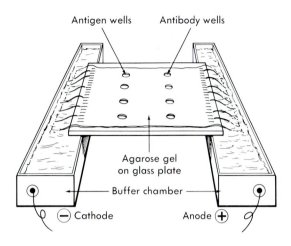

Figure 10.6
Apparatus for performing counterimmunoelectrophoresis.

equivalence occurs, and the antigen-antibody complexes form a visible precipitin band (Figure 10.7). The entire procedure usually takes about 1 hour. Any antigens for which antisera are available can be tested by CIE. The sensitivity appears to be less than that of agglutination, detecting approximately 0.01 to 0.05 mg/ml antigen, which translates to about 10^3 organisms per milliliter of fluid. Bands are often difficult to see, and the agarose gel may require overnight washing in distilled water to remove non-specific precipitin reactions. Testing positive and negative controls is especially critical, since sera may contain nonspecifically reacting agents that form nonstable complexes in the gel. CIE is more expensive (because of the initial capital outlay and the large quantities of antigen and antibody that must be used) than either latex particle agglutination or coagglutination.

10.5. *Limulus* Amebocyte Lysate (LAL) Assay

Within the hemolymph (bloodlike circulating fluid) of the horseshoe crab, *Limulus polyphemus*, are numerous circulating cells called amebocytes. It was found by Levin and Bang in 1964 that the lysate of these amebocytes would gel in the presence of minute amounts of lipopolysaccharide (endotoxin) from the cell walls of gram-negative bacteria. The test for gelation of this material, known as the *Limulus* amebocyte lysate (LAL) assay, has been used by industry to detect gram-negative bacterial contamination in a wide range of products, including injectables and

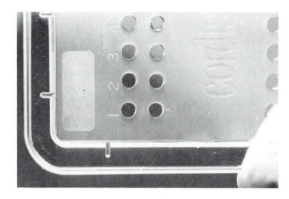

Figure 10.7
Precipitin band in row 1 formed between antigen well on left and antibody well on right.

other parenterally administered products, and has been modified for use with body fluids from patients to detect circulating endotoxin, a tangible sign of gram-negative bacterial infection. The gelation of the lysate is specific for endotoxin and sensitive to <0.1 ng of endotoxin per milliliter. Kits for performing the test, including special endotoxin-free tubes and diluent, are commercially available.

Fluids that have been tested by the LAL assay include cerebrospinal fluid, plasma and serum, joint fluid, urine, and cervical and urethral discharge from patients with gonorrhea. Problems of nonspecific positive reactions, particularly with plasma and serum, have precluded its routine use in most clinical laboratory situations. Performance of the LAL assay requires meticulous attention to technique, as any contaminating endotoxin (such as is found in almost all tap water and often in washed glassware) will yield a false-positive result.

10.6. Monoclonal Antibodies: Preparation and Utilization

One of the largest drawbacks to any of the systems that utilize antibodies as reagents has been the requirement for large quantities of rather pure, high avidity, high affinity antibody molecules. Previous technologies thus required immunization of either many small animals or several large animals with the antigen being sought, repeated bleedings, and subsequent purification of the antigen elicited. Different animals reacted with different antibody responses to the same antigen, resulting in a lack of uniform reagents and the necessity to continually retest the antibody for reactivity in a given system. Additionally, some antigens, such as *N. meningitidis* group B, were poor immunogens, and good antibodies were impossible to obtain in any quantity. The ability to create an immortal cell line, producing large quantities of a completely characterized and highly specific antibody, known as a **monoclonal antibody,** has revolutionized the science of immunologic testing. Monoclonal antibodies are produced by the daughter cells (clones) of a single hybrid cell, the product of fusion of an antibody-producing plasma cell and an immortal malignant antibody-producing myeloma cell from a plasma cell precursor. One technique for the production of such a clone of cells, called **hybridoma** cells, is illustrated in Figure 10.8. A mouse is immunized with the antigen for which an antibody is to be created. The animal responds by producing many antibodies to the antigenic determinants injected. The mouse's spleen, which contains antibody-producing plasma cells, is removed and emulsified so that single antibody-producing cells can be separated and placed into individual wells of a microdilution tray. These cells cannot remain viable in cell culture for very long. They must be fused together with cells that are able to survive and multiply in tissue culture, the immortal cells of **multiple myeloma** (malignant tumor of antibody-producing plasma cells). The special myeloma tumor cells used for hybridoma production possess a very important defect, however. They are deficient in the enzyme hypoxanthine phosphoribosyltransferase. This defect leads to their inability to survive in a medium containing hypoxanthine, aminopterin, and thymi-

dine (HAT medium). Antibody-producing spleen cells, however, possess the enzyme. Thus, fused hybridoma cells survive in the selective medium and can be recognized by their ability to grow indefinitely in the medium. Unfused antibody-producing lymphoid cells will die after several multiplications in vitro because they are not immortal, and unfused myeloma cells will die in the presence of the toxic enzyme substrates. The only surviving cells will be true "hybrids." The growth medium supernatant from the microdilution tray wells in which the hybridoma cells are growing is then tested for the presence of the desired antibody. Many such cell lines are usually examined before a suitable antibody is found, since it must be specific enough to bind only the type of antigen to be tested, but not so specific that it binds only the antigen from the particular strain with which the mouse was first immunized. When a good candidate antibody-producing cell is found, the hybridoma cells are either cultured in large numbers in cell cultures in vitro, or they are reinjected into the peritoneal cavities of many mice, where the cells multiply and produce large quantities of antibody in the ascitic fluid that is formed. Ascitic fluid can be removed from mice many times over the animal's lifetime. Since all of the cells are derived from a single cell producing one antibody molecule type, the antibody is called **monoclonal.**

Monoclonal antibodies have been successfully used in commercial systems for the detection of numerous infectious agents. For example, a monoclonal antibody to a protein of *Chlamydia. trachomatis* has been conjugated to a fluorescent dye, allowing the visual detection, under fluorescence microscopy, of the elementary bodies and inclusions present in clinical material from patients infected with chlamydiae. Monoclonal antibodies to the *N. meningitidis* group B capsular polysaccharide have been bound to latex particles to create a reagent that can detect the presence of this organism in cerebrospinal fluid, urine, and other body fluids. Many other commercial products utilizing monoclonal antibodies are available.

10.7. Genetic Probes: Preparation and Utilization

Potentially even more specific than antibody reagents are nucleic acid probes, discrete sequences of single-stranded DNA or RNA that form strong covalently bonded hybrids with the specific complementary strand of nucleic acid.[11] Methods are available that allow isolation of nucleic acid sequences

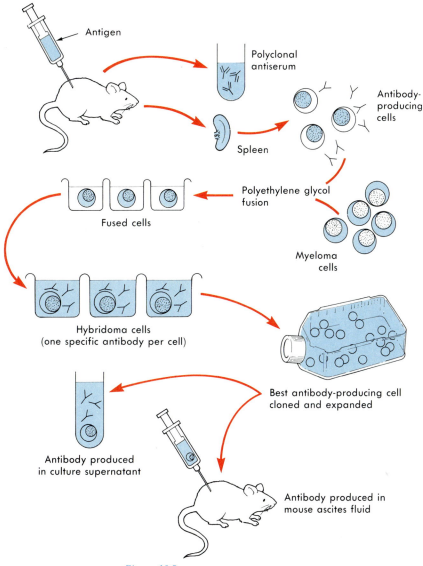

Figure 10.8
Production of a monoclonal antibody.

from cultures of clones of a known bacterial species that constitute a single gene or locus, specific for the whole species or a gene that is common to all pathogenic organisms within the species. An example of a method for preparation of a DNA probe for a segment of the chromosome of a virus is illustrated in Figure 10.9. The chromosomal nucleic acid from a prototype virus is released by lysing the virions. Bacterial endonuclease restriction enzymes are used to cut the DNA into small segments, which are inserted into a circular strand of plasmid DNA. The plasmid has been chosen for its ability to multiply to large numbers once it has entered the cytoplasm of its bacterial host cell. The expanded plasmids are released from the bacteria and isolated based on their molecular weight and charge. The particular fragments of DNA that match that found in the virus are then isolated by using the same restriction endonucleases, purified, and labeled with either a **radioisotope** (often ^{32}P) or **biotin,** a small molecule that can be covalently bound to the DNA without destroying its ability to hybridize with complementary DNA. The biotinylation method of labeling nucleic acid probes was developed as recently as 1981 by

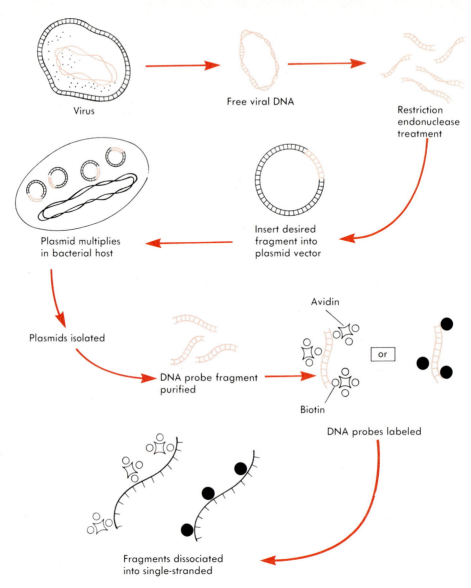

Virus

Free viral DNA

Restriction endonuclease treatment

Insert desired fragment into plasmid vector

Plasmid multiplies in bacterial host

Plasmids isolated

DNA probe fragment purified

Avidin

Biotin

or

DNA probes labeled

Fragments dissociated into single-stranded

Figure 10.9

Production of a radioactive or biotin-avidin–labeled single-stranded nucleic acid probe for a specific segment of DNA from a specific virus. The isolated viral DNA is inserted into a plasmid vector, which is expanded by multiplication within a bacterial host.

Langer and coworkers.[9] Bacterial or eukaryotic organism nucleic acid can be isolated and cloned as well. The material to be tested (either a culture of unknown microorganism or clinical material that may contain the organisms being sought) is usually affixed to a solid matrix, typically some sort of filter.[2] After the material suspected of containing the gene or nucleic acid sequence being sought has been applied, the filter is treated to render the double-stranded DNA single-stranded. The probe, a small piece of labeled single-stranded DNA, is then allowed to react with the material on the filter. If complementary sequences are present, the probe DNA will form strong bonds and remain on the filter, even when the filter is washed extensively to remove unbound DNA and nonspecifically bound DNA (Figure 10.10). The labeled DNA probe is now treated to allow visualization (Figure 10.11). If the

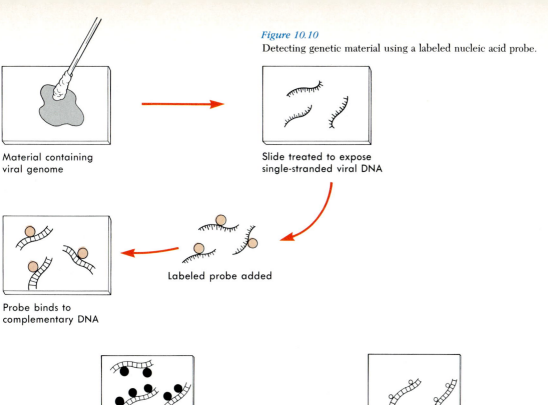

Figure 10.10
Detecting genetic material using a labeled nucleic acid probe.

Material containing
viral genome

Slide treated to expose
single-stranded viral DNA

Labeled probe added

Probe binds to
complementary DNA

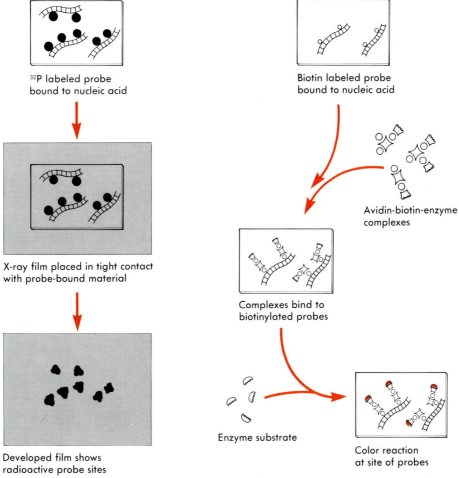

^{32}P labeled probe
bound to nucleic acid

X-ray film placed in tight contact
with probe-bound material

Developed film shows
radioactive probe sites

Biotin labeled probe
bound to nucleic acid

Avidin-biotin-enzyme
complexes

Complexes bind to
biotinylated probes

Enzyme substrate

Color reaction
at site of probes

Figure 10.11
Detection of labeled nucleic acid probe using radiography or colorimetric enzymatic detection system.

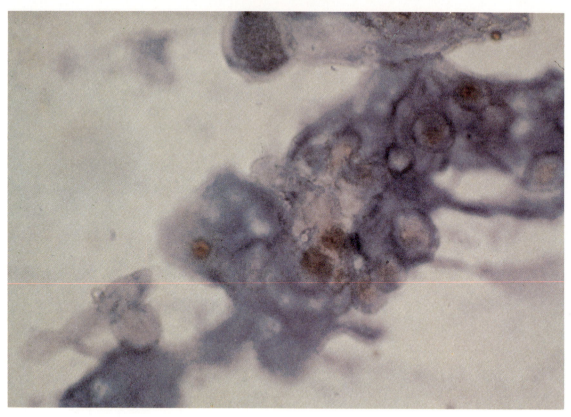

Figure 10.12
Direct detection of herpes simplex virus on a vaginal smear. A herpes simplex–specific biotinylated
DNA probe (Enzo Biochem) complexes to homologous viral DNA sequences in the nuclei of infected
cells. Avidin complexed to horseradish peroxidase serves as the visual marker, causing the nuclei of
infected cells to appear red. (Courtesy Enzo Biochem, Inc.)

label is radioactive, the filter is covered with a piece of film; the film develops a dark spot wherever the bound probe is present on the filter underneath. In the case of biotin-labeled probes, a second protein, avidin, which binds tightly to biotin, is added to the matrix. Avidin can be attached to a number of different marker materials, including enzymes such as horseradish peroxidase, alkaline phosphatase, fluorescent dyes, radioisotope-labeled molecules, or electron-dense markers like ferritin. Thus the exact location of the bound DNA probe can be determined by the visualization of the avidin-bound marker. Figure 10.12 illustrates the use of a biotin–avidin–horseradish peroxidase probe to detect the antigen of herpes simplex virus in infected cells on a filter.

Advantages of the nucleic acid probe systems include the ability of the DNA probe to detect se-quences among a mixture of many other genes and molecules, the stability of DNA (allowing the material to remain on the filter for a long period before the test must be performed), and the ability of the probe to detect DNA from nonviable material. For example, a drop of fecal material may be placed on a filter, allowed to dry, and the filter then can be carried or mailed to a distant laboratory for testing at some future date. Conversely, because growth is not necessary, the material can be tested immediately. The biotin-avidin system obviates the need for radioactive materials, but it is not as sensitive. Problems with cross-reactivity and sensitivity still exist.[1] Many workers are actively seeking ways to improve this technology, including the use of fluorogenic markers. One company has developed a new approach utilizing ribosomal RNA detection that has significantly increased sensitivity and speed, can

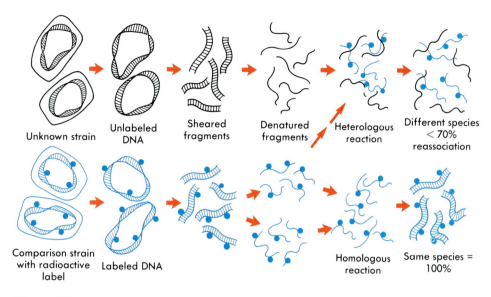

Figure 10.13
DNA-DNA hybridization to determine the amount of relatedness between the genomes of two bacterial clones.

give quantitative results, and does not require a solid matrix for testing.

10.8. Nucleic Acid Hybridization

Another development that utilizes much of the same technology as that described for genetic probes is DNA or nucleic acid hybridization. Used primarily to determine the relatedness of two different bacterial clones, this method exploits the ability of single-stranded DNA to bind to complementary sequences. Clones from a single colony of a known bacterium are grown in a medium containing radiolabeled substrates that are incorporated into the bacterial DNA during growth, often using a method called **nick translation**. These known bacteria are then lysed to release their DNA, which is treated with endonucleases to cleave it into small fragments. These fragments are then heated or chemically treated to cause them to dissociate and become single-stranded. The bacteria to be compared to the known strain are cloned, cultured in unlabeled media, and attached to a filter matrix and treated so that their double-stranded DNA also dissociates into single strands. The known labeled fragments of single-stranded DNA are allowed to react with the DNA of the unknown strain on the filter, and unbound DNA is washed off. The labeled DNA pieces will bind (or hybridize) only to DNA that is an exact

match, so the amount of labeled DNA left on the filter after washing will define how closely related the genetic material of the two strains is. One type of such an assay is called a *dot blot* hybridization assay. If both clones are derived from the same original colony, there should be 100% relatedness. Workers have defined a species as those bacteria with very similar morphologic and biochemical characteristics that exhibit $\geq$ 70% genetic relatedness by DNA-DNA hybridization (Figure 10.13).

DNA hybridization technology has been used extensively to determine the relatedness of bacterial clones. It is in this manner that many species of bacteria have been characterized and given new designations. As a consequence, several historically characterized species have been broken down into many different new species, such as some groups within the genus *Enterobacter*, and other species have been combined (for example, all *Salmonella* species have been shown to be so closely related genetically that they belong to a single species). By using these new tools, scientists will probably redefine many of the bacterial taxa that are familiar to microbiologists and physicians. It is likely that confusion over nomenclature will continue for years to come.

10.8.a. Southern blot assays. Very specific DNA sequences can be detected using hybridization techniques with an assay known as **Southern blot**. DNA to be hybridized is first cleaved by restriction endonucleases and then the pieces are separated on the basis of size and charge by **agarose gel electrophoresis**. These fragments are transferred to a nitrocellulose membrane that is laid over the gel. When this membrane is allowed to react with labeled probe, only the fragment containing the specific sequence of DNA that hybridizes the probe will be detected. This method is currently too difficult for routine clinical laboratory diagnosis, but a variation (the **Western blot**) is being used as a confirmatory test for HIV infection in many laboratories.

10.8.b. Western blot assays. The DNA (or RNA) of a particular etiologic agent is treated with endonucleases or the protein components of an agent are treated with proteinases to create fragments of different size. The nucleic acid or protein fragments are separated by agarose gel electrophoreses, and the patterns are then blotted onto nitrocellulose as in the Southern hybridization assay. The filter paper containing specific nucleic acids or proteins is then allowed to react with antiserum from a patient or animal suspected of containing antibodies against the agent. If present, antibodies will bind to the protein or nucleic acid against which they were created, and they can then be detected by visual methods for the detection of antibodies (such as enzyme-labeled probes and fluorescent markers). Very specific assays for the presence of antibodies have been developed using Western blot methodology.

10.9. Future Uses of New Technology

By using the technological methods described, either singly or in combination, microbiologists will be able to diagnose many infections without the time-consuming requirement of culturing the pathogen in the laboratory. The development of nucleic acid probes for gene-size sequences of DNA and the ability to create infinite amounts of antibody of great specificity offer to students of infectious diseases the promise of exquisitely sensitive and specific reagents. It is currently possible to detect the presence of the gene that codes for resistance to a particular antibiotic in nonviable bacteria that have been affixed to a filter. Even the ability of certain colonies of bacteria to produce a particular toxin can be detected with DNA probe methods.

Recently, microbiologists have begun to use dot-blot assays for detection of particular nucleic acid sequences in clinical material deposited on the filter paper matrix directly. Presence of organisms as diverse as *Mobiluncus* species, mycobacteria, and cytomegalovirus have been detected with dot-blot assays. The future of microbiology is certain to include a large number of non-growth-dependent rapid testing methods for the presence of pathogens in clinical specimens. Many of these methods will make use of the technological breakthroughs described, often combined with instruments to further automate the processes. Microbiologists, who have traditionally taken great pride in the fact that their judgment and interpretation are still necessary for laboratory diagnosis of infectious diseases, will have to learn to trust results obtained by nontraditional approaches, sacrificing the satisfaction of seeing colonies and cytopathic effect for the worthwhile goal of better patient care through more rapid diagnosis. However, there will always be a place for traditional microbiology.

REFERENCES

1. Ambinder, R.F., Charache, P., Staal, S., et al. 1986. The vector homology problem in diagnostic nucleic acid hybridization of clinical specimens. J. Clin. Microbiol. 24:16.
2. Carrow, E, and Folds, J.D. 1987. Recombinant DNA methods in diagnostic microbiology. Lab. Management March:31.
3. Carter, J.H. 1984. Enzyme immunoassays: practical aspects of their methodology. J. Clin. Immunol. 7:64.
4. Doyle, R.J, and Keller, K.F. 1986. Lectins in the clinical microbiology laboratory. Clin. Microbiol. Newsletter 8:157.
5. Grist, R. 1987. Fluorogenics: a new application of an old technology. Clin. Microbiol. Newsletter 9:57.
6. Hendry, R.M, and Herrmann, J.E. 1984. Immobilization of antibodies on nylon for use in enzyme-linked immunoassay. J. Immunol. Methods 67:21.
7. Jackson, J.B, and Balfour, H.H., Jr. 1988. Practical diagnostic testing of human immunodeficiency virus. Rev. Clin. Microbiol. 1:124.
8. Jorgenson, J.H. 1987. Instrument systems which provide rapid (3- to 6-hour) antibiotic susceptibility results. p. 85-97. In Jorgenson, J.H., editor. Automation in Clinical Microbiology, CRC Press, Boca Raton, Fla.
9. Langer, P.R., Waldrop, A.A, and Ward, D.C. 1981. Enzymatic synthesis of biotin-labeled polynucleotides: novel nucleic acid affinity probes. Proc. Natl. Acad. Sci. U.S.A. 78:6633.
10. Meier, F.A, and Hill, H.R. 1987. Automation of antigen detection in infectious disease diagnosis. p. 101-120. In Jorgenson, J.H., editor. Automation in Clinical Microbiology, CRC Press, Boca Raton, Fla.

11. Tenover, F.C. 1988. Diagnostic deoxyribonucleic acid probes for infectious diseases. Clin. Microbiol. Rev. 1:82.

12. Tilton, R.C. 1987. Microbial antigen detection. p. 693-702. In Wentworth, B.B., editor. Diagnostic Procedures for Bacterial Infections, ed. 7. American Public Health Association, Washington, D.C.

13. Welliver, R.C. 1988. Detection, pathogenesis, and therapy of respiratory syncytial virus infections. Rev. Clin. Microbiol. 1:27.

14. Yolken, R.H. 1985. Solid-phase enzyme immunoassays for the detection of microbial antigens in body fluids. In Lennette, E.H., Balows, A., Hausler, W.J., Jr, and Shadomy, H.J., editors. Manual of Clinical Microbiology, ed. 4. American Society for Microbiology, Washington, D.C.

BIBLIOGRAPHY

Berry, A.J, and Peter, J.B. 1984. DNA probes for infectious disease. Diagn. Med. 7:62.

Conway de Macario, E, and Macario, A.J.L. 1983. Monoclonal antibodies for bacterial identification and taxonomy. Am. Soc. Microbiol. News 49:1.

Edberg, S.C. 1987. Nucleic acid probes. pp. 715-726. In Wentworth, B.B., editor. Diagnostic procedures for bacterial infections, ed. 7. American Public Health Association Washington, D.C..

Tompkins, L.S. 1985. DNA methods in clinical microbiology. In Lennette, E.H., Balows, A., Hausler, W.J., Jr, and Shadomy, H.J., editors. Manual of clinical microbiology, ed. 4. American Society for Microbiology, Washington, D.C.

11

Principles of Automated Methods for Diagnostic Microbiology

Since Isenberg and colleagues[7] pioneered the development of an automated system for antimicrobial susceptibility testing in the 1960s, the acceptance and utilization of instrumentation for clinical microbiology have become realities. More than one third of all hospital microbiology laboratories now use an automated method (Bactec, Johnston Laboratories) for detecting positive blood cultures. Many other instruments for the identification and susceptibility testing of microorganisms, the detection of antigens and microbial products in human clinical material, and the measurement of antimicrobial agents in body fluids are being used in laboratories throughout the United States and Europe. Some of the more commonly used instruments with applications directly related to diagnostic microbiology are mentioned in this chapter. Since the field is expanding so rapidly, not all systems will be mentioned. In addition to outlining the principles employed by some of the new microbiology instruments, we will mention some of the promising new directions that are being explored for diagnosis of infectious diseases.

11.1. Basic Principles Employed by Common Automated Systems for Detection and Identification of Viable Pathogens (Table 11.1)

11.1.a. Turbidity as an indicator of growth. Pasteur initially made use of the fact that microbes would multiply in liquid medium until their presence could be detected visually as an increase in turbidity. Turbidity is actually the ability of particles in suspension to refract and deflect light rays passing through the

Table 11.1

Automated Microbiology Systems That Measure Growth or Metabolism

PRINCIPLE	APPLICATION(S)	INSTRUMENT(S)
Nephelometry or colorimetry (cuvettes)	Growth detection, identification, susceptibilities	Autobac IDX-C (Organon Teknika) AutoMicrobic System (Vitek Systems) MS-2 (Abbott Laboratories) Uniscept (Analytab Products) Quantum II (Abbott Laboratories)
Nephelometry or colorimetry (microdilution format)	Identification, susceptibilities	Micro-Coder (Micro-Media Systems) MicroScan, AutoScan, and TouchScan (Baxter/American MicroScan) Pasco (Difco Laboratories) Precept (Austin Biological Laboratories) Sceptor (Becton-Dickinson) Sensititre (Radiometer America/Sensititre) Uniscept (Analytab Products)
Video image analysis (cuvettes)	Identification, susceptibilities	Aladin (Analytab Products)
Radiometric or spectrophotometric detection of metabolites	Growth detection, identification, susceptibilities	Bactec (Johnston Laboratories) BacT-Alert (Organon-Teknika)
Impedance changes for detection of growth	Growth detection	Malthus AT (Radiometer America/Sensititre)

suspension, such that the light is reflected back into the eyes of the observer. Some of the instruments that measure turbidity determine the optical density (OD), a measurement of turbidity, by comparing the amount of light that passes through the suspension (the percent transmittance) to the amount of light passing through a control suspension without particles. A photoelectric sensor, or photometer, converts the light that impinges on its surface to an electrical impulse, which can be quantified. A second type of turbidity measurement is obtained by **nephelometry,** or light scatter. In this case, the photometers are placed at angles to the suspension, and the scattered light, generated by a laser or incandescent bulb, is measured. The amount of light scattered is dependent on the number and size of the particles in suspension. Turbidity measurements are used to determine whether an organism is present in a clinical specimen (such as in the detection of clinically significant urinary tract infections by the MS-2 and Avantage instruments of Abbott Laboratories, the AutoMicrobic System of Vitek Systems, and the Autobac IDX of Organon-Teknika) or to determine whether a particular strain of bacterium or yeast can grow in the presence of specific growth inhibitors, including antimicrobial agents. In the case of the Autobac IDX, the substrates are introduced into medium in cuvettes by elution from filter paper disks; the other systems use lyophilized substrates. Most automated susceptibility testing systems make use of turbidometric or nephelometric measurements of growth.

For measurement of turbidity of a suspension to be accurate, the particles must either remain in suspension or must be agitated before measurement if the photometers are aimed horizontally. Automated systems that utilize turbidity measurements usually must include an automated agitation device. The Autobac IDX, Avantage, and MS-2 systems, all of which use cuvettes containing growth medium, utilize an incubator-shaker module. Another way to circumvent the problem is to measure the turbidity in the medium from the bottom. Those susceptibility testing systems that employ microdilution plates have adopted this method. For example, the MicroScan system uses fiberoptics to deliver an equal amount of light to the bottom of each microdilution well; the light transmitted is determined by photometric measurements from above (Figure 11.1). Other systems may use a single light source and move all wells of the microdilution plate through its path.

Certain systems quantitate the number of microorganisms in the specimen by turbidity measurements. The AutoMicrobic System (Vitek Systems), for example, pulls body fluid such as urine into the

To signal processor

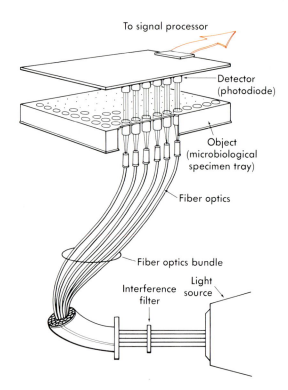

Detector (photodiode)

Object (microbiological specimen tray)

Fiber optics

Fiber optics bundle

Light source

Interference filter

Figure 11.1

Diagram of delivery of light to microdilution wells by fiberoptics, as utilized by MicroCoder identification and susceptibility testing system (MicroScan).

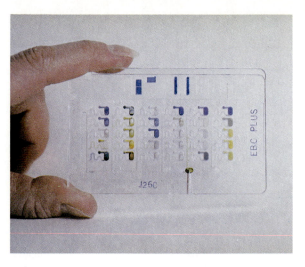

Figure 11.2

Plastic card containing dried substrate in tiny wells. The tray is filled with a suspension of urine or an organism by vacuum suction, incubated and interpreted automatically (AutoMicrobic System, Vitek Systems).

growth wells on a plastic card (Figure 11.2) by suction (another instrument is necessary to fill the cards). The wells are arranged in such a way that the body fluid is serially diluted as it fills successive wells. After a relatively short incubation period, the turbidity in the wells is measured and compared to wells containing no growth substances. The ability of an organism to grow in only certain wells is then used to determine the number of colony-forming units (CFU) present in the initial specimen. Susceptibilities can be determined by inoculating a suspension of the isolated organism into a second card of antimicrobial agent-containing wells and measuring turbidity after incubation. A classic 1975 paper by Thornsberry and others[21] describes parameters to examine in evaluating an automated susceptibility testing system.

11.1.b. Colorimetric determinations for microbial identification. Several systems use a modification of conventional biochemical testing that relies on the color changes of pH indicators in media to indicate the presence of metabolic end products. The

change in wavelength of light transmitted through the growth cuvette or well is measured by a photoelectric cell. Detection of microbial metabolism by measuring colored end products or indicators is called **colorimetry.** AutoMicrobic System cards with growth substance–containing wells are inoculated with clinical specimens (primarily urine) or bacterial or yeast suspensions made from pure cultures for identification. The UniScept Plus API overnight-incubation system utilizes color changes that indicate substrate utilization in plastic cuvettes, a small-volume modification of conventional biochemical testing. Makers of identification and susceptibility microdilution systems (such as MicroScan) have chosen to place turbidity and colorimetry determination tests on the same tray in some systems. Other manufacturers, including those of Micro-Coder I (Micro-Media Systems), Sceptor (BBL Microbiology Systems), Pasco (Difco Laboratories), Precept (Austin Biological Laboratories), and Sensititre (Gibco Laboratories) provide separate trays for identification and susceptibility testing.

In addition to the instrumentation required for automatic reading of results, several of these systems require a rehydrating apparatus. API 3600, Sensititre, and Sceptor systems are distributed dry, which increases shelf life and allows room-temperature

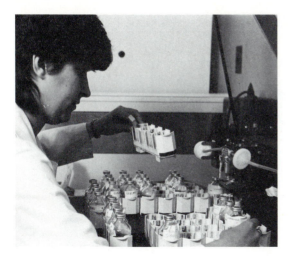

Figure 11.3
A technologist places blood culture bottles containing radioactive substrates on the Bactec instrument (Johnston Laboratories).

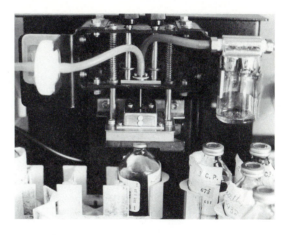

Figure 11.4
Detector module of the Bactec instrument, in which gas above the medium is removed and measured for radioactivity and fresh gas is substituted.

storage. Dry panels must be rehydrated, a task that is easily automated.

11.1.c. Detection of microbial growth by measuring carbon dioxide as a product of metabolic activity. The Bactec system (Johnston Laboratories) measures the production of carbon dioxide by metabolizing organisms. Either radioactive carbon dioxide gas produced as the final end product of metabolism of ^{14}C-labeled substrates (glucose, amino acids, and alcohols) is measured in an ionization chamber or, in a newer configuration of the system, unlabeled CO_2 is quantitated by infrared spectrophotometry. Blood (or sterile body fluid) for routine culture is inoculated into bottles that contain the substrates. The media are incubated and often agitated, preferably on a rotary shaker (also supplied by the manufacturer). At predetermined time intervals thereafter, the bottles are placed into the monitoring module (Figure 11.3), where they are automatically moved past a detector. The detector inserts two needles through a rubber septum seal at the top of each bottle (Figure 11.4) and draws out the gas that has accumulated above the liquid medium, replacing this headspace gas with fresh gas of the same mixture (aerobic or anaerobic). Any level of CO_2 (above a preset baseline that covers the metabolism of cellular elements in the blood) is considered to be suspicious for microbial growth. A computerized data-handling section of the instrument allows re-

cording of patient data and collates results. Microbiologists retrieve suspicious bottles and continue processing the culture.

Modifications of the basic principle have increased the capabilities of the Bactec system. The instrument has been used successfully to detect the presence of *Mycobacterium tuberculosis, Mycobacterium avium-intracellulare* complex, and other mycobacteria in clinical specimens.[13] A protective hood is placed over the module to prevent dissemination of aerosols. Sterile body fluids are inoculated directly, and urine and sputum specimens are inoculated after decontamination and concentration into Bactec bottles containing ^{14}C-labeled growth factors utilized only by mycobacteria, such as palmitic acid. Detection of products of metabolism of these substrates by mycobacteria may be possible within 10 days of inoculation. Because of certain technical considerations, it is still recommended that standard cultures on solid media be inoculated along with Bactec cultures. If growth is detected radiometrically, a subculture from the initial medium into a second medium that contains *p*-nitro-α-acetyl-β-hydroxy propiophenone (NAP) can differentiate *M. tuberculosis* and *Mycobacterium bovis*, which are susceptible to the agent, from other mycobacteria, which exhibit radiometric evidence of growth within 3 days. Mycobacterial susceptibility testing has also been performed acceptably using the radiometric

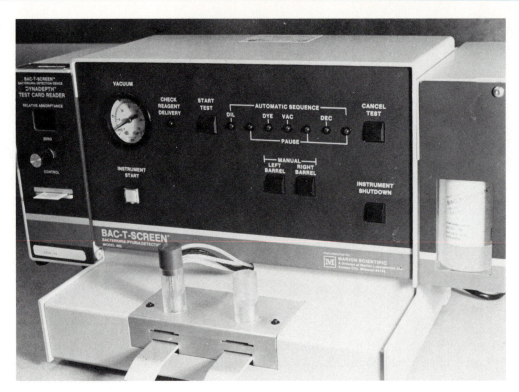

Figure 11.5
Bac-T-Screen bacteriuria detection instrument (Vitek Microbiology Systems).

Bactec system; this provides results more rapidly than conventional methods. The use of the Bactec instrument for mycobacteriology is discussed further in Chapter 41.

11.1.d. Bioluminescence assays for viable organisms. The glowing cold light produced in firefly tails is the end product of a chemical reaction, the conversion of the substrate luciferin to oxyluciferin and light, catalyzed by the enzyme luciferase, and driven by the dephosphorylation of adenosine triphosphate (ATP). The light generated by this reaction can be measured directly with a luminometer, similar to a photometer. The amount of light (measured in photons) produced by the reaction taking place in an excess of luciferin is directly proportional to the amount of ATP present in the solution. Unlike a photometric system, however, there is no need for an exogenous light source. ATP is present within all living cells, and by selectively releasing the ATP from bacterial cells only, the number of colony forming units in a clinical specimen can be estimated. At least three systems have employed this principle for screening urine specimens for bacteria: the Lumac Bacteriuria Screening System (3M Medical Prod-

ucts), the Monolight (Analytical Luminescence Laboratory), and the Turner Luminescent System (Turner Designs). Clinical microbiology laboratories have not adopted these systems at this writing, although some of them have been used for industrial applications and others are being modified for re-release. These systems require several steps, including the lysis of somatic cells to release nonbacterial ATP and the subsequent lysis of bacteria and measurement of the resulting bacterial ATP. Prototype systems have shown acceptable correlation with culture methods when 10^5 CFU/ml is chosen as the threshold number above which a urine is considered to be positive (and thus must be plated).[16] It should be noted that in certain types of urinary tract infection a threshold of 10^2 CFU/ml is appropriate; the luminescent systems currently available would not be satisfactory for screening urines in this category.

11.1.e. Colorimetric particle detection for urine screening. One of the newest technologies developed to rapidly determine whether a urine specimen contains significant numbers of bacteria is the Bac-T-Screen bacteriuria detection device (Figure 11.5; Vitek Microbiology Systems). With this system, a

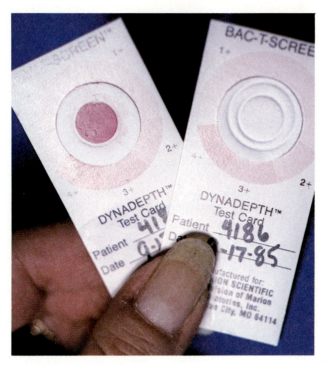

Figure 11.6
Filter paper used to detect pyuria and bacteriuria by staining trapped particles (Bac-T-Screen, Vitek Microbiology Systems). Amount of color yielded by specimen (center circle) is compared with control color samples around the edge of the specimen circle.

measured amount of urine is drawn through a paper filter by vacuum suction. Particles such as bacteria and white blood cells adhere to the filter. A stain is then passed through the filter imparting color, the depth of which is dependent on the number and type of stainable particles (Figure 11.6). The filter paper is then manually inserted into another section of the instrument, where a photometer compares the color to a preset standard. The filter may also be examined visually. Urines that stain at a level below the control can be considered negative and need not be processed further. This system has shown excellent correlation with clinical diagnoses of urinary tract infection, in part due to the positive staining characteristics of white blood cells present in urines from infected patients.[2]

11.1.f. Electrical impedance as an indicator of microbial growth. Although systems employing electrical impedance have not been used widely in clinical laboratories, there is a great theoretical advantage to being able to detect the presence of multiplying yeast or bacteria by measuring the changes in the flow of an electric current passing through the medium in which a specimen is being incubated (**impedance** changes). With continuous monitoring, the first sign of impedance change indicating microbial growth could be instantly recorded, unlike most of the other currently available systems that require periodic monitoring with manual or mechanical manipulation. Positive blood cultures, monitored by impedance, could be detected and reported in the middle of the night, without the presence of a technologist. Currently, trials are in progress with impedance devices produced in Scotland by Malthus Instruments and Bactomatic (Princeton, N.J.) for monitoring blood and urine specimens for bacteria.

11.1.g. Fluorophore-labeled substrate metabolism as an indicator of microbial growth. One commercial system, Sensititre (Radiometer America), utilizes substrate-fluorophore complexes. When microbial metabolic processes break down the substrates, the fluorogenic markers are freed to assume their fluorescent configuration. This system offers potentially greater sensitivity than is achievable with conventional substrate metabolism, which depends on a pH shift for detection; susceptibilities of some Enterobacteriaeceae have been measured at 4 and 5 hours with good agreement with subsequent overnight results.[5] Although this system is promising, there are concerns about detection of inducible cephalosporin resistance mutants, problems testing *Pseudomonas aeruginosa*, and quality control considerations that have yet to be fully satisfied.

11.1.h. Replica plating system for bacterial identifications and susceptibilities. The replica plating system (Cathra Repliscan II, MCT Medical, Inc.) makes use of the Steers-Foltz replicator (described in Chapter 13), a device that can deposit a standardized small inoculum of a suspension of bacteria in a discrete position on the surface of an agar plate. Inocula from approximately 35 separate bacterial suspensions can be deposited simultaneously on each of any number of agar plates, containing media for assessing substrate utilization as well as agar dilution susceptibilities. By recording, storing, and interpreting the results with the computer-assisted data system included with the product, technologists can perform rapid and cost-effective identifications and susceptibilities; this will be useful primarily for laboratories that must process large numbers of isolates daily.[15]

11.2. Automated Microbiology Support Systems

A number of instruments have been developed to aid microbiologists by automating certain tasks; often such automation increases reproducibility and consistency. For example, an automated agar sterilizer, Petri dish filler, liquid media dispenser, and colony counter are marketed by New Brunswick Scientific Co. Once the medium has been prepared, an automated plate inoculator (Spiral System Instruments) may be used to distribute the inoculum in a spiral pattern, producing isolated colonies near the outer edge. Spiral Systems Instruments is evaluating the use of their system for quantitative susceptibility testing, achieved by placing a graded concentration of antibiotic concentrically onto an agar plate and then streaking organisms from the center to the edge of the agar. The organism's line of growth would be inhibited at a defined distance from the edge of the plate depending on the concentration of antibiotic that is inhibitory. This manufacturer also markets a colony counter that uses computerized data processing.

Several companies produce devices that fill microdilution trays or make serial twofold dilutions in microdilution trays, including Dynatech, Bellco Glass, Cetus Corp., and Tomtec, Inc., which can be used for bacterial susceptibility testing and identification systems or for the new immunoassay methods (see section 11.4). Additional instruments have found niches in the practice of microbiology. Automatic Gram-staining devices, such as the instrument produced by Tomtec, Inc., can pay for themselves by reducing technologist time and reagent costs. Even pipetting has been automated with electrical vacuum-suction devices.

11.3. Antigen and Microbial Product Detection

In addition to identifying, quantifying, and determining susceptibilities of microorganisms, microbiologists are increasingly diagnosing disease by identifying microbial constituents (antigens) or products of microbial metabolism in specimens obtained from the infected host. Antimicrobial agents with sufficient toxicity to require therapeutic monitoring also require quantitation. Widely used methods for such studies that require instrumentation will be described here.

11.3.a. Gas-liquid chromatography (GLC). In **gas-liquid chromatography (GLC)** a liquid sample is passed through a matrix that differentially separates its constituents. The volatile components of the sample are carried along with a flow of specially prepared heated gas through a long, narrow column packed with resin or some other material that differentially slows down the rate of travel of the components based on their sizes, molecular weights, or charges. As the various components reach the end of the column, their presence is detected by a change in the temperature or ionization potential, and their relative amounts are plotted on a recording chart as peaks. GLC applications for diagnostic microbiology are increasing. GLC was first used by microbiologists to identify anaerobic bacteria by separating and identifying the metabolic end products (volatile fatty acids and nonvolatile organic acids) of carbohydrate fermentation or amino acid degradation. Different species of anaerobic bacteria yield different types or quantities of end products. The GLC patterns obtained from culture supernatants are often definitive (further discussed in the anaerobe laboratory manuals by Holdeman and coworkers[6] and by Sutter and coworkers.[20]) With the development of newer, more sensitive column materials, such as very long-fused silica capillary columns, whole cell fatty acids can now be analyzed to aid in identification of aerobic bacteria and mycobacteria.[9] Mayo Clinic workers use

GLC for routine identification of mycobacteria isolated from clinical specimens (Tisdall and coworkers[22]), and Centers for Disease Control experts have promoted use of such methods for identification of nonfermentative gram-negative bacilli.[1,14] Other uses proposed for GLC include the rapid detection of infection involving anaerobic organisms (with information on the specific organisms involved) directly from infected body fluids. Bacterial vaginosis, an infection of the vaginal tract characterized by decreased numbers of lactobacilli and increased numbers of anaerobes, often in concert with *Gardnerella vaginalis*, can be diagnosed by detecting an increased ratio of succinic to lactic acid in GLC profiles prepared from the foul-smelling vaginal discharge, as described by Spiegel and others.[18] Spiegel and others have also evaluated abdominal fluid for direct chromatographic analysis.[19] Any gas-liquid chromatograph instrument can be used for anaerobic microbiological assays, since the level of sensitivity required is not great. Martin and Schneider[11] present an overview of chromatographic methods. Computers may be used to start and stop the GLC analysis, to control the baseline, and to identify and quantify the peaks representing the various end products.

The combination of GLC and **mass spectrometry**, the separation and measurement of ions of a material to determine its structure and probable identification, gives microbiologists a very powerful tool for analysis of microorganisms. When this technology is applied to bacterial constituents or metabolic end products, very specific profiles can be generated that, compared with a data bank of known profiles, will facilitate identification of the substance or the organism. Such systems naturally require sophisticated computerized data handling. Applications of this technology are described by Larsson.[9]

11.3.b. High-performance liquid chromatography. The column packing material in **high-performance liquid chromatography (HPLC)** consists of special resins that bear a number of ion-exchange groups on their surfaces, such that constituents in the sample undergoing HPLC are preferentially retained in the column based on their affinity for the charged ionic groups. Components with the weakest attraction for the resin will flow through the column fastest and elute first. This process is known as **ion-exchange chromatography,** the same principle as that used to separate IgG from IgM by elution from a column (Chapter 12). HPLC, by using newly developed column packing material, high pressure to force the sample through the column, and liquid buffer carriers at room temperature instead of hot gas, has decreased analysis time and improved resolution compared with GLC. Uses of HPLC for microbiology are just being developed. It is currently being used by some medical centers to determine the levels of antimicrobial agents, including chloramphenicol, cephalosporins, flucytosine, vancomycin, aminoglycosides, and others, in body fluids, as well as for other therapeutic drug monitoring. Products of microbial metabolism may also be detected using HPLC.

11.4. Immunological Detection Methods for Antigen or Antibody

All of the automated immunological detection methods in use rely on the same principle, the ability of an antigen and its homologous antibody to bind to each other selectively and with high affinity. If either component is labeled in such a way that it can be recognized and quantified, the amount of the other component can be accurately determined. The methods are suitable for detection and quantitation of either antibodies to infectious agents or antigens of various sorts, not limited to microbial antigens. With the advent of monoclonal technology and the development of nonradioactive labels, the possibilities for sensitivity and broad applicability of immunologic methods are practically infinite.

11.4.a.   **Counterimmunoelectrophoresis.** The simplest method for determining the presence of cross-reacting antigen or antibody is to visually observe the product of the reaction between an antigen and its bound antibody. Originally performed in liquid with whole bacterial cells (agglutination), the procedure was modified by Ouchterlony for performance in a semisolid gel matrix. Antigen and antibody were placed in wells cut into the agarose or agar surface of the matrix and they slowly diffused toward each other. If they cross-reacted, they bound one another to form a precipitin reaction, visible as a white line in the gel somewhere between the two wells (Figure 11.7). Counterimmunoelectrophoresis merely adds an electric current to help move the antigen and antibody toward each other more quickly. Since there is really no automation involved in this technique, it is discussed in more depth in Chapter 10.

Counterimmunoelectrophoresis is specific, but it

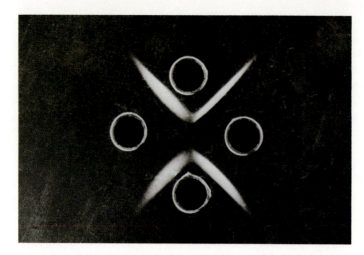

Figure 11.7
Ouchterlony gel diffusion reaction; antiserum in center well and antigens in outside wells. The continuous precipitin line indicates immunologic identity.

requires enough material to produce a visible reaction. In numerous situations, only minute amounts of the substance being sought are present in the patient. In other cases, the subject of the assay is a molecule too small to yield a visible precipitin reaction. Therefore, more sensitive immunoassays were developed.

11.4.b. **Nephelometry.** Antigen-antibody complexes in solution may be too small to see easily with the naked eye, but they do alter the turbidity of the suspension as measured photometrically. **Nephelometry** (described in section 11.1.a) measures the increased light scatter of a solution as the complexes form; the kinetics of this change can be determined quite quickly when the photometric results are analyzed by computer. Although more widely used in chemistry laboratories than in microbiology laboratories, nephelometry has been used to measure immune complexes and the presence of antibodies to several substances.

11.4.c. **Radioimmunoassay.** The main difference among various sophisticated immunoassay systems in use today is the choice of label. The first such methods employed radioisotopes, either tritium (^{3}H), iodine (^{125}I), cobalt (^{57}Co), or carbon (^{14}C), to label antigen molecules of the same substance being measured in the assay. **Radioimmunoassay (RIA),** as the method is called, relies on the competitive binding to antibody of labeled antigen, provided by the assay, and unlabeled antigen, present in the un-

known patient sample. When all three components are present in the system, an equilibrium exists, dependent on the amount of unlabeled antigen. The more unlabeled (patient) antigen that is added, the less the labeled antigen will be bound to the antibody. When the antigen-antibody complexes are precipitated out of solution and the amount of radioactive label in the precipitate is determined, the unlabeled antigen present in the sample being assayed can be quantified. In practice, a standard curve is first created by adding known amounts of unlabeled antigen to the system. The amount of radiolabel present in the precipitate of the test solution is compared with values obtained from the standard curve to provide quantitative results. Although RIA is an immunoassay procedure, it is used more widely for detection of circulating proteins, hormones, and drugs than for diagnosis of infectious diseases, and thus its primary application seems to be in chemistry laboratories. RIA is being used in a limited way in infectious disease diagnosis to detect antigens of and antibodies to the hepatitis viruses, enteroviruses, and *Legionella*, as well as to determine the presence of immune complexes and to measure the amount of antimicrobial agents in patients' body fluids. RIA techniques are highly specific and sensitive, but they require very expensive instruments and highly skilled technologists. The radioisotopes have a relatively short half-life. Additionally, the institution must be licensed and willing to deal with the use

Table 11.2
Automated Microbiology Systems That Use ELISA Technology

MATRIX	INFECTIOUS AGENT ANTIBODY (AB) OR ANTIGEN (AG)	MANUFACTURER(S)
Plastic bead	Gonococcal, chlamydial, hepatitis, rotavirus, respiratory syncytial virus, streptococcal ag; hepatitis, rubella, HIV, *Toxoplasma* ab	Quantum System (Abbott Laboratories)
Metal bead	*Entamoeba histolytica, Treponema, Toxoplasma,* rubella, cytomegalovirus, herpes, Epstein-Barr virus, varicella-zoster virus ab; rotavirus ag	Bio-Enzabead (Organon Teknika)
Microdilution	Rubella, cytomegalovirus, herpes, *Toxoplasma* ab; respiratory syncytial virus, varicella-zoster, herpesvirus, *Chlamydia* ag	Microwell Test System (Ortho Diagnostics)
	Toxoplasma, rubella, cytomegalovirus, herpes ab	Clin-ELISA (Clinical Sciences, Inc.)
	Epstein-Barr virus, HIV ab	EIA Plate Kit (DuPont Co.)
	Lyme spirochete, mumps, measles, herpes, rubella, cytomegalovirus, varicella-zoster, *Mycoplasma, Chlamydia, Toxoplasma* ab	EIA System (Whittaker M.A. Bioproducts)
	Rubella, cytomegalovirus, herpes, hepatitis, measles, mumps, varicella-zoster ab; rotavirus ag	Calbiochem-Behring
	HIV	LAV-EIA (Genetic Systems)
	Hepatitis, HIV, HTLV-I, Epstein-Barr virus ab	Summit (DuPont Co.)
Plastic paddle	*Toxoplasma, Borrelia burgdorferi*, rubella, cytomegalovirus, herpes, measles, varicella-zoster, *Mycoplasma* ab	FIAX (Whittaker M.A. Bioproducts)

HIV = human immunodeficiency virus; HTLV-I = human T-lymphotropic virus type I.

and disposal of radioactive substances. At least two alternatives to radioactive labels are being promulgated, as described below.

11.4.d. Enzyme-linked immunosorbent assay (ELISA). By using enzymes instead of isotopes as labels for antigen or antibody, many of the disadvantages of RIA can be overcome. Instead of a radioactive substance, the antigen (or antibody) is bound to an enzyme that can react with a substrate to yield a colored end product. Horseradish peroxidase and alkaline phosphatase (which yield yellow, orange, or blue precipitates depending on the substrates used) are often chosen. The use of biotin-avidin complexes (described in Chapter 10) for binding enzyme can greatly increase the affinity of the reactants and the speed and intensity of the result. The reagents have a long half-life, and the sensitivity of some assays approaches that of RIA.

Enzyme-linked immunosorbent assay (ELISA) systems are gaining wide usage in microbiology laboratories. The basic principles of ELISA assays that can be performed without automation are described in Chapter 10. For most clinical applications, how-

ever, the changes being detected are so subtle that computer analysis of results is required. Standard commercially produced immunoassay kits that rely on competitive binding, removal of free substrate from the bound complexes before measurement, and comparison of results to a standard curve, as in RIA, are available for the detection of antibodies to viruses, bacteria, and parasites. The most commonly used systems use a direct determination of the amount of bound, labeled substance after unbound constituents have been removed by a washing step. Sensitive photometers that can determine slight differences in color are coupled with computers to automatically compare results to standards. Most of the systems are prepared in microdilution plates, but other configurations are used. In many commercial systems, antigen-antibody complexes are bound to a solid phase, either the inside of the microdilution well, a plastic paddle, or a plastic bead. This simplifies washing and allows easier manipulation. Table 11.2 lists products available currently that employ automated ELISA technology for detection of microbial antigens or antibodies. In addition to the

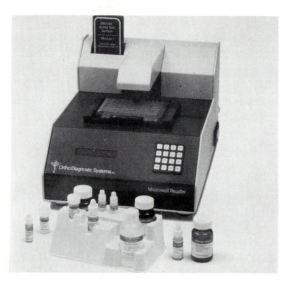

Figure 11.8
Spectrophotometric instrument adapted to read ELISA results in microbroth dilution format (BioTek Instruments).

ELISA readers provided by most manufacturers of the reagents, several companies, including Dynatech Laboratories, SLT Labinstruments, and Bio-Tek Instruments, produce computerized, programmable reader instruments for determining and printing results from any microdilution format assay system (Figure 11.8) and companion instruments, such as microdilution plate washers (Figure 11.9). According to Meier and Hill,[12] the use of automated washers can be justified by the improved reproducibility of ELISA assays.

A modification of ELISA assays is widely used for monitoring levels of drugs, including antimicrobials. The enzyme-multiplied immunoassay, marketed by Syva Company as EMIT, uses an enzyme bound to a molecule identical to the agent being sought as the third constituent in a competitive assay. The agent, if present in the patient's sample, will bind to antibody, allowing the free enzyme-agent complex to react with its substrate to produce a color change. If the patient's specimen contains only small amounts or none of the agent being tested for, the enzyme-agent complex is free to bind to the

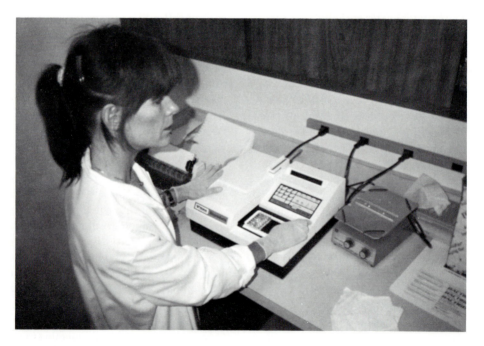

Figure 11.9
Microdilution plate washer for ELISA test systems (SLT Labinstruments).

antibody. When bound to antibody, the enzyme changes conformation, reducing enzyme activity. This commercial system, used to monitor aminoglycoside levels and to detect various proteins, is very specific and correlates well with RIA methods.

11.4.e. Fluorescent immunoassays (FIAs). Fluorescent molecules are also used as substitutes for radioisotope or enzyme labels in several automated systems. In contrast to ELISA systems, **fluorescent immunoassays (FIA)** require only minimal incubation times, no buffered substrate, and fewer washing steps. Current uses in microbiology encompass detection of antibodies to numerous viruses, a few parasites, antibodies directed against host tissue (autoantibodies), and some antigens (such as hepatitis virus determinants). Commercially available systems include the TDA (Ames Division of Miles Laboratories), which uses a fluorogenic substrate (umbelliferyl-β-D-galactoside) bound to molecules of the agent being assayed to compete with free molecules of the agent for antibody-binding sites. The more competing free agent (from patient serum), the more fluoroescence can be produced by an exogenous enzyme acting on the unbound substrate-agent complex. In another system, the FIAX system (Whittaker M.A. Bioproducts), fluorescent-labeled and patient-unlabeled substance compete for antibody (or antigen, if antibody is being assayed) bound to a plastic paddle. This relatively simple system has been formulated to detect antibodies to *Toxoplasma*, rubella virus, *Borrelia burgdorferi*, cytomegalovirus, and herpesvirus, as well as to other infectious agents and proteins (such as immunoglobulin subtypes and C-reactive protein). The TD$_x$ System from Abbott Laboratories uses a fluorescence polarization format for a competitive therapeutic drug-monitoring assay. A molecule identical to that being assayed is bound to fluorescein, a fluorescent dye. Under polarized light, the amount of fluorescence emitted is dependent on the amount of rotation of the fluorescein-drug complex; the more rotation, the less fluorescence. The conjugated drug and the free drug in the patient sample compete for antibody-binding sites. As the fluorescein complex is bound, it will fluoresce with greater polarization, since its rotation is slowed by the antibody. This sensitive and specific assay is available for monitoring levels of aminoglycosides and vancomycin, as well as many other compounds. Recently, a potentially more sensitive fluoroimmunoassay system that uses time-resolved immunofluorometry to detect very small amounts of antigens and other proteins, including hepatitis viral proteins, has been marketed. With this method, two substances, europium and a diketone (such as isothiocyanatophenyl-DTTA), are chelated together to act as a fluorophore. Because the europium emits fluorescent light for a relatively long time, the fluorometer can measure the light at a time period after all background fluorescence has faded, resulting in very sensitive and specific assay results.

The increasing sensitivity of newer enzyme and fluorescent immunoassays has accelerated the move away from radioactive markers and opened new areas for automation of the diagnosis of infectious diseases. It is anticipated that many applications in microbiology will be realized within the next few years.

11.5. Possible Future Directions in Clinical Microbiology

Every month suggestions for new ways to utilize technology for diagnosis of infectious disease or identification of pathogens are published. A few novel methods that have not yet been adopted for routine use are mentioned here.

The Aladin automated identification-susceptibility system developed by Analytab Products, Inc. analyzes growth in the bottom of a clear plastic cuvette by video image analysis. A camera produces an image of the well, which is projected onto a screen and broken up into discrete increments for computerized analysis. This process can theoretically detect subtle differences that turbidity measurements cannot evaluate and ultimately can produce a very precise result.[4] Aladin products are not yet widely distributed.

Flow cytometry has been explored for detection of bacteria in body fluids such as blood and urine.[10,23] In such methods, bacteria are stained with fluorescent dyes and passed through a detector module in a thin stream of liquid such that only a single organism is measured at any given moment. Based on the size, charge, and staining characteristics of the particles being detected, the number of bacteria per volume of fluid can be determined.

Another new approach for detection and identification of bacteria in clinical specimens is that of multiparameter light scattering.[17] Bacteria passing singly in a stream of fluid such as that used for flow cytometry are bombarded by polarized light; the angle of polarization is rotated as the object is measured. The scatter of the beam of light produced by passing through the object is then measured and compared with a data base of patterns generated from known organisms. Since light scatter is dependent on intracellular as well as surface characteristics, all species of bacteria may be expected to produce different patterns, specific for the species. This system, in development by Mesa Diagnostics, Albuquerque, N.M., is in the trial stages.

A final new technology that may find practical use in the diagnosis of infectious diseases is the **polymerase chain reaction**. Once the base pair composition of a specific gene or piece of a gene is known, a tiny amount of the gene in solution can be selectively amplified. Complementary gene sequences with primers for DNA polymerase are used as targets to bind to the sequence in question. If present, the double-stranded primer thus created serves as a template upon which further rounds of replication occur. This reaction has been speeded up dramatically because of the ability to automate the DNA denaturization and subsequent chain elongation steps based on discovery of a heat-stable polymerase, the Taq enzyme of a thermophilic bacterium, *Thermus aquaticus*, and the use of a microprocessor-controlled water bath (DNA Thermal Cycler, Perkin-Elmer-Cetus). Heating the mixture splits the DNA fragments and opens the ends for the next round of polymerase activity; cooling the mixture then activates the enzyme to begin chain elongation again. The average 30-cycle amplification takes approximately 3 hours to complete. The technique has been used for detection of tiny amounts of human immunodeficiency virus (HIV) antigen, malaria, and numerous genetic anomalies.

11.6. Computerization in Microbiology

Very few of the automated systems just described or described in other areas of the book would be possible without computerization. Microprocessor-controlled mechanical functions, such as moving a culture bottle into position for removing headspace gas or shining a beam of light through a solution in a plastic well to determine the turbidity of the solution, are integral to the new microbiology systems. Even more obvious is the computer-controlled recording and integration of data, which are stored and printed, often as directly reportable results. Aside from their important place as the central processing units of almost all automated instruments, however,

computers can perform an even more fundamental role in facilitating smooth functioning of the laboratory.

A microbiology computer or a laboratory computer with microbiology functions can perform multiple tasks.[8] Word processing programs can be used in microbiology for a number of administrative functions. Besides the obvious ones of facilitating correspondence and writing manuscripts, a word processor is invaluable for preparing and updating procedure manuals. Quality control recording sheets and records can be generated with such a program, changing parameters as necessary. Ongoing records of quality control discrepancies can be placed into the program and then printed out as a single report when needed. Programs are available for inventory control that can greatly reduce time and anxiety associated with ordering and maintaining supplies. The computer could be programmed to flag certain dates for checking on back orders or initiating inquiries. As supplies are received, they are logged into the system.

Computers can be used to calculate workload units such as those utilized by the College of American Pathologists. Raw data can be entered daily as numbers of specimens processed or numbers of tests performed and the calculations can be analyzed and stored for later retrieval. Cost accounting of procedures can be facilitated by computer-assisted data processing.

Computers can also directly decrease the manual labor involved in logging in new specimens by printing labels for culture media, printing up work cards, and notifying the laboratory if a request for processing a particular specimen is repeated within a specified number of days. A computer in the accessioning area can even perform automatic billing of tests. The maintenance of records of results, both identifications and susceptibilities, is critical for epidemiologic surveillance and for monitoring patient progress. Myriad computer systems have capabilities for data storage and retrieval. Reports can be generated that catalogue susceptibility results of isolates sorted by source, species, doctor, ward, and any other parameter. Unusual susceptibility patterns or those that do not match the supposed identification of the isolate can be flagged. Results of cultures can be studied in many ways, allowing microbiologists access to information that could be gathered previously only by great effort. Data analysis and storage by microcomputers has been outlined by Buck.[3]

In addition to handling management functions, the computer can aid in reporting results. Results immediately accessible to the patient units will have much greater impact on patient care, as well as cut down on communication lags and errors. It is estimated that systems in operation at several large institutions have saved at least one hour per physician per day. Physicians may even request tests by computer, which gains them time and reduces transcription errors. Laboratory computers that interface with hospital computers can deliver patient demographic data directly to the laboratory and provide direct billing capability. Epidemiologic data entered in the laboratory could be retrieved by nurse epidemiologists in another location for more efficient operation. In the ultimate computerized laboratory, results generated by instruments automatically would be updated to the patient's charts, even during the middle of the night.

REFERENCES

1. Alexander, H. 1987. Gas-liquid chromatography as an aid in identification of glucose-nonfermenting gram-negative bacilli. Microbiol. News 9:25.
2. Baron, E.J., Tyburski, M., Almon, R., et al. 1988. Visual and clinical analysis of Bac-T-Screen urine screen results. J. Clin. Microbiol. 26:2382.
3. Buck, G.E. 1987. The role of microcomputers for data analysis and storage. p. 177-187. In Jorgenson, J.H., editor. Automation in clinical microbiology, CRC Press, Boca Raton, Fla.
4. D'Amato, R.F., Isenberg, H.D., McKinley, G.A., et al. 1988. The novel application of video image processing to biochemical and antimicrobial susceptibility testing. J. Clin. Microbiol. 26:1492.
5. Doern, G.V., Staneck, J.L., Needham, C., et al. 1987. Sensititre autoreader for same-day breakpoint broth microdilution susceptibility testing of members of the family *Enterobacteriaceae*. J. Clin. Microbiol. 256:1481.
6. Holdeman, L.V., Cato, E.P. and Moore, W.E.C, editors, 1977. Anaerobe laboratory manual, ed. 4. Virginia Polytechnic Institute and State University, Blacksburg, Va.
7. Isenberg, H.D., Reichler, A., and Wiseman, D. 1971. Prototype of a fully automated device for determination of bacterial antibiotic susceptibility in the clinical laboratory. Appl. Microbiol. 22:980.
8. Jorgenson, J.H. 1987. Use of laboratory computer systems to facilitate reporting of instrument-generated microbiology results. p. 169-176. In Jorgenson, J.H., editor. Automation in clinical microbiology, CRC Press, Boca Raton, Fla.
9. Larsson, L. 1987. Gas chromatography and mass spectometry. p. 153-166. In Jorgenson, J.H., editor. Automation and clinical microbiology, CRC Press, Boca Raton, Fla.
10. Mansour, J.D., Robson, J.A., Arndt, C.W., et al. 1985. Detection of *Escherichia coli* in blood using flow cytometry. Cytometry 6:186.
11. Martin, R., and Schneider, W.A. 1987. Chromatography for the identification of microorganisms. p. 703-714. In Wentworth, B.B., editor. Diagnostic procedures for bacterial infections, ed. 7. American Public Health Association, Washington, D.C..
12. Meier, F.A., and Hill, H.R. 1987. Automation of antigen detection in infectious disease diagnosis. p. 101-120. In Jorgenson, J.H., editor. Automation in clinical microbiology, CRC Press, Boca Raton, Fla.
13. Morgan, M.A., and Roberts, G.D. 1987. Radiometric detection, identification, and antimicrobial susceptibility testing of mycobacteria. p. 31-38. In Jorgenson, J.H., editor. Automation in clinical microbiology, CRC Press, Boca Raton, Fla.
14. Moss, C.W., and Nunez-Monteil, O.I. 1982. Analysis of short-chain acids from bacteria by gas-liquid chromatography with a fused-silica capillary column. J. Clin. Microbiol. 15:308.
15. Murray, P.R. 1987. Rapid automated identification systems. p. 53-67. In Jorgenson, J.H., editor. Automation in clinical microbiology, CRC Press, Boca Raton, Fla.
16. Pezzlo, M. 1987. Instrument methods for detection of bacteriuria. p. 15-29. In Jorgenson, J.H., editor. Automation in clinical microbiology, CRC Press, Boca Raton, Fla.
17. Salzman, G.C., Griffith, J.K., and Gregg, C.T. 1982. Rapid identification of microorganisms by circular intensity differential scattering. Appl Environ Microbiol 44:1081.
18. Spiegel, C.A., Amsel, R., Eschenbach, D., et al. 1980. Anaerobic bacteria in non-specific vaginitis. N Engl J Med 303:601.
19. Spiegel, C.A., Malangoni, M.A., and Condon, R.E. 1984. Gas-liquid chromatography for rapid diagnosis of intraabdominal infection. Arch. Surg. 119:28.
20. Sutter, V.L., Citron, D.M., Edelstein, M.A.C., et al. 1985. Wadsworth anaerobic bacteriology manual, ed 4. Star Publishing Co., Belmont, Calif.
21. Thornsberry, C., Gavan, T.L., Sherris, J.C., et al. 1975. Laboratory evaluation of a rapid, automated susceptibility testing system: report of a collaborative study. Antimicrob. Agents Chemother. 7:466.
22. Tisdall, P.A., DeYoung, D., Roberts, G.D., et al. 1982. Identification of clinical isolates of mycobacteria with gas-liquid chromatography: a 10-month follow-up study. J. Clin. Microbiol. 16:400.
23. Van Dilla, M.A., Langlois, R.G., Pinkel, D., et al. 1983. Bacterial characterization by flow cytometry. Science 220:620.

BIBLIOGRAPHY

Ackerman, B.H., Berg, H.G., Strate, R.G., et al. 1983. Comparison of radioimmunoassay and fluorescent polarization immunoassay for quantitative determination of vancomycin concentrations in serum. J. Clin. Microbiol. 18:994.
Barry, A.L., Jones, R.N., and Gavan, T.L. 1978. Evaluation of the Micro-Media System for quantitative antimicrobial drug susceptibility testing: a collaborative study. Antimicrob. Agents Chemother. 13:61.

Buchanan, A.G., Witwicki, E, and Albritton, W.L. 1983. Serum aminoglycoside monitoring by enzyme immunoassay, biological, and fluorescence immunoassay procedures. Am. J. Med. Tech. 49:437.

Cohen, R.L. 1987. Instrument systems which utilize a conventional incubation period. p. 71-83. In Jorgenson, J.H., editor. Automation in clinical microbiology, CRC Press, Boca Raton, Fla.

Fitzgibbon, R.J. 1984. Clinical laboratory reference. Medical Economics Books, Oradell, N.J.

Gerson, B. 1984. Fluorescence immunoassay. J. Clin. Immunoassay 7:73.

Isenberg, H.D. 1984. Automated methods of bacterial susceptibility testing. Ann. N.Y. Acad. Sci. 428:236.

Isenberg, H.D., and D'Amato, R.F. 1984. Rapid methods for antimicrobic susceptibility testing. In Cunha, B.A., and Ristuccia, A.M., editors. Antimicrobial therapy. Raven Press, New York.

Isenberg, H.D., and D'Amato, R.F. 1985. New methods for the detection of bacteria and fungi. Lab. Med. 2:1.

Johnson, J.E. 1987. Instrument-based serodiagnostic methods. p. 139-150. In Jorgenson, J.H., editor. Automation in clinical microbiology, CRC Press, Boca Raton, Fla.

Looney, C.E. 1984. High-sensitivity light scattering immunoassays. J. Clin. Immunoassay 7:90.

Murray, P.R. 1987. Rapid automated identification systems. p. 53-67. In Jorgenson, J.H., editor. Automation in clinical microbiology, CRC Press, Boca Raton, Fla.

Murray, P.R. 1987. Overnight automated identification systems. p. 41-51. In Jorgenson, J.H., editor. Automation in clinical microbiology, CRC Press, Boca Raton, Fla.

Narayan, S. 1983. Chromatography. III. Ion-exchange chromatography. J. Clin. Lab. Automation 3:225.

Pezzlo, M. 1987. Instrument methods for detection of bacteriuria. p. 15-29. In Joorgenson, J.H., editor. Automation in clinical microbiology, CRC Press, Boca Raton, Fla.

Pfaller, M.A. 1987. Immunoassays for measurement of antimicrobial agents in body fluids. p. 121-137. In Jorgenson, J.H., editor. Automation in clinical microbiology, CRC Press, Boca Raton, Fla.

Shekarchi, I.C., Sever, J.L., Nerurkar, L., and Fuccillo, D. 1984. Comparison of enzyme-linked immunosorbent assay with enzyme-linked fluorescence assay with automated readers for detection of rubella virus antibody and herpes simplex virus. J. Clin. Microbiol. 21:92.

12 Diagnostic Immunological Principles and Methods

Infectious diseases can be definitively diagnosed in only three ways: (1) by documenting the presence in the patient of an agent known to cause the disease, either by visualizing the agent directly in clinical material obtained from the patient, by detecting antigens or genetic material specific for the agent, or by cultivating the agent in the laboratory (within an animal host or in vitro); (2) by detecting a specific product of the infectious agent in clinical material obtained from the patient, a product that could not have been produced without the agent's presence; and (3) by detecting an immunological response specific to the infecting agent in the patient's serum. Detection of the agent by visualization or cultivation is the focus of much of this text, covered extensively in Parts Two and Three. Detection of products or antigens of the agent is addressed in Chapter 10 and again as this diagnostic method relates to individual pathogens. Methods for documenting the presence of an immune response will be described in this chapter.

12.1. General Features of the Immune Response

12.1.a. Categories of immune responses. The human specific immune responses are simplistically divided into two categories. Cell-mediated immune responses, which are carried out by special lymphocytes of the T (thymus-derived) class, include production of activator chemicals that induce other cells to attack and kill pathogens readily as well as the direct attacking and killing of pathogens (or host cells damaged or infected by pathogens) by the T lymphocytes themselves. Although diagnosis of certain diseases may be aided by measuring the cell-mediated immune response to the pathogen, such tests entail skin tests performed by physicians or in vitro cell function assays, performed by specially trained immunologists. These tests are usually not within the repertoire of clinical microbiology laboratories and a discussion of their performance is beyond the scope of this book. Antibody-mediated immune responses are those produced by specific proteins generated by lymphocytes of the B (bone marrow—derived) class. Because these proteins have immunological function and because they fold into a globular structure in the active state, they are called **immunoglobulins.** Immunoglobulins, also called **antibodies,** since they are produced against a particular foreign structure or "body," attach to offending agents or their products and thus aid the host in removing the agents. These agents need not be pathogenic microorganisms, as the immune system is also effective against some tumor cells, transplanted (nonself) tissue, pollen, and other foreign substances. This chapter will deal only with the detection of antibodies produced against infectious agents, although many of the techniques employed may be used for the detection of other types of antibodies.

Antibodies are either secreted into the blood or lymphatic fluid (and sometimes other body fluids) by the B lymphocytes, or they remain attached to the surface of the lymphocyte or other effector cells. Because the mediators of this category of immune response chiefly circulate in the blood, this type of immunity is also called **humoral immunity.** For purposes of determining whether an antibody has been produced against a particular agent by a patient, the patient's **serum** (or occasionally the plasma) is tested for the presence of the antibody. The study of the diagnosis of disease by measuring antibody levels in serum is thus called *serology*.

12.1.b. Characteristics of antibodies. Antibodies are produced against a specific small chemically and physically defined substance recognized as foreign by the host, called an antigen or an antigenic determinant. By a genetically determined mechanism, normal humans are able to produce antibodies specifically directed against almost all the antigens with which they might come into contact throughout their lifetimes. Antigens may be part of the physical structure of the pathogen or they may be a chemical produced and released by the pathogen. One pathogen may contain or produce many different antigens

that the host will recognize as foreign, so that infection with one agent may cause a number of different antibodies to appear. *Streptococcus pyogenes* is an example of a pathogen that induces production of several different antibodies (Figure 12.1). In addition, some antigenic determinants of a pathogen may not be available for recognition by the host until the pathogen has undergone a physical change. For example, until a pathogenic bacterium has been digested by a human polymorphonuclear neutrophil, certain antigens deep within the cell wall are not "visible" to the host immune system. Once the bacterium is broken down, these new antigens are revealed and antibodies can be produced against them. For this reason, a patient may produce different antibodies at different times during the course of a single disease.

Antibodies function by attaching to the surface of pathogens and making the pathogens more amenable to ingestion by phagocytic cells (**opsonizing** antibodies) or by attaching to the surface of pathogens and contributing to their destruction by the lytic action of complement (complement-fixing antibodies). Although humans produce several different classes of antibodies, differentiated by their structures, diagnostic serologic methods have been primarily developed to measure only two antibody classes, **immunoglobulin M (IgM)** and **immunoglobulin G (IgG).** The basic structure of an antibody molecule is comprised of two mirror images, each made up of two identical protein chains. At the terminal ends are the antigen-binding sites, which specifically attach to the antigen against which the antibody was. produced. Depending on the specificity of the antibody, antigens of some similarity, but not identical, to the inducing antigen may also be bound. The complement-binding site is found in the center of the molecule in a structure that is similar for all antibodies of the same class. In most cases, the first antibody produced in response to a foreign agent is IgM. Thus, presence of IgM is usually indicative of recent infection and active infection. IgG antibody may persist long after infection has run its course. The IgM antibody type (Figure 12.2) consists of five identical proteins with the basic antibody structures linked together at the bases, leaving 10 antigen-binding sites available. The second antibody class, IgG, consists of one basic antibody molecule with two binding sites (Figure 12.3). The differences in the size and conformation between these two classes

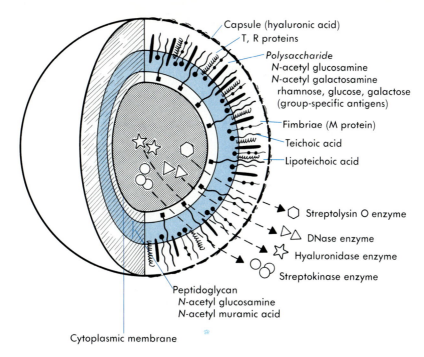

Figure 12.1
S. pyogenes contains many antigenic structural components and produces several antigenic enzymes, each of which may elicit a specific antibody response from the infected host.

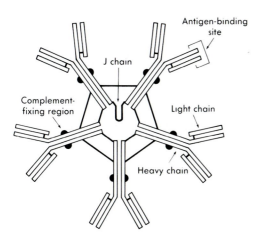

Figure 12.2
Structure of immunoglobulin M.

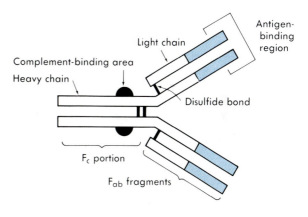

Figure 12.3
Structure of immunoglobulin G.

of immunoglobulins result in differences in activities and functions.

12.1.c. Features of humoral immune response useful in diagnostic testing. Normal humans produce both IgM and IgG in response to most pathogens. The larger number of binding sites on IgM molecules can help to more quickly clear the offending patho-

gen, even though each individual antigen-binding site may not be the most efficient for attaching the antigen. Over time, the cells that were producing IgM switch to producing IgG, often more specific for the antigen (also called more **avid**). The IgG has only two binding sites, but it can bind complement. When IgG has bound to an antigen, the base of the molecule may be left projecting out in the environment. Structures on the base attract and bind phagocytic cell membranes, increasing the chances of engulfment and destruction of the pathogen by the host cells. In most cases IgM is produced by a patient only after the first interaction with a given pathogen and is no longer detectable within a relatively short period afterward. For serologic diagnostic purposes, one important difference between IgG and IgM is that IgM cannot cross the placenta of pregnant women. Therefore, any IgM detected in the serum of a newborn baby must have been produced by the baby itself. IgM, because of its shape, cannot bind complement. Other differences between IgG and IgM are exploited to separate them so that the presence of one class of antibody in a patient's serum will not interfere with testing for the presence of the other class. A second encounter with the same pathogen will usually induce only an IgG response. Because the B lymphocytes retain memory of this pathogen, however, they can respond more quickly and with larger numbers of antibodies than at the initial interaction. This response is called the **anamnestic response.** Because the B cell memory is not perfect, occasional clones of memory cells will be stimulated by an antigen that is similar but not identical to the original antigen; thus, the anamnestic response may be polyclonal and nonspecific. For example, reinfection with cytomegalovirus may stimulate memory B cells to produce antibody against Epstein-Barr virus, which they encountered previously, in addition to antibody against cytomegalovirus. The relative humoral responses over time are diagramed in Figure 12.4.

12.1.d. Interpretation of serologic tests. A central dogma of serology is the concept of "rise in titer." The **titer** of antibody is the reciprocal of the highest dilution of the patient's serum in which the antibody is still detectable. Patients with large amounts of antibody have high titers, since antibody will still be detectable at very high dilutions of serum. Serum for antibody levels should be drawn during the acute phase of the disease (when it is first discovered or suspected) and again during convalescence (usually at least 2 weeks later). These specimens are called **acute** and **convalescent sera.** For some infections, such as Legionnaires' disease, hepatitis, and others, titers may not rise until months after the acute infection or may never rise. Accurate results useful for diagnosis of many infections are achieved only when acute and convalescent sera are tested concurrently in the same system, since variables inherent in the

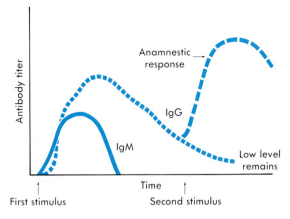

Figure 12.4
Relative humoral response to antigen stimulation over time.

procedures and laboratory error can easily result in differences of one doubling (or twofold) dilution in the results obtained from even the same sample tested at the same time.

Patients with intact humoral immunity will develop increasing amounts of antibody to a disease-causing pathogen over several weeks. If it is the patient's first encounter with the pathogen and the specimen has been obtained early enough, no antibody will be present at the onset of disease. In the case of a second encounter the patient's serum will usually contain measurable antibody during the initial phase of disease and the level of antibody will quickly increase, due to the anamnestic response. For most pathogens, an increase in the patient's titer of two doubling dilutions (for example, from a positive result at 1:8 to a positive result at 1:32) is considered to be diagnostic of current infection. This is called a fourfold rise in titer.

With most diseases, there exists a spectrum of responses in infected humans, such that a person may develop antibody from subclinical infection or after colonization by an agent without actually having disease. In these cases, the presence of antibody in a single serum specimen or a similar titer of antibody in paired sera may merely indicate past contact with the agent and cannot be used to accurately diagnose a recent disease. On the other hand, patients may respond to an antigenic stimulus by producing antibody that can cross-react with other antigens. These antibodies are nonspecific and thus they may cause misinterpretation of serologic tests. Therefore, for the vast majority of serologic procedures for diagnosis of recent infection, testing both acute and convalescent sera is the method of choice. Except for detecting the presence of IgM, the testing of a single serum can be recommended only in certain cases, such as for diagnosis of recent infection with *Mycoplasma pneumoniae* and viral influenza B, where high titers may indicate recent infection. Unfortunately, a certain proportion of infected individuals may never show a rise in titer, necessitating the use of other diagnostic measures. Cumitech 15, by Chernesky and others,[1] contains an excellent discussion on the collection and interpretation of paired sera for immunological testing. Because the delay inherent in testing paired acute and convalescent sera results in diagnostic information that arrives too late to influence initial therapy, increasing numbers of early serologic testing assays are being evaluated. More sensitive and specific measurements for IgM are often keys to these newer methods.

If the infecting or disease-causing agent is extremely rare and people without disease or prior immunization would have no chance of developing an immune response, such as the rabies virus or the toxin of botulism, the presence of specific antibody in a single serum specimen can be diagnostic. There are, in addition, a number of circumstances when serum is tested only to determine whether a patient is "immune," that is, has antibody to a particular agent either in response to a past infection or to immunization. These tests can be performed with a single serum sample. Correlation of the results of such tests with the actual immune status of individual patients must be performed to determine the level of detectable antibody present that corresponds to actual immunity to infection or reinfection in the host. For example, very sensitive tests can detect the presence of very tiny amounts of antibody to the rubella virus. Certain people, however, may still be susceptible to infection with the rubella virus with such small amounts of circulating antibody, and a higher level of antibody may be required to assure protection from disease. Depending on the etiologic agent, even low levels of antibody may protect a patient from pathologic effects of disease, although they may not prevent reinfection. As more sensitive testing methods are developed, and these types of problems become more common, microbiologists will need to work closely with clinicians to develop guidelines for interpreting serologic test results as they relate to the status of individual patients.

12.2. Principles of Serologic Test Methods

Antibodies can be detected in many different ways. In some cases, antibodies to an agent may be detected in more than one way, but the different antibody detection tests may not be measuring the same antibody. For this reason, the presence of antibodies to a particular pathogen as detected by one method may not correlate with the presence of antibodies to the same agent detected by another test method. This concept will become clearer after antibody detection methods have been discussed.

Slide agglutination tests are the easiest to perform and in some cases are the most sensitive tests currently available. Either artificial carriers, such as latex particles or treated red blood cells, or biological carriers, such as whole bacterial cells, can carry on their surface an antigen that will bind with antibody produced in response to that antigen when it was introduced to the host. Reagents for many of the following tests are commercially available; selected suppliers are listed in Appendix C.

12.2.a. Direct whole pathogen agglutination for antibody detection. The most basic tests for antibody are those that measure the antibody produced by a host to determinants on the surface of a bacterial agent in response to infection with that agent. Specific antibodies bind to surface antigens of the bacteria in a thick suspension and cause the bacteria to clump together in visible aggregates (Figure 12.5). Such antibodies are called agglutinating antibodies, and the reaction is called bacterial **agglutination**. Electrostatic and other forces influence the formation of aggregates in solutions, so that certain conditions are usually necessary for good results. Since most bacterial surfaces exhibit a negative charge, they tend to repel each other. Performance of agglutination tests in sterile physiologic saline (0.85% sodium chloride in distilled water), which has free positive ions present in the solution, will enhance the ability of antibody to cause aggregation of bacteria. Bacterial agglutination tests can be performed on the surface of glass slides or in tubes. Tube agglutination tests are often more sensitive, since a longer incubation period, allowing more antigen and antibody to interact, can be used. The small volume of liquid used for slide tests requires a rather rapid reading of the result, before the liquid has evaporated.

Examples of bacterial agglutination tests are the tests for antibodies to *Francisella tularensis* and *Bru-*

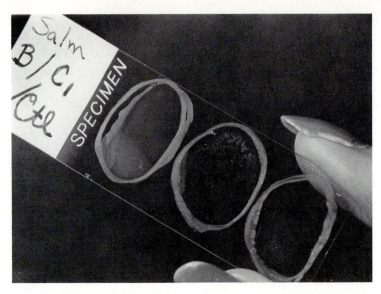

Figure 12.5
Example of a slide agglutination test. An organism that biochemically resembles a *Salmonella* species is emulsified in several drops of saline on a slide. Drops of antiserum prepared against specific *Salmonella* serotypes are added to the suspension; the organism agglutinates in the presence of homologous antiserum (center circle).

cella species, usually part of a panel of so-called "febrile agglutinin" tests. Bacterial agglutination tests are often used to diagnose diseases in which the bacterial agent is difficult to cultivate in vitro. Diseases commonly diagnosed by this technique include tetanus, yersiniosis, leptospirosis, brucellosis, and tularemia. The reagents necessary to perform many of these tests are commercially available, singly or as complete systems (Appendix C). Agglutination tests for certain diseases such as typhoid fever have become less useful with the ability of most laboratories to culture and identify the causative agent. Furthermore, the typhoid febrile agglutinin test (called the Widal test) is often positive in patients with infections caused by other bacteria, due to cross-reacting antibodies or to previous immunization against typhoid. We recommend that appropriate specimens from patients suspected of having typhoid fever be cultured for the presence of salmonellae (stool, urine, or blood, as appropriate) and that reliance not be placed on febrile agglutinins for diagnosis of this disease.

Whole cells of parasites, including *Plasmodium*, *Leishmania*, or *Toxoplasma gondii*, have also been used for direct detection of antibody by agglutination. In addition to using the actual infecting bacteria or parasites as the agglutinating particles for the detection of antibodies, certain bacteria may be agglutinated by antibodies produced against another infecting agent. Many patients infected with one of the rickettsiae produce antibodies that can agglutinate bacteria of the genus *Proteus*. Tests for these cross-reacting antibodies are called the **Weil-Felix tests.** Although these antibodies are also produced in response to bacterial infection, their presence has been used traditionally as presumptive serologic evidence of rickettsial disease. As newer, more specific serologic methods of diagnosing rickettsial disease become more widely available, the use of the *Proteus* agglutinating tests should be discontinued.

12.2.b. **Latex particle agglutination tests.** Numerous serologic procedures have been developed for the detection of antibody via the agglutination of an artificial carrier with antigen bound to its surface. As noted in Chapter 10, similar systems employing artificial carriers coated with antibodies are commonly used for detection of microbial antigens. Antigens of streptococci, *Cryptococcus neoformans*, agents of bacterial meningitis, and other etiologic agents can be detected using latex and staphylococcal particle agglutination systems. The size of the carrier enhances the visibility of the agglutination reaction, and the artificial nature of the system allows the antigen bound to the surface to be extremely specific. Complete systems for the use of latex or other particle agglutination tests are commercially available for the accurate and sensitive detection of antibody to cytomegalovirus and rubella virus. *Toxoplasma,* the heterophile antibody of infectious mononucleosis, teichoic acid antibodies against staphylococci, antistreptococcal antibodies, mycoplasma antibodies, and other systems are in the evaluation stage. Staphylococci containing protein A have occasionally been used as antibody-capture reagents, or to remove IgG from serum that also contains IgM. Although latex particle agglutination tests have been developed for detecting antibodies to gonococci, they have not been found to be as reliable as other tests for gonorrhea. Latex tests for antibodies to *Coccidioides, Sporothrix, Echinococcus,* and *Trichinella* are available, although they are not widely used because of the uncommon occurrence of the corresponding infection or its limited geographic distribution. Use of tests for *Candida* antibodies has not yet shown results reliable enough for diagnosis. Results of latex agglutination tests are dependent on several factors, including the amount and avidity of antigen conjugated to the carrier, the time of incubation together with patient's serum (or other source of antibody), and the microenvironment of the interaction (including pH, tonicity, protein concentration, and so forth).[4] Commercial tests have been developed as systems, complete with their own diluents, controls, and containers. For accurate results, they should be used as units, without modifications. If tests have been developed for use with cerebrospinal fluid, for example, they should not be used with serum unless the product insert or the technical representative has certified such usage.

12.2.c. **Hemagglutination tests for antibody detection.** Treated animal red blood cells have also been used as carriers of antigen for agglutination tests, called indirect **hemagglutination** or passive hemagglutination tests, since it is not the antigens of the blood cells themselves but the passively attached antigens that are being bound by antibody. The most widely used of these tests are the microhemagglutination test for antibody to *Treponema pallidum* (MHA-TP, so-called because it is performed in a microtiter plate), the hemagglutination treponemal test for syphilis (HATTS), the passive hemagglutination tests for antibody to extracellular antigens of streptococci, and the rubella indirect hemagglutination tests, all of which are available commercially. Certain reference laboratories, such as the Centers for Disease Control, also perform indirect hemagglutination tests for antibodies to some clostridia, *Pseudomonas pseudomallei, Bacillus anthracis, Corynebacterium diphtheriae, Leptospira,* and the agents of several viral and parasitic diseases.

12.2.d. **Flocculation tests for antibody detection.** In contrast to the aggregates formed when particulate antigens bind to specific antibody, the interaction of soluble antigen with antibody results in the formation of a precipitate, a concentration of fine particles, usually visible only because the precipitated product is forced to remain in a defined space within a matrix. Although the **precipitin test** is not used for serologic determinations directly, two variations are widely used. In **flocculation tests,** the precipitin end product forms macroscopically or microscopically visible clumps. The Venereal Disease Research Laboratory test, known as the **VDRL,** is the most widely used flocculation test. Patients infected with pathogenic treponemes, most commonly *T. pallidum,* the agent of syphilis, form an antibodylike protein called **reagin** that binds to the test antigen, cardiolipin-lecithin–coated cholesterol particles, causing the particles to flocculate. Since reagin is not a specific antibody directed against *T. pallidum* antigens, the test is not highly specific, but it is a good screening test, detecting over 99% of cases of secondary syphilis. Very early in the infection, the VDRL test is still negative. Conditions and infections other than syphilis can cause a patient's serum to yield a positive result in the VDRL test, called a "biologic false positive" test. The VDRL is the single most useful test available for testing cerebrospinal fluid in cases of suspected neurosyphilis, although it may be falsely positive in the absence of this disease. The performance of the VDRL test requires scrupulously clean glassware and exacting attention to detail, including numerous daily quality control checks. In addition, the reagents must be prepared fresh each time the test is performed, patients' sera must be inactivated by heating for 30 minutes at 56° C before testing, and the reaction must be read microscopically. For all these reasons, it is being supplanted in many laboratories by a qualitatively comparable test, the rapid plasma reagin, or **RPR** test.

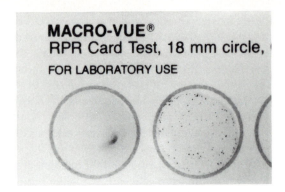

Figure 12.6
Rapid plasma reagin test for syphilis. (Courtesy Hynson, Westcott, & Dunning.)

The RPR test is commercially available as a complete system containing positive and negative controls, the reaction card, and the prepared antigen suspension. The antigen, cardiolipin-lecithin–coated cholesterol with choline chloride, also contains charcoal particles to allow for macroscopically visible flocculation. Sera are tested without heating, and the reaction takes place on the surface of a specially treated cardboard card, which is then discarded (Figure 12.6). The RPR test is not recommended for testing cerebrospinal fluid. All procedures are standardized and clearly described in product inserts, and these procedures should be adhered to strictly. The failure of the RPR test to detect minimally reactive sera in one statewide proficiency testing survey was shown to be due to deficiencies in technique used, rather than deficiencies in the reagents or the test system itself. An excellent set of guidelines for acceptable test performance was published by Neimeister and coworkers.[3] Overall, the RPR appears to be a more specific screening test for syphilis than the VDRL and it is certainly easier to perform. Flocculation tests are also performed to detect antibodies to *Trichinella*; reagents are commercially available.

12.2.e. Countercurrent immunoelectrophoresis for antibody detection. The second variation of the classic precipitin test has been widely used to detect small amounts of antibody. This test takes advantage of the net electric charge of the antigens and antibodies being tested in a particular test buffer. Because the antigen and antibody being sought migrate toward one another in a semisolid matrix under the influence of an electrical current, the method is called countercurrent immunoelectrophoresis, or simply **counterimmunoelectrophoresis (CIE)**. The principles of this test were outlined in Chapter 10; the same methodology is used to identify specific antigen or antibody. When antigen and antibody meet in optimal proportions, a line of precipitation will appear. Since all variables, such as buffer pH, type of gel or agarose matrix, amount of current, amounts and concentrations of antigen and antibody, size of antigen and antibody inocula, and placement of these inocula, must be carefully controlled for maximum reactivity, CIE tests are difficult to develop and perform. Other methods for detection of antibody to infectious agents are more commonly used in most diagnostic laboratories. A very sensitive, but not very specific, commercially available test employs CIE for detection of antibody to *Entamoeba histolytica* in patients suspected of having invasive, extraintestinal amebic disease, primarily liver abscess.

12.2.f. Immunodiffusion assays for detection of antifungal antibodies. Closely resembling the precipitin test is a method widely used for detecting antibodies directed against fungal cell components, the immunodiffusion assay (ID). Whole cell extracts or other antigens of the suspected fungus are placed in wells in an agarose plate and the patient's serum and a control positive serum are placed in adjoining wells. If the patient has produced specific antibody against the fungus, precipitin lines will be visible between the wells; their identity to similar lines from the control serum helps establish the results. The type and thickness of the precipitin bands may have prognostic as well as diagnostic value. Antibodies against *Histoplasma*, *Blastomyces*, *Coccidioides*, *Paracoccidioides*, and some opportunistic fungi are routinely detected by ID. Immunodiffusion tests usually require at least 48 hours and may require additional washing time to develop the bands.

12.2.g. Hemagglutination inhibition tests for viral antibodies. Many human viruses have the ability to bind to surface structures on red blood cells from different species. For example, rubella virus particles can bind to human type O, goose, or chicken erythrocytes and cause agglutination of the red blood cells. Influenza and parainfluenza viruses agglutinate guinea pig, chicken, or human O erythrocytes; many arboviruses agglutinate goose red blood cells; adenoviruses agglutinate rat or rhesus monkey cells;

mumps virus agglutinates chicken or goose cells; measles virus binds red blood cells of monkeys; and herpesvirus and cytomegalovirus agglutinate sheep red blood cells. Serologic tests for the presence of antibodies to these viruses exploit the agglutinating properties of the virus particles. Patients' sera that have been treated with kaolin or heparin-magnesium chloride (to remove nonspecific inhibitors of red cell agglutination and nonspecific agglutinins of the red cells) are added to a system that contains the virus suspected of causing disease. If antibodies to the virus are present, they will form complexes and block the binding sites on the viral surfaces. When the proper red cells are added to the solution, all of the virus particles will be bound by antibody, preventing the virus from agglutinating the red cells. Thus the patient's serum is positive for hemagglutination-inhibiting antibodies. As for most serologic procedures, a fourfold increase in such titers is considered diagnostic. The hemagglutination inhibition tests for most agents are performed only at reference laboratories. Procedures for performing such tests are delineated in the *Manual of Clinical Immunology* (American Society for Microbiology). Rubella antibodies, however, are often detected with this method in routine diagnostic laboratories. Several commercial rubella antibody detection systems are available.

12.2.h. Neutralization tests. To test for certain antibodies, the ability of a patient's serum to block the effect of the antigenic agent can be evaluated. In the case of viruses, antibody that destroys the infectivity of the virus is called "neutralizing antibody." The serum to be tested is mixed with a suspension of infectious virus particles of the same type as those with which the patient is suspected of being infected. A control suspension of viruses is mixed with normal serum. The virus suspensions are then inoculated into a cell culture system that supports growth of the virus. The control cells will display evidence of virus infection. If the patient's serum contains antibody to the virus, that antibody will bind the virus particles and prevent them from invading the cells in culture. The antibody has "neutralized" the infectivity of the virus. These tests are technically demanding and time-consuming and are performed only in those laboratories that routinely perform virus cultures.

Antibodies to bacterial toxins and other extracellular products that display measurable activities can be tested in the same way. The ability of a patient's serum to neutralize the erythrocyte-lysing capability of streptolysin O, an extracellular enzyme produced by *S. pyogenes* during infection, has been used for many years as a test for previous streptococcal infection. After pharyngitis with streptolysin O–producing strains, most patients show a high titer of the antibody antistreptolysin O (**ASO**). Streptococci also produce the enzyme deoxyribonuclease B (DNase B) during infections of the throat, skin, or other tissue. A neutralization test that prevents activity of this enzyme, the *anti-DNase B test*, has also been used extensively as an indicator of recent or previous streptococcal disease. The use of particle agglutination (latex or indirect hemagglutination) tests for the presence of antibody to many of the streptococcal enzymes has replaced the use of these neutralization tests in many laboratories.

12.2.i. Complement fixation for antibody detection. One of the classic methods for demonstrating the presence of antibody in a patient's serum has been the **complement fixation test (CF)**. This test consists of two separate systems, the first (the indicator system) consisting of a combination of sheep red blood cells, complement-fixing antibody (IgG) raised against the sheep red blood cells in another animal, and an exogenous source of complement (usually guinea pig serum). When these three components are mixed together in optimum concentrations, the anti–sheep erythrocyte antibody will bind to the surface of the red cells and the complement will then bind to the antigen-antibody complex, ultimately causing lysis of the red cells. For this reason, the anti–sheep red cell antibody is also called "hemolysin." The second system consists of the antigen suspected of causing the patient's disease and the patient's serum. These components are added to a suspension of the sheep erythrocytes, hemolysin, and a critical amount of complement. For the CF test, these two systems are tested in sequence (Figure 12.7). The patient's serum is first added to the putative antigen; then the limiting amount of complement is added to the solution. If the patient's serum contains antibody to the antigen, these antigen-antibody complexes will bind all of the complement added. In the next step, the sheep red blood cells and the hemolysin (indicator system) are added. Only if the complement has not been bound by a complex formed with antibody from the patient's serum will the complement be available to bind to

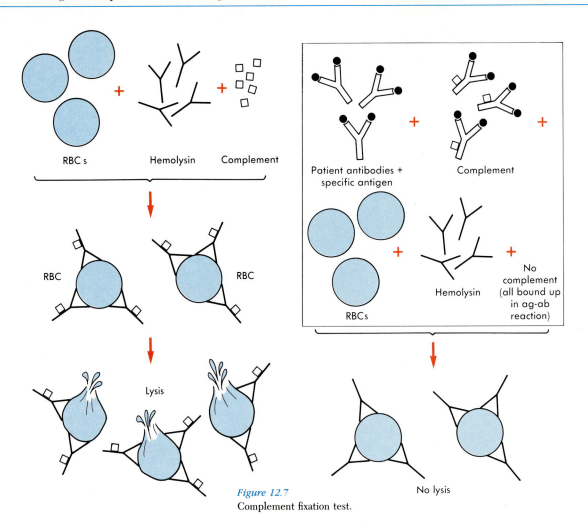

Figure 12.7
Complement fixation test.

the sheep cell–hemolysin complexes and cause lysis. A positive result, meaning the patient does possess complement-fixing antibodies, is revealed by failure of the red cells to lyse in the final test system. Lysis of the indicator cells indicates lack of antibody and a negative CF test.

This test has been used over the years for the detection of many types of antibodies, particularly antiviral, although it requires many manipulations, at least 48 hours for both stages of the test to be completed, and often yields nonspecific results. Many new systems both for improved recovery of pathogens or their products and for more sensitive and less demanding procedures for detection of antibodies, including particle agglutination, indirect fluorescent antibody tests, and ELISA procedures, described in this chapter and throughout the text,

have gradually been introduced to replace the CF test. At this time CF tests are performed chiefly for diagnosis of unusual infections; these tests are done primarily in reference laboratories. This test is still probably the most common method for diagnosis of infection due to some respiratory viruses, influenza A and B, parainfluenza, adenovirus, and arboviruses, some fungi, as well as for diagnosis of Q fever. It is recommended that laboratories without experience in performing these tests not adopt complement fixation tests for routine diagnostic testing when other, less demanding, procedures are available.

12.2.j. Enzyme-linked immunosorbent assays. The number of antibody detection tests developed utilizing **enzyme-linked immunosorbent assay (ELISA)** technology is expanding rapidly. ELISA methods for antibodies to infectious agents are sensitive and specific. As described more thoroughly in Chapter 10, the presence of specific antibody is detected by its ability to bind a second antibody conjugated to a colored or fluorescent marker. Various enzyme-substrate systems and the use of avidin-biotin to bind marker substances were also discussed in Chapter 10. The antigen to which the antibodies bind, if they are present in patients' sera, is either attached to the inside of wells of a microtiter plate, adherent to a filter matrix, or bound to the surface of beads or plastic paddles. Although the sensitivity of certain particle-agglutinating tests is greater than ELISA tests for antibody at the current time, ELISA methodology is being improved rapidly. The addition of membrane-bound ELISA components has improved sensitivity and ease of use dramatically. Once a few of the other disadvantages of this method have been overcome (some are mentioned later), it is probable that these systems will be the most commonly used antibody-detection systems. Currently, most ELISA test procedures require several incubation periods and washes. However, the complete automation of these procedures is possible, and much automation has already been introduced into commercial systems. Advantages are that tests can be performed easily on many serum samples at the same time and that the colored or fluorescent end products are easily detected by instruments, removing the element of subjectivity inherent in so many serologic procedures that rely on a technologist's interpretation of a reaction. Disadvantages include the need for some special equipment; the fairly long reaction times (usually hours instead of minutes); the relative end point of the test (that relies on measuring the amount of a visible end product that is not dependent on the original antigen-antibody reaction itself, but on a second enzymatic reaction), as compared with a directly quantitative result; and the requirement for batch processing to ensure that performance of the test is cost-effective. Possibly as a result of the measurement of the end point of a secondary reaction, ELISA methods do not generate a true titer result, another major disadvantage of the system. ELISA results thus may not correlate well with titers, a problem for those who are accustomed to interpreting serologic results as titers.

A general discussion of the principles of automated ELISA readers currently available is found in Chapter 11. Commercial microdilution systems are available for the detection of antibody specific for hepatitis virus antigens, herpes simplex viruses I and II, respiratory syncytial virus, cytomegalovirus, human immunodeficiency virus (HIV) (the etiologic agent of acquired immunodeficiency syndrome [AIDS]), rubella virus (both IgG and IgM), mycoplasmas, chlamydiae, the Lyme disease spirochete (*Borrelia burgdorferi*), *E. histolytica*, and *T. gondii*. Accuracy of the results of these tests is variable. ELISA systems with the solid phase represented by a bead of metal or glass are available for detection of antibody to rubella virus, cytomegalovirus, herpes simplex virus, *T. gondii*, *T. pallidum*, *E. histolytica*, HIV, and numerous other pathogens. Even when not available commercially, ELISA methods have been developed for detection of antibody to almost all microbial pathogens. The recent advances in ELISA methods, including membrane-fixed antibodies, fluorescent labels, more specific antibodies (discussed more completely in Chapter 10), and others have brought ELISA methodology to the forefront of serologic assay techniques in routine use today.

12.3. Indirect Fluorescent Antibody Tests and Other Immunomicroscopic Methods

Perhaps the serologic method most widely applied for the detection of diverse antibodies is that of indirect fluorescent antibody determination (**IFA**). For tests of this type, the antigen against which the patient makes antibody (such as whole *Toxoplasma* organisms or viruses in infected tissue culture cells) is affixed to the surface of a microscope slide. The patient's serum to be tested is diluted and placed on the slide, covering the area in which antigen was placed. If antibody is present in the serum, it will bind to its specific antigen. Unbound antibody is then removed by washing the slide. In the second stage of the procedure, antihuman globulin (which may be directed specifically against IgG or IgM) conjugated to a dye that will fluoresce when exposed to ultraviolet light (such as fluorescein) is placed on the slide. This conjugated marker for human antibody will bind to the antibody already bound to the antigen on the slide and will serve as a marker for the antibody when viewed under a fluorescence microscope (Figure 12.8). Commercially available systems include the slides with the antigens, positive and negative control sera, diluent for the patients' sera, and the properly diluted conjugate. As with other

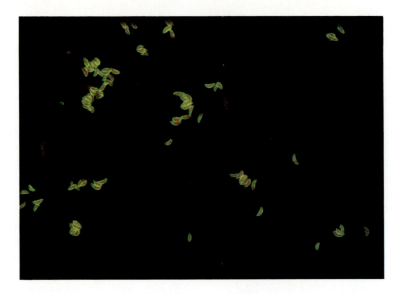

Figure 12.8
Indirect fluorescent antibody test for *T. gondii* antibodies. *Toxoplasma* organisms affixed to the slide
bind specific antibodies in the patient's serum. Antihuman antibody conjugated with fluorescein binds
in turn to the bound patient's antibodies, causing the organisms to fluoresce.

commercial products, IFA systems should be used as units, without modifying the manufacturers' instructions. After they have been stained, the slides are covered with a drop of buffered glycerol and a glass coverslip is applied. The fluorescence does not fade appreciably for several days if the slides are kept refrigerated in the dark, but it is best to examine them immediately after staining. Such slides cannot be used as permanent mounts, since the fluorescence does fade with time. Currently, commercially available IFA tests include those for antibodies to *Legionella* species; *B. burgdorferi*; *T. gondii*; varicella-zoster virus; cytomegalovirus; Epstein-Barr virus capsid antigen, early antigen, and nuclear antigen; herpes simplex viruses I and II; rubella virus; *M. pneumoniae*; *T. pallidum* (the fluorescent treponemal antibody absorption test, **FTA-ABS**); and several rickettsiae. Most of these tests, if performed properly, give extremely specific and sensitive results, although polyclonal antibodies often yield cross-reactive positive results; monoclonal antibody stains are usually less sensitive but more specific. Although proper interpretation of IFA tests requires experienced and technically competent technologists, these tests can be performed rapidly and are cost-effective with only a few samples, in contrast to ELISA.

Antibodies may be conjugated to other markers in addition to fluorescent dyes. This technology has been called "colorimetric immunologic probe detection." Recently, the use of enzyme-substrate marker systems has expanded. Horseradish peroxidase, alkaline phosphatase, and avidin-biotin–conjugated enzyme labels have all been used as visual tags for the presence of antibody. These reagents have the advantages of allowing the preparation of permanent mounts, since the reactions do not fade with storage, and of requiring only a standard light microscope for visualizing results.

12.4. Radioimmunoassay

This automated method of detecting antibodies is usually not performed in a serology laboratory, but in a chemistry laboratory. **Radioimmunoassay (RIA)** is primarily used to measure antigens (notably certain hormones or proteins) in serum samples. The techniques can be used to determine the quantity of antibody as well. For diagnosis of infectious diseases, RIA tests are primarily used to detect antibody to hepatitis B viral proteins. As described in Chapter 11, radioactively labeled antibody competes with the patient's unlabeled antibody for binding sites on a known amount of antigen. A reduction in radioactivity of the antigen-patient antibody complex compared with the radioactive counts measured in a control test with no antibody is used to quantitate the amount of patient antibody bound to the antigen. The development of new marker substances, such as enzyme and substrate systems, chemiluminescence, and fluorescence, is leading to availability of tests as sensitive as RIA without the hazards of radioactive reagents.

12.5. Fluorescence Immunoassays

Because of the inconveniences associated with radioactive substances and scintillation counters, **fluorescent immunoassays (FIA)** were developed. Using fluorescent dyes or molecules as markers instead of radioactive labels, these tests are based on the same principle as RIA. The primary difference is that in RIA systems the competitive antibody is labeled with a radioisotope and in FIA the antigen is labeled with a compound that will fluoresce under the appropriate light rays. Binding of patient antibody to a fluorescent-labeled antigen can reduce or "quench" the fluorescence, or binding can cause fluorescence by allowing conformational change in a fluorescent molecule. These principles and others can be employed for diagnostic tests. Chapter 11 describes the principles involved in the fluorescence immunoassay for microbiological determinations. Systems are commercially available to measure antibody developed against a number of infectious agents, as well as against self-antigens (autoimmune antibodies).

12.6. Separating IgM from IgG for Serologic Testing

Since IgM is usually produced only during a patient's first exposure to an infectious agent, the detection of specific IgM can help the clinician a great deal in establishing a diagnosis, especially for diseases that may have less well-characterized clinical presentations, such as toxoplasmosis, or those for which rapid therapeutic decisions may be required. Pregnant women who are exposed to rubella and develop a mild febrile illness can be tested for the presence of antirubella IgM. If positive, damage to the fetus is possible and the option of elective termination of pregnancy should be offered. An additional reason to measure IgM alone is for the diagnosis of neonatal infections. Since IgG can readily cross the placenta, newborn babies will carry titers of IgG nearly identical to those of their mothers. Accurate serologic

diagnosis of infection in neonates requires either demonstration of a rise in titer (which takes time to occur) or the detection of specific IgM directed against the putative agent. This IgM would have to be of fetal origin, since the molecule does not cross the placental barrier. Agents that are difficult to culture or those that adult females would be expected to have encountered during their lifetimes, such as cytomegalovirus, herpesviruses, *Toxoplasma*, rubella virus, or *T. pallidum*, are those for which specific identification of fetal IgM is most often used. The names of some of these agents have been grouped together with the acronym **TORCH** (*Toxoplasma*, rubella, cytomegalovirus, and herpes). These tests should be ordered separately, depending on the clinical illness of a newborn suspected of having one of these diseases. However, infected babies often appear clinically the same as those without any of these infections.

Several methods have been developed to measure only the specific IgM in sera that may also contain specific IgG. In addition to using a labeled antibody specific for only IgM as the marker in the assays described above, the immunoglobulins can be separated from each other by physical means. Centrifugation through a sucrose gradient, performed at very high speeds, has been used in the past to separate IgM, which has a greater molecular weight, from IgG. This method is time consuming and requires a very expensive ultracentrifuge. Many laboratories use a commercially available system that follows the principle of ion exchange (Figure 12.9). In the system's original format, serum was placed on a column of QAE-Sephadex A-50 (an ion-exchange resin that binds proteins on the basis of attracting molecules of opposite electrical charge).[2] Both immunoglobulins initially bind to the resin. A solution of buffer at pH 7.0 was run through the column, and IgG, because of its relatively lesser negative charge, was washed through (eluted) with the buffer. A second buffer of pH 4.2 was then run through the column to elute the more negatively charged IgM. A newer version of the column removes the required pH step but may recover slightly less IgM. The commercially available IgM isolation system (Isolab, Inc.) recovers more than 80% of the IgM present in the original serum, with a small amount of contaminating IgG. Since the serum must be washed through the column with buffer, the IgM solution in the eluate (fluid collected from the col-

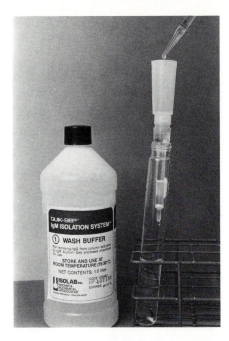

Figure 12.9
Separation of IgM from human serum by passing the serum through an ion-exchange column.

umn) is more dilute than in the original serum (usually 1:10, depending on the volume of serum originally placed on the column).

Other IgM separation systems available utilize the fact that certain proteins on the surface of staphylococci (protein A) and streptococci (protein G) will bind the Fc portion of IgG. A simple centrifugation then separates the particles and their bound immunoglobulins from the remaining mixture, which contains the bulk of the IgM. Other methods use antihuman IgG antibodies to remove IgG from sera containing both IgG and IgM. Different systems perform best under different circumstances and for recovery of specific immunoglobulins. An added bonus of IgM separation systems is that **rheumatoid factor,** IgM antibodies produced by some patients against their own IgG, will often bind to the IgG molecules being removed from the serum and consequently these IgM antibodies will be removed along with the IgG. Rheumatoid factor can cause nonspecific and interfering results with many serologic tests, and its presence should be taken into account. There are many cases in which serologic tests can yield false-positive and false-negative results. Other considerations, including patient history and clinical situation, must be employed in the diagnosis of neonatal infection. Culturing the agent from patient material from infants suspected of having herpesvirus or cytomegalovirus infection is still the most reliable diagnostic method.

REFERENCES

1. Chernesky, M.A., Ray, C.G., and Smith, T.F. 1982. In Drew, W.L., editor. Laboratory diagnosis of viral infections. Cumitech 15. American Society for Microbiology, Washington, D.C.
2. Johnson, R.B., and Libby, R. 1980. Separation of immunoglobulin M (IgM) essentially free of IgG from serum for use in systems requiring assay of IgM-type antibodies without interference from rheumatoid factor. J. Clin. Microbiol. 12:451.
3. Neimeister, R.P., Teschemacher, R., Yankevitch, I.J., and Cocklin, J. 1975. Proficiency testing, trouble shooting and quality control for the RPR test. Am. J. Med. Technol. 41:13.
4. Stevens, R.W. 1980. Particle agglutination tests in the rapid serodiagnosis of bacterial infections. Clin. Immunol. Newsletter 1:1.

BIBLIOGRAPHY

Carter, J.B., Biesecker, J.L., and Rippey, J.H. 1983. Immunoserology review or "the modern serology lab." p. 53. American Society of Clinical Pathologists, Commission on Continuing Education, Council on Immunopathology, Chicago.

Nichols, W.S., and Nakamura, R.M. 1980. Agglutination and agglutination inhibition assays. In Rose, N.R., and Friedman, H., editors. Manual of clinical immunology, ed. 2. American Society for Microbiology, Washington, D.C.

Noonan, K.D. 1984. Latex agglutination testing: the importance of the microenvironment. Clin. Microbiol. Newsletter **6:**20.

Palmer, D.F. 1980. Complement fixation test. In Rose, N.R., and Friedman, H., editors. Manual of clinical immunology, ed. 2. American Society for Microbiology, Washington, D.C.

Roitt, I.M., Brostoff, J., and Male, D.K. 1989. Immunology, ed. 2. Gower Medical Publishing, Ltd., London. (Distributed by The C.V. Mosby Co., St. Louis.)

Rose, N.R., Friedman, H., and Fahey, J.L., editors. 1986. Manual of clinical immunology, ed. 3. American Society for Microbiology, Washington, D.C.

Methods for Testing Antimicrobial Effectiveness

Isolating an infectious agent from a patient with disease is often not sufficient for determining proper therapy. Many bacteria and some fungi manifest resistance to antimicrobial agents and some viruses have already developed resistance to the newest antiviral agents. Patterns of resistance are constantly changing. Even the pneumococcus, which for decades was invariably susceptible to penicillin G at levels of less than 0.04 U/ml, has developed resistance to this drug in some strains.

Since the susceptibility of many bacteria, fungi, and viruses to antimicrobial agents cannot be predicted, testing individual pathogens against appropriate antimicrobial agents is often necessary. The appropriate agent (with the most activity against the pathogen, bactericidal activity when indicated, the least toxicity to the host, the least impact on normal flora, appropriate pharmacologic characteristics, and most economical) can then be chosen, allowing a more certain therapeutic outcome. Table 13.1 lists some commonly encountered organisms and the types of antimicrobial agents that are usually effective against them. The ultimate therapeutic outcome depends on many more variables, of course. The underlying disease and condition of the host, the use of indicated drainage, debridement, or other surgical procedures, the pharmacologic properties of the antimicrobial agent, additional therapeutic agents being given, and other factors will exert a strong influence on the ultimate outcome. In addition, the blood and tissue levels of an antimicrobial agent are dependent on the route of administration (oral versus parenteral).

Microbiologists can only recommend therapeutic agents based on their in vitro activities. The clinician

Table 13.1
Selected Bacteria and General Categories of Antimicrobial Agents Used to Treat Systemic Infection
Due to Them

GRAM-NEGATIVE ORGANISMS OTHER THAN *PSEUDOMONAS AERUGINOSA*	*P. AERUGINOSA*	GRAM-POSITIVE BACILLI AND STAPHYLOCOCCI	ENTEROCOCCI	ANAEROBES	NONENTEROCOCCAL STREPTOCOCCI
Aminoglycosides	Aminoglyco-	Cephalosporins	Penicillin and amino-	β-Lactam plus	Penicillins
Broad-spectrum	sides	Erythromycin	glycoside combination	β-lactamase in-	
penicillins	Broad-spec-	Penicillins	Vancomycin	hibitor	
Cephalosporins	trum	Vancomycin		Broad-spectrum	
Cotrimoxazole	penicillins			penicillins	
Imipenem	Cefoperazone			Cefoxitin	
Monobactams	Ceftazidime			Chloramphenicol	
Quinolones	Imipenem			Clindamycin	
	Monobactams			Imipenem	
	Quinolones			Metronidazole	

must make the final choice based on his or her knowledge of all the pertinent facts. At times, an antimicrobial agent that shows poor in vitro activity against an organism is used in a patient with good results; the opposite effect may also occur. One important concept that must be stressed is that in vitro susceptibility tests cannot be performed on mixed cultures; only pure cultures will yield valid results. With these caveats in mind, we have catalogued the antimicrobial susceptibility testing methods currently in widespread use among microbiologists in the United States.

The term **antibiotic** has been defined as a chemical produced by a microorganism that inhibits the growth of other microorganisms. Antibiotics modified by chemical manipulations are still considered to be antibiotics. An **antimicrobial** agent is active against microorganisms and may be produced either naturally by microorganisms or synthetically by scientists in laboratories. The term **chemotherapeutic** agent has been used to refer to synthetic and other antimicrobial agents and also to refer to agents that act against human cells, such as anticancer drugs. The subterms "antiviral agent" and "antifungal agent" are more specific terms that fall into the general category of antimicrobial agents as we refer to them here.

13.1. Nonautomated in Vitro Susceptibility Testing

During the days soon after the discovery of sulfonamides and penicillin, pathogenic organisms were

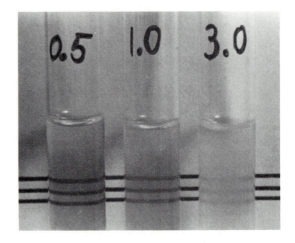

Figure 13.1
McFarland standards numbers 0.5, 1, and 3.

rarely tested for their susceptibility to drugs. Patients were treated empirically and the organisms were often susceptible. It was not until resistance began to emerge, soon after the agents were introduced, that microbiologists began to test an infecting organism against antimicrobial agents. The classic method used for in vitro testing was that of broth dilution, which yields a quantitative result for the amount of antimicrobial agent that is needed to inhibit growth of a specific microorganism.

For many types of susceptibility testing, a standard inoculum of bacteria must be used. The number of bacteria in a liquid medium can be determined in four ways:

Table 13.2

McFarland Nephelometer Standards

	TUBE NUMBER									
	0.5	**1**	**2**	**3**	**4**	**5**	**6**	**7**	**8**	**9**	**10**
Barium chloride (ml)	0.05	0.1	0.2	0.3	0.4	0.5	0.6	0.7	0.8	0.9	1
Sulfuric acid (ml)	9.95	9.9	9.8	9.7	9.6	9.5	9.4	9.3	9.2	9.1	9
Approx. cell density ($\times 10^8$/ml)	1.5	3	6	9	12	15	18	21	24	27	30

1. By counting individual cells in a microscopic counting chamber, called a Petroff-Hausser chamber
2. By measuring the optical density of a broth culture of the bacteria and comparing it to the number of colonies found on subculture to solid agar
3. By growing the organisms to stationary phase (when the number of bacteria levels out at approximately 1×10^9/ml)
4. By visually comparing the turbidity of the liquid medium to a standard that represents a known number of bacteria in suspension, the most practical method. Turbidity standards (Figure 13.1) can be prepared by mixing chemicals that precipitate to form a solution of reproducible turbidity. Such solutions, using barium sulfate, were developed by McFarland to approximate numbers of bacteria in solutions of equal turbidity, as determined by colony counts (Table 13.2). They are prepared as detailed in Procedure 13.1.

13.1.a. Bacterial broth dilution methods. A complete protocol for performing these tests is found in the National Committee for Clinical Laboratory Standards (NCCLS) publication, M7-T2.[11] We will describe the basics of the procedures, but the reader is referred to the NCCLS publications and other references cited at the end of this chapter for more complete details. For broth dilution methods, decreasing concentrations of the antimicrobial agent(s) to be tested, usually prepared in serial twofold dilutions, are placed in tubes of a broth medium that will support the growth of the test microorganism. The most commonly used broth for these tests is Mueller-Hinton (available commercially) supplemented with the magnesium and calcium cations

PROCEDURE 13.1

Preparation of McFarland Nephelometer Standards

Principle

A chemically induced precipitation reaction can be used to approximate the turbidity of a bacterial suspension.

Method

1. Set up 10 test tubes or ampules of equal size and of good quality. Use new tubes that have been thoroughly cleaned and rinsed.
2. Prepare 1% chemically pure sulfuric acid.
3. Prepare a 1.175% aqueous solution of barium chloride ($BaCl_2 \cdot 2 H_2O$).
4. Slowly, and with constant agitation, add the designated amounts of the two solutions to the tubes as shown in Table 13.2 to make a total of 10 ml per tube.
5. Seal the tubes or ampules. The suspended barium sulfate precipitate corresponds approximately to homogenous *E. coli* cell densities per milliliter throughout the range of standards, as shown in Table 13.2.
6. Store the McFarland standard tubes in the dark at room temperature. They should be stable for 6 months.

(From NCCLS M2-T4.[10])

Table 13.3

Solvents and Diluents for Preparation of Stock Solutions of Antimicrobial Agents

ANTIMICROBIAL	SOLVENT*	DILUENT*
Amoxicillin, Ticarcillin	Phosphate buffer, pH 6.0, 0.1 M	Phosphate buffer, pH 6.0, 0.1 M
Ampicillin	Phosphate buffer, pH 8.0, 0.1 M	Phosphate buffer, pH 6.0, 0.1 M
Cephalothin†	Phosphate buffer, pH 6.0, 0.1 M	Water
Chloramphenicol and erythromycin	Ethanol	Water
Moxalactam (diammonium salt)‡	0.04 N HCl (let sit for 1.5-2 h)‡	Phosphate buffer, pH 6.0, 0.1 M
Nalidixic acid	½ volume of water, then add NaOH 1 M, dropwise to dissolve	Water
Nitrofurantoin§	Phosphate buffer, pH 8.0, 0.1M	Phosphate buffer, pH 8.0, 0.1M
Rifampin	Methanol	Water (with stirring)
Sulfonamides	½ volume hot water and minimal amount of 2.5 M NaOH to dissolve	Water
Trimethoprim	0.05 N lactic or hydrochloric acid, 10% of final volume	Water (may require heat)

From National Committee for Clinical Laboratory Standards. 1986. Performance standards for antimicrobial susceptibility testing; Second informational supplement. M100-S2. Permission to reproduce this table has been granted by the Committee. NCCLS is not responsible for errors or inaccuracies. The most current edition of the standard is available from NCCLS, 771 E. Lancaster Ave., Villanova, PA 19085.

*These solvents and diluents are for making *stock solutions* of antimicrobial agents requiring other than water. They can be further diluted as necessary in water or broth. The products known to be suitable for water solvents and diluents are amikacin, azlocillin, carbenicillin, cefamandole, cefonicid, cefotaxime, cefoperazone, cefoxitin, ceftizoxime, ceftriaxone, ciprofloxin, clindamycin, gentamicin, kanamycin, methicillin, mezlocillin, nafcillin, netilmicin, oxacillin, penicillin G, piperacillin, tetracyclines, tobramycin, trimethoprim (if lactate), and vancomycin.

†Solubilize all other cephalosporins and cephamycins (unless manufacturer indicates otherwise) in phosphate buffer, pH 6.0, 0.1 M and further dilute in sterile distilled water. These include cephalothin, cefazolin, and cefuroxime.

‡The diammonium salt of moxalactam is very stable, but is almost pure R isomer. Moxalactam clinical is a 1:1 mixture of R and S isomers. Therefore, dissolve the salt in 0.04 N HCl and allow it to react for 1.5 to 2.0 hours to convert it to equal parts of both isomers.

§Alternatively, dissolve nitrofurantoin in dimethyl sulfoxide (DMSO).

(formulas in Appendix A). For broth dilution susceptibility testing of staphylococci against methicillin, oxacillin, or nafcillin, 2% sodium chloride must be added to the cation-adjusted Mueller-Hinton broth (CAMHB).

The antimicrobial agents are prepared in concentrated solution in diluent and then diluted to the appropriate concentrations in broth. The diluents used for the commonly tested antimicrobial agents are shown in Table 13.3. Preparation of the antimicrobial agents must take into consideration that the laboratory standard powder obtained from the manufacturer (some of these are listed in Table 13.4), usually at no cost, often does not consist of 100% active compound. The *specific activity* is the amount, in micrograms per milligram, of active antimicrobial agent in the powder. To make a solution containing 1280 μg/ml rifampin, assuming an activity of 950 μg/mg, a simple calculation is performed. First, determine how much powder will be necessary for the volume of diluent that you desire:

$$\text{Weight (mg)} = \frac{\text{volume (ml)} \times \text{concentration (μg/ml)}}{\text{potency (μg/mg)}}$$

$$\textit{Example: } \text{Weight (mg)} = \frac{20 \text{ ml} \times 1280 \text{ μg/ml}}{950 \text{ μg/ml}} = 26.9 \text{ mg}$$

Weigh out an amount of powder similar to the desired weight (usually slightly more) on an analytical balance. Then determine the exact amount of diluent necessary to achieve the required concentration:

$$\text{Volume (ml)} = \frac{\text{weight (mg)} \times \text{potency (μg/mg)}}{\text{concentration (μg/ml)}}$$

$$\textit{Example: } \text{Volume (ml)} = \frac{28 \text{ mg} \times 950 \text{ μg/mg}}{1280 \text{ μg/ml}} = 20.8 \text{ ml}$$

For every 1280 μg of active rifampin desired, 1347 μg of powder of 95% activity must be added

Table 13.4

Manufacturers of Commonly Used Antimicrobial Agents (Sources of Laboratory Reference Standard Powders)*

ANTIMICROBIAL AGENT	MANUFACTURER
Amikacin	Bristol Laboratories, Syracuse, N.Y.
Amoxicillin	Bristol Laboratories, Syracuse, N.Y.
	Beecham Laboratories, Bristol, Tenn.
Amphotericin	Squibb & Sons, Inc., Princeton, N.J.
Ampicillin	Bristol Laboratories, Syracuse, N.Y.
	Beecham Laboratories, Bristol, Tenn.
Ampicillin-sulbactam (see Unasyn)	
Augmentin (ampicillin-clavulanic acid)	Beecham Laboratories, Bristol, Tenn.
Azlocillin	Miles Pharmaceutical, West Haven, Conn.
Aztreonam	Squibb & Sons, Inc., Princeton, N.J.
Carbenicillin	Pfizer, Inc., Quality Control Section, Terre Haute, Ind.
Cefaclor, cefamandole, cefazolin	Lilly Research Laboratories, division of Eli Lilly & Co., Indianapolis, Ind.
	Smith, Kline & French Laboratories, Philadelphia, Pa.
Cefoperazone	Pfizer, Inc., Quality Control Section, Terre Haute, Ind.
Cefoxitin	Merck Institute for Therapeutic Research, Rahway, N.J.
Cefotaxime	Hoechst-Roussel, North Somerville, N.J.
Cefotetan	Stuart Pharmaceuticals, Wilmington, Del.
Ceftazidime, cefuroxime	Glaxo, Research Triangle Park, N.C.
Ceftizoxime, cefonicid	Smith, Kline & French Laboratories, Philadelphia, Pa.
Ceftriaxone	Hoffmann-LaRoche, Inc., Nutley, N.J.
Cephalexin, cephalothin	Lilly Research Laboratories, division of Eli Lilly & Co., Indianapolis, Ind.
Cephradine	Smith, Kline & French Laboratories, Philadelphia, Pa.
Chloramphenicol	Warner Lambert Co., Ann Arbor, Mich.
Ciprofloxacin	Miles Pharmaceuticals, West Haven, Conn.
Clindamycin	The Upjohn Company, Kalamazoo, Mich.
Cloxacillin	Bristol Laboratories, Syracuse, N.Y.
Dicloxacillin	Bristol Laboratories, Syracuse, N.Y.
Doxycycline	Pfizer, Inc., Quality Control Section, Terre Haute, Ind.
Erythromycin	Eli Lilly & Co., Indianapolis, Ind.
Flucytosine (5-fluorocytosine)	Hoffmann-LaRoche, Inc., Nutley, N.J.
Gentamicin	Schering Corporation, Bloomfield, N.J.
Imipenem	Merck Institute for Therapeutic Research, Rahway, N.J.
Kanamycin	Bristol Laboratories, Syracuse, N.Y.
Ketoconazole	Janssen Pharmaceutica, Inc., New Brunswick, N.J.
Methicillin	Bristol Laboratories, Syracuse, N.Y.
Metronidazole	G.D. Searle & Co., Skokie Ill.
Mezlocillin	Miles Pharmaceuticals, West Haven, Conn.
Moxalactam	Lilly Research Laboratories, division of Eli Lilly & Co., Indianapolis, Ind.
Nafcillin	Wyeth Laboratories, Inc., Philadelphia, Pa.
Nalidixic acid	Sterling-Winthrop Research Institute, Rensselaer, N.Y.
Neomycin	The Upjohn Company, Kalamazoo, Mich.
Netilmicin	Schering Corporation, Bloomfield, N.J.
Nitrofurantoin	Norwich Pharmacal Company, Norwich, N.Y.
Norfloxacin	Merck Institute for Therapeutic Research, Rahway, N.J.

*Powders may also be purchased from the United States Pharmacopeial Convention, Inc., Reference Standards Order Department, 12601 Twinbrook Parkway, Rockville, MD 20852.

Continued.

Table 13.4—cont'd

Manufacturers of Commonly Used Antimicrobial Agents (Sources of Laboratory Reference Standard Powders)*

ANTIMICROBIAL AGENT	MANUFACTURER
Nystatin	E.R. Squibb & Sons, Inc., Princeton, N.J.
Oxacillin	Bristol Laboratories, Syracuse, N.Y.
Penicillin	Wyeth Laboratories, Inc., Philadelphia, Pa.
	Bristol Laboratories, Syracuse, N.Y.
Piperacillin	Lederle Laboratories, Pearl River, N.Y.
Rifampin	Ciba Pharmaceutical Co., Summit, N.J.
Spectinomycin	The Upjohn Company, Kalamazoo, Mich.
Streptomycin	Pfizer, Inc., Quality Control Section, Terre Haute, Ind.
Sulfamethoxazole	Burroughs Wellcome Co., Research Triangle Park, N.C.
	Hoffmann-La Roche, Inc., Nutley, N.J.
Sulfisoxazole	Hoffmann-La Roche, Inc., Nutley, N.J.
Tetracycline	Bristol Laboratories, Syracuse, N.J.
	Lederle Laboratories, Pearl River, N.J.
Ticarcillin, Timentin (ticarcillin/clavulanic acid)	Beecham Laboratories, Bristol, Tenn.
Tobramycin	Lilly Research Laboratories, division of Eli Lilly & Co., Indianapolis, Ind.
Trimethoprim	Burroughs Wellcome Co., Research Triangle Park, N.C.
	Hoffmann-La Roche, Inc., Nutley, N.J.
Unasyn (ampicillin-sulbactam)	Pfizer, Inc., Quality Control Section, Terre Haute, Ind.
Vancomycin	The Upjohn Company, Kalamazoo, Mich.
	Lilly Research Laboratories, division of Eli Lilly & Co., Indianapolis, Ind.

to the diluent. The weight of powder greater than 1280 µg includes the inactive components. NCCLS M7-T2 and M100-2S also describe preparation of antimicrobial agent solutions.[11,15]

To perform the classic broth dilution susceptibility test, a standard inoculum of the microorganism (for example, organisms 1×10^6 ml, a 1:500 dilution of a suspension of turbidity equal to a McFarland standard 1.0, Table 13.2) is added to an equal volume (often 1 ml) of each concentration of antimicrobial agent and to a tube of the growth medium without antimicrobial agent, which serves as a growth control (Figure 13.2). Notice that adding a bacterial suspension will dilute both the suspension and the concentration of antimicrobial agent in the tube; this must be taken into account during preparation of the inoculum and of the dilutions of antimicrobial agents. An uninoculated tube of medium is incubated to serve as a negative growth control. After sufficient incubation (usually overnight), the tubes are examined for turbidity, indicating growth of the microorganism. The organism will grow in the control tube and in any other tube that does not contain enough antimicrobial agent to inhibit growth. The lowest concentration of the agent that inhibits growth of the organism, as detected by lack of visual turbidity (matching the negative growth control), is designated the **minimum inhibitory concentration (MIC).** If the concentration of antimicrobial agent represented by the MIC can be readily achieved in the *patient's serum* by normal routes of delivery, the organism is said to be *susceptible* to that agent. Most clinicians try to achieve a concentration of antimicrobial agent at the site of infection that is four times (or higher in the case of immunosuppressed patients) the in vitro MIC of the microorganism being tested although this is not always feasible or necessary. The level of agent attained in the urine, cerebrospinal fluid, other body fluid, or in an abscess may be very much different, however, and such differences must be considered when therapy is being chosen. If the MIC is above the achievable level or within a range toxic to the host, the microorganism is said to be *resistant* to the antimicrobial agent. Thus, susceptibility and resistance are functions of the site of the infection, the microorganism, and the antimicrobial agent being tested. The **breakpoint** of an antimicrobial agent is the concentration that can be achieved

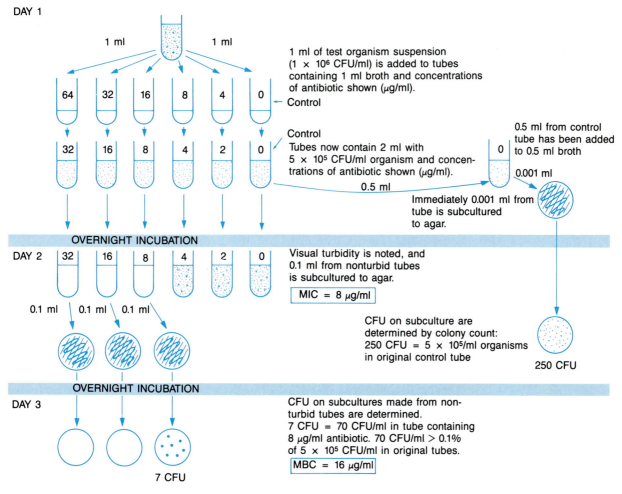

Figure 13.2
Determining MIC and MBC for one organism and one antibiotic.

in the serum with optimal therapy (Table 13.5). One can find several different versions of breakpoints.

Organisms with MICs at or below the breakpoint are considered "susceptible." An "intermediate" result indicates that the test result is equivocal and that susceptibility of that particular organism cannot be predicted. A "moderately susceptible" category also exists for certain organism-antibiotic combinations. In this case, the amount of drug given to the patient can be increased beyond standard dosages to obtain higher levels in the infected site. Certain antimicrobial agents are less active at an acid pH, such as might be found within an abscess. These

factors also contribute to the efficacy of treatment. The results of in vitro tests are subject to many variables, such as inoculum size, the rate of growth of the bacterium, the incubation period, the nature of the medium used, and the stability of the antimicrobial agent. By using standard methods, as detailed in NCCLS M7-T2, microbiologists can deliver consistent results that can serve to aid clinicians in their choices of therapeutic regimens. Figure 13.2 illustrates a procedure commonly used to determine the MIC of an antibiotic against a test organism.

The MIC measures the ability of the antimicrobial agent to inhibit multiplication of the organism.

Table 13.5
"Breakpoints"* for Activity of Antimicrobial Agents

DRUG	BREAKPOINT†
Amikacin	32
Ampicillin	16
Aztreonam	16
Carbenicillin, ticarcillin	128
Cefaclor	8
Cefamandole	32
Cefazolin	32
Cefoperazone	32
Cefotaxime	32
Cefotetan	32
Cefoxitin	32
Ceftazidime	16
Ceftizoxime	32
Cephalexin	8
Cephalothin	16
Chloramphenicol	16
Ciprofloxacin	2
Clindamycin	4
Doxycycline	4
Erythromycin	4
Gentamicin	8
Imipenem	8
Kanamycin	32
Metronidazole	16
Moxalactam	16
Oxacillin, nafcillin	12
Penicillin G	16
Piperacillin, mezlocillin, azlocillin	128
Tetracycline	8
Tobramycin	8
Vancomycin	16

*The term "breakpoint" as used here means a concentration of an antimicrobial agent in blood that can be achieved with maximal therapy.
†Levels expressed as micrograms of drug per milliliter, except for penicillin G, which is expressed as units of drug per milliliter.

Thus, organisms in the inoculum may be merely inhibited by the antimicrobial agent and will be able to recommence growing if the antimicrobial influence is removed. In that case the antimicrobial agent is said to be **bacteriostatic,** or inhibitory. For certain serious infections, such as endocarditis and meningitis, and perhaps osteomyelitis, and in patients who lack a well-functioning immune system, it may be important to determine the ability of an agent to actually kill the infecting organism.

To measure the ability of the antimicrobial agent to kill the microorganism, the **bactericidal** activity test is performed using a modification of the broth dilution susceptibility testing system. In reality, macrobroth dilution tests in tubes, as described above, are rarely performed for MICs alone, but a modification of the procedure is used to determine bactericidal levels for organism-antimicrobial combinations that cannot be tested by commercially available methods. When the initial microorganism suspension is being inoculated into the tubes of broth, a measured portion is removed from the growth control tube immediately after it was inoculated and this aliquot is plated to solid agar for determination of actual **colony** forming units (**CFU**) in the inoculum. The technologist determines this number by counting the number of colonies present after overnight incubation of the agar plate and multiplying times the dilution factor. For example, a 0.001 ml calibrated loop can be used to streak a plate for CFU from dilutions made from the growth control tube. If the organism concentration is $5 \times 10^5/$ml in the test tubes, there should be around 250 colonies on a subculture plate made from a 1:2 dilution of the growth control tube (0.001 ml of a suspension of 2.5×10^5 organisms contains 2.5×10^2 organisms). The 1:2 dilution is necessary in order to be able to count the colonies on the plate. It is possible to count colonies accurately numbering from 30 to 300 on a subculture plate, but counting a greater number of colonies is time-consuming and often inaccurate.

After the MIC has been determined, a known quantity (often 0.1 ml) of inoculum from each of the tubes of broth that showed no visible turbidity after overnight incubation is subcultured to solid agar plates. The small amount of the antimicrobial agent that is carried over with this inoculum is easily removed by diffusion into the agar, and the effect is negated by spreading the inoculum over a large area. The number of colonies that grow on this subculture after overnight incubation is then counted and compared to the number of CFU/ml in the original inoculum. Within those tubes that showed no turbidity, microorganisms were either still viable or they were killed by the antimicrobial agent. Since even bactericidal drugs do not always totally sterilize a bacterial population, the lowest concentration of antimicrobial agent that allowed less than 0.1% of the original inoculum to survive is said to be the **minimum bactericidal concentration** (**MBC**), also called the "minimum lethal concentration (MLC)" (illustrated in Figure 13.2). For our example, the MBC would be the tube from which less than 5 CFU (50 organisms per milliliter in the tube) grew. The technologist must be careful that the original inoculum

Table 13.6

Activity of Antimicrobial Agents Against Bacteria

AGENTS THAT ARE USUALLY BACTERICIDAL	AGENTS THAT ARE USUALLY BACTERIOSTATIC
Aminoglycosides	Chloramphenicol (also bactericidal in some cases)
Cephalosporins	
Cotrimoxazole	
Metronidazole	Erythromycin
Monobactams	Nalidixic acid
Penicillins	Sulfonamides
Quinolones	Tetracyclines
Rifampin	
Vancomycin	

Note: Erythromycin and clindamycin can act as bactericidal or bacteriostatic agents.

is great enough to measure a 99.9% lethal effect by the techniques being used in the test. For example, if the original inoculum contained only 10^4 CFU/ml, it would require the subculture of a 1 ml aliquot to yield the number of colonies (greater than 10 CFU) required to demonstrate less than 0.1% survival. One milliliter can be subcultured by pour plate, but it is a cumbersome task. NCCLS Publication M26-P describes this procedure. [16]

Certain antimicrobial agents are bactericidal in activity; they cause irreversible damage to bacteria. Other agents are known to be bacteriostatic, inhibiting growth by preventing multiplication, but not causing death. In some cases, drugs that are primarily bacteriostatic may be bactericidal against a given type of organism. The general category of certain antimicrobial agents is shown in Table 13.6. When an agent that has known bactericidal properties exhibits an in vitro MBC that is very much greater than its MIC (requires a great deal more antimicrobial agent to kill the bacteria than to merely inhibit growth; differences of 32 times are sometimes cited) against a bacterial strain, the strain is said to exhibit **tolerance.** Laboratory techniques play a large part in determining whether a bacterial strain is designated as tolerant, as has been pointed out by Taylor and others. [27] The clinical importance of tolerance, if any, has never been established and we do not recommend its use in routine clinical microbiology laboratories. In addition, truly reliable MBC determinations are difficult to achieve; modifications performed from microbroth dilution tray wells do not yield results as accurate as those obtained via ma-

crobroth dilution methods. MBC testing should be limited to those laboratories proficient in its performance and for those clinical situations in which such results are important (such as osteomyelitis, endocarditis, and immunosuppressed patients).

The MICs and MBCs of a given antimicrobial agent can be determined for any bacterium that is able to grow in liquid media. The optimal temperature for such tests is 35° C, since methicillin-resistant *Staphylococcus aureus* only exhibits that resistance at 35° C or below. Many bacteria require a medium different from cation-supplemented Mueller-Hinton broth or require special supplements added to the standard broth to achieve good growth. For example, streptococci are often tested in Todd-Hewitt broth. Certain fastidious bacteria require the addition of horse serum, lysed horse blood, rabbit serum, or special commercially produced nutrient supplements, such as Fildes' extract (Difco) or IsoVitaleX (BBL Microbiology Systems), as recommended by NCCLS M7-T2. [15] Organisms for which standardized procedures have not been agreed upon can be tested for in vitro susceptibility to selected agents. However, in the absence of standards, results should be interpreted with caution. Susceptibility testing of clinically important unusual organisms for which standard methods are not yet available should be performed only by reference laboratories that have experience in such procedures.

The methods outlined can be used to test many types of bacteria, aerobic and anaerobic, but they are time-consuming and very labor intensive. For each combination of bacterium and antimicrobial agent, a complete set of tubes must be prepared. It would be prohibitive to test more than a few antimicrobial agents against each isolate. Clinicians, however, have to choose from among numerous possible agents; a more practical method had to be adopted. The development of agar dilution (Section 13.1.c) and disk diffusion (Section 13.1.b) methods was one solution to the problem. A more recent innovation has been the adaptation of macrobroth dilution methods to a microbroth format, saving in reagents and technologist time.

The use of a microdilution format, which utilizes plastic microdilution trays (Figure 13.3), has made routine reporting of MIC results possible for many laboratories. Although a few large centers still prepare their own microdilution plates to save money and allow flexibility in the antimicrobial agents being tested, most laboratories buy commercially prepared

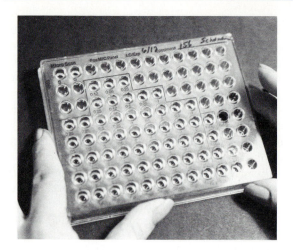

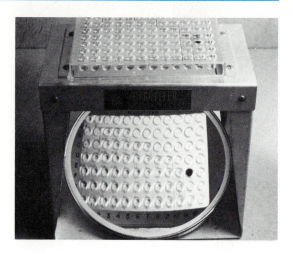

Figure 13.3
Plastic microdilution tray used for microbroth dilution antibiotic susceptibility testing. Antimicrobial agents are arranged in linear arrays of serial twofold dilutions.

Figure 13.4
Reading microbroth dilution results using a magnifying mirror reader.

plates. MIC microdilution trays purchased as commercial systems have the advantage of being prepared in great quantities under very strict quality control standards to assure consistent performance. Their disadvantages include high cost and a predetermined format. Even anaerobic susceptibility testing trays are commercially available. All plates are viewed manually on a light box or read from the bottom with a mirror reader (Figure 13.4). Automated readers are described in Chapter 11.

Some systems are prepared complete by the manufacturer, shipped frozen to the consumer, and stored in the freezer until thawed and used. Such systems are easy to inoculate, often including a disposable plastic inoculating apparatus that requires only one manipulation to inoculate simultaneously all 96 wells in the microdilution plate. However, they may suffer from degradation of the antimicrobial agents if major temperature variations are encountered during shipping and storage. A second type of commercial microbroth system consists of dried or lyophilized antimicrobials. The organism suspension or another diluent may be used to rehydrate the wells. If any number of such plates must be inoculated, some mechanical or instrumental device is necessary. Because of the small volume of medium in the wells, the incubating plates must be protected from dehydration by sealing them with a plastic tape, incubating them in a small humidified chamber (Figure 13.5), or stacking them.

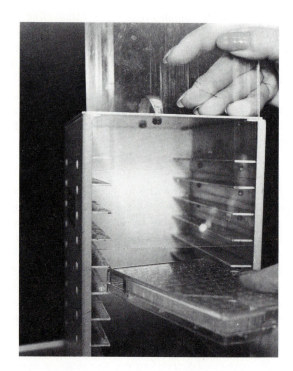

Figure 13.5
Incubating microdilution trays in a humidified chamber.

Although microdilution plates are prepared using the same growth medium and the same antimicrobial agent concentrations as macrobroth methods, there is one important difference. The true inoculum of bacteria, still 5×10^5/ml, is considerably decreased per microdilution well because of the small volume being tested. These wells usually hold only 0.1 ml, effectively reducing the final inoculum to 5×10^4 CFU per well. This number may not include a sufficient number of colony-forming units to allow expression of resistance shared by only a small proportion of the total organisms present in the primary isolate. The small inoculum also makes MBC testing difficult or impossible, as the numbers of CFU may not be great enough to determine 99.9% killing. NCCLS M26-P presents a method for performing MBCs with microdilution trays[16]; we do not recommend this as a routine procedure.

As for all laboratory tests, susceptibility test results must be monitored and evaluated using standard quality control strains of bacteria. By testing strains with known MICs, technologists can uncover breaks in technique or problems with media or reagents. NCCLS recommends routine testing of *Escherichia coli* American Type Culture Collection (ATCC) 25922, *Pseudomonas aeruginosa* ATCC 27853, *S. aureus* ATCC 29213, and *Streptococcus faecalis* ATCC 29212, since their MICs all fall within a measurable range and the results are consistent on repetitive testing. NCCLS M7-T2 discusses performance of quality control procedures, and M100-S2 lists the most recent recommendations.[11,15]

13.1.b. Bacterial disk diffusion methods. As more antimicrobial agents became available for treating a wide variety of bacteria, the limitations of the macrobroth dilution method became apparent. Before microdilution technology was available, methods were developed for testing an isolate against more than one antimicrobial agent, such as inoculating the surface of an agar plate with the organism to be tested, placing small glass or metal cylinders into the agar to create tiny wells above the agar surface, and placing suspensions of antimicrobial agents into the cylinders. The antimicrobial agent would diffuse into the medium in a circle around the cylinder, inhibiting the growth of the organism wherever the concentration of drug was high enough. Large zones indicated more effective antimicrobial activity or greater diffusibility of the drug or both. No zone indicated complete resistance. In this crude way, several agents could be tested against one isolate at the same time. This method was modified in 1947 by Bondi and others[3] by incorporating the antimicrobial agents into filter paper disks. Thus, a large number of identical disks could be prepared in ad-

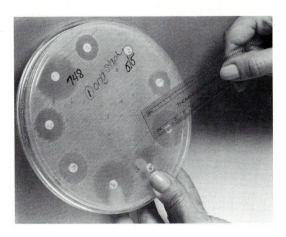

Figure 13.6
Measuring zones of inhibition on a disk diffusion susceptibility test plate.

vance and stored for future use. It was not until the landmark study by Bauer, Kirby, Sherris, and Turck in 1966 that the use of filter paper disks for susceptibility testing was standardized and correlated with MICs using a large number of bacterial strains.[2] The disk diffusion susceptibility test, as the method of Bauer, Kirby, Sherris, and Turck is designated, uses single high antibiotic content disks and yields qualitative results that correlate well with the quantitative results obtained by MIC tests.

These authors chose concentrations of antimicrobial agents to incorporate into the filter paper disks that showed the best results (clearest, within acceptable size, and most consistent zones of inhibition). They then tested many strains of rapidly growing bacteria, such as various Enterobacteriaceae and staphylococci, by both broth dilution and by spreading the bacteria on the surface of Mueller–Hinton agar plates, pressing the disks onto the inoculated plate surfaces, incubating the plates overnight at 35° C, and measuring the zone of inhibition of growth around each disk (Figure 13.6). For each combination of antimicrobial agent and bacterial species tested, a regression analysis was performed, plotting the zone size in millimeters against the $\log_2$ MIC (Figure 13.7). Breakpoint zone diameters were chosen that corresponded to the MICs that fell into the susceptible and resistant ranges, based on *achievable serum levels*.

In some cases, due to technical factors, the zone size did not correlate well with the MIC. For this

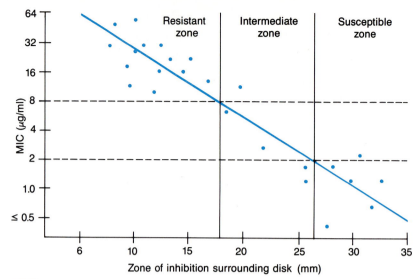

Figure 13.7

Example of a regression analysis plot used to determine zone sizes that correspond to susceptibility characteristics of the species of bacteria being tested. In this example the maximum achievable serum concentration is 8 μg/ml. Zone sizes ≤18 mm are interpreted as resistant; zone sizes ≥26 are interpreted as susceptible.

reason, zone sizes that fell within an arbitrarily selected middle range were designated "intermediate." For bacteria whose zones fall in this range, the extrapolated MIC should be considered equivocal and dilution tests may be indicated. The latest modifications of the agar disk diffusion testing procedure have been published in NCCLS M2-T4, the current state of the art in such matters; a "moderately susceptible" category has been established for certain drugs (penicillins and cephalosporins, in particular) in which higher levels of drug may be achieved in those body sites where the drugs are concentrated, for which a range of dosages might be possible, or for organisms that may require more aggressive therapy.[10]

The agar disk diffusion test is still used by many laboratories in the United States and around the world, for it is easy and inexpensive to perform and standardization is not difficult. The results can also be directly correlated to MIC values. Each time a new antimicrobial agent is developed and released for clinical use, a large number of organisms must be tested in the manner described here to establish interpretive zone sizes for the agent. Unless zone sizes have been specifically established for a species of bacterium, results achieved by the agar disk diffusion method may not be reliable. It must also be

remembered that the designations "susceptible" and "resistant" relate to achievable serum levels; antimicrobial agents that are excreted through the kidneys achieve much higher concentrations in urine than are obtainable in serum, such that an isolate from a urinary tract infection that is "resistant" by agar disk diffusion may be "susceptible" to the same antimicrobial agent in the urine. For the same reason, the zone sizes that have been established for antimicrobial agents that are used primarily or exclusively for treatment of urinary tract infections, such as nalidixic acid, cinoxacin, nitrofurantoin, trimethoprim, sulfonamides, and norfloxacin, correspond to levels of antimicrobial agent achievable in urine only. Special criteria have been established for other drugs, such as ceftizoxime, when they are being tested against urinary tract isolates. By the same token, drug levels in spinal fluid are commonly lower than in serum.

Interpretation of the results of the disk diffusion test depends on proper performance of the test. The variables that influence the outcome include the depth, pH, cation content, supplements, and source of the Mueller-Hinton agar; the age and turbidity of the bacterial inoculum; the way in which the inoculum is spread on the plate; the temperature, atmosphere, and duration of incubation; the method

Table 13.7

NCCLS Recommendations for Disk Diffusion Testing of Fastidious Aerobic Bacteria*

ORGANISM†	MEDIUM, SUPPLEMENT	DISK (CONTENT)	ZONE (mm) BREAKPOINT FOR	
			SUSCEPTIBLE	RESISTANT
H. influenzae	*H* Test Medium (HTM)‡ Mueller-Hinton agar 15 µg/ml NAD 15 µg/ml bovine hematin 5 mg/ml yeast extract pH 7.2 to 7.4	Amoxicillin-clavulanic acid (20/10 µg)	≥20	≤19 ≤21
		Ampicillin (10 µg)	≥25	
		Cefotaxime, ceftazidime, ceftriaxone, ceftizoxime (30 µg)	≥26	
		Cefuroxime (30 µg)	≥24	≤20
		Chloramphenicol (30 µg)	≥29	≤25
		Ciprofloxacin (5 µg)	≥21	
		Trimethoprim-sulfamethoxazole (1.25 and 23.75 µg)	≥16	≤10
			(standard break points appear to apply for chloramphenicol, tetracycline, and trimethoprim-sulfamethoxazole)	
S. pneumoniae	MHA, 5% sheep blood	Oxacillin (1 µg) (to screen for penicillin resistance)	≥20	≤19
N. gonorrhoeae	GC Agar Base (Difco), 1% IsoVitaleX or Supplement VX	Penicillin (10 U)	≥20	≤19

*As modified from NCCLS protocol M2-T4

†Inoculum preparation: Suspend overnight growth from plate into MHB to obtain turbidity equivalent to a McFarland 0.5 standard. Incubation: Overnight at 35°C in CO_2 for *N. gonorrhoeae*. CO_2 is usually not necessary for *H. influenzae* and *S. pneumoniae*.

‡To make *Haemophilus* Test Medium (HTM), first prepare a fresh hematin stock solution by dissolving 50 mg of powder in 100 ml of 0.01 N NaOH with heat and stirring until the powder is thoroughly dissolved. Add 30 ml of the hematin stock solution to 1 L of MHB with 5 g of yeast extract also added. After the solution has been autoclaved and cooled, cations are added aseptically, if needed as in CAMHB, and 3 ml of a NAD stock solution (50 mg of NAD dissolved in 10 ml of distilled water; filter-sterilized) also is aseptically added. If sulfonamides or trimethoprim is to be tested, 0.2 IU/ml thymidine phosphorylase should also be aseptically added to the medium. From Hindler, J. 1983. Strategies for antimicrobial susceptibility testing of fastidious aerobic bacteria. Am. J. Med. Tech. **49**:761.

of reading results; the antimicrobial content of the disks, their age and storage conditions; and more. For these reasons, performance of the test must strictly adhere to the NCCLS guidelines.

Laboratories should monitor their performance by periodically testing the recommended quality control strains *S. aureus* ATCC 25923, *E. coli* ATCC 25922, and *Pseudomonas aeruginosa* ATCC 27853. For monitoring disks that contain combinations of β-lactam agents plus β-lactamase inhibitors, such as amoxicillin plus clavulanic acid, *E. coli* ATCC 35218 is used.

Trimethoprim-sulfamethoxazole is tested with *S. faecalis* ATCC 29212 to determine that the Mueller-Hinton agar does not itself contain sulfonamide-inhibiting substances. The NCCLS publication M2-T4 describes all aspects of performance of this test.[10] An excellent trouble-shooting guideline for tracing

sources of error in the disk diffusion test was written by Miller and colleagues.[9]

Enterobacteriaceae, *Aeromonas*, *Acinetobacter*, *Pseudomonas*, staphylococci, enterococci, nonenterococcal streptococci, and *Listeria monocytogenes* can be tested against selected antimicrobial agents by the standard disk diffusion method.[10,15] If the organism is unable to grow satisfactorily after overnight incubation on Mueller-Hinton agar, 5% defibrinated sheep blood may be added to the agar without appreciably affecting the overall results. Modifications of the standard disk diffusion test have been adopted for testing several commonly isolated bacteria with unique growth characteristics: *Haemophilus* species, *Neisseria gonorrhoeae*, and *Streptococcus pneumoniae*. Table 13.7 summarizes some of these considerations and a recent publication by Thornsberry and others[28] details current recommendations. Detecting resistance of staphylococci to the penicillinase-resistant penicillins (oxacillin, methicillin, nafcillin, cloxacillin, and dicloxacillin) poses special problems. Plates should be incubated at 35° C or slightly lower for at least 24 hours, and zones of inhibition around methicillin and oxacillin disks should be examined carefully, using *transmitted* light, for a slight haze of growth; such a haze indicates a resistant subpopulation, and the organism should be reported as "resistant." Strains of staphylococci that demonstrate in vitro resistance to methicillin or oxacillin should be considered resistant to all β-lactam agents, including penicillins and cephalosporins, and should be reported as such.

Certain results obtained in vitro are known to be unreliable. Although *Salmonella typhi* is inhibited by aminoglycosides in vitro, these agents are ineffective for treating typhoid fever. Aminoglycosides may inhibit enterococci in vitro, but they are not ever recommended alone for the treatment of enterococcal infections. Disk diffusion susceptibility testing, while appearing to be deceptively simple, is a demanding test, fraught with pitfalls that, if not circumvented, can render the results less than totally reliable.

13.1.c. **Agar dilution methods.** In addition to broth dilution MIC's, another method for testing the MIC's of a large number of isolates against many concentrations of several antimicrobial agents is that of *agar dilution*. For this method, concentrations of antimicrobial agents are incorporated into agar plates, one plate for each concentration to be tested. The organisms to be tested are diluted to a slightly greater turbidity than that of a McFarland 0.5 standard, and an aliquot of each suspension is placed into one well of a replicating inoculator device (called a Steers-Foltz replicator, Figure 13.8). This device has metal prongs that are calibrated to pick up a small amount of the bacterial suspension (usually 0.001 ml) and deliver it to the agar surface. At least 25 different strains plus controls can be placed in the wells of the inoculator for delivery to each plate in a single manual movement. In this manner, approximately 1×10^4 CFU are delivered in a discrete drop to the surface of agar plates containing different concentrations of antimicrobial agents. After overnight incubation, the organisms will grow on those plates that do not contain enough antimicrobial agent to inhibit them. The lowest concentration of agent that allows no more than one or two CFU or only a slight haze to grow is the MIC. MBC results cannot be determined using this technique. NCCLS publication M7-T2 describes performance of this test in detail.[11]

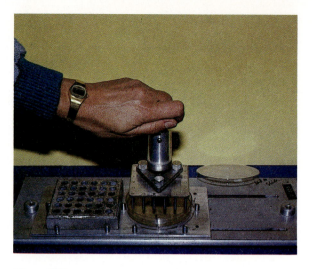

Figure 13.8
Steers-Foltz replicator apparatus used for performing agar dilution susceptibility tests.

Although agar dilution susceptibility testing is not commonly used by clinical laboratories for testing aerobic organisms, it is a good research laboratory technique for testing anaerobic bacteria and also is used as a reference method against which other methods are compared for testing anaerobic bacteria. As described in NCCLS publication M11-A,[12] the reference test is performed much like the aerobic test, with several important modifications. Agar plates must be prepared fresh the same day as they are inoculated, using Wilkins-Chalgren agar (available commercially). The bacterial suspensions are brought to the appropriate turbidity in *Brucella* broth or Schaedler broth before being placed in the inoculator wells. Plates are inoculated quickly and immediately placed into an anaerobic atmosphere for incubation (as described in Chapter 8) and MIC results are read after 48 hours' of incubation. It must be noted that this NCCLS procedure is a reference procedure and should *not* be used for testing susceptibility of clinical isolates for purposes of guiding therapy—not all anaerobes are able to grow on Wilkins-Chalgren agar, and some that do grow do not grow well. Accordingly, the inoculum is relatively small and the organisms may be susceptible to lower

Table 13.8

Antimicrobial Agents Used for Testing
Mycobacterial Susceptibilities

PRIMARY DRUGS	SECONDARY DRUGS
Isoniazid	Amikacin
Ethambutol	Ansamycin (for *M. avium-intracellulare*)
Streptomycin	Capreomycin
Rifampin	Cycloserine
Pyrazinamide	Ethionamide
	Kanamycin
	p-Aminosalicylic acid

Table 13.9

Concentrations of Antimicrobial Agents Used in
Middlebrook 7H11 Agar Quadrants for
Susceptibility Testing of Mycobacteria

PLATE	QUADRANT	ANTIMICROBIAL AGENT
1	I	None (control)
	II	Isoniazid (0.2 μg/ml)
	III	Isoniazid (1 μg/ml)
	IV	Ethambutol (10 μg/ml)
2	I	None (control)
	II	Streptomycin (2 μg/ml)
	III	Streptomycin (10 μg/ml)
	IV	Rifampin (1 μg/ml)
3	I	*p*-Aminosalicylic acid (2 μg/ml)
	II	*p*-Aminosalicylic acid (10 μg/ml)

levels of drug than when tested with other media. This procedure may be used with *Brucella* base blood agar to yield reliable results.[26] The Brucella base blood agar allows better growth and easier interpretation of end points.

13.1.d. Agar dilution susceptibility testing of mycobacteria. Although the frequency with which most bacterial populations produce a mutation that leads to resistance to an antimicrobial agent is usually 1 in 10^6, it is 10 times greater for *M. tuberculosis*. Thus, primary treatment of mycobacterial disease should include combinations of two or more agents and susceptibility testing methods should allow recognition of 1% resistance in the population. The antimicrobial agents tested against these organisms are listed in Table 13.8. Secondary agents are tested when an isolate is found to be resistant to the first-choice (primary) agents. The recommended method, the proportion method, is a modified agar dilution susceptibility test. Performance of this test is detailed in the book by Vestal.[30] Identical methods can be used to test *M. avium* complex, although this organism is unlikey to be susceptible to any one agent alone. Because of its importance in patients with AIDS, consideration of this group of organisms has become more important (see Chapter 41).

Since isolation of mycobacteria can take as long as several weeks and since primary resistance to the first-choice antimycobacterial agents is becoming more common, we recommend that susceptibility testing be performed directly on specimens that are discovered to harbor acid-fast bacilli, as seen on microscopic examination of the concentrate (detailed in Chapter 41). More commonly, however, the presence of mycobacteria will be discovered by isolation of the organisms on culture. The procedures for testing such isolates against primary drugs (*indirect susceptibility testing*) are included here, as well as modifications for *direct* testing of positive specimens.

For testing mycobacteria, Middlebrook 7H11 agar (Appendix A) containing antimicrobial agents is prepared in quantity, and 5 ml is poured into each section of divided Petri dishes (Felsen quadrant plates), as outlined in Table 13.9. A number of whole Petri plates are poured containing drug-free Middlebrook 7H11, to serve as growth controls for determining CFU. These plates can be stored refrigerated, tightly wrapped in plastic, for up to a maximum of 4 weeks before they are inoculated. As in preparing any solution of antimicrobial agent, the specific activity must be taken into account, as described in Section 13.1.a. Another method for incorporating antimycobacterial agents into agar is to pour the molten agar into the quadrants over antimicrobial agent–impregnated filter paper disks, as described by Wayne and Krasnow[31] and outlined in Table 13.10 (Figure 13.9). These plates must be incubated overnight to allow diffusion of the antimicrobial agent throughout the agar in the quadrant. They may then be refrigerated, but it is best to inoculate them within a few days after preparation. This technique of preparing antimicrobial agent solutions using filter paper–impregnated disks as the source of the drug is called "agar disk elution." Broth-disk elution, a similar method, is used for testing anaerobes (see Section 13.1.e).

Preparation of the inoculum for indirect myco-

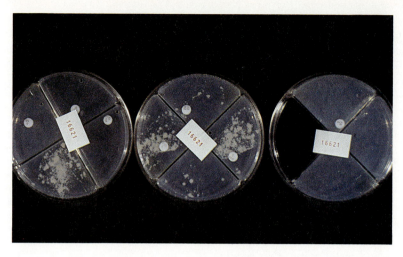

Figure 13.9
M. tuberculosis susceptibility test (organism is INH-resistant).

Table 13.10
Disk Contents for Preparation of Disk-Elution Mycobacterial Susceptibility Test Plates Using Middlebrook 7H11 Agar

PLATE	QUADRANT	DISK	FINAL CONCENTRATION (μg/ml)
1	I	None (control)	0
	II	Isoniazid (1 μl)	0.2
	III	Isoniazid (5 μl)	1
	IV	Rifampin (5 μl)	1
2	I	None (control)	0
	II	Ethambutol (25 μl)	5
	III	Streptomycin (10 μl)	2
	IV	Streptomycin (50 μl)	10
3	I	None (control)	0
	II	p-Aminosalicylic acid (10 μl)	2
	III	p-Aminosalicylic acid (50 μl)	10

bacterial susceptibility testing against the primary drugs is outlined in Procedure 13.2. Mycobacteria tend to grow in serpentine fashion, called "cords," consisting of many individual organisms bound together in parallel rows end to end. It is necessary to attempt to break up these cords as much as possible to determine accurately the number of resistant bacteria in a population. The use of Tween-containing media and glass beads for vortexing bacterial suspensions helps to break up the cords. As for all procedures involving mycobacteria, these manipu-

lations must be carried out within a biological safety cabinet. Only reference laboratories should test secondary drugs.

If acid-fast bacilli are seen on the concentrated direct smear, material from the concentrate can be diluted in Middlebrook 7H9, as shown in Table 13.11, and then inoculated onto quadrants for susceptibility testing as outlined in Procedure 13.2.

The report of results of drug susceptibility tests should include the following:

1. Type of test—direct or indirect

Indirect Mycobacterial Susceptibility Testing

Principle

Antimycobacterial agents can diffuse throughout an agar quadrant; on a solid agar surface quantitative susceptibility testing of mycobacteria can be done by direct inoculation of a known number of organisms.

Method

1. Suspend a wooden stickful or a loopful of growth in 5 ml of Middlebrook 7H9 broth (commercially available) containing five glass beads, 1 to 2 mm in diameter. Vortex for 15 s. Allow the solution to settle for 10 to 15 min after vortexing to discourage aerosol dissemination. Either adjust turbidity directly, if culture is fresh, or allow culture to incubate for 7 days.

2. Vortex several times for 15 s. each to break up cords. Adjust turbidity to that of a McFarland 0.5 standard.

3. Dilute this suspension 1:100 (0.05 ml into 5 ml) and then 1:100 again, to make a final dilution of 1:10,000 in Middlebrook 7H9 broth.

4. Inoculate 0.1 ml of each of the two dilutions (the 10^{-2} and 10^{-4}) onto each quadrant of the drug-containing plates and to two whole plates with drug-free media. Tilt the plates gently to spread the 0.1 ml drop around; do not allow it to pool up around the edges. By spreading the 0.1 ml onto the surface of a whole plate for the growth controls, the actual number of colonies can usually be counted. Leave the plates upright in the safety cabinet with tops slightly ajar for about 10 min to allow the inoculum to dry.

5. Tape the plates closed on two sides with clear cellophane tape to prevent accidental opening, and then place the plates, stacked two high, four plates each, into polyethylene plastic bags, sealed with tape. (Do not use Saran Wrap.)

6. Incubate the plates in 5% to 10% CO_2 at 37° C for a maximum of 3 weeks, or until colonies can be counted. Record growth as 4 + (>500 CFU), 3 + (200-500 CFU), 2 + (100-200 CFU), 1 + (50-100 CFU), or the actual number if <50 CFU.

7. Using the number of CFU on the growth control plates from the 10^{-4} dilution, estimate whether >1% of the inoculum grew on any drug-containing quadrant.

Quality control

A strain of *M. tuberculosis* susceptible to all antimicrobial agents (such as H37RV) should be tested concurrently with clinical isolates.

Expected results

The QC strain should not grow on agar containing antimicrobial agents but should grow on the control agar without antibiotics.

Performance schedule

QC should be performed each time the test is performed.

Modified from Vestal, A.L. 1975. Procedures for the isolation and identification of mycobacteria. DHEW publication no. (CDC) 77-8230. Centers for Disease Control, Atlanta, Ga.

Table 13.11
Dilution of Concentrate for Inocula

NO. OF ACID-FAST BACILLI PER OIL IMMERSION FIELD	CONTROL QUADRANT 1	CONTROL QUADRANT 2	DRUG QUADRANTS
Less than 1	Undiluted	10^{-2}	Undiluted
1-10	10^{-1}	10^{-3}	10^{-1}
More than 10	10^{-2}	10^{-4}	10^{-2}

2. Number of colonies on control quadrant
3. Number of colonies on drug quadrant
4. Concentration of drug in each quadrant

From these data, a rough approximation of the percentage of organisms resistant to the drug may be calculated as follows:

$$\frac{\text{Number of colonies on drug quadrant}}{\text{Number of colonies on control quadrant}} \times 100$$
$$= \% \text{ resistance at that drug concentration}$$

Radiometric growth detection (described in Chapter 11) has recently been modified for detection and susceptibility testing of *Mycobacterium tuberculosis* and other mycobacteria. Such testing yields results in several days, as compared with several weeks required for agar dilution methods. Antimicrobial agents are incorporated into bottles containing radioactive substrates (Johnston Laboratories) and growth of the mycobacteria, indicating resistance, is detected by measuring the amount of radioactive gas produced by the bacteria. Further discussion of radiometric detection of growth of mycobacteria is found in Chapter 41. Although the technology has not been adopted by large numbers of laboratories, those that can use the Bactec instrument cost-effectively report good results.

The rapidly growing mycobacteria *M. fortuitum* and *M. chelonae* can be tested by microbroth dilution in cation-supplemented Mueller-Hinton broth. The inoculum (McFarland 0.5 turbidity) is prepared from overnight growth in Mueller-Hinton broth plus 0.02% Tween 80. Plates are inoculated as above and incubated in air at 35° C for 72 hours before being read. Antibiotics suitable for testing in this way include aminoglycosides, cefoxitin, doxycycline, erythromycin, sulfonamides, and ciprofloxacin. [28]

13.1.e. Broth-disk elution methods. Using drug-impregnated filter paper disks as the source of antimicrobial agent for broth or agar dilution testing, disk elution is used not only for testing mycobacteria but also is commonly used for testing anaerobic bacteria. Anaerobes can also be tested by using macrobroth or microbroth dilution or agar dilution procedures. Additional details are in the *Wadsworth Anaerobic Bacteriology Manual*[26] and NCCLS publications.[12,14] For most laboratories, the broth-disk elution method or a microbroth procedure using commercially available frozen drug–containing trays would be most practical for susceptibility testing of anaerobes, although numerous isolates will not grow in the standard media without supplements. The broth-disk elution method, which is outlined in Procedure 13.3, is detailed in NCCLS M17-PA.[14]

At least two automated susceptibility testing systems, Autobac (Organon-Teknika) and Avantage (Abbott Laboratories), use the disk elution technique

Table 13.12

Preparation of Broth-Disk Elution Tubes for Anaerobic Susceptibility Testing

ANTIMICROBIAL AGENT	DISK CONTENT (µg)	NO. DISKS/5 ml	FINAL CONCENTRATION (µg/ml)
Ampicillin-sulbactam	10/10	8	16/16
Carbenicillin	100	6	120
Cefoperazone	75	2	30
Cefotaxime	30	5	30
Cefotetan	30	5	30
Cefoxitin	30	5	30
Chloramphenicol	30	3	18
Clindamycin	10	2	4
	2	10	4
Imipenem*	10	4	8
Mezlocillin	75	8	120
Moxalactam	30	5	30
Metronidazole	80	1	16
Penicillin G	10	8	16
Piperacillin	100	6	120
Ticarcillin	75	8	120

*Cannot be tested in thioglycollate broth. Use brain-heart infusion or other anaerobic broth and incubate anaerobically.

PROCEDURE 13.3

Anaerobic Susceptibility Testing by Broth-Disk Elution

Principle

Antimicrobial agents impregnated into filter paper disks can diffuse from the disk throughout a small volume of liquid medium (elute) and allow a single concentration to be tested in a modification of a macrobroth dilution procedure. By choosing the concentration to approximate the break point of the drug being tested, the presence of growth in the tube will indicate resistance.

Method

1. Prepare enriched (supplemented) thioglycollate broth without indicator (Appendix A) in 16 × 100 mm glass screw-cap test tubes, 5 ml broth per tube. Just before use, the media should be boiled for 5 min with cap loosened to drive off oxygen; the cap is then tightened, and the tube cooled to room temperature.
2. Add the appropriate number of drug-impregnated disks, as shown in Table 13.12. Although a 2-hour diffusion period was originally recommended, this has not been found to be essential for good results.
3. Prepare the inoculum directly from colonies on agar. Suspend enough growth in 5 ml of freshly boiled thioglycollate to approximate the turbidity of a 0.5 McFarland standard. If there are insufficient isolated colonies for direct inoculation, colonies may be incubated overnight in supplemented thioglycollate broth to achieve enough turbidity. Add two drops of inoculum to each tube of broth with disks and to one tube of drug-free broth as a growth control.
4. Tighten caps, gently invert tubes two or three times to mix, and incubate 18 to 24 hours at 37° C. (Occasionally, 48-hour incubation is required.) Interpret the anaerobic isolate to be resistant to all antimicrobial agents in which growth (measured by visual turbidity) is clearly visible, assuming turbid growth in the control tube. If the interpretation of the test is unclear for any single antimicrobial agent, repeat the test.

Quality control

Test appropriate susceptible anaerobic bacteria (*Bacteroides fragilis* ATCC 25285, *Clostridium perfringens* ATCC 13124, and *B. thetaiotaomicron* ATCC 29741) in the same manner as clinical isolates.

Expected results

The organisms should grow to easily visible turbidity in the control tube and should show no growth in antibiotic-containing tubes.

Performance schedule

Test QC organisms with each new lot number of thioglycollate broth and antimicrobial disks. Thereafter, test an organism of the same gram reaction as the clinical isolate each time a test is performed.

for susceptibility testing of aerobes. These instruments are described in Chapter 11. Automated susceptibility testing instruments are mentioned briefly in Section 13.4.

13.1.f. **In vitro fungal susceptibility testing methods.** Because fungi are large cells or hyphae with more variation in size than bacteria, preparation of a standard suspension of known CFU is difficult. For this reason and because of peculiar growth patterns, fungal susceptibility testing is difficult to perform and is thus much less standardized than are bacterial methods. Although possible for yeast, establishing a standardized inoculum for filamentous fungi is beyond the capability of most laboratories. Basically, fungi are tested by the macrobroth dilution method against amphotericin B and 5-fluorocytosine, the two most commonly used antifungal agents. Methods for testing the newer imidazoles, such as fluconazole, ketoconazole, miconazole, and clotrimazole, are described in NCCLS M20-CR.[13] Special media are necessary for fungal susceptibility testing; such testing is best left to a reference laboratory.

Disk diffusion tests for testing 5-fluorocytosine have been described by Utz and Shadomy.[29] A good discussion of current methods can be found in the chapter by Shadomy and others.[24]

13.1.g. In vitro viral susceptibility testing methods. Although not routinely performed, even by laboratories that perform routine viral cultures, viral susceptibility testing is a procedure that has been described and will undoubtedly become more widely used in the future. As shown by Howell and Miller,[7] routine testing of herpes simplex isolates against acyclovir can be accomplished without much difficulty. With increasing use of antiviral agents, such as amantadine for influenza A and the antiherpetic agents (such as acyclovir and ribavirin), the testing of viral isolates for resistance will undoubtedly become necessary to assist clinicians in choices of therapy. Briefly, supernatant from a tissue culture known to be producing infectious virus is inoculated into several wells of freshly passed tissue culture cells, some control wells without drug and some wells containing dilutions of the antiviral agent being tested. After sufficient incubation to produce cytopathic effect in the control wells, the wells containing antiviral agent are examined. The concentration of antiviral agent that eliminates cytopathic effect can be identified. Arbitrary numbers of infected cells can be chosen to approximate different levels of antiviral activity. For herpes cultures, results may be available as quickly as within 24 hours.

13.2. Serum Bactericidal Levels

In addition to determining in vitro susceptibility test results for isolates from patients receiving antimicrobial therapy, a laboratory can measure the activity of the patient's own serum (containing an antibacterial agent) against his or her specific pathogen. The lowest dilution of patient's serum that kills a standard inoculum of the organism is called the **serum bactericidal level** (**SBL**). Originally described by Schlichter and MacLean,[22] the test was used to measure the antibacterial level of serum from rabbits being treated with penicillin for experimental endocarditis. Still known as the **Schlichter test** in some laboratories, it has been modified to serve as a broad guideline to aid clinicians in deciding whether a patient is being given effective therapy for a serious infection, such as endocarditis or sepsis in a severely neutropenic patient.

Current recommendations include testing an inoculum of 10^5 CFU/ml of an actively growing suspension of organisms in both peak (one-half hour after delivery of antibiotic) and trough (immediately before the next antibiotic dose is given to the patient) sera in a diluent containing at least 50% normal, noninhibitory, pooled human serum. If a microbroth dilution format is used, the entire contents of wells showing no growth should be subcultured to agar plates (blood, chocolate, or Mueller-Hinton) for evidence of growth. Peak bactericidal serum titers $\geq 1:16$ and trough titers $\geq 1:8$ are considered desirable.

Often the results of tests of this type are not clear-cut. Each laboratory must decide how skipped tubes and inconsistent results should be handled. Possible strategies include performing tests in duplicate or repeating the entire procedure. The NCCLS has formed a subcommittee to establish standardized procedures for serum inhibitory and bactericidal testing procedures. M21-P[17] and the review by Stratton[25] contain excellent discussions of this test and include numerous relevant references.

13.3. In Vitro Synergism and Antagonism

When combinations of two or more antimicrobial agents provide more antimicrobial activity against a pathogen than the total additive effect of the agents given separately, the agents are said to exhibit **synergism.** Combinations of antimicrobial agents may be advisable for treating serious infections, for infections in hosts with compromised immune systems, for treating infections due to organisms known to readily develop resistance to one agent (*M. tuberculosis, P. aeruginosa,* and enterococci), and for certain mixed infections. However, when the infecting organism is known and there is a single agent highly active against it, there is probably no advantage to combination therapy except for organisms that readily develop resistance.

In contrast, when one agent diminishes the activity of a concurrently administered second antimicrobial agent, **antagonism** is said to occur. For instance, if a growth-inhibiting agent, such as chloramphenicol, is administered with an agent such as

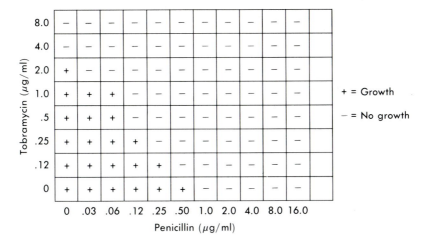

Figure 13.10
Checkerboard microdilution format used for testing synergism of two antimicrobial agents against a bacterium.

penicillin, which requires actively growing bacteria for bactericidal activity, the antagonism is primarily of the nature of *slower* bactericidal activity; such slowing of bactericidal activity may be significant in meningitis, for example.

Synergism and antagonism of two antimicrobial agents against a particular bacterium can be measured by performing an in vitro test using a checkerboard format, as illustrated in Figure 13.10. Two-fold dilutions of each antibiotic being tested are prepared in large volume and dispensed, one antibiotic in the horizontal rows and the other in the vertical columns of a microbroth dilution tray, beginning with a control well containing no antibiotic. Thus, wells in the upper right-hand corner of the tray contain the highest concentrations of both drugs, and the lower left-hand corner well contains no antibiotic. The wells along the left-hand column and the bottom row contain only the individual antibiotic placed in them (Figure 13.10). After inoculating all wells with the same inoculum of the organism being tested and incubating the tray appropriately, the presence of growth or no growth is recorded. If growth is inhibited by combinations of both antibiotics in concentrations fourfold or more less than that required by either antibiotic alone, the combination is said to be synergistic at those concentrations. Conversely, if the organism is able to grow better at combinations of concentrations fourfold or more higher than those required for inhibition when the agents are used singly, then the combination is said to be antagonistic. No difference in inhibition between either agent used alone and any combina-

tion of the two agents is called "indifference."

If only two agents are being assessed for synergism, *time-kill curves* may provide the most clinically relevant answer. In such tests, the antimicrobial agents are added to broth in fractions of the MIC, which was established in a previous test. For example, drug A is tested at one fourth of its MIC and drug B is added to drug A at one half, one fourth, and one eighth of its MIC (when tested separately). The definition of synergy is that the sum of the fractions for an effective combination is less than unity. The reverse combinations of antimicrobial agents are also tested, as are the antimicrobial agents alone. The inoculum is added as for MIC tests, and samples of the suspensions are removed at intervals over 24 hours for subculture to determine CFU. If there is a decrease of CFU corresponding to 1/100 of the CFU found on subculture from a tube containing the most effective drug tested singly, synergism is said to be demonstrated.

Serious infections caused by enterococci, the most penicillin-resistant streptococci, are often treated with combinations of a penicillin and an aminoglycoside. Although time-kill curves of the organism against combinations of the two antimicrobial agents being used would give the most specific information about synergism, a screening procedure has been employed effectively. By determining whether the isolate is resistant to a very high concentration of aminoglycoside, a prediction can be made as to the organism's probable response to such combination therapy. For example, the isolate is tested in a broth dilution system against 2000 µg/

ml of streptomycin. If the enterococcus is resistant to this amount, it can be assumed that there will be no synergism.

Synergism tests with three or more agents can be performed, but the methods are too cumbersome for routine use. Methods for synergism testing are described in the book edited by Lorian,[8] the review by Norden,[18] discussions by Edberg,[5] as well as in many other publications.

13.4. Rapid Tests for Antimicrobial Susceptibility

Certain bacteria are resistant to some penicillin and cephalosporin antibotics due to their production of **β-lactamase** enzymes. These enzymes bind to antibiotics that possess a β-lactam ring (Figure 13.11) and that, in most cases, ultimately opens the ring, inactivating the antibiotic. Although it is not the only resistance mechanism against β-lactam antibiotics, it is a very important one. The presence of β-lactamase, either in body fluid, culture supernatant, or directly within bacterial cells, can be demonstrated with a very rapid test, the "β-lactamase test." The substrate can be a penicillin or a cephalosporin, since both classes of antibiotic may be affected by these enzymes, although one may be affected much more than another. Several methods have been used to detect β-lactamases, as described in the *Manual of Clinical Microbiology*.[23] For example, products of penicillin breakdown can reduce iodine bound to starch, causing loss of the color of the starch-iodine compound. Hydrolysis of penicillin into acid products by the enzyme has been measured by a color change in a pH indicator (phenol red) from red to yellow.

The most sensitive method, however, is detection of the enzyme by its ability to hydrolyze the β-lactam ring of a **chromogenic** cephalosporin (a cephalosporin that is a yellow-colored compound in its intact state and red if the β-lactam ring is broken). The most commonly used compound, called nitrocefin (Glaxo), has a very high affinity for most bacterial β-lactamases. The compound is commercially available impregnated onto filter paper disks (Cefinase, BBL Microbiology Systems). A small amount of growth of the organism to be tested is rubbed on the moistened filter paper. Development of a red color within a maximum of 30 minutes indicates presence of β-lactamase. The test is most useful for testing *Haemophilus influenzae*, but it can also be used for gonococci, staphylococci, and all anaerobes. *Bacteroides*

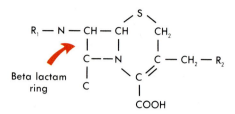

Figure 13.11
The β-lactam ring.

gracilis and some other anaerobes are often resistant to a number of β-lactam drugs but are nitrocefin negative; this resistance is not mediated by β-lactamases. Resistance of *Bacteroides fragilis* group strains to cefoxitin and imipenem is not usually detectable by the nitrocefin test. *H. influenzae*, gonococci, and other organisms may, of course, be β-lactam-resistant by a mechanism other than β-lactamase production and would thus be β-lactamase-negative. The nitrocefin test is the most sensitive β-lactamase test for all of the aforementioned species.

A second rapid test can be used to detect chloramphenicol resistance among *Haemophilus* species. If the organisms possess chloramphenicol acetyltransferase, the enzyme will modify a substrate (acetyl-S-coenzyme A), the breakdown product of which can induce a chromogenic indicator substance to turn yellow. The reagents for this test are commercially available as filter paper disks (C.A.T., Remel Laboratories).

Several other strategies can be used to determine susceptibility results more rapidly than is possible with conventional methods. Agar disk diffusion results on plates prepared in the standard manner may be read quite accurately after only 5 to 6 hours' incubation in many cases. Some workers have used tetrazolium dye, a compound that is reduced to a purple-colored compound by metabolizing bacteria, to delineate zones of inhibition on agar disk diffusion plates after 6 ½ hours' incubation. By increasing the initial inoculum, broth dilution tests may be modified to yield faster results. All of these approaches are not standardized. They should be confirmed by standard methods subsequently. The most radical method for obtaining rapid results, however, is the inoculation of susceptibility testing media with material from the clinical specimen itself. Although results using inocula from body fluids and urines have not correlated well with conventional methods, they do yield general information. Tests performed on positive blood culture broth, however, have given satisfactory results.[4] As detailed in Chapter 4, susceptibility tests may be set up directly or within a few hours of detection of a positive blood culture.

The most accepted methods for obtaining rapid susceptibility results are the automated systems. General principles of such systems are discussed in Chapter 11. New methods being developed include the use of fluorogenic compounds to measure growth, laser imaging of growth in wells, and fluorescence markers as probes for actively growing cells. The ability to deliver susceptibility determinations to the physician within the first few hours of discovery of the infectious process is the ultimate goal of such studies.

13.5. Measurement of Antimicrobial Agent Levels in Body Fluids

The measurement of the amount of antimicrobial agent in the serum or body fluid of a patient is performed for two reasons. First, it is the best method for determining whether an effective level of antimicrobial agent is being achieved. Although serum is usually tested, levels of agents in cerebrospinal fluid or other body fluids may be tested since they do not correlate with serum levels. For some drugs, impaired renal function and other conditions may lead to excessive serum levels with conventional dosage. Second, several agents, notably the aminoglycosides, are therapeutically effective at concentrations very close to those that may be toxic to the host. The administration of these agents should be carefully monitored by determining serum levels. The dosage can usually be adjusted to prevent toxicity while maintaining adequate therapeutic levels.

Methods for measuring the concentrations of these agents in body fluids are constantly being improved and refined. Originally, all assays were performed as *bioassays*, using an indicator strain of bacterium sensitive to the drug being evaluated. Known concentrations of the drug were impregnated into filter paper disks or placed in wells on the surface of an agar plate that had been seeded with an inoculum of an organism known to be sensitive to that drug. The patient's serum or other body fluid was also placed on similar disks or in similar wells in duplicate. By comparing the sizes of zones of inhibition of the bacterial strain around the known amounts of drug (setting up a standard curve) to the

zones formed around the patient specimen, the amount of the antimicrobial agent present in the specimen could be determined. This method worked well with single agents but became difficult to perform when a patient was receiving multiple agents. At first, organisms that were resistant to every antimicrobial agent except the one being tested were sought. Eventually, however, technological advances allowed the development of automated methods employing chemical or immunological procedures.

Most antimicrobial agent levels are now performed by gas-liquid chromatography, high-pressure liquid chromatography, fluorescence polarization immunoassay, radioimmunoassay or other type of competitive binding immunoassay, or some other form of immunoassay. Discussion of the principles of some of the instruments involved is found in Chapter 11.

The results of tests for levels of antimicrobial agents, also called "therapeutic drug monitoring (**TDM**)," are used to modify treatment being administered to patients with infectious diseases. The same automated test systems, however, are also used to monitor therapy with many other agents, including antiepileptic, antiarrhythmic, antineoplastic, and antidepressant compounds. For this reason, such testing is usually performed in the chemistry section of the laboratory, rather than microbiology. The immunoassays and chemical assays used for TDM are much more specific and easier to perform than were the bioassays, and they have the advantage of yielding results within hours, rather than requiring overnight incubation. Publications by Anhalt,[1] Edberg and others,[6] Pezzlo,[19] Pfaller,[20] and Saubolle[21] discuss various aspects of TDM testing.

REFERENCES

1. Anhalt, J.P. 1981. Liquid chromatographic assay of antibiotics. Clin. Microbiol. Newsletter 3:159.
2. Bauer, A.W., Kirby, W.M.M., Sherris, J.C., et al. 1966. Antibiotic susceptibility testing by a single disc method. Am. J. Clin. Pathol. 45:493.
3. Bondi, A., Spaulding, E.H., Smith, E.D., et al. 1947. A routine method for the rapid determination of susceptibility to penicillin and other antibiotics. Am. J. Med. Sci. 214:221.
4. Coyle, M.B., McGonagle, L.A., Plorde, J.J., et al. 1984. Rapid antimicrobial susceptibility testing of isolates from blood cultures by direct inoculation and early reading of disk diffusion tests. J. Clin. Microbiol. 20:473.
5. Edberg, S.C. 1988. Antibiotic interaction tests: Should they be performed? Clin. Microbiol. Newsletter 10:77.
6. Edberg, S.C., Barry, A.L. and Young, L.S. 1984. Cumitech

20. Therapeutic drug monitoring: antimicrobial agents. American Society for Microbiology, Washington, D.C.

7. Howell, C.L., and Miller, M.J. 1984. Rapid method for determining the susceptibility of herpes simplex virus to acyclovir. Diagn. Microbiol. Infect. Dis. 2:77.

8. Lorian, V., editor. 1986. Antibiotics in laboratory medicine, ed. 2. Williams & Wilkins, Baltimore.

9. Miller, J.M., Thornsberry, C., and Baker, C.N. 1984. Disk diffusion susceptibility test troubleshooting guide. Lab. Med. 15:183.

10. National Committee for Clinical Laboratory Standards. 1988. Performance standards for antimicrobial disk susceptibility test, ed. 4, M2-T4. NCCLS, Villanova, Pa. Order from NCCLS, 771 East Lancaster Ave., Villanova, PA 19085. Enclose check for $20 with your order, plus $5 for overseas postage.

11. National Committee for Clinical Laboratory Standards. 1988. Methods for dilution antimicrobial susceptibility tests for bacteria that grow aerobically, ed 2, tentative standard. M7-T2. NCCLS, Villanova, Pa. Order from NCCLS, 771 East Lancaster Ave., Villanova, PA 19085. Enclose check for $30 with your order, plus $5 for overseas postage.

12. National Committee for Clinical Laboratory Standards. 1985. Reference agar dilution procedure for antimicrobial susceptibility testing of anaerobic bacteria; approved standard, M11-A, NCCLS, Villanova, Pa. Order from NCCLS, 771 East Lancaster Ave., Villanova, PA 19085. Enclose check for $30 with your order, plus $5 for overseas postage.

13. National Committee for Clinical Laboratory Standards. 1985. Antifungal susceptibility testing; committee report. M-20-CR, NCCLS, Villanova, Pa. Order from NCCLS, 771 East Lancaster Ave., Villanova, PA 19085. Enclose check for $20 with your order, plus $5 for overseas postage.

14. National Committee for Clinical Laboratory Standards. 1989. Methods for antimicrobial susceptibility testing of anaerobic bacteria; ed. 2, tentative standard. M11-T2. NCCLS, Villanova, Pa. Order from NCCLS, 771 East Lancaster Ave., Villanova PA 19085. Enclose check for $20 with your order, plus $5 for overseas postage.

15. National Committee for Clinical Laboratory Standards. 1986. Performance standards for antimicrobial susceptibility testing; second informational supplement. M100-S2, NCCLS, Villanova, Pa. Order from NCCLS, 771 East Lancaster Ave., Villanova, PA 19085. Enclose check for $20 with your order, plus $5 for overseas postage.

16. National Committee for Clinical Laboratory Standards. 1987. Methods for determining bactericidal activity of antimicrobial agents; proposed guideline. M26-P, NCCLS, Villanova, Pa. Order from NCCLS, 771 East Lancaster Ave., Villanova, PA 19085. Enclose check for $20 with your order, plus $5 for overseas postage.

17. National Committee for Clinical Laboratory Standards. 1987. Methodology for the serum bactericidal test; proposed guideline. M21-P, NCCLS, Villanova, Pa. Order from NCCLS, 771 East Lancaster Ave., Villanova, PA 19085. Enclose check for $20 with your order, plus $5 for overseas postage.

18. Norden, C.W. 1982. Problems in determination of antibiotic synergism in vitro. Rev. Infect. Dis. 4:276.

19. Pezzlo, M. 1983. Assay of antimicrobial agents. Am. J. Med. Technol. 49:565.

20. Pfaller, M.A. 1987. Immunoassays for measurement of antimicrobial agents in body fluids. p 121-137. In Jorgenson, J.H., editor. Automation in clinical microbiology, CRC Press, Boca Raton, Fla.

21. Saubolle, M.A. 1987. Are assays for serum levels of antifungal agents routinely needed? Clin. Microbiol. Newsletter 9:113.

22. Schlichter, J.G., and MacLean, H. 1947. A method for determining the effective therapeutic level in the treatment of subacute bacterial endocarditis with penicillin: a preliminary report. Am. Heart J. 34:209.

23. Schoenknecht, F.D., Sabath, L.D., and Thornsberry, C. 1985. Susceptibility tests: special tests. In Lennette, E.H., Balows, A., Hausler, W.J. II, and Shadomy, H.J., editors. Manual of clinical microbiology, ed. 4. American Society for Microbiology, Washington, D.C.

24. Shadomy, S., Espinel-Ingroff, A., and Cartwright, R.Y. 1985. Laboratory studies with antifungal agents: susceptibility tests and bioassays. In Lennette, E.H., Balows, A., Hausler, W.J., Jr., and Shadomy, H.J., editors. Manual of clinical microbiology, ed. 4. American Society for Microbiology, Washington, D.C.

25. Stratton, C.W. 1988. Serum bactericidal test. Clin. Microbiol. Rev. 1:19.

26. Sutter, V.L., Citron, D.M., Edelstein, M.A.C., et al. 1985. Wadsworth anaerobic bacteriology manual, ed. 4. Star Publishing Co., Belmont, Calif.

27. Taylor, P.C., Schoenknecht, F.D., Sherris, J.C., et al. 1983. Determination of minimum bactericidal concentrations of oxacillin for *Staphylococcus aureus*: influence and significance of technical factors. Antimicrob. Agents Chemother. 23:142.

28. Thornsberry, C., Swenson, J.M., Baker, C.N., et al. 1988. Methods for determining susceptibility of fastidious and unusual pathogens to selected antimicrobial agents. Diagn. Microbiol. Infect. Dis. 9:139.

29. Utz, C., and Shadomy, S. 1977. Antifungal activity of 5-fluorocytosine as measured by disc diffusion susceptibility testing. J. Infect. Dis. 135:970.

30. Vestal, A.L. 1975. Procedures for the isolation and identification of mycobacteria DHEW Publication No. (CDC) 77-8230, Centers for Disease Control, Atlanta, Ga.

31. Wayne, L.G., and Krasnow, I. 1966. Preparation of tuberculosis susceptibility testing medium by means of impregnated discs. Am. J. Clin. Pathol. 45:769.

BIBLIOGRAPHY

Lorian, V., editor. 1986. Antibiotics in laboratory medicine, ed. 2. Williams & Wilkins, Baltimore.

Inderlied, C.B., and Hindler, J.A. 1987. Clinical significance of antimicrobial susceptibility testing. ASCP Check Sample Microbiology No. MB 87-7 (MB-168) 30:1-9. American Society for Clinical Pathology, Chicago, Ill.

Thornsberry, C., Swenson, J.M., Baker, C.N., et al. 1988. Methods for determining susceptibility of fastidious and unusual pathogens to selected antimicrobial agents. Diagn. Microbiol. Infect. Dis. 9:139.

Willett, H.P. 1988. Antimicrobial agents. pp. 128-160. In Joklik, W.K., Willett, H.P., and Amos, D.B., editors. Zinsser's Microbiology, ed. 19. Appleton & Lange, Norwalk, Conn.

Part Three

Etiologic Agents Recovered from Clinical Material

14 Microorganisms Encountered in the Blood

Microorganisms present in the circulating blood, whether continuously or transiently, are a threat to every organ in the body. Invasion of the bloodstream by microorganisms per se, aside from the problems of disseminating infection and involving and affecting the function of implanted foreign bodies (for example, artificial heart valves and joints), may have serious immediate consequences, including shock, multiple organ failure, disseminated intravascular coagulation (DIC), and death. Thus, bacteremia constitutes one of the most serious situations in infectious disease. The expeditious detection and identification of blood-borne pathogens is one of the most important functions of the microbiology laboratory. Positive blood cultures may help provide a clinical diagnosis as well as a specific etiologic diagnosis. Pathogens of all four major groups of microbes— bacteria, fungi, viruses, and parasites—may be found in circulating blood during the course of disease. Bacteria, on the other hand, may also be recovered from peripheral blood in the absence of disease. After any loss of the integrity of the capillary endothelial cells, a few bacteria may enter the bloodstream and live for a short time until the primary defense systems of a healthy host (phagocytic cells in the liver and spleen, polymorphonuclear leukocytes, and antibody and complement) destroy them. Eukaryotic parasites may also be found transiently in the bloodstream as they migrate to the environment of choice. Their presence, however, cannot be considered to be consistent with a state of good health. Table 14.1 shows the most common microorganisms isolated from blood during a 2-year period at one major medical center. The kinds of microorganisms isolated from blood cultures vary according to the patient population served by an institution.

Table 14.1

Microorganisms Isolated from Blood Cultures Monitored from 1975-1977 at the University of Colorado and the Denver Veterans Administration Hospitals

ORGANISM	NUMBER OF TRUE SEPTICEMIAS	NUMBER OF CONTAMINANTS	ORGANISM	NUMBER OF TRUE SEPTICEMIAS	NUMBER OF CONTAMINANTS
Escherichia coli	113	2	*Neisseria gonorrhoeae*	8	0
Staphylococcus aureus	68	23	*Corynebacterium* species	7	26
Streptococcus pneumoniae	43	0	*Peptococcus* species	7	1
Klebsiella pneumoniae	40	0	*Eubacterium* species	7	1
Pseudomonas aeruginosa	36	0	*Candida parapsilosis*	7	0
Bacteroides fragilis	30	0	*Listeria monocytogenes*	7	0
Enterococci	26	4	*Clostridium* species	6	3
Streptococcus pyogenes	18	1	*Cryptococcus neoformans*	6	0
Other Enterobacteriaceae	17	0	Other gram-negative rod nonfermenters	6	0
Candida albicans	15	0			
Other streptococci	14	3	Other *Candida* species	5	0
Torulopsis galbrata	14	1	*Bacteroides* species	5	0
Proteus mirabilis	14	0	*Fusobacterium necrophorum*	5	0
Viridans streptococci	13	12	*Acinetobacter calcoaceticus*	5	0
Serratia marcescens	13	1	*Haemophilus influenzae*	5	0
Enterobacter aerogenes	11	2	*Candida tropicalis*	3	4
Streptococcus agalactiae	11	0	*Propionibacterium acnes*	1	73
Staphylococcus epidermidis	10	153	*Mucor* species	1	0
Peptostreptococcus species	9	0	Other	8	8
Clostridium perfringens	8	8			

Modified from Weinstein, M.P., Reller, L.B., Murphy, J.R., and Lichtenstein, K.A. 1983. The clinical significance of positive blood cultures: a comprehensive analysis of 500 episodes of bacteremia and fungemia in adults. I. Laboratory and epidemiologic observations. Rev. Infect. Dis. 5:35.

14.1. Parasitic Infections

14.1.a. Pathogenic mechanisms. Parasites that infect cellular components may cause disease by disrupting the normal function of the infected cells. Invasion of the phagocytic cells of the reticuloendothelial system, as occurs in visceral leishmaniasis, renders those cells less able to fulfill their role as nonspecific immune responders. Proliferation of infected mononuclear phagocytes in the liver, spleen, and bone marrow leads to enlargement of the liver and spleen and contributes to the anemia and leukopenia seen in patients with this infection. Primary growth of *Trypanosoma cruzi* in the human host occurs in various host cells that are initially penetrated. When the parasites mature to the trypomastigote stage and burst out of the host cells, a generalized parasitemia results. Although able to multiply in any organ, the organisms prefer to invade muscle (including heart muscle) and nerve tissue; the cycle then repeats itself. Damage to the host is probably due both to its own inflammatory response attempting to localize or destroy infected tissue and to rupture of infected host cells during the release of trypomastigotes. The most important consequences of the disease are congestive heart failure and cardiac arrhythmias relating to cardiac muscle and its conducting tissue involvement, and dilation of the esophagus and colon, related to neuronal involvement.

Tachyzoites of the parasite *Toxoplasma gondii* may be found in circulating blood. They invade cells within lymph nodes and other organs, including lung, liver, heart, brain, and eye. The resulting cellular destruction accounts for the manifestations of toxoplasmosis. Malarial parasites invade host erythrocytes and hepatic parenchymal cells. Cerebral malaria is especially dangerous. The significant anemia and subsequent tissue hypoxia that may result from destruction of red cells by the parasite are a major cause of morbidity. The host's immunological response is to remove the parasites and damaged red blood cells; the immune response may also have deleterious effects. Although microfilariae are seen in peripheral blood during infection with *Dipetalo-*

nema, *Mansonella*, *Loa loa*, *Wuchereria*, or *Brugia*, it is the adult worm eliciting the inflammatory response, primarily in lymphatics, that causes the distinctive lesions of filariasis related to lymphatic obstruction.

14.1.b. Detection. Parasites in the bloodstream are usually detected by direct visualization. Those parasites for which diagnosis is routinely dependent on observation of the organism in peripheral blood smears include *Plasmodium*, *Trypanosoma*, and *Babesia*. Patients with malaria or filariasis may display a periodicity in their episodes of fever that allows the physician to time the collection of blood for visual examination for parasites for optimal results. Further discussion of life cycles of blood-borne parasites and techniques for examination of blood for their presence can be found in Chapter 44. Serologic tests for diagnosis of infection due to blood-borne parasites are also useful, as will be detailed in Chapter 44.

14.2. Virus Infections

14.2.a. Pathogenic mechanisms. Although many viruses do circulate in the peripheral blood at some stage of disease, the primary pathology relates to infection in the target organ or cells. Those viruses that preferentially infect blood cells are the Epstein-Barr virus and the cytomegalovirus, which invade lymphocytes; human immunodeficiency virus (HIV, which involves only certain T lymphocytes and perhaps macrophages); and other human retroviruses that attack lymphocytes. The pathogenesis of viral diseases of the blood is the same as that of viral diseases of any organ; by diverting the cellular machinery to create new viral components or by other means, the virus may prevent the host cell from performing its normal function. The cell may be destroyed or damaged by viral replication, and immunological responses of the host may also contribute to the pathology of the resulting disease.

14.2.b. Detection. Although many viral diseases have a viremic stage, recovery of virus particles or detection of circulating viruses has been used routinely in the diagnosis of only a few diseases. Detection of viral antigen by immunological methods has gained widespread use for diagnosis of hepatitis B. By using an enzyme-linked immunosorbent assay (ELISA) procedure, the surface antigen (HbsAg), core antigen (HbcAg), and early antigen (HbeAg) can be measured quantitatively in serum. Separation of the buffy coat cells from blood using a Ficoll-Hy-

paque gradient allows this virus-rich component to be inoculated into tissue culture for isolation of cytomegalovirus. Most recently, the discovery of a viral etiology for acquired immunodeficiency syndrome (AIDS) has led to the development of methods including ELISA, particle agglutination, and polymerase chain reaction for detection of HIV virus antigens or genes.

14.3. Fungal Infections

14.3.a. Pathogenic mechanisms. Fungemia is usually a serious condition, occurring primarily in immunosuppressed patients and in those with serious or terminal illness. The fungi do not invade blood cells, but their presence in the blood usually indicates a focus of infection elsewhere in the body. The large size and sterol-containing cell walls of molds make them particularly insensitive to the primary host defenses, antibody and phagocytic cells. Fungi in the bloodstream can be carried to all organs of the host, where they may grow, invade normal tissue, and elaborate toxic products. Fungi gain entrance to the circulatory system via loss of integrity of the gastrointestinal or other mucosa, through damaged skin, secondary to involvement of the lung or other organ, or by means of intravascular catheters. Several outbreaks of systemic *Rhizopus* infection were traced to the use of bandage material contaminated with spores of the fungus. Systemic fungal diseases that begin as pneumonia disseminate from the lungs, which serve as the portal of entry. Arthroconidia of *Coccidioides immitis* and microconidia of *Histoplasma capsulatum* and *Blastomyces dermatitidis* are ingested by alveolar macrophages in the lung. These macrophages carry the fungi to nearby lymph nodes, usually the hilar nodes. The fungi multiply within the macrophages and ultimately are released into the circulating blood, from which they go on to seed other organs or are destroyed by the body's defenses.

14.3.b. Culture. Even though all disseminated fungal disease is preceded by fungemia, recovery of the microorganisms from blood cultures has not been accomplished readily until recently. One reason for this may be that cultures were not often taken at the fungemia stage because presence of the disease had not yet been recognized. However, introduction of better methods for isolation of fungi from blood, including the lysis-centrifugation system described later, has resulted in increasing reports of recovery of fungi from peripheral blood and greater awareness by physicians to order fungal blood cultures.

Many fungi, particularly yeast, can be recovered in standard blood culture media if the bottle has been vented to allow sufficient oxygen in the atmosphere for fungal growth. Fungi may grow slowly and poorly in the media that best support bacterial growth, however, and the ideal temperature for certain fungal forms (30° C) is lower than that recommended for optimal bacterial isolation. Until recently, the best medium for the recovery of fungi from blood has been a biphasic system. The biphasic bottle contains an agar slant partially immersed in broth (Figure 14.1). Higher isolation rates and decreased time to recovery are achieved with brain-heart infusion agar and broth incubated at 30° C than with other media. The bottle requires adequate ventilation, since pathogenic fungi grow best at normal atmospheric oxygen tension. Even with such a system, optimal recovery rates for fungi have not been achieved. Several medical centers have now reported increased numbers of fungal isolations with the use of the commercially available lysis centrifugation system, the DuPont Isolator (Section 14.5.c).[6,7]

Blood specimens for detection of fungemia are collected in the same manner as for bacterial culture. Using conventional media, vented and incubated at 30° C, many yeasts will be isolated within a week. Faster detection may occur with the Bactec CO_2 detection system (discussed later). However, for recovery of blood-borne fungi, the lysis-centrifugation system has been most efficacious.[5]

14.3.c. Antigen detection. Because many patients with systemic or invasive fungal infections are immunosuppressed and do not produce appreciable antibodies, detection of circulating fungal antigens or other cell wall components may be a more fruitful diagnostic method than searching for the presence of antibodies. This procedure might also give positive results early in the illness, before there has been time for an antibody response. This concept is being explored for diagnosis of several of the common fungal diseases, and tests employing it have been marketed for aiding diagnosis of at least two mycotic diseases. The presence of mannan antigen, one of the polysaccharides found in *C. albicans* cell walls, has been noted in the serum of some severely ill patients with invasive disease. A commercially available latex agglutination test (Cand-Tec, Ramco Laboratories) can be used to detect circulating mannan

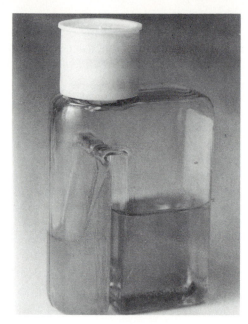

Figure 14.1
Biphasic blood culture bottle, containing an agar slant that can be immersed in broth if the bottle is tipped. (Courtesy GIBCO Laboratories.)

in serum, thus suggesting systemic infection with *C. albicans*. This test has yet to be validated clinically. A sensitive latex particle agglutination test is also available for detection of the polysaccharide capsular antigen of *C. neoformans* in serum or cerebrospinal fluid (Calas, Meridian Diagnostics, and Crypto-Test, M.A. Bioproducts). Quantitation of this antigen can be followed sequentially to determine the effectiveness of antifungal therapy and prognosis.

14.4. Bacterial Infections

14.4.a. Pathogenic mechanisms. Bacteria in the bloodstream, bacteremia, may indicate the presence of a focus of disease, such as pneumonia or liver abscess, or may merely represent transient release of bacteria into the bloodstream, such as occurs after vigorous toothbrushing by a normal person. Septicemia or sepsis indicates a situation in which bacteria or their products (toxins) are causing harm to the host. Unfortunately, clinicians often use the terms interchangeably. Signs and symptoms of septicemia may include fever or hypothermia, chills, hyperventilation and subsequent respiratory alkalosis, skin lesions, change in mental status, and diarrhea. More

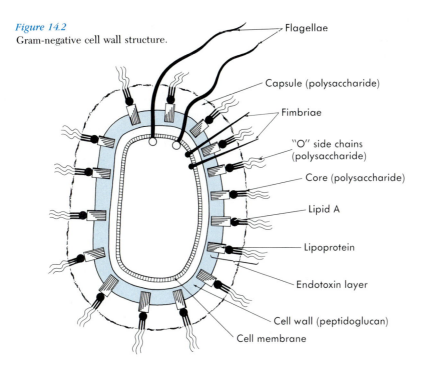

Figure 14.2
Gram-negative cell wall structure.

Flagellae

Capsule (polysaccharide)

Fimbriae

"O" side chains
(polysaccharide)

Core (polysaccharide)

Lipid A

Lipoprotein

Endotoxin layer

Cell wall (peptidoglucan)

Cell membrane

serious manifestations include hypotension or shock, disseminated intravascular coagulation (DIC), and major organ system failure.

Shock is the gravest complication of septicemia. In septic shock, the presence of bacterial products and the host's responding defensive components act to shut down major host physiologic systems. Manifestations include drop in blood pressure, rise in heart rate, impairment of function of vital organs (brain, kidney, liver, and lungs), acid-base problems, and bleeding problems. Gram-negative bacteria and certain other microorganisms contain a substance in their cell walls, endotoxin, that has a strong effect on several physiologic functions. This substance, a lipopolysaccharide (LPS) comprising part of the cell wall structure (Figure 14.2), may be released during the normal growth cycles of bacteria or after the destruction of bacteria by host defenses. Endotoxin (or the lipoidal disaccharide core of the LPS, lipid A) has been shown to mediate a number of systemic reactions, including a drop in circulating granulocytes, a febrile response, and the activation of complement and certain blood-clotting factors.

Although most gram-positive bacteria do not contain endotoxin, some produce exotoxins and, in any case, the effects of their presence in the bloodstream may be equally devastating to the patient. The disastrous complication of disseminated intravascular coagulation, in which numerous small blood vessels become clogged with clotted blood and bleeding may result from depletion of coagulation factors, can occur with septicemia involving any circulating pathogen, including parasites, viruses, and fungi, although it is most often a consequence of gram-negative bacterial sepsis.

14.4.b. Organisms commonly isolated from blood. The commonest portals of entry for septicemia are the genitourinary tract (25%), respiratory tract (20%), abscesses (10%), surgical wound infections (5%), biliary tract (5%), miscellaneous sites (10%), and uncertain sites (25%). The organisms most commonly isolated from blood are gram-negative rods, including the Enterobacteriaceae and *Pseudomonas* species, organisms most likely to be inhabitants of the hospital environment and thus to colonize the skin, oropharyngeal area, and gastrointestinal tract of hospitalized patients (Table 14.1). Factors contributing to initiation of such infections are immunosuppressive agents, widespread use of broad-spectrum antibiotics that suppress the normal flora and allow the emergence of resistant strains of bacteria, invasive procedures that allow bacteria access to the interior of the host, more extensive surgical procedures, and prolonged survival of debilitated and seriously ill patients.

With the ever-increasing use of intravenous catheters, intraarterial lines, and vascular prostheses, organisms found as normal (or hospital-acquired) inhabitants of the human skin are able to gain access to the bloodstream and to find a surface on which to multiply. Heart valves and vascular endothelium may represent such surfaces. When endocarditis occurs, colonies of bacteria embedded in fibrin (vegetations) occur on a heart valve. Constant shedding of fibrin particles and bacteria into the bloodstream is one of the usual consequences of endocarditis. In such a setting, *S. epidermidis* and other coagulase-negative staphylococci have been increasingly detected. The isolation of coagulase-negative staphylococci with the same biochemical and antibiotic susceptibility patterns from more than one blood culture from a patient should alert the clinician to the possibility of a clinically significant isolate. *S. epidermidis* is the most common etiologic agent of prosthetic valve endocarditis, with *S. aureus* the second most common. *S. aureus* is an important cause of septicemia without endocarditis, in association with other foci such as abscesses, wound infections, and pneumonia, as well as sepsis related to indwelling intravascular catheters.

Immunocompromised hospitalized patients tend to become colonized with bacteria that are relatively antibiotic-resistant, such as *S. marcescens*, *Enterobacter* species, *Enterococcus*, and *P. aeruginosa*. Another such bacterium, much less commonly recognized (perhaps because it is relatively fastidious), is *Corynebacterium* group JK (*C. jeikeium*). This organism should be suspected if a diphtheroidlike bacterium isolated from blood displays an unusually broad antibiotic resistance pattern, often being sensitive only to vancomycin. *Corynebacterium* JK is extremely virulent and must not be dismissed as a contaminant.

The primary causes of infectious endocarditis are the viridans streptococci, comprising a large number of species. These organisms are normal inhabitants of the oral cavity or gastrointestinal tract, often gaining entrance to the bloodstream because of gingivitis, periodontitis, or dental manipulation. Heart valves, especially those that have been previously damaged, present convenient surfaces for attachment of these bacteria. The resulting vegetations ultimately seed bacteria into the blood at a slow but

---

Common Agents of Infectious Endocarditis

Viridans streptococci
Nutritionally deficient streptococci
Enterococci
Streptococcus bovis
Staphylococcus aureus
Staphylococci (coagulase-negative)
Salmonella species
Serratia marcescens
Other Enterobacteriaceae
Pseudomonas species
Haemophilus species
Unusual gram-negative bacilli (*Actinobacillus*, *Cardiobacterium*, *Eikenella*, etc.)
Bacteroides fragilis
Other *Bacteroides* species
Fusobacterium species
Other anaerobes
Candida parapsilosis
Candida tropicalis
Other yeast species
Coxiella burnetii
Chlamydia species
Other (including polymicrobial infectious endocarditis)

---

constant rate. Identification of these streptococci may be useful, as certain species (such as *Streptococcus anginosus*), may be associated with increased frequency of metastatic abscess formation. *Streptococcus sanguis* I and II and *Streptococcus mutans* are most frequently isolated in streptococcal endocarditis. Common agents of infectious endocarditis are listed in the box.

The group D streptococci are normal gastrointestinal flora but may be found in the oral cavity as well. Their involvement in bacteremia is usually related to infection of the genitourinary tract or to intraabdominal infection involving bowel flora. The presence of *S. bovis*, a nonenterococcal group D streptococcus, is significantly associated with large bowel carcinoma; clinicians should be aware of this association when this organism is isolated from blood. Identification of this group D streptococcus as *S. bovis* is also important in that infection with this organism (including endocarditis) will respond to penicillin G, whereas enterococcal endocarditis requires a more aggressive therapeutic approach.

Septicemia occurs in 25% to 30% of patients with pneumococcal pneumonia and is often the most reliable way to establish the diagnosis. The prognosis is poorer in patients with pneumococcal pneumonia complicated by sepsis. Because the organisms produce an autolytic enzyme, early subculture of blood culture broths (before 18 hours) is necessary. *S. pneumoniae* grows extremely well in biphasic media, as described below.

H. influenzae infections may be accompanied by septicemia. The organism requires an enriched medium, such as chocolate agar, and 10% CO_2 enhances growth. *Haemophilus parainfluenzae* can also be recovered from blood, particularly as an etiologic agent of endocarditis. This organism grows as large clumps of filamentous rods, which may appear branched in the original stains from broth. Other *Haemophilus* species, including recently renamed *H. actinomycetemcomitans*, *H. aphrophilus*, and *H. paraphrophilus*, may also cause bacteremia and endocarditis. Major arterial embolization is relatively common in endocarditis involving *Haemophilus* species. All of the *Haemophilus* species grow sparsely in blood culture broth and often do not exhibit visually discernible turbidity. For this reason, blind stains or subcultures are essential. Unless such subcultures are made to a medium such as chocolate agar and incubated under 5%-10% CO_2, the organism can be overlooked.

L. monocytogenes is a cause of septicemia in immunosuppressed patients, alcoholics, and pregnant women. The bacterium may resemble a diphtheroid or coccus on Gram stain but grows on 5% sheep blood agar as a translucent, moderately β-hemolytic colony, resembling group B streptococci. *Listeria* must be distinguished from diphtheroids and from groups B and D streptococci. It displays a characteristic tumbling motility at room temperature but not at 35° C.

Anaerobic organisms also cause septicemia. *B. fragilis* is the most common anaerobe isolated from blood. *C. perfringens*, however, can cause rapidly fatal disease and must be presumptively identified by Gram stain appearance and gas and hemolysis in the bottle so that clinicians can be alerted to the possibility of the presence of this virulent bacterium in the bloodstream. In one large recently reported study, however, *C. perfringens* was judged to be a significant isolate (representing true infection) only

50% of the time.[14] The isolation of *Clostridium septicum* may be indicative of malignancy, particularly in the cecum or elsewhere in the gastrointestinal tract of the patient.

An organism associated with fulminant septicemia, often in splenectomized or immunocompromised patients, although rarely isolated, is DF-2. DF-2 is part of the normal oral flora of dogs; 12 of 20 reported cases of DF-2 infection were associated with dog contact or dog bites. A fastidious fermentative gram-negative bacillus, DF-2 will grow in conventional blood culture media. Subcultures may require as long as 4 days before colonies are visible. The organism is described in Chapter 29.

Almost every recognized bacterial species has been implicated as a cause of bacteremia; it is beyond the scope of this text to mention them all here. Certain organisms that require special techniques for isolation are mentioned below. Other bacteria that may grow in routine culture media include *Rothia dentocariosa*, *Campylobacter* species (especially *Campylobacter fetus*), *Alcaligenes* species, *Cardiobacterium hominis*, *Chromobacterium* species, *Eikenella corrodens*, *Flavobacterium* species, and *Mycoplasma*. If these less common organisms are suspected by the clinician, the laboratory should be alerted to hold the blood cultures for an extended period of time past the first week and to make blind subcultures to several media, including more supportive media such as buffered charcoal yeast extract.

Although *Yersinia pestis*, the agent of plague, and *Francisella tularensis*, the agent of tularemia, may grow in routine blood culture media, diagnosis by blood culture is not recommended for two reasons: (1) These organisms are fastidious in their growth requirements and often require prolonged incubation time for detection. The serious nature of the diseases, however, demands a more rapid method of diagnosis. Serologic methods are more reliable and rapid. If an organism resembling *Y. pestis* or *F. tularensis* is isolated from blood, the physician should be notified, and the organism should be forwarded to the nearest public health facility that can handle such an isolate. (2) These pathogens are classified as class three etiologic agents (extremely hazardous) and require special containment facilities for their manipulation.

14.4.c. Timing and quantity of blood for conventional culture. Conditions in which bacteria are only transiently present in the bloodstream include manipulation of infected tissues, instrumentation of contaminated mucosal surfaces, and surgery involving nonsterile sites. These backgrounds may also lead to significant septicemia. Incidental, transient bacteremia may occur spontaneously or with such minor events as chewing food. Bacteria can be found intermittently in the blood of patients with undrained abscesses. During early stages of typhoid fever, brucellosis, and leptospirosis, bacteria are continuously present in the bloodstream. The causative agents of meningitis, pneumonia, pyogenic arthritis, and osteomyelitis are often recovered from blood during the early course of these diseases. In the case of transient seeding of the blood from a sequestered focus of infection, such as an abscess, bacteria are released into the blood before the febrile episode. If a regular periodicity of fevers can be established, the most advantageous time to draw blood cultures will be just before the anticipated rise in temperature. In bacterial endocarditis and other endovascular infections, organisms are released into the bloodstream at a fairly constant rate so that timing of cultures is not important. Many studies have shown that the likelihood of recovering a pathogen is increased as the volume of blood cultured increases, provided that there is adequate dilution of such blood to negate the effect of normal antibacterial substances and antimicrobial agents that may be present. When a patient's condition requires institution of therapy as rapidly as possible, the luxury of time for the collection of multiple blood culture samples is lacking. A compromise that has been generally accepted is to collect 30 ml of blood at one time, 10 ml from each of *three separate venipunctures from three different sites, using three separate needles and syringes*, before the patient is given antimicrobial therapy. For initial evaluation of fever of unknown origin, four separate blood cultures, two drawn on each of 2 days, will detect most causative agents. The large study reported by Weinstein et al.[14] revealed that 99.3% of 500 episodes of septicemia were identified by the first two blood cultures, comprising 30 ml total volume of blood cultured. In another study, in 98% of patients with infective endocarditis who had not received antimicrobial agents, two blood cultures established the diagnosis. If therapy can be delayed, three separate blood collections of 10 ml each, and an additional blood culture or two taken on the second day (if necessary), will detect most etiologic agents of endocarditis,

even for patients who have received prior antibiotic therapy. This presumes use of setups adequate for growth of the organism involved. An excellent discussion on the rational use of blood cultures was presented by Aronson and Bor.[1]

It is not safe to take large samples of blood from children, particularly young infants. Fortunately, infants with more serious disease usually yield >10 colony-forming units (CFU) of bacteria per milliliter of blood. For infants and children, only 1 to 5 ml of blood can usually be drawn for bacterial culture.[10] Quantities less than 1 ml may not be adequate to detect pathogens, however, since one early study showed 23% of blood specimens from septic children yielded <5 CFU/ml of the organism.[3]

14.4.d. How to draw blood for conventional culture. Since the media into which blood specimens are placed have been developed as enrichment broths to encourage the multiplication of even one bacterium, it follows that these media will enhance the growth of any stray contaminating bacterium, such as a normal inhabitant of human skin. Because of the rising incidence of true infections caused by bacteria that normally are nonvirulent indigenous microflora of a healthy human host, interpretation of the significance of growth of such bacteria in blood cultures has become increasingly difficult. To help clinicians determine whether an *S. epidermidis*, other coagulase-negative staphylococcus, *Corynebacterium* species, or *P. acnes* is a true pathogen or an inadvertently introduced skin contaminant, blood cultures are drawn from separate sites, even when more than one blood culture is to be drawn at one time, such as before instituting emergency therapy. Only recovery of identical bacteria of these types from multiple cultures is considered to be indicative of infection. Quantitation of bacteremia, as is possible with the lysis-centrifugation system, may be helpful.

Another strategy is to reduce the risk of introducing contaminants into blood culture media by careful skin preparation. Procedure 14.1 details the steps necessary for drawing blood for culture. A publication from the National Committee for Clinical Laboratory Standards describes in more detail the mechanics of collection of blood by venipuncture.[9] Laboratories that recover "contaminants," as determined by clinical evaluation of the patients' conditions, at rates greater than 3% should suspect improper phlebotomy techniques and should institute

PROCEDURE 14.1

Drawing Blood for Culture

Principle

Organisms found in circulating blood can be enriched in culture for isolation and further studies. Blood for culture must be obtained aseptically. Once removed from the circulation, unclotted blood must be diluted in growth media.

Method

1. Choose the vein to be drawn by touching the skin before it has been disinfected.
2. Cleanse the skin over the venipuncture site in a circle approximately 5 cm in diameter with 70% alcohol, rubbing vigorously.
3. Starting in the center of the circle, apply 2% iodine (or povidone-iodine) in ever-widening circles until the entire circle has been saturated with iodine. Allow the iodine to dry on the skin for at least 1 min. The timing is critical; a watch or timer should be used.
4. If the site must be touched by the phlebotomist after preparation, the phlebotomist must disinfect the fingers used for palpation in identical fashion or must palpate through a sterile glove. (Universal Precautions dictates that phlebotomists wear gloves.)
5. Insert the needle into the vein and withdraw blood. Change needles before injecting the blood into the culture bottle.
6. After the needle has been removed, the site should be cleansed with 70% alcohol again, as many patients are sensitive to iodine.

Quality control

Blood culture results should be monitored regularly. If greater than 3% of isolates are judged on clinical grounds to be contaminants, then the aseptic techniques are inadequate and additional training should be initiated.

---

measures to reeducate the phlebotomists in proper skin preparation methods. It is undesirable to draw blood through a vascular shunt or catheter, since these prosthetic devices may harbor colonizing bacteria that are not present in the circulating blood of the patient, and blood obtained through the foreign material would yield false positive results. It is also recommended to draw blood below an existing intravenous line, if possible, since blood above the line will be diluted with the fluid being infused.

If the blood for culture is not being inoculated directly into broth media, it must be transported with an anticoagulant. Heparin, ethylenediaminetetraacetic acid (EDTA), and citrate have been found to be inhibitory to a number of organisms; thus, sodium polyanethol sulfonate (SPS, Liquoid) in concentrations of 0.025% to 0.03% is the best anticoagulant for blood.

14.4.e. How to culture intravenous catheter tips. When colonization of an indwelling catheter is suspected of being the focus for septicemia, the catheter tip may be cultured to determine its status. As first reported by Maki and coworkers,[8] the number of colony-forming units of bacteria on the catheter directly relates to whether it is the source of the infection. The skin around the catheter is carefully disinfected with an iodine preparation, and the catheter is removed. A short section (approximately 5 cm [2 in]), including the area directly beneath the skin, is aseptically cut off and sent to the microbiology laboratory in a sterile container without liquid. This section of catheter is rolled across the surface of an agar plate with sterile forceps (as shown in Figure 14.3). After overnight incubation, the colonies are counted. A finding of ≥15 CFU correlates well with the catheter tip's being the source of infection.

14.4.f. Conventional blood culture media, additives, and dilution factors. The diversity of bacteria that are recovered from blood requires an equally diverse armamentarium of media to enhance the growth of these bacteria. Basic blood culture media contain a nutrient broth and an anticoagulant. Numerous different broth formulations are available,

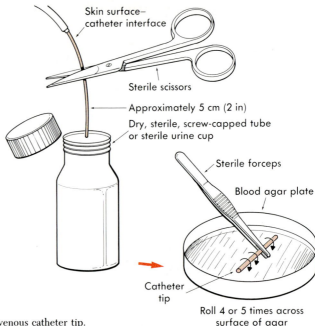

Skin surface–
catheter interface

Sterile scissors

Approximately 5 cm (2 in)

Dry, sterile, screw-capped tube
or sterile urine cup

Sterile forceps

Blood agar plate

Catheter
tip

Roll 4 or 5 times across
surface of agar

Figure 14.3
Method for culturing intravenous catheter tip.

including those that can be prepared by the laboratory in-house and those that are commercially prepared. Most blood culture bottles available commercially contain trypticase soy broth, brain-heart infusion agar, supplemented peptone, or thioglycollate broth. More specialized broth bases include Columbia or *Brucella* broth. Growth of cell wall–deficient bacteria may be enhanced by the addition of osmotic stabilizers such as sucrose, mannitol, or sorbose to create a hyperosmotic (hypertonic) medium. Media without such osmotic additives are known as isotonic. The hypertonic bottles are difficult to inspect visually for evidence of bacterial growth, as red cells in the media become partially lysed and no longer sediment to the bottom, giving a muddy appearance to the broth. Such media are more useful when blood culture systems do not rely on visual evidence of growth as the only indication for further examination, such as the automated growth detection system described later.

The anticoagulant in blood culture media must not harm the bacteria and must prevent clotting of the blood, which would entrap bacteria and prevent their detection. The most commonly used preparation in blood culture media today is 0.025% to 0.05% SPS. In addition to its anticoagulant properties, SPS is also anticomplementary, antiphagocytic, and interferes with the activity of certain antimicrobial

agents, the aminoglycosides. SPS may, however, inhibit the growth of a few microorganisms such as some strains of *Neisseria* species, *Gardnerella vaginalis*, *Streptobacillus moniliformis*, and all strains of *Peptostreptococcus anaerobius*. The addition of 1.2% gelatin has been shown to counteract this inhibitory action of SPS; however, a large series comparing Bactec media with and without added gelatin failed to show any advantage with gelatin-supplemented Bactec media for recovery of *Neisseria* species, *Haemophilus influenzae*, and *Candida albicans*. In addition, recovery of other organisms was decreased.[12]

Penicillinase may be added to blood culture media to specifically inactivate certain penicillins and other β-lactam antibiotics in the blood of patients. After addition of penicillinase, an equivalent amount of the penicillinase should be cultured on the surface of a chocolate agar plate to rule out the possibility that a contaminant has been introduced into the blood culture via the additive. The use of penicillinase has been largely superseded in recent years by the availability of a resin-containing medium that inactivates most antibiotics nonselectively by adsorbing them to the surface of the resin particles. Several studies have detailed faster and increased recovery of pathogens from patients receiving antibiotics when blood was cultured with the aid of resin-containing systems. When the Antimicrobial Removal Device (ARD, Becton-Dickinson), a resin-containing bottle into which blood from patients receiving antibiotics is drawn, is used with conventional manual blood culture systems, it is necessary to perform the additional manipulations of rotating the blood with the resin and then centrifuging the blood to remove the resin particles before inoculating the culture media. This device has been shown to remove at least 25 antimicrobial agents from blood[11]; its use may be associated with inhibition of some strains of bacteria, however, especially gram-negative rods. The Bactec system also offers several resin-containing media. Preliminary studies have shown one medium (Bactec Plus), which allows inoculation of a larger volume of blood (10 ml per bottle) to yield enhanced recovery of agents of septicemia in comparison with the DuPont Isolator system.[6a,7a] These bottles would have the added benefit of adequate conditions for recovery of anaerobes.

In addition to volume of blood cultured and type of media chosen, the dilution factor for the blood in the medium must be considered. To conserve space and materials, it is desirable to combine the largest feasible amount of blood from the patient (usually 10 ml) with the smallest amount of medium that will still encourage the growth of bacteria and dilute out or inactivate the antibacterial components of the system. For this purpose, a 1:10 ratio of blood to medium has been found to be convenient.

14.4.g. Incubation conditions for conventional blood cultures. The atmosphere in commercially prepared blood culture bottles is usually at a low oxidation-reduction potential, allowing most facultative and some anaerobic organisms to multiply. To encourage the growth of strict aerobes, such as yeast and *P. aeruginosa*, transient venting of the bottles with a sterile, cotton-plugged needle is necessary. For optimal recovery of pathogens, therefore, the use of two different bottles of blood culture media, one vented and the other unvented, is recommended.

14.4.h. Detecting growth in conventional blood cultures. Most clinical laboratories report a positive blood culture rate of greater than 8%. Five percent or more of positive blood cultures will yield anaerobic bacteria. Restricted patient populations may influence the rate of positive cultures reported from smaller hospitals and clinics.

After 6 to 18 hours of incubation, most bacteria are present in numbers large enough to detect by

blind subculture or acridine orange viable stain (discussed in Chapter 7). Constant agitation of the bottles during initial incubation will enhance the growth of most bacteria. Agitation does not allow the red cells to settle in the media, however, so that gross visual detection of growth is not possible soon after the initial incubation with agitation.

Blind subcultures after the first 6 to 12 hours of incubation are performed by aseptically removing a few drops of the well-mixed medium and spreading this inoculum onto a chocolate blood agar plate, which is incubated in 5% to 10% CO_2 at 35° C for 48 hours. Bottles are then reincubated without agitation for 7 days unless the patient's condition requires special consideration, as discussed later. Growth of anaerobic bacteria can be detected by visual inspection with such success that blind anaerobic subcultures are not recommended. After 48 hours' incubation, a second blind subculture or acridine orange stain may be performed.

Bottles should be examined visually at least daily. Growth is usually indicated by hemolysis of the red cells, gas bubbles in the medium, turbidity, or appearance of small colonies in the broth, on the surface of the sedimented red cell layer (Figure 14.4), or occasionally along the walls of the bottle. When macroscopic evidence of growth is apparent, a Gram stain of a drop of medium will be more rewarding. Methanol fixation of the smear preserves bacterial and cellular morphology, which may be especially valuable for detecting gram-negative bacteria among red cell debris. Examination of the positive broth under phase microscopy will reveal details of morphology and motility that may aid the clinician in making an early decision regarding treatment. As soon as a morphological description can be tentatively assigned to a pathogen detected in blood, the physician should be given all of the available information. Determining the clinical significance of an isolate is the physician's responsibility. If no organisms are seen on microscopic examination of a bottle that appears positive, subcultures should be performed anyway.

14.4.i. Procedures for handling positive blood cultures. Subcultures from blood cultures suspected of being positive, whether proved by microscopic visualization or not, should be made to a variety of media so as to be able to support the growth of most bacteria, including anaerobes. Initial subculture may include chocolate blood agar, 5% sheep blood agar, MacConkey agar (if gram-negative bacteria are

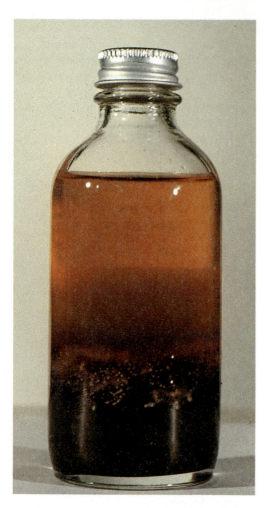

Figure 14.4
Many colonies of S. *aureus* on layer of settled red blood cells
in blood culture bottle.

seen), and supplemented anaerobic blood agar. The
incidence of polymicrobic bacteremia or fungemia
ranges from 3% to 20% of all positive blood cultures.
For this reason, samples must be streaked for isolated colonies. Restreaking positive bottles a second
time at the end of the incubation period to detect
further organisms after the original subculture is of
questionable value and is not recommended.

A number of rapid tests for identification and
presumptive antimicrobial susceptibilities can be
performed from the broth blood culture, if a uni-
microbic infection is suspected (based on microscopic evaluation). A suspension of the organism that
approximates the turbidity of a 0.5 McFarland standard, achieved directly from the broth, or by cen-

trifuging the broth and resuspending the pelleted
bacteria, can be used to inoculate Mueller-Hinton
agar plates for the Bauer-Kirby susceptibility test or
for performing dilution antimicrobial susceptibilities. These suspensions may also be used to set up
preliminary biochemical tests such as coagulase,
thermostable nuclease, esculin hydrolysis, bile solubility, or antigen detection by fluorescent-antibody
stain or agglutination procedures for gram-positive
bacteria and oxidase and rapid biochemicals such as
API Rapid E, Minitek, or Micro-ID for gram-negative bacteria. Presumptive results must be verified
with conventional procedures using pure cultures.
Chapter 4 includes some discussion of rapid methods
of handling positive blood cultures.

All isolates from blood cultures should be stored
for an indefinite period, preferably by freezing at
$-70°$ C in 10% skim milk. Storing an agar slant of
the isolate under sterile mineral oil at room temperature is a good alternative to freezing. It is often
necessary to compare separate isolates from the same
patient or isolates of the same species from different
patients, sometimes even months after the bacteria
were isolated.

14.4.j. **Culturing suspected contaminated banked
blood, plasma, or other infused fluids**. When an infusion is suspected of being the source of bacteremia
or fungemia, it must be cultured in a manner similar
to that used for blood. Since contamination is usually
random and rare, the routine monitoring of intravenous fluids and banked blood is not rational. However, in cases of suspected contamination, the fluid,
plasma, or other blood product is aseptically aspirated into a syringe and 5 to 10 ml is aseptically
introduced into each of two blood culture bottles.
One bottle is incubated at room temperature to enhance the growth of psychrophilic (cold-loving)
gram-negative bacilli, which have been implicated
as the cause of fatal transfusion reactions, and the
other bottle is incubated at $35°$ C. The normal visual
and cultural methods used to detect positive cultures
are then followed. The putative contaminated blood
product bag, tubing, and all isolates should be saved
until epidemiologic investigations are complete.

A number of infections have been documented
to be transmitted by blood transfusions or needle
contact, including malaria, trypanosomiasis, toxoplasmosis, cytomegalovirus disease, AIDS, hepatitis, and bacterial endocarditis. Gram-negative bacteria are most often implicated in contaminated in-

travenous fluids, although the possibility exists for any organism to multiply in a suitable environment and subsequently be injected into a compromised host. Recently, several episodes of *Yersinia entero-colitica* bacteremia, shock, and even death following transfusion of packed red blood cells were reported.[2] *Yersinia* can multiply to large numbers in red cells stored at refrigerator temperatures without showing visible evidence of their presence.

14.4.k. Special problems and unusual microorganisms. Special handling may be required for recovery of *Brucella* species from blood; septicemia occurs primarily during the first 3 weeks of illness. Best recovery is obtained with *Brucella* or trypticase soy broth, and the use of biphasic media may enhance growth of the bacteria. The bottles should be continuously vented and incubated in 10% CO_2 at 37° C for at least 4 weeks. Blind subcultures should be performed at 4 days and weekly thereafter onto *Brucella* blood agar plates incubated as described. *Brucella* species may grow slowly, so cultures must be incubated for longer than average time periods. Cultures should be handled in a biological safety cabinet. The use of the lysis-centrifugation method may enhance recovery. In some cases, only bone marrow cultures are positive.

Visualization in direct preparations is diagnostic for 70% of cases of febrile disease caused by *Borrelia* species. The organisms may be seen in direct wet preparations of a drop of anticoagulated blood diluted in saline as long, thin, unevenly coiled spirochetes that seem to push the red blood cells around as they move. Thick and thin smears of blood, prepared as for malaria testing (described in Chapter 44) and stained with Wright's or Giemsa stain, are also quite sensitive for the detection of *Borrelia*.

Leptospirosis can be diagnosed by isolating the causative spirochete from blood during the first 4 to 7 days of illness. Media with up to 14% (vol/vol) rabbit serum, such as Fletcher's, polysorbate 80 (Tween 80)–albumin, or Ellinghausen, McCullough, Johnson, Harris (EMJH) semisolid medium are recommended (described in Chapters 31 and Appendix A). After adding 1 to 3 drops of fresh or SPS-anticoagulated blood to each of several tubes with 5 ml of culture medium, the cultures are incubated for 5 to 6 weeks at 28° to 30° C in air in the dark. Leptospires will grow 1 to 3 cm below the surface, usually within 2 weeks. The organisms remain viable in blood with SPS for 11 days, allowing

for transport of cultures from distant locations. Direct darkfield examination of peripheral blood is not recommended, since many artifacts are present that may resemble spirochetes.

One of the agents of rat-bite fever, *Streptobacillus moniliformis*, may be recovered in blood cultures. Concentrations of SPS greater than 0.025% will inhibit the growth of this organism, however, so the addition of 1.2% gelatin to commercial media is recommended. These organisms will grow in conventional media after several days of incubation, visible as "puffball" colonies on the surface of the red cell layer. Cell wall–defective forms may require the use of hypertonic media for recovery.

Mycobacterium avium-intracellulare complex organisms have been isolated increasingly often from the blood of patients suffering from AIDS. By the time the infection is discovered, the bacteria are usually circulating in great numbers. The use of special media, such as Middlebrook 7H9 broth with 0.05% SPS or brain-heart infusion broth with 0.5% polysorbate 80, with or without a Middlebrook 7H11 agar slant, is recommended. The newer methods of detection, radiometric and lysis-centrifugation (described later), have been shown to shorten greatly the time required for mycobacterial cultures to become positive.

Certain streptococci are unable to multiply without the addition of 0.001% pyridoxal hydrochloride (also called thiol or vitamin B_6). These streptococci are known as "nutritionally variant" or "satelliting" streptococci. Although human blood introduced into the blood culture medium will provide enough of the pyridoxal to allow the organisms to multiply in the bottle, standard sheep blood agar plates may not support their growth. Subculturing the broth to a 5% sheep blood agar plate and overlaying a streak of *S. aureus* to produce the supplement will generally demonstrate colonies of the streptococci growing as tiny "satellites" next to the streak (see Figure 25.1). Some commercial media may be supplemented with enough pyridoxal (0.001%) to support growth of nutritionally variant streptococci.

14.5. New and Nonconventional Methods for Detecting Bacteremia

14.5.a. Antimicrobial removal device. Introduction of blood into a vial containing anticoagulant, a cationic resin, and a polymeric adsorbent resin will remove antimicrobial agents present in the blood before the blood is inoculated into culture media. The vial is commercially available (ARD, Marion Laboratories). Blood must be rotated in the vial with the resins for 15 minutes, centrifuged to remove the resins, and then inoculated into the media of choice. This device can remove up to 100 μg of most antibiotics. Although there are studies that imply no significant advantage with this system, most workers have found increased and faster isolation of pathogens from the blood of patients being treated with antimicrobial agents. Negative aspects include inhibition of the growth of some strains of gram-negative bacilli.

14.5.b. Detection of CO_2 end product of metabolism. More than one third of all hospital microbiology laboratories use the Bactec automated blood culture system (Johnston Laboratories) described in Chapter 11 for the radiometric or spectrophotometric detection of CO_2 produced by microbial metabolism and released into the airspace above the fluid medium. The blood cultures are always agitated during early incubation to facilitate the growth of aerobic and facultative organisms. Additionally, the growth index readings must be monitored, since a minimal amount of background in the culture medium is common. Resin-containing broth media are also available for the Bactec; enhanced recovery of fungi and fastidious bacteria have been reported. No further manipulations are required to use this medium after the blood has been introduced into the bottle.[7a]

Problems encountered with the Bactec system include false-positive findings due to inappropriate threshold values, false-positive findings due to carryover of organisms from positive bottles to adjacent culture bottles by inadequately sterilized sampling needles, false-negative findings due to failure of certain microorganisms to metabolize enough substrate, and the need for special disposal of the radioactive media (for the radiometric system) at the end of the incubation period. Regulations governing the disposal of the media vary among states.

Advantages of the Bactec system are more rapid detection time for many pathogens, availability of an antimicrobial-removal additive for the medium, the ability to monitor growth without visual inspection or subculture, the automated handling of large numbers of blood culture bottles, allowing the use of hypertonic media, and the potential to tie the system into a management information processing data base for monitoring results and generating statistical re-

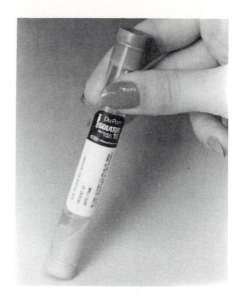

Figure 14.5
DuPont Isolator lysis-centrifugation tube.

ports for both historical and epidemiologic studies. Modified radiometric Bactec media have been used successfully for relatively rapid detection of circulating mycobacteria.

14.5.c. Lysis-centrifugation. In order to rapidly remove pathogens from the blood and its antibacterial properties and antimicrobial agents, Sullivan and coworkers[13] introduced a system that employed lysis of blood cells and filtration of the hemolyzed suspension to trap the bacteria on the filter. Although the technology was cumbersome, the results were rewarding. This filtration system was the forerunner of the lysis-centrifugation system developed by Dorn and coworkers,[4] commercially available as the Isolator (E. I. DuPont de Nemours & Co.). The Isolator consists of a stoppered tube containing saponin to lyse blood cells, polypropylene glycol to decrease foaming, SPS as an anticoagulant, EDTA to chelate calcium ions and thus inhibit the complement cascade and coagulation, and a small amount of an inert fluorochemical (Fluorinert, 3M Co., St. Paul, Minn.) to cushion and concentrate the microorganisms during 30-minute centrifugation at 3000 × g (Figure 14.5). The sediment is cushioned by Fluorinert. After centrifugation, the supernatant is discarded, the sediment containing the pathogens is vigorously vortexed, and the entire sediment is plated to solid agar.

Benefits of this system include the more rapid and greater recovery of certain microorganisms, the presence of actual colonies for direct identification and susceptibility testing after initial incubation, the ability to quantify the colony-forming units present in the blood, rapid detection of polymicrobial bacteremia, increased recovery of filamentous fungi and yeasts, dispensing with the need for a separate antibiotic-removal step, the ability to choose special media for initial culture setup based on clinical impression (such as direct plating onto media supportive of *Legionella* species or *Mycobacterium* species), and possible greater recovery of intracellular microorganisms due to lysis of host cells. Shortcomings of the system seem to be a relatively high rate of plate contamination, necessitating manipulation inside a laminar flow biosafety cabinet, and failure of the system to detect certain bacteria, such as *S. pneumoniae*, *L. monocytogenes*, and anaerobic bacteria, as well as conventional systems. The combination of an Isolator tube and an anaerobic broth blood culture bottle should recover most pathogens.

14.5.d. Self-contained subculture. Recent modifications of the biphasic blood culture medium are the Septi-Chek system (Roche Diagnostics) and the Vacutainer Agar Slant system (Becton-Dickinson), consisting of a conventional blood culture broth bottle with an attached chamber containing a slide coated with agar or several types of agars (Figure 14.6). To subculture, the entire broth contents are allowed to contact the agar surface by inverting the bottle, a simple procedure that does not require opening the bottle or using needles. The large volume of broth that is subcultured and the ease of subculture allow faster detection time for many organisms than is possible with conventional systems. The Septi-Chek system appears to enhance the recovery of *S. pneumoniae*, but such systems do not efficiently recover anaerobic isolates.

14.5.e. Detection of microorganisms through changes in electrical impedance. The passage of electric current through a liquid medium can be measured. Electrodes placed in the broth can continuously monitor electrical impedance, even overnight when no technologists are present. The Bactometer is currently the only commercially available instrument in the United States for this purpose. Initial impedance changes occur at a microbial colony count of approximately 5×10^5, the same level of growth at which turbidity is first discernible. This

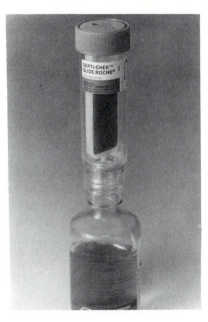

Figure 14.6
Self-contained subculture system for blood cultures.

system and others that detect microbial growth through changes in electrical conductivity or microcalorimetry (heat given off during bacterial metabolism) have not enjoyed wide use in clinical laboratories yet.

14.5.f. Nonculture methods for detecting bacteremia. Circulating antigens can be detected by latex agglutination procedures, available for some yeasts, group B streptococci, *H. influenzae* type b, *S. pneumoniae*, staphylococcal teichoic acids, and *Neisseria meningitidis*. These techniques are discussed in Chapter 10.

The lysate from amebocytes of *Limulus polyphemus*, the horseshoe crab, will gel in the presence of as little as 0.1 ng of endotoxin. This highly sensitive test, the *Limulus* amebocyte lysate assay, can be used to detect circulating lipopolysaccharides (LPS) in patients with gram-negative bacteremia. Sites of gram-negative bacterial infection other than blood may also cause a positive test result with serum. Although often used as an emergency test to diagnose gram-negative bacterial meningitis, the amebocyte lysate assay is not commonly used to diagnose bacteremia, in part because of its nonspecific nature in blood testing.

Detecting the presence of metabolic end products of microbial activity in serum using gas-liquid chromatography (GLC) has been explored. Some success in detecting products of anaerobic metabolism has been reported. A promising use of GLC may be its ability to detect metabolic products of mycobacteria, organisms whose diagnosis by conventional methods is extremely time-consuming.

Lysis-filtration of blood and subsequent staining of the filter surface, either with traditional stains or with new molecular reagents, may prove to be a very sensitive and rapid method for detection of circulating microorganisms. New methods are in development for exploiting nucleic acid probe reagents for detection of pathogens in blood.

REFERENCES

1. Aronson, M.D., and Bor, D.H. 1987. Blood cultures. Ann. Intern. Med. 106:246.
2. CDC 1988. *Yersinia enterocolitia* bacteremia and endotoxin shock associated with red blood cell transfusion—United States, 1987-1988. MMWR 37:577.
3. Dietzman, D.E., Fischer, G.W., and Schoenknecht, F.D. 1974. Neonatal *Escherichia coli* septicemia—bacterial counts in blood. J. Pediatr. 85:128.
4. Dorn, G.L., Haynes, J.R., and Burson, G.G. 1976. Blood culture technique based on centrifugation: developmental phase. J. Clin. Microbiol. 3:251.
5. Guerra-Romero, L., Edson, R.S., Cockerill, F.R., et al. 1987. Comparison of DuPont Isolator and Roche Septi-Chek for detection of fungemia. J. Clin. Microbiol. 25:1623.
6. Henry, N.K., Grewell, C.M., VanGrevenhof, P.E., et al. 1984. Comparison of lysis-centrifugation with a biphasic blood culture medium for the recovery of aerobic and facultatively anaerobic bacteria. J. Clin. Microbiol. 20:413.
6a. Kelly, M., Roberts, F., Henry, D., et al. 1989. Comparison of Bactec 660 resin media to Isolator for detection of bacteremia. Abstr. Ann. Meeting, Amer. Soc. Clin. Microbiol., C-228, p. 431.
7. Kiehn, T.E. 1988. Isolators versus broth for blood cultures. Clin. Microbiol. Newsletter 10:53.
7a. Koontz, F., Chavez, A., and Pfaller, M.A. 1989. Comparison of the Bactec Plus (high blood volume) system to the DuPont Isolator in patients at high risk for fungal sepsis. Abstr. Ann. Meeting, Amer. Soc. Clin. Microbiol., C-226, p. 431.
8. Maki, D.G., Weise, C.E., and Sarafin, H.W. 1977. A semi-quantitative culture method for identifying intravenous catheter–related infection. N. Engl. J. Med. 296:1305.
9. NCCLS procedures for the collection of diagnostic blood specimens by venipuncture, ed. 2. National Committee for Clinical Laboratory Standards, Villanova, Pa.
10. Neal, P.R., Kleiman, M.B., Reynolds, J.K., et al. 1986. Volume of blood submitted for culture from neonates. J. Clin. Microbiol. 24:353.
11. Rodriguez, F., and Lorian, V. 1985. Antibacterial activity in blood cultures. J. Clin. Microbiol. 21:262.
12. Stratton, C.W., Weinstein, M.P., Mirrett, S., et al. 1988. Controlled evaluation of blood culture medium containing gelatin and V-factor-analog for detection of septicemia in children. J. Clin. Microbiol. 26:747.
13. Sullivan, N.M., Sutter, V.L., and Finegold, S.M. 1975. Practical aerobic membrane filtration blood culture technique: development of procedure. J. Clin. Microbiol. 1:30.
14. Weinstein, M.P., Reller, L.B., Murphy, J.R., et al. 1983. The clinical significance of positive blood cultures: a comprehensive analysis of 500 episodes of bacteremia and fungemia in adults. I. Laboratory and epidemiologic observations. Rev. Infect. Dis. 5:35.

BIBLIOGRAPHY

Balows, A., and Sonnenwirth, A.C. 1983. Bacteremia: laboratory and clinical aspects. Charles C Thomas, Springfield, Ill.

Balows, A., and Tilton, R.C., editors. 1983. Proceedings of a symposium. Body fluids and infectious diseases: clinical and microbiologic advances. Am. J. Med. 75:1.

Blazevic, D.J., McCarthy, L.R., and Morello, J.A. 1982. Minimum guidelines for blood cultures. Clin. Microbiol. Newsletter 4:85.

Farrar, W.E. 1985. Leptospira species (leptospirosis). In Mandell, G.L., Douglas, R.G., Jr., and Bennett, J.E., editors. Principles and practice of infectious diseases, ed. 2. John Wiley & Sons, New York.

Reller, L.B., Murray, P.R., and MacLowry, J.D. 1982. Cumitech IA. Blood cultures II, American Society for Microbiology, Washington, D.C.

Scheld, W.M., and Sande, M.E. 1985. Endocarditis and intravascular infections. In Mandell, G.L., Douglas, R.G., Jr., and Bennett, J.E., editors. Principles and practice of infectious diseases, ed. 2. John Wiley & Sons, New York.

Tilton, R.C. 1982. The laboratory approach to the detection of bacteremia. Annu. Rev. Microbiol. 36:467.

Washington, J.A. II. 1978. The detection of septicemia, CRC Press, West Palm Beach, Fla.

15 Microorganisms Encountered in the Cerebrospinal Fluid

15.1. Anatomy of the Meninges and Choroid Plexus; Cerebrospinal Fluid

Fully surrounding the brain and spinal cord, the cerebrospinal fluid (CSF) has several functions. It cushions the bulk of the brain and provides buoyancy, reducing the effective weight of the brain by a factor of 30. The CSF, through its circulation around the entire brain, ventricles, and spinal cord, carries essential metabolites into the neural tissue and cleanses the organs of wastes. Every 3 to 4 hours, the entire volume of CSF is exchanged. The CSF is produced by the choroid plexus, specialized secretory cells located centrally within the brain in the third and fourth ventricles (fluid-filled cavities within the brain). The fluid travels around the ouside areas of the brain within the subarachnoid space, driven primarily by the pressure produced initially at the choroid plexus. The subarachnoid space is the intervening space between the pia mater, the tissue layer immediately covering the brain, and the arachnoid, a membrane loosely covering the brain and part of the spinal cord. Attachment between these two membranes is mediated by a thin network of fibers. The membranes surrounding the brain, the pia mater and the arachnoid, are collectively called the leptomeninges. All of the membranes surrounding the brain, including the dura, which covers the leptomeninges, are called the meninges. The portion of the arachnoid that covers the top of the brain contains special structures, arachnoid villi, that absorb the spinal fluid and allow it to pass into the blood.[5]

Infection within the subarachnoid space or throughout the leptomeninges is called **meningitis.** With bacterial meningitis, cerebrospinal fluid usually contains large numbers of inflammatory cells (greater than $1000/mm^3$), primarily polymorphonuclear neutrophils, shows a decreased glucose level relative to the serum glucose level (the normal ratio of CSF to serum glucose is approximately 0.6), and shows an increased protein concentration (normal protein is 15 to 50 mg/dl in adults and as high as 170 mg/dl, with an average of 90 mg/dl, in newborns). Most infectious agents reach the leptomeninges via hematogenous spread, entering the subarachnoid space through the choroid plexus or through other blood vessels of the brain. Meningitis can be either acute, usually caused by an encapsulated bacterial species, or chronic, caused by *Mycobacterium tuberculosis*, other bacteria, or fungi. Some of the more common causes of acute meningitis are listed in the box. Inflammation of the brain parenchyma, called **encephalitis,** is usually a result of viral infection. Concomitant inflammation of the meninges often occurs with this condition, which is then called *meningoencephalitis*, although the cellular infiltrate is more likely to be lymphocytic in this situation. Early in the course of viral encephalitis or when much tissue damage occurs as a part of encephalitis, however, the nature of the inflammatory cells found in the cerebrospinal fluid is no different from that associated with bacterial meningitis; typically, cell counts are much lower.

In the past, patients who showed symptoms of meningitis and yielded cerebrospinal fluid samples that failed to grow a bacterial agent in culture were said to be suffering from "aseptic meningitis." The other possibility to consider in the case of a patient who had received antibiotics previously, of course, is that of partially treated bacterial meningitis. With the advent of improved technology and availability of viral and other special cultures, many instances of "aseptic meningitis" can now be assigned a viral, leptospiral, or other etiology. Aseptic meningitis may also be due to tumor, cysts, chemicals, sarcoidosis, or other noninfectious causes.

15.2. Pathogenesis and Epidemiology of Meningeal Infections

Most cases of meningitis caused by bacteria or encephalitis caused by viruses share the same pathogenesis. The etiologic agent impinges on the mucous membranes of the nasopharynx and oropharynx, attaches with the aid of an adherence mechanism (discussed in Chapter 16), and multiplies at the initial

---

Etiologic Agents of Acute Meningitis

Acute bacterial meningitis

Streptococcus pneumoniae
Haemophilus influenzae
Neisseria meningitidis
Streptococcus agalactiae (group B streptococci)
Gram-negative bacilli, including *Flavobacterium meningosepticum*
Listeria monocytogenes
Staphylococci
Leptospira
Treponema pallidum
Mycobacterium tuberculosis

Acute nonbacterial meningitis

Cryptococcus neoformans
Naegleria or *Acanthamoeba*
Candida
Viruses (usually enteroviruses)
Angiostrongylus cantonensis
Toxoplasma gondii

---

site. The organism somehow invades or is carried across tissue into the bloodstream, where it disseminates throughout the system during a bacteremic or viremic phase. Humoral immunity presumably intervenes at this stage in patients who are protected; the antibodies bind to the bacterial capsules and promote phagocytosis by opsonization. The microorganism enters the CSF through loss of capillary integrity, or through some other mechanism, and multiples within the CSF, initially free of harmful antibodies or phagocytic cells. Organisms that can adhere to mucosal epithelium and evade destruction by possessing an antiphagocytic capsule are the best pathogens. In patients with impaired host defenses, other etiologic agents can gain a foothold and cause disease. Patients with prosthetic devices, particularly central nervous system shunts, are at increased risk of developing meningitis due to less "virulent" species, such as organisms that comprise the normal skin flora, aerobic and anaerobic diphtheroids, and *Staphylococcus epidermidis*. Staphylococci may possess specialized virulence factors that allow them to colonize artificial surfaces. The "slime" or noncapsular polysaccharide produced by some staphylococci seems to help these bacteria adhere to smooth plastic and glass surfaces.

Viruses may enter the central nervous system through the bloodstream, but they may also travel along the nerves that lead to the brain (for example, herpes simplex, adenovirus). Infections adjacent to the brain such as sinusitis and subdural abscess, may also lead to meningitis or may simulate it (parameningeal focus). Patients with meningitis or encephalitis may present with fever, stiff neck, headache, nausea and vomiting, neurologic abnormalities, and change in mental status.

Which etiologic agents are involved as the cause of any occurrence of bacterial meningitis is dependent on several factors, but age of the patient is most prominent. Ninety-five percent of all cases in the United States occur in children less than 5 years. In children in the United States between the ages of 1 month and 6 years, *Haemophilus influenzae* type b is the most common agent. From age 6, patients are more likely to develop meningococcal or pneumococcal meningitis. Ninety-five percent of all cases are due to *H. influenzae* type b, *Neisseria meningitidis*, and *Streptococcus pneumoniae*.

The age group with the highest prevalence of meningitis is that of the newborn, with a concomitant increased mortality rate (as high as 20%). Organisms causing disease in the newborn are different from those that affect other age groups; many of them are acquired by the newborn during passage through the mother's vaginal vault. Neonates are likely to be infected with, in order of incidence, group B streptococci, *Escherichia coli*, other gram-negative bacilli, *Listeria monocytogenes*, and other organisms. The prevalence of these organisms is probably due to the immature immune system of neonates, the organisms present in the colonized female vaginal tract, as well as to the increased permeability of the blood-brain barrier of newborns. *Flavobacterium meningosepticum* has been associated with nursery outbreaks of meningitis. The organism is presumably acquired nosocomially, since it is a normal inhabitant of water in the environment. Isolation of *Staphylococcus aureus* or other unusual organism from the CSF of a child should alert the clinician to look for congenital anatomic defects that might account for the entry of such an organism.

Lack of demonstrable humoral antibody against *H. influenzae* type b in children has been associated with increased incidence of meningitis. Most children develop measurable antibody by age 5. The importance of antibody is also a factor in adults, since military recruits without antibody to *N. meningitidis* are more likely to develop disease. *N. meningitidis* has been associated with epidemic meningitis among young adults in crowded conditions (for example, military recruits and college dormitory mates). Meningococcal meningitis is endemic in certain areas of central Africa and Nepal. The *Morbidity and Mortality Weekly Report*, published by the Centers for Disease Control, furnishes physicians with an annual guide to recommendations for precautions to be taken by travelers.

Factors that predispose adults to meningitis are often the same factors that increase the likelihood that the adult will develop pneumonia or other respiratory tract colonization or infection, since the respiratory tract is the primary portal of entry for many etiologic agents of meningitis. Alcoholism, splenectomy, diabetes mellitus, prosthetic devices, and immunosuppression contribute to increased risk. Important causes of meningitis in the adult, in addition to the meningococcus in young adults, include pneumococci, *L. monocytogenes*, and, less commonly, *S. aureus* and various gram-negative bacilli. The latter organisms lead to meningitis via hematogenous seeding from various sources, including urinary tract infections.

The sequelae of acute bacterial meningitis in children are frequent and serious. Seizures occur in 20% to 30% of patients seen at large urban hospitals, and other neurologic changes are common. Acute sequelae include cerebral edema, hydrocephalus, cerebral herniation, and focal neurologic changes. Permanent sensorineural deafness occurred in 10% of children who recovered from bacterial meningitis studied at one institution. It has also been reported that more subtle physiologic and psychologic sequelae follow an episode of acute bacterial meningitis. It can be appreciated that even though the mortality from such infections has dropped from 90% to 100% in the preantibiotic era to 3% to 30% today, the morbidity associated with meningitis today is still significant.[10]

Chronic meningitis often occurs in those patients who are immunocompromised in some way, although this is not always the case. The various etiologic agents of chronic meningitis are listed in the box on p. 216.

Etiologic Agents of Chronic Meningitis

Mycobacterium tuberculosis
Cryptococcus neoformans
Coccidioides immitis
Histoplasma capsulatum
Blastomyces dermatitidis
Candida species
Miscellaneous other fungi
Nocardia
Actinomyces
Treponema pallidum
Brucella
Salmonella
Rare parasites—*Toxoplasma gondii*, cysticercus, *Paragonimus westermani*, *Trichinella spiralis*

Patients experience an insidious onset of disease, with some or all of the following: fever, headache, stiff neck, nausea and vomiting, lethargy, confusion, and mental deterioration. Symptoms may persist for a month or longer before treatment is sought. The CSF usually manifests an abnormal number of cells (usually lymphocytic), elevated protein, and some decrease in glucose content. The pathogenesis of chronic meningitis is similar to that of acute disease.[11]

Brain abscesses may occasionally cause changes in the CSF and clinical symptoms that mimic meningitis. Brain abscesses may also rupture into the subarachnoid space, producing a severe meningitis with high mortality. If anaerobic organisms or viridans streptococci are recovered from CSF cultures, the diagnosis of brain abscess must be entertained; however, CSF culture is usually negative in brain abscess. Immunosuppressed patients and diabetics with ketoacidosis may show a rapidly progressive fungal infection (phycomycosis) of the nasal sinuses or palatal region that travels directly to the brain.

Viral encephalitis, which cannot always be distinguished from meningitis clinically, is common in the warmer months. The primary agents are enteroviruses (coxsackieviruses A and B, echoviruses), mumps virus, herpes simplex virus, and arboviruses (togavirus, bunyavirus, equine encephalitis, St. Louis encephalitis, and other encephalitis viruses). Other viruses, such as measles, cytomegalovirus, lymphocytic choriomeningitis, Epstein-Barr virus, hepatitis, varicella-zoster virus, rabies, and myxoviruses, and paramyxoviruses, are less commonly encountered. The preceding viral illness and exposure history are important considerations in establishing a cause by clinical means.

Parasites can cause meningoencephalitis, brain abscess, or other central nervous system infection via two routes. The free-living amebae, *Naegleria fowleri* and *Acanthamoeba* species, invade the brain via direct extension from the nasal mucosa. These organisms are acquired by swimming or diving in natural freshwater ponds and lakes, especially those with stagnation. Other parasites reach the brain via hematogenous spread. Immunosuppressed patients are likely to acquire toxoplasmosis, the agent of which grows intracellularly and destroys brain parenchyma. Toxoplasmosis is a common central nervous system affliction in patients with acquired immuno deficiency syndrome (AIDS; discussed further in Chapter 23). *Entamoeba histolytica* and *Strongyloides stercoralis* have been visualized in brain tissue, and the larval form of *Taenia solium* (the pork tapeworm), called a "cysticercus," can travel to the brain via the bloodstream and grow in that site. Amebic brain infection and cysticercosis cause changes in the CSF that mimic meningitis.[11]

15.3. Collection, Transport, and Initial Handling of Specimens

CSF is usually collected by aseptically inserting a needle into the subarachnoid space at the level of the lumbar spine. Three or four tubes of CSF should be collected and immediately labeled with the patient's name. Tube 3 or 4 is used for cell count and differential. If a small capillary blood vessel is inadvertently traversed during the spinal tap (lumbar puncture), blood cells picked up from this source will usually be absent from the last tube collected; comparison of counts between tubes 1 and 4 is usually of interest. The other tubes can be used for both microbiological and chemical studies. In this way, a larger proportion of the total fluid can be concentrated, facilitating detection of infectious agents present in low numbers, and the supernatant can still be used for other required studies. Microbiologists should periodically monitor the sterile tubes used in lumbar puncture kits prepared at their institutions by processing filter-sterilized negative

CSF as a quality control check. CSF collecting tubes have been known to harbor nonviable bacteria, which can cause false-positive Gram stain results.

The volume of CSF is critical for detection of certain microorganisms, such as *M. tuberculosis* and *C. neoformans*. At least 10 ml of CSF is recommended for analysis of CSF suspected of containing these pathogens by centrifugation and subsequent culture. When an inadequate volume of CSF is received, the physician should be consulted as to the order of priority of laboratory studies.[8]

CSF should be hand-delivered *immediately* to the laboratory. Specimens should never be refrigerated. If they are not being processed immediately, they should be incubated or left at room temperature. One exception to this rule involves CSF for viral studies. These specimens may be refrigerated for up to 24 hours after collection or frozen at $-70°$ C if a longer delay is anticipated until they are inoculated. CSF for viral studies should never be frozen at temperatures that are warmer than $-70°$ C. Certain agents, such as *S. pneumoniae*, may not be detectable after an hour or longer unless antigen detection methods are used. Prompt examination by microbiologists can often determine the etiologic agent within as short a time as 30 minutes, helping the clinician to direct or correct therapy. CSF is one of the few specimens handled by the laboratory for which information promptly relayed to the clinician can directly affect therapeutic outcome. Such specimens should be processed immediately upon receipt in the laboratory and all results should be telephoned to the physician as soon as they are available.

Initial processing of CSF for bacterial, fungal, or parasitic studies includes centrifugation of all specimens greater than 1 ml in volume for at least 15 minutes at $1500 \times g$.[8] Specimens in which cryptococci or mycobacteria are suspected must be handled differently. Discussions of techniques for culturing CSF for fungi are found in Chapter 43, and methods for isolating mycobacteria are detailed in Chapter 41. The supernatant is decanted into a sterile tube, leaving approximately 0.5 ml fluid in which to suspend the sediment by vortexing before it is inoculated to media or examined visually. This mixing of the sediment is critical. Laboratories that use a sterile capillary pipette to remove portions of the sediment from underneath the supernatant will miss a significant number of positive specimens. The sediment must be thoroughly mixed *after* the super-

natant has been removed. Either vortexing or forcefully aspirating the sediment up and down into a sterile pipette several times will adequately disperse the organisms that remained adherent to the bottom of the tube after centrifugation. The supernatant can be used to test for the presence of antigens or for chemistry evaluations (protein, glucose, lactate, for example). Even if there is no immediate use for the supernatant, it should be kept as a safeguard. Later, supernatants from culture-negative CSF can be pooled, filter-sterilized, and used as a diluent for other tests or for quality control.

Communication between physician and microbiology laboratory is essential, since the results of hematologic and chemical tests directly relate to the probability of infection. Among 555 cerebrospinal fluids from patients older than 4 months of age tested at UCLA, only two showed normal cell count and protein in the presence of bacterial meningitis.[6] Thus, the diagnosis of acute bacterial meningitis can be excluded in patients with normal fluid parameters in almost all cases, precluding further expensive and labor-intensive microbiological processing beyond a standard smear and culture (which must be included in all cases).

15.4. Visual Detection of Etiologic Agents of Meningitis

15.4.a. Direct wet preparation. Amebas are best observed by examining thoroughly mixed sediment as a wet preparation under phase-contrast microscopy (Chapter 7). If a phase-contrast microscope is not available, observing under light microscopy with the condenser closed slightly is an alternative technique. Amebas are recognized by typical slow, methodical movement in one direction by advancing pseudopodia. The organisms may require a little time under the warm light of the microscope before they begin to move. They must be distinguished from motile macrophages, which occasionally occur in CSF. Following up a suspicious wet preparation, a trichrome stain (Chapter 44) can help differentiate amebas from somatic cells (Figure 15.1) The pathogenic amebas can be cultured on a lawn of *Klebsiella pneumoniae*, as outlined in Chapter 44.

15.4.a. (1). India ink stain. C. neoformans, because of the large polysaccharide capsule, can often be visualized by the India ink stain, although latex agglutination testing for capsular antigen is more sensitive and extremely specific. The strains of *C.*

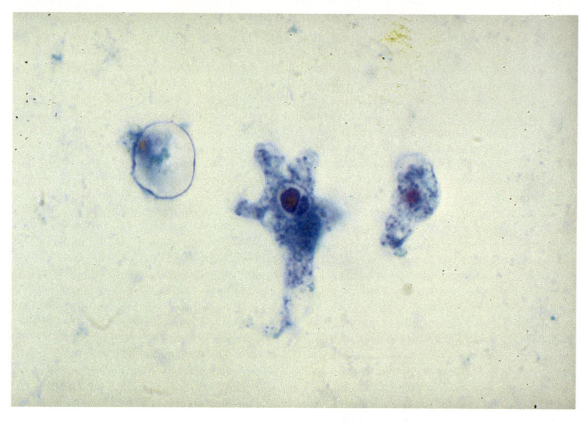

Figure 15.1
Trichrome-stained preparation of *N. fowleri* isolated from cerebrospinal fluid and grown on a lawn of Enterobacteriaceae.

neoformans that infect patients with AIDS may not possess detectable capsules, so culture is also essential. To perform the India ink preparation, a drop of CSF sediment is mixed with one third volume of India ink (Pelikan Drawing Ink, Block, Gunther, and Wagner; available at art supply stores). The India ink can be protected against contamination by adding 0.05 ml thimerosal (Merthiolate, Sigma Chemical Co.) to the bottle when it is first opened. After mixing the CSF and ink to make a smooth suspension, a coverslip is applied to the drop and the preparation is examined under high-power magnification (400×) for characteristic encapsulated yeast cells, which can be confirmed by examination under oil immersion (1000×) (Figure 15.2). The inexperienced microscopist must be careful not to confuse white blood cells with yeast. The presence of encapsulated buds, smaller than the mother cell, is diagnostic. All requests for India ink preparations should automati-

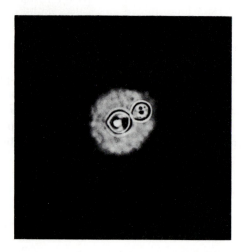

Figure 15.2
Encapsulated budding cells of *C. neoformans* seen in an India ink preparation made from infected cerebrospinal fluid (1000×).

cally include performance of a cryptococcal latex agglutination test, as outlined below.

15.4.a. (2) Quellung reaction. A test rarely performed today is the Quellung reaction, in which spinal fluid sediment is mixed with antisera against the suspected organism (*H. influenzae* type b, *N. meningitidis*, or *S. pneumoniae*) and a drop of saturated aqueous methylene blue dye. If the organism is present, the antibody combining with the capsular polysaccharide will cause apparent capsular swelling, which can be visualized under the microscope.

15.4.b. Stained smear of sediment. The Gram stain must be performed on all CSF sediments. After thoroughly mixing the sediment, a heaped drop is placed on the surface of a sterile or alcohol-wiped slide. Applying a second heaped drop in the same area after the first drop has dried will increase the concentration of material that can be thoroughly examined. The sediment should never be spread out on the slide surface, as this increases the difficulty of finding small numbers of microorganisms. False-positive smears have resulted from inadvertent use of contaminated slides. The use of a steel autoclavable slide holder is recommended (Figure 15.3). The drop of sediment is allowed to air dry, is heat- or methanol-fixed, and is stained by either Gram or acridine orange stain (Chapter 7). The acridine orange fluorochrome stain may allow faster examination of the slide under high-power magnification (400×), and thus a more thorough examination. The brightly fluorescing bacteria will be easily visible. All suspicious smears can be restained by the Gram stain (directly over the acridine orange stain) to confirm morphology of any organisms seen. Based on demographic and clinical patient data and Gram stain morphology, the etiology of the majority of cases of bacterial meningitis can be presumptively determined within the first 30 minutes after receiving the specimen. Acid fast smears are handled differently, as discussed in Chapter 41. Several workers have reported enhanced sensitivity of the Gram stain by spinning the CSF onto the slide in a cytocentrifuge (Cytospin, Shandon-Southern), a device that concentrates material directly on the slide surface and allows excess liquid to be absorbed.

15.5. Syphilis Serology

Diagnosis of neurosyphilis is based on several parameters, including the number and types of white and red cells present in the patient's CSF, patient

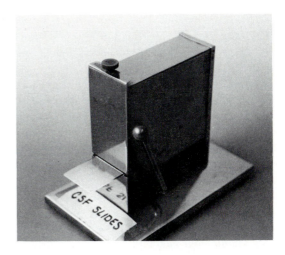

Figure 15.3
Stainless steel autoclavable glass microscope slide holder, suitable for autoclaving cleaned slides.

history and epidemiologic factors, levels of protein and glucose, and the VDRL test. The VDRL test is the only useful test for detecting antibodies directed against *T. pallidum* in CSF, although new technological developments promise better methods in the future. A positive CSF VDRL is still not diagnostic in itself, as patients with successfully treated neurosyphilis may retain a positive CSF VDRL even years later.

15.6. Detection of Antigen in CSF

Reagents and complete systems for the rapid detection of antigen in CSF have been available for several years. Countercurrent immunoelectrophoresis (CIE), although the first widely accepted method for rapid antigen detection from CSF, has been largely replaced by the more sensitive and simpler techniques of latex agglutination and coagglutination, although CIE may be used in some laboratories for detection of antigen to *L. monocytogenes*, for which no latex tests are available. All of the commercial systems utilize the principle of an antibody-coated particle that will bind to specific antigen, resulting in macroscopically visible agglutination. The soluble capsular polysaccharide produced by the most common etiologic agents of meningitis and the group B streptococcal polysaccharide are well suited to serve as bridging antigens. The systems differ in that certain antibodies are polyclonal and others are monoclonal, and not all systems detect all antigens.

With the exception of latex tests for cryptococcal antigen, the use of these reagents is somewhat controversial, and they should be used as an adjunct to standard procedures.[3]

Reagents for the detection of the polysaccharide capsular antigen of *C. neoformans* are available from M.A. Bioproducts and Meridian Diagnostics. CSF specimens that yield positive results for cryptococcal antigen should be tested with a second latex agglutination test for rheumatoid factor. A positive rheumatoid factor test renders the cryptococcal latex test uninterpretable, and the results should be reported as such, unless the rheumatoid factor antibodies can be diluted out. The commercial test systems incorporate rheumatoid factor testing in their protocol. Undiluted specimens that contain large amounts of capsular antigen may yield a false-negative reaction due to a prozone phenomenon.

In general, the commercial systems have been developed for use with CSF, urine, or serum, although results with serum have not been as useful diagnostically as those with CSF. Soluble antigens from *S. agalactiae* and *H. influenzae* may concentrate in the urine. Urine, however, does seem to produce a higher incidence of nonspecific reactions than either serum or CSF. The manufacturers' directions must be followed for performance of antigen detection test systems for different specimen types. Although some of the systems require pretreatment of samples, usually heating for 5 minutes, not all manufacturers recommend such a step. The reagents, however, may yield false-positive or cross-reactions unless specimen pretreatment is performed. Interference by rheumatoid factor and other substances, more often present in body fluids other than CSF, has also been reported. The method of Smith and coworkers[9] has been shown to effectively reduce a substantial portion of nonspecific and false-positive reactions, at least for tests performed with latex particle reagents. This pretreatment, called rapid extraction of antigen procedure (REAP; Procedure 15.1), is recommended for those laboratories that use commercial body fluid antigen detection kits. Certain commercial systems have such an extraction procedure included in their protocols.

Using a direct antigen detection system, confirmation of identification of organisms seen on Gram stain as well as the detection of an etiologic agent in smear-negative specimens or those from previously treated patients can be accomplished. The systems

PROCEDURE 15.1

Rapid Extraction of Antigen Procedure (REAP)

Principle

Removal of nonspecific cross-reactive material can improve the specificity of direct antigen detection particle agglutination tests. Ethylene-diaminetetraacetic (EDTA) complexes cross-reactive materials and they are removed from the reaction mixture by centrifugation.

Method

1. Pipette 0.05 ml fluid to be tested (CSF, serum, or urine) into a 1.5 ml plastic conical microcentrifuge tube.
2. Add 0.15 ml of 0.1 M EDTA (Sigma Chemical) to the microcentrifuge tube, close the cap tightly, and vortex the tube.
3. Heat in a dry bath (available from instrument supply companies) for 3 minutes at 100° C.
4. Centrifuge the tubes for 5 minutes at 13,000 × g in a tabletop microcentrifuge. Be certain that the instrument used achieves the required centrifugal force.
5. Remove the supernatant with a capillary pipette and use one drop of this solution as the test sample in the antigen detection test, following the manufacturer's instructions for performance of the test.

Quality control

Test the reagents using filter-sterilized known negative CSF.

Expected results

Agglutination should not occur.

Performance schedule

Test reagents once when each new batch is prepared and after every positive test result.

Modified from Smith, L.P., Hunter, K.W., Jr., Hemming, V.G., et al. 1984. J. Clin. Microbiol. 20:981.

are not substitutes for properly performed smears and cultures because they provide less than 100% sensitivity and specificity, but they provide an additional diagnostic test to aid clinicians in initial management of serious meningitis.[1,4] The standard procedures and empiric therapeutic decisions of clinicians served by a laboratory will determine whether these types of tests are cost-effective.[2,7]

15.7. Culture for Etiologic Agents of CSF Infection

After vortexing the sediment and preparing smears, several drops of the sediment should be inoculated to each medium. Routine bacteriologic media should include a chocolate agar plate, 5% sheep blood agar plate, and an enrichment broth, usually thioglycolate without indicator. The plates should be incubated at 37° C in 5% to 10% CO_2 for at least 72 hours. If a CO_2 incubator is not available, a candle jar (Chapter 8) can be used. The broth should be incubated in air at 37° C for at least 5 days. The broth cap must be loose to allow free exchange of air. If organisms morphologically resembling anaerobic bacteria are seen on the Gram stain and in suspected brain abscess, an anaerobic blood agar plate may be inoculated additionally. If the Gram stain revealed large, regular gram-negative rods, a MacConkey plate should be added to the initial media. These media will support the growth of almost all bacterial pathogens and several fungi. The authors of Cumitech 14[8] recommend that penicillinase (Difco Laboratories or BBL Microbiology Systems) be added to culture media if patients have received prior antibiotic therapy.

Cultures for detection of fungi or mycobacteria are handled in a biological safety cabinet. The symptoms of chronic meningitis that prompt a physician to request fungal cultures are the same as those for tuberculous meningitis, which should always be sought by the laboratory if chronic or fungal meningitis is suspected. Two drops of the well-mixed sediment should be inoculated to a non blood containing medium (brain-heart infusion with gentamicin and chloramphenicol) plate or slant and a brain-heart infusion or inhibitory mold agar slant or plate. Addition of a third medium such as Mycosel or Mycobiotic (selective agar, Chapter 8) is recommended. The material can be deposited on the agar surface without spreading for isolation. Fungal media should be incubated in air at 30° C for 4 weeks. If possible, it is best to inoculate two sets of media

and incubate one set at 30° C and one set at 35° C. As discussed in Chapter 41, centrifugation may not effectively sediment mycobacteria; other methods are suggested.

The free-living amebas can be cocultivated on artificial media if they are supplied with a living nutrient, such as *K. pneumoniae*. This procedure should be tried if amebic meningoencephalitis is suspected (Chapter 44).

CSF may be inoculated directly to tissue culture for detecton of viral agents. Diagnosis of viral encephalitides is often accomplished by isolation of the virus from a throat culture, feces, or blood, so these specimens should be submitted in addition to CSF for identification of an etiologic agent. Methods for cultivation of viruses from such specimens are discussed in detail in Chapter 42. Briefly, 0.25 ml of CSF per tube is inoculated into tubes of primary monkey kidney, Hep-2 continuous cell line, and human fetal diploid foreskin fibroblast cell cultures. These culture systems are incubated at 35° C in air for varying amounts of time, depending on the cell culture system.

15.8. Other Diagnostic Techniques

Certain agents of encephalitis or meningitis can be detected only by histopathologic examination of brain biopsy material. Direct smears (touch preparations) can be stained with fluorescein or enzyme conjugated antibodies for rapid detection of herpesviruses, varicella-zoster, rabies, and *T. gondii*. Conventionally stained smears can be used to visualize *T. gondii* and other parasites, as well as the characteristic inclusions of cytomegalovirus and herpes virus. These diagnostic procedures are usually performed by pathologists rather than microbiologists.

Other new approaches are being explored for diagnosis of meningitis. ELISA procedures are being manufactured for detection of *H. influenzae*, *S. pneumoniae*, and *N. meningitidis* antigens. An ELISA system has been shown to reliably detect antigens of *M. tuberculosis* in CSF. Because of the slow growth of this organism and the lack of any rapid procedures for its detection, such tests are highly desirable. No commercial systems are currently available. Gas-liquid chromatography, with electron-capture and other detectors, and mass spectrometry have been evaluated for rapid detection of etiologic agents of disease in CSF. Although reports are promising, these methods are not yet available for routine testing.

REFERENCES

1. College of American Pathologists. 1987. Rapid microbial detection of 1987 survey, Set 1D-B. Final critique. The College, Chicago.
2. Dagbjartsson, A., and Ludvigsson, P. 1987. Bacterial meningitis: diagnosis and initial antibiotic therapy. Pediatr. Clin. North Am. 34:219.
3. Gerber, M.A. 1985. Critical appraisal of the clinical relevance of rapid diagnosis in pediatrics. Diagn. Microbiol. Infect. Dis. 4:39S.
4. Granoff, D.M., Murphy, T.V., Ingram, D.L., et al. 1986. Use of rapidly generated results in patient management. Diagn. Microbiol. Infect. Dis. 4:157S.
5. Greenlea, J.E. 1985. Anatomic considerations in central nervous system infections. In Mandell, G.L., Douglas, R.G., Jr., and Bennett, J.E., editors. Principles and practice of infectious diseases, ed. 2. John Wiley & Sons, New York.
6. Hayward, R.A., Shapiro, M.F., and Oye, R.K. 1987. Laboratory testing on cerebrospinal fluid, a reappraisal. Lancet 1:1.
7. McCracken, G.H., Nelson, J.D., Kaplan, S.L., et al. 1987. Consensus report: Antimicrobial therapy for bacterial meningitis in infants and children. Pediatr. Infect. Dis. 6:501.
8. Ray, C.G., Wasilauskas, B.L. and Zabransky, R.J. 1982. Laboratory diagnosis of central nervous system infections. In McCarthy, L.R., editor. Cumitech 14, American Society for Microbiology, Washington, D.C..
9. Smith, L.P., Hunter, K.W., Jr., Hemming, V.G., et al. 1984. Improved detection of bacterial antigens by latex agglutination after rapid extraction from body fluids. J. Clin. Microbiol. 20:981.
10. Swartz, M.N. 1984. Bacterial meningitis: more involved than just the meninges. N. Engl. J. Med. 311:912.
11. Wilhelm, C., and Ellner, J.J. 1986. Chronic meningitis. Neurol Clin 4:115.

BIBLIOGRAPHY

Conly, J.M., and Ronald, A.R. 1983. Cerebrospinal fluid as a diagnostic body fluid. Am. J. Med. 75:102.

McGee, Z., and Kaiser, A.B. 1985. Acute meningitis. In Mandell, G.L., Douglas, R.G., Jr., and Bennett, J.E., editors. Principles and practice of infectious diseases, ed. 2. John Wiley & Sons, New York.

Neu, H.C. 1985. CNS infection: first things first. Hosp. Pract. 20:69. In Swartz, M.N. 1984. Bacterial meningitis: more involved than just the meninges. N. Engl. J. Med. 311:912.

16

Microorganisms Encountered in the Respiratory Tract

16.1. General Considerations, Anatomy, and Normal State of Respiratory Tract

The respiratory tract begins with the nasal or oral passages and extends past the nasopharynx and oropharynx to the trachea and then into the lungs. The trachea divides into bronchi, which subdivide into bronchioles, the smallest branches of which terminate in the alveoli. Several mechanisms nonspecifically protect the respiratory tract from infection: the nasal hairs and convoluted passages and mucus lining of the nasal turbinates; secretory IgA and nonspecific antibacterial substances (lysozyme) in respiratory secretions; the cilia and mucus lining of the trachea; and reflexes such as coughing, sneezing, and swallowing. These mechanisms prevent foreign objects or organisms from entering the bronchi and gaining access to the lungs, which should be sterile in the healthy host. Once particles that have escaped the airflow turbulence and the mucociliary sweeping activity enter the alveoli, alveolar macrophages ingest them and carry them to the lymphatics. In addition, normal flora of the nasopharynx and oropharynx help to prevent colonization of the upper respiratory tract by pathogenic microorganisms.

16.2. Flora of Respiratory Tract

Those bacteria that can be isolated as part of the normal flora of healthy hosts are listed in the box on p. 224, as well as many species that may cause disease under certain circumstances but that are often isolated from the respiratory tracts of healthy persons. Under certain circumstances, for unknown reasons—perhaps because of previous damage by a viral infection, loss of some host immunity, or because

---

Organisms Commonly Present in Nasopharynx and Oropharynx of Healthy Humans

Rarely pathogens

Nonhemolytic streptococci
Staphylococci
Micrococci
Corynebacterium species
Coagulase-negative staphylococci
Neisseria species, other than *N. gonorrhoeae* and *N. meningitidis*
Lactobacillus species
Veillonella species
Spirochetes

Possible pathogens

Acinetobacter
Viridans streptococci
β-Hemolytic streptococci
Streptococcus pneumoniae
Staphylococcus aureus
Corynebacterium diphtheriae
Neisseria meningitidis
Cryptococcus neoformans
Mycoplasma species
Haemophilus influenzae
Haemophilus parainfluenzae
Branhamella catarrhalis
Candida albicans
Herpes simplex virus
Enterobacteriaceae
Mycobacterium species
Pseudomonas species
Filamentous fungi
Klebsiella ozaenae
Eikenella corrodens
Bacteroides species
Peptostreptococcus species
Actinomyces species

Respiratory Tract Pathogens

Definite respiratory tract pathogens

Corynebacterium diphtheriae (toxin-producing)
Neisseria gonorrhoeae
Mycobacterium tuberculosis
Mycoplasma pneumoniae
Chlamydia trachomatis
Chlamydia (TWAR) pneumoniae
Bordetella pertussis
Legionella species
Pneumocystis carinii
Nocardia species
Histoplasma capsulatum
Coccidioides immitis
Cryptococcus neoformans (may also be recovered from patients without disease)
Blastomyces dermatitidis
Viruses (respiratory syncytial virus, adenoviruses, enteroviruses, herpesviruses, influenza and parainfluenza viruses, rhinoviruses)

Rare respiratory tract pathogens

Francisella tularensis
Bacillus anthracis
Yersinia pestis
Pseudomonas pseudomallei
Coxiella burnetti
Chlamydia psittaci
Brucella species
Salmonella species
Pasteurella multocida
Klebsiella rhinoscleromatis
Parasites

---

of physical damage to the respiratory epithelium (from smoking, for example)—these colonizing organisms go on to cause disease. Organisms isolated from normally sterile sites in the respiratory tract by methods that avoid contamination with normal flora should be definitively identified and reported to the clinician.

Certain microorganisms are considered to be etiologic agents of disease if they are present in any numbers in the respiratory tract because they possess virulence factors that are expressed in every host. These are listed in the box above. Many selective media have been designed to isolate these organisms, even in the presence of normal flora. This chapter discusses such methods, as well as strategies to follow for handling of specimens received from the respiratory tract.

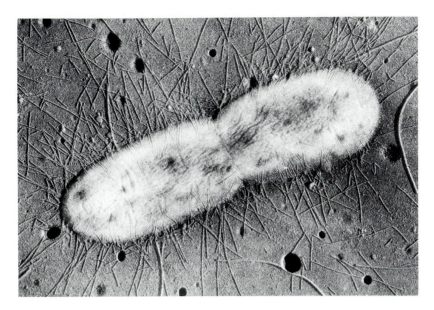

Figure 16.1
Fimbriae of *Escherichia coli*, extending as thin projections from the cell periphery. (Courtesy A. Ryter, Institut Pasteur. From Boyd, R.F. 1984. General microbiology. The C.V. Mosby Co., St. Louis.)

16.3. Pathogenic Mechanisms Used by Agents of Respiratory Tract Infections

Microorganisms primarily cause disease by only a few pathogenic mechanisms. As these mechanisms relate to respiratory tract infections, they will be discussed briefly. For any organism to cause disease, it must first be able to gain a foothold within the respiratory tract in order to grow to sufficient numbers to produce symptoms. Therefore most etiologic agents of respiratory tract disease must first adhere to the mucosa of the respiratory tract. The presence of normal flora and the overall state of the host affect the ability of microorganisms to adhere. Surviving or growing on host tissue without causing overt harmful effects is called "colonization." Except for those microorganisms that are breathed directly into the lungs, all etiologic agents of disease must first colonize the respiratory tract to some degree before they can cause harm.

Bacteria that possess specific adherence factors include *Streptococcus pyogenes*, whose cell wall contains lipoteichoic acids and certain proteins (M protein and others), visible as a thin layer of fuzz surrounding the bacteria. Other bacteria that possess lipoteichoic acid adherence complexes are *Staphylococcus aureus* and certain viridans streptococci. Many gram-negative bacteria, particularly Enterobacteriaceae, *Legionella* species, *Pseudomonas* spe-

cies, *Bordetella pertussis*, and *Haemophilus* species (and *Actinomyces* species, which are gram positive), adhere by means of proteinaceous fingerlike surface structures called **fimbriae** (Figure 16.1). Fimbriae are often also called **pili,** although this is technically the term for a similar structure that participates in sexual interaction rather than just adherence. Viruses possess either a hemagglutinin (influenza viruses) or other protein that mediates their attachment to host epithelium.

The production of extracellular toxin was one of the first pathogenic mechanisms discovered among bacteria. It has been appreciated more recently that certain fungi may also produce toxins that may play a role in human disease, but there have been no proven toxins among those fungi that cause respiratory disease. *Corynebacterium diphtheriae* is a classic example of a bacterium that produces disease through the action of an extracellular toxin. Once the organism colonizes the upper respiratory epithelium, it elaborates a toxin that is disseminated systemically, adhering preferentially to central nervous system cells and muscle cells of the heart. Systemic disease characterized by myocarditis and local disease leading to respiratory distress can follow, as can peripheral neuritis. Growth of *C. diphtheriae* causes necrosis of the epithelial mucosa, producing a "diphtheritic (pseudo) membrane," which may extend from the anterior nasal mucosa to the bronchi or be limited to any area between, most often to the tonsillar and peritonsillar areas. The membrane may cause sore throat and interfere with respiration and swallowing. Although nontoxic strains of *C. diphtheriae* can cause disease, it is much milder than the version mediated by toxin. The toxin gene is carried into the bacteria by phage (Chapter 33).

Some strains of *Pseudomonas aeruginosa* produce a toxin very similar to diphtheria toxin. Whether this toxin actually contributes to the pathogenesis of respiratory tract infection with *P. aeruginosa* has not been verified. *B. pertussis*, the agent of whooping cough, also produces toxins. The role of these toxins in production of disease is not clear. They may act to inhibit the activity of phagocytic cells or to damage cells of the respiratory tract. *S. aureus* and β-hemolytic streptococci produce extracellular enzymes that act to damage host cells or tissues. Extracellular products of staphylococci aid in production of tissue necrosis and destruction of phagocytic cells, contributing to the commonly seen phenomenon of abscess formation associated with infection caused by this organism. Although *S. aureus* can be recovered from throat specimens, it has not been proven to cause pharyngitis. Enzymes of streptococci, including hyaluronidase, allow rapid dissemination of the bacteria. Many other etiologic agents of respiratory tract infection also produce extracellular enzymes and toxins.

In addition to adherence and toxin production, pathogens cause disease by merely growing in host tissue, interfering with normal tissue function and attracting host immune effectors, such as neutrophils and macrophages. Once these cells begin to try to destroy the invading pathogens and repair the damaged host tissue, an expanding reaction ensues with more nonspecific and immunological factors being attracted to the area, increasing the amount of host tissue damage. Respiratory viral infections usually progress in this manner, as do many types of pneumonias, such as those caused by *Streptococcus pneumoniae*, *S. pyogenes*, *Staphylococcus aureus*, *H. influenzae*, *Neisseria meningitidis*, *Branhamella catarrhalis*, *Mycoplasma pneumoniae*, and most gram-negative bacilli. Aspiration of minor amounts of oropharyngeal material, as occurs often during sleep, plays an important role in the pathogenesis of many types of pneumonia.

The ability to evade host defense mechanisms is another virulence mechanism that certain respiratory tract pathogens possess. *S. pneumoniae*, *N. meningitidis*, *H. influenzae*, *Klebsiella pneumoniae*, mucoid *P. aeruginosa*, *Cryptococcus neoformans*, and others possess polysaccharide capsules that serve both to prevent engulfment by phagocytic host cells and to protect somatic antigens from being exposed to host immunoglobulins. The capsular material is produced in such abundance by certain bacteria, such as pneumococci, that soluble polysaccharide antigen particles can bind host antibodies, blocking them from serving as opsonins. Proof that the capsular polysaccharide is the principal virulence mechanism of *H. influenzae*, *S. pneumoniae*, and *Neisseria meningitidis* was established when vaccines consisting of capsular antigens alone were shown to protect individuals from disease.

Some respiratory pathogens evade the host immune system by multiplying within host cells. *Chlamydia trachomatis*, *Chlamydia psittaci*, and all viruses replicate within host cells. They have evolved methods for being taken in by the "nonprofessional" phagocytic cells of the host to achieve their required environment, which is protected from host humoral immune factors and other phagocytic cells until the host cell becomes sufficiently damaged that it is recognized as foreign and attacked. A second category of agents of respiratory tract disease is actively taken up by phagocytic host cells, usually macrophages, within which they are able to multiply. *Legionella*, *Listeria*, some *Salmonella* species, *Pneumocystis carinii*, and *Histoplasma capsulatum* are some of the more common intracellular parasites.

Mycobacterium tuberculosis is the classic representative of an intracellular pathogen. In primary tuberculosis the organism is carried to an alveolus in a **droplet nucleus**, a tiny aerosol particle containing a few tubercle bacilli (the minimum infective dose is quite small). There it is phagocytized by alveolar macrophages, which carry it to the nearest lymph node, usually in the hilar or other mediastinal chains. In the node the organisms slowly multiply within macrophages, destroying them and being taken up by other phagocytic cells in turn. Within the protected environment of the macrophages, which are somehow prevented by the bacteria from accomplishing lysosomal fusion, tubercle bacilli multiply to a critical mass, which spills out of the destroyed macrophages through the lymphatics into the bloodstream, producing bacteremia and carrying tubercle bacilli to many parts of the body. In most cases, the host immune system reacts sufficiently at this point to kill most of the bacilli; a small reservoir of live bacteria may be left, usually in the apical portion of the lung. These bacilli are walled off, and a subsequent insult to the host, either immunological or physical, may cause breakdown of the focus of latent tubercle bacilli, allowing active multiplication and disease (secondary tuberculosis). In certain patients with primary immune defects of some type, the initial bacteremia seeds bacteria throughout a host that is unable to control them, leading to disseminated or **miliary** tuberculosis. Growth of the bacteria within host macrophages and histiocytes in the lung causes an influx of more effector cells, including lymphocytes, neutrophils, and histiocytes, eventually resulting in granuloma formation, then tissue destruction and cavity formation. The lesion is characteristically a semisolid, amorphous tissue mass resembling semisoft cheese, from which it receives the name **caseation necrosis.** The infected tissue or organisms from it can extend into bronchioles and bronchi, from which bacteria are disseminated via respiratory secretions, coughing, or other forms of transmission, to the next victim and also to other portions of the patient's own lungs.

16.4. Upper Respiratory Tract Infections

Microorganisms that cause disease in the upper respiratory tract, the nasopharynx, and the pharynx must come into contact with the mucosal epithelium, adhere, and multiply. They are carried in by aerosols in the case of *N. meningitidis, B. pertussis, C. diphtheriae,* and many viruses. They may be passed in secretions, either by intimate contact or through crowded conditions or poor hygiene. *Mycoplasma* species and *S. pyogenes* are often passed in this way. Although a large number of species of bacteria and fungi may be isolated from specimens taken from the upper respiratory tract, very few organisms have been shown to cause true disease in that area.

16.4.a. Etiologic agents of nasopharyngeal and oropharyngeal infections. The most commonly sought bacterial pathogen is *S. pyogenes,* or group A β-hemolytic streptococcus, the agent that leads to poststreptococcal sequelae such as acute rheumatic fever and glomerulonephritis. The organism not uncommonly causes suppurative (pyogenic) infections (**suppurations**) of the tonsils, sinuses, and middle ear and cellulitis as secondary pyogenic sequelae after an episode of pharyngitis. Accordingly, streptococcal pharyngitis is usually treated to prevent both the suppurative and nonsuppurative sequelae, as well as

to decrease morbidity. Cases of pharyngitis caused by groups B, C, and G and by nonhemolytic members of these groups of streptococci (including group A) have been reported. Although bacteria other than group A streptococci may cause pharyngitis, this occurs only rarely, and laboratories should not look routinely for other agents except in special circumstances and after discussion with the clinician involved.

Although much less common than streptococcal pharyngitis, *C. diphtheriae* can still be isolated from patients with sore throat, as well as more serious systemic disease. Other *Corynebacterium* species (*C. ulcerans, C. hemolyticum,* and *C. pyogenes*) can cause pharyngitis with or without membrane formation or associated rash, but such infections are rare. *N. meningitidis* can be recovered from the nasopharynx of carriers, although it does not cause significant disease at this site. *Neisseria gonorrhoeae,* however, can cause an exudative pharyngitis that is especially prevalent among men who engage in oral-genital practices. In disseminated gonococcal disease, the organism may be isolated from throat cultures as well. Gonococcal pharyngitis is not always symptomatic. Although *H. influenzae, S. aureus,* and *S. pneumoniae* are frequently isolated from nasopharyngeal and throat cultures, they have not been shown to cause pharyngitis. Carriage of any of these organisms, as well as *N. meningitidis,* may have clinical importance for some patients or their contacts. Especially in patients with cystic fibrosis, throat cultures may yield etiologic agents of pneumonia that cannot be isolated from sputum because of overgrowth by other bacteria. As in all other situations, communication between microbiologists and physicians clarifies the relevance of such findings. Cultures of specimens obtained from the anterior nares often yield *S. aureus* organisms. The carriage rate for this organism is especially high among health care workers.

M. pneumoniae may, rarely, cause pharyngitis and can be isolated from nasopharyngeal swabs. Such a swab may also be the most easily collected specimen for isolation of *C. trachomatis* from suspected cases of pneumonia, especially in very young babies. A number of viruses cause exudative pharyngitis or rhinitis, including rhinoviruses, adenoviruses, respiratory syncytial virus, influenza and parainfluenza viruses, coronaviruses, coxsackieviruses, cytomegalovirus, and Epstein-Barr virus. Nasopharyngeal washings or tracheal secretions are the specimens of choice. Additionally, *H. influenzae* (and occasionally other organisms) causes a serious epiglottitis that can rapidly lead to airway obstruction if not treated. The combined efforts of certain anaerobic oral flora causes an exudative pharyngitis known as **Vincent's angina** that may be characterized by a membrane-type lesion similar to that of diphtheria (the foul odor noted in patients with Vincent's angina helps to differentiate the two syndromes). Peritonsillar abscess is a common feature of this syndrome. Evidence suggests that *Fusobacterium necrophorum* is a key pathogen in this setting, but other anaerobes may also be involved.

Immunosuppressed patients, including very young babies, may develop oral candidiasis, called **thrush.** Oral thrush can extend to produce esophagitis, a common finding in AIDS and other immunosuppressed patients. Oral mucositis or pharyngitis in the granulocytopenic patient may be caused by Enterobacteriaceae, *S. aureus,* or *Candida* species. It is manifested by erythema, sore throat, and possibly exudate or ulceration. Herpes simplex virus can cause painful lesions in the mouth and the oropharynx, another condition that is also prevalent among immunosuppressed patients.

A rare form of chronic, granulomatous infection of the nasal passages, including the sinuses and occasionally the pharynx and larynx, is rhinoscleroma. Associated with *Klebsiella rhinoscleromatis,* the disease is characterized by nasal obstruction appearing over a long period of time, caused by tumorlike growth with local spread. Another species, *Klebsiella ozaenae,* can also be recovered from upper respiratory tract infections. This organism may contribute to the condition called "ozaena," characterized by a chronic, mucopurulent nasal discharge (often foul-smelling, due to secondary low-grade anaerobic infection).

16.4.b. Collection and transport of specimens. Although the general concepts of collection and transport of specimens were covered in Chapter 6, a few specific comments are appropriate here. Either cotton-, Dacron-, or calcium alginate–tipped swabs are suitable for collection of most upper respiratory tract microorganisms. Calcium alginate may be toxic, however, to some *Chlamydia* species. If the swab remains moist, no further precautions need to be taken for specimens that are inoculated within 4 hours of collection. After that period, some kind of transport medium to maintain viability and prevent

overgrowth by contaminants should be used. Swabs for detection of group A streptococci only are the exception. This organism is highly resistant to desiccation and will remain viable on a dry swab for as long as 48 hours. Throat swabs of this type can be placed in glassine paper envelopes for mailing or transport to a distant laboratory. Throat swabs are adequate for recovery of adenoviruses and herpesviruses, *C. diphtheriae, Mycoplasma, Chlamydia,* yeast, and *Haemophilus* species.

Nasopharyngeal swabs are better suited for recovery of respiratory syncytial virus, parainfluenza virus, *B. pertussis, Neisseria* species, and the viruses causing rhinitis. Although modified Stuart's transport medium, as is often used in commercially produced swab systems, will preserve most viruses for a short time, nasopharyngeal swabs should ideally be transported in veal infusion broth or other protein-containing fluid if they are not being cultured within a few hours. They should be refrigerated, *not frozen.* Recovery of *C. diphtheriae* is enhanced by culturing both throat and nasopharynx. Transport media should be used as discussed in Chapter 6. Aspirated nasopharyngeal secretions collected in a soft rubber bulb are the best specimens for *B. pertussis.* Specimens for *B. pertussis* ideally should be inoculated directly to fresh culture media at the patient's bedside. If this is impossible, transport for less than 2 hours in 1% casamino acid media is acceptable.

16.4.c. Direct visual examination of upper respiratory tract specimens. A Gram stain of material obtained from upper respiratory secretions or lesions can do very little to help with diagnosis. Yeastlike cells can be identified, helpful in identifying thrush, and the characteristic pattern of fusiforms and spirochetes of Vincent's angina may be visualized. Plain Gram's crystal violet (allowed to remain on the slide for 1 minute before rinsing with tap water) can be used to identify the agents of Vincent's angina as well as the Gram stain. For other causes of pharyngitis, Gram stains are unreliable. Direct smears of exudate from membranelike lesions to differentiate diphtheria from other causes of such membranes are not reliable and are not recommended. Fungal elements, including yeast cells and pseudohyphae, may be visualized with a 10% potassium hydroxide (KOH) preparation or with calcofluor white fluorescent stain. Direct examination of material obtained from the nasopharynx of suspected cases of whooping cough using a fluorescent antibody stain (Chapter 29) has been shown to yield some early positive results.[1]

Direct fluorescent antibody smears have been used to identify group A β-hemolytic streptococci in throat specimens. This technology has largely been supplanted by direct detection of antigen, for which a large number of commercial products are available. Direct antigen detection systems will be discussed in Section 16.4.e. Fluorescent antibody stain reagents are also commercially available for detection of herpes simplex antigen, influenza virus (rarely used), adenovirus, parainfluenza virus, and respiratory syncytial virus (RSV). Particularly for RSV, direct fluorescent antibody stain methods have been shown to be superior to culture.

16.4.d. Culturing upper respiratory tract specimens. Classically, throat swabs have been plated onto 5% sheep blood agar (trypticase soy base). Other animal blood cells will serve to provide the necessary nutrients required by the usual pathogens being sought (primarily *S. pyogenes*), but sheep blood does not support growth of the β-hemolytic bacteria *Haemophilus haemolyticus* and *Haemophilus parahaemolyticus*. Thus these organisms will not be mistaken for possible β-hemolytic streptococci if sheep blood agar is used. The use of a sheep blood agar plate for isolation of *S. pyogenes* has the drawback of requiring overnight growth for colony formation and further manipulations of β-hemolytic growth for definitive identification. If sufficient numbers of pure colonies are not available for antigenic typing, a subculture requiring additional growing time is necessary. New selective agars (such as Strep Selective Agar, mentioned in Chapter 8) have been developed that suppress the growth of almost all normal flora and β-hemolytic streptococci except for groups A and B. By placing a 0.04 unit differential bacitracin filter paper disk (Taxo A, BBL or Bacto Bacitracin, Difco Laboratories) directly on the area of initial inoculation, presumptive identification of *S. pyogenes* can be made after overnight incubation (Figure 16.2; all group A and a very small percentage of group B streptococci are susceptible). If preferred, direct antigen detection tests (coagglutination or latex agglutination) or PYR test (Chapter 25) can also be carried out from the more isolated β-hemolytic colonies that appear after overnight incubation on selective agar.

Cultures for *C. diphtheriae* should be plated onto

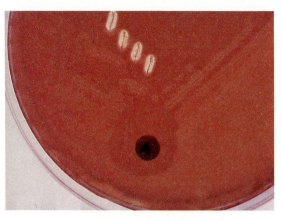

Figure 16.2
Primary streptococcal selective agar (BBL Microbiology Systems) culture plate from a throat specimen that contained many group A β-hemolytic streptococci. Growth of the bacteria is inhibited in zone surrounding the 0.04-unit bacitracin disk.

sheep blood agar or streptococcal selective agar as well as onto special media for recovery of the agent of diphtheria, since streptococcal pharyngitis is in the differential diagnosis of diphtheria and since dual infections do occur. These special media include a Loeffler's agar slant and a cystine-tellurite agar plate. Identification of the organism is discussed in Chapter 33. Recovery of this organism is enhanced by culturing specimens from both throat and nasopharynx of infected patients.

Freshly prepared Bordet-Gengou agar is the medium of choice for isolation of *B. pertussis*. A modified medium designed for isolation of *Legionella* species, buffered charcoal yeast extract agar with 3 μg/ml lincomycin and 80 μg/ml anisomycin has also been shown to yield good recovery of *B. pertussis*, as reported by workers at the Centers for Disease Control.[5] Jones and Kendrick[7] have also reported excellent recovery on a blood-free medium containing charcoal, heart infusion base, 2% agar, and 0.3 U/ml penicillin. Stauffer and others[14] showed best recovery of *B. pertussis* when this medium was supplemented with 40 μg/ml cephalexin. The charcoal medium developed for *Legionella* is more readily available and is a useful substitute. Specimens should be plated directly onto media, if possible, as the organisms are extremely delicate. Technologists should utilize both fluorescent antibody smears and cultures to achieve maximum detection. The yield of positive isolations from clinical cases of pertussis seems to vary from 20% to 98%, depending on the stage of disease, previous treatment of the patient, and laboratory techniques.

Specimens received in the laboratory for isolation of *N. meningitidis* (for detection of carriers) or for *N. gonorrhoeae* should be plated to a selective medium, either modified Thayer-Martin or Martin-Lewis agar. After 48 hours incubation in 5% to 10% CO_2, typical colonies of *Neisseria* species will be visible.

Clinical specimens from cases of epiglottitis (swabs obtained by a physician) should be plated to sheep blood agar, chocolate agar (for recovery of *Haemophilus* species), and a streptococcal selective medium if desired. Since *S. aureus* and *S. pneumoniae* may, rarely, cause this disease, their presence must be sought.

16.4.e. Nonculture methods for detecting agents of pharyngitis. One of the major improvements in clinical microbiology in recent years has been the development of rapid methods for antigen detection that obviate the need for culture. Identification of group A streptococcal antigen in throat specimens has benefitted greatly from these developments. At least 40 commercial products are available, employing latex agglutination or enzyme immunoassay technologies, that allow detection of group A streptococcal antigen within as short a time as 10 minutes. Although the specific procedures vary with the products, several generalizations can be made. Throat swabs are incubated in some type of acid reagent or enzyme to extract the group A–specific carbohydrate antigen. It seems that Dacron swabs are most efficient at releasing antigen, although other types of swabs may yield acceptable results. Wooden handles seem to interfere with extraction. It is best to follow the recommendations of the manufacturer of the extraction kit to achieve optimal results.

In most laboratory comparisons between a rapid method and conventional culture methods for detecting the presence of group A streptococci in throat swabs, the commercial kits have shown good sensitivity (> 90%) and exquisite specificity. There have been doubts expressed, however, about their overall ability to detect all clinically important streptococcal infections. Such systems are discussed further in Chapter 25. In those situations in which rapid results are important (such as outpatient clinics), information about the presence of other organisms is not required, and the number of positive results allows the test to be cost-effective. A commercial screening test for group A streptococci in throats may be the method of choice in selected situations. Rapid nonmicroscopic detection methods for most other agents of upper respiratory tract infections are not so well developed as those for *S. pyogenes* and those for many agents of lower respiratory tract disease, discussed below.

16.5. Acute Lower Respiratory Tract Infections

The etiologic agents of community-acquired pneumonia vary with the age and state of health of the patient. Pneumonias among patients with various types of immunosuppressive factors are discussed in Chapter 23. Among previously healthy patients 2 months to 5 years old, viruses, including respiratory syncytial, parainfluenza and influenza, and adenoviruses, are the most common etiologic agents of lower respiratory tract disease. In addition to pneumonia, which indicates involvement of the lung parenchyma, viruses cause bronchiolitis and bronchitis. The latter infections may manifest as croup. Presumably, growth of viruses in host cells disrupts the function of the latter and encourages the influx of nonspecific immune effector cells that exacerbate the damage. Damage to host epithelial tissue by virus infection is known to predispose patients to secondary bacterial infection, as reviewed by Mills.[11] Children suffer less commonly from bacterial pneumonia, usually caused by *H. influenzae*, pneumococci, or *S. aureus*. Neonates may acquire lower respiratory tract infections with *C. trachomatis* or *P. carinii* (which may indicate an immature immune system or other immune defect).

The most common etiologic agent of lower respiratory tract infection among adults younger than 30 years old is *M. pneumoniae*. This organism is transmitted via close contact. Contact with secretions seems to be more important than inhalation of aerosols for dissemination. Once they contact respiratory mucosa, *Mycoplasma* organisms are able to adhere to and colonize respiratory mucosal cells. Both a protein adherence factor and gliding motility may be determinants of virulence. Once oriented in their preferred site between the cilia of respiratory mucosal cells, *Mycoplasma* organisms multiply and somehow destroy ciliary function. Cytotoxins produced by *Mycoplasma* organisms may account for the cell damage they inflict. A recently described species of *C. pneumoniae* (originally called *Chlamydia TWAR*) has been seen as the third most common agent of lower respiratory tract infection in young adults, after mycoplasmas and influenza viruses; it also affects older individuals. Chlamydiae are intracellular parasites; thus their ability to disrupt cellular function and cause respiratory disease is similar to that of viruses.

Lower respiratory tract infections in older patients are due most commonly to bacterial infection, with *S. pneumoniae* most prevalent (causing 80% of all community acquired bacterial pneumonia). Aspiration pneumonia occurs in the community setting and involves primarily oral anaerobes and viridans streptococci but may also involve *S. aureus* or gram-negative rods such as *K. pneumoniae*, other Enterobacteriaceae, and *Pseudomonas* species, particularly in patients with recent hospital or nursing home experience. *H. influenzae*, *Legionella* species, *Acinetobacter*, *B. catarrhalis*, *C. pneumoniae*, meningococci, and other agents may also be implicated.[10,12] In the hospital setting, pneumonia involves many of these same agents. Aspiration pneumonia is probably the major type of hospital-acquired pneumonia. It is followed by pneumococcal disease. *Legionella* has been implicated in a number of hospital outbreaks.

Aspiration of oropharyngeal contents, often not overt, plays an important role in the pathogenesis of many different types of pneumonia. Aided by gravity and often by loss of some host nonspecific protective mechanism, the organisms reach lung tissue, where they multiply and attract host responder cells. Other mechanisms include inhalation of aerosolized material and hematogenous seeding. The buildup of cell debris and fluid contributes to the loss of lung function and thus to the pathology. Agents with polysaccharide capsules, such as pneumococci, *Klebsiella* species, *Haemophilus* species, certain *S. aureus*, and cryptococci, seem more able to avoid phagocytosis and thus are more likely to cause pneumonia in patients without adequate humoral immunity in the form of specific antibody.

Adults may suffer from viral pneumonia caused by influenza, adenovirus, cytomegalovirus, parainfluenza, varicella, rubeola, or respiratory syncytial virus, particularly during epidemics. After viral pneumonia, especially influenza, secondary bacterial disease caused by β-hemolytic streptococci, pneumococci, *S. aureus*, *B. catarrhalis*, *H. influenzae*, *C. pneumoniae*, and *N. meningitidis* is more likely. Unusual causes of acute lower respiratory tract in-

fection include *Actinomyces* and *Nocardia* species; the agents of plague, tularemia, melioidosis (*Pseudomonas pseudomallei*), *Brucella*, *Salmonella*, *Coxiella burnetti* (Q fever), *Bacillus anthracis*, and *Pasteurella multocida*. *Paragonimus westermani*, *Entamoeba histolytica*, *Ascaris lumbricoides*, and *Strongyloides* species (the latter may cause fatal disease in immunosuppressed patients) may be recovered from sputum rarely. A high index of suspicion by the clinician is usually a prerequisite to a diagnosis of parasitic pneumonia in the United States. Psittacosis should be ruled out as a cause of acute lower respiratory tract infection in patients who have had recent contact with birds. *Histoplasma capsulatum*, *Blastomyces dermatitidis*, *Paracoccidioides brasiliensis*, *Coccidioides immitis*, and *Cryptococcus neoformans*, and, occasionally, *Aspergillus fumigatus* may cause acute pneumonia. In the immunosuppressed patient, these fungi, as well as other *Aspergillus* species, *Candida*, zygomycetes, and other fungi, may cause pulmonary infection.

As noted, pneumonia secondary to aspiration of gastric or oral secretions is rather common. It happens most often during a loss of consciousness as might occur with anesthesia or a seizure or after alcohol or drug abuse, but other patients, particularly among geriatric groups, may also develop aspiration pneumonia. Neurologic disease or esophageal pathology and periodontal disease or gingivitis are other important background factors. The oral black-pigmenting *Bacteroides* and *Porphyromonas* species, *Bacteroides oris*, *B. buccae*, *B. disiens*, *B. gracilis*, fusobacteria, and anaerobic and microaerophilic streptococci, are the most common agents, but, as noted, *S. aureus*, various Enterobacteriaceae, and *Pseudomonas* may also be acquired in this way. The anaerobic agents possess many factors that may enhance their ability to produce disease, such as extracellular enzymes and capsules. It is their presence, however, in an abnormal site within the host and lowered oxidation-reduction potential secondary to tissue damage that probably contribute most to their pathogenicity.

Nonaspiration pneumonia in hospitalized patients is associated most commonly with *P. aeruginosa*, *S. aureus*, *Klebsiella* species, and other Enterobacteriaceae. Some of these pneumonias are secondary to sepsis, and some are related to contaminated inhalation therapy equipment. Other aspects of pneumonia in hospitalized patients, as well as other groups at increased risk of developing respiratory tract disease, are discussed in Chapter 23.

16.6. Chronic Lower Respiratory Tract Infections

Mycobacterium tuberculosis is the most likely etiologic agent of chronic lower respiratory tract infection, but fungal infection and anaerobic pleuropulmonary infection may also run a subacute or chronic course. Mycobacteria other than *M. tuberculosis* (MOTT) may also cause such disease, particularly *M. avium-intracellulare* and *M. kansasii*. Although possible causes of acute, community-acquired lower respiratory tract infections, fungi and parasites are more commonly isolated from patients with chronic disease. *Actinomyces* and *Nocardia* may also be associated with gradual onset of symptoms. Agents of chronic disease in compromised hosts are discussed in Chapter 23. The pathogenesis of many of the infections caused by agents of chronic lower respiratory tract disease is characterized by the requirement for some breakdown of cell-mediated immunity in the host or the ability of these agents to avoid being destroyed by host cell-mediated immune mechanisms. This may be by an effect on macrophages, by the ability to mask foreign antigens, sheer size, or by some other factor, allowing them to grow within host tissues without eliciting an overwhelming local reaction.

16.7. Laboratory Diagnosis of Lower Respiratory Tract Infections

16.7.a. Collection and transport of specimens. Lower respiratory tract secretions will be contaminated with upper respiratory tract secretions, especially saliva, unless they are collected using some invasive technique. For this reason, sputa are among the least clinically relevant specimens received for culture in microbiology laboratories, as well as being among the most numerous and time consuming. When hospital laboratories began to reject some sputum samples based on visual examination of predominant cell types (as discussed in Section 16.7.b), the numbers of acceptable specimens received by the laboratory increased significantly. It is possible, therefore, for microbiologists and clinicians to influence the quality of specimens received for culture. Good sputum samples are dependent on thorough patient education and the presence of a health care worker to oversee all phases of the collection process. Patients should be instructed to provide a deep cough specimen. The material should be expelled into a sterile container, with an attempt to minimize contamination with saliva. Specimens should be transported to the laboratory immediately, as even a moderate amount of time at room temperature can result in loss of some etiologic agents of respiratory tract infection.

Patients who are unable to produce sputum may be assisted by respiratory therapy technicians, who can use postural drainage and thoracic percussion to stimulate production of acceptable sputum. Alternatively, an "aerosol-induced specimen" may be collected. Particularly useful for obtaining material suitable for isolation of the agents of mycobacterial or fungal disease and recently extolled for their high yield in cases of *Pneumocystis carinii* pneumonia, aerosol-induced specimens are collected by allowing the patient to breathe aerosolized droplets of a solution of 15% sodium chloride and 10% glycerin for approximately 10 minutes, or until a strong cough reflex is initiated. The lower respiratory secretions obtained in this way appear watery, resembling saliva, although they often contain material directly from alveolar spaces. They are usually adequate for culture and should be accepted in the laboratory without prescreening. Obtaining such a specimen may obviate the need for a more invasive procedure in many cases.

Another specimen, exclusively for isolation of acid fast bacilli, that may be collected from patients who are unable to produce sputum, particularly young children, is the **gastric aspirate.** Before the patient has arisen in the morning, a nasogastric tube is inserted into the stomach and contents are withdrawn (on the assumption that acid fast bacilli from the respiratory tract were swallowed during the night and will be present in the stomach). The relative resistance of mycobacteria to acidity allows them to remain viable for a short period. Gastric aspirate specimens must be delivered to the laboratory immediately so that the acidity can be neutralized. Due to the presence of mycobacteria in tap water, acid-fast smears from gastric aspirates are often falsely positive and ordinarily should not be examined. A physician may be able to pass a long, soft catheter into the tracheobronchial tree and obtain a "tracheal aspirate" by suctioning with a syringe.

Patients with tracheostomies are unable to produce sputum in the normal fashion, but nurses can

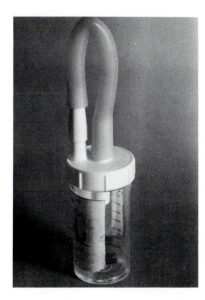

easily collect lower respiratory tract secretions in a Lukens trap (Figure 16.3). These specimens (called "tracheostomy aspirates") should be treated as sputum (without microscopic screening, discussed in Section 16.7.b) by the laboratory. Patients with tracheostomies rapidly become colonized with gram-negative bacilli and other nosocomial pathogens. Such colonization per se does not necessarily have clinical relevance, but these organisms may be aspirated and cause pneumonia. Thus there is real confusion for microbiologists and clinicians trying to ascertain the etiologic agent of disease in these patients.

When pleural empyema is present, thoracentesis may be used to obtain infected fluid for direct examination and culture. This constitutes an excellent specimen that accurately reflects the bacteriology of an associated pneumonia. Laboratory examination of such material is discussed in Chapter 21. Blood cultures, of course, should always be obtained from patients with pneumonia. Physicians sometimes attempt to obtain more representative specimens via a bronchoscope than are possible with noninvasive techniques. Bronchial secretions are often obtained by instilling a small amount of sterile physiologic saline into the bronchial tree and withdrawing the fluid when purulent secretions are not visualized. Such **bronchial washing** specimens will still be contaminated with upper respiratory tract flora, such as

viridans streptococci and *Neisseria* species. Recovery of potentially pathogenic organisms from bronchial washings should be attempted, however, since such specimens may be more diagnostically relevant than sputa.

A deeper sampling of desquamated host cells and secretions is also obtained via bronchoscopy by bronchoalveolar lavage (**BAL**). Lavages are especially suitable for detecting *Pneumocystis* cysts and fungal elements. The collection methods and handling of the specimen are well described by Bartlett and others.[2] Recent publications document the value of this technique, with quantitative culture, for diagnosis of most major respiratory tract pathogens, including bacterial pneumonia.[8,15] These authors found significant correlation between acute bacterial pneumonia and greater than 10^4 bacterial colonies per milliliter of BAL fluid.

The specimen obtained by only moderately invasive means that is best suited for microbiological studies, particularly in aspiration pneumonia, is that obtained via a *protected catheter bronchial brush*. A small brush that holds 0.01 to 0.001 ml of secretions is placed within a double cannula. The end of the outermost tube or cannula is closed with a displaceable plug made of polyethylene glycol. Once the cannula has been inserted to the proper area, the inner cannula is pushed out, dislodging the protective plug as it is extruded. Then the brush is extended beyond the inner cannula. The specimen is collected and the brush is withdrawn into the inner cannula, which is withdrawn into the outer cannula to prevent contamination as it is removed. The contents of the bronchial brush may be suspended in 1 ml of broth solution with vigorous vortexing and then inoculated onto culture media by technologists using a 0.01 ml calibrated inoculating loop. Specimens obtained via double lumen protected catheters have been stated by some workers to be suitable for anaerobic as well as aerobic cultures. Colony counts of greater than 1000 organisms per milliliter in the broth diluent (or 10^6/ml in the original specimen) have been considered to correlate with infection, as reported by Pollock and associates.[13] However, other studies question the validity of this procedure, even when cultures are done quantitatively. Furthermore, the tiny sample and its aeration are problems with the technique.

Several invasive procedures are used to collect specimens when definitive results are necessary or when anaerobic bacteria are being sought. Percutaneous **transtracheal aspirates (TTA),** as mentioned in Chapter 6, are obtained by inserting a small plastic catheter into the trachea via a needle previously inserted through the skin and cricothyroid membrane. This invasive procedure, although somewhat uncomfortable for the patient and not suitable for all patients (it cannot be used in uncooperative patients, in patients with bleeding tendency, or with poor oxygenation) guarantees a specimen uncontaminated by upper respiratory tract flora and undiluted by added fluids, provided that care is taken to keep the catheter from being coughed back up into the pharynx. Anaerobic agents of actinomycosis and aspiration pneumonia can best be isolated from transtracheal aspirate specimens.

For patients with pneumonia, a thin needle aspiration of material from the involved area of the lung may be performed percutaneously, often without fluoroscopy. If no material is withdrawn into the syringe after the first try, approximately 3 ml of sterile saline can be injected and withdrawn into the syringe. Patients with emphysema, uremia, thrombocytopenia, or pulmonary hyptertension may be at increased risk of complication (primarily pneumothorax or bleeding) from this procedure. The specimens obtained are very small in volume, and protection from aeration is usually impossible.

Transbronchial biopsies are used more for histologic diagnosis than for culture. Direct examination of biopsy specimens for agents such as *Pneumocystis* often shows positive findings.

The most invasive procedure for obtaining respiratory tract specimens is the "open lung biopsy." Performed by surgeons, this method is used to procure a wedge of lung tissue. Biopsy specimens are extremely helpful for diagnosis of severe viral infections, such as herpes pneumonia, for rapid diagnosis of *Pneumocystis* pneumonia, and for other hard-to-diagnose or life-threatening pneumonias. Ramifications of this and all other specimen collection techniques are discussed in Cumitech 7A, Laboratory Diagnosis of Lower Respiratory Tract Infections.[2]

16.7.b. Direct visual examination of lower respiratory tract specimens. Lower respiratory tract specimens can be examined by direct wet preparation for some parasites and by special procedures (see below) for *Pneumocystis*. Fungal elements can be visualized under phase microscopy with 10% KOH or under UV light with calcofluor white. If

pneumococci or *H. influenzae* type b is suspected, a portion of purulent material may be mixed with an equal amount of antiserum for performance of the Quellung test.

For most other evaluations, the specimen must be fixed and stained. Bacteria and yeasts can be recognized on Gram stain. One of the most important uses of the Gram stain, however, is to evaluate the quality of expectorated sputum received for routine bacteriologic culture.[9] A portion of the specimen consisting of purulent material is chosen for the stain. One enterprising group showed that the smear can be evaluated adequately even before it is stained, thus negating the need for Gram stain of specimens later judged unacceptable.[17] An acceptable specimen will yield less than 10 squamous epithelial cells per low-power field ($100\times$). The number of white cells may not be relevant, since many patients are severely neutropenic. On the other hand, the presence of greater than or equal to 25 polymorphonuclear leukocytes per $100\times$ field, together with few squamous epithelial cells, assures one of an excellent specimen (Figure 16.4). Only expectorated sputa are suitable for rejection based on microscopic screening. However, it is important to realize that in *Legionella* pneumonia, sputum may be scant and watery with few or no host cells. Such specimens may still often be positive by direct fluorescent antibody stain and culture and should not be subjected to screening procedures. Respiratory secretions may need to be concentrated before staining. The cytocentrifuge instrument has been used successfully for this purpose, concentrating the cellular material in an easily examined monolayer on a glass slide. Alternatively, specimens are centrifuged and the sediment is used for visual examinations and cultures. For screening purposes, the presence of ciliated columnar bronchial epithelial cells, goblet cells, or pulmonary macrophages in specimens obtained by bronchoscopy or BAL is indicative of a specimen from the lower respiratory tract.

In addition to the Gram stain, respiratory specimens may be stained for acid fast bacilli with either the classic Ziehl-Neelsen or the Kinyoun carbolfuchsin stain. Auramine or auramine-rhodamine is also used for detection of acid-fast organisms. Because they are fluorescent, these stains are more sensitive than the carbolfuchsin formulas and are preferable for rapid screening. Slides may be restained with the classic stains directly over the fluo-

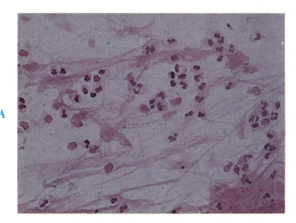
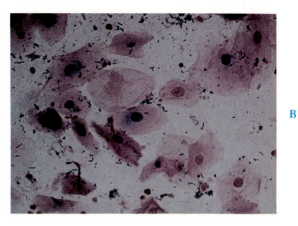

A   B

Figure 16.4
Gram stain of sputum specimens (400×). **A,** This specimen contains numerous polymorphonuclear
leukocytes and no visible squamous epithelial cells, indicating that the specimen is acceptable for
routine bacteriologic culture. **B,** This specimen contains numerous squamous epithelial cells and rare
polymorphonuclear leukocytes, indicating an inadequate specimen for routine bacteriologic culture.

rochrome stains as long as all of the immersion oil
has been removed carefully with xylene. When results are needed urgently, material may be stained
unconcentrated, as described in Chapter 7. All of
the acid-fast stains will also reveal *Cryptosporidium*
species if they are present in the respiratory tract,
as may occur in immunosuppressed patients.

Immunosuppressed patients are often at risk of
infection with *P. carinii*. Although the modified Gomori methenamine silver stain procedure (Chapter
44) has been chosen traditionally and is the easiest
to interpret for identification of nocardiae, actinomyces, fungi, and parasites, it takes approximately
1 hour of technologist time to perform and may not
be suitable as an emergency procedure, especially
on nights or weekends. A fairly rapid stain, toluidine
blue O, has been used in many laboratories with
great success. It stains not only *Pneumocystis* but
also *Nocardia asteroides* and some fungi. This stain
is described in Chapter 44. A new monoclonal antibody stain for *Pneumocystis* shows great promise
as a specific and sensitive stain (Chapter 44).

Direct fluorescent antibody stain has been used
for detection of *Legionella* species in lower respiratory tract specimens. Sputum, pleural fluid, aspirated material, and tissue are all suitable specimens. Polyclonal antibody reagents and a monoclonal antibody directed against all serotypes of
Legionella pneumophila are used, since there are so
many different serotypes of legionellae. A radioac-

tively labeled nucleic acid probe capable of detecting
all species of *Legionella* is also available commercially and has been shown to yield results comparable to those of direct fluorescent antibody (DFA).
DFA results should not be relied on in lieu of culture,
which remains the gold standard for legionellae.

DFA reagents (commercially available) are also
used to detect antigens of a number of viruses, including herpes simplex, cytomegalovirus, adenovirus, and respiratory syncytial virus.[4,6] Commercial
suppliers of reagents provide procedure information
for each of the tests available. Monoclonal and polyclonal fluorescent stains for *C. trachomatis* are
available and may be useful for staining respiratory
secretions of infants with pneumonia.[3]

**16.7.c. Culture of lower respiratory tract speci-
mens.** Most of the commonly sought etiologic agents
of lower respiratory tract infection will be isolated
on the commonly used media: 5% sheep blood agar,
MacConkey agar, and chocolate agar. Because of contaminating oral flora, sputum specimens, specimens
obtained by bronchial washing and lavage, tracheal
aspirates, and tracheostomy or endotracheal tube aspirates are not inoculated to enrichment broth or
incubated anaerobically. Only specimens obtained
by percutaneous aspiration (including transtracheal
aspiration) and perhaps by protected bronchial brush
are suitable for anaerobic culture; the latter must be
done quantitatively. Transtracheal and percutaneous
lung aspiration material may be inoculated to en-

riched thioglycollate as well as to solid media. For suspected cases of Legionnaire's disease, buffered charcoal yeast extract (BCYE) agar and selective BCYE are inoculated. Pertussis media, as mentioned in Section 16.4.d, may also be inoculated.

Contaminated specimens received for isolation of mycobacteria must be decontaminated and concentrated before they are inoculated to media (see Chapter 41). The radiometric detection system (Bactec, Johnston Laboratories) has been used with good success for more rapid detection of growth of mycobacteria, especially *M. avium-intracellulare*, than can be achieved with conventional cultures. Specimens are inoculated to special media for mycoplasma isolation (Chapter 38).[3] For isolation of the dimorphic fungi, material should be inoculated to brain heart infusion agar as well as to infusion or Sabouraud's heart infusion agar (SABHI) with sheep blood and Mycobiotic or Mycosel (or some inhibitory mold agar), as discussed in Chapters 8 and 43.

Patients with cystic fibrosis may yield such numerous colonies of mucoid *Pseudomonas aeruginosa* that other growth is obscured.[16] For such specimens, selective agar, mentioned in Chapter 23, should be inoculated. The isolation of *Haemophilus* species in specimens containing large numbers of normal flora can be facilitated by placing a 10-U bacitracin disk in the area of the primary inoculum on the chocolate agar plate (George Tortora, personal communication). This may be particularly valuable with sputum specimens received from patients with cystic fibrosis.

Viruses and chlamydiae require tissue culture techniques,[4] detailed in Chapters 38 and 42. Specimens for viral culture should be placed in a protein-containing transport medium such as Minimum Essential Medium in Eagle's Buffered Salt Solution (commercially available) with amphotericin B or veal infusion broth and refrigerated (never frozen) until they can be cultured. Chlamydia cultures are transported in 2-sucrose phosphate (2SP) or other transport medium (Chapter 38).

16.7.d. **Nonculture methods for diagnosing lower respiratory tract infections.** In addition to direct fluorescent antibody staining of lower respiratory tract secretions, several other nonculture techniques have been utilized. Traditional serology, of course, is valuable for retrospective diagnosis of re-

spiratory tract infections. A recently introduced enzyme immunoassay for the detection of *B. pertussis* antibodies (Labsystems) may be helpful in timely diagnosis of pertussis. Gas-liquid chromatography has been used to analyze fluids for the presence of metabolites of pneumococci and other pathogens (see Chapter 11). Gas-liquid chromatography, electron-capture gas chromatography, and gas-chromatography mass spectroscopy have been evaluated for diagnosis of tuberculosis. Although the ideas are promising, there are no practical schemes in general use for diagnosing lower respiratory tract infection in this way. Elevated pleural fluid lactic acid levels are indicative of bacterial empyema, but there is a little overlap with malignant pleural effusion.

Testing clinical material directly for antigens of common pathogens, an approach that has succeeded for detection of group A streptococci in throat swabs, shows promise for diagnosis of pneumonia. The problems of nonspecific reactivity and masking of reactions by mucus and other factors have not been fully resolved. At least one commercially available **radioimmunoassay (RIA)** procedure, detection of antigens of *L. pneumophila* in urine of patients with legionellosis (DuPont), has been found to be approximately as sensitive as direct fluorescent antibody stains of sputum. Electron microscopy has been used for detection of virus particles, although this procedure is limited to a few very specialized laboratories. DNA hybridization, a promising technique for detection of viral and other microbial gene sequences in clinical material, discussed in Chapter 10, has been used by a number of workers. **In situ hybridization** procedures utilizing biotinylated or other DNA probes have successfully visualized herpes simplex, varicella-zoster, adenovirus, and cytomegalovirus-infected cells in sections from lungs and in cell layers.

DNA probes for hybridization tests performed in liquid are available from GenProbe (San Diego) for detection of RNA sequences from *Legionella* species, *Mycoplasma pneumoniae*, *Mycobacterium tuberculosis*, *M. avium*, and *M. intracellulare* using an iodinated probe and for *C. trachomatis* using a chemiluminescent probe. Although some of these reagents, notably those for mycobacteria, have not proved sensitive enough for routine use, others are successfully employed in several laboratories.

REFERENCES

1. Anhalt, J.P. 1981. Flourescent antibody procedures and counterimmunoelectrophoresis. In Washington, J.A. II, editor. Laboratory procedures in clinical microbiology, Springer-Verlag, New York.
2. Bartlett, J.G., Ryan, K.J., Smith, T.F., et al. 1987. Cumitech 7A, Laboratory diagnosis of lower respiratory tract infections, American Society for Microbiology, Washington, D.C.
3. Clyde, W.A. Jr., Kenny, G.E., and Schachter, J. 1984. Cumitech 19. In Drew, W.L., editor. Laboratory diagnosis of chlamydial and mycoplasmal infections. American Society for Microbiology, Washington, D.C.
4. Greenberg, S.B., and Krilov, L.R. 1986. Cumitech 21, In Drew, W.L., editor. Laboratory diagnosis of viral respiratory disease. American Society for Microbiology, Washington, D.C.
5. Hayes, P.S., Feeley, J.C., Johnson, S.E., et al. 1985. Use of charcoal yeast extract agar for the isolation of *Bordetella pertussis*, American Society for Microbiology, Washington, D.C.
6. Hildreth, S.W., Hall, C.B. and Menegus, M.A. 1983. Respiratory syncytial virus. Clin. Microbiol. Newsletter 5:93.
7. Jones, G.L., and Kendrick, P.L. 1969. Study of a blood-free medium for transport and growth of *Bordetella pertussis*. Health Lab. Sci. 6:40.
8. Kahn, F.W., and Jones, J.M. 1987. Diagnosing bacterial respiratory infection by bronchoalveolar lavage. J. Infect. Dis. 155:862.
9. Lentino, J.R. 1987. The nonvalue of unscreened sputum specimens in the diagnosis of pneumonia. Clin. Microbiol. Newsletter 9:70.
10. Marrie, T.J., Grayston, T., Wang, S.-P., et al. 1987. Pneumonia associated with the TWAR strain of *Chlamydia*. Ann. Intern. Med. 106:507.
11. Mills, E.L. 1984. Viral infections predisposing to bacterial infections. Annu. Rev. Med. 35:469.
12. Parker, R.H. 1983. Hemophilus influenzae respiratory infection in adults: recognition and incidence. Postgrad. Med. 73:179.
13. Pollock, H.M., Hawkins, E.L., Bonner, J.R., et al. 1983. Diagnosis of bacterial pulmonary infections with quantitative protected catheter cultures obtained during bronchoscopy. J. Clin. Microbiol. 17:255.
14. Stauffer, L.R., Brown, D.R. and Sandstrom, R.E. 1983. Cephalexin-supplemented Jones-Kendrick charcoal agar for selective isolation of *Bordetella pertussis*: comparison with previously described media. J. Clin. Microbiol. 17:60.
15. Thorpe, J.E., Baughman, R.P., Frame, P.T., et al. 1987. Bronchoalveolar lavage for diagnosing acute bacterial pneumonia. J. Infect. Dis. 155:855.
16. Welch, D.F. 1984. Clinical microbiology of cystic fibrosis. Clin. Microbiol. Newsletter 6:39.
17. Wetterau, L.M., Zeimis, R.T., and Hollick, G.E. 1986. Direct examination of unstained smears for the evaluation of sputum specimens. J. Clin. Microbiol. 24:143.

BIBLIOGRAPHY

Browning, R.J. 1983. Diagnosing pulmonary diseases: a clinician's perspective. Diagn. Med. 6:39; 6:62.

McDougall, J.K., Beckman, A.M., Galloway, D.A., et al. 1985. Defined viral probes for the detection of HSV, CMV, and HPV. In Kingsbury, D.T., and Falkow, S., editors. Rapid detection and identification of infectious agents. Academic Press, New York.

von Graevenitz, A. 1983. Which bacterial species should be isolated from throat cultures? (Editorial.) Eur. J. Clin. Microbiol. 2:1.

17 Microorganisms Encountered in the Gastrointestinal Tract

17.1. Anatomy and General Features of Gastrointestinal Tract

The gastrointestinal tract (Figure 17.1) is actually in continuation with the external environment. Ingested material that enters the gastrointestinal tract passes through the esophagus into the stomach, through the duodenum, the jejunum, the ileum, and finally through the cecum and colon to the anus. During passage, fluids and other components are both added to this material (as secretory products of individual cells and as enzymatic secretions of glands and organs) and removed from this material by absorption through the gut epithelium. The duodenum, jejunum, and ileum are collectively called the "small intestine," and the cecum and colon comprise the "large intestine." The nature of the epithelial cells lining the gastrointestinal tract varies with the segment; the small intestine is lined with small projections, called **villi,** that greatly increase the surface area. The function of villi is to absorb fluids and nutrients from the intestinal contents. Other cells of the small intestine secrete fluids and metabolites into the lumen. Many of the cells in the lining of the large intestine are mucus secreting, and there are no villous projections into the lumen. The remaining excess fluid within the gastrointestinal tract is reabsorbed by the cells lining the large intestine before waste is finally discharged through the anus. The lining of the gastrointestinal tract is called the **mucosa.** Because of the differing nature of the mucosal surfaces of various segments of the bowel, different infectious disease processes tend to occur in each segment. The appendix, a long, narrow tube of bowel tissue, extends from the cecum near the

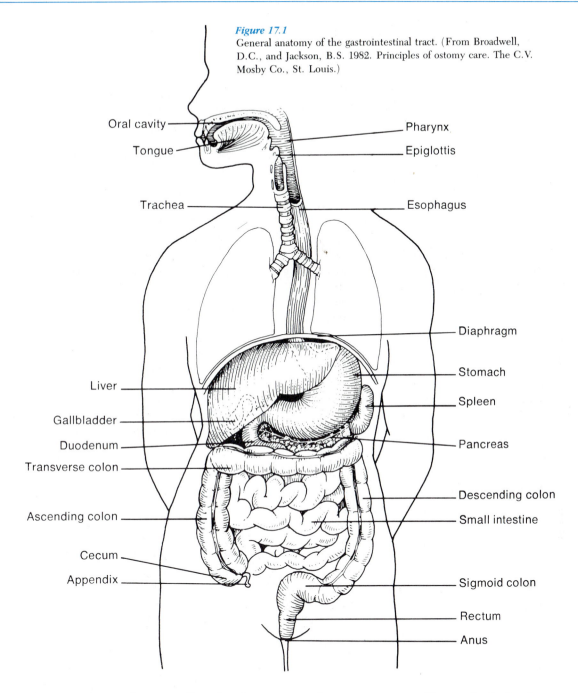

Figure 17.1
General anatomy of the gastrointestinal tract. (From Broadwell, D.C., and Jackson, B.S. 1982. Principles of ostomy care. The C.V. Mosby Co., St. Louis.)

Oral cavity

Tongue

Trachea

Liver

Gallbladder

Duodenum

Transverse colon

Ascending colon

Cecum

Appendix

Pharynx

Epiglottis

Esophagus

Diaphragm

Stomach

Spleen

Pancreas

Descending colon

Small intestine

Sigmoid colon

Rectum

Anus

ileum. The appendix may become inflamed and even gangrenous when there is stasis within its lumen or when there is an adjacent inflammatory process. Appendicitis is the most common initial event leading to intra-abdominal abscess in children. Infections of the appendix are discussed in Chapter 20.

The gastrointestinal tract contains a vast and diverse normal flora. Although the acidity of the stomach prevents any significant colonization in a normal host, many species can survive passage through the stomach to become resident within the lower intestinal tract. Normally, the upper small intestine also contains only a sparse flora (bacteria, primarily streptococci, lactobacilli, and yeasts, 10 to 10^3/ml), but by the time the distal ileum is reached, counts are about 10^6 to 10^7/ml, and Enterobacteriaceae and

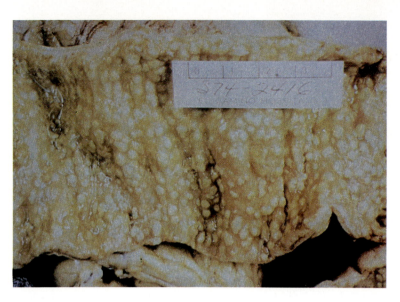

Figure 17.2
Autopsy specimen of colon showing multiple yellow, elevated plaques indicative of the inflammatory exudate of pseudomembranous colitis.

Bacteroides are present. In the case of certain types of pathology (for example, bleeding or obstructing peptic ulcer) there may be much higher bacterial counts and a more diverse flora in the stomach and duodenum. This has implications in the case of a patient who suffers a perforated peptic ulcer. Babies usually are colonized by normal human epithelial flora (staphylococci, *Corynebacterium* species, and so forth) and other gram-positive organisms (bifidobacteria, clostridia, lactobacilli, streptococci) within a few hours of birth. Over time, the content of the intestinal flora changes. The normal flora of the adult large bowel, predominantly anaerobic species, including *Bacteroides, Clostridium, Peptostreptococcus, Bifidobacterium, Eubacterium,* and others, is established relatively early in life. The anaerobes outnumber the aerobes, which include primarily *Escherichia coli*, other Enterobacteriaceae, enterococci, and other streptococci, by 1000:1. The number of bacteria per gram material within the lumen of the bowel increases steadily as material approaches the sigmoid colon (the last segment). Eighty percent of the dry weight of feces from a healthy human consists of bacteria, which can be present in numbers as high as 10^{11} to 10^{12}/g. After antimicrobial therapy, the large bowel may become colonized with nosocomial pathogens such as *Staph-*

ylococcus aureus, Pseudomonas aeruginosa, and other resistant gram-negative bacilli. This influences the flora of any subsequent intra-abdominal infection.

17.2. Pathophysiology of Gastrointestinal Infections

17.2.a. Role of normal flora in host defense. The normal flora is an important factor in the response of the host to introduction of a potentially harmful microorganism. It has been shown that whenever a reduction in normal flora occurs, due to antibiotic treatment or to some host factor, resistance to gastrointestinal infection is significantly reduced. The most common example of the protective effect of normal flora is the development of the syndrome **pseudomembranous colitis (PMC).** Caused by the toxins of the anaerobic organism *Clostridium difficile* and occasionally other clostridia and *S. aureus*, this inflammatory disease of the large bowel (Figure 17.2) seldom occurs except after antimicrobial or antimetabolite treatment has altered the normal flora. Almost every antimicrobial agent and several chemotherapeutic agents have been associated with the development of cases of PMC. *C. difficile*, either present in small numbers in the normal host or resident in the hospital environment, from which it colonizes hospitalized patients, is suppressed by normal flora. When normal flora are reduced, *C. difficile* is able to multiply and produce its toxins. Thus, this syndrome is also known as "antibiotic-associated colitis." Other microorganisms that may gain a foothold when released from selective pressure of normal flora include *Candida* species, staphylococci, *Pseudomonas* species, and various Enterobacteriaceae.

17.2.b. **Nonspecific host defense mechanisms.** Several other factors contribute to host resistance to disease. The acidity of the stomach effectively restricts the number and types of organisms that enter the lower gastrointestinal tract. Normal peristalsis helps to move organisms along, interfering with their ability to adhere to the mucosa. The mucus layer coating the epithelium entraps microorganisms and helps to propel them along. The normal flora, of course, prevents colonization by potential pathogens. Secretory IgA and phagocytic cells within the gut help to destroy etiologic agents of disease, as do eosinophils (particularly active against parasites). For a microorganism to cause gastrointestinal infection, it must possess one or more factors that allow it to overcome these host defenses, or it must enter the host at a time when one or more of the innate defense systems is inactive. For example, certain stool pathogens are able to survive gastric acidity only if the acidity has been reduced by bicarbonate or other buffer or by cimetidine and similar medications. Pathogens taken in with milk have a better chance of survival, since milk neutralizes stomach acidity. Organisms such as *Mycobacterium tuberculosis* and *Shigella* are able to withstand exposure to gastric acids, and thus require much smaller infectious inocula than acid-sensitive organisms such as *Salmonella*.

17.2.c. **Pathogenic mechanisms of agents of gastrointestinal infections.** Etiologic agents of gastrointestinal infection are known to cause disease in only four ways:

1. By producing a toxin that affects fluid secretion, cell function, or neurologic function
2. By growing within or close to intestinal mucosal cells and destroying them, thus disrupting function
3. By invading the mucosal epithelium, causing cellular destruction and occasionally invading the bloodstream and going on to systemic disease
4. By adhering to intestinal mucosa, thus preventing the normal functions of absorption and secretion.

Since the normal adult gastrointestinal tract receives up to 8 L of fluid daily in the form of ingested liquid and the secretions of the various glands that contribute to digestion (salivary glands, pancreas, gallbladder, and stomach), of which all but a small amount must be reabsorbed, it is obvious that any disruption of the normal flow or resorption of fluid will have a profound effect on the host.

"Food poisoning" may occur as a result of the ingestion of toxins produced by microorganisms. The microorganisms usually produce their toxins in consumables before they are ingested; thus the patient ingests *preformed* toxin. Although strictly speaking these syndromes are not gastrointestinal infections but intoxications, they are acquired by ingestion of microorganisms or their products and will be considered in this chapter. It is possible, particularly in staphylococcal food poisoning and botulism, that the causative organisms are not present in the bowel of the patient at all.

17.2.d. **Gastrointestinal or systemic diseases associated with toxin-producing microorganisms.** One of the most potent neurotoxins known is produced by the anaerobic organism *Clostridium botulinum*. This toxin acts to prevent the release of the neurotransmitter acetylcholine at the cholinergic nerve junctions, causing flaccid paralysis. The toxin acts primarily on the peripheral nerves but also on the autonomic nervous system. Patients exhibit descending symmetrical paralysis and ultimately die from respiratory paralysis unless they are given mechanical ventilation. In most cases, adult patients who develop botulism have ingested the preformed toxin in food (home-canned tomato products and canned cream-base foods are often implicated) and the disease is considered to be an intoxication, although *C. botulinum* has been recovered from the stools of a number of adult patients. *Wound botulism* also occurs, but it is rare. A relatively recently recognized syndrome, *infant botulism*, is a true gastrointestinal infection. It is probable that the flora of the normal adult bowel usually prevent colonization by *C. botulinum*, whereas the organism is able to multiply and produce toxin in the infant bowel. Infant botulism is not uncommon; babies acquire the organism by ingestion, although the source of the bacterium is not always clear. There has been an association with honey and corn syrup; it is recommended that babies under 9 months of age not be fed honey. The effect of the toxin is the same, whether it is ingested in food or produced within the bowel.

Other bacterial agents of food poisoning that produce neurotoxins include *S. aureus* and *Bacillus cereus*. Toxins produced by these organisms cause vomiting, independent of other actions on the gut mucosa. Staphylococcal food poisoning is one of the most commonly reported categories of food-borne disease. The organisms grow in warm food, primarily meat or dairy products, and produce the toxin. Onset of disease is usually within 2 to 6 hours of ingestion. *B. cereus* produces two toxins, one of which is preformed, called the **emetic** toxin, because it produces vomiting. The second type, probably involving several enterotoxins (discussed below), causes diarrhea. Often acquired from rice, *B. cereus* has also been associated with cooked meat, poultry, vegetables, and desserts. Perhaps the most common cause of food poisoning is type A *Clostridium perfringens*, which produces toxin in the host after ingestion. It causes a relatively mild, self-limited (usually 24 hours) gastroenteritis, often in outbreaks in hospitals. Meats and gravies are common offending foods. Clinical symptoms of *B. cereus* and *C. perfringens* food-borne disease occur 8 to 14 hours after ingestion. Investigations of outbreaks of food poisoning due to preformed toxin ingestion are carried out by public health laboratories and should not be attempted by clinical laboratories.

The second category of toxins, **cytotoxins,** acts to disrupt the structure of individual intestinal epithelial cells. When these cells are destroyed, they slough from the surface of the mucosa, leaving it raw and unprotected. The secretory or absorptive functions of the cells are no longer performed. The damaged tissue evokes a strong inflammatory response from the host, further inflicting tissue damage. Patients often shed numerous polymorphonuclear neutrophils and blood into the stool and experience pain, cramps, and an urgent need to defecate even though there is little material in the bowel (tenesmus). The term **dysentery** refers to this destructive disease of the mucosa, almost exclusively occurring in the colon. Cytotoxin has not yet been shown to be the sole virulence factor for any etiologic agent of gastrointestinal disease; most agents produce a cytotoxin in conjunction with another factor.

E. coli strains seem to possess virulence mechanisms of many types[6]; some strains produce a cytotoxin that destroys epithelial cells and blood cells. Certain strains produce a cytotoxin that affects Vero cells (African green monkey kidney cells) and resem-

bles the cytotoxin produced by *Shigella dysenteriae* (Shiga toxin); such strains of *E. coli* are associated with hemorrhagic colitis and hemolytic uremic syndrome.

C. difficile produces a cytotoxin, the presence of which is a most useful marker for diagnosis of PMC. (The *C. difficile* cytotoxin assay is discussed in Section 17.6.) *S. dysenteriae*, *Staphylococcus aureus*, *C. perfringens*, and *Vibrio parahaemolyticus* produce cytotoxins that probably contribute to the pathogenesis of diarrhea, although they may not be essential for initiation of disease. Other vibrios, *Aeromonas hydrophila*, a relatively newly described agent of gastrointestinal disease, and *Campylobacter jejuni*, the most common cause of gastrointestinal disease in many areas of the United States, have been shown to produce cytotoxins. The role that these toxins actually play in the pathogenesis of the disease syndromes is not yet delineated. With the exception of tests for the cytotoxin of *C. difficile*, tests for cytotoxins are not routinely performed.

Enterotoxins cause an alteration in the metabolic activity of intestinal epithelial cells, resulting in an outpouring of electrolytes and fluid into the lumen. They act primarily in the jejunum and upper ileum, where the majority of the fluid transport takes place. The stool of patients with enterotoxic diarrheal disease involving the small bowel is profuse and watery, and polymorphonuclear neutrophils and blood are not prominent features. The classic example of an enterotoxin is that of *Vibrio cholerae*, called "choleragen" (Figure 17.3). This toxin consists of two subunits, A and B.[10] The A subunit is composed of one molecule of A_1, the toxic moiety, and one molecule of A_2, which binds an A_1 subunit to five B subunits. The B subunits bind the toxin to a receptor (a ganglioside, an acidic glycolipid) on the intestinal cell membrane. Once the toxin binds, it acts on adenylate cyclase enzyme, which catalyzes the transformation of adenosine triphosphate (ATP) to cyclic adenosine monophosphate (cAMP). Increased levels of cAMP stimulate the cell to actively secrete ions into the intestinal lumen; to maintain osmotic stabilization, the cells then secrete fluid into the lumen. The fluid is drawn from the entire fluid store of the body. Patients therefore can become dehydrated very rapidly, as mentioned in Chapter 30. Oral fluid replacement with a glucose-containing electrolyte solution will adequately treat most patients with

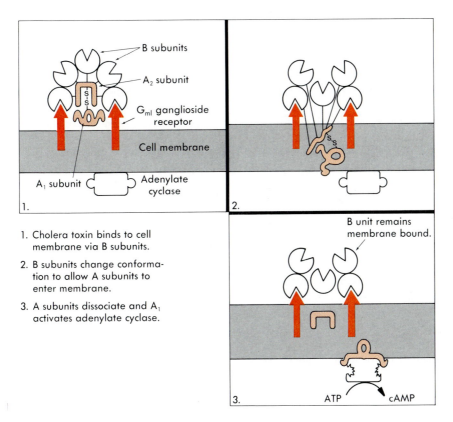

1. Cholera toxin binds to cell membrane via B subunits.

2. B subunits change conformation to allow A subunits to enter membrane.

3. A subunits dissociate and A_1 activates adenylate cyclase.

Figure 17.3
Diagrammatic representation of the structure and action of cholera toxin.

cholera, since fluid reabsorption can be coupled to glucose transport into the cells. *V. cholerae* must be able to multiply to sufficient numbers to produce toxin in the infected host. To this end, the bacteria possess motility and adherence factors, as discussed in Section 17.2.g. *V. cholerae* inhabit sea and stagnant water and are spread in contaminated water. They have been isolated from coastal waters of several states, and there have been a few cases of cholera reported that were acquired in the United States in recent years.

Other organisms also produce a choleragen-like enterotoxin. A group of vibrios similar to *V. cholerae* but serologically different, known as the *noncholera vibrios*, produce disease clinically identical to cholera, effected by a very similar toxin. The heat labile toxin (LT) elaborated by certain strains of *E. coli*, called **enterotoxigenic** *E. coli* (ETEC), is similar to choleragen, sharing cross-reactive antigenic determinants. The enterotoxins of some *Salmonella* species (including *S. arizonae*), *Vibrio parahaemolyticus*, the *C. jejuni* group, *C. perfringens*, *C. diffi-*

cile, *B. cereus*, *Aeromonas*, *S. dysenteriae*, and many other Enterobacteriaceae also cause positive reactions in at least one of the tests for enterotoxin. The exact contribution of these enterotoxins to the pathogenicity of each of these stool pathogens remains to be elucidated.

Certain strains of *E. coli*, in addition to producing a heat-labile toxin similar to choleragen (LT), also produce a heat stable toxin (ST) with other properties. Although ST also promotes fluid secretion into the intestinal lumen, its effect is mediated by activation of guanylate cyclase, resulting in increased levels of cyclic guanylate monophosphate (GMP), which yields the same net effect as increased cAMP. Tests for ST include enzyme-linked immunosorbent assay (ELISA), immunodiffusion, and the classic suckling mouse assay, in which culture filtrate is placed into the stomach of a suckling mouse and the intestinal contents are later measured for fluid volume increase.

Several tests are available for the detection of enterotoxin, although these are not performed routinely in diagnostic microbiology laboratories. The classic test is the "ligated rabbit ileal loop test." For this test, portions of rabbit ileum are tied off and injected with culture filtrate being tested and known toxin-positive control material. Within a period of hours, the rabbit is sacrificed and the intestinal loops are examined. Those loops that received toxin are found to be distended with fluid that has been secreted into the loop, whereas the loops without enterotoxin will show no distention, resembling the control loops. Several different fluids may be tested for enterotoxin in the same rabbit.

Other tests for enterotoxin include the Chinese hamster ovary (CHO) cell assay and the Y-1 adrenal cell assay, tissue culture assays in which a tissue culture consisting of CHO cells or Y-1 adrenal cells, known to be sensitive to the action of enterotoxin, are exposed to test fluids and examined for evidence of damage (rounding up). Since enterotoxins are toxigenic, homologous antibodies can be used to identify them specifically. Immunodiffusion type, ELISA, and latex agglutination tests are all available. Molecular probes have also been developed for research use.

17.2.e. Gastrointestinal infections associated with destruction of cell function without toxins. Organisms that multiply within certain cells of the mucosa, disrupting normal function of those cells, can cause diarrheal disease. Viruses probably act in this manner, multiplying within cells of the small bowel. Diarrhea of viral etiology is not associated with the presence of blood and white cells. Hepatitis A, B, non-A non-B, rotavirus, Norwalk-like agents, and occasionally adenovirus have been associated with diarrheal symptoms in infected patients, whereas the role of other viruses, such as coxsackievirus and echoviruses, in the etiology of diarrhea has not been established. Viral diarrhea may be the second most common infectious disease among people in the United States (after upper respiratory tract infections). Nursery and day-care center outbreaks of rotavirus diarrhea have been reported. Although young children are at most risk, close adult contacts may also become infected. Rotaviruses and Norwalk-like agents are both visualized by electron microscopy within the absorptive cells at the ends of the intestinal villi, where they multiply and destroy cellular function. The villi become shortened and inflammatory cells infiltrate the mucosa, further contributing to the pathologic condition. Hepatitis vi-

ruses have not been found in intestinal cells, but it is possible that some multiplication occurs there, since diarrhea is a common early symptom of hepatitis. Other viruses, particularly enteroviruses, can be recovered from feces, although the disease-producing activity occurs in other sites. The etiology of diarrhea associated with an overgrowth of *Candida* species in the bowel, especially in patients taking broad spectrum antibiotics, has not been established. It is not due to *Candida* and probably is similar to other types of antibiotic-associated diarrhea without PMC. Filamentous fungi may, on occasion, be associated with altered gastrointestinal function, particularly in immunosuppressed patients.

17.2.f. Gastrointestinal infections associated with invasive microorganisms. Certain parasites, particularly *Entamoeba histolytica* and *Balantidium coli*, invade the intestinal epithelium of the colon as a primary site of infection. The ensuing amebic dysentery is characterized by blood and *numerous white blood cells*, and the patient experiences cramping and tenesmus. Other parasites that are acquired by ingestion, such as *Schistosoma* species and *Trichinella*, may cause transient bloody diarrhea and pain during migration through the intestinal mucosa to their preferred sites within the host.

Bacteria that invade the epithelial cells also produce symptoms of dysentery. The most common etiologic agent is *Shigella*, although strains of *E. coli* called **enteroinvasive** may be associated with an identical syndrome. The bacteria penetrate the superficial layers of the mucosa, rarely passing into deeper host tissues. Invasiveness, then, is a virulence factor for these organisms. The classic test for invasiveness is the **Sereny test,** in which a suspension of the organism is placed within the conjunctival sac of a guinea pig or rabbit. Within a short time, an invasive organism will penetrate the epithelial cells, causing a purulent and exudative conjunctivitis. Although tissue culture methods for determining invasiveness have been described, this factor is not tested for in routine clinical laboratories.

Other bacteria not only invade superficial epithelia but also may invade the blood vessels to disseminate systemically. Certain *Salmonella* serotypes, such as *S. typhi* and *S. choleraesuis*, are more likely to do this. *S. typhi* and *S. choleraesuis* are etiologic agents of **enteric fever,** systemic diseases characterized by fever, headache, vomiting, and sometimes constipation (rather than diarrhea). The organisms can be recovered from the blood, stool, and, occasionally, the duodenal fluid of patients with this syndrome. Invasiveness is also thought to contribute to the pathogenesis of disease associated with species of vibrios, campylobacters, *Yersinia enterocolitica*, *Plesiomonas shigelloides*, and *Edwardsiella tarda*.

17.2.g. Gastrointestinal infections associated with adherent microorganisms. *Giardia lamblia* has become increasingly more common as an etiologic agent of gastrointestinal disease in the United States. Excreted into fresh water by natural animal hosts such as the beaver, the organism can be acquired by drinking stream water or even city water in some localities, particularly in the Rocky Mountain states, as well as throughout the world. The organism, a flagellated protozoan, adheres to the intestinal mucosa of the small bowel, possibly by means of a ventral sucker, destroying the ability of the mucosal cells to participate in normal secretion and absorption. There is no evidence of invasion or toxin production.

Yet another virulence mechanism for *E. coli* may be adherence. Certain strains have been implicated as etiologic agents of malabsorption diarrhea; the strains have no other detectable pathogenic mechanisms, but are able to multiply in close proximity to the intestinal epithelial cells. This has been documented by electron microscopic studies in both rabbits and humans. *Cryptosporidium* and *Isospora* species, etiologic agents of diarrhea in animals and poultry and more recently recognized as causing human disease, probably also act by adhering to intestinal mucosa and disrupting function. Cryptosporidia are often seen in the diarrhea of patients with acquired immunodeficiency syndrome (AIDS), as well as in travelers' diarrhea, day-care epidemics, and diarrhea in people with animal exposure; both cryptosporidia and *Isospora* may cause severe, protracted diarrhea in AIDS patients. Other coccidian parasites such as microsporidia produce diarrhea by destroying intestinal cell function.

17.2.h. Other infectious causes of gastrointestinal disease. The curved organism associated with gastritis, called *"Campylobacter pylori,"* is seen on the surface of gastric epithelial cells of patients with gastritis and peptic ulcer. This organism is recovered from gastric biopsy material obtained endoscopically and not from stool.

Unusual agents and those that have not been cul-

tured, such as the mycobacteria that may be associated with Crohn's disease and the bacteria associated with Whipple's disease, are also candidates as etiologic agents of gastrointestinal disease. Occasionally, stool cultures from patients with diarrheal disease yield heavy growths of organisms such as *Pseudomonas* species or *Klebsiella pneumoniae*, not usually found in such numbers as normal flora. There is no definitive evidence that these organisms actually contribute to the pathogenesis of the diarrhea.

Agents of sexually transmitted disease may cause gastrointestinal symptoms when they are introduced into the colon via sexual intercourse. *Mycobacterium avium-intracellulare* may be transmitted in this way, going on to cause systemic disease in patients with AIDS. Homosexual practices predispose people to infections such as gonococcal and herpetic proctitis, syphilis, and others. Chapter 23 contains further discussion of patients at risk for these and other causes of gastrointestinal disease. The pathogenesis of infections due to *Blastocystis hominis* (a possible coccidian etiologic agent of human diarrheal disease) is not well documented, although these organisms are associated with gastrointestinal symptoms.

17.3. Collection and Transport of Stool Specimens

Specimens that can be delivered to the laboratory within 1 hour may be collected in a clean waxed cardboard or plastic container. Stool for direct wet mount examinations, *C. difficile* toxin assays, concentration for detection of ova and parasites, immunoelectron microscopy for detection of viruses, and ELISA or latex agglutination test for rotavirus must be sent to the laboratory without any added preservatives or liquids. Volume of stool at least equal to the size of a walnut is necessary for most procedures. If a delay longer than 2 hours is anticipated for stools for bacterial culture, the specimen should be placed in transport medium. For bacterial culture, Cary-Blair transport medium has been shown to preserve best the viability of intestinal pathogens, including *Campylobacter* and *Vibrio* species. Some workers recommend reducing the agar content of Cary-Blair medium from 0.5% to 0.16% for maintenance of *Campylobacter*. Buffered glycerol transport medium does not maintain these bacteria. Several manufactureres produce a small vial of Cary-Blair with a self-contained plastic scoop suitable for collecting samples. *Shigella* species are delicate; best recovery is obtained by inoculating media (brought to room temperature) directly at the bedside. If direct plating is not convenient, a transport medium of equal parts of glycerol and 0.033 M phosphate buffer (pH 7.0) will support viability of *Shigella* better than will Cary-Blair. For this purpose, maintenance of the glycerol transport medium at refrigerator or freezer temperatures will yield better results.

For detection of ova and parasites, polyvinyl alcohol (PVA) fixative is recommended (Chapter 44). One part fecal material should be added to three parts PVA. PVA vials are available commercially. Stools for virus culture must be refrigerated if they are not inoculated to media within 2 hours. A rectal swab, transported in modified Stuart's transport medium, is adequate for recovery of most viruses from feces. Stools received for detection of *C. difficile* cytotoxin should be refrigerated for a maximum of 48 hours until they are tested. The stool-free filtrate can be frozen without seriously affecting the qualitative results (although there is some loss of titer). Freezing whole stool will result in fewer positive results.

If an etiologic agent is not isolated with the first culture or visual examination, two additional specimens should be submitted to the laboratory over the next few days. Since organisms may be shed intermittently, collection of specimens at different times over several days should enhance recovery. Certain infectious agents, such as *Giardia*, may be difficult to detect, requiring the processing of multiple specimens over many weeks, duodenal aspirates (in the case of *Giardia*), or alternative methods.

If stool is unavailable, a rectal swab may be substituted as a specimen for bacterial or viral culture but it is not as good, particularly for diagnosis in adults. For suspected intestinal infection with *Campylobacter*, the swab must be placed in transport medium immediately to avoid drying. Swabs are not acceptable for detection of parasites or viral antigens. The swab should be placed in Cary-Blair transport medium. Further discussion of handling of stool can be found in an article by Sack et al.[12]

Other specimens that may be obtained for diagnosis of gastrointestinal tract infection include duodenal aspirates (usually for detection of *Giardia* or *Strongyloides*), which should be examined immediately by direct microscopy for presence of motile trophozoites, cultured for bacteria, and placed into PVA fixative. The laboratory should be informed in advance that such a specimen is going to be collected, so that the specimen can be processed and examined effectively. The "string test" has proven useful for diagnosis of duodenal parasites such as *Giardia* and for isolation of *S. typhi* from carriers and patients with acute typhoid fever. A weighted gelatin capsule containing a tightly wound length of string is swallowed by the patient, leaving the end of the string protruding from the patient's mouth (and taped to the cheek). After a predetermined time period, during which the capsule reaches the duodenum and dissolves, the string is pulled back out, covered with duodenal contents. This string must be delivered immediately to the laboratory. In the laboratory, the technologist strips the mucus and secretions that are attached to the string with sterile gloved fingers, depositing some material on slides for direct examination, some material into fixative for preparation of permanent stained mounts, and inoculating some material to appropriate media for isolation of bacteria.

Biopsy material and material from mucosal lesions may be obtained from patients during proctoscopy or sigmoidoscopy. Such material is often fixed for histological and pathological examinations. Microbiologists should handle such material as if it were feces, staining or culturing as requested. For detection of "*C. pylori*," biopsy material should be transported to the laboratory without diluent, ground in dextrose phosphate broth, and inoculated to culture media within 1 hour of collection.[8]

17.4. Direct Detection of Agents of Gastroenteritis in Feces

A direct wet mount of fecal material, particularly with liquid or unformed stool, is the fastest method for detection of motile trophozoites of *Dientamoeba fragilis*, *Entamoeba*, *Giardia*, and other intestinal parasites (that may not contribute to disease, but may alert the microbiologist to the possibility of finding other parasites), such as *Entamoeba coli*, *Endolimax nana*, *Chilomastix mesnili*, and *Trichomonas hominis*. Occasionally, the larvae or adult worms of other parasites may be visualized. Experienced observers can also see the refractile forms of cryptosporidia and many types of cysts on the direct wet mount. Examination of a direct wet mount of fecal material taken from an area with blood or mucus, with the addition of an equal portion of Loeffler's methylene blue, is helpful for detection of fecal leukocytes, which may aid in differentiating among the various types of diarrheal syndromes. If they are plentiful, the ova of intestinal parasites will be seen. Under phase-contrast and darkfield microscopy, the darting motility and curved forms of *Campylobacter* may be observed in a warm sample. Water, which will immobilize *Campylobacter*, should not be used. Trained observers working in endemic areas can recognize the characteristic appearance and motility of *V cholerae*.

Immunoelectron microscopy is a very rapid method for detecting rotavirus and Norwalk-like agents. Details of the procedures are discussed in Chapter 42. For most laboratories, electron microscopy is unavailable, and rotavirus is detected using a solid phase ELISA procedure or a latex agglutination test. Several manufacturers produce systems for detection of the antigen of rotavirus, including microbroth dilution well systems, plastic bead systems, and latex agglutination systems. For the immunoassay systems, the feces are diluted to suspend the viral antigens, the solid material is removed by filtration or centrifugation, and the filtrate is added to the immunoassay solid phase on which antibody to rotavirus has been adsorbed. After an attachment step, excess material is washed off and an enzyme-conjugated antibody is added. If viral antigens were present, the conjugate will adhere to the solid phase as well. With the addition of the proper substrate, the enzyme will effect a visible color change (further discussed in Chapter 12). Instructions for each of the commercial systems vary, but the results have been uniformly good, with detection of rotavirus by ELISA comparable to electron microscopy in sensitivity. The latex agglutination test exhibits similar sensitivity with a much less complex system. This high sensitivity is probably a result of the huge numbers of virus particles that are shed in the feces of patients with infection. ELISA methods are also available now for detection of antigens of *G. lamblia*. Because this organism is often difficult to detect visually, the commercial ELISA may prove to be a welcome diagnostic alternative to direct visualization, even when one considers the added sensitivity of monoclonal fluorescent stain reagents. ELISA methods have been evaluated for detection of certain bacterial pathogens.[7]

DNA probe technology is available commercially for detection of at least two fecal pathogens, *Cam-pylobacter* species and rotavirus. After the cells are lysed in stool, nucleic acids are extracted and fixed to a filter paper matrix, and target sequences are detected by enzyme-labeled probes (SNAP [synthetic nucleic acid probes], Molecular Biosystems). This technology is still in its infancy, although the concept is promising. Probes for *Salmonella*, *Shigella*, and *Yersinia* are being evaluated. Disadvantages with probe technology are that the organism itself is not available for susceptibility testing, important for certain bacterial pathogens for which susceptibility patterns vary.

Feces may be Gram-stained for detection of certain etiologic agents. Although gram-negative bacilli cannot be differentiated, sheets of polymorphonuclear neutrophils and many clumps of typical gram-positive cocci are indicative of staphylococcal infection (Figure 17.4). Many thin, comma-shaped gram-negative bacilli may indicate *Campylobacter* infection (if vibrios have been ruled out), and large numbers of gram-positive bacilli, large and thin with parallel walls, may be suggestive (but not reliable enough for routine use[2]) of overgrowth by *C. difficile* (Figure 17.5). An acid-fast stain should be used to detect *Cryptosporidium* species and mycobacteria. *Isospora* are also acid-fast. Examination of fixed fecal material for parasites by trichrome or other stains is thoroughly covered in Chapter 44. It is recommended that a permanent stained preparation be made from all stool specimens received in the laboratory for detection of parasites.

Giardia and cryptosporidia can easily and unequivocally be visualized with a monoclonal antibody fluorescent stain (Meridian Diagnostics). This stain is recommended for specimens from patients in whom these parasites are very likely or for specimens that yield suspicious results by standard methods.

17.5. Culture of Fecal Material for Isolation of Etiologic Agents of Gastrointestinal Disease

As outlined in Chapter 6, fecal specimens for culture should be inoculated to several media for maximum yield, including solid agar and broth. The choice of media is arbitrary and based on the particular requirements of the clinician and the laboratory. Recommendations are given in Section 17.5.a.

17.5.a. Cultures for bacterial etiologic agents. Stools received for routine culture in most clinical laboratories in the United States should be examined for the presence of *Campylobacter*, *Salmonella*, and

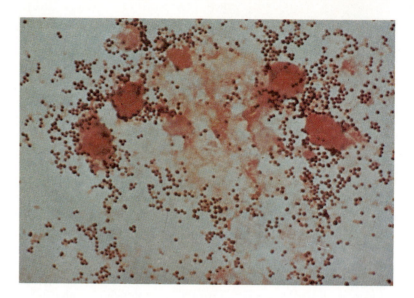

Figure 17.4
Gram stain of stool with staphylococcal
enterocolitis.

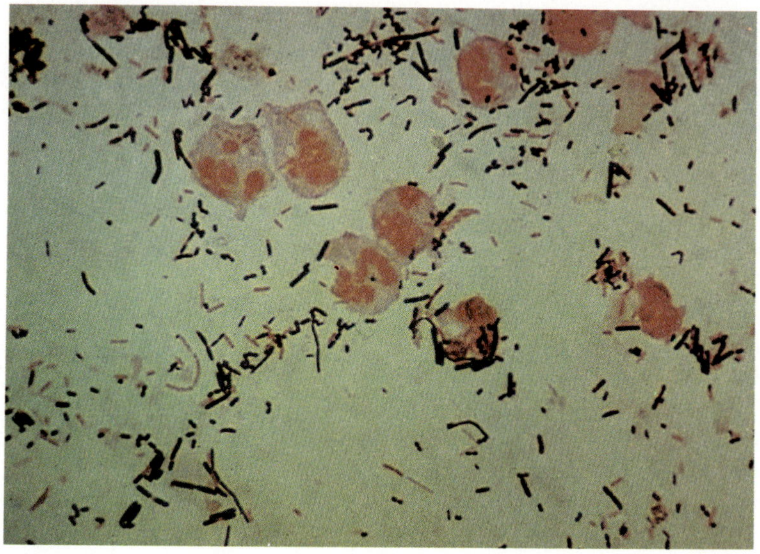

Figure 17.5
Gram stain of stool with *C. difficile*
pseudomembranous colitis.

Shigella species under all circumstances. An argument can also be made for performing procedures for detection of rotavirus as part of the standard protocol. If the incidence of *Y. enterocolitica* gastroenteritis is high enough in the area served by the laboratory, this agent should also be sought routinely. Special procedures for detection of vibrios, *C. difficile*, Verotoxin-producing *E. coli*, and mycobacteria should be carried out on request. *Vibrio* disease has become increasingly prevalent among travelers, as well as among individuals living in high risk areas of

the United States (seacoasts). We recommend, in addition, that detection of *Aeromonas* species should be incorporated into the routine stool culture procedures.

Specimens received for detection of the most commonly isolated Enterobacteriaceae, *Salmonella* and *Shigella* species, should be plated to a supportive medium, a slightly selective and differential medium, and a moderately selective medium. A highly selective medium does not seem to be cost effective for most microbiology laboratories. Blood agar (tryp-

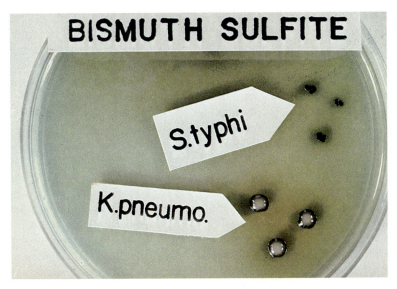

Figure 17.6
Appearance of colonies of *S. typhi* on bismuth sulfite agar.

tic soy agar with 5% sheep blood) is an excellent general supportive medium. Blood agar medium will allow growth of yeast species, staphylococci, and enterococci, in addition to gram-negative bacilli. If there is a predominance of a gram-positive organism, it will be detected on the blood agar. For routine cultures, use of an additional selective medium for detection of small numbers of gram-positive organisms does not seem warranted. Another benefit of blood agar is that it will allow oxidase testing of colonies. We recommend that several colonies (that do not resemble *Pseudomonas*) from the third or fourth quadrant be routinely screened for production of cytochrome oxidase. If large numbers of *Aeromonas*, *Vibrio*, or *Plesiomonas* species are present, they will be detected by their positive oxidase reaction.

The moderately selective agar should support growth of most Enterobacteriaceae, vibrios, and other possible pathogens, MacConkey agar seems to work very well. Some laboratories use eosin-methylene blue (EMB), which is slightly more inhibitory. All lactose-negative colonies should be tested further, ensuring adequate detection of most vibrios and most pathogenic Enterobacteriaceae. Lactose-positive vibrios (*V. vulnificus*), pathogenic *E. coli*, some *Aeromonas*, and *Plesiomonas* species will not be distinctive on MacConkey agar.

The specimen should also be inoculated to a mod-

erately selective agar such as Hektoen enteric (HE) or xylose-lysine desoxycholate (XLD) media. These media inhibit growth of most Enterobacteriaceae, allowing *Salmonella* and *Shigella* species to be detected. Colony morphologies of lactose-negative, lactose-positive, and H_2S-producing organisms are outlined in Chapter 8. The highly selective brilliant green (BG) or bismuth sulfite (BS) media may be used for detection of *Salmonella* species; they should be heavily inoculated, since they are quite inhibitory. *S. typhi* will often display silver metallic colonies with black halos surrounding them on BS (Figure 17.6), whereas salmonellas show pink colonies on BG. Other potential pathogens do not survive on these agars. All these media are incubated at 35° to 37° C in air and examined at 24 and 48 hours for suspicious colonies.

Verotoxin-producing *E. coli* serotype O157:H7 can be detected by screening on a sorbitol-containing selective medium (sorbitol-MacConkey, which contains 1% D-sorbitol instead of lactose), since these strains are unable to ferment sorbitol and 95% of other *E. coli* are sorbitol-positive. Suspicious colonies should be serotyped by slide and tube agglutination tests.[4] Final identification of Verotoxin-producing *E. coli* depends on the detection of Verotoxin by cell culture assay. Alternatively, stool filtrate may be tested for toxin production in Vero cells. Comprehensive and practical methods are described by Karmali[4] and a simpler approach is presented by Haldane and others.[3]

Cultures for isolation of *C. jejuni* and *Campylobacter coli* should be inoculated to Campy-blood agar (further discussed in Chapter 30). *Brucella* broth base has yielded less satisfactory recovery of *Campylobacter* species. Commercially produced agar plates for isolation of campylobacters are available from several manufacturers. These plates are incubated in a microaerophilic atmosphere at 42° C and examined at 24 and 48 hours for suspicious colonies (Chapter 30). Other campylobacters associated with gastrointestinal disease, such as *C. laridis*, *C. hyointestinalis*, and *C. fetus* ss. *fetus*, grow best at 37° C. Tenover and Gebhart[13] recommend that one selective agar be inoculated with fresh stool and one nonselective agar (trypticase-soy blood agar) be inoculated with stool filtrate that has been passed through a cellulose acetate filter of 0.65 or 0.8 µm pore size. The selective agar should be incubated at 42° C and the filtered stool on nonselective agar at 37° C. Although common campylobacters will be detected at 48 hours, incubating plates for 72 hours or longer will yield better recovery.

"*C. pylori*," associated with gastritis and possibly with peptic ulcer disease, can be isolated from gastric biopsy tissue by inoculating the specimen onto Skirrow agar or other Campylobacter agar containing blood and appropriate antimicrobial agents (cefoperazone is recommended) and incubating microaerophilically at 37° C in high humidity for up to 7 days. The organism may grow on chocolate, modified Thayer-Martin, or gonococcal agar base without supplements from some commercial suppliers; however, not all agars with the same formulas will support growth of "*C. pylori*." Alternatively, a small piece of tissue may be placed directly into urea broth base or onto a Christensen's urea agar slant. Demonstration of urease activity (often within 30 minutes but may take as long as 24 hours) is presumptive evidence of the presence of this organism.

Vibrios that are etiologic agents of gastroenteritis may be detected by screening all oxidase-positive colonies growing on blood agar. Many vibrios are β-hemolytic. For specific detection of *V. cholerae* and other vibrios, thiosulfate-citrate-bile salts–sucrose (TCBS) agar is recommended. The agar is heavily inoculated with feces, as are the moderately selective media, and incubated in air at 35° to 37° C

for up to 48 hours. Either large, flat, yellow or olive green colonies should be tested further.

A special medium has been developed for recovery of *Y. enterocolitica*. Often called CIN agar, this medium is made from a peptone agar base with mannitol, neutral red, crystal violet, and the antimicrobial agents cefsulodin, 3, 3′, 4′, 5-tetrachlorosalicylanilide (irgasan), and novobiocin. CIN agar is available commercially as powder or plates. The specimen is streaked on the agar, and the plate is incubated at room temperature for 48 hours. Colonies of *Y. enterocolitica* appear bright pink with a red center. Very few other organisms will grow on CIN agar, although some *Aeromonas* species have been found to grow very well on some formulations of this medium. If *Aeromonas* is suspected as the etiologic agent of diarrheal disease, we recommend inoculation of CIN agar at 37° C in addition to other media. A blood agar medium containing ampicillin has been used for selective recovery of *Aeromonas* with good success.

Enrichment broths are often used for enhanced recovery of *Salmonella*, *Shigella*, and *Campylobacter*, although *Shigella* will not survive enrichment. Gram-negative broth (Hajna GN) or selenite F broth yields good recovery. Campy-thioglycolate enrichment broth increases the yields of positive cultures for *Campylobacter* species, although it is not necessary for routine use. Enrichment broths for Enterobacteriaceae should be incubated in air at 35° C for 12 to 18 hours, and then several drops should be subcultured to at least two selective medium plates. A commercial system that allows such broth to be tested for antigen of *Salmonella* or *Shigella* directly has been described. Stool would be inoculated to broth only initially; those broths that tested negative could be discarded without subculturing. These systems have not been fully evaluated yet.

Enrichment broth for *Campylobacter* is refrigerated overnight or for a minimum of 8 hours before a few drops are plated to Campylobacter agar and incubated at 42° C in a microaerophilic atmosphere. *Y. enterocolitica* also can be "cold-enriched." A swab of fecal material is inoculated to a tube of 5 ml of phosphate-buffered saline (pH 7.2), and the tube is refrigerated for up to 21 days. A few drops are subcultured to CIN agar every 4 days and incubated in air at room temperature for up to 3 days. Such a cold enrichment procedure is most useful for epidemiologic studies, since results may not be known soon enough to benefit an individual patient. Alkaline peptone water (see Appendix A) has been shown to adequately enrich for vibrios. After 8 hours incubation, several drops from the broth should be inoculated to TCBS agar and incubated in air at 35° to 37° C.

C. difficile may be recovered by plating stool to cycloserine cefoxitin egg fructose agar (CCFA). Two or three drops (or 0.1 g) of stool are inoculated to CCFA and streaked for isolation. Plates are incubated anaerobically for 48 hours and examined for the characteristic large (4 mm diameter) yellow colonies with an opalescent sheen. *C. difficile* is one of the most oxygen-sensitive of the clinically important clostridia. For this reason, it may fail to grow from material inoculated to plates in the air and incubated in an anaerobic jar or plastic bag. Best recovery is obtained on freshly prepared plates inoculated with fecal material in an anaerobic chamber. *C. difficile* colonies will fluoresce yellow-green under ultraviolet light, and they exhibit a strong horse manure–like odor. *C. difficile* can be presumptively identified on the basis of colony and Gram stain morphology. Definitive identification is outlined in Chapter 35. Detection of *C. difficile* in stool of patients with diarrhea may be suggestive of PMC; however, this method is not specific, as up to 20% of hospitalized adult patients may be colonized with the organism, and the carriage rate in asymptomatic infants is high. At least one additional test (discussed in Section 17.6) should be performed for a more specific laboratory diagnosis. A good case can be made for not culturing for *C. difficile* in the clinical laboratory unless this is needed for epidemiologic reasons.

M. avium-intracellulare complex organisms may be isolated from the stool of patients with AIDS, and intestinal tuberculosis may still be suspected in some unusual cases. Methods for culturing acid fast bacilli from feces are discussed in Chapter 41. It is not recommended that clinical microbiology laboratories process stool for *M. tuberculosis,* since the procedure is so cumbersome. Reference laboratories are better equipped for such requests.

17.5.b. Cultures for viral etiologic agents. In addition to the viral agents of gastroenteritis, rotavirus, and Norwalk-like agent, whose detection is by latex agglutination, enzyme immunoassay, or electron microscopy, many viral agents of disease are routinely sought in feces. Fresh feces or rectal swabs are inoculated to antibiotic-containing media for 30 minutes before inoculating to tissue culture. Choice of tissue culture is determined by the etiologic agents sought, but feces are usually inoculated to primary monkey kidney, human fetal diploid fibroblast, and a human epithelial continuous cell line (Chapter 42).

17.6. Laboratory Diagnosis of *C. difficile*– Associated Diarrhea

The definitive diagnosis of *C. difficile*–associated diarrhea is based on clinical criteria. Visualization of characteristic pseudomembrane or plaque (Figure 17.2) on endoscopy is diagnostic for pseudomembranous colitis and, with the appropriate history of prior antibiotic usage, meets the criteria for diagnosis of antibiotic-associated pseudomembranous colitis. No one laboratory test will establish that diagnosis unequivocally; three tests are currently available for routine use. Culture on CCFA medium will detect the organism in most cases of *C. difficile*–associated diarrhea, although this test is not specific, and culture plates cannot be examined until after 48 hours of anaerobic incubation. Detection of cytotoxin by tissue culture is probably most closely associated with disease, although this test also suffers from false-positive and false-negative results in some patients, and results are not available for 48 hours. The tissue culture assay can be performed using any of several cell lines. Although it is possible to maintain a cell line in the laboratory, cell lines are also available commercially. Recently, a prepared microdilution tray containing tissue culture cells has been made available for the *C. difficile* toxin assay (Bartels Immunodiagnostics, Baxter Healthcare Systems). With the availability of this system, the cytotoxicity assay is within the ability of most clinical microbiology laboratories. A procedure for passage and maintenance of Hep-2 cells, a recommended cell line for the cytotoxic assay, is detailed in Chapter 42.

A very rapid latex agglutination assay for detection of a *C. difficile*–associated protein has shown good correlation with clinical diagnoses of *C. difficile*–associated disease. We recommend that microbiologists decide which tests best suit the needs of their clinicians and offer more than one test, perhaps in a reflexive panel. Several workers have published in this area,[1,5,9] and current knowledge is summarized in a reference volume.[11] Since both the cytotoxin and an enterotoxin have been shown to be important virulence factors for development of disease, laboratory tests to detect these toxins might prove more reliable for diagnosis. ELISA assays are being developed for this purpose, although they have not yet been released for routine use.

REFERENCES

1. Baron, E.J. 1989. Laboratory diagnosis of *Clostridium difficile*–associated diarrhea. Clin. Microbiol. Newsletter 11:118.
2. Gerding, D.N., Olson, M.M., Peterson, L.R., et al. 1986. Prospective case-controlled epidemiologic study of *Clostridium difficile*–associated diarrhea and colitis in adults. Arch. Intern. Med. 146:95.
3. Haldane, D.J.M., Damm, M.A.S., and Anderson, J.D. 1986. Improved biochemical screening procedure for small clinical laboratories for Vero (Shiga-like)-toxin–producing strains of *Escherichia coli* O157:H7. J. Clin. Microbiol. 24:652.
4. Karmali, M.A. 1987. Laboratory diagnosis of verotoxin-producing *Escherichia coli* infections. Clin. Microbiol. Newsletter 9:65.
5. Kelly, M.T., Champagne, S.G., Sherlock, C.H., et al. 1987. Commercial latex agglutination test for detection of *Clostridium difficile*–associated diarrhea. J. Clin. Microbiol. 25:1244.
6. Levine, M.M. 1987. *Escherichia coli* that cause diarrhea: enterotoxigenic, enteropathogenic, enteroinvasive, enterohemorrhagic, and enteroadherent. J. Infect. Dis. 155:377.
7. Pál, T., Páscsa, A.S., Emödy, L., et al. 1985. Modified enzyme-linked immunosorbent assay for detecting enteroinvasive *Escherichia coli* and virulent *Shigella* strains. J. Clin. Microbiol. 21:415.
8. Parsonnet, J., Welch, K., Compton, C., et al. 1988. Simple microbiologic detection of *Campylobacter pylori*. J. Clin. Microbiol. 26:948.
9. Peterson, L.R., Holter, J.J., Shanholtzer, C.J., et al. 1986. Detection of *Clostridium difficile* toxins A (enterotoxin) and B (cytotoxin) in clinical specimens (evaluation of a latex agglutination test). Am. J. Clin. Pathol. 86:208.
10. Ribi, H.O., Ludwig, D.S., Mercer, K.L., et al. 1988. Three-dimensional structure of cholera toxin penetrating a lipid membrane. Science 239:1272.
11. Rolfe, R.D., and Finegold, S.M., editors. 1988. *Clostridium difficile*: its role in intestinal disease, Academic Press, Orlando, Fla.
12. Sack, R.B., Tilton, R.C., and Weissfeld, A.S. 1980. Laboratory diagnosis of bacterial diarrhea. In Rubin, S.J., editor. Cumitech 12, American Society for Microbiology, Washington, D.C..
13. Tenover, F.C., and Gebhart, C.J. 1988. Isolation and identification of *Campylobacter* species. Clin. Microbiol. Newsletter 10:81.

BIBLIOGRAPHY

Brenden, R.A., Miller, M.A., and Janda, J.M. 1988. Clinical disease spectrum and pathogenic factors associated with *Plesiomonas shigelloides* infections in humans. Rev. Infect. Dis. 10:303.

Du Pont, H.L., and Pickering, L.K. 1980. Infections of the gastrointestinal tract. In Greenough, W.B., and Merigan, T.C., editors. Current topics in infectious disease. Plenum Publishing Co., New York.

George, W.L., Nakata, M.M., Thompson, J., and White, M.L. 1985. *Aeromonas*-related diarrhea in adults. Arch. Intern. Med. 145:2207.

Gradus, M.S. 1986. Public health criteria for the diagnosis of foodborne illness. Clin. Microbiol. Newsletter 8:85.

Guerrant, R.L. 1985. Principles and definition of syndromes of gastrointestinal infections and food poisoning. In Mandell, G.L., Douglas, R.G., Jr., and Bennett, J.E., editors. Principles and practice of infectious diseases, ed. 2. John Wiley & Sons, New York.

Guerrant, R.L. 1985. Inflammatory enteritides. In Mandell, G.L., Douglas, R.G., Jr., and Bennett, J.E., editors. Principles and practice of infectious diseases, ed. 2. John Wiley & Sons, New York.

Guerrant, R.L., and Hughes, J.M. 1985. Nausea, vomiting, and noninflammatory diarrhea. In Mandell, G.L., Douglas, R.G., Jr., and Bennett, J.E., editors. Principles and practice of infectious diseases, ed 2. John Wiley & Sons, New York.

Holmberg, S.D., Schell, W.L., Fanning, G.R., et al. 1986. Aeromonas intestinal infections in the United States. Ann. Intern. Med. 105:683.

Holmberg, S.D., Wachsmuth, I.K., Hickman-Brenner, F.W., et al. 1986. Plesiomonas enteric infections in the United States. Ann. Intern. Med. 105:690.

Middlebrook, J.L., and Dorland, R.B. 1984. Bacterial toxins: cellular mechanisms of action. Microbiol. Rev. 48:199.

Nelson, J.D. 1985. Etiology and epidemiology of diarrheal diseases in the United States. Amer. J. Med. 78(6B):76.

18 Microorganisms Encountered in the Urinary Tract

18.1. General Considerations, Anatomy, and Normal Flora

The urinary tract consists of the kidneys, the ureters, the bladder, and the urethra (Figure 18.1). Although the urethra hosts a resident microflora that colonizes its transitional epithelium, consisting of coagulase-negative staphylococci, viridans and nonhemolytic streptococci, lactobacilli, diphtheroids (*Corynebacterium* species), nonpathogenic *Neisseria* species, transient gram-negative aerobic bacilli (including Enterobacteriaceae), anaerobic cocci, *Propionibacterium* species, anaerobic gram-negative cocci and bacilli, commensal *Mycobacterium* species, commensal *Mycoplasma* species, and occasional yeasts, all areas of the urinary tract above the urethra in a healthy human are sterile. Because noninvasive methods for collecting urine must rely on a specimen that has passed through a contaminated milieu, special steps must be taken with collection, and interpretation of the results of cultures of such specimens requires that some discriminatory criteria be used. The use of quantitative cultures for diagnosis of urinary tract infections, first popularized by Kass,[5,6] has been modified to include separate quantitative criteria to be applied to different types of patients. Quantitative cultures of urine are still critical for diagnosis of urinary tract infection (UTI); however, the classical criterion of greater than 105 colony-forming units of bacteria per milliliter of urine as highly indicative of infection must be modified for different patient categories. This chapter will deal with various aspects of UTI and its laboratory diagnosis.

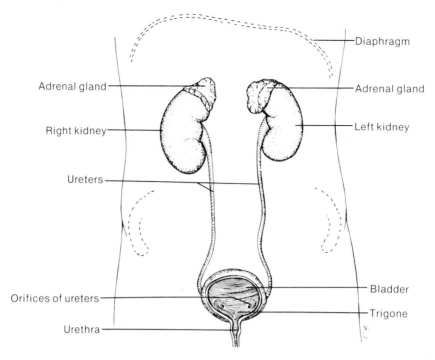

Figure 18.1

Overview of the anatomy of the urinary tract. (From Potter, P.H., and Perry, A.G. 1985. Fundamentals of nursing. The C.V. Mosby Co., St. Louis.)

18.2. Epidemiology and Pathogenesis of Urinary Tract Infections

UTIs are primarily of two types: cystitis, which is infection of the bladder, and pyelonephritis, which is infection of the renal parenchyma. Perinephric abscess is, as the name implies, an abscess adjacent to the kidney. Pyelitis and ureteritis do occur but are not commonly diagnosed as such. Urethritis, which is very common, is generally discussed as a sexually transmitted disease (Chapter 19), although the acute urethral syndrome (see below) is not usually placed in the sexually transmitted category, strictly speaking. UTIs are more common in women than in men, at least partially because of the short female urethra and its proximity to the anus. Additionally, sexual activity serves to increase the chances of bacterial contamination of the female urethra, pregnancy causes anatomic and hormonal changes that favor development of UTIs, and changes in the genitourinary tract mucosa related to menopause may play a role. Colonization of the introitus by coliforms is a major background factor for recurrent bladder infection in females. It is esti-

mated that approximately 20% of all women have a UTI at least once, with the incidence increasing with age. Among *asymptomatic* females of childbearing age or older, a culture yielding greater than 10^5 organisms per milliliter of a single bacterial species is very likely to correspond to UTI. If a repeat specimen also yields the same result with the same organism, presence of infection is 95% certain.

The incidence of UTI among males is low until after age 60; prostatic hypertrophy then contributes to development of UTI. Bacterial prostatitis is the key background factor for the problem of recurrent cystitis in males. Any anatomic barrier to free flow of urine through the urinary tract contributes to development of UTI; involved are prostatic hypertrophy, neurogenic disorders, tumors, and stones. Previous infection with certain urea-splitting organisms, notably *Proteus* and related species, is often associated with the formation of urinary stones, which further predispose the patient to infection. The introduction of a foreign body into the urinary tract, especially one that remains in place for a time (such as a Foley catheter), carries a substantial risk of leading to infection, particularly if obstruction is present. As many as 20% of all hospitalized patients who receive short-term catheterization develop a UTI. Consequently, UTI is the most common nosocomial infection in the United States and the infected urinary tract is the most common source of bacteremia.

Most infections involving the kidneys are acquired by the *ascending route* (bacteria migrate from the bladder to reach the tissues of the kidneys). However, yeast (usually *Candida albicans*), *Mycobacterium tuberculosis*, *Salmonella* species, *Leptospira* species, or *Staphylococcus aureus* in the urine often indicate pyelonephritis acquired via **hematogenous** spread, or the *descending route.*

Among the bacteria most commonly isolated from patients (overwhelmingly women) suffering from community-acquired acute cystitis are *Escherichia coli*, *Klebsiella* species, other Enterobacteriaceae, and *Staphylococcus saprophyticus*. Hospitalized patients are most likely to be infected by *E. coli*, *Klebsiella* species, *Proteus mirabilis*, other Enterobacteriaceae, *Pseudomonas aeruginosa*, and enterococci. Other less commonly isolated agents are other gram-negative bacilli such as *Acinetobacter* and *Alcaligenes* species, other *Pseudomonas* species, *Citrobacter* species, *Gardnerella vaginalis*, β-hemolytic streptococci, and *Neisseria gonorrhoeae*. *Trichomonas vaginalis* may occasionally be observed in urinary sediment and *Schistosoma haematobium* can lodge in the urinary tract and release eggs into the urine.

In most hospitalized patients, UTI is preceded by urinary catheterization or other manipulation of the urinary tract. Although the pathogenesis of catheter-associated UTI is not fully understood, certain possibilities have been discussed. It is certain that soon after hospitalization, patients become colonized with bacteria endemic to the institution, often gram-negative aerobic and facultative bacilli carrying resistance markers. These bacteria colonize patients' skin, gastrointestinal tract, and mucous membranes, including the anterior urethra. With insertion of a catheter, the bacteria may be pushed along the urethra into the bladder or, in the case of an indwelling catheter, may migrate along the track between the catheter and the urethral mucosa, gaining access to the bladder. There has been some suggestion that nosocomial UTIs caused by certain bacteria, notably *Serratia marcescens*, are more likely to result in secondary bacteremia.

Certain women are more likely to suffer from chronic or recurrent UTIs. Several studies by Leffler and Svanborg-Eden[7] and Svanborg-Eden and Jodal[12] have shown stronger binding of *E. coli* isolated from infected urine to the genitourinary tract epithelial cells of infection-prone women than to noninfected controls. The organisms themselves may have adherence mechanisms that allow them to adhere well. Mechanisms by which other common etiologic agents of UTI produce disease are not yet well understood. It is probable that their presence induces an inflammatory response, which in turn causes tissue destruction and the characteristic pain, burning, and urinary frequency of acute cystitis. Damage to renal parenchyma that occurs in pyelonephritis results in flank pain, fever and other systemic symptoms, or sometimes no symptoms until much damage has occurred.

Another urinary tract infection that has only recently been defined is the **acute urethral syndrome,** studied by Stamm.[11] Women, primarily young, sexually active women, experience dysuria, frequency, and urgency but yield fewer organisms than 10^5/ml urine on culture. As many as one third of all women who seek medical attention for complaints of symptoms of acute cystitis fall into this group. Although *Chlamydia trachomatis* and *N. gonorrhoeae* urethritis, anaerobic infection, genital herpes, and vaginitis account for some cases of acute urethral syndrome, most of these women are infected with organisms identical to those that cause cystitis, but in numbers less than 10^5/ml urine. One must use a cutoff of 10^2/ml, rather than 10^5/ml, in this group, but must insist on concomitant pyuria. The leukocyte esterase test (discussed in Section 18.4) is not sensitive enough for determining pyuria in these cases. Approximately 90% of these women have pyuria, an important discriminatory feature of infection. Recognition of this large class of patients with UTI that do not fit into classic categories has led to a reexamination of the criteria used to discriminate between urine specimens from patients with infection and those specimens from which culture results indicate only contamination.

Patients with true UTIs whose urine may yield fewer numbers of bacteria than the classic 10^5/ml include infants and children, males, catheterized patients, patients who have received antibacterial agents previously, patients who consume large amounts of liquid and thus dilute bladder urine, symptomatic patients (usually with pyuria), patients with urinary obstruction that may prevent organisms from being excreted, and patients with pyelonephritis acquired from hematogenous spread (particularly yeast, *S. aureus*, and *M. tuberculosis* infections). For this reason, good communication between clinicians and microbiologists is essential for proper interpretation of urine culture results. If laboratorians also quantitate polymorphonuclear neutrophils in urine, as they should, the diagnostic value of a urine specimen is increased significantly, just as it is for sputum or other specimens.

18.3. Collection and Transport of Urine Specimens

Prevention of contamination by normal vaginal, perineal, and anterior urethral flora is the most important consideration for collection of a clinically relevant urine specimen. The least invasive procedure, that of the *clean-catch, midstream urine specimen collection*, must be performed carefully for optimal results, especially in females. Good patient education is essential. A method for collection of such a specimen is detailed in Chapter 6. Uncleansed first-void specimens from males were shown to be as sensitive as (but less specific than) midstream urine specimens.[8] If the clinician wishes to determine whether UTI in a male is localized to the bladder or the prostate using a noninvasive procedure, the three-glass collection procedure may be used. The first specimen collected is the initial 5 to 10 ml voided; this represents the "urethral" specimen. The next ounce or so of voided urine is discarded, and then an additional 10 ml is collected (the "midstream" specimen). After the bladder has been emptied, the patient is given a prostatic massage and the third specimen is the next 10 ml of urine and that will include prostate secretions that accumulate. A higher count of organisms in the third specimen of urine than in the first indicates prostatic infection. Some physicians prefer to culture expressed prostatic secretions separately and then obtain another 10-ml urine specimen following this.

Slightly more invasive, urinary catheterization may allow collection of bladder urine with less urethral contamination. There is the risk, however, that urethral organisms will be introduced into the bladder with the catheter. **Suprapubic bladder aspiration,** withdrawal of bladder urine directly into a syringe through a percutaneously inserted needle, ensures a contamination-free specimen. This procedure can be performed with little risk in infants, small children, and adults with full bladders.

Collection of specimens from patients with indwelling catheters requires scrupulous aseptic technique. Health care workers who manipulate a urinary catheter in any way should wash their hands before and after the procedure or, preferably, should wear gloves. The catheter port or wall of the tubing should be cleaned vigorously with 70% ethanol and urine should be aspirated via a needle and syringe; the integrity of the closed drainage system must be maintained to prevent the introduction of organisms into the bladder. Specimens obtained from the collection bag are inappropriate, as organisms can multiply there, obscuring the true relative numbers.[17] Cultures should be obtained when patients are ill; routine monitoring does not yield clinically relevant data.[2]

Urine, being an excellent supportive medium for growth of most bacteria, must be immediately refrigerated or preserved. Bacterial counts in refrigerated (4° C) urine remain constant for as long as 24 hours. A urine transport tube, B-D Urine Culture Kit (Becton Dickinson Vacutainer Kits) containing boric acid, glycerol, and sodium formate, has been shown to preserve bacteria without refrigeration for as long as 24 hours when greater than 100,000 organisms per milliliter were present in the initial urine specimen, as reviewed by Weinstein.[15] The system may inhibit the growth of certain organisms, and it must be used with 3 to 5 ml of urine. Another preservative system (Sage Products) may be less toxic to bacteria, although counts failed to remain completely stable for periods longer than 4 hours. A new lyophilized system may prove to be more beneficial, but for populations of patients from whom colony counts of organisms of less than 100,000/ml might be clinically significant, the current preservative is not recommended. None of the kits has any advantage whatever over refrigeration except, perhaps, convenience.

18.4. Rapid Screening Tests and Nonculture Tests for UTI

As many as 60% to 80% of all urine specimens received for culture by the average hospital laboratory may contain only contaminants or no etiologic agents of infection. Procedures developed to quickly identify those urine specimens that will be "negative" on culture, to thus circumvent excessive use of media, technologist time, and the overnight incubation period, are discussed in this section. The Gram stain is the easiest and least expensive, and probably the most sensitive and reliable, screening method for identifying urine specimens that contain $>10^5$ colony-forming units (CFU) per milliliter. As outlined by Washington et al.,[14] a drop of well-mixed urine is allowed to air dry. The smear is stained and examined under oil immersion $(1,000\times)$. Presence of at least one organism per field (examining 20 fields) correlates with significant bacteriuria $(>10^5$ CFU/ml). The Gram stain should not be relied on for detecting polymorphonuclear leukocytes in urine.[1] Most microbiologists are unwilling to adopt this procedure as part of the routine laboratory examination of urine specimens, probably because of the low number of positive results.

Several chemical tests, impregnated onto paper strips, can be used to assess parameters that may indicate UTI. The "Griess test" for presence of nitrate-reducing enzymes, produced by the most common urinary tract pathogens, has been incorporated onto a paper strip that also tests for leukocyte esterase, an enzyme produced by polymorphonuclear neutrophils. These strips are available commercially (LN Strip and Chemstrip 9, Bio-Dynamics). Triphenyltetrazolium chloride is reduced by a number of commonly encountered urinary tract pathogens and can be impregnated into a strip test, but this test has not achieved wide usage. The sensitivity of these screening tests is not great enough to recommend their use (as a stand-alone test) in most circumstances.

Two automated methodologies have been used for screening urine specimens. The detection of bacterial adenosine triphosphate (ATP) by measuring light emitted by the reaction of luciferin-luciferase has been exploited by several companies (Chapter 11). After somatic cell ATP is removed by selectively disrupting somatic cells enzymatically, the bacterial cells are lysed and the released ATP is allowed to drive the light-producing reaction. Photons are measured, correlating with the numbers of bacteria present in the sample. Systems may require measurements to be made before and after a short incubation period, which allows bacteria to multiply; or they may measure the amount of ATP in the bacteria in the sample directly. These systems are somewhat expensive and do take time, and therefore are not suitable for every laboratory. Improvements in the ease of their use and decreasing test time will serve to make the luminescent tests more attractive to laboratories for screening urine specimens in the future.

The Bac-T-Screen Bacteriuria Detection Device (Vitek Systems, Inc.) uses a different approach (Chapter 11, Figure 11.5). Urine is forced through a filter paper, which retains microorganisms, somatic cells, and other particles. A dye is then added to the filter paper to visualize the particulate matter that has adhered. The intensity of color relates to the number of particles (Figure 11.6). This procedure, which takes approximately 1 minute, has been shown to detect greater than 90% of all positive urine specimens, even if 100 organisms per milliliter are considered to be significant.[1,9,10] The detection of somatic cells and particles as well as bacteria and yeast probably accounts for the increased sensitivity of this system at low numbers of CFU.[1,16] Organisms likely to be associated with false-negative results include enterococci and *P. aeruginosa*; the reason for this is not known.

Screening of urine can also be accomplished simply by enumerating polymorphonuclear neutrophils (PMNs) in uncentrifuged specimens, which correlates fairly well with the number of PMNs excreted per hour, the best indicator of the state of the host. Patients with more than 400,000 PMNs excreted into the urine per hour are likely to be infected, and the presence of more than 8 PMNs/mm^3 correlates well with this excretion rate and with infection.[3] This test can be performed using a hemocytometer, but it is not easily incorporated into the workflow of most microbiology laboratories. The standard urinalysis (usually done in hematology or chemistry sections) includes an examination of the *centrifuged* sediment of urine for enumeration of PMNs, results of which do not correlate well with either PMN excretion rate or the presence of infection.

Given the importance of the 10^2/ml count and the PMN count, no screening test should be used indiscriminately. In general, there is a cost advantage to screening only in laboratories receiving a large number of inappropriate specimens; accordingly, education of physicians is one important approach. Good medical practice and cost-effective microbiology dictate that only urine from patients with symptoms of UTI plus a selected group expected to have asymptomatic bacteriuria (for example, patients in the first trimester of pregnancy) should be cultured. Other situations in which patients with no symptoms of UTI might be cultured include bacteremia of unknown source, patients with urinary tract obstruction, follow-up after removal of an indwelling urinary catheter, and follow-up of previous therapy. It must also be remembered that screening may delay culture results, especially if one of the rapid, automated instruments for urine culturing is used.

Developed in 1974, the "antibody-coated bacteria test" is used to localize the site of infection to the bladder (cystitis) or renal tissue (pyelonephritis), using a noninvasive technique. Previous methods required collection of urine directly from the renal pelvis (an invasive procedure), bilateral ureteral catheterization after bladder washout, or direct tissue biopsy. Since simple bladder infection can usually be treated effectively by administration of a single large dose of an appropriate antimicrobial agent, it is important to be able to differentiate such an infection from one that requires more prolonged therapy. Incidentally, many clinicians use response to single-dose treatment as a means of distinguishing between upper and lower tract infection. The antibody-coated bacteria test consists of washing the centrifuged sediment of urine containing bacteria and then staining the washed bacteria with fluorescein-conjugated antihuman globulin. The bacterial cells are again washed to remove nonspecifically bound conjugate and the bacteria are examined under ultraviolet light. If at least one fourth of the bacteria are fluorescent, indicating the presence of human immunoglobulin on their surface, the test is considered positive and the patient is considered to have a more deep-seated infection than cystitis.[13] Although not difficult to perform, lack of standardization among laboratories and lack of uniformly available reagents have caused confusion in interpretation of results among different laboratories. Furthermore, there may be both false-positive and false-negative results. This test seems to be useful in certain settings but, in its present state, is not warranted for general testing.

18.5. Methods for Culturing Urine and Interpretive Criteria

18.5.a. Routine culture. Once it has been determined that a urine specimen should be cultured for isolation of the common agents of UTI, a measured amount of urine is inoculated to each of the appropriate media. The urine should be mixed thoroughly before plating. The plates can be inoculated using disposable sterile plastic tips with a displacement pipetting device, calibrated to deliver a constant amount, but this method is somewhat cumbersome. Most commonly, microbiologists use a **calibrated loop** designed to deliver a known volume, either 0.01 or 0.001 ml of urine. We recommend the larger volume to detect lower numbers of organisms that may be important in patient groups discussed in Section 18.2. These loops, made of platinum or other material, can be obtained from a number of laboratory supply companies (Appendix C). They must be inserted into the urine in a cup *vertically* or they will pick up more than the desired volume of urine. A widely used method is described in Procedure 18.1.

The choice of which media to inoculate is dependent upon the patient population served and the preference of the microbiologist. The use of a 5% sheep blood agar plate and a MacConkey agar plate will allow detection of most gram-negative bacilli and staphylococci. Enterococci and other streptococci, however, may be obscured by heavy growth of Enterobacteriaceae. The addition of a selective plate for gram-positive organisms, such as Columbia colistin-nalidixic acid agar (CNA) or phenylethyl alcohol agar may add discriminatory capability but also adds cost to the procedure. A recommended approach is to inoculate routine urine specimens to a MacConkey and a CNA plate. Any urine specimens received from female patients (who may be infected with *S. saprophyticus*, which is somewhat inhibited on CNA), from patients presenting diagnostic dilemmas, or that were collected by any technique other than clean-catch, midstream urine collection should be inoculated additionally to sheep blood agar.

18.5.b. Specimens from patients with indwelling catheters. The numbers of patients in hospitals and nursing homes with long-term indwelling urinary catheters continues to increase. These patients ultimately develop bacteriuria, which predisposes them to more severe infections. York and Brooks[17] suggest that urine be cultured quantitatively by allowing a 0.05 ml drop of mixed urine to run down the center of each half of a biplate containing blood agar and CNA and estimating CFU by comparing growth patterns to photographs. Additional urine is plated to a supportive and selective, differential agar biplate and streaked to obtain isolated colonies. All bacterial species in numbers greater than 10^2 CFU/ml, with the exception of normal skin or genital flora, are identified and susceptibilities are performed on gram-negative bacilli and *S. aureus*. Other methods that allow detection and identification of small numbers of organisms and separation of species in mixed culture are acceptable for specimens from patients with indwelling catheters.

18.5.c. Interpreting culture results. Growth of more than three species is usually considered indicative of contamination in routine urine cultures. For such cultures, the organisms are minimally identi-

fied (such as lactose-positive gram-negative rods and coagulase-negative staphylococci) and enumerated. Susceptibility tests are not performed. Plates from such cultures are held, however, as there are situations in which growth of more than three organisms may be significant (for example, patients with Foley catheters) and the physician always should have the option of calling the laboratory to request more de-

---

PROCEDURE 18.1

Inoculating Urine with a Calibrated Loop

Principle

The number of microorganisms per milliliter recovered on urine culture can aid in the differential diagnosis of UTI. Plastic or wire loops, available commercially, have been calibrated to deliver a known volume of liquid when handled correctly, thus enabling the microbiologist to estimate numbers of organisms in the original specimen based on CFU/ml growth on cultures.

Method

1. Flame a wire calibrated inoculating loop. Allow it to cool without touching any surface. Alternatively, aseptically remove a plastic calibrated loop from its package.
2. Mix the urine thoroughly and remove the top of the container. If the urine is in a small diameter tube, the surface tension will alter the amount of specimen picked up by the loop. A quantitative pipette should be considered if the urine cannot be transferred to a larger container.
3. Insert the loop vertically into the urine (Figure 18.2) to allow urine to adhere to the loop.
4. Spread the loopful of urine over the surface of the agar plate as shown in Figure 18.3. A standard quadrant streaking technique is also acceptable.
5. Without reflaming, insert the loop vertically into the urine again for transfer of a loopful to a second plate. Repeat for each plate.
6. Incubate plates for at least 18 hours at 35° to 37° C in air. Colonies are counted on each

plate. The number of CFU is multiplied by 1000 (if a 0.001-ml loop was used) or by 100 (if a 0.01-ml loop was used) to determine the number of microorganisms per milliliter in the original specimen.
7. Reincubate plates with no growth or tiny colonies for an additional 24 hours, because antimicrobial treatment or other factors may inhibit initial growth, before discarding plates.
8. It is desirable to store the loop (handle down) in a test tube taped to the wall, rather than flat on the bench, in order to prevent bending, which would destroy the calibration.

Quality control

Calibrated loops should be tested for proper volume delivery by using the loop to add dye to a measured volume of distilled water and then reading the optical density of the suspension spectrophotometrically, as described in Cumitech 2A.[3]

Expected results

The loops should dispense the correct volume ± 10%.

Performance schedule

Wire loops should be tested monthly, as they tend to bend and become encrusted and lose accuracy. Plastic loops may be tested once for each new lot number, although once a manufacturer's product has been determined to be accurate, it is unlikely to change much.

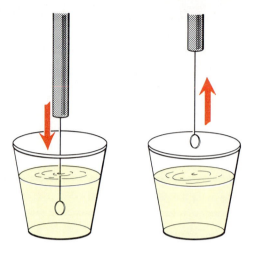

Figure 18.2
Method for inserting a calibrated loop into urine to ensure that the proper amount of specimen will adhere to the loop.

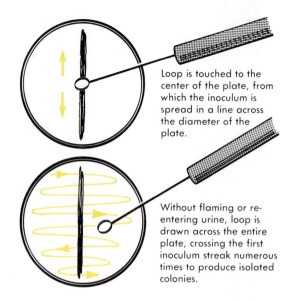

Loop is touched to the center of the plate, from which the inoculum is spread in a line across the diameter of the plate.

Without flaming or re-entering urine, loop is drawn across the entire plate, crossing the first inoculum streak numerous times to produce isolated colonies.

Figure 18.3
Method for streaking with calibrated urine loop to produce isolated colonies and countable CFUs of organisms.

finitive studies. Specimens from patients with long-term indwelling catheters yield an average of five species, each in numbers greater than 10^5 CFU/ml.[4] Because of the polymicrobic nature of infection in these patients, all species except skin and genital commensals should be evaluated.

Growth of less than 10,000 CFU/ml of one or two organisms may indicate infection. A CFU $>10^3$/ml has been shown to be significant in males.[8] The organisms are identified, but susceptibility studies are not performed unless the clinician notifies the laboratory to do so. One or two strains growing in numbers greater than 10,000/ml from routine urine specimens are identified and tested for antimicrobial susceptibilities. A pure culture of *S. aureus* is considered to be significant regardless of the number of CFU, and susceptibility tests are performed. The presence of yeast in any number is reported to physicians, and pure cultures of a yeast may be identified as to species.

18.5.d. Unusual etiologic agents of UTI. Culture methods for isolation of mycobacteria, *Haemophilus influenzae, Leptospira, Gardnerella vaginalis, T. vaginalis*, and other more rarely encountered agents of UTI are discussed in appropriate other areas of this book. *Salmonella* are recovered during the early stages of typhoid fever; their presence should be immediately reported to the physician. If anaerobes are suspected, percutaneous bladder tap should be done by the physician unless urine can be obtained from the upper urinary tract (for example, from a nephrostomy tube). Most important for detecting such agents is communication to the laboratory by the clinician that such an agent is suspected. However, the laboratory can exert some initiative here as well. In cases of "sterile pyuria," Gram stain may reveal unusual organisms with distinctive morphology (*H. influenzae* and anaerobes, for example). Presence of any organisms on smear that do not grow in culture is an important clue to the cause of the infection. The laboratory can then take the action necessary to optimize chances for recovery, whether it includes inoculating a special medium or examining a spun sediment under phase-contrast microscopy.

18.6. Automated Nonscreening Methods for Laboratory Diagnosis of UTI

Several instruments have been developed for the "hands-off" detection of bacteriuria. The principles employed by these systems are described in Chapter 11. The Autobac (Organon-Teknika Corp.) uses nephelometric determinations to identify numbers of bacteria in urine. The urine specimen is introduced to the instrument in a cuvette, which allows the urine to be diluted out into growth media containing different substrates. During incubation with shaking, growth in the cuvette is periodically monitored by measuring the amount of light scatter that occurs in the growth wells compared with a control well. An internal computer processes the information. Within 6 hours, most negative urine specimens can be identified. Those urine specimens that contain significant counts of bacteria (CFU $>10^5$/ml) are usually identified within 3 hours. Preliminary identification of the organisms is achieved by determining in which substrates growth occurred. Note that urine containing less than 10^5 CFU/ml will not be considered positive with such a system.

The AutoMicrobic System (Vitek Systems) is the most labor-free screening system. Once the urine is introduced into the tiny wells of a plastic substrate card by vacuum suction and the card is placed into the instrument, it is incubated and examined periodically by measuring the amount of light that passes through the individual wells. The wells contain substrates that can be utilized by only certain etiologic agents of UTI. After 6 to 8 hours, microorganisms will grow in the appropriate substrate wells and be detected by increased turbidity. The internal computer issues a colony count and a preliminary identification of the agent or agents identified. In this system as well, low counts of bacteria or yeast will be considered negative urine cultures.

The MS-2 and the Avantage (Abbott Laboratories Diagnostics Division) use a cuvette system similar to that of the Autobac. Urine specimens can be screened within 3 hours, as is true in most cases for the other automated systems, although positive results are reported more quickly with the MS-2.

Since most clinical laboratories receive more urine specimens than specimens of any other type, it is important that laboratories develop an efficient, cost-effective way of handling them. It seems that some form of preliminary screening system to rule out negative cultures, combined with a standard method for quantifying and identifying significant etiologic agents of UTI, will be of most benefit to the patients being served. Strategies employed by laboratories in hospitals that must cut costs without sacrificing patient-relevant quality are discussed in Chapter 4.

REFERENCES

1. Baron, E.J., Tyburski, M.B., Almon, R., and Berman, M. 1988. Visual and clinical analysis of Bac-T-Screen urine screen results. J. Clin. Microbiol. 26:2382.
2. Breitenbucher, R.B. 1984. Bacterial changes in the urine samples of patients with long-term indwelling cathethers. Arch. Intern. Med. 144:1585.
3. Clarridge, J.E., Pezzlo, M.T., and Vosti, K.L. 1987. Laboratory diagnosis of urinary tract infections. In Weissfeld, A.S., coordinating editor, Cumitech 2A. American Society for Microbiology, Washington, D.C.
4. Damron, D.J., Warren, J.W., Chippendale, G.R., and Tenney, J.H. 1986. Do clinical microbiology laboratories report complete bacteriology in urine from patients with long-term urinary catheters? J. Clin. Microbiol. 24:400.
5. Kass, E.H. 1956. Asymptomatic infections of the urinary tract. Trans. Assoc. Am. Physicians 69:56.
6. Kass, E.H. 1960. The role of asymptomatic bacteriuria in the pathogenesis of pyelonephritis. In Quinn, E.L., and Kass, E.H., editors: Biology of pyelonephritis. Little, Brown & Co., Boston.
7. Leffler, H., and Svanborg-Eden, C. 1981. Glycolipid receptors for uropathogenic *Escherichia coli* on human erythrocytes and uroepithelial cells. Infect. Immun. 34:920.
8. Lipsky, B.A., Ireton, R.C, Fihn, S.D., et al. 1987. Diagnosis of bacteriuria in men: specimen collection and culture interpretation. J. Infect. Dis. 155:847.
9. Murray, P.R., Niles, A.C., Heeren, R.L., and Pikul, F. 1988. Evaluation of the modified Bac-T-Screen and FiltraCheck-UTI urine screening systems for detection of clinically significant bacteriuria. J. Clin. Microbiol. 26:2347.
10. Pfaller, M., Ringenberg, B., Rames, L., et al. 1987. The usefulness of screening tests for pyuria in combination with culture in the diagnosis of urinary tract infection. Diagn. Microbiol. Infect. Dis. 6:207.
11. Stamm, W.E. 1980. Causes of the acute urethral syndrome in women. N. Engl. J. Med. 303:409.
12. Svanborg-Eden, C., and Jodal, U. 1979. Attachment of *Escherichia coli* to urinary sediment epithelial cells from UYIT-prone and healthy children. Infect. Immun. 26:837.
13. Thomas, V.L. 1983. The antibody-coated bacteria test: uses and findings. Lab. Management 21:39.
14. Washington, J.A. II, White, C.M., Laganiere, M., and Smith, L.H. 1981. Detection of significant bacteriuria by microscopic examination of urine. Lab. Med. 12:294.
15. Weinstein, M.P. 1983. Evaluation of liquid and lyophilized preservatives for urine culture. J. Clin. Microbiol. 18:912.
16. Wright, D.N., Saxon, B., and Matsen, J.M. 1986. Use of the Bac-T-Screen to predict bacteriuria from urine specimens held at room temperature. J. Clin. Microbiol. 24:214.
17. York, M.K., and Brooks, G.F. 1987. Evaluation of urine specimens from the catheterized patient. Clin. Microbiol. Newsletter 9:76.

BIBLIOGRAPHY

Edberg, S.C. 1981. Methods of quantitative microbiological analyses that support the diagnosis, treatment, and prognosis of human infection. CRC Crit. Rev. Microbiol. 8:339.

Fihn, S., and Stamm, W.E. 1983. Management of women with acute dysuria. In Rund, D.A., and Wolcott, B.W., editors: Emergency medicine annual, vol 2. Appleton-Century-Crofts, East Norwalk, Conn.

Gabre-Kidan, T., Lipsky, B.A., and Plorde, J.J. 1984. *Haemophilus influenzae* as a cause of urinary tract infections in men. Arch. Intern. Med. 144:1623.

Kunin, C.M. 1987. Detection, prevention, and management of urinary tract infections, ed. 4. Lea & Febiger, Philadelphia.

Platt, R. 1983. Quantitative definition of bacteriuria. Am. J. Med. 75:44.

Stamm, W.E. 1983. Interpretation of urine cultures. Clin. Microbiol. Newsletter 5:15.

Stamm, W.E. 1983. Measurement of pyuria and its relation to bacteriuria. Am. J. Med. 75:53.

Stamm, W.E., and Turck, M. 1983. Urinary tract infection. Year Book Medical Publishers, Chicago.

Wright, D.N., and Matsen, J.M. 1984. Diagnosing urinary tract infection. Diagn. Med. 7:44.

19

Genital and Sexually Transmitted Pathogens

19.1. Normal and Pathogenic Flora of the Genital Tract

The lining of the normal human genital tract is a mucosal layer made up of transitional, columnar, and squamous epithelial cells. A variety of species of commensal bacteria colonize these surfaces, causing no harm to the host except under abnormal circumstances, and helping to prevent the adherence of pathogenic organisms. Normal urethral flora include coagulase-negative staphylococci and corynebacteria, as well as a number of anaerobes. The vulva and penis, especially the area underneath the prepuce (foreskin) of the uncircumcised male, may harbor *Mycobacterium smegmatis* along with other gram-positive bacteria. The flora of the female genital tract (Figure 19.1) varies with the pH and estrogen concentration of the mucosa, which is dependent on the age of the host. Prepubescent and postmenopausal women harbor primarily staphylococci and corynebacteria, the same flora present on surface epithelium, while women of reproductive age may harbor large numbers of facultative bacteria such as Enterobacteriaceae, streptococci, and staphylococci, as well as anaerobes such as lactobacilli, anaerobic non–spore-forming bacilli and cocci, and clostridia. The numbers of anaerobic organisms remain constant throughout the monthly cycle. Many women carry group B β-hemolytic streptococci *(Streptococcus agalactiae)*, which may be transmitted to the neonate as it passes through the birth canal and may cause devastating systemic disease. Treatment of the mother to prevent carriage of the organism is not feasible, and whether a colonized infant will become ill cannot be predicted. Although yeasts (acquired from the gastrointestinal tract) may

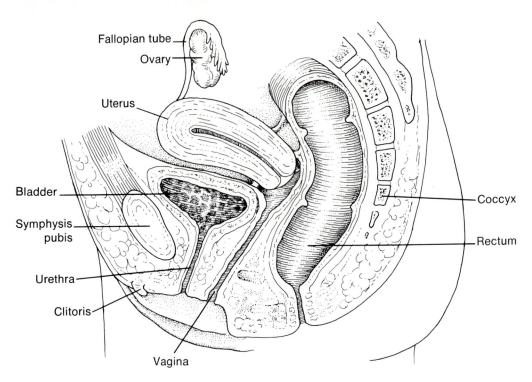

Diagrammatic representation of the female genital tract. (From Broadwell, D.C., and Jackson, B.S. 1982. Principles of ostomy care. The C.V. Mosby Co., St. Louis.)

be transiently recovered from the female vaginal tract, they are not normal flora of the genital tract. Lactobacilli are the predominant organisms in secretions from normal, healthy vaginas (Figure 19.2).

Infections of the genital tract in normal females above or below childbearing age are often a result of irritation or a foreign body and are caused by the same organisms that cause skin wound infections. Genital tract infections caused by sexually transmitted agents in children (preadolescents) are most often the result of sexual abuse. The laboratory should treat specimens from such patients with extreme care, carefully identifying and documenting all isolates, since medicolegal implications exist.

Chlamydia trachomatis, Gardnerella vaginalis, Neisseria gonorrhoeae and *meningitidis, Treponema pallidum, Ureaplasma urealyticum, Mycoplasma hominis*, other mycoplasmas, human papillomavirus, herpesvirus, and other organisms may be acquired as people engage in sexual activity. Some of these organisms may exist in the genital tract in the absence of any noticeable pathology. *C. trachomatis*, however, is the most prevalent agent of mucopu-

rulent cervicitis (and of all sexually transmitted diseases [STDs]) in the United States. It is clearly associated with pelvic inflammatory disease, subsequent infertility, and preterm births.[2,10] Although the role of *M. hominis* in the pathogenesis of genital infection is unclear, it has been associated with infections in females, such as pelvic inflammatory disease, pyelonephritis, and postpartum fever; and with morbidity and stillbirths in infants.[7,11,12] *Ureaplasma urealyticum*, but not *M. hominis*, has been associated causally with the acute urethral syndrome in women and with reproductive failure.[18,19] *U. urealyticum* may be related to nongonococcal urethritis in males and to low birth weight of the babies of infected females.[11,12]

The syndrome of **bacterial vaginosis**, consisting of copious, malodorous vaginal discharge, has recently been implicated in the etiology of premature labor and low birth weight.[5,10] Thus, diagnosis of this entity has taken on greater importance. Organisms recovered from the genital tract that have been implicated as pathogens are listed in the box on p. 265.

Figure 19.2
Predominance of lactobacilli in Gram stain from healthy vagina.

Genital Tract Pathogens

Bacteria

Chlamydia trachomatis
Gardnerella vaginalis
Haemophilus ducreyi
Mycoplasma hominis
Mycoplasma genitalium
Neisseria gonorrhoeae
Neisseria meningitidis
Ureaplasma urealyticum

Fungi

Candida species
Other yeast

Viruses

Cytomegalovirus
Herpes simplex virus

Protozoans

Trichomonas vaginalis

In addition, a number of other agents cause genital tract disease but are not routinely isolated from clinical specimens; included are the human papillomaviruses of molluscum contagiosum, genital warts (condylomata acuminata), and associated with cervical carcinoma; *Calymmatobacterium granulomatis*; *Treponema pallidum*; and ectoparasites such as scabies and lice. Infections with more than one agent are not uncommon. Such dual or concurrent infections should always be considered.

Homosexual practices and increasingly common heterosexual practices of anal-genital intercourse have required that a number of gastrointestinal and systemic pathogens also be considered etiologic agents of STDs. The intestinal protozoa *Giardia lamblia*, *Entamoeba histolytica*, and *Cryptosporidium* sp. are significant causes of STD, especially among homosexual populations. In the same group of patients, fecal pathogens such as *Salmonella*, *Shigella*, and *Campylobacter* are often transmitted sexually. Oral-genital practices probably allow *N. meningitidis* to colonize and infect the genital tract. Viruses shed in secretions or present in blood (cytomegalovirus, hepatitis B, C, and non-A non-B, human-T-lymphotropic virus type 1 (HTLV I), and human immunodeficiency virus (HIV) of AIDS are increasingly being spread by sexual practices. The spectrum of diseases (not previously considered to be sexually transmitted) that accompanies AIDS is discussed in Chapter 23.

Certain pathogens are usually sought in specimens from lesions on surface epithelium of or near the genital tract. These include herpes simplex virus, *H. ducreyi*, and *T. pallidum*. *C. granulomatis* is recovered from biopsy material taken from beneath the characteristic lesion. Collection of specimens from lesions will be discussed in Section 19.6.

19.2. Collection and Transport of Specimens from the Urethra and Vagina

Urethral discharge may occur in both males and females infected with certain pathogens, such as *N. gonorrhoeae* and *T. vaginalis*. Because the discharge is usually less profuse and may be masked more easily in the female by vaginal secretions, the presence of infection is more likely to be asymptomatic in females. *U. urealyticum* and *C. trachomatis* can also be isolated from male urethral discharge.

A urogenital swab designed expressly for collection of such specimens should be used. These swabs are made of cotton or rayon that has been treated with charcoal to adsorb material toxic to gonococci, wrapped tightly over one end of a thin wooden stick that has also been treated to remove resins and toxic chemicals (Chapter 6). Certain wooden sticks may be toxic to mycoplasmas and chlamydiae; plastic sticks are generally less toxic. Rayon-tipped swabs on thin wire may also be used for collection of specimens for isolation of mycoplasmas and chlamydiae. Calcium alginate swabs are generally more toxic for herpesvirus, gonococci, and mycoplasma than are treated cotton swabs. Rare lots of calcium alginate swabs have been toxic for chlamydiae.

The swab is inserted approximately 2 cm into the urethra and rotated gently before withdrawing. Since chlamydiae are intracellular pathogens, it is important to remove epithelial cells (with the swab) from the urethral mucosa. Separate samples for cultivation of gonococci and chlamydiae or ureaplasma are required. In cases where there is profuse urethral discharge, particularly in males, the discharge may be collected externally without inserting a sampling device into the urethra.

Since *T. vaginalis* may be present in urethral discharge, material for culture should be collected by swab as just described, but a swab should also be placed into a tube containing 0.5 ml of sterile physiologic saline and hand-delivered to the laboratory immediately. Direct wet mounts and cultures can be performed from this specimen. Commercial media for culture of trichomonas are available. The first few drops of voided urine may also be a suitable specimen for recovery of trichomonas from infected males, if it is inoculated into culture media immediately. Alternatively, material may be smeared onto a slide for later performance of a fluorescent antibody stain.

Organisms that cause purulent vaginal discharge (vaginitis) include *T. vaginalis*, yeast, gonococci, and, rarely, β-hemolytic streptococci. The same organisms that cause purulent infections in the urethra may also infect the epithelial cells in the cervical opening (os), as can herpes simplex virus. Mucus is removed by gently rubbing the area with a cotton ball. A special swab (the urethral swab just described) is inserted into the cervical canal and rotated and moved from side to side for 30 seconds before removal. A small, nylon-bristled brush (cytology brush or cytobrush) may be used to assure collection of cellular material, but its use is associated with some discomfort and bleeding. Reports indicate that the cytobrush may result in better specimens, at least for detection of *Chlamydia*.[3] The cytology brush is contraindicated in pregnant patients. Swabs are handled as urethral swabs for isolation of *Trichomonas* and gonococci. Chlamydiae cause a mucopurulent cervicitis with much discharge. Endocervical specimens are obtained after the cervix has been exposed by insertion of a speculum, which allows visualization of vaginal and cervical architecture. The speculum is moistened with warm water, since many lubricants contain antibacterial agents. Because the normal vaginal secretions contain great quantities of bacteria, care must be exercised to avoid or minimize contaminating swabs for culture by contact with these secretions. Swabs of Bartholin gland exudate, carefully collected, may also be obtained for culture.

In addition to cervical specimens, which are particularly useful for isolation of herpes, gonococci, *Mycoplasma*, and chlamydiae, vaginal discharge specimens may be collected. Organisms likely to cause vaginal discharge include *Trichomonas*, yeast, and the agents of bacterial vaginosis (presumably combinations of *G. vaginalis* and various anaerobic bacteria). The absence of inflammatory cells in the vaginal discharge is suggestive of bacterial vaginosis (formerly called nonspecific vaginitis). Swabs are

PROCEDURE 19.1

Preparation of Sucrose Buffer (2-SP) for transport of Chlamydia and Mycoplasma Specimens

Principle

Sucrose acts as an osmotic stabilizer and phosphates act as pH buffers to maintain viability of cell-wall fragile organisms, including *Mycoplasma* and *Chlamydia* species.

Method

Preparation of stock sucrose buffer

1. Dissolve 68.5 g sucrose in 100 ml distilled water.
2. Dissolve 2.1 g K_2HPO_4 in 60 ml distilled water.
3. Dissolve 1.1 g KH_2PO_4 in 40 ml distilled water.
4. Mix all three solutions and add distilled water to 1 L total volume.
5. Boil the solution for 30 min.
6. Cool to room temperature before preparing transport medium.

Modified from Mårdh, P.-A. 1984. In Holmes, K.K., Mårdh, P.-A., Sparling, P.F., and Wiesner, P.J., editors. Sexually transmitted diseases. McGraw-Hill Book Co., New York; and Gordon, F.B., Harper, I.A., Quan, A.L., et al. 1969.

Preparation of 2-SP

7. To 100 ml stock sucrose buffer, add 10 ml fetal calf serum (commercially available), 2 mg gentamicin powder, 0.5 mg amphotericin powder, and 10 mg vancomycin powder (suppliers listed in Chapter 13).
8. Dispense in 1 ml amounts into sterile, screw-topped plastic disposable test tubes, 16 × 150 mm.
9. Store at $-20°$ C for up to 6 months.

Quality control

Media should be incubated overnight to test for sterility. Tests for support of viability of the organisms are beyond the scope of most laboratories.

Expected results

Media should be sterile. Specimens from at least 50% of sexually active females should yield *U. urealyticum*.

Performance schedule

Test media each time a new batch is prepared.

---

dipped into the fluid that collects in the posterior fornix of the vagina.

Swabs collected for isolation of gonococci may be transported to the laboratory in modified Stuart's or Amies charcoal transport media, held at room temperature until inoculated to culture media. Good recovery of gonococci is possible if swabs are cultured within 24 hours of collection. Material that must be held longer than 24 hours should be inoculated directly to one of the commercial systems designed for recovery of gonococci, described in Section 19.4. Swabs for isolation of chlamydiae and *Mycoplasma* are best transported in sucrose buffer with antibiotics (2-SP), as described in Procedure 19.1. If the specimens are not going to be inoculated to cell culture within several hours, they should be refrigerated but *never frozen*.

19.3. Direct Microscopic Examination

In addition to culture, urethral discharge may be examined by Gram stain for the presence of gram-negative intracellular diplococci (Figure 19.3), usually indicative of gonorrhea in males. After inoculation to culture media, the swab is rolled over the surface of a glass slide, covering an area of at least 1 cm². If the Gram stain is characteristic, cultures of urethral discharge need not be performed. In homosexual males, however, *N. meningitidis* has been increasingly isolated from such specimens, so that the assumption that gram-negative diplococci are gonococci may no longer be valid for that patient population. Urethral smears from females may also be examined, but presumptive diagnosis of gonorrhea from vaginal smears is only reliable if the microscopist is experienced, since normal vaginal flora

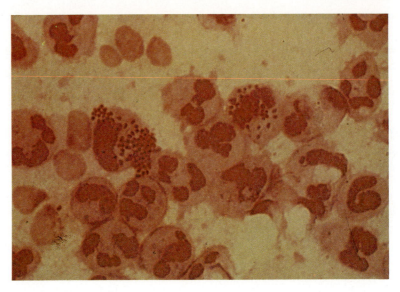

Figure 19.3
Gram-negative intracellular diplococci; diagnostic for gonorrhea in urethral discharge.

such as *Veillonella* or occasional gram-negative coccobacilli may resemble gonococci. If extracellular organisms resembling *N. gonorrhoeae* are seen, the microscopist should continue to examine the smear for intracellular diplococci for a longer time period than if no suspicious bacteria are seen. Cultures or an alternative antigen detection method should always be performed on specimens from females. Some strains of *N. gonorrhoeae* are sensitive to the amount of vancomycin present in selective media. If suspicious organisms seen on smear fail to grow in culture, reculture on chocolate agar without antibiotics may be warranted.

Within the last several years, very sensitive fluorescein-conjugated monoclonal antibody reagents have been developed for visualization of the inclusions of *C. trachomatis* in cell cultures and elementary bodies in urethral and cervical specimens containing cells (further discussed in Chapter 38). The reagents are available commercially in complete collection and test systems (Figure 19.4). Some authors have advocated the use of antibodies directed against the outer membrane protein for better results.[4] The swab is rolled over the surface of a special glass slide and the material is fixed with acetone. In some studies, the sensitivity of visual detection of chlamydiae with these newer reagents has been similar to that of culture, although such comparative

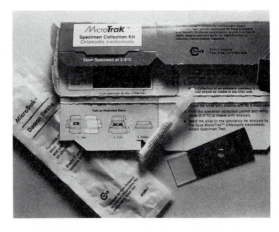

Figure 19.4
Commercial collection and monoclonal antibody stain test system for chlamydiae (MicroTrak, Syva Co.).

results are obtained only by technologists who are experienced in fluorescent techniques and when the slides are examined quite thoroughly.[9] False positive results should not occur if at least 10 morphologically compatible fluorescing organisms are seen on the entire smear. No direct visual methods exist for detection of mycoplasma at this time, but nucleic acid probes have been evaluated.

Direct microscopic examination of a wet prepa-

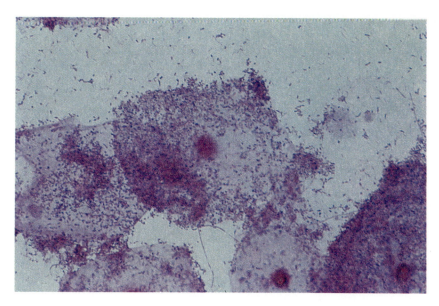

Figure 19.5
"Clue cells" in vaginal discharge, suggestive of bacterial vaginosis.

ration of vaginal discharge provides the simplest rapid diagnostic test for *T. vaginalis* when such a specimen is available, although use of a monoclonal fluorescent antibody stain has been reported to detect more positive specimens.[16] Motile trophozoites of *Trichomonas* can be visualized in a wet preparation performed by a proficient technologist in two thirds of cases, and budding cells and pseudohyphae of yeast can also be easily identified. The addition of 10% potassium hydroxide (KOH) to a separate preparation serves two functions: by dissolving host cell protein, it enhances the visibility of fungal elements, and by causing the discharge to become alkaline, it elicits the fishy, aminelike odor associated with bacterial vaginosis.[5]

Bacterial vaginosis, characterized by a foul-smelling discharge, can be diagnosed microscopically or clinically. The discharge is primarily sloughed epithelial cells, many of which are completely covered by tiny, gram-variable rods and coccobacilli. These cells are called "clue cells" (Figure 19.5). *G. vaginalis* has been associated with the syndrome historically, but the synergistic activity of a number of anaerobic organisms, including non–*Bacteroides fragilis Bacteroides* species, anaerobic streptococci, and perhaps *Mobiluncus* species (curved, motile rods), seems to contribute to the pathology.[15] Although *G. vaginalis* can be cultured on a human blood bilayer plate and isolated colonies can be iden-

tified within 1 hour, a clinical diagnosis of bacterial vaginosis is best made using three or more of the following criteria: homogeneous, gray discharge; clue cells seen on wet mount or Gram stain; amine or fishy odor elicited by the addition of a drop of 10% KOH to the discharge on a slide or on the speculum; and pH greater than 4.5.[5]

The absence of a predominance of lactobacilli on Gram stain, present in the normal vagina (Figure 19.2), is another sign of bacterial vaginosis.[17] A grading system for Gram stains of vaginal discharge has been developed by Hillier and others (Procedure 19.2). Using these criteria, the sensitivity of Gram stain for diagnosis of bacterial vaginosis (diagnosed clinically) was 93% to 97%, better than culture for *G. vaginalis* (sensitivity 95%).[5] The Gram stain is more specific than the wet mount for detection of clue cells and the smear can be saved and reexamined later. Additionally, *Mobiluncus* species, recently implicated in this syndrome, can be detected best on Gram stain because of their distinctive curved morphology.[15]

19.4. Direct Inoculation and Laboratory Handling of Urethral and Vaginal Specimens

Samples for isolation of gonococci may be inoculated directly to culture media, obviating the need for

PROCEDURE 19.2

Scoring Vaginal Gram Stains for Bacterial Vaginosis

1. Roll the swab of vaginal discharge over the surface of a slide.
2. Allow the smear to air dry, methanol-fix, and stain.
3. Scores are assigned as follows:

Organism morphotype	Number/oil immersion field	Score
Lactobacillus	>30	0
(parallel-sided gram-positive rods)	5-30	1
	1-5	2
	<1	3
	0	4
Gardnerella-like	>30	
Bacteroides-like	5-30	3
(tiny, gram-variable coccobacilli and rounded, pleomorphic gram-negative rods with vacuoles)	1-5	2
	<1	1
	0	0
Mobiluncus-like	5-30	2
(curved gram-negative rods)	Any-5	1
	0	0

4. Add up total score and interpret as follows:

Score	Interpretation
0-3	Normal
4-6	Intermediate, repeat test later
7-10	Bacterial vaginosis

From Hillier, S.L., Krohn, M.A., and Nugent, R.P. 1987. The relationship of vaginal microorganisms and clinical signs to a bacterial vaginosis score based on vaginal Gram smear. Abstract. 27th Interscience Conference on Antimicrobial Agents and Chemotherapy, p. 102.

transport. Several commercially produced systems have been developed for this purpose, and many clinicians inoculate standard plates directly if convenient access to an incubator is available. Modified Thayer-Martin medium is most commonly used, although New York City (NYC) medium has the added advantage of supporting the growth of mycoplasma as well as gonococci. A modification of NYC medium has been shown to yield comparable results for growth of *N. gonorrhoeae* but costs as much as 70% less.[1] These media contain numerous supplements, however, and are not suitable for preparation in most routine clinical laboratories. Excellent recovery of gonococci is the rule when specimens are inoculated directly to any of these media or their modifications in Transgrow bottles or onto the surface of Jembec plates (Figure 19.6 and Chapter 6, Figure 6.1). Media are commercially available. The swab containing material is rolled across the agar with constant turning to expose all surfaces to the medium. Transgrow bottles are filled with an atmosphere of increased CO_2, so they must be held upright during inoculation, a procedure often forgotten by busy clinicians. The Jembec plate, which generates its own increased CO_2 atmosphere by means of a tablet of sodium bicarbonate, is inoculated in a W pattern. It may be cross-streaked with a sterile loop in the laboratory (Figure 19.7).

T. vaginalis may be cultured in Diamond's medium (available commercially) from discharge material, direct wet preparations may be examined for the presence of motile trophozoites, or a direct fluorescent antibody (DFA) stain (Meridian Diagnostics) may be used. Smith found DFA to be second to culture in sensitivity.[16]

Specimens must be inoculated to other media in addition to gonococcal selective agar for isolation of yeast, streptococci, mycoplasmas, and *G. vaginalis*. Yeast will grow well on Columbia agar base with 5% sheep blood and colistin and nalidixic acid (CNA), as will most strains of *Gardnerella*, although more selective media are available (see Chapter 39). Most yeast and the streptococci will also grow on standard blood agar; thus, the addition of special fungal media such as Sabouraud's brain heart infusion agar (SABHI) is unwarranted.

A7 agar or a commercially available biphasic Mycoplasma culture system (Mycotrim, Hana Biologicals) can be used to culture mycoplasmas and *U. urealyticum*.[22] *M. genitalium* may not grow on commercial media because of the presence of thallium acetate.[21]

19.5. Infections of Female Pelvis and Male Internal Genital Organs

Pelvic inflammatory disease is often caused by the same organisms that cause cervicitis or by organisms that comprise normal flora of the vaginal mucosa.

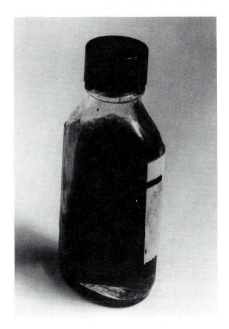

Figure 19.6
Transgrow bottle, a self-contained agar medium and CO_2
atmosphere for culture and transport of *N. gonorrhoeae*. The
physician holds the bottle upright while rolling a swab across
the agar surface to inoculate the medium. CO_2, which is
heavier than air, thus remains in the bottle to enhance growth
of the organism.

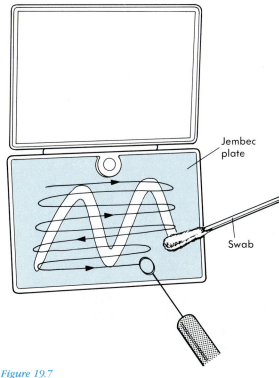

Jembec
plate

Swab

Figure 19.7
Method of cross-streaking Jembec plate after original specimen
has been inoculated by rolling the swab over the surface of the
agar in a W pattern.

Because of the profuse normal flora of the vaginal
tract, species of which may be involved in peritoneal
infection, specimens must be collected in such a way
as to prevent vaginal flora contamination. Aspirated
material collected by needle and syringe represents
the best specimen. If this cannot be obtained at the
time of surgery or laparoscopy, culdocentesis, following decontamination of the vagina by povidone-
iodine, is satisfactory. Aspirated material should be
placed into an anaerobic transport container. The
presence of either mixed anaerobic flora, gonococci,
or both can be rapidly detected from a Gram stain.
Direct examination with fluorescent monoclonal antibody stain may also detect chlamydiae. All such
specimens should be inoculated to media that allow
the recovery of anaerobic, facultative, and aerobic
bacteria, gonococci, fungi, mycoplasmas, and chlamydiae. All material collected from normally sterile
body sites in the genital tract should be inoculated
to chocolate agar and placed into a suitable broth
such as chopped meat medium or thioglycolate, in
addition to the other types of media noted.

Infections of the male prostate, epididymis, and
testes are usually bacterial. In younger men, chlamydiae predominate as the cause of epididymitis
and possibly of prostatitis. Urine or discharge collected via the urethra is the specimen of choice unless an abscess is drained surgically or by needle and
syringe. Urine (the first few milliliters of voided
urine) may be collected before and after prostatic
massage to try to pinpoint the anatomic site of the
infection. Cultures are inoculated to support the
growth of anaerobic, facultative, and aerobic bacteria, as well as gonococci. In patients with suspected
AIDS or other immunosuppression-related systemic
cytomegalovirus disease, semen or urine can be cultured for the virus. The specimen is transported immediately to the virology laboratory for culture. Refrigeration may preserve the virus for several hours;
specimens that must be held longer should be
placed into viral transport media, as is discussed in
Chapter 42.

19.6. Specimens Obtained from Skin and Mucous Membrane Lesions

External genital lesions are usually either vesicular or ulcerative in nature. Causes of lesions can be determined by physical examination, histological examination, or microscopic examination or culture of exudate. *Since any genital lesion may be highly contagious, all manipulations of lesion material should be carried out by clinicians wearing gloves.*

19.6.a. Examination of vesicular lesions. Vesicles in this area are almost always attributable to viruses, and herpes simplex is the most common cause. Material from the base of a vesicle may be spread onto the surface of a slide and examined for the typical multinucleated giant cells of herpes or stained by immunofluorescent antibody stains for viral antigens. Additionally or alternatively, the material is transported for culture of the virus, as outlined in Procedure 19.3.

There are several commercial fluorescein-conjugated monoclonal and polyclonal antibodies directed against herpetic antigens of either type 1 or 2. When fluorescent-antibody-stained lesion material containing enough cells is viewed under ultraviolet light, the diagnosis can be made in 70% to 90% of cases. Laboratories that routinely process genital material for herpes should be using immunofluorescent staining reagents in situations where a rapid answer is desirable; otherwise, culture, which is generally positive in 2 days, is the method of choice. Nonfluorescent markers such as biotin-avidin-horseradish peroxidase or alkaline phosphatase have also been conjugated to these specific antibodies, often allowing earlier detection of herpes-infected cells in tissue culture monolayers. Such reagents have been developed for use directly on clinical material, although their sensitivity is not great enough to forego culture if a definitive diagnosis is necessary.

19.6.b. Examination of ulcerative lesions. Ulcerative lesions are usually one of the following: a syphilitic chancre (caused by *T. pallidum*), the chancroid of *H. ducreyi*, later stages of herpetic vesicles, the ulcer of granuloma inguinale (also known as donovanosis, caused by *C. granulomatis*), an infected traumatic ulcer, or the result of some other rare infectious disease or even a noninfectious process. Macroscopically, lesions of syphilis are usually clean, with an even, indurated edge.[20] Only 30% of syphilitic chancres are tender. Lesions of chancroid are

---

PROCEDURE 19.3

Collection of Material from Suspected Herpetic Lesions

Principle

Herpes virus is best recovered from the base of active lesions in the vesicle stage. The older the lesion, the less likely it will yield viable virus.

Method

1. Open the vesicles with a small gauge needle or Dacron-tipped swab.
2. Rub the base of the lesion vigorously with a small cotton- or Dacron-tipped swab to recover infected cells.
3. Place the swab into viral transport medium (described in Chapter 42) and refrigerate until inoculated to culture media. Specimens in media may be stored at −70° C for extended periods without loss of viral yield.
4. If large vesicles are present, material for culture may be aspirated directly by needle and syringe.
5. Material from another lesion can be applied directly to a glass slide for a Tzanck preparation (histology) with Wright-Giemsa or fluorescent antibody stain for detection of multinucleated giant cells.

---

usually ragged, necrotic, painful, and are often found in pairs where material from the first lesion autoinoculated a second area in close contact ("kissing lesions"). The beefy red nonpainful lesion of donovanosis is characterized by a white border. These lesions can usually be differentiated from the painful, erythematous-bordered lesions of herpes, which usually begin as vesicles and occur in groups. Lesions suggestive of syphilis should be examined by darkfield microscopy, as described in Chapter 7. Collection of material for darkfield is outlined in Procedure 19.4.

All lesions suspected of infectious etiology may be Gram stained in addition to the procedures described. The smear of lesion material from a chan-

Collection of Material for Darkfield Examination for Syphilis

GLOVES SHOULD ALWAYS BE WORN

Principle

Numerous motile treponemes are present in a fresh lesion (chancre) of syphilis. Their characteristic motility can aid in presumptive diagnosis of this infection before a serologic response can be detected. Darkfield microscopy is necessary because the organisms are too thin to be visible under phase microscopy.

Method

1. Cleanse the area around the lesion with a sterile gauze pad moistened with sterile saline.
2. Abrade the surface of the ulcer with a sterile, dry gauze pad until some blood is expressed.
3. Continue to blot the blood until there is no further bleeding; then squeeze the area until serous fluid is expressed.
4. Touch the surface of a very clean glass slide or coverslip to the exudate and immediately cover the material on the slide with a coverslip or place the inoculated coverslip face-down onto a slide. If there was only very little material expressed, a drop of sterile physiologic saline may be added.

5. Immediately examine the material under darkfield microscopy (400×, high dry magnification) for the presence of motile spirochetes. Treponemes are very long (8-10 μg) slightly longer than a red blood cell, and consist of 8 to 14 tightly coiled, even spirals (Figure 19.8). They may bend slightly in the middle as they slowly move about. Once characteristic forms are seen, they should be verified by examination under oil immersion magnification (1000×).

Quality control

Proper setup of the microscope can be ascertained by making a wet preparation of a scraping of the inside of your cheek (mucosal surface).

Expected results

Numerous thin, fusiform and spirochetal organisms should be seen darting about.

Performance schedule

Test a cheek cell scraping each time the darkfield procedure is performed.
Note: All slides and materials should be handled as infectious, since syphilitic lesions may contain large numbers of infectious treponemes.

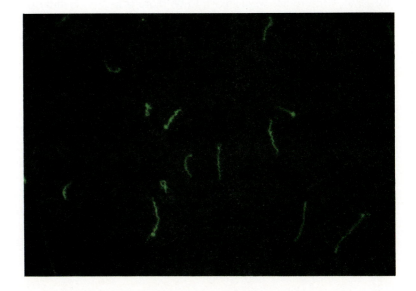

Figure 19.8
Appearance of fluorescent antibody–stained *T. pallidum*. Organisms appear to bend only near the center.

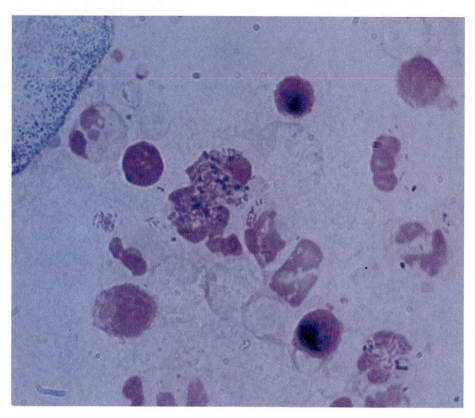

Figure 19.9
Gram stain of genital lesion showing typical "school-of-fish" formation of pleomorphic gram-negative bacilli characteristic of *H. ducreyi* infection.

croid patient may show many small, pleomorphic gram-negative rods and coccobacilli arranged in chains and groups, characteristic of *H. ducreyi* (Figure 19.9). Culture has been shown to be more sensitive for diagnosis of this agent, however. Material collected on cotton or Dacron swabs may be transported in modified Stuart's medium until it is inoculated to culture media. A special agar, consisting of chocolate agar enriched with 1% IsoVitaleX (BBL Microbiology Systems) and vancomycin 3 µg/ml, has yielded good isolation if cultures are incubated in 5% to 7% CO_2 in a moist atmosphere, such as a candle jar. Inoculation of a duplicate sample from each patient to a second agar, fetal bovine serum agar with vancomycin, has been suggested by Greenwood and Robertson to increase chances for recovery.[8]

Diagnosis of granuloma inguinale is achieved by staining a crushed preparation of a small piece of biopsy tissue from the edge of the base of the ulcer with Wright's or Giemsa stain and finding characteristic Donovan bodies (bipolar staining rods intracellularly within macrophages). Cytologists or pathologists usually examine such specimens, rather than microbiologists. No acceptable media for isolation of *C. granulomatis* are available.

19.7. Examination of Material from Buboes

Buboes, swollen lymph glands that occur in the inguinal region, are often evidence of a genital tract infection. Buboes are common in patients with primary syphilis, genital herpes, lymphogranuloma venereum, and chancroid. Patients suffering from AIDS may show generalized lymphadenopathy. Other diseases that are not sexually transmitted, such as plague, tularemia, and lymphoma, can also produce buboes. Those diseases will not be discussed further here. Material from buboes may be

PROCEDURE 19.5

Aspiration of Bubo Material

TO BE DONE BY PHYSICIAN

Principle

The etiologic agent of swollen inguinal lymph glands is often visible in material aspirated from the gland itself.

Method

1. Wipe overlying skin with an iodophore, allowing it to remain on the skin for at least 1 min.
2. Vigorously wash off the iodophore with 70% alcohol, allowing it to dry.
3. Introduce a 21-gauge needle with an attached 5-ml syringe through the skin into the node.
4. If the node is nonfluctuant, as in syphilis, the needle is plunged gently in various directions within the node while continuous suction is applied to the syringe.
5. Material aspirated from nonfluctuant nodes is examined under darkfield microscopy for spirochetes.
6. Material from fluctuant nodes is obtained by applying suction. If no pus is aspirated, the needle is left in place and a syringe containing at least 1 ml of nonbacteriostatic physiologic sterile saline is exchanged for the initial empty syringe. This saline is injected into the node and withdrawn. Rigorous aseptic technique is important.
7. Pus is cultured on chocolate and 5% sheep blood agars, special media for *H. ducreyi*, and in broth such as thioglycollate, and is Gram-stained.
8. Lesion material is also placed into sucrose buffer for chlamydial culture and examined by fluorescein-conjugated monoclonal chlamydial antibody stain.

aspirated for microscopic examination and culture as described in Procedure 19.5.

19.8. Infections of Human Products of Conception

Certain infectious agents are known to cause fetal infection and even abortion. *Listeria monocytogenes*, although usually causing only mild flulike symptoms in the mother, can cause extensive disease and abortion of the fetus if infection occurs late in the pregnancy, as discussed in Chapter 33. A recent California outbreak traced to contaminated Jalisco Mexican-style cheese resulted in several deaths among pregnant women. The organism can be isolated from the placenta and from tissues of the fetus. Other agents that cross the placental barrier to infect a developing fetus include *Toxoplasma gondii*, rubella, cytomegalovirus, herpes simplex virus, parvovirus, and *T. pallidum*.

Infections that can be acquired by infants as they pass through an infected birth canal include herpes, cytomegalovirus (CMV) infection, gonorrhea, group B streptococcal sepsis, chlamydial conjunctivitis and pneumonia, and *Escherichia coli* or other neonatal meningitis. Laboratory diagnosis of these infections is accomplished by culturing for the agents where possible and by performing serologic tests, especially for the presence of specific IgM directed against the agent in question. Specific IgM tests are commercially available for the TORCH agents (*Toxoplasma*, rubella, cytomegalovirus, and herpes) as discussed in Chapter 12. Unless serum IgM is separated from IgG, the IgM tests for neonatal rubella, CMV, and herpes are unreliable. Cytomegalovirus infection is best diagnosed by culture of the virus from urine. The most reliable diagnostic tests for neonatal herpes infection are demonstration of the antigen in clinical specimens by direct fluorescent antibody stain or recovery of the virus in tissue culture.

19.9. Nonculture Methods for Diagnosis of Diseases of the Genital Tract

19.9.a. Serologic tests for syphilis. Diagnosis of syphilis rests on demonstration of the organism in a lesion, a difficult and insensitive test, or demonstration of specific antibodies to the treponemes. Although a complete discussion of diagnosis of syphilis is beyond the scope of this text, certain tests will be mentioned here. The classic serologic tests for syphilis measure the presence of two types of antibodies: "treponemal" and "nontreponemal." Treponemal antibodies are produced against the antigens of the organisms themselves, whereas nontreponemal antibodies, often called **reaginic antibodies,** are produced by infected patients against components of mammalian cells. These antibodies, although almost always produced by patients with syphilis, are also produced by patients with a number of other infectious diseases such as leprosy, tuberculosis, chancroid, leptospirosis, malaria, rickettsial disease, trypanosomiasis, lymphogranuloma venereum (LGV), measles, chickenpox, hepatitis, and infectious mononucleosis; noninfectious conditions such as drug addiction; autoimmune disorders including rheumatoid disease; and such nondiseases as old age, pregnancy, and recent immunization. When a positive serologic test for syphilis occurs in a patient without syphilis, it is called a *biologic false-positive (BFP) test*.

The two most widely used nontreponemal serologic tests are the **VDRL (Venereal Disease Research Laboratory)** test and the **RPR (rapid plasma reagin)** test. Each of these tests is a flocculation (or agglutination) test, in which soluble antigen particles are coalesced to form larger particles that are visible as clumps when they are aggregated by antibody. The principles of these tests were discussed in Chapter 12.

Specific treponemal serologic tests include the **FTA-ABS (fluorescent treponemal antibody absorption)** test and the **MHA-TP (microhemagglutination)** test. Another test, the **TPI (*Treponema pallidum* immobilization)** test, is rarely performed these days, since it requires the maintenance of viable treponemes by passage in rabbit testicles.

The FTA-ABS test is performed by overlaying whole treponemes fixed to a slide with serum from patients suspected of having syphilis because of a previous positive VDRL or RPR test. The patient's serum is first absorbed with non–*T. pallidum* treponemal antigens (sorbent) to reduce nonspecific cross-reactivity. Fluorescein-conjugated antihuman antibody reagent is then applied as a marker for specific antitreponemal antibodies in the patient's serum. This test should not be used as a primary screening procedure. The MHA-TP test utilizes treated erythrocytes from a turkey or other animal that are coated with treponemal antigens. The presence of specific antibody causes the red cells to agglutinate and form a flat mat across the bottom of the microdilution well in which the test is performed. The serologic tests for syphilis can be used to determine quantitative titers of antibody, which are useful for following response to therapy. The relative sensitivity of each test is shown in Table 19.1. To confirm that a positive nontreponemal test result is due to syphilis rather than one of the other infections or biological false-positive conditions mentioned, a specific treponemal test should be performed.[20] Enzyme-linked immunosorbent assay (ELISA) tests for syphilis antibodies are available. Although not widely used yet, they should offer a sensitive and specific alternative to existing methods.

19.9.b. Other serologic tests for genital pathogens. As mentioned in the chapters that deal with individual pathogens, many conventional serologic tests for antibodies to genital pathogens are in use. Complement fixation and microimmunofluorescence are both used with excellent sensitivity for detection of antibodies to chlamydiae and mycoplasmas, although ELISA tests are probably more sensitive. ELISA tests are also primary choices for detection of antibodies to herpes and cytomegaloviruses, and a latex particle agglutination test (Hynson, Westcott & Dunning) for CMV is sensitive and simpler. Serologic tests for gonorrhea by antibody detection are not satisfactory in that they do not distinguish between past and current infection, nor between gonococcal and meningococcal infection. For patients whose serum contains antibody to HIV-1, as detected by ELISA tests, a Western blot nucleic acid hybridization test is used to confirm the diagnosis.

19.9.c. Antigen detection tests for genital tract pathogens. In addition to the fluorescent microscopic methods mentioned and described in more detail in the chapters relating to individual pathogens, several ELISA systems are currently available for detection of antigens of etiologic agents involved in STDs without ulture.

Table 19.1

Sensitivity of Commonly Used Serologic
Tests for Syphilis

Test*	Stage		
	1°	2°	LATE
Nontreponemal (reaginic tests)			
Venereal Disease Research Laboratory (reaginic) test (VDRL)	70%	99%	1%†
Rapid plasma-reagin card test (RPR)	80%	99%	
Automated reagin test (ART)			0%
Specific treponemal tests			
Fluorescent treponemal antibody absorption test (FTA-ABS)	85%	100%	98%
T. pallidum hemagglutination assay (TPHA-TP)	65%	100%	95%
Treponemal immobilization test (TPI)	50%	97%	95%

* Percentage of patients with positive serologic tests in treated or untreated primary or secondary syphilis.
† Treated late syphilis.
Reproduced from Tramont, E. 1985. *Treponema pallidum* (syphilis). In Mandell, G.L., Douglas, R.G., Jr., and Bennett, J.E., editors: Principles and practice of infectious diseases, ed. 2. John Wiley & Sons, New York.

Numerous commercial ELISA systems for detection of antigens of *C. trachomatis* are available and have been evaluated. ELISA systems suffer from being unable to assess specimen quality, an important parameter when an intracellular organism is being sought. Sensitivities vary greatly, depending on the patient population, skill of clinicians, and test system. Overall, sensitivity seems to be similar to that of the direct fluorescent antibody stain. Although no single test (culture, DFA, or ELISA) will detect all infections, laboratories are urged to perform at least one chlamydial test on cervical material. The public health consequences of this infection are too great to bypass any opportunity to detect infected patients.[2]

An *N. gonorrhoeae* ELISA test exists also (Gonozyme, Abbott Laboratories). The Gonozyme test has been shown to be similar to culture for detection of gonococcal urethritis and especially useful for screening asymptomatic females (although less sensitive than culture). It is not useful for detection of pharyngeal or rectal infection.

Systems are also being perfected for direct detection of herpes antigen by latex agglutination and membrane-fixed solid-phase immunoassay systems, although none are as sensitive as culture, which is still the method of choice for herpes. Polyclonal and monoclonal antibodies conjugated to either a fluorescent stain or to a biotin-avidin-enzyme marker are available for staining clinical material. They have been evaluated favorably, particularly for diagnosis of herpes meningoencephalitis from brain biopsy tissue.

19.9.d. Other tests. A new nucleic acid hybridization assay (PACE, Gen-Probe) utilizes a chemiluminescent marker for hybridized sequences of chlamydial ribosomal RNA and labeled homologous DNA probe. Test results are available within 2 hours and early evaluations are promising. This hybridization system is an attractive alternative because it does not require a radioactive marker and because the use of ribosomal nucleic acid as target allows greater sensitivity than DNA-based hybridization assays. A DNA-hybridization immunoperoxidase assay for herpes nucleic acid in cell culture and direct specimen material is available (Enzo Biochem). This system is not as sensitive or specific as culture as yet and results require more labor than fluorescent antibody stain methods.

Limulus lysate for detection of endotoxin has been used to diagnose gonococcal infections.[13,14] Although seemingly reliable for patients visiting STD clinics, the method has not been well accepted.

Systems for detection and typing of papillomavirus DNA by hybridization have been released recently (Life Technologies; Enzo Biochem). The relationship between these viruses and cervical cancer can be better elucidated once these tests are being used more routinely. Of course, the virus genome can be identified in genital warts, but the warts can be visualized directly and treated without resorting to expensive and laborious laboratory procedures. Dot-blot enzyme immunoassays for chlamydial antigen have been developed. They are too cumbersome for routine use.

Bacterial vaginosis can be diagnosed by an increased succinic:lactic acid ratio in vaginal secretions, as detected by direct gas liquid chromatography. The Gram stain, however, is equally sensitive and more readily available.

We expect that rapid, reliable, nonculture antigen-detection methods will soon be available for diagnosis of all significant STDs so that patients can be diagnosed and treated very soon after being examined. The rapid specific therapeutic intervention thus made possible will contribute greatly to minimizing spread of STDs and to a decrease in the morbidity that those infections currently produce.

REFERENCES

1. Anstey, R.J., Gun-Munro, J., Rennie, R.P., et al. 1984. Laboratory and clinical evaluation of modified New York City medium (Henderson formulation) for the isolation of *Neisseria gonorrhoeae*. J. Clin. Microbiol. 20:905.

2. CDC. 1985. *Chlamydia trachomatis* infections: policy guidelines for prevention and control. M.M.W.R. 34(Suppl.):53S.

3. Ciotti, R.A., Sondheimer, S.J., and Nachamkin, I. 1988. Detecting *Chlamydia trachomatis* by direct immunofluorescence using a Cytobrush sampling technique. Genitourin. Med. 64:245.

4. Cles, L.D., Bruch, K., and Stamm, W.E. 1988. Staining characteristics of six commercially available monoclonal immunofluorescence reagents for direct diagnosis of *Chlamydia trachomatis* infections. J. Clin. Microbiol. 26:1735.

5. Eschenbach, D.A., Hillier, S., Critchlow, C., et al. 1988. Diagnosis and clinical manifestations of bacterial vaginosis. Am. J. Obstet. Gynecol. 158:819.

6. Gordon, F.B., Harper, I.A., Quan, A.L., et al. 1969. Detection of chlamydiae (*Bedsonia*) in certain infections in man: I. Laboratory procedures: comparison of yolk-sac and cell culture for detection and isolation. J. Infect. Dis. 120:451.

7. Gravett, M.G., Hummel, D., Eschenbach, D.A., and Holmes, K.K. 1986. Preterm labor associated with subclinical amniotic fluid infection and with bacterial vaginosis. Obstet. Gynecol. 67:229.

8. Greenwood, J.R., and Robertson, C.A. 1983. *Haemophilus ducreyi*. Microbiol. No. MB 83-8. Check sample. Am. Soc. Clin. Pathol., vol 26, no 8. Chicago, Ill.

9. Lefebvre, J., Laperriere, H., Rousseau, H., and Masse, R. 1988. Comparison of three techniques for detection of *Chlamydia trachomatis* in endocervical specimens from asymptomatic women. J. Clin. Microbiol. 26:726.

10. Martius, J., Krohn, M.A., Hillier, S.L., et al. 1988. Relationship of vaginal *Lactobacillus* species, cervical *Chlamydia trachomatis*, and bacterial vaginosis to preterm birth. Obstet. Gynecol. 71:89.

11. Moller, B.R. 1983. The role of mycoplasmas in the upper genital tract of women. Sex. Transm. Dis. 10(Suppl.):281.

12. Oriel, J.D. 1983. Role of genital mycoplasmas in nongonococcal urethritis and prostatitis. Sexual. Transm. Dis. 10(Suppl.):263.

13. Prior, R.B., and Spagna, V.A. 1981. Application of a *Limulus* test device in rapid evaluation of gonococcal and non-gonococcal urethritis in males. J. Clin. Microbiol. 14:256.

14. Prior, R.B., and Spagna, V.A. 1982. Rapid evaluation of female patients exposed to gonorrhea by the use of the *Limulus* lysate test. J. Clin. Microbiol. 16:57.

15. Roberts, M.C., Hillier, S.L., Schoenknecht, F.D., and Holmes, K.K. 1985. Comparison of Gram stain, DNA probe, and culture for the identification of species of *Mobiluncus* in female genital specimens. J. Infect. Dis. 152:74.

16. Smith, R.F. 1986. Detection of *Trichomonas vaginalis* in vaginal specimens by direct immunofluorescence assay. J. Clin. Microbiol. 24:1107.

17. Spiegel, C.A., Amsel, R., and Holmes, K.K. 1983. Diagnosis of bacterial vaginosis by direct Gram stain of vaginal fluid. J. Clin. Microbiol. 18:170.

18. Stamm, W.E., Running, K., Hale, J., and Holmes, K.K. 1983. Etiologic role of *Mycoplasma hominis* and *Ureaplasma urealyticum* in women with the acute urethral syndrome. Sex. Trans. Dis. 10(Suppl.):318.

19. Toth, A., Lesser, M.L., Brooks, C., and Labriola, D. 1983. Subsequent pregnancies among 161 couples treated for T-mycoplasma genital-tract infection. N. Eng. J. Med. 308:505.

20. Tramont, E. 1985. *Treponema pallidum* (syphilis). In Mandell, G.L., Douglas, R.G., Jr., and Bennett, J.E., editors: Principles and practice of infectious diseases, ed. 2. John Wiley & Sons, New York.

21. Tully, J.G., Taylor-Robinson, D., Rose, D.L., et al. 1983. *Mycoplasma genitalium*, a new species from the human urogenital tract. Int. J. Syst. Bacteriol. 33:387.

22. Wood, J.C., Lu, R.M., Peterson, E.M., et al. 1985. Evaluation of Mycotrim-GU for isolation of *Mycoplasma* species and *Ureaplasma urealyticum*. J. Clin. Microbiol. 22:789.

BIBLIOGRAPHY

Eschenbach, D., Pollock, H.M., and Schachter, J. 1984. Laboratory diagnosis of female genital tract infections. In Rubin, S.J., Coordinating Editor, Cumitech 17. American Society for Microbiology, Washington, D.C.

Kramer, D.G., and Brown, S.T. 1984. Sexually transmitted diseases and infertility. Int. J. Gynaecol. Obstet. 22:19.

La Scolea, L.J. 19Chlamydial infections: the mother-infant connection. Clin. Microbiol. Newsletter 8:77.

Ledger, W.J. 1985. Infections of the female pelvis. In Mandell, G.L., Douglas, R.G., Jr., and Bennett, J.E., editors: Principles and practice of infectious diseases, ed. 2. John Wiley & Sons, New York.

Mårdh, P.-A. 1984. Laboratory diagnosis of sexually transmitted diseases. In Holmes, K.K., Mårdh, P.-A., Sparling, P.F., and Wiesner, P.J., editors: Sexually transmitted diseases. McGraw-Hill Book Co., New York.

Paavonen, J., Critchlow, C.W., DeRouen, T., et al. 1986. Etiology of cervical inflammation. Am. J. Obstet. Gynecol. 154:556.

Phillips, R.S., Aronson, M.D., Taylor, W.C., and Safran, C. 1987. Should tests for *Chlamydia trachomatis* cervical infection be done during routine gynecologic visits? Ann. Intern. Med. 107:188.

Rein, M.F. 1985. Urethritis, In Mandell, G.L., Douglas, R.G., Jr., and Bennett, J.E., editors: Principles and practice of infectious diseases, ed. 2. John Wiley & Sons, New York.

20 Microorganisms Encountered in Wounds, Abscesses, Skin, and Soft Tissue Lesions

Infections in the categories covered in this chapter are commonly encountered clinically and therefore commonly sent to the laboratory for culture. A wide variety of bacteria, fungi, and viruses may be involved. Parasites (*Trichinella*, *Taenia solium*, and *Toxoplasma*) may be involved in myositis but are not sought in the usual processing of specimens in the clinical laboratory; biopsy and serologic procedures are typically employed. The bacterial flora involved in bite infections and clenched fist injuries usually originates in the oral cavity and thus is often polymicrobic and includes anaerobes. Tissue obtained by debridement or biopsy (Chapter 21) may be an important source of information on the infections discussed in this chapter. Venereal diseases of certain types produce skin and soft tissue lesions; these are discussed in Chapter 19. Other agents of skin infections are also discussed elsewhere in the book (*Bacillus anthracis*, *Corynebacterium diphtheriae*, mycobacteria, viruses, and fungi, for example).

A number of the agents involved in the infections covered in this chapter are fastidious; accordingly, careful attention to specimen transport and culture techniques, including the use of specialized media, will be important. The potential for introduction of indigenous and transient skin flora into the specimen is great; therefore, proper specimen collection is critical for laboratory diagnosis of these infections. In some cases, the amount of material available for direct examination and culture will be very small. The use of more than one swab (swabs may be the only practical collection device in such cases) and careful specimen transport will help ensure reliable bacteriologic results. Biopsy, if feasible, will provide the best materials. Discussion between the microbiologist and the clinician will result in better specimen collection and transport and should provide the microbiologist with important information that will be of great assistance in selecting optimum culturing and processing procedures. For example, information on exposure of the patient to seawater or ingestion by the patient of raw shellfish would alert the laboratory to look for *Vibrio vulnificus*. Information that the specimen is from a necrotic palatal lesion in a patient with diabetic ketoacidosis would indicate the need to look carefully for *Aspergillus, Mucor, Rhizopus, Rhizomucor,* and *Absidia*. Clinical evidence of a necrotizing fasciitis would indicate the likely presence of group A streptococcus, *Staphylococcus aureus*, or various anaerobic bacteria. An excellent reference for more information is the Cumitech by Simor et al.[8]

20.1. Wound Infections, Abscesses

Wound infections and abscesses occur as complications of surgery, trauma, or disease that may interrupt a mucosal or skin surface. The nature of the infecting flora will depend on the underlying problem and the location of the process. In the case of a perforated appendix, the flora will be that of the indigenous flora of the lower gastrointestinal tract— *Escherichia coli*, streptococci, *Bacteroides* (*B. fragilis* group and others), *Peptostreptococcus* sp., and *Clostridium* sp., for the most part. In the case of postoperative wound infection following perforated peptic ulcer in a patient who was hospitalized for 2 weeks before the perforation and who has been receiving antimicrobial therapy for an unrelated process (for example, pneumonia), nosocomial pathogens, such as *S. aureus, Klebsiella, Enterobacter,* and *Pseudomonas aeruginosa,* are likely to be involved, in addition to oral flora (streptococci of the viridans group, oral anaerobes) and flora related to the underlying peptic ulcer disease (in the presence of obstruction or bleeding, there is often colonization of the stomach with *E. coli* and other elements typical of the colonic flora, including the *B. fragilis* group). Thus, knowledge of the indigenous flora of a viscus or an area, of the way in which this flora may be modified by disease or antimicrobial agents, and of the environmental flora permits one to make an educated guess as to the likely etiologic agents, and even their antimicrobial susceptibility patterns.

Organisms Generally Encountered in Wound Infections and Abscesses

Staphylococcus aureus
Streptococcus pyogenes
Escherichia coli
Bacteroides sp.
Fusobacterium sp.
Proteus, Morganella, Providencia
Other Enterobacteriaceae
Pseudomonas sp.
Clostridium sp.
Peptostreptococcus sp.
Microaerophilic streptococci
Enterococci
Non-spore-forming   anaerobic   gram-positive rods
Candida sp.

The clinician, of course, uses this approach (along with certain clinical features that may indicate the presence of one organism or another) to choose empirical therapy before availability of microbiological data; information from Gram stain or other direct examination is taken into account as well. The microbiologist uses this type of information to be certain that appropriate media, culture conditions, and so forth are employed. The organisms generally encountered are listed in the box above.

Since anaerobic bacteria are involved in many or most infections of this type, collection of specimens so as to avoid indigenous flora and specimen transport under good anaerobic conditions (which will not interfere with recovery of even obligate aerobes) is particularly important. Blood cultures, including special fungal blood cultures, should be taken since bacteremia or fungemia is encountered in a number of patients with wound infection or abscess. Unusual organisms associated with postsurgical wound infections include *Mycoplasma hominis, Mycobacterium chelonae, Mycobacterium fortuitum,* and even *Legionella* species. These organisms should not be overlooked.

Quantitative or semiquantitative reporting of culture results is desirable. This provides some information on the relative importance of the various organisms present in a mixed infection (the typical situation with wounds and abscesses). It may also provide information on the response of the infection to therapy. Quantitative culture results are particularly important for burn wound infections, where the number of organisms is indicative of the severity of disease.[8] Chapter 21 covers this topic in more detail.

20.2. Extremity Infections Related to Vascular and Neurologic Problems

The classic patient with one of these common infections has diabetes mellitus, poor arterial circulation (often there is both large- and small-vessel disease), and peripheral neuropathy. Such individuals traumatize their feet readily (often just by virtue of wearing a new pair of shoes) without being aware of it (loss of sensation because of the neuropathy). The traumatized area develops into an ulcer that does not heal readily because of the poor vascular supply and often becomes infected.[1] The infections tend to be chronic and difficult to clear up, manifesting primarily as purulent discharge and necrotic tissue in the base of the ulcer, often with a foul odor. Extension to the underlying bone to produce a difficult-to-manage osteomyelitis is very common. Periodically, there may be an acute cellulitis and lymphangitis engrafted on the chronic low-grade infection. This infection may make control of the patient's diabetes difficult. Peripheral vascular disease unrelated to diabetes mellitus may also predispose to this problem but is usually less difficult to manage because there is no associated neuropathy. Venous insufficiency, particularly when it leads to stasis ulcers, also predisposes to infection, again primarily of the lower extremities (in this case, often in the area of the calf or lower leg, rather than the foot).

Infections related to poor blood supply often involve *S. aureus* and *Streptococcus pyogenes*. Those with open ulcers often become colonized with Enterobacteriaceae and *P. aeruginosa*, which may or may not play a role in the infection. Less well appreciated is the fact that anaerobes are commonly involved in the infectious process, particularly in diabetics or others with peripheral vascular disease. The poor blood supply, of course, contributes to anaerobic conditions. Various anaerobes may be recovered, including the *Bacteroides fragilis* group and pigmented *Bacteroides* and *Porphyromonas*, *Peptostreptococcus* sp., and, less frequently, *Clostridium* sp.[8]

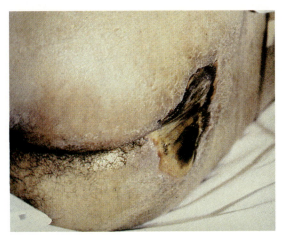

Figure 20.1
Sacral decubitus ulcer.

Another common type of infection in this general category, especially with the elderly or very ill bedridden patient, is infected **decubitus ulcer** (pressure sore) (Figure 20.1). Anaerobic conditions are present in such lesions due to necrosis of tissue. Because the majority of these lesions are located in proximity to the anus and because so many of these patients are relatively helpless, the ulcers become contaminated with bowel flora, which leads to chronic infection. This contributes to further death of tissue and enlargement of the decubitus ulcer. Bacteremia is not an uncommon complication; the *B. fragilis* group is often involved, along with clostridia and enteric bacteria. The ulcers themselves yield a variety of anaerobes and nonanaerobes characteristic of the colonic flora; nosocomial pathogens such as *S. aureus* and *P. aeruginosa* may also be recovered.

Collection and transport of specimens are important factors in laboratory diagnosis of this type of infection. Specimen collection is particularly difficult because many of these lesions are open and therefore readily colonized by nosocomial pathogens that often are not involved in the infection. In the event of an underlying osteomyelitis or a collection of pus in the subcutaneous tissues, attempts should be made to obtain a bone biopsy (for histology as well as smear and culture) or to drain the abscess by needle and syringe aspiration, in both cases traversing only normal skin to get to the underlying infected area, if possible. Bacteremia does not usually accompany this type of infection (with the major exception of

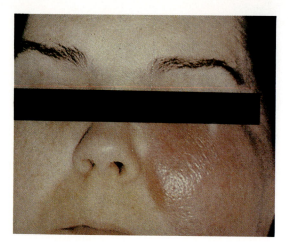

Figure 20.2
Erysipelas caused by S. *pyogenes*.

Organisms Seen in Vesicles and Bullae

Staphylococcus aureus
Group A streptococci
Pseudomonas aeruginosa
Other gram-negative bacilli
Clostridium sp.
Varicella-zoster virus
Herpes simplex virus
Other viruses

---

infected decubitus ulcers) unless there is an acute lymphangitis as part of the picture.

20.3. Pyoderma, Cellulitis

In this category are infections of the skin and subcutaneous tissue, including impetigo, folliculitis, furuncles, carbuncles, paronychia, cellulitis, erysipelas (Figure 20.2), and similar lesions. S. *aureus* and group A streptococci are the most common infecting organisms, with *Candida* and *P. aeruginosa* seen less frequently. Various non-spore-forming anaerobes are encountered more often than had been realized in the past.[3] Bacteremia is not a common accompaniment of this type of infection. A recent study identified diabetics and patients with underlying hematologic (especially plasma cell) malignancy as those more likely to have positive results from fine needle aspiration of cellulitis sites.[2,7]

20.4. Vesicles, Bullae

This type of fluid-filled lesion characteristically involves certain organisms predictably so that if the laboratory is aware of the nature of the lesion the microbiologist can anticipate the flora and use appropriate techniques to ensure recovery of the agent(s). The organisms seen in these lesions are listed in the box above.

The material in the blisterlike lesion varies from serous fluid to serosanguineous or hemorrhagic fluid. Large bullae permit withdrawal of 0.5 to 1 ml of fluid by needle and syringe aspiration. Some vesicles are

quite tiny so that one must use a swab for specimen collection. The clinician can usually readily anticipate whether the lesion is viral or bacterial in nature; recovery of the agent will be facilitated if this information is imparted to the microbiologist. Bullous lesions are caused by bacteria and are often associated with sepsis so that blood cultures are mandatory. With this type of lesion as well, the clinician may often be able to suspect a particular type of organism based on the clinical picture. In the case of an immunosuppressed patient with acute leukemia, for example, *P. aeruginosa* would be a common cause of bullous lesions (a type of ecthyma gangrenosum, Figure 20.3). One may see bronzed skin with bullous lesions in gas gangrene (Figure 20.4), an entity with a very distinctive clinical picture; *Clostridium perfringens* and other clostridia are the key pathogens. Gram stain of the fluid from such lesions typically reveals the etiologic agent and provides the clinician with additional valuable information on which to base initial therapy.

20.5. Draining Sinuses, Fistulas

The most common situation in which one finds draining sinuses is a deep-seated infection that spontaneously drains itself externally, most often a chronic osteomyelitis. Unfortunately, this type of drainage does not usually cure the underlying process, so that such sinuses themselves tend to be chronic. The organisms most often involved in sinuses with an underlying osteomyelitis are S. *aureus*, various Enterobacteriaceae, *P. aeruginosa*, anaerobic gram-negative bacilli, anaerobic gram-positive cocci, and occasionally other anaerobes. In the case of actinomycotic bone involvement, of course, one would ex-

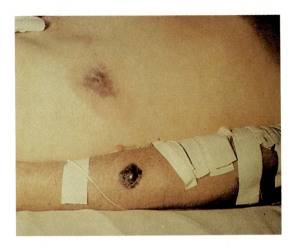

Figure 20.3
Ecthyma gangrenosum caused by *P. aeruginosa*.

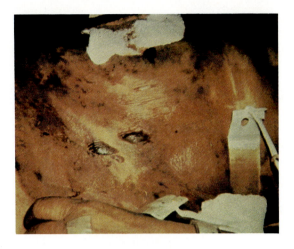

Figure 20.4
Gas gangrene, abdominal wall. Note bronze discoloration and fluid-filled blisters (bullae).

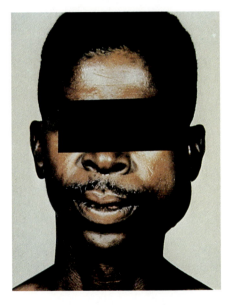

Figure 20.5
Actinomycosis. Note "lumpy" jaw.

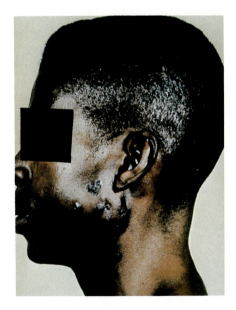

Figure 20.6
Actinomycosis, side view. Note sinuses in skin of face and neck.

pect to recover *Actinomyces* sp. (including former *Arachnia*), pigmented *Bacteroides* or *Porphyromonas* and other non-spore-forming anaerobes, and perhaps *Actinobacillus actinomycetemcomitans*. In the case of other types of draining sinuses, such as that associated with recurrent breast abscess of the subareolar type, the organisms involved will depend on the nature of the underlying process. In the ex-

ample of the breast abscess cited, non-spore-forming anaerobic bacteria are commonly isolated.

Other situations in which chronic draining sinuses are found typically include actinomycosis (cervicofacial [Figures 20.5 and 20.6], thoracic, abdominal, or pelvic), tuberculosis and atypical mycobacterial infection, *Nocardia* infection, and certain infections associated with implanted foreign bodies.

Fistulas (abnormal communications between a hollow viscus and the exterior) are difficult management problems. They also pose problems that are often insurmountable in terms of collection of meaningful specimens since the viscus (such as the bowel) that has the abnormal communication to the skin surface often has its own profuse indigenous flora. Examples are perirectal fistulas and enterocutaneous fistulas from the small bowel to the skin in association with Crohn's disease or chronic intra-abdominal infection. When the bowel is involved, only cultures for specific key organisms such as mycobacteria or *Actinomyces* are meaningful. One should always attempt to rule out specific underlying causes such as tuberculosis, actinomycosis, and malignancy; biopsy is most useful.

20.6. Suppurative Lymphadenitis

Lymphadenopathy may be seen in a variety of infectious processes, but the clinical microbiology laboratory is not usually involved directly in diagnosis of the underlying problem except for serologic testing (for example, in infectious mononucleosis syndromes). In the case of suppurative breakdown of a lymph node, material aspirated from the node will be submitted for direct examination and culture. Agents that may cause suppuration in a lymph node include group A streptococci, *S. aureus, Mycobacterium tuberculosis, Mycobacterium scrofulaceum, Yersinia pestis, Francisella tularensis, Pseudomonas pseudomallei, Pseudomonas mallei, Sporothrix, Coccidioides, Chlamydia trachomatis*, and the agent of cat-scratch disease.

20.7. Myositis

Involvement of muscle occurs with a wide variety of infectious agents. The nature of the pathologic process is variable, sometimes involving extensive necrosis of muscle, as in gas gangrene or clostridial myonecrosis, *necrotizing cutaneous* myositis or *synergistic nonclostridial anaerobic myonecrosis*, anaerobic streptococcal myonecrosis, myonecrosis due to *Bacillus* sp., or myonecrosis due to *Aeromonas*, and sometimes presenting with focal collections of suppuration in muscle (staphylococcal pyomyositis).[6] Muscle involvement may also manifest as a vasculitis in muscle tissue *(V. vulnificus)*, and sometimes as an inflammatory myositis presenting clinically as a benign myalgia (but occasionally with myoglobinuria secondary to muscle breakdown [rhabdomyolysis], as occurs in influenza and other viral infections, rick-

ettsial infections, infective endocarditis, bacteremia, *Legionella* infection [perhaps related to sepsis], toxoplasmosis, trichinosis, and cysticercosis). Abscess in the psoas muscles may involve *M. tuberculosis, S. aureus*, or various facultative gram-negative bacilli. Serious vascular problems may lead to death of muscle due to loss of blood supply; such muscle may become secondarily infected (infected vascular gangrene) but this is usually a low-grade process. Blood cultures should always be drawn from patients with significant myonecrosis. Transport of material (tissue is always better than pus, which is, in turn, better than a swab) should be under anaerobic conditions. In the course of setting up anaerobic cultures, consideration should be given to setting up a Nagler plate (Chapter 34) directly from the clinical specimen in order to rapidly detect *Clostridium perfringens* presumptively (in 12 to 18 hours). Similarly, *Bacteroides* bile esculin agar plates should be set up in the case of synergistic nonclostridial anaerobic myonecrosis; this permits rapid presumptive identification of the *B. fragilis* group (18 to 24 hours). Obviously, very early presumptive identification requires examination of plates at frequent intervals and much sooner than the usual 48-hour interval used conventionally. This may be accomplished readily if the laboratory has an anaerobic chamber that contains an incubator or by use of a single-plate anaerobic pouch system; these approaches avoid exposing the plates to air before it is determined that there is adequate growth. Organisms producing myositis or other muscle pathology are listed in the box on p. 285.

20.8. Serious Soft Tissue and Skin Infections

This category is used for a miscellaneous collection of infections, some extensive and some localized, but all serious or potentially serious. Anthrax and cutaneous diphtheria are discussed elsewhere, as noted previously. An often fatal, but fortunately rare, infection known as mucormycosis or phycomycosis is found in patients with diabetes, acidosis, or with hematologic neoplasms or other conditions requiring corticosteroid or cytotoxic therapy. Necrotic lesions of the palate or nasal mucous membranes are often noted first, but lesions may also spread to the brain or involve other deep organs early in the illness. The fungi most commonly involved are *Mucor, Rhizopus, Absidia*, and *Rhizomucor*, but occasionally other fungi of the order Mucorales may be involved; *Aspergillus* species and *Pseudallescheria boydii* may

---

Organisms Producing Myositis or Other Muscle Pathology

Clostridium perfringens	*Staphylococcus aureus*
C. novyii	Group A streptococci
C. septicum	*Pseudomonas mallei*
C. bifermentans	*P. pseudomallei*
C. histolyticum	*Vibrio vulnificus*
C. sordellii	*Mycobacterium tuberculosis*
C. sporogenes	*Salmonella typhi*
Bacillus sp.	*Legionella* sp.
Aeromonas sp.	*Rickettsia*
Peptostreptococcus sp.	Viruses
Microaerophilic streptococci	*Trichinella*
Bacteroides sp.	*Taenia solium*
Enterobacteriaceae	*Toxoplasma*

---

produce similar clinical pictures. Material should be obtained by biopsy of the necrotic tissue for direct examination and culture.

Necrotizing fasciitis is a serious infection that is more common than mucormycosis but is still relatively uncommon. The basic pathology is infection involving the fascia overlying muscle groups, often with concomitant involvement of the overlying soft tissue. At the fascial level there is no barrier to spread of infection so that fasciitis may extend widely and rapidly to involve huge areas of the body in short periods. This process, once known as hospital gangrene, commonly involves group A streptococci or *S. aureus*. Necrotizing fasciitis also commonly involves anaerobic bacteria, especially *Bacteroides* and *Clostridium* species. Many or most cases of perineal gangrene or phlegmon (Fournier's gangrene) and of necrotizing dermogenital infection are forms of necrotizing fasciitis, although some involve only the more superficial soft tissues (and thus are not as dangerous).

Progressive bacterial synergistic gangrene is usually a chronic gangrenous condition of the skin most often encountered as a postoperative complication, particularly after abdominal surgery requiring retention sutures or after thoracic surgery. The lesions may be extensive and, in the case of involvement of the abdominal wall, may lead to evisceration. As the name suggests, this is typically a mixed infection with microaerophilic streptococci and *S. aureus*. At times there may be a number of organ-isms other than *S. aureus*, including anaerobic streptococci, *Proteus*, and other facultative and anaerobic bacteria. If only the purulent or necrotic material from the central portion of the wound is cultured, the microaerophilic streptococcus will be missed (as may happen since this infection is very uncommon and the clinician may not recognize the usually distinctive clinical features) and the nature of the lesion may not be appreciated. Cultures should be taken from the advancing outer edge of the lesion.

Chronic undermining ulcer or *Meleney's ulcer* is a slowly progressive infection of the subcutaneous tissue with associated ulceration of portions of the overlying skin. The causative organism is classically a microaerophilic streptococcus, but anaerobic streptococci and, occasionally, other organisms may be involved.

Anaerobic cellulitis is an acute anaerobic infection of soft tissue that is much more common than the other infections in this category. It is most often found in the extremities and is particularly common in diabetics. It may also involve the neck, the abdominal wall, the perineum, or connective tissue in other areas. Anaerobic cellulitis also may occur as a postoperative problem. Although the onset and spread of this lesion are not usually rapid and the patients do not show impressive systemic effects at first, it is not an illness to be taken lightly. The organisms are almost always mixed aerobic and anaerobic. The aerobes include *E. coli*, α-hemolytic or nonhemolytic streptococci, and *S. aureus* predom-

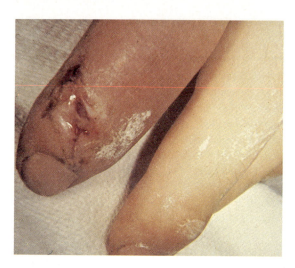

Figure 20.7
Human bite infection.

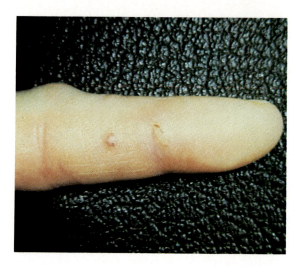

Figure 20.8
Animal bite infection caused by *Pasteurella multocida*.

inantly, but group A streptococci and other Entero-bacteriaceae are encountered as well. The anaerobes are typically found in greater numbers and in more variety than the aerobes; *Peptostreptococcus* sp., *B. fragilis* group strains, pigmented *Bacteroides* and *Porphyromonas*, other *Bacteroides*, clostridia, and occasional *Fusobacterium* sp. are encountered. Bacteremia is not usually present. Good anaerobic transport and culture techniques are important.

20.9. Burn Infections

Infection of burn wounds is essentially universal, not uncommonly is associated with bacteremia, may carry a significant mortality, and interferes with the acceptance of skin grafts. Many organisms are capable of infecting the eschar of a burn. Those most commonly encountered are various streptococci, *S. aureus*, *Staphylococcus epidermidis*, Enterobacteriaceae, *Pseudomonas* species, other gram-negative bacilli, *Candida*, and *Aspergillus*. The setting would seem to be ideal for anaerobic bacteria, and clostridia and *Bacteroides* have been recovered occasionally; very likely a carefully done study would reveal that anaerobes are more commonly involved than has been appreciated to date.

20.10. Bite Infections

Human bites (Figure 20.7), including clenched fist injuries, yield, among the aerobic or facultative flora, α-hemolytic streptococci, *S. aureus*, group A streptococcus, and *Eikenella corrodens*, in that order of frequency. Anaerobes recovered include, in order of frequency, *Peptostreptococcus*, pigmented *Bacteroides* and *Porphyromonas*, *Bacteroides oris*, *Bacteroides buccae*, and *Fusobacterium nucleatum*.[4] In infected animal bite wounds (Figure 20.8), the most commonly encountered aerobic and facultative bacteria are α-hemolytic streptococci, *S. aureus*, *Pasteurella multocida* and *Enterobacter cloacae*.[5] Predominant anaerobes in the animal bites are anaerobic gram-positive cocci, *Fusobacterium* sp., and *Bacteroides* sp.[4,5]

Oral and nasal fluids from dogs yield CDC groups II-J and EF-4, *P. multocida*, and *Staphylococcus intermedius* (with much smaller numbers of *S. aureus*).[9] *Simonsiella* is found in the oral cavity of most dogs and is also found in the oral cavity of humans, cats, and other animals. The oral flora of snakes contains various gram-negative bacilli including *Pseudomonas*, *Klebsiella*, *Proteus*, and *E. coli*. Clostridia may also be recovered from snakebite wounds.

Fastidious gram-negative bacilli designated as DF-2 (now called *Capnocytophaga canimorsus*) and DF-3 by CDC have been responsible for a number of serious infections, including bacteremia, endocarditis, and meningitis. Most of these patients had a history of dog bite and most had underlying diseases that impair host defense mechanisms. The organisms grow slowly on blood and chocolate agar (it does best with a heart infusion agar), and growth may be enhanced by rabbit serum and increased CO_2 tension. *C. canimorsus* (DF-2) is often recovered from blood cultures. It is typically resistant to aminoglycosides and is susceptible to penicillin G.

Bite wound infections usually involve relatively small lesions and minimal exudate so that a swab technique with anaerobic transport will usually be needed. Surrounding skin should be thoroughly cleansed before the specimen is obtained.

20.11. Uncommon But Important Causes of Skin and Soft Tissue Infection

There are a number of organisms that may cause infection with serious consequences that are encountered uncommonly or rarely. Included are *Clostridium tetani* (tetanus), *Clostridium botulinum* (wound botulism), *F. tularensis* (tularemia), various mycobacteria, *Erysipelothrix rhusiopathiae* (erysipeloid), *Actinomyces, Nocardia, Vibrio alginolyticus* (cellulitis in marine wound infection), *V. vulnificus* (wound infection), *Sporothrix schenckii* (sporotrichosis), and dematiaceous fungal agents of phaeohyphomycosis, chromoblastomycosis, and mycetoma. Various other systemic fungi, such as *Coccidioides immitis* and *Blastomyces dermatitidis*, may involve skin and subcutaneous tissue either as a primary inoculation infection or, more commonly, as part of the process of dissemination.

20.12. Miscellaneous Skin and Soft Tissue Infections of Mild to Moderate Severity

Erythrasma is a very mild and superficial skin infection; the causative organism is *Corynebacterium minutissimum*. The clinical picture is distinctive, with infected lesions fluorescing coral red under long-wave ultraviolet light. Skin scrapings may be cultured in media containing serum, but imprint smears of the lesion should reveal gram-positive pleomorphic rods, precluding the necessity for culture. There are numerous superficial mycoses involving skin, nails, and hair. They are discussed in Chapter 43, but it is well to be aware that on rare occasions under unusual circumstances, organisms such as *Pityrosporum orbiculare* (also called *Malassezia furfur*) or *Trichosporon* can cause systemic in-

fection. *Mycobacterium marinum* causes "swimming pool" or "fishbowl" granuloma. Hidradenitis suppurativa is a chronic, troublesome, annoying infection of the obstructed apocrine glands in the axillae and genital and perianal areas with intermittent discharge of pus (often foul smelling), draining sinuses at times, and scarring. Subareolar breast abscess probably involves this type of pathology. Secondary infection involves anaerobic gram-negative rods, anaerobic cocci, staphylococci, streptococci, and various aerobic and facultative gram-negative rods. Infected pilonidal cysts almost invariably yield anaerobic bacteria, sometimes to the exclusion of other types of bacteria. The anaerobes involved include the *B. fragilis* group, other *Bacteroides, Fusobacterium*, anaerobic gram-positive cocci, and clostridia. Various nonanaerobes, especially Enterobacteriaceae, enterococci, and other streptococci, may also be recovered. Infected "inclusion" or "sebaceous" cysts often yield anaerobic cocci or *Bacteroides*; staphylococci and streptococci are also found commonly in such cysts.

20.13. Skin Lesions as Part of Systemic Infection

Cutaneous manifestations of systemic infection such as bacteremia or endocarditis are not uncommon; they may be important clues for the clinician and they may present an opportunity for direct or cultural demonstration of the presence of a particular organism. For example, one may be able to scrape petechiae in cases of meningococcemia and demonstrate gram-negative diplococci. In other cases, the skin lesion represents a more impressive type of metastatic infection. The lesions of ecthyma gangrenosum in *P. aeruginosa* sepsis are prominent. In *V. vulnificus* sepsis, dramatic-appearing cutaneous ulcers with necrotizing vasculitis may be found. In some cases, skin lesions may actually represent a noninfectious complication of a local or systemic infection. Examples would be the rashes of scarlet fever and toxic shock syndrome. Various organisms that may be involved in systemic infection with cutaneous lesions are listed in the box on p. 288.

Organisms Involved in Systemic Infection with Cutaneous Lesions

Viridans streptococci	*Mycobacterium tuberculosis*
Staphylococcus aureus	*M. leprae*
Enterococci	*Treponema pallidum*
Group A and other β-hemolytic streptococci	*Leptospira*
Neisseria gonorrhoeae	*Streptobacillus moniliformis*
N. meningitidis	*Spirillum minus*
Haemophilus influenzae	*Bartonella bacilliformis*
Pseudomonas aeruginosa	*Rickettsia*
P. mallei	*Candida* sp.
P. pseudomallei	*Cryptococcus neoformans*
Listeria monocytogenes	*Blastomyces dermatitidis*
Vibrio vulnificus	*Coccidioides immitis*
Salmonella typhi	*Histoplasma capsulatum*

REFERENCES

1. Amin, N. 1988. Infected diabetic foot ulcers. Am. Fam. Physician 37:283.
2. Epperly, T.D. 1986. The value of needle aspiration in the management of cellulitis. J. Fam. Pract. 23:337.
3. Finch, R. 1988. Skin and soft-tissue infections. Lancet 1:164.
4. Goldstein, E.J.C., Reinhardt, J.F., Murray, P.M., and Finegold, S.M. 1987. Outpatient therapy of bite wounds: demographic data, bacteriology, and a prospective, randomized trial of amoxicillin/clavulanic acid versus penicillin + /- dicloxacillin. Int. J. Dermatol. 26:123.
5. Goldstein, R.W., Goodhart, G.L., and Moore, J.E. 1986. *Pasteurella multocida* infection after animal bite. N. Engl. J. Med. 315:460.
6. Isaacs, R.D., Paviour, S.D., Bunker, D.E., and Lang, S.D.R. 1988. Wound infections with aerogenic *Aeromonas* strains: a review of twenty-seven cases. Eur. J. Clin. Microbiol. Infect. Dis. 7:355.
7. Kielhofner, M.A, Brown, B., and Dall, L. 1988. Influence of disease process on the utility of cellulitis needle aspirates. Arch. Intern. Med. 148:2451.
8. Simor, A.E., Roberts, F.J., and Smith, J.A. 1988. Infections of the skin and subcutaneous tissues. In Smith J.A., Coordinating Editor. Cumitech 23. American Society for Microbiology, Washington, D.C.
9. Talan, D.A., Staatz, D., Staatz, A., et al. 1989. *Staphylococcus intermedius* in canine gingiva and canine-inflicted wound infections: laboratory characterization of a newly recognized zoonotic pathogen. J. Clin. Microbiol. 27:78.

BIBLIOGRAPHY

Bonner, J.R., Coker, A.S., Berryman, C.R., et al. 1983. Spectrum of *Vibrio* infections in a gulf coast community. Ann. Intern. Med. 99:464.
Chow, A.W., Galpin, J.E., and Guze, L.B. 1975. Clinical experience with clindamycin in sepsis caused by decubitus ulcers. J. Infect. Dis. 135:S65.
Churchill, M.A., Geraci, J.E., and Hunder, G.G. 1977. Musculoskeletal manifestations of bacterial endocarditis. Ann. Intern. Med. 87:754.
Davison, A.J., and Rotstein, O.D. 1988. The diagnosis and management of common soft-tissue infections. Can. Assoc. Gen. Surg. 31:333.
Finegold, S.M. 1977. Anaerobic bacteria in human disease. Academic Press, New York.
Meislin, H.W., Lerner, S.A., Graves, M.H., et al. 1977. Cutaneous abscesses. Anaerobic and aerobic bacteriology and outpatient management. Ann. Intern. Med. 87:145.
Sapico, F.L., Canawati, H.N., Witte, J.L., et al. 1980. Quantitative aerobic and anaerobic bacteriology of infected diabetic feet. J. Clin. Microbiol. 12:413.
Swartz, M.N. 1985. Skin and soft tissue infections. In Mandell, G.L., Douglas, R.G., Jr., and Bennett, J.E., editors. Principles and practice of infectious diseases, ed. 2. John Wiley & Sons, New York.

21

Microorganisms Encountered in Solid Tissue, Bone, Bone Marrow, and Body Fluids

Etiologic agents of disease from all four categories (bacteria, fungi, viruses, and parasites) may be found within the tissues of the body and in body fluids. This chapter will discuss the types of microorganisms likely to be recovered from specimens of tissue, bone marrow, bone, and "sterile" body fluids. Bacteria, fungi, and viruses can be identified by microbiological techniques practiced in routine clinical laboratories, and the discussion that follows will focus on those agents. Because even one colony of a potential pathogenic microorganism could be significant and because these specimens often undergo more handling in the laboratory than do other types of specimens, we recommend that all manipulations of the specimens, transferring material, and inoculating media be performed by a technologist wearing gloves and working within a *biological safety cabinet*.

In most cases, the detection of parasites in tissue is accomplished by observing characteristic morphological structures in stained histological sections; examination of tissue for parasites is usually done by pathologists. *Pneumocystis carinii*, however, is often diagnosed in lung biopsy material by microbiologists. Occasionally a wet preparation of pleural fluid may reveal *Entamoeba histolytica*. *E. histolytica* may also be identified in material from the wall of an amebic liver abscess. Other tissues may be cultured for parasites such as *Leishmania* and trypanosomes.

21.1. Sterile Body Fluids

In response to infection, fluid may accumulate in any body cavity. Infected solid tissue often presents

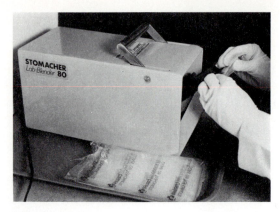

Figure 21.1
A mechanical tissue grinder (Stomacher Lab-blender 80, Tekmar Co.) Tissue is placed in 2 ml sterile broth in plastic bags. The action of two paddles serves to homogenize the tissue or drive the bacteria from the tissue into the broth.

as a phlegmon or cellulitis or with abscess formation (Chapter 20). Areas of the body from which fluids are commonly sent for microbiological studies (in addition to blood and cerebrospinal fluids, covered in Chapters 14 and 15) include the thorax (thoracentesis fluid [also called pleural fluid]), abdominal cavity (also called paracentesis fluid [ascitic fluid or peritoneal fluid]), joints, and pericardium (pericardial fluid). Techniques for laboratory processing of all sterile body fluids are somewhat similar. Clear fluids may be concentrated by centrifugation or filtration, while purulent material can be inoculated directly to media. Any body fluid that is received in the laboratory already clotted must be homogenized to release trapped bacteria and minced or cut to release fungal cells. Either processing such specimens in a tissue homogenizer (Stomacher Lab-blender 80, Tekmar Co.; Figure 21.1) or grinding them manually in a mortar and pestle or glass tissue grinder will allow better recovery of bacteria. Grinding may lyse fungal elements, therefore it is not recommended for specimens for fungi. Small amounts of whole material from a clot should be aseptically cut with a scalpel and placed directly onto media for isolation of fungi.

21.1.a. **Pleural fluid.** Pleural fluid or pleural effusion is a collection of fluid in the pleural space, extending between the lung and the chest wall. The fluid may contain few or no cells and be of a consistency similar to that of serum (but with a lower protein content). This type of effusion, called a **tran-**sudate,** is often the result of cardiac, hepatic, or renal disease. Pleural effusion that contains numerous white blood cells and other evidence of an inflammatory response is usually due to infection, but malignancy, pulmonary infarction, or autoimmune diseases in which an antigen-antibody reaction initiates an inflammatory response may also be responsible. Such an effusion, called an **exudate,** is the usual specimen submitted to microbiology laboratories. This pleural effusion is collected from the patient by needle aspiration (thoracentesis) and submitted to the laboratory as "pleural fluid," "thoracentesis fluid," or "empyema fluid." Exudative pleural effusions that contain numerous polymorphonuclear neutrophils, particularly those that are grossly purulent, are called **empyema** fluids. Empyema usually occurs secondary to pneumonia, but other infections near the lung (subdiaphragmatic infection, for example) may seed microorganisms into the pleural cavity.

The bacteria that may be recovered from pleural fluid include those that are associated with pneumonia, such as *Streptococcus pneumoniae, Staphylococcus aureus, Haemophilus influenzae,* Enterobacteriaceae, *Pseudomonas,* and anaerobes. Anaerobic organisms in pleural fluid or empyema occur secondary to aspiration pneumonia or its complications, such as lung abscess. Less commonly, other streptococci, *Mycobacterium tuberculosis* or nontuberculous mycobacteria, *Actinomyces* species, *Nocardia* species, fungi, and rarely mycoplasma or viruses may be recovered from empyema cultures.

Pleural fluid, as with other body fluids from sterile sites, should be transported to the laboratory in a sterile tube or vial that excludes oxygen. From 1 to 5 ml of specimen is adequate for isolation of most bacteria, but the larger the specimen the better, particularly for isolation of *M. tuberculosis* and fungi. Anaerobic transport vials are available from several sources, as mentioned in Chapter 6 and Appendix C. These vials are prepared in an oxygen-free atmosphere and are sealed with a rubber septum or short stopper through which the fluid is injected. Fluid may be transported quickly to the laboratory in a syringe capped with a sterile rubber stopper, but this method is a less desirable alternative to proper containers. Most clinically significant anaerobic bacteria survive adequately in nonanaerobic transport containers (such as syringes and sterile screw-capped tubes) for short periods if the specimen is frankly purulent and of some volume.

Specimens that are received in anaerobic transport vials or syringes should be inoculated to routine aerobic and anaerobic media as quickly as possible. Gram stains should be examined. If long, thin, gram-positive branching rods are seen, a second smear should be prepared and stained with the modified acid-fast stain for *Nocardia*. Non-acid-fast branching rods are usually *Actinomyces* species; other possibilities are discussed in Chapter 33.

Specimens for recovery of only fungi or mycobacteria may be transported in sterile, screw-capped tubes. At least 10 to 15 ml of fluid is required for adequate recovery of small numbers of organisms. Those specimens that are thin enough are concentrated by centrifugation at $1500 \times$ *g* for at least 15 minutes. The supernatant is aseptically decanted or aspirated with a sterile pipette, leaving approximately 1 ml liquid in which to mix the sediment thoroughly. Vigorous vortexing or drawing the sediment up and down into a pipette several times will adequately resuspend the sediment. This procedure should be done in a biological safety cabinet, of course. The suspension is used to inoculate media and prepare smears. Specimens for fungi should be examined by direct wet preparation in addition to Gram stain. Either 10% potassium hydroxide (KOH) or calcofluor white is recommended for visualization of fungal elements. In addition to hyphal forms, material from the thoracic cavity may contain spherules of *Coccidioides* or budding yeast cells. Specimens are inoculated to the primary media that support the growth of fungi, including brain heart infusion agar supplemented with sheep blood and inhibitory mold agars. Although *Legionella* species are seldom recovered from pleural fluid, special media for isolation of these organisms may be inoculated if clinically indicated. The physician should notify the laboratory to culture the specimen for *Legionella*.

21.1.b. Peritoneal fluid. The peritoneal cavity contains or abuts the liver, pancreas, spleen, stomach and intestinal tract, bladder, and fallopian tubes and ovaries. The kidneys occupy a retroperitoneal position. Within the healthy human peritoneal cavity is a small amount of fluid that maintains moistness of the surface of the peritoneum. Normal peritoneal fluid may contain as many as 300 white blood cells per milliliter, but the protein content and specific gravity of the fluid are low. Agents of infection gain access to the peritoneum either through a perforation of the bowel, infection within abdominal viscera, by way of the bloodstream, or by external inoculation (as in surgery or trauma). On occasion, as in pelvic inflammatory disease (PID), organisms travel through the natural channels of the fallopian tubes into the peritoneal cavity. In primary **peritonitis**, no apparent focus of infection is evident. Secondary peritonitis involves a rupture of a viscus or other known source of infection. During an infectious or inflammatory process, increased amounts of fluid accumulate in the peritoneal cavity. The fluid, often called "ascites" or **ascitic fluid**, contains an increased number of inflammatory cells and an elevated protein level.

The organisms likely to be recovered from specimens from patients suffering from primary peritonitis vary with the age of the patient. The most common etiologic agents in children are *S. pneumoniae* and group A streptococci. Enterobacteriaceae, other gram-negative bacilli, and staphylococci may also be isolated. In adults, *Escherichia coli* is the most common bacterium recovered, followed by *S. pneumoniae* and group A streptococci. Polymicrobic peritonitis is unusual when only aerobic bacteria are associated with disease. Among sexually active young women, *Neisseria gonorrhoeae* and *Chlamydia trachomatis* are common etiologic agents of peritoneal infection, often in the form of a perihepatitis (inflammation of the surface of the liver, called **Fitz-Hugh-Curtis syndrome**). Tuberculous peritonitis is uncommon in the United States today. It is more likely to be found among recent arrivals from South America, Southeast Asia, or less-developed areas of the world. Fungal causes of peritonitis are not common, but *Candida* species may be recovered from immunosuppressed patients and patients on prolonged antibacterial therapy. *Coccidioides immitis* is an uncommon cause of peritonitis found in patients who live in or have visited endemic areas such as the southwestern United States.

Secondary peritonitis is a sequel to a perforated viscus, surgery, traumatic injury, loss of integrity of bowel wall due to destructive disease (for example, ulcerative colitis, carcinoma), obstruction, or a preceding infection (liver abscess, salpingitis, septicemia, and so forth). The nature, location, and etiology of the underlying process govern the agents that will be recovered from peritoneal fluid. With pelvic inflammatory disease as the background, gonococci, anaerobes, or chlamydia will be isolated. In the case of peritonitis or intra-abdominal abscess, anaerobes will generally be found in peritoneal fluid, usually together with Enterobacteriaceae and enterococci or other streptococci. In patients whose bowel flora has been altered by antimicrobial agents, of course, more resistant gram-negative bacilli and S. aureus may be encountered. Since anaerobes outnumber aerobes in the bowel by 1000 fold, it is not surprising that anaerobic organisms play a prominent role in intra-abdominal infection, perhaps acting synergistically with facultative bacteria. The organisms likely to be recovered include E. coli, the *Bacteroides fragilis* group, enterococci and other streptococci, other *Bacteroides* species, other anaerobic gram-negative bacilli, anaerobic gram-positive cocci, and clostridia.

Specimens are collected by percutaneous needle aspiration (**paracentesis**) or at the time of surgery and sent to the laboratory for smears and appropriate cultures. Transport should be in an anaerobic vial. Usually 1 to 5 ml of fluid is sufficient for the diagnosis of peritonitis, but, again, a larger volume is desirable. Material should be inoculated as soon as possible, as should all specimens that may contain anaerobes. If a large volume of clear or serosanguineous fluid is received, it may be concentrated by centrifugation at $1500 \times g$ for ≥ 15 minutes. Bacteriologic media should include chocolate or other medium for recovery of gonococci and the occasional *Haemophilus* species. Appropriate procedures for isolation of fungi, *Chlamydia*, and viruses should be used when such tests are ordered.

21.1.c. Peritoneal dialysis fluid. Over 5000 patients with end-stage renal disease are maintained on chronic ambulatory peritoneal dialysis (**CAPD**); fluid injected into the peritoneal cavity and subsequently removed allows exchange of salts and water and removal of various wastes in the absence of kidney function. The average incidence of peritonitis in these patients is approximately two episodes per year per patient. Peritonitis is diagnosed clinically by the presence of cloudy dialysate with or without abdominal pain or abdominal pain alone.[10,11] Although white blood cells are usually plentiful (leukocytes >100/ml is usually indicative of infection), the number of organisms is usually too low for detection on Gram stain of the peritoneal fluid sediment; fungi are more readily detected. Most infections originate from the patient's own skin flora; *Staphylococcus epidermidis* and S. aureus are the most common etiologic agents, followed by streptococci, aerobic or facultative gram-

negative bacilli, *Candida* species, *Corynebacterium* species, and others. The oxygen content of peritoneal dialysate is usually too high for development of anaerobic infection. Among the gram-negative bacilli isolated, *Pseudomonas* species, *Acinetobacter* species, and the Enterobacteriaceae are common. Contaminated dialysis machinery may also contribute to peritoneal dialysis infections.

Fluid is usually received in the laboratory in a sterile tube or urine cup; less than 10 ml is unacceptable. Almost all patients with peritonitis have cloudy peritoneal dialysis fluid, with a white cell count of over $100/mm^3$.[12] If fluid is received in the original bag, the bag should be entered only once with a sterile needle and syringe to withdraw fluid for culture. Fluid may be processed directly by inoculation into blood culture bottles (at least 20 ml, 10 ml in each of two culture bottles, should be cultured).[13] For other culture methods, the fluid should be concentrated, either by centrifugation, as for other clear, sterile body fluids, or by filtration. A recent study has shown that lysis of leukocytes prior to concentration enhanced recovery significantly.[7] Filtration through a 0.45 μm pore size membrane filter allows a greater volume of fluid to be processed and will usually yield better results. Since the numbers of infecting organisms may be quite low (<1/10 ml fluid), a large quantity of fluid must be processed. Sediment obtained from at least 50 ml fluid is recommended.[2] Gram stains or acridine orange stains should be performed, even though the yield may be low. If the specimen is filtered, the filter should be cut aseptically into three pieces, one of which is placed on chocolate agar for incubation in 5% CO_2, one of which is placed on MacConkey agar, and the other of which is placed on a blood agar plate for anaerobic incubation. Commercial filtration-culture systems have been evaluated.[9] Sediment should be inoculated to aerobic media and thioglycollate or similar broth, although anaerobic media are unnecessary.

A study has documented the sensitivity of culturing the entire contents of a patient's dialysis exchange bag.[3] Processing dialysis fluid in this way may yield more positive cultures than does processing small amounts of dialysate, although the method is somewhat cumbersome.

21.1.d. Pericardial fluid. The heart and contiguous major blood vessels are surrounded by a protective tissue, the pericardium. The area between the epicardium (the membrane surrounding the heart muscle) and the pericardium, the pericardial space, normally contains 15 to 20 ml clear fluid. If an infectious agent is present within the fluid, the pericardium may become distended and tight, and eventually interference with cardiac function and circulation can ensue (called "tamponade"). Agents of **pericarditis** (inflammation of the pericardium) are usually viruses. Parasites, bacteria, certain fungi, and noninfectious causes are also associated with this disease. Inflammation of the heart muscle itself, **myocarditis,** may accompany pericarditis. The pathogenesis of disease involves the host inflammatory response contributing to fluid buildup and cell and tissue damage. The most common etiologic agents of pericarditis and myocarditis are enteroviruses, primarily coxsackieviruses A and B. Echoviruses, adenoviruses, influenza viruses, and other viruses play a lesser role. Among nonviral agents, *Mycoplasma pneumoniae, Chlamydia, M. tuberculosis, S. aureus, S. pneumoniae,* Enterobacteriaceae, other aerobic gram-negative bacilli, anaerobic bacteria, *C. immitis, Aspergillus* species, *Candida* species, *Cryptococcus neoformans, Histoplasma capsulatum, E. histolytica,* and *Toxoplasma gondii* may be found. Other bacteria, fungi, and parasitic agents have been recovered from pericardial effusions, however, and all agents should be sought. Patients who develop pericarditis due to agents other than viruses are often compromised in some way.

Collection of pericardial effusion is performed by needle aspiration with electrocardiographic monitoring or as a surgical procedure. The laboratory personnel should be alerted in advance so that the appropriate media, tissue culture media, and stain procedures are available immediately. Fluid should be processed in the same way as other sterile body fluids, as discussed above.

21.1.e. Joint fluid. Infectious arthritis may involve any joint in the body. It usually occurs secondary to hematogenous spread of bacteria or, less commonly, fungi, and it may occur as a direct extension of infection of the bone. It may also occur following injection of material (especially corticosteroids) into joints or after insertion of prosthetic material (for example, total hip replacement). Although infectious arthritis usually occurs at only one site (**monoarticular),** a preexisting bacteremia or fungemia may seed more than one joint to establish **polyarticular** infection. Knees and hips are the most commonly affected joints.

In addition to active infections associated with viable microorganisms within the joint, sterile, self-limited arthritis due to antigen-antibody interactions may follow an episode of infection, such as meningococcal meningitis. When an etiologic agent cannot be isolated from an inflamed joint fluid specimen, either the absence of viable agents or inadequate transport or culturing procedures can be blamed. For example, even under the best circumstances, *Borrelia burgdorferi* is isolated from the joints of less than 20% of patients with Lyme disease. Nonspecific test results, such as increased white blood cell count, decreased glucose, or elevated protein, may seem to implicate an infectious agent, but they are not conclusive. A role has been postulated for the persistence of bacterial L-forms (cell-wall-deficient forms) in joint fluid after systemic infection, but such organisms have not generally been recovered.

S. aureus is the most common etiologic agent of septic arthritis, accounting for approximately 70% of all such infections. In adults less than 30 years old, however, *N. gonorrhoeae* is isolated most frequently. *H. influenzae* is the most common agent of bacteremia in children less than 2 years of age, and consequently it is the most common cause of infectious arthritis, followed by *S. aureus.* Streptococci, including groups A and B, pneumococci, and viridans streptococci are prominent among bacterial agents associated with infectious arthritis in patients of all ages. *Bacteroides,* including *B. fragilis,* may be recovered, as may *Fusobacterium necrophorum,* which commonly involves more than one joint in the course of sepsis. Among people living in certain endemic areas of the United States and Europe, infectious arthritis is a prominent feature of Lyme disease. Some of the more commonly encountered etiologic agents of infectious arthritis are listed in the box on p. 294.

Most of these agents act to stimulate a host inflammatory response, which is ultimately responsible for the pathology of the infection. Arthritis is also a symptom associated with infectious diseases caused by certain agents, such as *Neisseria meningitidis* and *Streptobacillus moniliformis,* in which the agent cannot be recovered from joint fluid. Presumably, antigen-antibody complexes formed during active infection accumulate in a joint, initiating an inflammatory response that is responsible for the ensuing damage. Other agents, such as viruses, yeasts, and mycoplasmas, are unusual causes of infectious arthritis.

Commonly Encountered Etiologic Agents of Infectious Arthritis

Bacterial

Staphylococcus aureus
β-Hemolytic streptococci
Streptococci (other)
Haemophilus influenzae
Haemophilus sp. (other)
Bacteroides sp.
Fusobacterium sp.
Neisseria gonorrhoeae
Pseudomonas sp.
Salmonella sp.
Pasteurella multocida
Moraxella osloensis
Kingella kingae
Branhamella catarrhalis
Capnocytophaga sp.
Corynebacterium sp.
Clostridium sp.
Peptostreptococcus sp.

Eikenella corrodens
Actinomyces sp.
Mycobacterium sp.
Mycoplasma sp.
Ureaplasma urealyticum
Borrelia burgdorferi

Fungal

Candida sp.
Cryptococcus neoformans
Coccidioides immitis
Sporothrix schenckii

Viral

Hepatitis B
Mumps
Rubella
Other viruses (rarely)

Infections in prosthetic joints are usually associated with different etiologic agents than those in natural joints. Following insertion of the prosthesis, organisms that gained access during the surgical procedure slowly multiply until they reach a critical mass and produce a host response. This may occur long after the initial surgery; approximately one half of all prosthetic joint infections occur more than 1 year after surgery. Skin flora are the most common etiologic agents, with *Staphylococcus epidermidis*, other coagulase negative staphylococci, *Corynebacterium* species, and *Propionibacterium* species predominating. Alternatively, organisms may reach joints during hematogenous spread from distant infected sites.[8]

Specimens are collected by aspiration with a sterile needle and syringe, as are most other "sterile" body fluids. The specimen should be injected into an anaerobic transport vial to preserve viability of anaerobes, which are probably present more often than has been appreciated. It may also prove beneficial to inoculate one bottle of blood culture medium with some of the initial specimen, particularly if the specimen cannot be delivered to the laboratory immediately. This culture is processed as a blood culture, facilitating the recovery of small numbers of organisms and diluting out the effects of antibiotics. Citrate or sodium polyanetholesulfonate may be used as an anticoagulant. If the fluid contains a clot, it must be homogenized or ground up to release organisms, which tend to become trapped in clots. Gonococci may be recovered from joint fluids that have been incubated in hyperosmotic medium, such as sucrose-containing broth. Very purulent specimens are plated directly to several agars, including one that supports the growth of fastidious organisms, such as chocolate agar, and an enriched broth such as thioglycolate. Material should also be inoculated onto primary anaerobic media as discussed in Chapter 34. If fungi or mycobacteria are suspected, appropriate media for their isolation should also be inoculated. Methods for isolation of viruses and mycoplasma are described in Chapters 38 and 42. Direct Gram stains, KOH or calcofluor white preparations for fungi, and acid-fast stain for mycobacteria are also performed.

21.2. Bone Marrow Aspiration or Biopsy

Diagnosis of certain diseases, including brucellosis, histoplasmosis, and leishmaniasis, can sometimes be made only by detection of the organism in the bone marrow. *Brucella* species can be isolated on culture, as can fungi, but parasitic agents must be visualized in smears made from bone marrow material. Bone marrow is aspirated from the interstitium of the iliac crest or the sternum in a small, cylindrical plug. Some of the material may be inoculated directly into blood culture media for recovery of bacteria. Some laboratories report good recovery from bone marrow material that has been injected into a Pediatric Isolator tube (DuPont Co.; described in Chapter 14) as a collection and transport device. The lytic agents within the Isolator tube are thought to lyse cellular components, presumably freeing intracellular bacteria for enhanced recovery. Clotted specimens must be homogenized or ground up to release trapped microorganisms; specimens are inoculated to the same media as for other sterile body fluids. A special medium for enhancement of growth of *Brucella* species and incubation under 10% CO_2 may be used. A portion of the specimens may be inoculated directly to fungal media, as described in Chapter 43. Smears are made for fixation, staining, and examination (usually by pathologists) for the presence of fungal or parasitic agents.

21.3. Bone Biopsy

A small piece of infected bone is occasionally sent to the microbiology laboratory for determination of the etiologic agent of **osteomyelitis** (infection of bone). It has been shown that cultures taken from open wound sites above infected bone or material taken from a draining sinus leading to an area of osteomyelitis may not reflect the actual etiologic agent of the underlying osteomyelitis. Patients develop osteomyelitis from hematogenous spread of an infectious agent, invasion of bone tissue from an adjacent site of infection, such as joint infection or dental infection, or by breakdown of tissue due to trauma or surgery or lack of adequate circulation followed by colonization with microorganisms. Parasites are rarely, if ever, etiologic agents of osteomyelitis. Once established, infections in bone may tend to progress toward chronicity, particularly if there is a lack of effective blood supply to the affected area.

S. *aureus*, seeded during bacteremia, is the most common etiologic agent of osteomyelitis among people of all age groups. The toxins and enzymes produced by this bacterium, as well as its ability to adhere to smooth surfaces and produce a protective glycocalyx coating, seem to contribute to its pathogenicity. Among young persons, osteomyelitis is usually associated with a single agent, S. *aureus*. Such infections are usually of hematogenous origin. Other organisms that have been recovered from hematogenously acquired osteomyelitis include *Salmonella* species, *Haemophilus* species, Enterobacteriaceae, *Pseudomonas* species, *F. necrophorum*, and yeast species. S. *aureus* or *Pseudomonas aeruginosa*, as well as other gram-negative bacilli including *Eikenella corrodens*, is often recovered from drug addicts, whereas a preceding animal bite may lead to *Pasteurella multocida* infection and a human bite may lead to *Eikenella* infection.

Bone biopsies from infections that have spread to a bone from a contiguous source or that are associated with poor circulation (especially in diabetics) are more likely to yield multiple isolates. *M. tuberculosis* is presently an uncommon cause of osteomyelitis. Gram-negative bacilli are increasingly common among hospitalized patients; a break in the skin (surgery or intravenous line) may precede establishment of gram negative osteomyelitis. Breaks in skin from other causes (bite wound, trauma) also may be the initial event that leads to underlying bone infection. Poor oral hygiene may lead to osteomyelitis of the jaw with *Actinomyces* species, *Capnocytophaga* species, and other oral flora, particularly anaerobes. Pigmented *Bacteroides* and *Porphyromonas*, other *Bacteroides*, *Fusobacterium*, and *Peptostreptococcus* species are commonly involved. Pelvic infection in the female may lead to mixed aerobic and anaerobic osteomyelitis of the pubic bone.

Patients with poor circulation to the extremities, notably diabetics who commonly have neuropathy as well and therefore are subjected to trauma that they cannot feel, will develop ulcers on the toes and feet that do not heal, become infected, and may eventually progress to involve underlying bone. These infections are usually polymicrobial, involving anaerobic and aerobic bacteria.[1] Commonly encountered are the pigmented *Bacteroides* or *Porphyromonas*, other gram-negative anaerobes including the *B. fragilis* group, *Peptostreptococcus* species, S. *aureus*, and group A and other streptococci.

Bone removed at surgery or by percutaneous biopsy is sent to the laboratory in a sterile container. It is very difficult to break up bones; grinding them in a mortar and pestle may break off some pieces. It is sometimes possible to scrape off aseptically small shavings from the most necrotic-looking areas, which can be inoculated to media. Pieces should be placed directly into fungal media for recovery of fungi. Small bits of bone can be ground with sterile broth to form a suspension for bacteriological and mycobacterial cultures. If anaerobes are to be recovered, all manipulations should ideally be performed in an anaerobic chamber. If such an environment is unavailable, microbiologists should work quickly within a biosafety cabinet to inoculate anaerobic plates and broth with material from the bone.

21.4. Tissue

Pieces of tissue are removed from patients during surgical or needle biopsy procedures or are collected at autopsy. Any agent of infection may cause disease in tissue, and laboratory practices should be adequate to recover bacteria, fungi, and viruses and to detect the presence of parasites. Fastidious organisms, such as *Brucella* species, and agents of chronic disease such as systemic fungi and mycobacteria, may require special media and long incubation periods for isolation. Some agents that require special supportive or selective media are listed in the box below.

The conditions required for their isolation are discussed in the appropriate chapters. This chapter will not attempt to delineate all possible etiologic agents that can be recovered from tissue specimens, but will discuss general techniques for laboratory

handling of such material. It is the responsibility of the clinician or pathologist to inform the microbiologist of any suspected etiologic agent, since the appropriate procedures can then be initiated once the specimen reaches the laboratory. Often the physician will consult the microbiologist about possible agents to search for in advance of removing the tissue. The optimal diagnostic services are rendered when such dialogue is a constant and important part of the practice of clinical medicine and laboratory microbiology. Tissue specimens are obtained after careful preparation of the skin site. It is critical that biopsy specimens be collected aseptically. The best specimen is that collected aseptically at the time of surgery and submitted to the microbiology laboratory in a sterile container. A wide-mouthed, screw-capped bottle or plastic container is recommended. Anaerobic organisms will survive within infected tissue long enough to be recovered from culture. A small amount of sterile nonbacteriostatic saline may be added to keep the specimen moist.

NOTE: *Legionella* species may be inhibited by saline; a section of lung should be submitted without saline for *Legionella* isolation.

If anaerobic organisms are a particular concern, a small amount of tissue can be placed into a loosely capped wide-mouthed plastic tube and sealed into an anaerobic pouch system, which also seals in moisture enough for survival of organisms in tissue until the specimen is plated. The surgeon should take responsibility for seeing that a second specimen is submitted to pathology for histological studies. Formaldehyde-fixed tissue is not very useful for recovery of viable microorganisms, although some organisms can be recovered for short periods. Therefore an attempt should be made to subculture from tissue in formalin if that is the only specimen available. Material from draining sinus tracts should include a portion of the wall of the tract, obtained by deep curettage. Material from infective endocarditis should contain a portion of the valve and vegetation if the patient is undergoing valve replacement or autopsy examination is done.

Occasionally it is important to ascertain the number of organisms present per gram of tissue. Particularly for burn patients, greater than 10^5 colony-forming units (CFU) per gram of tissue is considered to be indicative of infection, whereas less than that number probably indicates only colonization. Although rarely required, a laboratory should be able

---

Infectious Agents in Tissue Requiring Special Media

Actinomyces sp.
Brucella sp.
Legionella sp.
Listeria monocytogenes (not fastidious)
Systemic fungi
Mycoplasma
Mycobacteria
Viruses

to perform quantitative cultures of tissue. Procedure 21.1 describes one method.

In some instances *contaminated* material may be submitted for microbiological examination. Specimens such as tonsils, autopsy tissue, or similar material may be surface-cauterized with an electric soldering iron or heated spatula or blanched by immersing in boiling water for 5 to 10 seconds to reduce surface contamination. The specimen may then be dissected with sterile instruments to permit culturing of the *center* of the specimen, which will not be affected by the heating.

Because surgical specimens are obtained at great risk and expense to the patient and because supplementary specimens cannot be obtained easily, it is important that the laboratory save a portion of the original tissue (if enough material is available) in a small amount of sterile broth in the refrigerator and at 70° C (or, if necessary, at −20° C) for at least 4 weeks in case additional studies are indicated. If the entire tissue must be ground up for culture, a small amount of the suspension should be placed into a sterile tube and refrigerated. Refrigeration is also used to recover *Listeria monocytogenes* from tissue (cold enrichment) (Procedure 21.2).

Tissue should be manipulated within a laminar flow biological safety cabinet by an operator wearing gloves. Processing tissue within an anaerobic chamber is best. The microbiologist should cut through the infected area (often discolored) with a sterile scalpel blade. The pathologist or clinician can help select a good area to sample. One half of the specimen can then be used for fungal cultures and the other for bacterial cultures. Both types of agents

---

PROCEDURE 21.1

Quantitative Bacteriologic Culture of Tissue

1. Cut a small piece of tissue, several millimeters cubed, aseptically onto a small, preweighed piece of sterile aluminum foil.
2. Determine the weight of the tissue by subtracting the weight of the aluminum foil from the total weight.
3. Place the specimen and 1 ml sterile nutrient broth in a glass tissue grinder or sterile plastic homogenizer bag and macerate the specimen.
4. Prepare six serial dilution tubes of 4.5 ml sterile physiologic saline. Make 1:10 serial dilutions of the macerated specimen by adding 0.5 ml of the original suspension to the first dilution tube, vortexing vigorously, and then adding 0.5 ml of this dilution to the second tube of saline. Repeat this procedure until all six dilutions have been made. Discard 0.5 ml from the last tube. This process can be done in an anaerobic chamber or alternatively in a biosafety cabinet.
5. Inoculate 0.1 ml from each of the six dilutions onto a blood agar plate, a Columbia colistin–nalidixic acid agar plate, an anaerobic blood agar plate (if indicated), and into thioglycollate broth. Spread the inoculum on the plates with a sterile glass spreading rod or a loop. Additional plates may be inoculated after the results of the Gram stain are known, but not all dilutions need to be plated on selective media.
6. Incubate plates in 5% to 10% CO_2 overnight and count the colonies of bacteria on the plate that contains between 30 and 300 CFU.
7. Calculate the number of CFU per gram of tissue with the formula: Number of CFU × Reciprocal of dilution (10^{-3} or 10^{-4}, etc.) × 10 (the inoculation of only 0.1 ml per plate) divided by the weight of the tissue.

For example, for tissue that weighed 0.02 g, 68 CFU were observed on the plate that received the 10^{-3} dilution of suspension:

$$\frac{68 \times 10^3 \times 10}{0.02} = \frac{6.8 \times 10^5}{0.02} = 3.4 \times 10^7 \text{ CFU/g}$$

Modified from a method published by Loebl et al.[6]

should be sought in all tissue specimens. Some sample should be saved for histology, if this has not already been done. Specimens should be cultured for viruses or acid-fast bacilli when such tests are requested. If material is to be cultured for parasites, it is finely minced or teased before inoculation into broth (Chapter 44). Direct examination of stained tissue for parasites is performed by pathologists. Imprint cultures of tissues yielded bacteriological results identical to homogenates in one study.[5]

Additional media may be inoculated for incubation at lower temperatures, which may facilitate recovery of certain systemic fungi and mycobacteria (Chapters 41 and 43). It is possible to obtain reliable microbiological information from tissues after a body has been embalmed. Bacteria and fungi may survive the embalming fluids.

Tissue may be inoculated to virus tissue culture media for isolation of viruses. Brain, lung, and blood are most useful. Tissue may be examined by immunofluorescence for the presence of herpes, cytomegalovirus, or rabies viral particles. Lung tissue should be examined by direct fluorescent antibody test for *Legionella* species. Fluorescent reagents are also available for detection of agents of plague, anthrax, and certain *Bacteroides* species, although most laboratories do not routinely perform such procedures. Visual detection of other etiologic agents of disease is usually performed by pathologists.

The tissues of all fetuses, premature infants, and young babies who have died from an infectious process should be cultured for listeriae (Procedure 21.2). Specimens of the brain, liver, and spleen are most likely to contain the organism. The isolation procedure is given in detail by Seeliger and Cherry.[14]

PROCEDURE 21.2

Isolation of Listeria *Species from Tissue*

1. Add 5-10 ml of ground tissue to each of two flasks of infusion broth.
2. Incubate one flask at 35° C for 24 h, and inoculate a drop of this to a blood agar plate and a tellurite blood agar plate. Incubate these in a candle jar or CO_2 incubator for at least 48 h, along with the original broth flask.
3. Store the second flask in a refrigerator at 4° C. If the 35° C subcultures (step 2) are unsuccessful, subculture material from the refrigerated flask at weekly intervals for at least 1 month.
4. Identify isolates as detailed in Chapter 33.

21.5. Autopsy Cultures

Several concepts about the microbiology of autopsy specimens are important. Most internal organs of previously uninfected patients remain sterile for approximately 20 hours after death. A significant portion of positive necropsy cultures, therefore, are due to contamination from the autopsy room or autopsy personnel. It is estimated that only half of all autopsies should yield positive cultures and that 75% of all tissues obtained at necropsy should be sterile. Procedures modified from studies by De Jongh et al.[4] and Silver and Sonnenwirth[15] are outlined in Procedure 21.3.

Collection of Postmortem Specimens for Microbiological Studies

General Tenets

1. Use fresh sterile instruments for each tissue sample collected.
2. Change to fresh sterile gloves if the current gloves become wet.
3. Sear outside of tissue to dryness before tissue is resected with sterile scalpel or scissors. Handle tissue aseptically from collection to delivery to the laboratory.
4. Bring material for culture to microbiology laboratory as soon as possible after collection.

Preparation of Body

Critical if Microbiological Data are Significant for Determination of Cause of Death or Adequacy of Treatment Before Death.

1. Shave anterior trunk
2. Thoroughly scrub body with povidone-iodine (5 min) followed by 70% alcohol (5 min).
3. Autopsy technicians and pathologists scrub for 10 min with hexachlorophene-containing soap. Personnel don sterile masks, gowns, gloves, and boots, just as for surgery.
4. Drape body in sterile plastic drapes and cover skin with adhesive plastic sterile drape.

Blood Cultures

Make usual Y-shape incision, but draw blood cultures first before any additional manipulation. Reflect skin and subcutaneous tisue over thorax and sear third intercostal space next to the sternum on the left side with a red-hot spatula. If seared tissue is not completely moisture-free, it must be seared a second time. Insert a sterile 18-gauge needle with attached 30-ml syringe into the heart (right ventricle). Withdraw as much blood as possible, up to 20 ml. Thoroughly and vigorously wipe the rubber septa of the blood culture containers with 70% alcohol. Change needles on the syringe, and inject 3 to 5 ml blood into each of two blood culture bottles (aerobic and anaerobic) for bacterial cultures and 10 ml into Isolator tube for fungal and acid-fast bacterial cultures.

Collection of Material from Peritoneal Cavity

Peritoneal fluid should be collected on a swab immediately after entering the peritoneal cavity. If intra-abdominal or other abscess is encountered, the outside of the abscess should be seared to dryness with a red-hot spatula, if feasible, and a sterile needle and syringe should be used to collect pus through intact cavity walls. Vigorously scrub the rubber top of an anaerobic transport vial with 70% alcohol, change needles, and inject aspirated material suspected of harboring anaerobes through the rubber septum into the anaerobic transport vial. All other fluid may be collected on standard transport swabs, with the exception of urine. If there is a significant amount of peritoneal fluid, it should be collected in a 20-ml syringe. For collection of urine, sear the bladder surface and collect bladder urine with a needle and syringe. Remove the needle and expel the urine into a sterile urine cup.

Collection of Tissue Specimens for Culture

Avoid sectioning any large vessels before adequate tissue specimens for culture are obtained. Be certain that the gloves of the prosector are dry and cannot drip onto the tissue. Sear a large area of the surface of the tissue to complete dryness, using a 5×5 cm red-hot bent spatula tip. Using fresh sterile scissors and forceps for each tissue specimen obtained, cut a 1 cm^3 block of tissue from the center of the seared area and place it immediately into a sterile Petri dish or sterile screw-cap urine cup, which is quickly covered up again.

Abscesses: Special Considerations

In addition to the aspirated material, the abscess wall may be the only site from which certain organisms, such as *Nocardia* and *Actinomyces*, may be recovered. Submit a small (1 cm^2) section of the abscess wall.

Collection of Material from Thoracic Cavity

Change to fresh, dry, sterile gloves and collect fluid from the pericardium, pleural cavity, and so on by needle and syringe or on swabs if necessary. Collect purulent or necrotic material with a needle and syringe, as described for abdominal abscess. Submit such material in an anaerobic transport vial. Tissue specimens are collected as described above.

REFERENCES

1. Amin, N.M. 1988. Infected diabetic foot ulcers. Am. Family Pract. 37:283.
2. Buggy, F.P. 1986. Culture methods for continuous ambulatory peritoneal dialysis-associated peritonitis. Clin. Microbiol. Newsletter 8:12.
3. Dawson, M.S., Harford, A.M., Garner, B.K., et al. 1985. Total volume culture technique for the isolation of microorganisms from continuous ambulatory peritoneal dialysis patients with peritonitis. J. Clin. Microbiol. 22:391.
4. De Jongh, D.S., Loftis, J.W., Green, G.S., et al. 1968. Postmortem bacteriology: a practical method for routine use. Am. J. Clin. Pathol. 49:424.
5. Fung, J.C., Sun, T., Kilius, I., and Gross, S. 1983. Print cultures for postmortem microbiology. Ann. Clin. Lab. Sci. 13:83.
6. Loebl, E.C., Marvin, J.A., Heck, E.L., et al. 1974. The method of quantitative burn wound biopsy cultures and its routine use in the care of the burned patient. Am. J. Clin. Pathol. 61:20.
7. Ludlam, H.A., Price, T.N., Berry, A.J., and Phillips, I. 1988. Laboratory diagnosis of peritonitis in patients on continuous ambulatory peritoneal dialysis. J. Clin. Microbiol. 26:1757.
8. Maderazo, E.G., Judson, S., and Pasternak, H. 1988. Late infections of total joint prostheses. Clin. Orthop. Rel. Res. Apr.(229):131.
9. Males, B.M., Walshe, J.J., Garringer, L., et al. 1986. Addi-Chek filtration, BACTEC, and 10-ml culture methods for recovery of microorganisms from dialysis effluent during episodes of peritonitis. J. Clin. Microbiol. 23:350.
10. Males, B.M., Walshe, J.J., and Amsterdam, D. 1987. Laboratory indices of clinical peritonitis: total leukocyte count, microscopy, and microbiologic culture of peritoneal dialysis effluent. J. Clin. Microbiol. 25:2367.
11. Rubin, J., Rogers, W.A., Taylor, H.M., et al. 1980. Peritonitis during continuous ambulatory peritoneal dialysis. Ann. Intern. Med. 92:7.
12. Rubin, S.J. 1984. Continuous ambulatory peritoneal dialysis: dialysate fluid cultures. Clin. Microbiol. Newsletter 6:3.
13. Ryan, S., and Fessia, S. 1987. Improved method for recovery of peritonitis-causing microorganisms from peritoneal dialysate. J. Clin. Microbiol. 25:383.
14. Seeliger, H.P.R., and Cherry, W.B. 1957. Human listeriosis: its nature and diagnosis. U.S. Government Printing Office, Washington, D.C.
15. Silver, H., and Sonnenwirth, A.C. 1969. A practical and efficacious method for obtaining significant postmortem blood cultures. Am. J. Clin. Pathol. 52:433.

BIBLIOGRAPHY

Brewer, N.S., and Weed, L.A. 1976. Diagnostic tissue microbiology methods. Hum. Pathol. 7:141.

Minshew, B.H. 1983. Are quantitative wound cultures worthwhile? Clin. Microbiol. Newsletter 5:51.

O'Toole, W.F., Saxena, H.M., Golden, A., and Ritts, R.E. 1965. Studies of postmortem microbiology using sterile autopsy technique. Arch. Pathol. 80:540.

Steigbiegel, R.T., and Cross, A.S. 1984. Infections associated with hemodialysis and chronic peritoneal dialysis. In Remington, J.S., and Swartz, M.N., editors. Current clinical topics in infectious diseases, ed. 5. McGraw-Hill Book Co., New York.

Young, E.J., and Sugarman, B. 1988. Infections in prosthetic devices. Surg. Clin. North Am. 68:167.

22

Infections of the Head and Neck

22.1. General Considerations, Anatomy

The head and neck have a rich vascular supply that promotes rapid healing after trauma or surgery and permits rapid mobilization of host defenses. Conversely, the rich venous drainage may facilitate the spread of infection throughout the body, in particular to the central nervous system. The mastoids and sinuses are unique air-filled cavities within the head (Figure 22.1). These structures, as well as the eustachian tube, the middle ear, and the respiratory portion of the pharynx, are lined by respiratory epithelium. The clearance of secretions and contaminants depends on normal ciliary activity and mucus flow. The maxillary sinuses are close to the roots of the upper teeth so that dental infections can extend into these sinuses. The fascias (firm, fibrous covering of muscles) of the neck behave like cylinders surrounding the important muscles, and other, deeper fascias surround the important structures of the neck (pharynx, trachea, and major salivary glands). These fascias communicate; they create neck spaces that tend to confine infection to specific areas within the neck. Unfortunately, spread to the mediastinum is not always prevented.

The delicate intraocular structures are enveloped in a tough collagenous coat. The eyes themselves are enclosed within the bony orbits, four-sided pyramids. Three of the four walls of the orbit are contiguous with the paranasal (facial) sinuses. The roof of the orbit is contiguous with the frontal sinus, the floor of the orbit forms the top wall of the maxillary sinus, and the ethmoid sinuses run along the medial aspect of the orbit. Thus, sinus infections may extend directly to the periocular orbital structures. The con-

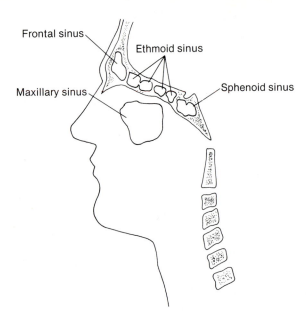

Figure 22.1
Location of the paranasal sinuses. (From Milliken, M.E., and
Campbell, G. 1985. Essential competencies for patient care.
The C.V. Mosby Co., St. Louis.)

junctival membranes line the eyelids and extend onto the surface of the eye itself. The eyelashes tend to prevent entry of foreign material into the eye. The lids blink 15 to 20 times per minute, during which time secretions of the lacrimal glands and goblet cells wash away bacteria and foreign matter. Lysozyme and IgA are secreted locally and serve as part of the natural defense mechanisms of the eye.

22.2. Microbial Flora of the Head and Neck

There is a rather sparse indigenous flora in the conjunctival sac. *Staphylococcus epidermidis* and *Lactobacillus* sp. are the most commonly encountered organisms; *Propionibacterium acnes* may also be present. *Staphylococcus aureus* is found in from 0% to 30% of people and *Haemophilus influenzae* in from 0.4% to 25%. *Branhamella catarrhalis*, various Enterobacteriaceae, and various streptococci (*Streptococcus pyogenes*, *Streptococcus pneumoniae* and α- and γ-hemolytic forms) are found in a very small percent of subjects. The normal flora of the external ear canal is also rather sparse. It is very much like that of the conjunctival sac qualitatively except that pneumococci, *P. acnes*, *S. aureus*, and Enterobacteriaceae are encountered somewhat more often and *Pseudomonas aeruginosa* is found on occasion. *Candida* sp. (non–*C. albicans*) are common.

The normal respiratory tract flora is discussed in Chapter 16. In addition to the organisms listed there, the oral flora may contain *Leptotrichia buccalis*, *Selenomonas*, *Wolinella*, *Stomatococcus mucilaginosus*, *Campylobacter*, and the following organisms that would be more likely to be involved in infection—*Clostridium perfringens* (found irregularly), *Eikenella corrodens*, *Capnocytophaga*, *Actinobacillus actinomycetemcomitans*, and *Haemophilus aphrophilus* and closely related species. Two protozoa, *Entamoeba gingivalis* and *Trichomonas tenax*, are found as normal flora but are rarely involved in infectious processes. We must also be concerned with indigenous flora of animals in the case of bite infections (Chapter 20). *Pasteurella multocida* is commonly involved in infection following dog and cat bites. A particularly virulent organism encountered in relation to dog bites, especially in immunocompromised patients, is a fastidious gram-negative bacillus now called *Capnocytophaga canimorsus* (DF-2).

22.3 Pathogenic Mechanisms

Much of the discussion of pathogenic mechanisms in Chapter 16 is pertinent to this chapter as well. *Capnocytophaga* (which includes organisms formerly called *Bacteroides ochraceus* and DF-1) has been shown to release lysosomal enzymes from human polymorphonuclear leukocytes. A sonic extract of these bacteria inhibits migration of phagocytes and suppresses the proliferation of human fibroblasts. One species of *Capnocytophaga* (*C. sputigena*) shows relatively weak endotoxin activity. Cell envelopes of *Capnocytophaga* exhibit several types of immunomodulating activity and evoke dermatoxic reactions on rabbit skin. The pathogenicity of *Clostridium perfringens* is discussed in Chapter 35.

22.4. Eye Infections

22.4.a. Conjunctivitis. *Chlamydia trachomatis* is responsible for one of the most important types of conjunctivitis, trachoma, one of the leading causes of blindness in the world. *C. trachomatis* acquired by the neonate during passage through an infected vaginal canal is also one of the causes of acute conjunctivitis in the newborn.

Bacterial conjunctivitis is the most common type of infectious conjunctivitis.[6] In adults, the most common organisms cultured are *S. pneumoniae*, *S. aureus*, and *S. epidermidis*. However, there is dispute as to the significance of isolates of the latter two organisms since they are commonly recovered from noninfected eyes. In children, the most common causes of conjunctivitis are *H. influenzae*, *S. pneumoniae*, and perhaps *S. aureus*.[3] *S. pneumoniae* and *H. influenzae* (especially subsp. *aegyptius*) have been responsible for epidemics of conjunctivitis. Gonococcal conjunctivitis may be quite destructive. With the common practice of instilling antibiotic drops into the eyes of newborns in the United States, the incidence of gonococcal and chlamydial conjunctivitis has dropped dramatically. Diphtheritic conjunctivitis may occur in conjunction with diphtheria elsewhere in the body. *Moraxella lacunata* produces a localized angular conjunctivitis with little discharge from the eye. Distinctive clinical pictures may also occur with conjunctivitis due to *Mycobacterium tuberculosis*, *Francisella tularensis*, *Treponema pallidum*, and *Yersinia enterocolitica*. A number of other bacteria have been isolated from cases of conjunctivitis. Fungi may also be responsible for this type of infection, often in association with a foreign body in the eye or an underlying immunological problem.

Viruses are an important cause of conjunctivitis; 20% of such infections were due to adenoviruses in one large American study. Adenoviruses types 4, 3, and 7A are common. Worldwide, enterovirus 70 and coxsackie A24 are responsible for outbreaks and epidemics of acute hemorrhagic conjunctivitis.[2] Puerto Rico suffered an epidemic due to coxsackie A24 recently.[1] It is likely that patients with this agent will soon be seen in the continental United States.

22.4.b. Keratitis. Keratitis, or inflammation of the cornea, may be caused by a wide variety of infectious agents, usually only after some type of trauma produces a defect in the ocular surface. Keratitis should be regarded as an emergency situation since corneal perforation and loss of the eye can occur within 24 hours when organisms such as *P. aeruginosa* or *S. aureus* are involved. The most common symptom of keratitis is pain, usually accompanied by some decrease in vision, but typically with no discharge from the eye. Bacteria account for 65% to 90% of corneal infections.

In the United States, the most common infecting organisms are *S. aureus*, *S. pneumoniae*, *P. aeruginosa*, *Moraxella*, and herpes simplex virus. The first three organisms listed account for over 80% of all bacterial corneal ulcers. A toxic factor known as exopeptidase has been implicated in the pathogenesis of corneal ulcer produced by *S. pneumoniae*. In the case of *P. aeruginosa*, proteolytic enzymes are responsible for the corneal destruction. The gonococcus may cause keratitis in the course of inadequately treated conjunctivitis. *Acinetobacter*, which may look identical microscopically to the gonococcus and is resistant to penicillin and many other antimicrobial agents, can cause corneal perforation. Many other organisms, including mycobacteria, *T. pallidum*, *Nocardia*, *C. trachomatis*, several viruses other than herpes simplex virus, and a large number of fungi may cause keratitis. Fungal keratitis is usually a complication of trauma. The organisms can be seen in scrapings from the lesion.

A previously rare etiologic agent of corneal infections is becoming more common in users of soft and extended-wear contact lenses. *Acanthamoeba* species can survive in improperly sterilized cleaning fluids and be introduced into the eye with the contact lenses. Other bacterial and fungal causes of infections in such patients have been traced to inadequate cleaning of lenses. The organism can often be recovered from the contact lens cleaning and storage containers.

22.4.c. Endophthalmitis. Surgical trauma, nonsurgical trauma (uncommonly), and hematogenous spread from distant sites of infection are the background factors in endophthalmitis. The infection may be limited to specific tissues within the eye or may involve all of the intraocular contents. Pain, especially on movement of the eye, is a prominent aspect of the clinical picture. Bacteria are the most common infectious agents responsible for endophthalmitis. Bacterial endophthalmitis develops suddenly and progresses rapidly.

Following surgery or trauma, evidence of the disease is found within 24 to 48 hours. Postoperative infection involves primarily bacteria from the ocular surface microflora. *S. aureus* is responsible for 50% of cases of endophthalmitis following cataract extraction. *S. aureus* and *Pseudomonas* usually lead to fulminating infection early in the postoperative period. Any bacterium, including those considered to be primarily saprophytic, may cause endophthalmitis. In hematogenous endophthalmitis, a septic focus elsewhere is usually evident before onset of the intraocular infection. *Bacillus cereus* has caused endophthalmitis following transfusion with contaminated blood and in narcotic addicts. Endophthalmitis associated with meningitis may involve various organisms, including *H. influenzae*, streptococci, and *Neisseria meningitidis*. *Nocardia* endophthalmitis may follow pulmonary infection with this organism. Endophthalmitis may be seen in the course of miliary tuberculosis and in syphilis.

Mycotic infection of the eye has increased significantly over the past three decades because of increased use of antibiotics, corticosteroids, antineoplastic chemotherapy, addictive drugs, and hyperalimentation. Fungi generally considered to be saprophytic are important causes of endophthalmitis. Fungi recovered from postoperative infection include *Volutella* sp., *Neurospora sitophila*, *Monosporium apiospermum*, *Candida parapsilosis*, *Trichosporon cutaneum*, *Paecilomyces lilacinus*, *Cephalosporium*, and *Candida glabrata*. Endogenous mycotic endophthalmitis is most commonly due to *C. albicans*. Patients with diabetes and underlying disease are most at risk. Other causes of hematogenous ocular infection include *Aspergillus*, *Cryptococcus*, *Coccidioides*, *Sporothrix*, and *Blastomyces*; *Histoplasma* is rarely involved.

Viral causes of endophthalmitis include herpes simplex I, herpes zoster, cytomegalovirus, and measles viruses. The most common parasitic cause is *Toxocara*. *Toxoplasma gondii* is a well-known cause of chorioretinitis. Thirteen percent of patients with cysticercosis have ocular involvement. *Onchocerca* usually produces keratitis, but intraocular infection also occurs.

22.4.d. Periocular infections. Included in this category are infections of the eyelids, of the lacrimal apparatus, and of the orbit. Lid infections include blepharitis (inflammation of the lid margins), hordeolum or the common sty, and chalazion. Most eyelid infections are due to bacteria, especially S. *aureus* and S. *epidermidis*. Other organisms that may be encountered include *Proteus mirabilis* and *Moraxella*, molluscum contagiosum, and herpes simplex viruses.

The three infections of the lacrimal apparatus are canaliculitis (chronic inflammation of the lacrimal canals), dacryocystitis (inflammation of the lacrimal sac), and dacryoadenitis (inflammation of the main lacrimal gland). Canaliculitis is usually due to *Actinomyces* or *Arachnia*, *Pityrosporum pachydermatis*, or *Fusobacterium*. Infection of the lacrimal sac may involve *Aspergillus*, *C. albicans*, or *Actinomyces*. Other causes are S. *pneumoniae*, mixed bacterial infection, and *C. trachomatis*. Dacryoadenitis often involves pyogenic bacteria such as S. *aureus* and streptococci, but gonococci and *Cysticercus cellu-*

losae have been reported. Chronic infections of the lacrimal gland occur in tuberculosis, syphilis, leprosy, and schistosomiasis. Acute inflammation of the gland may occur in the course of mumps and infectious mononucleosis.

Orbital cellulitis is an acute infection of the orbital contents that is most commonly caused by bacteria. It is a serious infection because it may spread posteriorly to produce cavernous sinus thrombosis. Most cases involve spread from contiguous sources such as the paranasal sinuses. In children, blood-borne bacteria, notably *H. influenzae*, may lead to orbital cellulitis. Intrauterine infections may be a background factor in newborns. S. *aureus* is the most common etiologic agent; S. *pyogenes* and S. *pneumoniae* are also common. Anaerobes may be involved secondary to chronic sinusitis, primarily in adults. Mucormycosis of the orbit is a serious, invasive infection seen particularly in diabetics with poor control of their disease, patients with acidosis due to other causes, and patients with malignant disease receiving cytotoxic and immunosuppressive therapy. *Aspergillus* may produce a similar infection in the same settings but also can cause mild, chronic infections of the orbit.

Newer surgical techniques involving the ocular implantation of prosthetic or donor lenses have resulted in increasing numbers of iatrogenic infections. Isolation of *P. acnes* may have clinical significance here, in contrast to many other sites in which it is usually considered to be a contaminant.

22.5. Ear, Nose, and Throat Infections

22.5.a. Pharyngitis, tonsillitis, peritonsillar abscess. The various forms of pharyngitis and tonsillitis, including diphtheria, are discussed in Chapter 16. The predominant organisms in peritonsillar abscess are non-spore-forming anaerobes including *Fusobacterium* (especially *F. necrophorum*), *Bacteroides* (including the *B. fragilis* group), and anaerobic cocci. S. *pyogenes* and viridans streptococci may also be involved. Vincent's angina, or anaerobic tonsillitis, involves pseudomembrane formation on tonsil surfaces; the infection is relatively rare today, but it is a very serious disease because it is commonly complicated by jugular septic thrombophlebitis, bacteremia, and widespread metastatic infection. Anaerobes, especially *F. necrophorum*, are implicated in this syndrome.

22.5.b. Dental and oral infections. Oral infection with herpes simplex virus, gonococci, and *Candida* has been discussed in Chapter 16. Oral lesions may be encountered in secondary syphilis (see Chapter 19 for a discussion of darkfield preparations and syphilis serology). A large spirochete seems to be a key pathogen in acute necrotizing ulcerative gingivitis (Vincent's gingivitis); clinical microbiology laboratories are not asked to do bacteriologic studies for diagnosis of this condition. The three dental problems in which help may be requested from clinical laboratories are root canal infections, with or without periapical abscess; orofacial odontogenic infections, with or without osteomyelitis of the jaw; and perimandibular space infections. The bacteriology is similar in all of these situations, involving only anaerobic bacteria and streptococci except for perimandibular space infections, which may also involve staphylococci and *E. corrodens* in about 15% of cases. The streptococci are microaerophilic or facultative and are usually α-hemolytic; they are usually found in 20% to 30% of infections of the preceding types of dental infection. Members of the *B. fragilis* group are found in root canal infections, orofacial odontogenic infections, and bacteremia secondary to dental extraction in 5% to 10% of cases. Anaerobic cocci (both *Peptostreptococcus* and *Veillonella*), pigmented *Bacteroides* and *Porphyromonas*, the *Bacteroides oralis* group, and *Fusobacterium* are found in about 20% to 50% of the three conditions mentioned above, as well as in postextraction bacteremia. Bacterial stomatitis is rarely seen now in the United States. It is characterized by superficial (and sometimes deep) tissue necrosis with pseudomembrane formation and a fetid odor. Anaerobes are clearly involved, but bacteriologic studies are unsatisfactory; spirochetes may be important. Oral bacteria are clearly important in other dental processes such as caries, periodontal disease (pyorrhea), and localized juvenile periodontitis, but clinical laboratories are not involved in culturing in such cases.

22.5.c. Salivary gland infections. Acute suppurative parotitis is seen in very ill patients, especially those that are dehydrated, malnourished, elderly, or recovering from surgery. It is associated with painful, tender swelling of the parotid gland; there may be purulent drainage evident at the opening of the duct of the gland in the mouth. *S. aureus* is the major pathogen, but on occasion viridans streptococci and oral anaerobes may play a role. A chronic bacterial parotitis has been described that usually involves *S. aureus*. Less commonly, other salivary glands may be involved with a bacterial infection; this is usually because of ductal obstruction. The mumps virus is the major viral agent involved in parotitis, but the influenza virus and enteroviruses may also cause this. Diagnosis of viral parotitis is usually done serologically. Uncommonly, *M. tuberculosis* may involve the parotid gland in conjunction with pulmonary tuberculosis.

22.5.d. Sinusitis. Acute sinusitis is usually due to bacterial infection; it tends to be self-limited, usually lasting 1 to 3 weeks. Most often it follows a common cold or other viral upper respiratory infection. Complications include local extension into the orbit, skull, meninges, or brain and development of chronic sinusitis. Most studies of the microbiology of acute sinusitis have dealt with maxillary sinusitis because this is the most common type and the one most accessible for puncture and aspiration. Bacterial cultures are positive in about three fourths of patients. In a recent study involving young adults, *H. influenzae* was recovered from 50% and *S. pneumoniae* from 19% of patients. *S. pyogenes* and *B. catarrhalis* were also found, in addition to contaminating normal skin flora including *P. acnes*. Anaerobes were considered pathogens in 2% of cases.[4] Among children, *S. pneumoniae*, *H. influenzae*, and *B. catarrhalis* are most common.[8] Rhinovirus is found in 15% of patients, influenza virus in 5%, parainfluenza virus in 3%, and adenovirus in <1%. Bacteria, particularly anaerobes, are commonly involved in chronic sinusitis in adults. A recent study by Tinkelman and Silk has shown *B. catarrhalis* to be an important agent in chronic sinusitis in children.[7] The primary problems are inadequate drainage, impaired mucociliary clearance, and mucosal damage. Ordinarily, surgery or drainage is required for successful management.

22.5.e. External ear infections. Otitis externa is similar to skin and soft tissue infections elsewhere, but there is the unique problem of a narrow, tortuous ear canal. There are several types of external otitis. Acute localized disease occurs in the form of a pustule or furuncle and is due to *S. aureus*. Erysipelas caused by group A streptococci may involve the external ear canal and the soft tissue of the ear itself. Acute diffuse otitis externa (swimmer's ear) is related to maceration of the ear from swimming or hot, humid weather. Gram-negative bacilli, particularly *P.*

aeruginosa, play an important role. A severe, hemorrhagic external otitis due to *P. aeruginosa* has been related to hot tub use.

Chronic otitis externa is due to the irritation of drainage from the middle ear in patients with chronic, suppurative otitis media and a perforated eardrum. Rarely, this condition may be caused by tuberculosis, syphilis, yaws, or leprosy. Malignant otitis externa is a necrotizing infection that spreads to adjacent areas of soft tissue, cartilage, and bone. It may progress to a life-threatening situation by spreading into the central nervous system or vascular channels. *P. aeruginosa*, in particular, and anaerobes are frequently associated with this process, which is seen in diabetics with small blood vessel disease of the tissues overlying the temporal bone; the poor local perfusion of tissues results in a milieu for invasion by bacteria. On occasion, external otitis will extend into the cartilage of the ear; this usually requires surgical intervention. Certain viruses may infect the external auditory canal, the soft tissue of the ear, or the tympanic membrane; influenza A virus is a suspected but not an established cause. Varicella-zoster virus may cause painful vesicles within the soft tissue of the ear and the ear canal. *Mycoplasma pneumoniae* is definitely implicated as a cause of bullous myringitis (a painful infection of the eardrum with hemorrhagic bullae); the ear canal itself may be involved.

22.5.f. Middle ear infection (otitis media) and mastoiditis. Acute otitis media may begin as a viral infection, but bacterial infection typically supervenes. In children (in whom the disease is most common), pneumococci (33% of cases) and *H. influenzae* (20%) are the usual etiologic agents; group A streptococci (8%) are the third most frequently encountered agents. Other organisms, encountered in only 1% to 3% of cases, include *B. catarrhalis, S. aureus,* gram-negative enteric bacilli, and anaerobes. Viruses, chiefly respiratory syncytial virus and influenza virus, have been recovered from middle ear fluid of 4% of children with acute or chronic otitis media. *C. trachomatis* has been isolated from middle ear aspirates occasionally and *M. pneumoniae* rarely.

Chronic otitis media and its complication, mastoiditis, yields a predominantly anaerobic flora with *Peptostreptococcus* sp., *B. fragilis* group, pigmented *Bacteroides* and *Porphyromonas*, other *Bacteroides* sp., and *Fusobacterium nucleatum* as the principal pathogens; less commonly present are *S. aureus,*

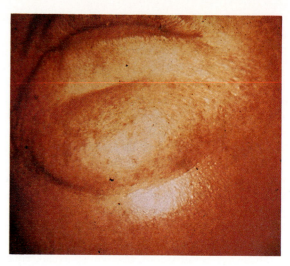

Figure 22.2
Ludwig's angina.

P. aeruginosa, Proteus sp., and other gram-negative facultative bacilli. *M. tuberculosis* may also cause a chronic otitis media and mastoiditis.

22.6. Neck Space Infections

Infections of the deep spaces of the neck are potentially serious because they may spread to critical structures such as major vessels of the neck or to the mediastinum, leading to mediastinitis, purulent pericarditis, and pleural empyema. One of these infections, Ludwig's angina (Figure 22.2), may lead to airway obstruction. The oral flora is responsible for these infections. Accordingly, the predominant organisms are anaerobes—*Peptostreptococcus*, various *Bacteroides* and *Fusobacterium* species, and *Actinomyces* for the most part. Streptococci, chiefly of the viridans variety, are also important, and *S. aureus* and various gram-negative non-anaerobic bacilli may be recovered, particularly from patients developing these problems in the hospital setting.

22.7. Collection and Transport of Specimens

Purulent material from the surface of the lower conjunctival sac and inner canthus of the eye is collected on a sterile swab for cultures of conjunctivitis. Both eyes should be cultured separately. Chlamydial cultures are taken with a dry calcium alginate swab; this is placed in 2-SP transport medium. An additional swab may be rolled across the surface of a slide, fixed with methanol, and sent for direct fluorescent antibody stain.

In the case of keratitis, an ophthalmologist should obtain scrapings of the cornea with a heat-sterilized platinum spatula. Multiple inoculations with the spatula are made to blood agar, chocolate agar, an agar for fungi, thioglycollate broth, and an anaerobic blood agar plate. Other special media may be used if indicated. For culture of herpes simplex virus and adenovirus, corneal material is transferred to viral transport media.

Cultures of endophthalmitis specimens are inoculated with material obtained by the ophthalmologist from the anterior chamber of the eye, the vitreous, wound abscesses, and wound dehiscences. Lid infection material is collected on a swab in a conventional manner. For microbiological studies of canaliculitis, concretions from the lacrimal canal should be transported under anaerobic conditions. Aspiration of fluid from the orbit is contraindicated in cases of orbital cellulitis. Since sinusitis is the most common background factor, the assistance of an otolaryngologist in obtaining material from the sinuses by antral puncture is helpful. Blood cultures should be obtained. Tissue biopsy is essential for microbiological diagnosis of mucormycosis; cultures are usually negative and the diagnosis is made by histological examination.

For laboratory diagnosis of external otitis, the external ear should be cleansed with a mild germicide such as 1:1000 aqueous solution of benzalkonium chloride to reduce the contaminating skin flora before obtaining the culture. Material from the ear, especially that obtained after spontaneous perforation of the eardrum or by needle aspiration of middle ear fluid (tympanocentesis), should be collected by an otolaryngologist, using sterile equipment and a sterile cotton or polyester swab. Cultures from the mastoid are generally taken on swabs during surgery; they should be transported anaerobically.

The problem in collecting oral and dental infection material is to avoid or minimize contamination with oral flora. For collection of material from root canal infection, the tooth is isolated by means of a rubber dam. A sterile field is established, the tooth is swabbed with 70% alcohol, and after the root canal is exposed, a sterile paper point is inserted, removed, and placed into semisolid, nonnutritive anaerobic transport medium. Alternatively, needle aspiration can be used if there is sufficient material. Defining the flora of such infections is beyond the scope of routine clinical microbiology laboratories.

Specimens from neck space infections can usually be obtained with a syringe and needle by the surgeon. Transport must be under anaerobic conditions.

22.8. Direct Visual Examination

All material submitted for culture should always be smeared and examined directly by Gram stain or other appropriate technique. In bacterial conjunctivitis, polymorphonuclear leukocytes will predominate; in viral infection, the host cells will be primarily lymphocytes and monocytes. Specimens in which chlamydia are suspected can be stained immediately with monoclonal antibody-conjugated fluorescein for detection of elementary bodies or inclusions. Using histological stains, basophilic intracytoplasmic inclusion bodies are seen in epithelial cells. Cytologists and pathologists usually perform this test.

Direct examination of conjunctivitis specimens using histological methods (Tzanck smear) may reveal multinucleated epithelial cells typical of herpes infections; immunoelectron microscopy and immunofluorescent techniques may also aid in diagnosing viral conjunctivitis. In the case of keratitis, scrapings are examined by Gram, Giemsa, periodic acid–Schiff (PAS), and methenamine silver stains. If *Acanthamoeba* or other amebae are suspected, a direct wet preparation should be examined for motile trophozoites and a trichrome stain should be added to the regimen. Transmission electron microscopy may establish viral etiology. In the case of endophthalmitis, material is also examined by Gram, Giemsa, PAS, and methenamine silver stains. When ophthalmic specimens are submitted in large volumes of fluid, they must be concentrated by centrifugation before further studies are performed.

Material aspirated from the maxillary sinus, from middle ear or mastoid infections, from neck space infections, and from bite infections is also examined directly for bacteria and fungi. The calcofluor white fluorescent stain reveals fungal elements unambiguously. Methenamine silver stains have the added efficiency of staining most bacterial, fungal, and several parasitic species.

22.9. Culturing

Because of the constant washing action of the tears, the number of organisms recovered from cultures of certain eye infections may be relatively low. Unless the clinical specimen is obviously purulent, it is recommended that a relatively large inoculum and a variety of media be used to ensure recovery of an etiologic agent. At a minimum, one should use blood agar and chocolate agar plates incubated under increased carbon dioxide tension. Since potential pathogens may be present in an eye without causing infection, it may be very helpful to the clinician, when only one eye is infected, to culture both eyes. When *Moraxella lacunata* (the Morax-Axenfeld bacillus) is suspected, Loeffler's medium may prove useful; the growth of the organism often leads to proteolysis and pitting of the medium, although there are nonproteolytic strains. If diphtheritic conjunctivitis is suspected, Loeffler's or cystine-tellurite medium should be used. For more serious eye infections such as keratitis, endophthalmitis, and orbital cellulitis, one should always include, in addition to the media just noted, a reduced anaerobic blood agar plate, a medium for fungi, and a broth such as thioglycolate broth. Blood cultures are also essential in the case of serious eye infections.

Cultures of material for *Chlamydia* and viruses should be inoculated to appropriate media from transport broth. Cycloheximide-treated McCoy cells for *Chlamydia* isolation and human embryonic kidney, primary monkey kidney, and Hep-2 cell lines for virus isolation should be inoculated. For recovery of some coxsackieviruses, suckling mice may be required.

A number of the other infections discussed in this chapter, such as peritonsillar abscess, oral and dental infections, chronic sinusitis, chronic otitis media and mastoiditis, and neck space infections, commonly involve anaerobic bacteria. The anaerobes involved typically originate in the oral cavity and are often more delicate than anaerobes isolated from other clinical material. Very careful attention must be paid to providing optimum techniques of anaerobic cultivation, as well as transport.

22.10. Noncultural Detection Methods

Although acute and convalescent serologic tests for viral agents might be used in the event of epidemic conjunctivitis, these are not generally done since the infections are self-limited. Enzyme-linked immunosorbent assay (ELISA) tests have been evaluated for detection of *C. trachomatis* in cervicitis and urethritis, but few studies on their efficacy for diagnosis of inclusion conjunctivitis have been published. An immune dot blot test may be useful for this purpose.[5]

It is anticipated that the direct antigen tests should perform well, particularly since so many eyes have been partially treated before culture. An ELISA test of aqueous humor is available for diagnosis of *Toxocara* infection.

REFERENCES

1. Centers for Disease Control. 1988. Acute hemorrhagic conjunctivitis caused by coxsackie A24 variant—Puerto Rico. M.M.W.R. 37:123.
2. Chou, M.Y., and Malison, M.D. 1988. Outbreak of acute hemorrhagic conjunctivitis due to coxsackie A24 variant—Taiwan. Am. J. Epidemiol. 127:795.
3. Gigliotti, F., Williams, W.T., Hayden, F.G., et al. 1981. Etiology of acute conjunctivitis in children. J. Pediatr. 98:531.
4. Jousimies-Somer, H.R., Savolainen, S., and Ylikoski, J.S. 1988. Bacteriologic findings of acute maxillary sinusitis in young adults. J. Clin. Microbiol. 26:1919.
5. Mearns, G., Richmond, S.J., and Storey, C.C. 1988. Sensitive immune dot blot test for diagnosis of *Chlamydia trachomatis* infection. J. Clin. Microbiol. 26:1810.
6. Seal, D.V., Barrett, S.P., and McGill, J.I. 1982. Aetiology and treatment of acute bacterial infection of the external eye. Br. J. Ophthalmol. 66:357.
7. Tinkelman, D.G., and Silk, H.J. 1989. Clinical and bacteriologic features of chronic sinusitis in children. Am. J. Dis. Child. 143:938.
8. Wald, E.R., Milmoe, G.J., Bowen, A., et al. 1981. Acute maxillary sinusitis in children. N. Engl. J. Med. 304:749.

BIBLIOGRAPHY

Bartlett, J.G., and Gorbach, S.L. 1976. Anaerobic infections of the head and neck. Otolaryngol. Clin. North Am. 9:655.

Baum, J.L. 1978. Ocular infections. N. Engl. J. Med. 299:28.

Brook, I. 19Microbiology of human and animal bite wounds in children. Pediatr. Infect. Dis. J. 6:29.

Brook, I., and Finegold, S.M. 1979. Bacteriology of chronic otitis media. J.A.M.A. 241:488.

Farr, B., and Gwaltney, J.M., Jr. 1989. Acute and chronic sinusitis. In Pennington, J.E., editor. Respiratory infections: diagnosis and management, ed 2. Raven Press, New York.

Finegold, S.M. 1977. Anaerobic bacteria in human disease. Academic Press, New York.

Hirst, L.W., Thomas, J.V., and Green, W.R. 1985. Conjunctivitis; keratitis; endophthalmitis; and periocular infections. In Mandell, G.L., Douglas, R.G. Jr., and Bennett, J.E., editors: Principles and practice of infectious diseases. John Wiley & Sons, New York.

Klein, J.O. 1989. Otitis media. In Pennington, J.E., editor. Respiratory infections: diagnosis and management, ed 2. Raven Press, New York.

Newman, M.G., and Goodman, A.D., editors. 1984. Guide to antibiotic use in dental practice. Quintessence Publishing Co., Chicago.

Sutter, V.L., Citron, D.M., Edelstein, M.A.C., and Finegold, S.M. 1985. Wadsworth anaerobic bacteriology manual, ed. 4. Star Publishing Co., Belmont, Calif.

23 Infections in the Vulnerable Host

An individual may be at increased risk of acquiring an infectious disease either because of inherent host factors, such as age or disease, environmental factors, manipulations performed as part of medical practice, or combinations of these factors (see box on p. 310). One of the ironies of modern medicine is that as treatments are improved to prolong the survival of patients suffering from many types of disease, these patients become more vulnerable to infectious diseases. Exposure to certain agents, such as viruses, may be related to occupation or life-style. This chapter focuses on some of the categories of patients who are at a greater risk of acquiring infections than are normal hosts and on some likely etiologic agents of these infections. In most cases, diagnosis of infectious disease is handled in the same way for compromised patients as for any infected host, as described in the preceding chapters. When special considerations are appropriate, they will be mentioned in this chapter. A discussion of all conditions that predispose a person to acquiring an infectious disease is beyond the scope of this text.

23.1. Infections Related to Age

23.1.a. **Infections in neonates**. As a fetus develops within the uterus, it is effectively protected from most environmental influences, including infectious agents, by the placenta and the amniotic fluid. The human immune system does not become wholly competent until several months after birth. Immunoglobulins that cross the placental barrier, primarily IgG, serve to protect the newborn from many agents until the infant begins to produce immunoglobulins of his or her own in response to antigenic stimuli. This unique environmental niche, however,

---

Factors Contributing to Increased Risk of Acquiring Infectious Disease

Host factors

- Age: very young or very old
- Anatomic defects: congenital or acquired, such as meningocele or benign prostatic hypertrophy
- Disease: cystic fibrosis, diabetes, cancer, sickle cell anemia, viral or other concomitant infections
- Immune system abnormalities
- Poor nutritional state

Environmental factors

- Iatrogenic causes: antibiotic or myelosuppressive therapy, foreign implants, surgery, access conduits such as catheters
- Tissue damage: trauma or surgery
- Life-style: sexual behavior, travel, eating habits, alcohol, drugs
- Occupation
- Proximity to other infected hosts, animal or human

Etiologic Agents of Congenital and Neonatal Infections

Viruses

  *Cytomegalovirus
  Enteroviruses
  *Hepatitis B virus
  *Herpes simplex virus
  Measles virus
  Parvovirus
  *Rubella virus
  Vaccinia virus
  Varicella-zoster virus

Bacteria

  Bacteroides fragilis
  Borrelia
  Brucella
  Campylobacter
  *Chlamydia
  *Escherichia coli
  Francisella
  Gardnerella
  Haemophilus influenzae
  Klebsiella
  Leptospira
  *Listeria
  Mycobacterium
  Mycoplasma
  Neisseria gonorrhoeae
  Salmonella
  Staphylococcus
  *Streptococcus, group B
  *Treponema

Fungi

  *Candida
  Coccidioides

Parasites

  Leishmania
  Plasmodium
  Pneumocystis
  *Toxoplasma
  Trypanosoma

* More commonly recognized agents or infection.
Modified from Peter, Cherry, and Bryson. 1982. Diagn. Med. 5:61.

---

does expose the vulnerable fetus to pathogens present in the mother. Infections in infants are of two unique types: **congenital,** acquired by the fetus as a result of a maternal infectious agent that crosses the placenta; and **neonatal,** acquired during passage through the birth canal or immediately postpartum.

The most common agents of congenital infection in the United States are *Toxoplasma gondii*, rubella, cytomegalovirus, and herpes simplex virus, the so-called **TORCH** agents. Congenital disease may also be caused by a number of other agents (see box opposite). Of these, *Treponema pallidum* (syphilis) and *Listeria monocytogenes* (neonatal listeriosis or abortion) are probably the most common.

Suspected congenital infection can be diagnosed culturally or serologically. Because maternal IgG crosses the placenta, serologic tests are often difficult to interpret. If the presence of IgG is the only available test, serum samples from both mother and baby must be tested simultaneously and the baby's titers must be observed to rise over several weeks, indicating that antigenic stimulation of active antibody production occurred as a result of infection. For culturable agents, the most definitive diagnoses involve recovery of the pathogen in culture. Rubella, herpes simplex, varicella zoster, enteroviruses, and cytomegalovirus can be cultured easily, as can most bacterial agents. Nasal and urine specimens offer the greatest yield for viral isolation, while blood, cerebrospinal fluid, and lesion material can also be productive. Systemic neonatal herpes without lesions may be difficult to diagnose unless tissue biopsy material is examined, since the viruses may not shed into cerebrospinal fluid or blood. Bacteria and fungi can be isolated from lesion sites, blood, and occasionally from other sources.

Determination of the presence of fetal IgM directed against the agent in question establishes the serologic diagnosis of congenital infection. Until recently, ultracentrifugation was required for separation of IgM from IgG, the only definitive means of preventing false positive results due to maternal IgG or fetal rheumatoid factor. Ion-exchange chromatography columns, antihuman IgG, and bacterial proteins that bind to IgG specifically are now commercially available for removing cross-reactive IgG and rheumatoid factor to obtain more homogeneous IgM for differentiation of fetal antibody. Indirect fluorescent antibody and enzyme-linked immunosorbent assay (ELISA) test systems are commercially available for detection of IgM against *T. gondii*, rubella, cytomegalovirus (CMV), herpes simplex, and varicella-zoster. Interference by rheumatoid factor is still a consideration in most of the commercial IgM test systems. Our ability to detect viral inclusions in tissue, conjunctival scrapings, and vesicular lesions, traditionally performed with Giemsa stain, has been improved by availability of monoclonal and polyclonal fluorescent antibody reagents, described in the chapters that discuss individual agents.

Unfortunately, the incidence of congenital syphilis, whose United States levels were at an all-time low in 1978, has been rising steadily over the last 8 years. If an infant is born to a mother with both a positive VDRL and FTA-ABS, the diagnosis of congenital syphilis is presumptive and treatment is begun. With VDRL positive mothers who were adequately treated for their disease in the past, diagnosis of a congenitally infected baby due to maternal reinfection may be more difficult. Congenital syphilis may be diagnosed by either darkfield examination of lesions or serologically. Since antitreponemal IgM

tests may be unreliable, infants should be tested sequentially over several months.

The Sabin-Feldman dye test has been the standard against which all other serologic tests for toxoplasmosis are measured; however, it is performed in only a few specialized laboratories and new methods have been developed with equal or better sensitivity. Commercial latex agglutination and ELISA tests have been shown to be adequate for detection of IgG against *Toxoplasma*, a useful screening test for women before they become pregnant. A fourfold rise in titer during pregnancy is indicative of a newly acquired infection. Laboratory serologic diagnosis of congenital disease, however, requires demonstration of specific IgM in fetal serum by either conventional ELISA, indirect immunofluorescent stain, or a reverse-capture IgM ELISA, which is the most sensitive and specific test available today. Because of the serious consequences of congenital toxoplasmosis, including deafness, microcephaly, and low IQ,[12] detection of high-risk pregnant women is very important so that prenatal therapy can be instituted.[3] For the parasitic agents of congenital infection other than *T. gondii*, visual evidence of the agent in fetal circulation is diagnostic.

Hepatitis B can be transmitted to fetuses of chronically infected mothers, and a significant number of such infected infants will themselves become chronic carriers of hepatitis B. Laboratory diagnosis of congenital hepatitis requires demonstration of hepatitis B surface antigen (HBsAg) in fetal serum, usually accomplished by performing an ELISA or a radioimmunoassay test.

Neonatal infections are often related to a difficult labor, premature birth, premature rupture of membranes, maternal genital infection, or other event. Meningitis with Enterobacteriaceae, usually *Escherichia coli*, sepsis with group B streptococci or *Listeria*, or herpes infections (often systemic) are the most common types encountered.[11] Infections with *Haemophilus influenzae*, *Gardnerella vaginalis*, *Bacteroides fragilis* or other anaerobic bacteria, sepsis due to mycoplasma that infect the genital tract, ophthalmia neonatorum caused by *Neisseria gonorrhoeae*, and inclusion conjunctivitis and pneumonia caused by *Chlamydia trachomatis* also occur, although less often. Diagnosis of these infections is usually based on recovery of the agent, but direct examination of conjunctival smears by Giemsa, fluorescent antibody stain, or Gram stain can allow a much more rapid determination of the etiology of purulent discharge from the infant's eye. Direct antigen detection tests are available for gonococci, herpes, cytomegalovirus, *Chlamydia*, and group B streptococci. The appropriate specimens (cerebrospinal fluid, serum, pus, tracheal aspirate, and so forth) should be examined immediately with these reagents. For all other agents, culture of blood, nasopharyngeal secretions, or stool will produce the greatest yield. Routine body surface cultures of infants in intensive care has not been shown to be helpful for predicting subsequent disease.[5]

23.1.b. Infections in the elderly. Pneumonia is the most common infection in aged patients; it is the fourth leading cause of death in patients older than 75 years in the United States. Factors such as decreased mucociliary function, decreased cough reflex, decreased level of consciousness, periodontal disease, and decreased general mobility probably contribute to a greater incidence of pneumonia in aged patients. Such patients have been found to be more frequently colonized with gram-negative bacilli than are younger people, perhaps due to poor oral hygiene, decreased saliva, or decreased epithelial cell turnover. When these patients are institutionalized, their oral colonization rate is higher and their chances of acquiring gram-negative bacterial pneumonia are enhanced. Mortality due to bacterial pneumonia following respiratory viral infections, influenza in particular, is greater in elderly patients. The bacteria associated with pneumonia in the elderly are *Streptococcus pneumoniae*, *Legionella* species, oral anaerobes, *Staphylococcus aureus*, the Enterobacteriaceae, and *Pseudomonas* species (especially in hospitalized patients). Reactivation tuberculosis occurs relatively often in elderly patients. The incidence of atypical mycobacterial disease is low, and the species of organisms involved may vary depending on the locality.

Urinary tract infections pose significant problems for elderly patients. Women may suffer from cystocele, loss of pelvic muscle tone, and changes in urinary tract mucosa, which predispose them to infection, whereas prostatic disease in males is the most common condition contributing to urinary tract infection in that group. It is possible that due to loss of somatic tissue integrity and poorer immune response associated with age, urinary tract infections in elderly patients are more likely to lead to sepsis. Important factors include obstructive uropathy and manipulation of the urinary tract (for example, catheterization). Gram-negative bacteremia, as a result of another focus of infection (often in the urinary tract), is an important problem infection seen in the elderly.

Other infections likely to be encountered among older patients include peritonitis or intra-abdominal abscess, often initiated by gastrointestinal tract disorders such as cholecystitis, obstruction, diverticulosis, peptic ulcer, or malignancy. Circulating bacteria may colonize heart valves, leading to endocarditis. The loss of some immune functions and of vascular integrity with age may predispose older patients to serious varicella-zoster infections (including pneumonia), infectious arthritis, meningitis, and skin and soft tissue infections. The specimens required for diagnosis and the handling of those specimens are no different from those used to diagnose infections in any patient, as described in previous chapters.

23.2. Infections in Patients with Underlying Disease

Diseases that alter the body's normal metabolism can affect the "steady-state" of the host, rendering the patient more vulnerable to infection. In addition, a number of diseases affect the immune system itself, preventing functional activity that serves to protect a normal host from many etiologic agents. A few of the more notable diseases that predispose the sufferer to infection are mentioned here.

23.2.a. Cystic fibrosis. Patients with cystic fibrosis may present as young adults with chronic respiratory tract disease, as well as the more common presentation in children that may also include gastrointestinal problems and stunted growth. A very mucoid *Pseudomonas* species, characterized by production of copious amounts of extracellular capsular polysaccharide, can be isolated from the sputum of almost all cystic fibrosis patients older than 18 years, becoming more prevalent with increased age of the patient after the age of 5 years. Even if cystic fibrosis has not been diagnosed, isolation of a mucoid *P. aeruginosa* of this type from sputum should alert the clinician to the possibility of such an underlying disease. Microbiologists should always report this unusual morphological feature if it is encountered. In addition to the mucoid *Pseudomonas*, cystic fibrosis patients are likely to harbor *S. aureus*, *H. influenzae*, and *Pseudomonas cepacia*. Respiratory syncytial virus and *Aspergillus* are also important pathogens in this population.[10] Sputum specimens from patients known to have cystic fibrosis should be inoculated to selective agar, such as mannitol salt for recovery of *S. aureus* and selective horse blood-bacitracin, incubated anaerobically and aerobically, for recovery of *H. influenzae* that may be obscured by the mucoid *Pseudomonas* on general media. The use of a selective medium for *P. cepacia* is also recommended.

23.2.b. Diabetes mellitus. Diabetes mellitus, especially in older patients, seems to predispose sufferers to several infectious diseases. Lack of adequate peripheral circulation (via both small and large vessels) and peripheral neuropathy lead to tissue necrosis and the commonly encountered diabetic foot ulcer (Chapter 20). Chronic soft tissue infections, often of mixed bacterial etiology, including anaerobic and facultative bacteria (including *S. aureus*), can lead to osteomyelitis (Chapter 21). Diabetics are also at risk of developing various other forms of anaerobic cellulitis and fasciitis (Chapter 20), synergistic necrotizing cellulitis caused by mixed aerobic and anaerobic bacteria, malignant otitis externa, and streptococcal cellulitis. Acidosis predisposes patients to fungal infection. Rhinocerebral mucormycosis and candidiasis are relatively frequent in patients with diabetes.

23.2.c. Sickle cell disease. Circulating antibodies of patients with sickle cell disease seem to display impaired ability to opsonize certain bacteria, particularly *S. pneumoniae* and *Salmonella* species. These patients suffer from defective complement activity and lack of a functional spleen, which may also contribute to their increased risk for infection. Primary pneumococcal sepsis, peritonitis, and meningitis are common in patients with sickle cell disease. *Salmonella* is the cause of 80% of osteomyelitis cases in patients with sickle cell disease; this is usually secondary to sepsis. Other gram-negative bacilli account for the other 20%.

23.2.d. Congenital immunodeficiency diseases. A number of children are born with defects of the immune system, either cellular or humoral, or combined immunodeficiency syndromes that involve components of each of the immune effector systems. Additional defects include lack of certain complement components. Infections that are easily handled by the normal host become problems in the immunodeficient host. For example, patients with antibody deficiencies are often plagued by infections

caused by encapsulated bacteria such as pneumococci, meningococci, and *H. influenzae*. Patients who lack certain elements of the complement cascade are more likely to contract infections with meningococci and gonococci. Children with chronic granulomatous disease, a disease with polymorphonuclear neutrophil (PMN) dysfunction, have gram-negative bacterial and staphylococcal infections. A complete discussion of the infectious consequences of inherited immunological defects is beyond the scope of this book.

23.2.e. Neoplastic diseases and bone marrow transplant recipients. Patients with cancer are more likely to become infected, and the nature of the malignancy often determines the etiologic agent(s). Table 23.1 contains a list of etiologic agents associated with certain malignancies. Hodgkin's disease affects the cell-mediated immune response that normally helps to protect the body from intracellular pathogens such as herpes, mycobacteria, *Salmonella*, *Brucella*, *Nocardia*, and *Listeria*. Even before chemotherapy, patients with Hodgkin's-type lymphoma are likely to become infected with these and other agents normally handled by the cellular immune system. Treatment with certain chemotherapeutic agents and with corticosteroids also impairs cellular immunity. Other malignancies may affect the humoral immune response, which contributes to protection against agents such as viruses, *Pneumocystis*, *Giardia*, staphylococci, and encapsulated bacteria.

Cancer patients are likely to be undergoing treatment for their disorder, and a discussion of infection in such hosts must consider the effects of therapy as a necessary consequence of the disease. Although a few infectious agents are associated with certain carcinomas irrespective of therapy, such as *S. bovis* and *C. septicum* bacteremia in patients with bowel malignancy, most infections in cancer patients are at least partially a result of the loss of immunological effector cells, either as a part of the disease process or as a consequence of chemotherapy.

Allogeneic bone marrow transplantation is performed commonly for patients (particularly young persons) with hematologic malignancies and for other indications. Destruction of host immune effectors predisposes the patient to gram-negative infection from endogenous bowel flora and gram-positive infections due to skin flora. Subsequent graft-versus-host disease can lead to systemic viral infec-

Table 23.1

Infectious Agents Commonly Associated with Certain Malignancies

MALIGNANCY (SITES AND TYPES OF INFECTIONS)	PATHOGENS
Acute nonlymphocytic leukemia (pneumonia, oral lesions, cutaneous lesions, urinary tract infections, hepatitis, most commonly sepsis without obvious focus)	Enterobacteriaceae *Pseudomonas* Staphylococci *Corynebacterium JK* *Candida* *Aspergillus* *Mucor* Hepatitis (non-A, non-B)
Acute lymphocytic leukemia (pneumonia, cutaneous lesions, pharyngitis, disseminated disease)	Streptococci (all types) *Pneumocystis carinii* Herpes simplex Cytomegalovirus Varicella-zoster
Lymphoma (disseminated disease, pneumonia, urinary tract, sepsis, cutaneous lesions)	*Brucella* *Candida* (mucocutaneous) *Cryptococcus neoformans* Herpes simplex (cutaneous) Herpes zoster Cytomegalovirus *Pneumocystis carinii* *Toxoplasma gondii* *Listeria monocytogenes* Mycobacteria *Nocardia* *Salmonella* Staphylococci Enterobacteriaceae *Pseudomonas* *Strongyloides stercoralis*
Multiple myeloma (pneumonia, cutaneous lesions, sepsis)	*Haemophilus influenzae* *Streptococcus pneumoniae* *Neisseria meningitidis* Enterobacteriaceae *Pseudomonas* Herpes varicella-zoster *Candida* *Aspergillus*

tions. After immune function has returned via donor tissue, the transplant patient is at risk for infection associated with encapsulated bacteria, fungi, and systemic viral disease.[13]

A critical factor that determines whether an immunosuppressed patient will suffer increased risk of infection is the number of circulating granulocytes, primarily PMNs. Patients with severe **granulocytopenia** (markedly decreased numbers of circulating granulocytes, PMNs $<500/mm^3$ and particularly those with less than PMNs $100 < mm^3$) are the most likely to develop infections.[15] Gram-negative facultative organisms and staphylococci are the most common etiologic agents. Gram-negative anaerobic organisms and fungi are encountered less often. The authors of one major study found that routine surveillance cultures of nose, throat, urine, and stool were not helpful for predicting those patients at risk for septicemia or for determining empiric therapy once the patients became febrile.[7] Follow-up daily blood cultures drawn on febrile patients after they had been started on empiric therapy, however, were helpful for identifying an etiologic agent and ultimately for guiding therapy. By drawing such blood cultures into resin-containing media to remove antibiotics from the milieu or into the Isolator system, microbiologists should increase the chances of recovering an organism from a patient receiving antibiotics. Persistent fever in the granulocytopenic patient on antibiotics suggests the presence of a fungal infection, particularly *Candida* or *Aspergillus* and less often *Mucor*. Diagnosis of such fungal infections is difficult, and direct visual examination of specimens should always accompany culture, which may be negative in these cases.[9]

23.3. Infections in Hospitalized Patients (Nosocomial Infections)

Patients are at increased risk for acquiring infections merely by being hospitalized. Approximately 2 million people (5% or greater of all hospitalized patients) acquire a **nosocomial** infection (an infection that occurs at least 72 hours after admission and was not present at the time of admission) each year. The cost of increased antibiotics, increased length of hospital stay, and loss of work due to nosocomial infections is staggering. Factors that contribute to the risk of acquiring a nosocomial infection include the poor state of health of many patients, the use of immunosuppressive therapy, extensive surgery, invasive diagnostic tests, use of indwelling catheters in veins, arteries, and the bladder, indwelling tubes in the respiratory and gastrointestinal tract, infusion of contaminated intravenous fluids, contaminated respiratory therapy equipment, and the widespread use of broad-spectrum antibiotics, which leads to the prevalence of antibiotic-resistant strains of bacteria in the hospital environment. Protein malnutrition, not uncommon in surgical and other hospitalized patients, contributes to such patients' increased risk of infection.[4]

Pneumonia is the leading cause of death among nosocomial infections (as high as 50% mortality in intensive care unit patients), although urinary tract infections are the most prevalent type of nosocomial infection. Etiologic agents recovered from nosocomial urinary tract infections include *E. coli*, enterococci, *Pseudomonas aeruginosa*, *Klebsiella* species, and *Proteus* species. Urinary tract, surgical wound, and lower respiratory tract infections account for more than 70% of all nosocomial infections. Hospitalized patients are often colonized in the respiratory tract, gastrointestinal tract, and the skin by endemic hospital strains of bacteria within several days of admission.[8] The nosocomial infection rate is highest among patients admitted to the surgery service (where most patients experience a breakdown of skin barriers), and the lowest rates are found among neonates and pediatric patients. Surgical wound infections are most commonly caused by *S. aureus*, *E. coli*, other Enterobacteriaceae, anaerobes, *P. aeruginosa*, and enterococci. Intra-abdominal and burn infections often lead to bacteremia secondary to the primary infection.[4] The most common isolates are *Bacteroides* species, *Serratia* species, *S. aureus*, *Acinetobacter* species, *Streptococcus agalactiae*, and *Providencia* species.

Nosocomial pneumonia is a risk for any hospitalized patient, and in particular for intubated patients. Organisms associated with these infections include *Klebsiella* species, other Enterobacteriaceae, *S. aureus*, anaerobes, *S. pneumoniae*, *Legionella*, and *P. aeruginosa*. Other agents have been associated with nosocomial outbreaks, including influenza virus. Viruses such as respiratory syncytial virus, adenovirus, and influenza A are often implicated as causes of nosocomial pneumonia among hospitalized children. Hospitalized patients are at increased risk of aspirating upper respiratory flora into the lungs (because of anesthesia, stroke, depressed sensorium, for example). "Aspiration pneumonia," as it is called, is usually caused by mixed anaerobic oral bacteria and aerobic streptococci. In the hospital setting, *S. aureus* and various gram-negative bacteria may also be involved. Material introduced into the lungs of patients via contaminated fluids or equipment during respiratory therapy has led to infections with *P. aeruginosa*, *Acinetobacter* species, *Serratia* species, and other gram-negative bacteria. Bronchoalveolar lavage and the protected specimen brush technique are useful for diagnosis of most nosocomial pneumonias (with quantitative culture), although transtracheal aspiration may be necessary for optimal recovery of anaerobes.

Antibiotic treatment, by altering normal flora and thus removing the protective effect of such flora, can select for multiply resistant strains of bacteria or allow fungal agents to multiply within the susceptible host. Such colonizing organisms may become involved in a variety of hospital-acquired infections. Alteration of the gastrointestinal flora may allow overgrowth of toxin-producing *Clostridium difficile*. This may lead to a syndrome called antibiotic-associated **pseudomembranous colitis (PMC)**, definitively diagnosed by visualizing (by sigmoidoscopy or colonoscopy) typical pseudomembrane or plaques made up of necrotic epithelial cells and pus cells on the mucosal surface of the lower gastrointestinal tract. Chapter 17 contains further information about this syndrome and its diagnosis.

23.4. Infections in Patients with Grafts, Shunts, Intravenous Cathethers, or Prosthetic Devices

Production of an artificial opening in the surface epithelium and then insertion of a plastic catheter into a blood vessel of a patient compromises the skin's ability to exclude pathogens and allows such agents direct access to the bloodstream. Devices such as intravenous catheters, heparin locks, hemodialysis shunts, total parenteral nutrition catheters, and arterial catheter lines expose patients to increased risk of infection. The agents present on the skin surface near the site of access are the most prevalent isolates from nosocomial infections; included are *S. aureus* and coagulase negative staphylococci, gram-negative bacilli, *Candida albicans*, other *Candida* species, *Candida glabrata*, and *Corynebacterium* JK. *S. aureus* is the most common etiologic agent of infected hemodialysis shunts, and *Staphylococcus epidermidis* is most commonly associated with peritonitis in patients undergoing ambulatory peritoneal dialysis.

S. epidermidis is the most common etiologic agent of infected intravenous catheters, heparin locks, and cerebrospinal fluid shunts. Other skin flora, including diphtheroids, micrococci, *Propionibacterium acnes*, and colonizing gram-negative bacilli, are common causes of infection associated with catheters and shunts. Patients receiving parenteral nutrition via a Broviac, Hickman, or other catheter are at risk of developing infections due to *Candida* species, including *C. glabrata*, staphylococci, or gram-negative bacilli. It is important to culture the blood and the catheter tip to document catheter-associated septicemia (described in Chapter 14). Semiquantitative cultures of catheter tips have been validated as useful for diagnosis of catheter-associated bacteremia.[2] Contaminated intravenous fluids have been documented as a cause of serious nosocomial sepsis on occasion. The most common agents have been gram-negative rods, including *Citrobacter freundii*, *Enterobacter agglomerans*, *P. aeruginosa*, *P. cepacia*, *Klebsiella* species, and *Serratia* species.

Prosthetic devices often present a surface on which bacteria and fungi can adhere and multiply. Accordingly, a small percentage of patients receiving vascular grafts, prosthetic heart valves, cardiac pacemaker devices, and joint prostheses become infected with bacteria or fungi. The time until presentation of infection may vary from 1 week to 2 years. Staphylococci again dominate as the most important etiologic agents of such infections.[14] The role of extracellular "slime" produced by coagulase negative staphylococci as an adherence mechanism is controversial. Prosthetic heart valve infections may also be caused by diphtheroids, gram-negative bacilli, *C. albicans*, and *Aspergillus* species, particularly in the early postoperative period. In addition, enterococci and viridans streptococci can cause late-appearing (after 60 days) infections in patients with prosthetic valves. *Mycobacterium chelonae* and fungi have been rare causes of porcine valve infection.

23.5. Infections in Drug Abusers

Drug abusers are at increased risk of acquiring infectious disease for several reasons: they may inject contaminated foreign material or their own cutaneous or oral flora into their bloodstreams along with the drug; they may be malnourished or inattentive to proper hygiene; they may suffer from lapses of consciousness and thus be at risk of aspirating oral secretions into their lungs; and they may contract viral infections (such as hepatitis and acquired immunodeficiency syndrome [AIDS]) via contaminated needles.

Sites of injection of drugs are often infected, most commonly with *S. aureus*, which is carried on the skin of most drug abusers. Streptococci are also common etiologic agents of cutaneous and subcutaneous

infections, and severe necrotizing fasciitis and pyomyositis following introduction of mixed aerobic and anaerobic oropharyngeal flora have been seen occasionally in "skin poppers." Injection of microorganisms directly into the bloodstream often results in endocarditis among drug abusers. The most common agents include *S. aureus*, streptococci, enterococci, *P. aeruginosa*, *Serratia marcescens*, other gram-negative bacilli including *Eikenella corrodens*, and *Candida* species. Staphylococcal involvement of the tricuspid valve is particularly common.

Drug addicts, due to drug-induced stupor and depressed cough reflex, may aspirate oropharyngeal flora into the lungs, causing lung abscess, aspiration pneumonia, and empyema. Organisms associated with these syndromes are black-pigmented and other *Bacteroides* species, *Peptostreptococcus* species, microaerophilic and facultative streptococci, fusobacteria, *S. aureus*, and various gram-negative rods. General poor health and depressed respiratory defense mechanisms predispose such patients to the more common agents of pneumonia, including *S. pneumoniae*, *H. influenzae*, viruses, and mycoplasma. As mentioned earlier, most addicts are positive for hepatitis B surface antigen, and many will suffer from hepatitis (either hepatitis B or non-A, non-B) at least once. Sexually transmitted diseases (STDs) are common among drug abusers, particularly women, who may turn to prostitution to support their habit. Those drug abusers who are homosexual, bisexual, or who develop AIDS are at even greater risk of acquiring infections, as outlined below.

23.6. Infections in Homosexual Males

Homosexuality per se does not predispose a person to infectious disease, and homosexual women are at no greater risk than heterosexual women of becoming infected. Many common practices among some homosexual men, however, including oral-genital, anal-genital, and oral-anal activities, as well as interacting with multiple partners over a relatively short time period, predispose these men to a number of infectious diseases. As might be suspected, acquisition of the standard STDs is facilitated by participating in sexual activity with increased numbers of partners. Gonorrhea, syphilis, and genital herpes infection are more prevalent among homosexuals than heterosexuals of similar demographic groups. In addition to the usual genital sites of infection, gonococci and herpes are often isolated from oropharyngeal lesions and as causes of proctitis. Oral-genital practices may predispose some patients to unusual oral presentation of STDs. Frequent isolation of *Neisseria meningitidis* from the oropharynx, anus, and urethra of homosexual men is probably also a consequence of oral-genital contact.

Anal-genital and anal-oral practices predispose participants to a number of infections that are usually transmitted by the fecal-oral route. Non-B hepatitis (as well as type B) is prevalent among homosexual males. A group of agents has been found to comprise the most common causes of inflammatory, diarrheal, or ulcerative bowel disease in homosexual men, collectively called the "gay bowel syndrome." Diarrhea is usually caused by *Entamoeba histolytica, Giardia lamblia, Cryptosporidium, Salmonella* species, *Shigella* species, or *Campylobacter jejuni*. Painful lesions may be caused by herpes, gonococci, meningococci, *Chlamydia* (both LGV and non-LGV strains), *Haemophilus ducreyi, Calymmatobacterium granulomatis*, or *Candida* species. The primary chancre of syphilis may occur within the rectum. In addition to hepatitis virus, cytomegalovirus, human immunodeficiency virus (HIV-I), and human T-lymphotropic virus type I (HTLV-I) may be transmitted sexually. Homosexual males are one of the largest risk groups in the United States for contracting AIDS, a devastating disease of the cell-mediated immune system marked by destruction of a subclass of T lymphocytes and other cells by the HIV virus.

23.7. Infections in Patients with AIDS

Since 1981, when the first cluster of cases of pneumonia caused by the rare pathogen *Pneumocystis carinii* was reported among young homosexuals, more than 80,000 Americans have developed AIDS. Although numbers of cases among homosexuals has leveled off, there has been a slow increase in cases among drug abusers and their contacts, including children of drug abusers. Because a primary site of cellular destruction is the host immune system, AIDS patients suffer from numerous infections. Patients often develop pneumonia, meningoencephalopathy and neurologic dysfunction, mucocutaneous candidiasis, mycobacterial and other systemic infections, and diarrhea.[6] Common infectious complications of AIDS are listed in the box opposite. Other infectious organisms reported in AIDS patients include pneumococci, *Legionella* species, *C. jejuni*, other unusual *Campylobacter* species, *Salmonel-*

la species, *Isospora belli*, varicella-zoster virus, *Histoplasma* and *Coccidioides* species, and other fungi.

The HIV of AIDS, a retrovirus, has been better studied since its discovery in 1983 than has any other virus, yet understanding of the pathogenesis of disease is not complete. The virus, an enveloped RNA virus that carries its own reverse transcriptase, adheres preferentially to helper T (T4 surface antigen) lymphocytes, to macrophages and perhaps certain other cells (such as those in brain tissue), from which it enters the host cell and either transforms it or destroys it. HIV can alter its antigenic composition to avoid immune destruction while it undermines the host's immunologic capabilities, hence the preponderance of opportunistic infections in patients with AIDS. It is known that the virus itself contrib-

---

Common Infectious Agents and Syndromes Associated with AIDS

Bacterial

Mycobacterium avium-intracellulare complex
M. tuberculosis
Other mycobacteria

Fungal

Esophageal candidiasis
Disseminated aspergillosis
Cryptococcosis

Parasitic

Chronic cryptosporidiosis
Pneumocystis carinii pneumonia
Strongyloidosis, intestinal and disseminated
Toxoplasmosis (pneumonia or central nervous system infection)

Viral

Disseminated cytomegalovirus infection
Chronic (>1 month) or disseminated herpes simplex infection
Progressive multifocal leukoencephalopathy (JC virus)
Condylomata acuminata

utes directly to the neurologic symptoms seen commonly in AIDS patients, but it also predisposes to infection by a number of other pathogens in the central nervous system.

Prevention has focused on alteration of life-styles (by education) and treatment or screening of blood products to prevent transmission. The complexity of the virus suggests that a vaccine will not be developed quickly. Amelioration of some symptoms can be achieved with azidothymidine (AZT), but this drug is not without side effects, including bone marrow suppression. Numerous other treatments are in developmental stages.

23.7.a. Epidemiology of AIDS. New York, New Jersey, Washington, D.C., Florida, and California have the highest incidence of AIDS in the United States. Homosexual and bisexual men, intravenous drug abusers, Haitians, recipients of transfused blood and blood products, hemophiliacs who received factor VIII concentrate, and sexual contacts and children of people within risk groups are at risk of acquiring AIDS. Males greatly outnumber females. Recently, increasing numbers of patients in the United States with only heterosexual exposure are developing AIDS. This form of exposure is the primary mode of transmission in underdeveloped countries, such as those in central Africa, where AIDS is a major health crisis and there are no sex-related differences in prevalence. The overall long-term mortality of AIDS seems to approach 100%. Patients with Kaposi's sarcoma alone have the best prognosis for survival; those with an opportunistic infection have the worst prognosis. Although cases have occurred in health care workers, occupational transmission has been documented only rarely. Involvement of children is directly related to congenital spread or subsequent sexual abuse or use of narcotics.

In addition to patients with infectious diseases or neoplasms suggestive of an underlying immune disorder, there are a number of patients with HIV antibody whose primary evidence of disease is lymphadenopathy. These patients may also complain of malaise, weight loss, and fever. These symptoms are indicative of the **AIDS-related complex, ARC** and signify a prodrome of AIDS. HIV has been cultured from peripheral blood and, on occasion, saliva of patients with ARC. Recently it has been shown that another retrovirus, HIV-2, can also cause AIDS. Although the prevalence of this virus is very low in the United States, early protective measures, including screening the blood supply for HIV-2 antibody, are being instituted to prevent an additional nationwide epidemic.

ELISA and Western blot tests for detection of the HIV antibody and ELISA tests for HIV-1 are used to screen all donated blood. This screening is highly sensitive and specific but does miss those patients with recent acquisition of infection who have not yet produced detectable antibodies. Through screening, numbers of individuals with no symptoms are identified. The ultimate fate of such persons is not yet known, although some have gone on to develop ARC or AIDS.

Literature concerning all aspects of AIDS is readily available; books, newsletters, and reviews abound. A complete discussion of this disease is beyond the scope of this book. Readers are referred to the publications listed in the bibliography of this chapter as an initial resource for more information.

23.7.b. Laboratory diagnosis of HIV infection. Diagnostic testing for the HIV agent encompasses antibody and antigen detection systems. ELISA tests (at least eight commercial tests are approved by the Food and Drug Administration [FDA]) are the first screening test of choice for HIV antibodies. These tests usually yield less than 1% false-negative results but may show false-positive results in as many as 25% of some patient groups. The Western blot confirmatory test helps to weed out false-positives, although a gold standard of criteria for a positive test has not been determined. Patients who have been infected recently and produce only IgM may test negative in these tests. Immunofluorescent assay (IFA) tests are used with reliability by the California State Health Department and other centers as a supplement to ELISA; these tests are not available commercially. Radioimmunoprecipitation (RIPA) is a relatively new test for HIV that utilizes radioactively labeled viral proteins that bind to specific serum antibodies. The pattern of antibodies is then determined. RIPA is available only as a research test, although it is probably more specific and sensitive than the commercially available tests. Double-antibody sandwich ELISA tests for HIV antigen are also available.

Commercially available antigen detection by ELISA is not yet sensitive enough for routine use, although specific tests for the p24 antigen (most prevalent in patients with HIV infection) are promising. Amplification methods, however, improve the sensitivity of antigen tests. Polymerase chain reaction (PCR) systems show much promise for detection of even small amounts of viral DNA in patient specimens. Once the viral target nucleic acid is amplified, it can be detected easily using hybridization techniques. Finally, culture of the virus from peripheral blood monocytes in a cocultivation system seems to detect most positive reactions. Detection of either reverse transcriptase activity or HIV antigen denotes a positive culture result. Cultures are expensive and time-consuming but may be the only positive test in some stages of HIV infection.

23.7.c. **Laboratory diagnosis of infections associated with AIDS.** Standard methods for diagnosis of infections should be used for this purpose in AIDS patients. Some additional measures that have been useful in diagnosing opportunistic infections in AIDS patients are mentioned here. Patients with bacteremia due to *Mycobacterium avium-intracellulare* complex often have large numbers of circulating bacteria, and blood cultures are often positive, particularly with a lysis-centrifugation system (DuPont Isolator) or when blood is cultured directly using a radiometric procedure developed for that purpose (Johnston Laboratories). Blood is allowed to remain at room temperature for approximately 1 hour in the Isolator tube before centrifugation and plating. Presumably this time period allows the white cells to be lysed, releasing viable mycobacteria that would not have been detected if the white cells were to remain intact. Additionally, numbers of circulating organisms can be quantitated by using the Pediatric 1.5 ml Isolator tube in a manner similar to that used for the standard Isolator. Quantitation of this sort can help to monitor the patient's response to therapy.

A number of procedures, including open lung biopsy, transbronchial biopsy, and bronchoalveolar lavage, are useful in diagnosing *P. carinii* pneumonia, although even sputum may often be positive in AIDS patients. A rapid stain such as toluidine blue O or the monoclonal fluorescent antibody for detection of *P. carinii* should be used on respiratory specimens. A silver stain will reveal fungal elements in addition to *Pneumocystis*. Other agents of pulmonary infection can be detected by standard methods. Acid fast stains of stool, as well as sputum, may be helpful in detecting mycobacteria and also *Cryptosporidium*.

Bone marrow cultures have proved valuable for diagnosis of infections in febrile AIDS patients.[1] One must carefully examine all specimens from AIDS patients with an open mind since unusual pathogens and unusual presentations of infectious diseases are not uncommon.

REFERENCES

1. Bishburg, E., Eng, R.H., Smith, S.M., and Kapila, R. 1986. Yield of bone marrow culture in the diagnosis of infectious diseases in patients with acquired immunodeficiency syndrome. J. Clin. Microbiol. 24:312.
2. Collignon, P.J., Soni, N., Pearson, I.Y., et al. 1986. Is semiquantitative culture of central vein catheter tips useful in the diagnosis of catheter-associated bacteremia? J. Clin. Microbiol. 24:532.
3. Daffos, F., Forrestier, F., Capella-Pavlosky, M., et al. 1988. Prenatal management of 746 pregnancies at risk for congenital toxoplasmosis. N. Engl. J. Med. 318:271.
4. Deitch, E.A. 1988. Infection in the compromised host. Surg. Clin. North Am. 68:181.
5. Evans, M.E., Schaffner, W., Federspiel, C.F., et al. 1988. Sensitivity, specificity, and predictive value of body surface cultures in a neonatal intensive care unit. JAMA 259:248.
6. Janoff, E.N., and Smith, P.D. 1988. Perspectives on gastrointestinal infections in AIDS. Gastroenterol. Clin. North Am. 17:451.
7. Kramer, B.S., Pizzo, P.A., Robichaud, K.J., Witebsky, F., and Wesley, R. 1982. Role of serial microbiologic surveillance and clinical evaluation in the management of cancer patients with fever and granulocytopenia. Am. J. Med. 72:561.
8. Larson, E.L., McGinley, K.J., Foglia, A.R., et al. 1986. Composition and antimicrobic resistance of skin flora in hospitalized and healthy adults. J. Clin. Microbiol. 23:604.
9. McGowan, K.L. 1987. Practical approaches to diagnosing fungal infections in immunocompromised patients. Clin. Microbiol. Newsletter 9:33.
10. McGowan, K.L. 1988. The microbiology associated with cystic fibrosis. Clin. Microbiol. Newsletter 10:9.
11. Peter, J.B., Cherry, J.D., and Bryson, Y.J. 1982. Improving diagnosis of congenital infections. Diagn. Med. 5:61.
12. Sever, J., Ellenberg, J.H., Ley, A.C., et al. 1988. Toxoplasmosis: maternal and pediatric findings in 23,000 pregnancies. Pediatrics 82:181.
13. Tutschka, P.J. 1988. Infections and immunodeficiency in bone marrow transplantation. Pediatr. Infect. Dis. J. 7:S22.
14. Young, E.J. and Sugarman, B. 1988. Infections in prosthetic devices. Surg. Clin. North Am. 68:167.
15. Young, L.S. 1988. Antimicrobial prophylaxis in the neutropenic host: lessons of the past and perspectives for the future. Eur. J. Clin. Microbiol. Infect. Dis. 7:93.

BIBLIOGRAPHY

Centers for Disease Control. 1987. Update: acquired immunodeficiency syndrome—United States. M.M.W.R. 36:522.
Inderlied, C.B., and Young, L.S. 1985. Clinical microbiology of acquired immune deficiency syndrome. J. Med. Technol. 2:167.

Jackson, J.B., and Balfour, H.H., Jr. 1988. Practical diagnostic testing for human immunodeficiency virus. Clin. Microbiol. Rev. 1:124.

Mandell, G., Douglas, R.G. Jr., and Bennett, J.E., editors. 1985. Principles and practice of infectious diseases, ed. 2. Part IV: Special problems. Section A: Nosocomial infections and Section B: Infections in special hosts. John Wiley & Sons. New York.

Ostrow, D.G. 1984. Homosexuality and sexually transmitted diseases. In Holmes, K.K., Mårdh, P.-A., Sparling, P.F., and Wiesner, P.J., editors. Sexually transmitted diseases. McGraw-Hill Book Co., New York.

Quinn, T.C., and Holmes, K.K. 1984. Proctitis, proctocolitis, and enteritis in homosexual men. In Holmes, K.K., Mårdh, P.-A., Sparling, P.F., and Wiesner, P.J., editors. Sexually transmitted diseases. McGraw-Hill Book Co., New York.

Rankin, J.A., Coliman, R., and Daniele, R.P. 1988. Acquired immune deficiency syndrome and the lung. Chest 94:155.

Remington, J.S., and Klein, J.O., editors. 1983. Infectious diseases of the fetus and newborn infant. W.B. Saunders Co., Philadelphia.

Sen, P., Kapila, R., Chmel, H., Armstrong, D.A., and Louria, D.B. 1982. Superinfection: another look. Am. J. Med. 73:706.

Steigbigel, R.T., and Cross, A.S. 1984. Infections associated with hemodialysis and chronic peritoneal dialysis. In Remington, J.S., and Swartz, M.N., editors. Current clinical topics in infectious diseases. McGraw-Hill Book Co., New York.

Yoshikawa, T.T. 1983. Geriatric infectious diseases: an emerging problem. J. Am. Geriatr. Soc. 31:34.

Part Four

Methods for Identification
of Etiologic Agents of
Infectious Disease

24

Micrococcaceae: Staphylococci, Micrococci, and Stomatococci

The genera *Staphylococcus*, *Micrococcus*, *Stomatococcus*, and *Planococcus* are members of the family Micrococcaceae. The majority of planococci and micrococci are free-living saprophytes, but the natural habitat of staphylococci and *Stomatococcus* species is the surface of primates and other mammals. Their presence as endogenous flora allows many species of staphylococci the opportunity to cause infection under certain circumstances. Staphylococci, *Stomatococcus* sp., and micrococci have been isolated from clinically significant sources.

Staphylococcus aureus (usually coagulase-positive staphylococci, described in Section 24.1) has been recognized historically as a virulent and important human pathogen; its capacity to produce human disease has not diminished with the introduction of antibiotics. Reviews by Sheagren[22] and Kaplan and Tenenbaum[13] are excellent sources of information about this ubiquitous pathogen. *Staphylococcus intermedius*, another coagulase-positive species, has recently been identified as an important agent of dog-bite wound infections; it was isolated four times more frequently than *S. aureus* from the oral cavity of 135 dogs.[23] This species has probably been misidentified as *S. aureus* when isolated from such infections. *Staphylococcus hyicus* is also coagulase-positive, but it has not yet been implicated as a human pathogen. During the last several years, coagulase-negative staphylococci have surfaced as important pathogens, preying primarily on compromised hosts, especially patients with some sort of prosthetic or indwelling device. Pfaller and Herwaldi[18] and Archer[2] have reviewed current thought on these organisms.

Specimens that may harbor clinically important Micrococcaceae come from almost any source. The organisms are hardy and do not require special collection procedures other than those outlined in Chapter 6. *S. aureus* is recovered from a variety of infections including skin lesions such as furuncles and carbuncles, various abscesses, wound infections, pneumonia, and so forth. From these sites organisms can invade the bloodstream and seed metastatically, appearing in the urine or forming abscesses in various body organs, or producing septic shock or endocarditis. The organism can also be recovered from the anterior nares, perineum, and other skin sites from as many as 10% to 15% of healthy people and a significantly greater percentage of people in the hospital setting. This **carrier** state can serve as a reservoir for infection of hospitalized patients, but most carriers do not disseminate the organism and are not a risk to others. Although it is also an important source of food poisoning, *S. aureus* is usually not isolated from the patient suffering from this intoxication, and clinical laboratories usually do not attempt to culture pathogens from food. Coagulase-negative staphylococci are a common cause of bacteremia in neutropenic patients; of infections related to indwelling catheters, shunts, and prosthetic devices; and of urinary tract infections in young, sexually active women. Micrococci become pathogens during accidental introduction into a susceptible host. They may cause endocarditis and other diverse syndromes. It appears that they are less virulent than the staphylococci. *Stomatococcus mucilaginosus* is part of the normal oral flora and is an opportunistic pathogen.

24.1. Morphology and General Characteristics

Micrococcaceae are spherical cocci with gram-positive cell walls; they are nonmotile, aerobic or facultatively anaerobic, and, except for stomatococci, are catalase-positive. During binary fission, Micrococcaceae divide along both longitudinal and horizontal planes, forming pairs, tetrads, and ultimately irregular clusters (Figure 24.1). The Greek word *staphyle*, meaning a "bunch of grapes," is the descriptive stem for the genus name. Very old cells may lose their ability to retain crystal violet and thus may be more easily decolorized in a Gram stain than young cells.

Micrococcaceae will grow on most laboratory me-

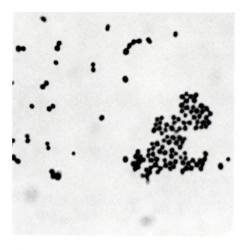

Figure 24.1
Appearance of Micrococcaceae in Gram stain.

dia that support gram-positive organisms, yielding circular, opaque, smooth colonies. The growth is usually **butyrous** (like butter) and colonies can be emulsified in water easily to form a smooth suspension. Hemolysis on blood agar and color of the colony are variable. Since yeast colonies can resemble Micrococcaceae and may be catalase-positive, all colonies should be examined microscopically by wet mount or Gram stain before further tests are performed. Mannitol salt agar is commonly used to isolate staphyloccoci from clinical material. This medium contains a high salt concentration, mannitol, and phenol red pH indicator. *S. aureus* will yield colonies surrounded by a yellow halo. Other staphylococci (particularly *S. saprophyticus*) may ferment mannitol and thus resemble *S. aureus* on mannitol salt agar.

Once an organism isolated from a clinical specimen has been characterized as a gram-positive, catalase-positive coccoid bacterium, it is further identified in a series of steps, the first of which involves the coagulase test. *S. aureus* is identified on the basis of presence of the enzyme *coagulase,* which binds plasma fibrinogen, causing the organisms to agglutinate or plasma to clot. A rapid screening slide test for the production of *clumping factor* (cell-bound coagulase) that is positive with over 95% of strains of *S. aureus* is described in Chapter 9. Isolates that do not produce clumping factor must be tested for the ability to produce extracellular coagulase (*free*

PROCEDURE 24.1

Tube Coagulase Test

Principle

Only *S aureus*, the most virulent species, and *S. intermedius* and *S. hyicus* (both rarely isolated from humans) produce coagulase enzyme able to clot rabbit plasma, differentiating them from the rest of the Micrococcaceae.

Method

1. Prepare coagulase reagent, rabbit plasma with EDTA (Difco Laboratories and BBL Microbiology Systems) in 0.5 ml amounts in 13 × 100 mm glass or plastic tubes. The tubes can be prepared in large numbers and refrigerated for 10 days, or frozen at −20° C for several months.
2. Emulsify a visible portion of growth from isolated colonies (grown on supportive medium) in the plasma by rubbing the material on the side of the tube while holding the tube at an angle. Straighten the tube, causing the plasma level to cover the site of inoculation.
3. Incubate the suspension for 1 to 4 h at 35° to 37° C and observe for the presence of a gel or clot that cannot be resuspended by gentle shaking (Figure 24.2). If no clot forms after 4 h, the tube should be incubated at room temperature overnight. Rare isolates require such extended incubation.
4. Organisms that fail to clot the plasma within 24 h are considered coagulase-negative and must be identified by other methods.

Quality control

Inoculate coagulase tubes with fresh subcultures of *S. aureus* ATCC 25923 and *S. epidermidis* ATCC 14990 and proceed as above.

Expected results

The *S. aureus* should clot the plasma in 4 h; the *S. epidermidis* should not clot the plasma even after overnight incubation.

Performance schedule

Test each new lot of coagulase plasma when it is received and weekly thereafter.

coagulase). This enzyme will cause clotting of plasma after 1 to 4 hours of incubation at 37° C. The tube coagulase test for free coagulase is described in Procedure 24.1. Coagulase plasma with citrate is not suitable for use in this test because citrate-utilizing organisms may yield false-positive results. A positive coagulase test is sufficient for naming an isolate *S. aureus* in most cases, although other staphylococcal species do produce clumping factor (Table 24.1). *S. intermedius*, a rare human isolate (usually from canine bite wounds) that also produces coagulase, is positive for the enzyme pyroglutamyl-β-naphthylamide aminopeptidase (the PYR test, described in Chapter 9), which distinguishes it from PYR-negative *S. aureus*.

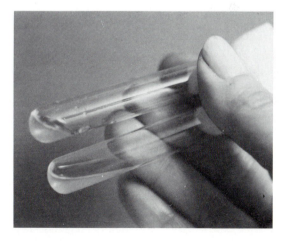

Figure 24.2

Tube coagulase test. Presence of clot (tube on top) indicates a positive coagulase result.

Table 24.1
Selected Characteristics of Coagulase-negative *Staphylococcus* Species Isolated From Humans

SPECIES	PYR HYDROLYSIS	CLUMPING FACTOR	UREASE	ACID PRODUCED AEROBICALLY FROM		ZONE OF INHIBITION*		
				MANNITOL	SUCROSE	BACITRACIN (10 U) <11 mm	POLYMYXIN B (300 U) <10 mm	NOVOBIOCIN (5 µg) <12 mm
capitis	−	−	−	+	+^{d}	−	−	−
cohnii	−	−	−/+^{w}	+/+^{w}	−	+/−	−	+
epidermidis	−	−	+	−	+	−	+	−
haemolyticus	+	−	−	+/−	+	+	−	−
hominis	−	−	+	−/+	+^{d}	−	−	−
lugdunensis	−	+	−	−	+	−	−	−
saccharolyticus	−	−	NT	−	−	−	−	−
saprophyticus	−	−	+	+/−	+	−/+	−	+
schleiferi	+	+	−	−	−	−	−	−
simulans	+	−	+	+/+^{w}	+	−	−	−
warneri	−	−	+	+/−	+	−	−	−
xylosus	+	−	+	+/+^{w}	+	−/+	−	+

+ = 90% strains positive; − = 90% strains negative; +/− = variable, results more often positive; −/+ = variable, results more often negative; w = weak; d = delayed; NT = not tested.

*Cotton swab is rinsed in McFarland 1.0 suspension in trypticase soy broth, pressed against side of tube to remove excess moisture, and streaked onto trypticase soy agar in one direction. After agar has dried, disks are placed on surface of agar. Plates are incubated at 35° C for 24 hours.

Table 24.2
Differences Between *Staphylococcus* and *Micrococcus* Genera

GENUS	RESISTANT TO LYSOSTAPHIN (200 µg/ml)	MODIFIED OXIDASE AND BENZIDINE	RESISTANT TO BACITRACIN (0.04 U)
Micrococcus	+	+	−
Staphylococcus	−	−	+

24.2. Differentiation Among Coagulase-Negative Staphylococci, Micrococci, and *Stomatococcus mucilaginosus*

Catalase-positive, coagulase-negative organisms may be either staphylococci or micrococci. Catalase-negative organisms that resemble staphylococci by Gram stain and colony morphology may be S. *mucilaginosus*, described in Section 24.5. The micrococci are resistant to lysostaphin (an enzyme produced by certain staphylococci), are benzidine-positive, are susceptible to 0.04 units of bacitracin (Procedure 24.2), and contain cytochrome C, as determined by a positive modified oxidase test (Procedure 24.3).[8,9,21] Differentiation of coagulase-negative staphylococci from micrococci (considered to be less virulent) is outlined in Table 24.2.[9,21] Two methods recommended for routine laboratories are detailed in Procedures 24.2 and 24.3. Commercial reagents are available for the lysostaphin test (Remel Laboratories; Roche Products Ltd). Using a combination of these tests, microbiologists should easily be able to differentiate staphylococci and micrococci likely to be found in clinical material.

24.3. *Staphylococcus aureus*

24.3.a. **Structure and extracellular products.** Because of its structure, S. *aureus* is uniquely suited to be a human pathogen. The cell wall is composed of tightly crosslinked peptidoglycan and teichoic acid moieties that protect the organism from lysis under harsh osmotic conditions and probably aid in attachment of the bacteria to mucosal cell receptor sites. Certain strains produce a polysaccharide capsule that

PROCEDURE 24.2

Bacitracin Susceptibility

Principle

All coagulase-negative staphylococci are resistant to 0.04 U bacitracin, which differentiates them from micrococci and stomatococci.

Method

1. Growth from the colony to be tested is inoculated into 1 ml of trypticase soy broth to a turbidity equal to that of a McFarland 0.5 standard.
2. Using a cotton swab saturated with the test suspension, the microbiologist must streak a small (90 mm diameter) Mueller-Hinton or trypticase soy agar plate in three directions, exactly as if preparing the inoculum for agar disk diffusion susceptibility testing.
3. Place a 0.04 U bacitracin-impregnated filter paper disk (Taxo A, BBL Microbiology Systems, or Bacto Group A Differential Disk, Difco) on the surface of the plate.
4. Incubate the plate at 35° C in air for 18 h and observe for any zone of inhibition around the disk. Micrococci will yield zones of inhibition, and staphylococci will be resistant, showing growth up to the disk. If an organism fails to grow, it is probably a micrococcus.

Quality control

S. epidermidis ATCC 14990 and a *Micrococcus luteus* strain should be tested as above.

Expected results

The micrococcus should yield a zone of inhibition around the bacitracin disk, usually greater than 10 mm, whereas the staphylococcus should grow up to the disk.

Performance schedule

Each new lot of bacitracin disks should be tested, and control organisms should be run with each test.

Modified from Falk and Guering[8] and Hebert et al.[12]

PROCEDURE 24.3

Modified Oxidase Test

Principle

The cytochrome oxidase system of micrococci (and the rare *Staphylococcus sciuri*) contains cytochrome C, which yields a colored end product in the presence of the oxidase reagent.

Method

1. A visible amount of a colony from a 15- to 24-h-old 5% sheep blood agar plate is smeared onto a piece of filter paper as for the standard oxidase test (Chapter 9). Colonies from other media or colonies older than 24 h will give aberrant results.
2. A drop of modified oxidase reagent (6% tetramethylphenylenediamine hydrochloride [Eastman Kodak Co.] in dimethyl sulfoxide [DMSO, Sigma Chemical Co.]) is added to the bacteria on the filter paper. Disks impregnated with this reagent are available from Remel Laboratories.
3. Oxidase-positive organisms turn dark blue within 2 min. All oxidase-positive organisms are micrococci, with the exception of rare *S. sciuri* (which has been isolated only from animals).

Quality control

Test *Staphylococcus epidermidis* ATCC 14990 and a *Micrococcus luteus* strain as described above.

Expected results

The micrococcus should yield a blue color on the filter paper within 2 min; the staphylococcus spot should remain colorless.

Performance schedule

Test the reagent with each new batch made and weekly thereafter.

Modified from Faller and Schleifer.[9]

helps to protect them from phagocytosis by polymorphonuclear neutrophils (PMNs). In addition, most strains possess a cell wall protein, protein A, that binds the Fc segment of IgG, preventing antibody-mediated phagocytosis by PMNs. In the bloodstream, aggregates of IgG bound to protein A on staphylococcal surfaces will fix complement, causing complement-mediated tissue damage to the host.

S. aureus produces a number of enzymes and toxins that contribute substantially to its ability to cause disease. In addition to coagulase, S. aureus produces the enzymes phosphatase, thermostable deoxyribonuclease, lipase, gelatinase, protease, and fibrinolysin. Another enzyme, hyaluronidase, may contribute to the spread of infection involving S. aureus. Among the toxins elaborated by S. aureus are alpha, beta, gamma, and delta toxins and leukocidin, which act on the red and white blood cell membranes of some species. The role of these toxins in the pathogenesis of disease is unclear.

Toxins that have been shown clearly to contribute to certain disease syndromes are enterotoxins, exfoliative toxin, and the toxins associated with toxic shock syndrome. S. aureus produces at least six different enterotoxins, some of which are implicated in food poisoning and antibiotic-induced pseudomembranous colitis. In the case of food poisoning, toxins are elaborated by the organisms growing in food and then are ingested by the patient. Staphylococcal scalded skin syndrome, often affecting newborns, is caused by an exfoliative toxin called *exfoliatin* (which cleaves the middle layers of the epidermis, allowing the surface skin to peel). The most recently described toxin-mediated staphylococcal disease is **toxic shock syndrome,** a systemic disease characterized by fever, hypotension, and multiorgan involvement but negative blood cultures.[24] The disease is caused by toxins, one of which is called toxic shock syndrome toxin-1 (TSST-1), which is elaborated by certain S. aureus strains growing in a localized focus of infection or colonization. Many cases have occurred in menstruating young females who were vaginal carriers of S. aureus and who used tampons. Any site, however, such as an abscess or wound, may harbor the toxin-producing organisms. The clinical laboratory may be asked to isolate S. aureus from suspected sites of infection; a reverse passive latex agglutination test for TSST-1 toxin is available commercially (Oxoid USA).

24.3.b. Identification. S. aureus is coagulase-positive, which is its most distinguishing characteristic. For the rare isolate suspected of being S. aureus that fails to produce coagulase, an even more specific test for thermostable deoxyribonuclease can be performed.[16] One method requires that suspensions of overnight broth cultures of the organisms be boiled for 15 minutes and an aliquot placed into wells punched into thermostable nuclease test agar (Remel Laboratories or Edge Diagnostics). A pink halo surrounding the well after 1 to 4 hours' incubation at 37° C indicates presence of the nuclease.[25]

Madison and Baselski[15] used 1 ml of the culture supernatant from blood culture bottles showing positive cocci in clusters for a rapid modification of the thermostable nuclease test described in the preceding paragraph. The supernatant was boiled for 15 minutes and placed into 3-mm diameter wells cut into the surface of thermonuclease agar plates. Correlation with standard methods was 100% and only 2 hours' incubation was needed before results could be interpreted. Another very similar rapid method for performing a thermostable nuclease test directly from blood culture broth was described in Chapter 9. The source of the test agar was critical for reliable results; thermonuclease (not DNase) agar must be used.

Commercial particle agglutination tests are available for rapid differentiation of S. aureus from other staphylococci. Staphylatex (American Scientific Products), Staphylochrome (Innovative Diagnostics), Sero-STAT (Scott Laboratories), Bacto Staph Latex (Difco Laboratories), Staphaurex (Wellcome Diagnostics), and Accu-Staph (Carr-Scarborough Microbiologicals) use latex particles; Hemastaph (Remel Laboratories) and Staphyloslide (BBL Microbiology Systems) use sensitized sheep erythrocytes as particles. Although these systems are quite accurate, there may be a small percentage of false-negative results, particularly with methicillin-resistant strains.[14] Methicillin-resistant strains of S. aureus are often slide coagulase-negative as well, suggesting that a common cell wall structure contributes to both clumping factor expression and methicillin resistance. The rapid commercial tests can be used in most institutions with confidence if microbiologists confirm the identity of methicillin-resistant strains by tube coagulase. However, the slide test for clumping factor yields approximately the same results as the tests mentioned and can be performed as rapidly and is less expensive than tests using commercial reagents. Tube coagulase should be used to confirm all slide test negative results on clinically significant isolates in either case; detection of thermostable nuclease is the definitive test for *S. aureus*.

Strains of *S. aureus* may be identified for epidemiologic purposes by phage typing. Characterizing strains by phage type, biotype, plasmid profile, and slime production may help to delineate the path of spread of strains among hospitalized patients, the environment, and the attending medical staff. Used primarily for investigation of nosocomial outbreaks of *S. aureus* infection, phage typing schemes have also been developed for coagulase-negative staphylococci. In some cases, possession of virulence factors can be traced to particular phage types. This time-consuming procedure is performed by a small number of laboratories in the United States, Canada, and England.

24.3.c. **Susceptibility.** Most strains (85% to 90%) of *S. aureus*, even those acquired in the community, are penicillin-resistant. In most cases this resistance is attributable to β-lactamase production and is effected by extrachromosomal plasmids. Some staphylococci that are penicillin-resistant are also resistant to the newer β-lactamase-resistant semisynthetic penicillins such as methicillin, oxacillin, and nafcillin. This resistance is due partially to the presence of an unusual penicillin-binding protein in the cell wall of resistant strains; the genetic determinants are chromosomal.[3] Clinically significant methicillin-resistant *S. aureus* is being isolated with greater frequency in the United States, often posing problems as causes of nosocomial infections. It has been shown that these strains, although they may exhibit susceptibility to cephalosporins in vitro, cannot be treated effectively with either cephalosporins or β-lactamase-resistant penicillins.

Strategies for susceptibility testing and reporting of *S. aureus* are described in Chapter 13. In particular, the use of both methicillin (5 μg) and oxacillin (1 μg) disks, the addition of 2% NaCl to cation-supplemented Mueller-Hinton broth or 4% NaCl to Mueller-Hinton agar, incubation at temperatures no greater than 35° C (preferably 30° C), and incubation for a full 24 hours before reading results have been shown to increase the chances of detecting methicillin-resistant *S. aureus*. A screening test for methicillin-resistant staphylococci incorporating 10 μg/ml methicillin or 6 μg/ml oxacillin in 4% NaCl-supplemented Mueller-Hinton agar, inoculated with a spot of a McFarland 0.5 turbidity suspension of the organism to be screened, and incubated for 24 hours at 35° C will accurately detect resistant strains as those that grow on the agar. A simple broth-disk elution modification of this screening test has been developed.[17] An additional procedure for detecting resistance should be used with any automated susceptibility system, none of which can reliably detect all methicillin-resistant strains of staphylococci.[3] Collopy and others[5] have suggested that methicillin-resistant strains are less likely to be associated with severe infections, but once established, they are more difficult to eradicate. All staphylococci are still susceptible to vancomycin, and many or most strains are susceptible to rifampin. Certain *S. aureus* strains exhibit in vitro tolerance (minimum bactericidal concentration [MBC] at least 32 times greater than minimum inhibitory concentration [MIC]) to some antimicrobial agents because of clones of bacteria that are killed more slowly than the majority of cells in the population. There is no definitive evidence that tolerance is of clinical significance.

24.3.d. **Nonculture methods for diagnosing *Staphylococcus aureus* infections.** Tests for staphylococcal antigen have not been shown to aid in diagnosis of disease. However, some workers believe that detection of circulating antibodies to the teichoic acid component of the *S. aureus* cell wall is useful for monitoring the course of infection and for differentiating long-standing or deep-seated infections from lesser infections. Although radioimmunoassay, enzyme-linked immunosorbent assay (ELISA), crossed immunoelectrophoresis, agar-gel diffusion, and immunoprecipitation methods have all been used to detect such antibodies successfully, many of these methods are too sensitive to differentiate between patients with more serious or less serious infections. Almost all human sera can be found to contain antibodies against staphylococcal teichoic acid if a sensitive enough assay is used for detection. One use of detection of such antibodies is for confirmation of a diagnosis of toxic shock syndrome.[1] Diagnostic applications of tests for teichoic acid antibody, including evaluation of a new commercial immunodiffusion kit (Endo-Staph, Meridian Diagnostics), are being developed.

24.4. Coagulase-Negative Staphylococci

Coagulase-negative staphylococci vary in pathogenic potential.[18] As is true for many other resident human flora of relatively low virulence, these organisms are more likely to cause infection in compromised hosts, particularly cancer patients. *Staphylococcus epidermidis* is known to cause infection of native heart valves and intravascular prostheses, including intravenous catheters and artificial heart valves. It can cause peritonitis in patients receiving peritoneal dialysis. *S. epidermidis*, usually introduced via a break in the patient's skin, also causes infections in prosthetic joints, central nervous system shunts, and has been isolated from subcutaneous infections. *S. saprophyticus* is isolated most frequently from uncomplicated urinary tract infections in nonhospitalized patients, notably sexually active young women. The incidence of *S. saprophyticus* urinary tract infection varies considerably among the patient populations served by institutions and in different geographic areas. Species that are less commonly implicated as pathogens include *S. cohnii*, *S. haemolyticus*, *S. haemolyticus*, *S. hominis*, *S. lugdunensis*, *S. saccharolyticus*, *S. schleiferi*, *S. simulans*, and *S. warneri*. Those species rarely isolated from patients are *S. auricularis*, *S. capitis*, *S. carnosus*, *S. lentus*, and *S. xylosus*. Coagulase-negative staphylococci isolated only from animal sources to date include *S. arlettae*, *S. caprae*, *S. carnosus*, *S. caseolyticus*, *S. chromogenes*, *S. equorum*, *S. gallinarum*, *S. hyicus* (coagulase- variable), *S. kloosii*, *S. lentus*, and *S. sciuri*.[10,12,18]

24.4.a. Morphology and extracellular products. Morphologically similar to *S. aureus*, coagulase-negative staphylococci may possess many of the same virulence properties. Although they do not produce the number of extracellular products that *S. aureus* does, many species produce hemolysins and some seem to possess an antiphagocytic capsule. In addition, the production of slime may correlate with pathogenicity, particularly in foreign body-associated infection where slime may mediate bacterial adherence.[4,7]

24.4.b. Identification. The majority of coagulase-negative staphylococci isolated from clinically significant sources are *S. epidermidis*. These isolations may merely reflect its prevalence as the most common strain on human skin. Since any of the other species can cause disease, coagulase-negative staphylococci cannot arbitrarily be reported as *S. epider-*

midis without further biochemical tests. For those laboratories that do not identify this group to species, a report of "coagulase-negative staphylococci" is sufficient.

Isolates obtained from the urinary tract of nonhospitalized patients are usually *S. saprophyticus*. It may be involved in recurrent infection and in stone formation. This species is resistant to the antibiotic novobiocin, as are *S. cohnii*, *S. lentus*, *S. sciuri*, and *S. xylosus*. The latter four species, however, are rarely isolated from patients. We recommend that for coagulase-negative staphylococcal isolates from sources other than blood, body fluids, or other sterile sites, a *presumptive* identification of *S. saprophyticus* should be reported based on the broth disk elution novobiocin test[11] (Procedure 24.4) or novobiocin resistance, as indicated by a zone of inhibition of ≤16 mm diameter surrounding a 5-μg novobiocin disk, in an agar disk diffusion test performed in the same way as the disk diffusion susceptibility test. Phosphatase production, as described by Pickett and Welch,[19] can also be used to distinguish between *S. saprophyticus* (negative) and *S. epidermidis* (positive).[19]

Table 24.2 shows some of the biochemical reactions used to differentiate coagulase-negative staphylococci. Many other reactions may be used to identify these organisms, but the tests require specialized media and may be difficult to perform. Commercial identification kits, including API Staph-Ident (Analytab Products), API Staph-Trac (Analytab Products), American MicroScan Staph ID system (American Hospital Supply/Baxter), Sceptor (Johnston Laboratories), and Vitek GPI (Vitek Microbiology Systems) have been shown to identify coagulase-negative staphylococci with accuracies varying from 65 to 95%, depending on the species studied.[18] A simplified scheme for identification of these organisms using susceptibility to five antimicrobial agents, PYR test, adherence to glass, and synergistic hemolysis has been developed recently by Hebert and others.[12]

24.4.c. Susceptibility. Unlike *S. aureus*, coagulase-negative staphylococci have no predictable patterns of susceptibility. Strains associated with nosocomial infections are likely to be multiply resistant and may carry resistance plasmids that serve to spread antimicrobial resistance among other bacterial strains. Like *S. aureus*, coagulase-negative staphylococci resistant to penicillinase-resistant pen-

PROCEDURE 24.4

Rapid Novobiocin Test

Principle

S. saprophyticus, because of its importance as a urinary tract pathogen, should be distinguished from *S. epidermidis* on the basis of resistance to novobiocin. Broth disk elution allows antibiotic impregnated in a filter paper disk to diffuse throughout a liquid medium to create a standard concentration of the drug. This method bypasses the problem of obtaining and measuring antibiotic powder to make broth solutions.

Method

1. Inoculate growth from isolated colonies into two tubes containing 3 ml each of trypticase soy broth. The inoculum should be extremely light, such that there is no visible turbidity.
2. Immediately add one 5-μg novobiocin filter paper disk, such as those used for agar diffusion susceptibility testing, to one of the tubes and shake the tube gently for 10 s to disperse the antibiotic.
3. Incubate both tubes at 37 ° C for up to 5 h, or until the control tube (without novobiocin) reaches the turbidity of a McFarland 0.5 standard.

Modified from Harrington and Gaydos.[11]

4. Observe the tube containing the novobiocin disk for turbidity. Novobiocin-resistant organisms, presumptively identified as *S. saphrophyticus*, yield turbidity equal to that of the control tube. Most other human isolates of coagulase-negative staphylococci are novobiocin susceptible and show no visible turbidity after 5 h of incubation.

Quality control

Test stock isolates of *S. epidermidis* ATCC 14990 and *S. saprophyticus* ATCC 13518 as described above.

Expected results

S. epidermidis will be inhibited by novobiocin and will show no turbidity; *S. saprophyticus*, because of its resistance to novobiocin, will show turbidity equal to the control tube.

Performance schedule

Test control organisms when each new batch of antibiotic disks is received and weekly thereafter.

---

icillins in vitro may also fail to respond in infections treated with cephalosporins. Strains exhibiting oxacillin resistance (tested in the same manner as for *S. aureus*) should be reported as cephalosporin-resistant regardless of in vitro susceptibilities to cephalosporins. Unlike the other coagulase-negative staphylococci, *S. saprophyticus* is usually susceptible to most antimicrobial agents with the exception of the urinary tract agent nalidixic acid (which is active only against gram-negative bacilli). There are presently no diagnostic methods for disease caused by coagulase-negative staphylococci that do not require isolation of the bacteria.

24.5. *Stomatococcus* Species

Several recent reports have focused on recovery of *S. mucilaginosus*, an encapsulated Micrococcaceae species that occurs as normal oral flora, from clinically important sites. The organism has been recovered from compromised patients, particularly drug abusers, as an agent of endocarditis and septicemia. Stomatococci morphologically (colony and microscopic appearance) resemble staphylococci but may adhere to the agar because of their capsule. They are catalase-negative and may be vancomycin-resistant. Inability of stomatococci to grow in media containing 5% NaCl further distinguishes them from all other Micrococcaceae.[6,20] Susceptibility to penicillins, penicillinase-resistant penicillins, and cephalosporins has been reported; penicillins are the drug of choice for initial therapy.

24.6. Micrococci

Rarely identified as causes of infection, micrococci are saprophytic, often pigmented members of the Micrococcaceae. Species include *M. agilis*, *M. kristinae*, *M. luteus*, *M. lylae*, *M. nishinomiyaensis*, *M. roseus*, *M. sedentarius*, and *M. varians*. Hospital microbiology laboratories should not attempt identification of species of these bacteria. Isolates of micrococci that are unequivocally implicated as causes of infection should be sent to a reference laboratory for further studies.

REFERENCES

1. Abramson, C., Bergdoll, M.S., and Wheat, L.J. 1987. Immunoserology of staphylococcal disease. In Abramson, C., editor. Cumitech 22, American Society for Microbiology, Washington, D.C.
2. Archer, G.L. 1984. *Staphylococcus epidermidis*: the organism, its diseases, and treatment. In Remington, J.S., and Swartz, M.N., editors. Current clinical topics in infectious diseases 5, McGraw-Hill Book Co., New York.
3. Chambers, H.F. 1988. Methicillin-resistant staphylococci. Clin. Microbiol. Rev. 1:173.
4. Christensen, G.D., Parisi, J.T., Bisno, A.L., et al. 1983. Characterization of clinically significant strains of coagulase negative staphylococci. J. Clin. Microbiol. 18:258.
5. Collopy, B.T., Dalton, M.F., Wright, C., et al. 1984. Comparison of the clinical significance of methicillin-resistant and methicillin-sensitive *Staphylococcus aureus* isolations. Med. J. Aust. 140:211.
6. Coudron, P.E., Markowitz, S.M., Mohanty, L.B., et al. 1987. Isolation of *Stomatococcus mucilaginosus* from drug user with endocarditis. J. Clin. Microbiol. 25:1359.
7. Davenport, D.S., Massanari, R.M., Pfaller, M.A., et al. 1986. Usefulness of a test for slime production as a marker for clinically significant infections with coagulase-negative staphylococci. J. Infect. Dis. 153:332.
8. Falk, D., and Guering, S.J. 1983. Differentiation of *Staphylococcus* and *Micrococcus* spp. with the Taxo A bacitracin disk. J. Clin. Microbiol. 18:719.
9. Faller, A., and Schleifer, K.H. 1981. Modified oxidase and benzidine tests for separation of staphylococci and micrococci. J. Clin. Microbiol. 13:1031.
10. Freney, J., Brun, Y., Bes, M., et al. 1988. *Staphylococcus lugdunensis* sp. nov. and *Staphylococcus schleiferi* sp. nov., two species from human clinical specimens. Int. J. System. Bacteriol. 38:168.
11. Harrington, B.J., and Gaydos, J.M. 1984. Five-hour novobiocin test for differentiation of coagulase negative staphylococci. J. Clin. Microbiol. 19:279.
12. Hebert, G.A., Crowder, C.G., Hancock, G.A., et al. 1988. Characteristics of coagulase-negative staphylococci that help differentiate these species and other members of the family *Micrococcaceae*. J. Clin. Microbiol. 26:1939.
13. Kaplan, M.H., and Tenenbaum, M.J. 1982. *Staphylococcus aureus*: cellular biology and clinical application. Am. J. Med. 72:248.
14. Lairscey, R., and Buck, G.E. 1987. Performance of four slide agglutination methods for identification of *Staphylococcus aureus* when testing methicillin resistant staphylococci. J. Clin. Microbiol. 25:181.
15. Madison, B.M., and Baselski, V.S. 1983. Rapid identification of *Staphylococcus aureus* in blood cultures by thermonuclease testing. J. Clin. Microbiol. 18:722.
16. Menzies, R.E. 1977. Comparison of coagulase, deoxyribonuclease (DNase), and heat-stable nuclease tests for identification of *Staphylococcus aureus*. J. Clin. Pathol. 30:606.
17. Otero, J.R., Amor, E., Martin-Rabadan, P., et al. 1987. A simple broth-disk elution test for screening methicillin-resistant (heteroresistant) staphylococci. Diagn. Microbiol. Infect. Dis. 7:279.
18. Pfaller, M.A., and Herwaldi, L.A. 1988. Laboratory, clinical, and epidemiological aspects of coagulase-negative staphylococci. Clin. Microbiol. Rev. 1:281.
19. Pickett, D.A., and Welch, D.F. 1985. Recognition of *Staphylococcus saprophyticus* in urine cultures by screening colonies for production of phosphatase. J. Clin. Microbiol. 21:310.
20. Relman, D.A., Ruoff, K., and Ferraro, M.J. 1987. *Stomatococcus mucilaginosus* endocarditis in an intravenous drug abuser. J. Infect. Dis. 155:1080.
21. Schleifer, K.H., and Kloos, W.E. 1975. A simple test system for the separation of staphylococci from micrococci. J. Clin. Microbiol. 1:337.
22. Sheagren, J.N. 1984. *Staphylococcus aureus*, the persistent pathogen. N. Engl. J. Med. 309:1368.
23. Talan, D.A., Staatz, D., Staatz, A., et al. 1989. *Staphylococcus intermedius* in canine gingiva and canine-inflicted human wound infections: laboratory characterization of a newly recognized zoonotic pathogen. J. Clin. Microbiol. 27:78.
24. Todd, J.K. 1988. Toxic shock syndrome. Clin. Microbiol. Rev. 1:432.
25. Zarzour, J.Y., and Belle, E.A. 1978. Evaluation of three test procedures for identification of *Staphylococcus aureus* from clinical sources. J. Clin. Microbiol. 7:133.

BIBLIOGRAPHY

Hindler, J.A., and Inderlied, C.B. 1985. Effect of the source of Mueller-Hinton agar and resistance frequency on the detection of methicillin-resistant *Staphylococcus aureus*. J. Clin. Microbiol. 21:205.

Scand. J. Infect. Dis. Suppl. 41, 1983. Entire issue devoted to *S. aureus* organisms and disease.

Selepak, S.T., and Witebsky, F.G. 1984. Beta-lactamase detection in nine staphylococcal species. J. Clin. Microbiol. 20:1200.

25

Streptococci and Related Genera

Members of the genus *Streptococcus* are catalase-negative gram-positive cocci that tend to grow in chains in liquid media. Streptococci form large quantities of lactic acid as the end product of carbohydrate metabolism, and they are facultatively anaerobic. They are not only normal flora of humans, but some species are the etiologic agents of several devastating diseases, including pneumococcal pneumonia, meningitis, sepsis, bacterial endocarditis, streptococcal exudative pharyngitis, cellulitis, wound infection, and visceral abscesses. Acute rheumatic fever and poststreptococcal glomerulonephritis are secondary sequelae of infection caused by *Streptococcus pyogenes* and occasional other species. *Enterococcus* species, also normal animal mucous membrane flora, are the agents of urinary tract and wound infections and are important in bacterial endocarditis, as well as being important secondary pathogens in patients receiving antibiotics.

A number of other related genera have recently been implicated in human disease. *Leuconostoc* sp. has been reported as the etiologic agent of septicemia and meningitis.[13,20,34] *Lactococcus garviae* and *Pediococcus* sp. have been recovered from patients with sepsis. Vancomycin resistance, characteristic of *Leuconostoc* and *Pediococcus* sp., may be important in the pathogenesis of disease associated with these organisms. The single species of *Aerococcus*, *A. viridans*, is included in the family Streptococcaceae. *Aerococcus* is an opportunistic pathogen, probably occurring naturally in the environment. It has been isolated from cases of bacteremia, endocarditis, meningitis, and osteomyelitis. Both *Aerococcus* and *Gemella* species resemble streptococci on gross inspection of colonies, although in Gram stains made from cultures grown in broth they tend to form packets and tetrads and no chains. The genus *Gemella* has not been well characterized; however, the streptococcus species *S. morbillorum* has recently been transferred to the *Gemella* genus, requiring that methods for identification of these organisms be implemented.

The streptococci can be identified in the laboratory by several different processes. The methods most commonly used in clinical microbiology laboratories involve preliminary grouping of isolates based on the hemolysis of colonies growing on blood agar. In the United States, 5% sheep blood agar is commonly used. Originally used primarily for cultures of inflamed throats because it inhibits growth of hemolytic *Haemophilus* species, whose presence would complicate the recognition of hemolytic streptococci, 5% sheep blood agar is now used routinely for initial cultivation of almost all types of clinical specimens. Horse blood, which exhibits similar hemolytic reactions, is commonly used for initial processing in Europe. In discussions about epidemiology and pathogenesis in this chapter, clinically important streptococci are grouped according to hemolytic patterns or species. β-Hemolytic streptococci include *S. pyogenes*, *S. agalactiae*, and a number of other species. α-Hemolytic streptococci include *S. pneumoniae* and, of course, the viridans species. *Enterococcus* sp., now recognized as a separate genus, are primarily α-hemolytic or nonhemolytic (and occasionally β-hemolytic). These organisms differ from the streptococci by their resistance to salt and broader antibiotic resistance.

25.1. Epidemiology and Pathogenic Mechanisms

25.1.a. *Streptococcus pneumoniae.* *S. pneumoniae*, a bile-sensitive α-hemolytic streptococcus, is found as normal nasopharyngeal and oropharyngeal flora in as many as 15% of children and approximately 5% of adults. It is also found in the upper respiratory tract of animals, but not in the inanimate environment. Organisms are presumably passed from person to person via respiratory secretions and aerosols. The organisms are surrounded by an antiphagocytic capsule composed of polysaccharide antigens useful in strain typing; more than 80 types have been described. *S. pneumoniae*, also called the "pneumococcus," is an etiologic agent of the second most common cause of bacterial meningitis, often preceded by pneumonia. Pneumococcal pneumonia is

the most common type of community-acquired bacterial pneumonia; the fatality rate of uncomplicated pneumococcal pneumonia is still relatively high (5% to 7%), even with prompt institution of appropriate therapy. In addition to pneumonia and meningitis, *S. pneumoniae* is an etiologic agent of otitis media, purulent sinusitis, and, occasionally, peritonitis, especially in young patients with nephrotic syndrome.

Pneumococci cause disease in the presence of a predisposing host condition, often a preceding viral respiratory tract infection. Individuals with other compromising conditions of the respiratory tract, such as chronic obstructive pulmonary disease, silicosis, anthracosis, treatment with anesthetic agents, and alcoholism, are at increased risk. The pathogenesis of pneumonia was discussed in Chapter 16. For *S. pneumoniae*, the capsular polysaccharide plays a key role in allowing the establishment of infection. The organisms enter the alveoli via the bronchial tree in the face of impaired host defenses that normally include the cough reflex, ciliary movement, and secretory immunoglobulin. Once within alveoli, they resist phagocytosis by macrophages, multiply, and induce an inflammatory response that impairs lung function. Patients usually experience an abrupt onset of fever following a shaking chill. Sputum is often purulent and may appear rusty-colored.

The best evidence that capsular polysaccharide is the primary virulence factor is that antibody to the capsular antigen is protective. Recovery from pneumococcal pneumonia in a nonimmune individual is accompanied by a rise in capsular antibody titer, whereas presence of circulating antibodies prevents establishment of the disease. This fact has spurred development of a pneumococcal vaccine, containing antigens of 23 serotypes, the most commonly recognized etiologic serotypes in the United States and Europe. Patients with chronic respiratory tract disease, those without spleens, immunosuppressed patients, elderly patients, and others deemed to be at increased risk have all been cited as those for whom vaccine is warranted, although not all will respond optimally to it. *S. pneumoniae* produces other factors that may play a role in virulence, including pneumolysin O, an oxygen-sensitive toxin that is cytolytic for cells, and a neuraminidase, an enzyme that degrades surface structures of host tissue. The cell wall of pneumococci contains C-substance, a teichoic acid that reacts with a certain serum protein (C-reactive protein, CRP), resulting in the activation of some nonspecific host immune responses.

25.1.b. *Streptococcus pyogenes.* Most streptococci that contain cell wall antigens of Lancefield group A (discussed in Section 25.2.a) are known as *S. pyogenes*. Members of this species are almost always β-hemolytic. They are found in the respiratory tract of humans and are always considered to be potential pathogens. A number of persons, particularly children, however, do carry the organism without signs of illness. The numbers of organisms isolated from such asymptomatic carriers are usually low. Because numbers of colony-forming units (CFU) seen on primary culture plates is dependent on many factors, including the presence of competing normal oral flora, the skill with which the specimen was obtained, the way in which the culture medium was inoculated, culture medium incubation conditions, and the culture medium itself, the likely presence or absence of streptococcal infection should not be assessed entirely on the numbers of colonies recovered. Infection is spread by aerosols and respiratory secretions, although food-borne and milk-borne epidemics do occur. Members of this species are among the etiologic agents of pharyngitis, cellulitis, scarlet fever, erysipelas, **pyoderma** (a purulent skin infection), puerperal fever (uncommonly seen today), and other purulent (or suppurative) infections. *S. pyogenes* may also be involved alone or with other bacteria, particularly *Staphylococcus aureus*, in impetigo (a form of pyoderma). Infections that extend from the pharynx into the paranasal sinuses, tonsils, and other parts of the respiratory tract can lead to abscesses, pneumonia, otitis media, and other suppurative processes. With the decline of rheumatic fever in the United States, treatment of streptococcal pharyngitis is often initiated for prevention of these other sequelae.

In terms of human morbidity and mortality worldwide, however, the role of *S. pyogenes* in the subsequent development of acute rheumatic fever and poststreptococcal glomerulonephritis is more important. Both diseases are most prevalent among children. Rheumatic fever and subsequent valvular heart disease are problems of major importance in developing nations throughout the world. In the United States rheumatic fever is uncommon, although an upsurge of cases has been reported in several areas, including Utah, Pennsylvania, and Ohio, beginning in 1985.[3-5,23] Acute rheumatic fever

and poststreptococcal glomerulonephritis are considered to be "nonsuppurative," because the organism itself and a purulent inflammatory response are not present in the affected organs (heart, joints, blood vessels, kidneys). Although the pathogenesis of these diseases has not been entirely clarified, it seems certain that they are autoimmune phenomena. It is believed that cross-reactive antibodies, originally directed against streptococcal cell membranes, specifically bind to myosin in human heart muscle cells; other cross-reactive antibodies bind to components of the glomerular basement membrane, forming immune complexes at the affected site. These antigen-antibody complexes attract host reactive cells and enzymes that ultimately cause the damage. Patients with previous rheumatic heart disease (as a result of rheumatic fever) are at significantly increased risk of developing cardiac malfunction and endocarditis at a later time. Patients who develop streptococcal glomerulonephritis are also at risk of developing later renal failure.

Not all infections with *S. pyogenes* lead to nonsuppurative sequelae. Acute rheumatic fever occurs only after upper respiratory tract infection. The development of this disease is dependent on host factors, such as histocompatibility-linked antigen (HLA; chromosome constituent) type, immunoglobulin secretory status, and immune responsiveness; and organism factors, such as adherence mechanisms and cell wall carbohydrate components. Glomerulonephritis, on the other hand, occurs after pharyngitis or after suppurative skin infection (pyoderma). Acute glomerulonephritis is more commonly associated with a limited number of serotypes. These serotypes are defined by antisera against a protein component of the cell wall, the M protein, which is also mentioned below in connection with virulence.

S. pyogenes produces a number of extracellular products and toxins that probably enhance virulence (see Figure 12.1). Erythrogenic toxin, elaborated by scarlet fever–associated strains, is responsible for the characteristic rash. Group A streptococci also produce DNase, hyaluronidase (also known as spreading factor), which breaks down host cell connective tissue, and streptokinase, an enzyme that dissolves clots. NADase, proteinases, and other enzymes are secreted. Mucoid strains possess a large hyaluronic acid capsule that acts to inhibit phagocytosis. The two hemolysins, streptolysin O, an oxygen-labile enzyme, and streptolysin S, oxygen-stable, can lyse human and other erythrocytes, as well as the cell membranes of polymorphonuclear neutrophils, platelets, and other cells. There are, however, pathogenic strains of *S. pyogenes* that do not produce hemolysins, which makes them extremely difficult to recognize on primary blood agar culture plates. The cell wall lipoteichoic acids serve to effect adherence of the organism to host cell respiratory epithelium, an essential first step in the development of infection (Chapter 16). In association with the hyaluronic acid capsule, cell wall M protein serves to prevent phagocytosis, another essential virulence mechanism. The M protein is the major virulence factor of the bacteria since strains of *S. pyogenes* that lack M protein cannot cause disease.

25.1.c. *Streptococcus agalactiae*. These β-hemolytic streptococci possess Lancefield group B capsular polysaccharide antigens and are normal flora in the genitourinary tract of humans and other mammals. They are the only streptococci in which specific morphological criteria (ability to hydrolyze hippurate; positive CAMP test, Procedure 25.1) are associated with a single Lancefield group. Group B streptococci are an important etiologic agent of bovine mastitis, from which they can be transmitted in milk. They are destroyed by pasteurization. From their carriage site in the human vagina, they can colonize neonates; *S. agalactiae* is currently the most common etiologic agent of neonatal sepsis and meningitis, accounting for over one third of all cases (*Escherichia coli* still accounts for another third).[2] Postpartum fever and sepsis, not surprisingly, are also commonly associated with *S. agalactiae*. This organism has been found to be the etiologic agent in cases of sepsis in nonparturient women and in men, in joint infection, osteomyelitis, urinary tract infection, and wound infection. *S. agalactiae* is associated with endocarditis, pneumonia, and pyelonephritis in immunosuppressed patients.

25.1.d. Other β-hemolytic streptococci. Non–group B β-hemolytic streptococci can be divided into groups based initially on colony size. Small or "minute" colony types (<1 mm diameter) have been placed into the genus *Streptococcus anginosus*, which may include nonhemolytic streptococci of former species "*S. milleri*," *S. constellatus*, *S. intermedius*, and *S. anginosus*.[30-32] At this time confusing and conflicting results generated from taxonomic studies make it impossible to recommend a practical identification scheme for clinical laboratories that

would correlate with the genetic description of this group of streptococci. Additional genera and species will probably be recognized. For convenience, we suggest that the minute-colony-forming β-hemolytic streptococci that possess A, C, G, or F group antigens be called *S. anginosus*, group A, C, G, or F. These organisms have been implicated in the production of abscesses and other purulent infections in internal organs. Production of hyaluronidase, DNase, and other extracellular enzymes may contribute to their pathogenicity.[17,30,31] *S. anginosus* recovered from throats does not possess human immunoglobulin receptors and is not thought to be associated with pharyngitis.[8,21]

Large colony-forming β-hemolytic streptococci of serologic group C (*S. equisimilis*, *S. zooepidemicus*, and *S. equi*) may cause a severe pharyngitis, often followed by bacteremia and metastatic infection.[8,31] One species of group C (*S. zooepidemicus*) has been associated with poststreptococcal glomerulonephritis, acquired after drinking milk from a cow with mastitis.[1] Certain group C strains recovered from throats were found to possess human antibody receptors, thought to be a virulence factor for these organisms.[21] Group C and G streptococci may cause suppurative infection in humans, including postpartum sepsis, erysipelas, pharyngitis, and bacteremia. Endocarditis is rare. β-Hemolytic large-colony-forming group G streptococci isolated from human wound infections are related to group L and group C strains.[10] They are included in the species *S. dysgalactiae* by some authors. Species of groups C and G may additionally colonize the human gastrointestinal tract and vagina. Acute glomerulonephritis in a human due to a group G streptococcus has been reported.[16] Group G animal strains, now called *S. canis*, are pathogens in dogs and cows.[10]

Large colony-forming β-hemolytic strains not containing group antigens are very rarely etiologic agents of human disease. Those possessing group antigens other than A, B, C, and G have been isolated only from animals or environmental sources. They are carried as normal flora of the pharynx, vagina, or skin of wild and domestic animals.

25.1.e. Viridans and nonenterococcal group D streptococci. Species of streptococci that are not β-hemolytic (with rare exceptions), do not possess Lancefield group B or D cell wall antigens, are not *S. pneumoniae* (which are bile-soluble and inhibited by the antipneumococcal agent optochin), and cannot grow in broth containing 6.5% sodium chloride are considered to belong to the general category of "viridans streptococci." Viridans was derived from the Latin word *viridis*, meaning "green." Most species in this group are α-hemolytic and produce a "green" discoloration in blood agar, probably due to the production of hydrogen peroxide. Numerous characteristics of this group of streptococcal species are variable, including cell wall carbohydrates and biochemical and morphological characteristics. Many of the streptococci in the viridans group are able to grow better under anaerobic or microaerophilic conditions than when incubated in air; thus they are also called "microaerophilic" streptococci. Because the taxonomy of this group of streptococci is in a very active state of flux, we recommend that isolates be identified presumptively only when deemed to be important clinically, such as isolates from blood. Coykendall has recently reviewed the current taxonomy of this group of streptococci.[8a]

The viridans streptococci are normal inhabitants of the oral, respiratory, and gastrointestinal mucosa of humans and animals. They are opportunistic pathogens and have generally been thought to be of low virulence. Viridans streptococci are, however, the major etiologic agents of bacterial endocarditis in the United States. Patients who develop streptococcal endocarditis usually possess a previously damaged heart valve (from previous rheumatic fever or other cause). Gingival disease or dental manipulations, including dental prophylaxis, are often predisposing factors in the development of endocarditis.

Viridans streptococci are able to adhere to epithelial and endothelial cells, and adherence is probably a key factor in their ability to cause disease. *Streptococcus mutans* has been definitively established as a major etiologic agent of dental caries in addition to being a cause of endocarditis. Extracellular sugars, called dextrans, serve as attachment mediators for tooth surfaces as well as heart valves. The viridans streptococci are also associated (often in combination with anaerobic or other bacterial species) with brain abscess, perioral abscess, aspiration pneumonia, liver abscess, and other suppurative infections. Some species of viridans streptococci produce extracellular enzymes and toxins similar to those produced by β-hemolytic streptococci. The role of these products in virulence is not known. In all series, *S. sanguis* I, *S. sanguis* II, and *S. mutans* are the most common etiologic agents of endocarditis. Since the organisms are normal oral flora, isolation of viridans streptococci from a single blood culture may not be indicative of an ongoing infectious process, although it usually is. Cultivation of the same organism from more than one blood culture is highly suggestive of endocarditis, abscess, or other serious infection.

Two species of streptococci possess group D cell wall teichoic acid antigens and are unable to grow in media with a high salt concentration. Although *S. equinus* is rarely, if ever, encountered, *S. bovis* may be responsible for as many as one third of all cases of viridans streptococcal endocarditis. The presence of *S. bovis* bacteremia, associated with endocarditis or not, is almost always indicative of a loss of integrity of the gastrointestinal mucosa. A strong correlation exists between isolation of *S. bovis* from blood and colon cancer. Since detection of this organism may be the first evidence of such a malignancy, this may be an impelling reason for identification of streptococci (at least those isolated from blood) to species.[34a]

25.1.f. Nutritionally variant streptococci. A group of streptococci, first described in the early 1960s, has been found to be significant etiologic agents of endocarditis. These organisms, called "nutritionally deficient," "pyridoxal-dependent," "satelliting streptococci," or "thiol-requiring," are presumably normal flora. At New York Hospital, 5% to 6% of all cases of endocarditis were caused by such streptococci.[29] Nutritionally variant streptococci require vitamin B_6, or pyridoxal, for growth. Consequently, standard 5% sheep blood agar plates do not support growth of these organisms. Commercial lots of chocolate agar vary with respect to their ability to support growth.[27] Subcultures from blood culture broth media (which usually support growth because the human erythrocytes provide the necessary growth factor) must be made to plates known to support growth of such organisms. It was shown that addition of pyridoxal to all blood agar plates would inhibit growth of other commonly encountered bacteria.[28] Alternatively, subcultures can be made to a blood agar plate cross-streaked with a *S. aureus* strain (Figure 25.1). *S. aureus* provides the necessary growth factor that allows development of satelliting colonies of the streptococci in a zone surrounding the staphylococcus. It is for this reason that the nutritionally variant streptococci have also been called the satelliting streptococci. When pyridoxal is used to supplement biochemical media, these strains can be identified as species of viridans streptococci.

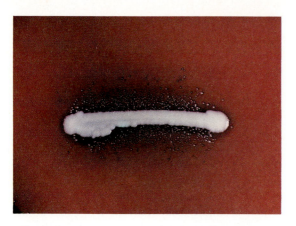

Figure 25.1
Nutritionally variant streptococci growing as satelliting colonies surrounding growth of *S. aureus*.

25.1.g. Enterococci. Enterococci possess group D teichoic acid antigen, are able to grow in 6.5% sodium chloride and in 40% bile, and exhibit resistance to some β-lactam agents, such as penicillin G. They are part of the normal fecal flora of all warm-blooded animals, including humans.[11] *Enterococcus faecalis* and *E. faecium*, the most common human isolates among the enterococci, are encountered as etiologic agents of urinary tract infections, wound infections, and intraabdominal abscesses. They must possess some virulence factors, but these have not been characterized. Superinfection with enterococci, including bacteremia, is a relatively common occurrence in patients being treated with a third generation cephalosporin, as they are resistant to these agents as well as to penicillin. Other enterococci, *E. durans*, *E. gallinarum*, *E. avium*, *E. casseliflavus*, *E. malodoratus*, *E. mundtii*, *E. raffinosus*, *E. pseudoavium*, *E. solitarius*, and *E. hirae*, have been isolated less frequently from clinically significant human infections.[15]

25.1.h. Related genera. *Leuconostoc* species are vancomycin-resistant gram-positive cocci that resemble streptococci morphologically and biochemically, making recognition difficult. They have been isolated from blood and wound infections.[13,20,34] Another vancomycin-resistant genus, *Pediococcus*, is normal fecal flora but is also involved in human infection.[13,34] Recently, streptococci of Lancefield group N have been transferred to the new genus *Lactococcus*. At least one species, *L. garviae*, has been implicated in human disease. The lactococci

are susceptible to vancomycin, nonmotile, catalase-negative, PYR-negative (except for *L. garviae*), α-hemolytic or nonhemolytic, and otherwise resemble viridans streptococci. Catalase-negative *Aerococcus* and *Gemella*, whose colonies may be mistaken for streptococci, yield gram-positive cocci in tetrads and clusters, rather than chains. Since the majority of these groups have been described recently, their virulence mechanisms and their role in human disease are not known. Once microbiologists begin to fully characterize the streptococcus-like organisms isolated from infectious processes, the extent of their involvement will be better understood.

25.2. Laboratory Identification of Streptococci

Streptococci grow on standard laboratory media containing blood or blood products, such as trypticase soy agar with 5% sheep blood and chocolate agar, as well as the selective agars Columbia agar with colistin and nalidixic acid (CNA) and phenylethyl alcohol agar (PEA). Blood culture media support the growth of streptococci. For those streptococci that require pyridoxal, subculture may require a staphylococcal cross-streak or media containing the necessary growth factors, as discussed in Section 25.1.f. The identification scheme recommended here is not likely to produce definitive species identification of all strains, but it should suffice for the majority of clinically important strains encountered in a clinical laboratory. When identification of unusual strains, such as those isolated from normally sterile sites or clearly implicated as pathogens, is required, the isolate should be sent to a reference laboratory or identified using published criteria.*

25.2.a. Initial characterization of streptococci and related groups. Because most laboratories incubate all blood agar plates (except the anaerobic plates) in 5% to 10% CO_2, colony morphology of streptococci from that environment will be described. The streptococci are facultative anaerobes and will grow very well anaerobically (often better than they will aerobically). Those organisms that grow better in reduced oxygen tension are sometimes called **microaerophilic** streptococci; they are usually identified as members of the viridans streptococci. Those streptococci that grow as obligate anaerobes, *Peptostreptococcus* species, are covered in Chapters 34 and 37. Visualization of β-hemolytic

---

*References 8a, 13, 15, 32, 34, 34a, and 37.

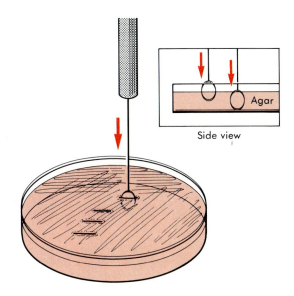

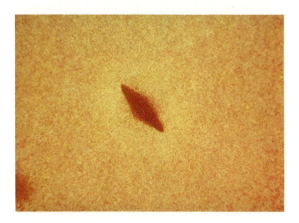

Figure 25.3
α-Hemolysis surrounding the elliptical subsurface colony of an isolate of viridans streptococcus growing in a pour plate of 5% sheep blood agar, as seen by examining the colony microscopically under low power (100× magnification). Notice that the red blood cells are intact.

Figure 25.2
Stabbing the inoculating loop vertically into the agar after streaking the blood agar plate allows subsurface colonies to display hemolysis due to streptolysin O.

streptococcal colonies from throat specimens, as well as recovery of group A β-hemolytic streptococci, is enhanced by anaerobic incubation. Detection of group A β-hemolytic streptococci in pharyngeal cultures will be discussed separately.

Identification of streptococci should be initiated by careful examination of colony morphology and hemolytic pattern on 5% sheep blood agar. Hemolysis is enhanced by stabbing the inoculating loop into the agar several times (Figure 25.2). Colonies can then grow throughout the depth of the agar, producing subsurface oxygen-sensitive hemolysins (streptolysin O) if they are able to. Streptococci grow on the agar surface as translucent to milky, circular, small (≤1 mm diameter) colonies with a shiny surface. Colony variants are common, however, including rough, umbonate, dull matte, and spreading morphologies. *Aerococcus* colonies are gray-white, convex, and circular. All streptococci, leuconostocs, and lactococci are catalase-negative. Occasional enterococci and *Aerococcus* species produce a pseudocatalase that yields a very weak positive test. Pediococci may be catalase-positive. *S. pneumoniae*, *Aerococcus viridans*, and many species of viridans streptococci, enterococci, and other group D streptococci will show a zone of α-hemolysis surrounding the colony. α-Hemolysis, macroscopically ap-

pearing as a green discoloration of the medium surrounding the colony, is characterized by the presence of intact erythrocytes, visible by observing the medium surrounding the colony through the low power of a microscope (Figure 25.3). An unusual type of α-hemolysis produced by some viridans streptococci is called "wide-zone α-hemolysis." Colonies are surrounded by a zone of incomplete hemolysis of erythrocytes (Figure 25.4), but a wider zone further out consists of completely lysed red cells, as seen in true β-hemolysis (Figure 25.5). Wide-zone α-hemolysis macroscopically resembles β-hemolysis. If the presence of hemolysis is uncertain, it may be detected by moving the colony aside with a loop and examining the area of medium directly beneath the original colony site. Plates are always examined by holding them in front of a light source (Figure 25.6).

Microscopically, streptococci are gram-positive, round or oval-shaped, occasionally forming elongated forms that resemble pleomorphic corynebacteria or lactobacilli. Streptococci may occasionally appear gram-negative if cultures are old or if there has been treatment with antibiotics. Differentiation between streptococci and lactobacilli may be difficult, especially if the lactobacilli are catalase-negative strains. A Gram stain of growth just outside the zone of inhibition surrounding a 10-U penicillin disk placed on a blood agar plate inoculated with a lawn of the organism will reveal long bacilli if the organism

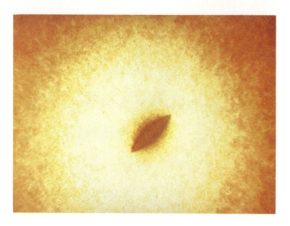

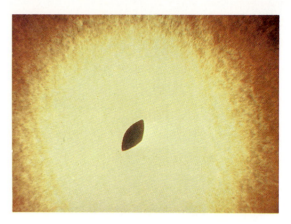

Figure 25.4

Wide zone α-hemolysis surrounding the elliptical subsurface colony of a streptococcus growing in a pour plate of 5% sheep blood agar, as seen by observing the colony microscopically under low power (100× magnification). Notice that there is a narrow zone of intact red blood cells, seen as a red haze, immediately surrounding the colony and a wider zone containing no intact red cells extending further out from the colony.

Figure 25.5

β-Hemolysis surrounding the elliptical subsurface colony of a β-hemolytic streptococcus growing in a pour plate of 5% sheep blood agar, as seen by observing the colony microscopically under low power (100× magnification). Notice that there are no intact red blood cells in the vicinity of the colony.

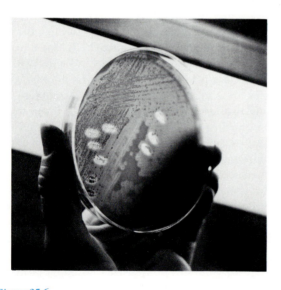

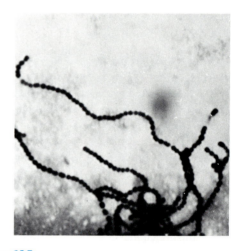

Figure 25.7

Chains of streptococci seen in Gram stain prepared from broth culture.

Figure 25.6

Observing hemolysis on sheep blood agar plates by viewing the plates in front of a light source.

is a *Lactobacillus* and spherical forms if it is a *Streptococcus*. Additionally, growth in thioglycollate broth usually induces streptococci to form long chains of cocci (Figure 25.7). Growth in broth should always be used for determination of cellular morphology. *Aerococcus*, *Gemella*, and *Pediococcus* species will grow in thioglycollate as large, spherical cocci arranged in tetrads and pairs, and individual cells rather than chains. Lactobacilli will grow as rods and filaments.

A screening test for vancomycin susceptibility should be performed to differentiate nonstreptococcal isolates. The organism is suspended in broth to the turbidity of McFarland 0.5 and spread onto the surface of Mueller-Hinton-blood agar as for the Bauer-Kirby disk diffusion test. A 30-μg vancomycin disk is placed on the agar surface and the plate is incubated overnight in 5% CO_2. All streptococci, aerococci, gemellas, lactococci, and most entero-cocci (a few isolates resistant to vancomycin have been described recently) are susceptible to vanco-mycin; whereas pediococci, leuconostocs, and most lactobacilli are typically resistant.

Serologic typing of cell wall components has clas-sically been used to separate streptococci into spe-cies. Recent DNA homology studies have shown that this is not possible. However, it is still a very useful practice to aid in the identification of clinical isolates and thus in the management of infected patients. For performance of the serologic test developed by Rebecca Lancefield, the "Lancefield precipitin test," cell wall antigens must be extracted, either physi-cally by heating or by chemical or enzymatic ex-traction of a cell suspension grown overnight in Todd-Hewitt broth. A small amount of antiserum (previously produced by hyperimmunizing rabbits with fixed cells of the appropriate serogroup) is drawn up into a microcapillary tube (1.5 mm di-ameter) and the bacterial cell extract is drawn into the tube below the antiserum. After approximately 10 minutes, a positive reaction is visible as a diffuse white precipitate that forms at the juncture of the two materials. The precipitin line may vanish quickly, so tubes should be inspected often. A sep-arate tube is needed for each serogroup being tested. The extraction procedures and performance of the precipitin test are described in the American Society for Microbiology *Manual of Clinical Microbiology*, fourth edition (see Bibliography). Modifications of the precipitin test include counterimmunoelectro phoresis or gel diffusion detection of antigen-anti-body reactions. For unusual group antigens and for group D antigens, the Lancefield test in some form is still used in reference laboratories.

Fluorescent antibody stains for groups A and B streptococci have also been used for identification (Figure 25.8), although they are infrequently used in routine clinical laboratories today, because of the availability of commercially produced reagents for rapid serogrouping of β-hemolytic streptococci.

25.2.b. Identification of β-hemolytic streptococci (Figure 25.9). β-Hemolysis is characterized by com-plete lysis of erythrocytes, as determined by ex-amining the medium microscopically (Figure 25.5). Large-size (>0.5 mm diameter) β-hemolytic colo-nies may rarely be *E. faecalis*, *E. durans*, or *S. mu-tans*, but they are almost always groupable with Lancefield antisera to cell wall carbohydrates of groups A, B, C, or G. Colonies of *S. pyogenes* are

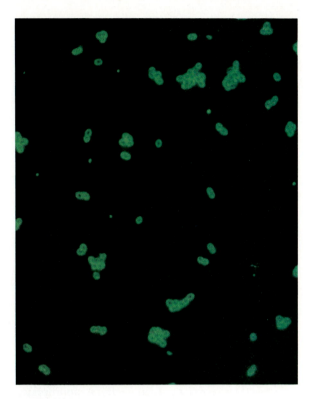

Figure 25.8
Group A streptococci stained with fluorescein-conjugated anti-group A antibody, examined with ultraviolet light under oil immersion (1000× magnification). Notice that the organisms stain as rings, with dark centers.

transparent to translucent, convex, entire, circular, shiny, and surrounded by a rather wide zone of β-hemolysis. They are Lancefield group A and PYR-positive. The PYR test, hydrolysis of L-pyrrolidonyl-β-naphthylamide, described in Chapter 9, is positive for *S. pyogenes*, all *Enterococcus* species, *L. garviae*, nutritionally variant streptococci, and *Gemella* spe-cies. Modifications of the PYR test, including a broth test that can be read within 4 hours of incubation, and even more rapid chromogenic substrates and fluorescent systems are commercially available.

Group B streptococci, *S. agalactiae*, yield larger, more translucent to opaque, whitish gray, soft, smooth colonies surrounded by a much smaller zone of β-hemolysis. The colonies of *S. agalactiae* resem-ble those of *Listeria* species, which are catalase-pos-itive. *S. agalactiae* strains are positive in the CAMP test (Procedure 25.1) and able to hydrolyze hippur-ate (Chapter 9). Named for the originators, Christie, Atkins, and Munch-Peterson,[7] the CAMP test re-

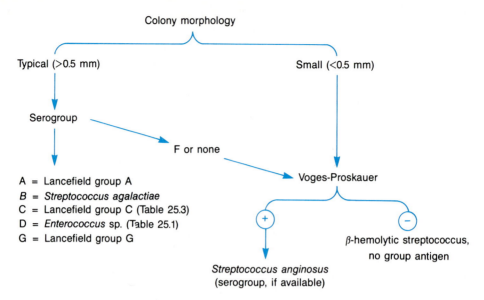

Figure 25.9
Presumptive identification of β-hemolytic streptococci.

quires overnight incubation, but it is much less expensive than serologic typing. If an appropriate staphylococcus is unavailable, a commercial CAMP factor-impregnated filter paper disk can be used.

The minute-colony β-hemolytic streptococci are all likely to be *S. anginosus*.[12] Those possessing group A, C, or G can be verified with a positive Voges-Proskauer test. All Lancefield group F β-hemolytic streptococci are *S. anginosus*. Nongroupable minute colony-forming β-hemolytic streptococci must be identified biochemically.[30] β-Hemolytic large-colony type streptococci other than groups A, B, and F may be identified by serogroup and further characterized biochemically. Group C streptococci can be differentiated into species and subspecies by carbohydrate fermentation (Table 25.1). The use of highly sensitive polyclonal antibody reagents and monoclonal antibodies, conjugated to carrier particles, latex beads, or staphylococci, has greatly facilitated the ability of microbiologists to rapidly and specifically type β-hemolytic streptococcal colonies by latex agglutination or coagglutination methods. Numerous systems are available commercially that yield satisfactory serogroup identifications as compared with the Lancefield precipitin standard. Some of these methods require an extraction step, which may take an hour or longer, whereas others do not. Identification can usually be accomplished with one or two isolated colonies,

Table 25.1
Identification of Group C Streptococci

| SPECIES | ACID FROM | |
	TREHALOSE	SORBITOL
equi	−	−
equi supsp. *zooepidemicus*	−	+
dysgalactiae subsp. *equisimilis*	+	−

shortening the laboratory turnaround time by at least 24 hours. As with all commercial systems, manufacturers' instructions should be followed exactly, and substitutions of reagents or specified equipment are not acceptable.

25.2.c. Identification of α-hemolytic and nonhemolytic streptococci and related genera. Vancomycin-susceptible, α-hemolytic streptococci are preliminarily identified as shown in Figure 25.11. The colony morphology of *S. pneumoniae* is usually distinctive, with very mucoid and glistening colonies that tend to dip down in the center and resemble a doughnut after increased incubation time because of the action of autolytic enzymes (Figure 25.12). Suspicious colonies must be tested for either bile solubility (Chapter 9) or susceptibility to optochin (Procedure 25.2).

PROCEDURE 25.1

CAMP Test

Principle

Group B streptococci produce a proteinlike compound called the "CAMP factor" that is able to act synergistically with the beta toxin produced by some strains of *S. aureus* to produce even more potent hemolysis.

Method

1. Inoculate a streak of beta toxin-producing *S. aureus* down the center of a 5% sheep blood agar plate.
2. Inoculate straight lines of the isolates to be tested at right angles to the staphylococcal streak, stopping just before the staphylococcal line is reached. Several different isolates can be tested on one plate.
3. Incubate plates at 35° to 37° C overnight in air or for 6 h in 5% to 10% CO_2. Air incubation will increase the specificity of the test, since

Modified from Washington. 1985. In Washington, J.A. II, editor. Laboratory procedures in clinical microbiology, ed. 2. Springer-Verlag, New York.

fewer non–group B streptococci will be positive in an air atmosphere.

4. Observe for an arrowhead-shaped zone of enhanced hemolysis at the juncture between positive streptococci and the staphylococcus (Figure 25.10). Approximately 95% of group B streptococci, as well as rare strains of other groups, are CAMP-positive.

Quality control

Inoculate *S. agalactiae* ATCC 27956 and *S. pyogenes* ATCC 19615 as described above.

Expected results

The *S. agalactiae* should display enhanced hemolysis in an arrowhead pattern (Figure 25.10) and the *S. pyogenes* should not.

Performance schedule

Test both quality control strains each time a CAMP test is performed.

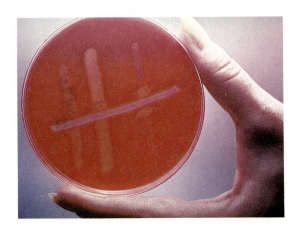

Figure 25.10
The CAMP test for presumptive identification of group B streptococci. The *S. agalactiae* (group B streptococcus) streaked down the right side of the plate exhibits the enhanced zone of hemolysis in an "arrow" shape near the *S. aureus* streak. The β-hemolytic streptococcal isolates streaked down the left and center of the test plate are not group B.

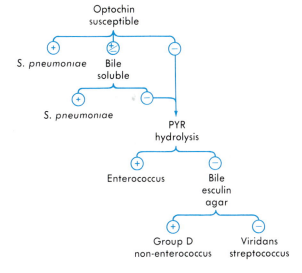

Figure 25.11
Flow chart for preliminary identification of α-hemolytic streptococci.

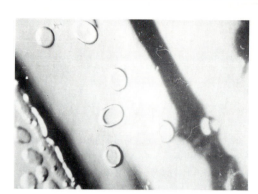

Figure 25.12
Colony morphology of pneumococci after 24 hours incubation
($20\times$).

Once it has been determined that an α-hemolytic streptococcus is not *S. pneumoniae*, it is treated as an enterococcus or viridans streptococcus. Vancomycin-susceptible, nonhemolytic (sometimes called "gamma" hemolytic) colonies are usually enterococci or "viridans" streptococci. α-Hemolytic and nonhemolytic colonies are screened as *Enterococcus* species by the PYR test. All enterococci are PYR-positive and clinically important strains are further characterized biochemically (Table 25.2). Additionally, all enterococci can grow in the presence of 6.5% NaCl in trypticase soy broth, a characteristic shared by rare strains of viridans streptococci. Nonenterococcal α-hemolytic and nonhemolytic streptococci are serogrouped. Group D are *S. bovis* or *S.*

PROCEDURE 25.2

Optochin Susceptibility Test

Principle

S. pneumoniae is susceptible to the antibacterial agent ethylhydrocupreine hydrochloride, (optochin), which is impregnated in a filter paper disk. Performance of the test is similar to that of the disk diffusion susceptibility test.

Method

1. Streak one quadrant or one half of a 5% sheep blood agar plate with an inoculum from a pure isolate of the organism to be tested.
2. Place an optochin disk (Taxo P, BBL Microbiology Systems, or Bacto Optochin disk, Difco Laboratories) in the center of the inoculum.
3. Incubate overnight at 35° C in 5% to 10% CO_2 or a candle jar. Observe for zones of inhibition surrounding the disk. Zones ≥14 mm surrounding a 6-mm diameter disk and zones ≥16 mm surrounding a 10-mm diameter disk are considered positive, presumptive identification of *S. pneumoniae*. Zone sizes between 6 and 14 mm (6-mm disk) and 10 and 16 mm (10-mm disk) are equivocal, and those isolates should be tested for bile solubility.

Quality control

Test *S. pneumoniae* ATCC 27336 and a viridans streptococcus (laboratory strain) as described above.

Expected results

The pneumococcus should yield a positive test result and the viridans streptococcal species should grow right up to and under the optochin disk.

Performance schedule

Test each new batch of optochin disks and monthly thereafter.

Modified from Facklam, R.R., and Carey, R.B. 1985. Streptococci and aerococci. In Lennette, E.H., Balows, A., Hausler, W.J. Jr., and Shadomy, H.J., editors. Manual of clinical microbiology, ed. 4. American Society for Microbiology, Washington, D.C.

Table 25.2
Differentiation Among *Enterococcus* Species

SPECIES	YELLOW PIGMENT	MOTILITY	ACID PRODUCED FROM							ARGININE DIHYDROLASE
			MAN-NITOL	SOR-BITOL	SORBOSE	ARAB-INOSE	RAFFI-NOSE	SUCROSE	LACTOSE	
faecalis*	−	−	+	+	−	−	NA†	NA	+	+
avium	−	−	+	+	+	+	−	NA	NA	−
faecium	−	−	+	+/−	−	+	NA	NA	+	+
raffinosus	−	+	+	+	+	+	+	NA	NA	−
gallinarum	−	−	+	+/−	−	+	NA	NA	+	+
hirae	−	+	−	−	−	NA	+/−	+/−	NA	+
casseliflavus	+	+	+	+/−	−	+	NA	NA	+	+
durans	−	−	−	−	−	NA	−	−	NA	+
solitarius	−	−	+	+/−	−	−	NA	NA	−	+
mundtii	+	−	+	+/−	−	+	NA	NA	+	+
malodoratus	−	−	+	+	+	−	+	NA	NA	−
pseudoavium	−	−	+	+	+	−	−	NA	NA	−

*An asaccharolytic variant of *E. faecalis* has been described.

†NA = Not applicable; + = 90% strains positive; − = 90% strains negative; +/− = variable, more often positive; −/+ = variable, more often negative.

Modified from Facklam, R.R., and Collins, M.D. 1989. Identification of *Enterococcus* species isolated from human infections by a conventional test scheme. J. Clin. Microbiol. 27:731.

PROCEDURE 25.3

Rapid Tests for Presumptive Identification of S. anginosus

Principle

S. anginosus, a cause of purulent infections in humans, can be nonhemolytic, β-hemolytic (minute colony morphology), rarely α-hemolytic, and possess Lancefield antigens A, C, F, or G. Differentiation from other streptococci is based on biochemical reactions.

Method

A. Voges-Proskauer (VP) test
   1. Place 0.2 ml MR-VP broth (available commercially) into a small (10 × 75 mm) tube and inoculate with a heavy suspension of the organism to be tested.
   2. Incubate for 5 h at 35° C.
   3. Add one drop each of 0.5% aqueous creatine (Sigma and other suppliers), 5% α-naphthol in absolute ethanol (Sigma; VP reagent A as described in Chapter 27), and 40% aqueous potassium hydroxide (Sigma; VP reagent B as described in Chapter 27).
   4. Shake or vortex thoroughly and observe for 15 min for development of a pink color.
B. Arginine hydrolysis test
   1. Place 0.2 ml Moeller decarboxylase broth base and Moeller base with arginine (available commercially) into small (10 × 75 mm) tubes and inoculate each with a heavy suspension of the organism to be tested.
   2. Overlay each tube with mineral oil and incubate for 5 h at 35° C.
   3. Observe for color change. Purple indicates hydrolysis of arginine. Organisms that do not hydrolyze arginine will still be able to ferment glucose in the medium, creating

acid by-products and a yellow color change in the pH indicator.
C. Sorbitol fermentation test
   1. Place 0.2 ml sorbitol-containing phenol red carbohydrate broth (available commercially) into small (10 × 75 mm) tubes and inoculate each with a heavy suspension of the organism to be tested.
   2. Overlay each tube with mineral oil and incubate for 5 h at 35° C.
   3. Observe for color change. Yellow or orange indicates sorbitol fermentation; red or orange colors are indicative of negative results.

Quality control

Inoculate *S. anginosus* ATCC 12393, *S. mitis* ATCC 6249, and *E. faecalis* ATCC 19433 and test as described above.

Expected results

S. anginosus will be positive for acetoin production (VP-positive, pink or red), able to hydrolyze arginine (yellow in base broth and purple in arginine broth), and negative for sorbitol fermentation (red or orange). *S. mitis* should yield a negative VP reaction, negative arginine hydrolysis (yellow in both Moeller tubes), and negative sorbitol fermentation. *E. faecalis* should yield a positive VP test, positive arginine hydrolysis, and positive sorbitol (yellow).

Performance schedule

Test all quality control strains each time new reagents are prepared.

Modified from Ruoff and Ferraro.[33]

Table 25.3

Presumptive Differentiation Among Viridans Streptococci

| SPECIES | VOGES-PROSKAUER | ARGININE DIHYDROLASE | HIPPURATE HYDROLYSIS | ACID FROM | | | |
				MANNITOL	INULIN	DEXTRAN	LEVAN
bovis I	+	−	−	+	+ / −	−	+
bovis II	+	−	−	−	−	−	−
intermedius-milleri group	+	+	−	−	−	−	−
mitis-oralis-sanguis II group	−	− / +	−	−	−	− / +	−
mutans	+	−	−	+	+ / −	+	−
sanguis I	−	+ / −	−	−	+	+	−
uberis	−	− / +	+ / −	+	+ / −	−	−
salivarius	+	−	−	−	+	−	+

+ = 90% strains positive; − = 90% strains negative; + / − = variable, more often positive; − / + variable, more often negative.
* Data from R. R. Facklam (personal communication).

equinus.[32] *S. equinus* is rarely isolated from humans. Because of the associations of *S. bovis* with gastrointestinal malignancy, blood culture isolates of veridans streptococci should be identified at least to rule out *S. bovis.*[34a]

The ability to hydrolyze esculin in the presence of bile is a positive characteristic among all group D streptococci and enterococci, although 5% to 10% of the viridans group may also hydrolyze esculin in the presence of bile. This test, "bile esculin," is performed by inoculating a slant or plate of bile esculin agar (available commercially), incubating in air for as long as 4 days, and observing for a blackening of the agar, indicating the presence of the end product of esculin hydrolysis combined with iron in the medium.

Some authors suggest presumptive identification of *S. anginosus* based on acetoin production (V-P test), arginine hydrolysis, and sorbitol fermentation (Procedure 25.3).[33] Negative hippurate hydrolysis, production of alkaline phosphatase, and ability to ferment trehalose are also characteristic for *S. anginosus.* Other nonenterococcal α-hemolytic and nonhemolytic streptococci (viridans group) can be identified by the tests listed in Table 25.3. It is critical that biochemical reagents be prepared according to methods described in Procedure 25.4. Only bromcresol purple broths, prepared as in Procedure 25.4, should be used for carbohydrate utilization tests. Esculin hydrolysis is performed on slants of esculin medium without bile, which are available commercially (dry powder is also available commercially).

The arginine hydrolysis test is described in Procedure 25.3. Commercial biochemical systems and rapid kits are available.

25.3. Rapid Methods and Commercial Systems for Identification of Streptococci

β-Hemolytic streptococci have classically been identified based on their serologic group, rather than biochemically. Numerous commercial systems utilizing either latex agglutination or coagglutination are available (Pharmacia Diagnostics, Wellcome Diagnostics, Scott Laboraties, Meridian Diagnostics, API Analytab Products, Diagnostics Products Corp., BBL Microbiology Systems, Difco Laboraties, and others). As long as Voges-Proskauer negative strains are tested, reliable results should be achieved with all commercial systems. The PYR test, which is faster and less expensive than serologic typing, should be used to separate *S. pyogenes.* Group B can be identified economically and quickly by a rapid CAMP test. CAMP factor has been impregnated into filter paper disks (Pasco Laboratories; Remel) that yield accurate identification of *S. agalactiae* from colonies on a primary blood agar plate within 30 minutes.[26]

Identification of *S. pneumoniae* can be made rapidly with the Quellung test. Addition of specific capsular antibody to a wet preparation of sample containing the organism, either from an isolated colony or in the actual clinical material (sputum or cerebrospinal fluid), results in an antigen-antibody response, visible as apparent capsular swelling (Figure

PROCEDURE 25.4

Preparation and Use of Media for Identification of Viridans Streptococci

A. Carbohydrate fermentation media
1. Prepare carbohydrate utilization broths as follows:

Brain heart infusion broth	900 ml
10% carbohydrate in H_2O	100 ml
Bromcresol purple (1.6% in 95% ethanol)	1 ml

   Carbohydrates to be used include inulin, mannitol, lactose, trehalose, raffinose, and sorbitol. Dispense 3 ml each into 12 × 75 mm glass screw cap tubes and autoclave at 121° C for 10 min. Unlike other carbohydrate broths, these carbohydrate media are autoclaved containing the carbohydrates. Certain carbohydrates, such as inulin and starch, will not completely dissolve in the water. Gentle heating may help but will not entirely clear the solutions. Do not boil them to try to clear them, but merely agitate them thoroughly immediately before adding to the brain heart infusion broth.

2. Inoculate broths with pure isolates and incubate in air for up to 4 days. Positive results (acid production) are visualized by a change in the indicator to yellow.

B. Production of extracellular polysaccharide (glucan)
1. Prepare 5% sucrose broth by mixing together two separate solutions, autoclaved before mixing, as follows:

Thioglycollate broth base (Difco)	28.5 g
K_2HPO_4	10 g
Sodium acetate	12 g
Distilled water	500 ml

Mix together in a 1000 ml flask:

Sucrose	50 g
Distilled water	500 ml

Prepare each solution in a separate 1000 ml flask. Autoclave the two solutions at 121° C for 15 min. Cool both to 55° C and aseptically mix them by pouring the contents of one flask into the other. Dispense aseptically in 5 ml amounts into 16 × 125 mm sterile glass test tubes with screw caps. Store refrigerated.

2. Inoculate a pure culture of the organism; incubate in air at 35° C for up to 1 week, and observe for gelation of the medium. Glucan production is indicated by formation of complete or partial gel in the broth (observed by gently tipping the tube back and forth). If the broth is merely thickened, this is not glucan production but may suggest slime produced by *S. bovis*.

C. Colony morphology on sucrose agar
1. Prepare 5% sucrose agar as follows:

Brain-heart infusion agar (Difco)	40 g
Sucrose	50 g
Distilled water	1000 ml

Mix together, autoclave for 15 min at 121° C, cool to 55° C, and pour into 90-mm diameter Petri plates, at least 20 ml per plate. Allow to set, and store tightly wrapped in polyethylene bags in the refrigerator. Plates are good for several weeks.

2. Inoculate plates with pure cultures of the organisms to be tested. Incubate in air for a maximum of 4 days. Examine for colony morphology. *S. sanguis* and *S. mutans*, both glucan producers, form very dry, adherent, refractile colonies that are difficult to move with a loop. Levan producers, such as *S. salivarius*, yield opaque, very gummy (gumdrop-like), but nonadherent colonies. Growth can be scraped up and lifted (in a glob) from the agar surface. Organisms that produce no extracellular polysaccharides, such as *S. uberis*, *S. mitis*, and *S. (Gemella) morbillorum*, produce mucoid, nonadherent colonies.

Modified from Rubin. 1984. Lab. Med. 15:171, using data from original work by Facklam.[33]

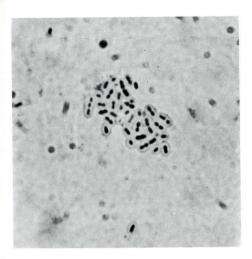

llung reaction with S. *pneumoniae*, showing apparent
ular swelling.

13). The capsules become more visible and re-
ctile because of antibody attachment. Omniserum
ailable from Statens Serum Institute or DAN-
um Inc.) will react with the most common se-
ypes of pneumococci. Difco produces a less in-
sive serum reagent. Latex reagents are available
pneumococci, as described for detection of pneu-
coccal meningitis (Wellcome Diagnostics, Phar-
cia Diagnostics, BBL Microbiology Systems, and
ers). A coagglutination reagent (Phadebact by
armacia Diagnostics) and latex agglutination re-
nt (Pneumoslide, BBL Microbiology Systems)
 also available for rapid identification from cul-
e.

Several systems have been developed for bio-
mical or enzymatic identification of viridans
ptococci and enterococci (American MicroScan,
alytab Products, Inc., BBL Microbiology Sys-
s, Carr-Scarborough, Innovative Diagnostics,
 Vitek Systems). These were reviewed by Wau-
uskas.[36] The Rapid Strep system (Analytab Prod-
s, Inc.) was used reliably by Coykendall and
ers[9] for identification of *S. anginosus* and by Ruoff
 others[34a] for identification of *S. bovis* and *S.
ivarius*, You and Facklam[37] reported favorably on
ults using RapID STR (Innovative Diagnostics).
wever, it is apparent that with the recent changes
taxonomy of *Enterococcus* and viridans strepto-
ci, all of these systems will need additional de-
opment and evaluation.

25.4. Screening Methods for Specific Streptococcal Species

25.4.a. **Detection of *S. pyogenes* in throat swab
specimens.** Detection of *S. pyogenes* in throat cultures is important for clinicians. When specimens
are positive, therapy can be initiated to prevent sequelae and the spread of infection to others. In addition, prompt initiation of therapy can significantly
shorten the duration of symptoms of pharyngitis.
Since pharyngitis caused by streptococci cannot always be distinguished from that due to viruses (the
most common etiologic agents) on clinical grounds,
microbiological procedures are necessary. A large
number of commercial kits for rapid detection of
group A streptococcal antigen, utilizing latex agglutination, coagglutination, or enzyme-linked immunosorbent assay (ELISA) technologies, are currently
available. These reagents have been reported to be
very specific.[14] Sensitivity, however, is dependent
on a number of variables, and reports have ranged
from approximately 60% sensitivity to greater than
95%. Membrane-bound ELISA test systems are
probably the most sensitive currently. Whether
some false-positive results might be due to detection
of group A–carrying *S. anginosus* strains has not
been explored. Strict adherence to manufacturers'
recommendations, including close monitoring of incubation temperatures by using a water bath or heat
block, is necessary for proper results. It has been
found that personnel must be carefully trained in the
correct interpretation of these tests.

We recommend that two swabs be collected from
each throat to be tested. If the first swab tests positive by a direct antigen method, the second swab
can be discarded (avoiding the cost of plates for these
specimens). During streptococcal season, as many
as 25% of patients are likely to test positive in a direct
antigen test. For those specimens in which the rapid
antigen test yielded a negative result, a blood agar
or selective streptococcal blood agar plate should be
inoculated with the second swab. Selective streptococcal agar detects the most positive results and
should be used unless organisms other than *S. pyogenes* are being sought. None of the current rapid
antigen detection products is sensitive enough to use
alone, prompting the suggestion by several prominent pediatricians of an algorithm that includes both
rapid tests and cultures, depending on severity of
illness, risk factors for rheumatic fever, and social
factors.[25]

Considerations for the adult patient with pharyngitis are different from those for children. One approach advocates treating certain adult patients based on clinical signs and symptoms alone and, for those patients who require laboratory testing, treat only those with positive rapid test results and perform no cultures.[6] The availability of rapid tests for antigen detection has generated significant controversy; no one philosophy is generally accepted. Streptococcal selective media can be used for presumptive identification of *S. pyogenes* in throat specimens after overnight incubation by placing a bacitracin disk on the initial inoculum. Most streptococci other than *S. pyogenes* are resistant to this antibiotic. The use of selective media is not universally accepted; many clinicians believe that it distorts the true picture of the relative numbers of different bacterial species present in the throat culture. For laboratories wishing to use only one blood agar plate, placing a bacitracin disk contiguous to a trimethoprim-sulfamethoxazole susceptibility disk on the heavily inoculated area of a 5% sheep blood agar plate allows presumptive identification of the majority of group A streptococci after overnight incubation in CO_2 (Figure 25.14). The sulfa combination inhibits most normal flora, allowing growth of groups A and B streptococci, whereas the bacitracin inhibits only group A streptococci. β-Hemolytic colonies in numbers too small to evaluate must be subcultured for further studies.

Other considerations for identification of *S. pyogenes* from throats are collection and transport of the specimen. Unlike most bacteria, streptococci are very resistant to drying. Swabs may be placed in paper, or material may even be transferred to filter paper for transport without significant loss of recovery.

25.4.b. Detection of group B streptococci in vaginal specimens and specimens from infected neonates. For diagnosis of neonatal sepsis and meningitis due to group B streptococci, several commercial antigen detection kits are available that have good sensitivity and specificity. Developed for use on serum, urine, or cerebrospinal fluid, the best results have been achieved with cerebrospinal fluid so far. Latex agglutination procedures appear to be the most sensitive.

Because neonates acquire group B infection during passage through a colonized vagina, much interest has been generated recently in detection of

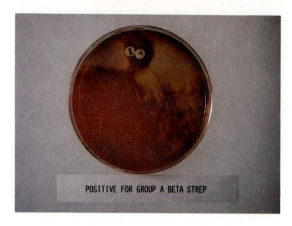

POSITIVE FOR GROUP A BETA STREP

Figure 25.14
Placement of a bacitracin disk and a trimethoprim-sulfamethoxazole disk next to each other in the primary inoculated area of a throat culture plated to 5% sheep blood agar. The sulfa drug inhibits most normal flora and the bacitracin inhibits group A beta streptococci.

S. agalactiae in the vagina before delivery. At least one group has reported successful prevention of neonatal disease by treating (with ampicillin) colonized mothers during labor and delivery.[2]

One screening approach uses enrichment broth for initial growth of group B streptococci and subsequent serogrouping of broth supernatant.[22] Enrichment broths are superior to direct plating for detection of this organism in contaminated specimens.[24] Direct extraction and latex particle agglutination for antigen detection have not been sensitive enough for use alone as a screening test.[35] A solid-phase immunoassay for direct detection from swab specimens has been introduced (Equate, Binax) but not yet evaluated in clinical trials.

25.5. Serologic Diagnosis of Group A Streptococcal Infection

Individuals with disease due to *S. pyogenes* produce antibodies against many of the extracellular products mentioned at the beginning of this chapter. For determining whether a patient has recently suffered streptococcal infection, several tests are usually performed. The diagnostic usefulness of such tests is likely to increase, especially with the decline of rheumatic fever in the United States. They should be used only for diagnosis of nonsuppurative sequelae of streptococcal infection. The most common of these is the **ASO,** determination of presence and titers of

Table 25.4

Products Available for Determining
Antistreptococcal Antibody Titers

TEST	MANUFACTURER
ASO Latex Test	ICL Scientific
ASO Quantum	Sclavo
ASO Test	American Dade
LEAP Strep test	Cooper Biomedical
Rapitex ASO Kit	Behring Diagnostics
SerImmSure	Analytab Products
Strep-phile	BioDiagnostics Systems
Streptonase	Wampole Laboratories
Streptozyme	Wampole Laboratories

antistreptolysin O antibodies. Anti-DNAse B, anti-streptokinase, and antihyaluronidase have all been used to diagnose streptococcal infection retrospectively. Pharyngitis seems to be followed by rises in antibody titers against all three antigens, whereas the ASO titers of patients with pyoderma are frequently not above normal. Anti-DNAse B titers, however, do increase after pyoderma, and thus this test is the most sensitive. Commercial products are available for detection of these antibodies, using latex agglutination or whole red blood cell agglutination methodologies (Table 25.4). LEAP Strep was not sensitive enough for routine screening in one evaluation.[18] Streptozyme, which detects a mixture of antibodies, has consistently shown the highest sensitivity for detection of ASO but yielded low sensitivity for detection of anti–DNase B in at least one study.[19] There are false positive results associated with its use. No commercial system has been shown to accurately detect all streptococcal antibodies likely to be present in serum of patients with prior infection. Serum obtained as long as 2 months after infection will usually demonstrate increased antibodies. As with other serologic tests, an increasing titer over time is most useful for diagnosing previous streptococcal infection.

25.6. Treatment of Streptococcal Infections

Penicillin is still the drug of choice for most streptococcal infections. With the exception of rare *S. pneumoniae* and the enterococci, most streptococci (including nonenterococcal group D organisms) are susceptible to penicillins, which can be given in high dosage. For penicillin-allergic patients, erythromy-cin or vancomycin may be used. Erythromycin resistance has been reported.

The enterococci are uniquely antibiotic-resistant. They are resistant to penicillin, aminoglycosides, cephalosporins, clindamycin, and numerous other agents. Synergism between a penicillin and an aminoglycoside (usually gentamicin) has been repeatedly demonstrated, however, and this combination is the therapy of choice. Vancomycin is also typically effective. High level resistance to streptomycin, indicating in vivo resistance to the combination of penicillin and streptomycin, can be detected by testing the enterococcus isolate against 2000 μg of streptomycin. Growth in the presence of this quantity of antibiotic indicates that synergism with a β-lactam agent will be absent. Continuous infusion ampicillin therapy may be useful but ampicillin resistance has also been encountered.

REFERENCES

1. Barnham, M., Thornton, T.J., and Lange, K. 1983. Nephritis caused by *Streptococcus zooepidemicus* (Lancefield group C). Lancet 1:8331.
2. Boyer, K.M., and Gotoff, S.P. 1986. Prevention of early-onset neonatal group B streptococcal disease with selective intrapartum chemoprophylaxis. N. Engl. J. Med. 314:1665.
3. Centers for Disease Control. 1987. Acute rheumatic fever—Utah. M.M.W.R. 36:108.
4. Centers for Disease Control. 1988. Acute rheumatic fever among army trainees—Fort Leonard Wood, MO, 1987-1988. M.M.W.R. 37:519.
5. Centers for Disease Control. 1988. Acute rheumatic fever at a Navy training center—San Diego, CA. M.M.W.R. 37:101.
6. Centor, R.M., Meier, F.A., and Dalton, H.P. 1986. Throat cultures and rapid tests for diagnosis of group A streptococcal pharyngitis. Ann. Intern. Med. 105:892.
7. Christie, R., Atkins, N.E., and Munch-Peterson, E. 1944. A note on the lytic phenomenon shown by group B streptococci. Aust. J. Exp. Biol. 22:193.
8. Cimolai, N., Elford, R.W., Bryan, L., et al. 1988. Do the beta-hemolytic non-group A streptococci cause pharyngitis? Rev. Infect. Dis. 10:587.
8a. Coykendall, A.L. 1989. Classification and identification of the viridans streptococci. Clin. Microbiol. Rev. 2:315.
9. Coykendall, A.L., Wesbecher, P.M., and Gustafson, K.B. 1987. "*Streptococcus milleri,*" *Streptococcus constellatus,* and *Streptococcus intermedius* are later synonyms of *Streptococcus anginosus.* Int. J. System. Bacteriol. 37:222.
10. Devriese, L.A., Hommez, J., Kilpper-Balz, R., et al. 1986. *Streptococcus canis* sp. nov.: a species of group G streptococci from animals. Int. J. System. Bacteriol. 36:422.
11. Devriese, L.A., Van de Kerckhove, A., Killper-Balz, R., et al. 1987. Characterization and identification of *Enterococcus* species isolated from the intestines of animals. Int. J. System. Bacteriol. 37:257.

12. Ezaki, T., Facklam, R.R., Takeuchi, N., et al. 1986. Genetic relatedness between the type strain of *Streptococcus anginosus* and minute-colony-forming beta-hemolytic streptococci carrying different Lancefield grouping antigens. Int. J. System. Bacteriol. 36:345.

13. Facklam, R., Hollis, D., and Collins, M.D. 1989. Identification of gram-positive coccal and coccobacillary vancomycin-resistant bacteria. J. Clin. Microbiol. 27:724.

14. Facklam, R.R. 1987. Specificity study of kits for detection of group A streptococci directly from throat swabs. J. Clin. Microbiol. 25:504.

15. Facklam, R.R., and Collins, M.D. 1989. Identification of *Enterococcus* species isolated from human infections by a conventional test scheme. J. Clin. Microbiol. 27:731.

16. Gnann, J.W., Jr., Gray, B.M., Griffin, F.M., Jr., et al. 1987. Acute glomerulonephritis following group G streptococcal infection. J. Infect. Dis. 156:411.

17. Gossling, J. 1988. Occurrence and pathogenicity of the *Streptococcus milleri* group. Rev. Infect. Dis. 10:257.

18. Heath-Fracica, L.A., and Estevez, E.G. 1987. Evaluation of a new latex agglutination test for detection of streptococcal antibodies. Diagn. Microbiol. Infect. Dis. 8:25.

19. Hostetler, C.L., Sawyer, K.P., and Nachamkin, I. 1988. Comparison of three rapid methods for detection of antibodies to streptolysin O and DNase B. J. Clin. Microbiol. 26:1406.

20. Isenberg, H.D., Vellozzi, E.M., Shapiro, J., et al. 1988. Clinical laboratory challenges in the recognition of *Leuconostoc* spp. J. Clin. Microbiol. 26:479.

21. Lebrun, L., Guibert, M., Wallet, P., et al. 1986. Human Fc(gamma) receptors for differentiation in throat cultures of group C "*Streptococcus equisimilis*" and group C "*Streptococcus milleri*." J. Clin. Microbiol. 24:705.

22. Lim, D.V., Morales, W.J., and Walsh, A.F. 1987. Lim group B strep broth and coagglutination for rapid identification of group B streptococci in preterm pregnant women. J. Clin. Microbiol. 25:452.

23. Marcon, M.J., Hribar, M.M., Hosier, D.M., et al. 1988. Occurrence of mucoid M-18 *Streptococcus pyogenes* in a central Ohio pediatric population. J. Clin. Microbiol. 26:1539.

24. Persson, K.M.-S., and Forsgren, A. 1987. Evaluation of culture methods for isolation of group B streptococci. Diagn. Microbiol. Infect. Dis. 6:175.

25. Radetsky, M., Solomon, J.A., and Todd, J.K. 1987. Identification of streptococcal pharyngitis in the office laboratory: reassessment of new technology. Pediatr. Infect. Dis. 6:556.

26. Ratner, H.B., Weeks, L.S., and Stratton, C.W. 1986. Evaluation of spot CAMP test for identification of group B streptococci. J. Clin. Microbiol. 24:296.

27. Reimer, L.G., and Reller, L.B. 1981. Growth of nutritionally variant streptococci on common laboratory and 10 commercial blood culture media. J. Clin. Microbiol. 14:329.

28. Reimer, L.G., and Reller, L.B. 1983. Effect of pyridoxal on growth of nutritionally variant streptococci and other bacteria on sheep blood agar. Diagn. Microbiol. Infect. Dis. 1:273.

29. Roberts, R.B, Krieger, A.G., Schiller, N.L., et al. 1979. Viridans streptococcal endocarditis: the role of various species, including pyridoxal-dependent streptococci. Rev. Infect. Dis. 1:955.

30. Ruoff, K.L. 1988. *Streptococcus anginosus* ("*Streptococcus milleri*"): the unrecognized pathogen. Clin. Microbiol. Rev. 1:102.

31. Ruoff, K.L. 1988. *Streptococcus anginosus* ("*Streptococcus milleri*"). Clin. Microbiol. Newsletter 10:65.

32. Ruoff, K.L. 1988. An update on streptococcal taxonomy. Clin. Microbiol. Newsletter 10:1.

33. Ruoff, K.L., and Ferraro, M.J. 1986. Presumptive identification of "*Streptococcus milleri*" in 5 h. J. Clin. Microbiol. 24:495.

34. Ruoff, K.L., Kuritzkes, D.R., Wolfson, J.S., et al. 1988. Vancomycin-resistant gram-positive bacteria isolated from human sources. J. Clin. Microbiol. 26:2064.

34a. Ruoff, K.L., Miller, S.I., Garner, C.V., et al. 1989. Bacteremia with *Streptococcus bovis* and *Streptococcus salivarius*: clinical correlates of isolates. J. Clin. Microbiol. 27:305.

35. Wald, E.R., Dashefsky, B., Green, M., et al. 1987. Rapid detection of group B streptococci directly from vaginal swabs. J. Clin. Microbiol. 25:573.

36. Wausilauskas, B.L. 1987. Viridans streptococci: methods and rationale for species identification. Clin. Microbiol. Newsletter 9:125.

37. You, M.S., and Facklam, R.R. 1986. New test system for identification of *Aerococcus*, *Enterococcus*, and *Streptococcus* species. J. Clin. Microbiol. 24:607.

BIBLIOGRAPHY

Auckenthaler, R., Hermans, P.E., and Washington, J.A. II. 1983. Group G streptococcal bacteremia: clinical study and review of the literature. Rev. Infect. Dis. 5:196.

Bisno, A.L. 1985. Nonsuppurative poststreptococcal sequelae: rheumatic fever and glomerulonephritis. In Mandell, G.L., Douglas, R.G., Jr., and Bennett, J.E., editors. Principles and practice of infectious diseases, ed. 2. John Wiley & Sons, New York.

Carey, R.B. 1984. Handling the nutritionally deficient streptococci in the diagnostic laboratory. Clin. Microbiol. Newsletter 6:131.

Facklam, R.R., and Carey, R.B. 1985. Streptococci and aerococci. p. 154-175. In Lennette, E.H., Balows, A., Hausler, W.J., Jr., and Shadomy, H.J., editors. Manual of clinical microbiology, ed. 4. American Society for Microbiology, Washington, D.C.

Fernandez, C., Daasch, V.N., and Folds, J.D. 1983. Streptococcal serology. Clin. Microbiol. Newsletter 5:73.

Klein, J.O., Dashefsky, B., Norton, C.R., and Mayer, J. 1983. Selection of antimicrobial agents for treatment of neonatal sepsis. Rev. Infect. Dis. 5(Suppl 1):S55.

Krisher, K., and Cunningham, M.W. 1985. Myosin: a link between streptococci and heart. Science 227:413.

Schleifer, K.H., Kraus, J., Dvorak, C., et al. 1985. Transfer of *Streptococcus lactis* and related streptococci to the genus *Lactococcus* gen. nov. System. Appl. Microbiol. 6:183.

Senitzer, D., and Freimer, E.H. 1984. Autoimmune mechanisms in the pathogenesis of rheumatic fever. Rev. Infect. Dis. 6:832.

Washington, J.A. II, editor. 1985. Laboratory procedures in clinical microbiology, ed. 2. Springer-Verlag, New York.

26

Aerobic Gram-Negative Cocci (*Neisseria* and *Branhamella*)

The family Neisseriaceae contains the genera *Acinetobacter*, *Kingella*, *Moraxella*, which includes *Branhamella*, and *Neisseria*; those to be discussed in this chapter include *Neisseria* and *Branhamella*. Other genera within the family are discussed in Chapters 28 and 29. Although the latest edition of *Bergey's Manual of Systematic Bacteriology* has classified *Branhamella* as a subgenus of *Moraxella*, we chose to discuss the *Branhamella* species in this chapter, because their morphology and biochemical identification parameters most closely resemble those of *Neisseria*. These organisms are oxidase-positive gram-negative cocci (with the exception of *N. elongata*). They are normal flora of the respiratory, alimentary, and genitourinary mucosal surfaces of humans. Although any of the normally commensal *Neisseria* species can cause disease in a debilitated host, the organisms most commonly responsible for disease in this group are *N. gonorrhoeae* (gonococcus), the agent of gonorrhea, and *N. meningitidis* (meningococcus), the agent of meningococcal meningitis and septicemia. The pathogenesis of infections due to the *Neisseria* species is discussed in the sections that relate to the diseases they cause, particularly Chapters 15 and 19. Recently, *Branhamella catarrhalis* has been recognized more frequently as a cause of respiratory tract disease.

26.1 Morphology

Organisms appear as kidney bean-shaped diplococci on Gram stain. In smears made from clinical material, groups of *Neisseria* and *Branhamella* are often seen within polymorphonuclear neutrophils, sometimes in large numbers (Figure 26.1). This morphological appearance is known as GNID (gram-

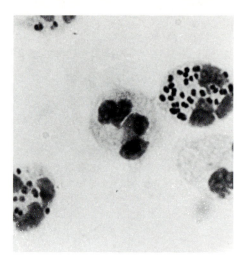

Figure 26.1
Gram-negative intracellular diplococci, typical of *Neisseria* or *Branhamella* species, within polymorphonuclear neutrophils.

negative intracellular diplococci) and helps the microbiologist to identify a true infection. *N. elongata*, which has been isolated from throats of patients with pharyngitis, is rod-shaped and will extend into long forms under antibiotic pressure.[11]

26.2 General Growth Characteristics

Neisseria and *Branhamella* grow best on enriched media in a humid atmosphere of 2% to 8% CO_2. *N. gonorrhoeae* requires the added nutrients of chocolate agar or special enrichments, while *N. meningitidis*, other *Neisseria* species, and *B. catarrhalis* can grow on blood agar. The commensal *Neisseria* species and *Branhamella* are able to grow at room temperature, but some strains of the pathogenic *Neisseria* are very sensitive to temperature variations; for this reason, clinical specimens sent to the laboratory for recovery of these organisms must be guarded from the cold and inoculated to growth media as soon as possible after collection. Although holding media at refrigerator temperature will not inhibit recovery, culturing *Neisseria* on media brought to room temperature will facilitate luxuriant growth.[5]

26.3. *Neisseria gonorrhoeae*

26.3.a. Specimen collection. Specimens to be collected for the isolation of *N. gonorrhoeae* include material from genital sources such as the urethra, cervix, and anal canal, as well as specimens from

sites of extragenital infection such as the oropharynx, skin lesions, inflamed joints, blood, and pelvic inflammatory disease. Sterile body fluids are collected in blood culture bottles or in syringes, in which they may be transported immediately to the laboratory.

Neonates may become infected during passage through the birth canal of an infected mother; a particularly virulent conjunctivitis, *gonococcal ophthalmia neonatorum*, is often the result. With the requirement that silver nitrate, erythromycin, or penicillin drops be instilled in the eyes of all infants at birth, this disease has become quite uncommon. Swabs of discharge from the eye may be collected for culture.

The use of nontoxic cotton swabs (treated with charcoal to absorb toxic fatty acids) or calcium alginate swabs will allow the best recovery of organisms. Specimens that are not inoculated immediately to culture media should be transported and held at room temperature in a protective carrying medium that prevents or minimizes overgrowth of nonpathogens, preferably Amie's charcoal transport medium. It is better to refrigerate genital specimen swabs in transport media for a maximum of 3 hours than to incubate the swabs. The best method for culture and transport of *N. gonorrhoeae* is to inoculate agar immediately after specimen collection and to place the medium in an atmosphere of increased CO_2 for transport. Specimens can be inoculated to selective or nonselective agar plates (depending on the source of the specimen) and then placed immediately into a candle extinction jar (see Section 26.3.b). Specialized packaged media consisting of selective agar in plastic trays that contain a CO_2 generating system (Jembec plates, Neigon plates, and Transgrow bottles) are also available.

26.3.b. Culture media and methods. Since gonococci must often be recovered from sites that contain large numbers of organisms from the commensal flora, such as the genital tract, and even from sites that may harbor nonpathogenic *Neisseria* species, such as the oropharynx, special selective media have been developed to aid in the detection of *N. gonorrhoeae*. The first of these was Thayer-Martin medium, chocolate agar with an enrichment supplement and the antibiotics colistin (to inhibit gram-negative bacilli), nystatin (to inhibit yeast), and vancomycin (to inhibit gram-positive bacteria). Modifications of this medium include the addition of trimethoprim lactate to inhibit swarming of *Proteus* species (modified Thayer-Martin medium, [MTM]) and the substitution of anisomycin, an antifungal agent with a longer half-life, for nystatin (Martin-Lewis medium). A transparent medium containing buffered proteose-peptone with many supplements and the same antibiotics as Thayer-Martin medium (New York City medium, [NYC]) has been employed with similar results for the recovery of gonococci.[7] As many as 5% of gonococci are inhibited by the concentrations of antibiotics (particularly vancomycin) in the selective media commonly used, so the use of a nonselective medium is warranted in suspect cases that are culture-negative and for specimens not contaminated with normal flora.

The increased CO_2 necessary for the growth of gonococci can be attained by incubating inoculated media in an incubator that regulates the flow of extraneously provided gas from a commercially purchased gas cylinder or by incubating inoculated media in a closed glass jar (such as a commercial mayonnaise jar) in which a small white candle has been allowed to burn to extinction, called a **candle jar** (see Chapter 6, Figure 6.2), thus removing atmospheric oxygen (to approximately 3%) and creating a bit of extra water vapor.

Sites to culture and techniques to apply for maximum recovery of *N. gonorrhoeae* from genital sites are discussed in Chapter 19. Chapter 16 mentions methods of obtaining material for recovery of gonococci from the oropharynx. Special methods for recovery of gonococci from blood in cases of disseminated disease are mentioned in Chapter 14. The recovery of *N. gonorrhoeae* from normally sterile body fluids does not require any special methods other than those routinely used for such specimens, except that they should be plated onto enriched chocolate agar (in addition to other media) and incubated for 48 hours at 36° to 37° C in a humidified atmosphere of 5% to 10% CO_2. Joint fluids rarely yield isolates, even in definite cases of gonococcal arthritis. The use of a lysis-centrifugation system for such fluids may increase recovery.

26.3.c. Preliminary identification. After 24 to 48 hours incubation, colonies of *N. gonorrhoeae* appear as small (0.5 to 2 mm), translucent, grayish, convex, shiny colonies with entire margins. They will often lift off the agar surface as whole colonies and may appear to be mucoid or sticky. Since the organisms produce an active autolytic enzyme, they must not be exposed to room air for too long.

Colonies on chocolate or selective agar that resemble those of *N. gonorrhoeae* can be screened for the presence of the enzyme indophenol oxidase either by removing a portion of a colony to a piece of filter paper for the Kovacs' test (as described in Chapter 9) or by dropping the fresh reagent (tetramethyl-*p*-phenylenediamine dihydrochloride) directly onto the colony on the agar surface. Oxidase-positive colonies will turn purple, darkening with time (Figure 26.2). These colonies must be subcultured immediately, since the oxidase reagent will rapidly render them nonviable. A Gram stain of the oxidase-positive organism will show typical gram-negative diplococci, with adjacent sides flattened. It has been recommended that the isolation of oxidase-positive, gram-negative diplococci on selective agar such as Thayer-Martin medium from genital sites of infection may be reported presumptively as *N. gonorrhoeae*. However, several recent reports have documented the increasing incidence of gonorrhea-like infections in genital sites caused by *N. meningitidis*, and misidentification of other *Neisseria* as *N. gonorrhoeae*, indicating that the reporting of gonococcal disease based on presumptive criteria is no longer valid.[4,6] Definitive biochemical identification methods and newer identification techniques are discussed in Sections 26.7 and 26.8. It cannot be assumed that an organism with diplococcal morphology that grows on a selective medium is a pathogenic *Neisseria* species, since other organisms, including *Kingella dentrificans*, *B. catarrhalis*, and *Neisseria cinerea*, will grow on these media.

26.3.d. Colony morphology variation. On translucent agar, at least five distinct types of colony morphology can be distinguished.[10] Types T1 and T2, small, bright reflective colonies typical of fresh isolates from cases of gonorrhea, differ from the larger, flatter, nonreflecting colonies of types T3, T4, and T5 that develop from fresh isolates after in vitro passage (Figure 26.3). The T1 and T2 colony types, which are virulent for human volunteers, possess multiple hairlike projections extending from the cell membrane, called fimbriae or pili. The T3, T4, and T5 organisms fail to cause infection in human urethras and do not have fimbriae. These proteinaceous structures are thinner and shorter than flagella, which they resemble (Figure 26.4). The pili function in adherence of bacteria to mucosal cell surfaces, as well as for the conjugal transfer of genetic material between bacteria. It seems likely that virulence,

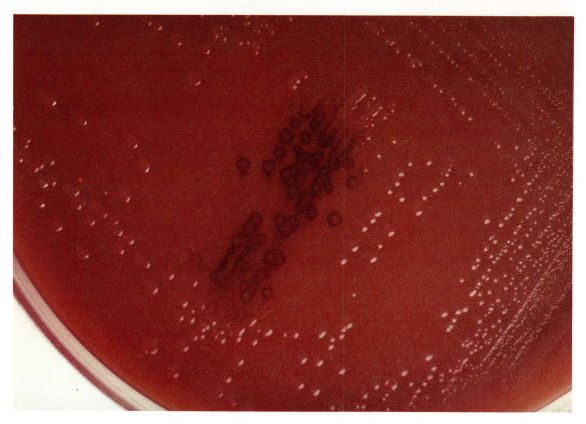

Figure 26.2
Colonies of *Neisseria* species on Thayer-Martin agar after addition of oxidase reagent. Oxidase-positive organisms turn purple within several seconds.

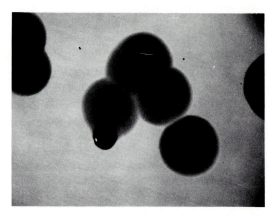

Figure 26.3
Colony morphology variants of *N. gonorrhoeae*. The large colonies (type T3 or T4) represent nonpiliated organisms, whereas the small colonies (T1 or T2) indicate that the organisms possess pili and are more virulent. (Courtesy D. S. Kellogg, Jr., Centers for Disease Control.)

ability to adhere to host surfaces by virtue of possession of pili, and colony morphology of the gonococci are all interrelated.

26.3.e. **Nutritionally variant gonococci.** Another feature of *N. gonorrhoeae* that deserves mention is the phenomenon of "auxotypes." Certain strains, or auxotypes, of gonococci require the addition of particular defined nutrients to grow on artificial media. Those strains that require arginine, hypoxanthine, and uracil (AHU-dependent auxotypes) are usually sensitive to penicillin, resistant to the bactericidal activity of human serum, and more likely to cause asymptomatic urethritis in males and disseminated gonococcal disease in females. Although at least 30 auxotypes have been described, the methods are not yet readily available for routine epidemiologic studies.

26.3.f. **Antibiotic resistance.** Penicillin-resistant *N. gonorrhoeae* have been causing disease in the

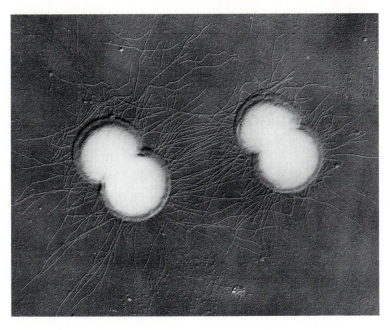

Figure 26.4
N. gonorrhoeae with pili extending from their surfaces. (Courtesy Chuen-mo To and C. C. Brinton, Jr., University of Pittsburgh.)

United States for more than 30 years, but the incidence of such strains has increased in certain areas. The number of reported cases in the United States jumped from 16,000 in 1986 to 25,000 in 1987. The ability to hydrolyze the β-lactam ring of penicillin-like antibiotics is mediated by a bacterial plasmid harboring the gene for the enzyme β-lactamase. **PPNG**, "penicillinase-producing *N. gonorrhoeae*," can be easily detected using a rapid test for hydrolysis of a chromogenic cephalosporin, nitrocefin, as described in Chapter 13. We recommend that all isolates of *N. gonorrhoeae* be tested by this method and reported as "β-lactamase positive" or "β-lactamase negative." Of course, penicillin resistance can occur in non-β-lactamase-producing strains as well. Disk diffusion on GC agar base plus 1% IsoVitaleX is recommended; a zone ≥25 mm surrounding a 10-U penicillin disk is considered susceptible.

26.4. Neisseria meningitidis

26.4.a. **Specimen collection.** *N. meningitidis* is a normal inhabitant of the human nasopharynx, with carriage rates as high as 44% in some populations. The presence of meningococci in the upper respiratory tract of a normal host has not been shown to predispose the host to meningococcal disease; thus isolation of the organism from nasopharyngeal cultures has no clinical significance. However, close contacts (persons who eat and sleep together) of a patient with known meningococcal meningitis have as much as 1000 times greater risk of developing meningococcal disease than others; therefore, carriage of *N. meningitidis* by a close contact of a patient has significance—this carrier should be given prophylaxis, often rifampin. Since the organism is not normal oropharyngeal flora, it may be significant if recovered with polymorphonuclear neutrophils in the absence of other pathogens (especially if found intracellularly) from sputum in large numbers. It is definitely significant if recovered from a transtracheal aspirate or material from percutaneous needle aspirate of the lung infiltrate from a patient with pneumonia. Definitive diagnosis of meningococcal bacteremia, meningitis, or other serious disease is usually accomplished by isolation of the organism from a normally sterile body fluid, such as blood, cerebrospinal fluid, synovial fluid or pleural fluid, or from aspirates of petechiae. Other specimens may also yield meningococci; included are material from eyes, the genital tract, and the anus. Methods for isolation of the *Neisseria* species from blood are discussed in Chapter 14. Handling of other specimens for recovery of meningococci must minimize exposure to air and cool temperatures, as well as prevent dehydration.

26.4.b. Culture media and methods. Body fluids for isolation of all bacteria are treated as outlined in Chapter 21. Any volumes of clear fluid greater than 1 ml are centrifuged at room temperature at $1500 \times g$ for 15 minutes. The supernatant is removed to a sterile tube (and may be utilized for direct detection of soluble antigens) and the sediment is vigorously vortexed, inoculated onto an enriched supportive medium, such as enriched chocolate agar, into a supportive broth medium, such as thioglycolate, and a direct Gram stain is prepared from the last drop of sediment. Purulent fluids may be handled directly without concentrating. All media are immediately incubated in a moist atmosphere of 5% to 10% CO_2 at 36° to 37° C for at least 5 days before discarding as negative.

N. meningitidis strains are able to grow on blood agar as well as on chocolate agar, unlike the gonococcus, although both organisms grow better in increased CO_2 concentration. Specimens from sites with contaminating normal flora may be inoculated to Thayer-Martin or NYC media for selective isolation.

26.4.c. Preliminary identification. The same techniques that are used for preliminary identification of gonococci are useful for the meningococci. A positive oxidase test combined with typical gram-negative diplococcal morphology defines those isolates that require further identification, either with the biochemical tests described below or with the use of one of the new techniques to be discussed. As with gonococci, it is important that these organisms be fully identified.

26.4.d. Serologic classification. Nine serogroups of *N. meningitidis* (A, B, C, D, X, Y, Z, 29E, and W135) have been defined on the basis of differing capsular polysaccharides. The most important serogroups in the United States are A, B, C, and Y. Interestingly, group B polysaccharide is a very poor immunogen for humans and animals, leading to difficulty in developing an effective vaccine against this strain and limiting the development of serologic reagents prepared in animals for laboratory diagnostic tests. Only since the development of techniques for the preparation of monoclonal antibodies has a consistently good immunological reagent for identification of group B meningococci become widely available.

26.4.e. Rapid detection of *N. meningitidis* antigen in body fluids. The sometimes rapidly fulminant course of meningococcal meningitis has spurred the development of several rapid methods for the detection of capsular polysaccharide antigen in body fluids (urine, serum, and cerebrospinal fluid) before culture results are available. Although counterimmunoelectrophoresis (CIE) was the first of these methods to be developed, it has been shown to be less sensitive (and more time-consuming) than particle agglutination techniques such as latex and coagglutination. These reagents are able to detect minute amounts of antigen, often in the absence of viable organisms due to previous treatment or dilution. The latex particles have been the most sensitive in direct assays for antigen, although a thoroughly studied Gram stain is still the most definitive rapid diagnostic method. Due to a small but significant number of false-positive and false-negative results in the commercially available rapid antigen tests, clinicians rarely rely exclusively on such data.

26.5. Other *Neisseria* Species

Neisseria cinerea has recently been recognized as a pathogen associated with bacteremia, conjunctivitis, nosocomial pneumonia, and proctitis.[2,4,12] *N. cinerea* is part of the normal oropharyngeal and genital tract flora. The recognition of this species is largely due to its biochemical resemblance to, and consequent confusion with, *N. gonorrhoeae*. Rare strains of *N. cinerea* have been found to metabolize glucose when tested by more than one system. To prevent misidentification, all strains of glucose and oxidase-positive gram-negative diplococci recovered from noninhibitory media (such as chocolate agar) should be plated to trypticase soy or Mueller-Hinton agar, which support growth of *N. cinerea* but not *N. gonorrhoeae*, and to selective agar such as modified Thayer-Martin, on which growth of *N. cinerea* is inhibited. As another differential test, *N. cinerea* is susceptible to colistin, in contrast to *N. gonorrhoeae* and *N. meningitidis*. *Neisseria mucosa*, also normal flora in the human respiratory tract, has been isolated in association with meningitis, endocarditis, cellulitis, and, most recently, neonatal conjunctivitis.[6] Colonies are mucoid and opaque and the organism is able to grow on nutrient agar.

Certain strains of *Neisseria* exhibit biochemical characteristics of *N. gonorrhoeae* and serologic characteristics of *N. meningitidis*. These strains have been termed *N. gonorrhoeae* subspecies *kochii*.

Originally isolated from conjunctivitis specimens from patients in Egypt, a similar strain has been described from a vaginal specimen in Canada.[9,11]

Neisseria polysaccharea, a newly described commensal in the nasopharynx, resembles *N. meningitidis* morphologically. It may be isolated from selective media, such as Thayer-Martin agar; most strains produce acid from glucose and maltose, whereas sucrose oxidation is variable. This nonpathogenic species is distinguished by its production of large amounts of polysaccharides (visible as precipitation after 3 days of growth) when grown on 1% or 5% sucrose agar or in 1% or 5% sucrose broth.[1]

Other commensal *Neisseriae* include *N. flavescens*, *N. lactamica*, *N. sicca*, and the *N. subflava* biovars: *subflava*, *flava*, and *perflava*. Knapp suggests that *N. flavescens* was of historical importance but is no longer extant.[11] Except for *N. lactamica* and *N. flavescens*, these organisms do not grow on gonococcal selective media and colonies are usually opaque and often yellow-pigmented. They can be distinguished from pathogenic species biochemically.

26.6. *Branhamella catarrhalis*

Although classified as a member of the *Moraxella* genus on the basis of DNA homology studies, *Branhamella* morphologically and biochemically resembles the *Neisseria* species (Table 26.1). It is normal flora of the upper respiratory tract, but it has been isolated as the causative agent of disease, including septicemia, meningitis, endocarditis, otitis media, conjunctivitis, sinusitis, laryngitis, pneumonia, and bronchitis. The majority of patients are elderly and many have predisposing pulmonary disease.[8] Any gram-negative diplococci recovered in large numbers from the lower respiratory tract of a patient with bronchitis or pneumonia should be identified. *Branhamella* is asaccharolytic, commonly β-lactamase positive, and the only DNase-positive species within the group.

26.7. Definitive Biochemical Identification

26.7.a. Traditional biochemical identification. The extent to which identification of isolates resembling *Neisseria* species is carried out is dependent on the source of the specimen. Obviously, an isolate from a child must be identified unequivocally because of the medicolegal ramifications of those results. Isolates from genital sites of adult patients at risk of sexually transmitted disease can be identified

presumptively; this is a good setting for one of the new, rapid methods mentioned in Section 26.8.a. We recommend complete identification of isolates from normally sterile body fluids.

Isolated bacterial colonies on selective media to be characterized by biochemical confirmatory tests must be subcultured to a nonselective medium, such as chocolate agar, for purification and amplification. Subcultures are incubated for a maximum of 48 hours before inoculation to carbohydrates. Cystine trypticase soy agar (CTA) base, pH 7.6, with the addition of 1% filter-sterilized carbohydrate solutions, has been used traditionally. Interpretable results may be obtained with a very heavy inoculum scraped from a plate on a cotton swab, which is swirled vigorously in the top one fourth inch of the medium. CTA carbohydrates, as all carbohydrates, are incubated in air. To overcome some of the problems associated with the growth-dependent CTA medium test, detection of carbohydrate oxidation patterns may be enhanced by inoculating an extremely heavy suspension of the organism into a small volume of buffered, low-peptone substrate, described in Procedure 9.10, Rapid Carbohydrate Utilization test. Table 26.1 shows the reactions used to differentiate members of the Neisseriaceae and *Kingella*, with which they may be confused. The superoxol test, production of gas bubbles from 30% H_2O_2, is positive only for *N. gonorrhoeae*, a useful rapid screening test. *Kingella*, being a true rod, will elongate and form filaments under the influence of penicillin: this can be visualized by staining the growth near a 10-Unit penicillin disk placed on the surface of an agar plate streaked with the organism being tested.

26.7.b. Commercial biochemical systems. Several commercial identification systems that employ biochemical or enzymatic substrates are available for identification of the *Neisseria* species and *Branhamella* or for *N. gonorrhoeae* alone (RapID NH, Innovative Diagnostic Systems; Identicult-Neisseria, Scott Laboratories; Gonochek II, DuPont; RIM-Neisseria kit, Austin Biological Laboratories; Minitek, BBL Microbiology Systems; GONOCHEK II, DuPont Co.; QuadFERM; Analytab Products; *Neisseria-Haemophilus* Identification Card, Vitek Systems; and the HNID Panel, MicroScan Division of Baxter/American Scientific Products). These products usually use the ability of preformed enzymes to act on substrates (conventional or chromogenic) to form a colored end product as the indicator system. A heavy inoculum of the organism is nec-

Table 26.1

Characteristics of Human *Neisseria* spp., *B. catarrhalis*, and *K. denitrificans*[a]

SPECIES	PIGMENT[b]	SUPEROXOL[c]	GLUCOSE	MALTOSE	FRUCTOSE	SUCROSE	LACTOSE (ONPG)
N. gonorrhoeae	−	+	+	−	−	−	−
N. meningitidis	−	−	+	+	−	−	−
N. lactamica	−	−	+	+	−	−	+
N. cinerea	−	−	−[h]	−	−	−	−
N. polysaccharea	−	−	+	+	−	−	−
N. kochii	−	+	+	−	−	−	−
N. flavescens	+	−	−	−	−	−	−
N. sicca	d	−	+	+	+	+	−
N. subflava[j]							
Biovar *subflava*	+	−	+	+	−	−	−
Biovar *flava*	+	−	+	+	+	−	−
Biovar *perflava*	+	−	+	+	+	+	−
N. mucosa	+	−	+	+	+	+	−
B. catarrhalis	−	−	−	−	−	−	−
K. denitrificans	−	−	+	−	−	−	−

[a]ONPG, *o*-Nitrophenyl-β-D-galactopyranoside; DNase, deoxyribonuclease; MTM, modified Thayer-Martin medium; ML, Martin-Lewis medium; NYC, New York City medium. +, Most strains (≥90%) positive; −, most strains (≥90%) negative; d, some strains positive, some strains negative.

[b]Pigment observed in colonies on nutrient agar. Strains of *N. cinerea* and *N. lactamica* are yellow-brown and yellow-pigmented when growth is harvested on a cotton applicator or smeared on filter paper.

[c]All *Neisseria* species and *B. catarrhalis* give a positive catalase test with 3% H_2O_2; *N. gonorrhoeae* strains give strong reactions with 30% H_2O_2 (superoxol), whereas other species are negative.

[d]Some strains may be inhibited by 5% sucrose; reactions may be obtained on a starch-free medium containing 1% sucrose. Strains of *N. gonorrhoeae*, *N. meningitidis*, and *N. kochii* do not grow on this medium.

[e]Results for tests in 0.1% (wt/vol) nitrite; *N. gonorrhoeae* strains of some other species that are negative in 0.1% nitrite can reduce 0.01% (wt/vol) nitrite.

essary for proper reactions, although viable organisms may not be necessary. More reliable identifications result from systems that combine enzymatic and other substrates. Manufacturers' instructions must be followed exactly; several systems were developed only for strains isolated on selective media and should not be used to test other gram-negative diplococci.

26.8. Nonbiochemical Detection and Identification Methods

26.8.a. Identification methods. Both monoclonal and polyclonal fluorescent antibody stains are commercially available (Difco Laboratories; Syva) for *N. gonorrhoeae* culture confirmation. Because of a large number of cross-reacting organisms in urethral or other discharge, these stains are not particularly useful for direct examination of such specimens.

Once an oxidase-positive organism morphologically consistent with gonococci has been isolated on selective media, however, fluorescent stain may provide rapid identification; equivocal reactions must be confirmed by some other method. Good fluorescent reagents are not available for other members of the Neisseriaceae.

Antibody-based particle-agglutination identification systems available include GonoGen (New Horizons Diagnostics), Phadebact (Pharmacia), and Meritec-GC (Meridian Laboratories).

Ortho Diagnostics has developed a biotinylated DNA probe for identification of *N. gonorrhoeae* in 10 minutes. Preliminary results have yielded 100% accuracy with fresh, viable pure cultures of gonococci. Probes have not been developed for other members of Neisseriaceae. The measurement of radioactive end products of metabolism from labeled

POLYSAC-CHARIDE FROM ≥1% SUCROSE[d]	REDUCTION OF		DNase	EXTRA CO2 NEEDED[f]	GROWTH ON		
	NO3	NO2[e]			MTM, ML, OR NYC MEDIUM	CHOCOLATE, BLOOD AGAR AT 22° C	NUTRIENT AGAR AT 35° C
−	−	−	−	VI	+[g]	−	−
−	−	d	−	I	+	−	+
−	−	d	−	d	+	−	+
−	−	+	−	d	−[i]	−	+
+	−	d	−	d	+	−	+
−	−	−	−	No	+	−	+
+	−	−	−	I	+	−	+
+	−	+	−	No	−	+	+
−	−	+	−	No	−	+	+
−	−	+	−	No	−	+	+
+	−	+	−	No	−[k]	+	+
+	+	+	−	No	−	+	+
−	+	−	+	No	d	+	+
−	+	−	−	I	+	−	−

[f] Extra CO2: VI, very important; I, important for growth; No, not needed for growth.

[g] ≥90% of vancomycin-susceptible strains of *N. gonorrhoeae* may not grow on TM or MTM medium.

[h] Some strains of *N. cinerea* may give a weak reaction in glucose in some rapid tests for the detection of acid from carbohydrates.

[i] Some strains of *N. cinerea* have been isolated on gonococcal selective medium, but are colistin susceptible and will not grow when subcultured on selective media. Colistin-resistant mutants of *N. cinerea* have not been described.

[j] Strains of *N. subflava* biovars give consistent patterns of acid production when tested in appropriate media.

[k] Some strains of *N. subflava* biovar *perflava* grow on gonococcal selective media in primary culture, are colistin resistant, and grow on selective media on subculture.

From Knapp, J.S.: Historical perspectives and identification of *Neisseria* and related species. Clin. Microbiol. Rev. 1:41, 1988.

substrates in fluid medium has also been used as a method for identification of *Neisseria* species. Use of the Bactec system was detailed in Chapter 11.

26.8.b. Direct detection of gonococci in specimens. A commercial enzyme-linked immunosorbent assay (ELISA) system (Gonozyme, Abbott Laboratories) has been shown to be very sensitive and specific for the detection of gonococcal antigen in the urethral and endocervical discharge from suspected cases of gonorrhea, although no more sensitive than a Gram stain of male urethral discharge. The test is much more rapid than culture and is suitable for large-scale screening programs among sexually active people.[3] The ELISA tests have not been particularly useful for rapid diagnosis of meningitis, perhaps because of the time required to perform the assays (often 4 to 6 hours). Studies are exploring ways to speed up the end point determination, which may allow the ELISA systems to serve better as diagnostic tests for antigen in cerebrospinal fluid.

Gen-Probe has developed a liquid-probe system with a chemiluminescent detection system for direct detection of gonococci in genital specimens. Preliminary tests have shown its sensitivity to be equal to that of the ELISA system, with the possibility of greater specificity.

The Limulus test for endotoxin may be useful for detection of meningitis caused by meningococci, especially if organisms are present at $>10^3/cm^3$. The gel formation of the lysate is nonspecific, however, and will occur in the presence of endotoxin from any organism, such as gram-negative bacteria. Surprisingly, this assay has been found to be useful as a diagnostic test for gonococcal infection in women, as well as men. Material collected on swabs from the endocervical canal of women with gonorrhea, including early cases and asymptomatic cases, may yield positive *Limulus* amebocyte lysate tests.

REFERENCES

1. Boquete, M.T., Marcos, C., and Saez-Nieto, J.A. 1986. Characterization of *Neisseria polysacchareae* sp. nov. (Riou, 1983) in previously identified noncapsular strains of *Neisseria meningitidis*. J. Clin. Microbiol. 23:973.

2. Boyce, J.M., Taylor, M.R., Mitchell, E.B. Jr., et al. 1985. Nosocomial pneumonia caused by a glucose-metabolizing strain of *Neisseria cinerea*. J. Clin. Microbiol. 21:1.

3. Demetriou, E., Sackett, R., Welch, D.F., et al. 1984. Evaluation of an enzyme immunoassay for detection of *Neisseria gonorrhoeae* in an adolescent population. J.A.M.A. 252:247.

4. Dossett, J.H., Appelbaum, P.C., Knapp, J.S., et al. 1985. Proctitis associated with *Neisseria cinerea* misidentified as *Neisseria gonorrhoeae* in a child. J. Clin. Microbiol. 21:575.

5. Evans, K.D., Peterson, E.M., Curry, J.I., et al. 1986. Effect of holding temperature on isolation of *Neisseria gonorrhoeae*. J. Clin. Microbiol. 24:1109.

6. Gini, G.A. 1987. Ocular infection in a newborn caused by *Neisseria mucosa*. J. Clin. Microbiol. 25:1574.

7. Greenwood, J.R., Voss, J., Smith, R.F., et al. 1986. Comparative evaluation of New York City and modified Thayer-Martin medium for isolation of *Neisseria gonorrhoeae*. J. Clin. Microbiol. 24:1111.

8. Hager, H., Verghese, A., Alvarez, S., et al. 1987. *Branhamella catarrhalis* respiratory tract infections. Rev. Infect. Dis. 9:1140.

9. Hodge, D.S., Ashton, F.E., Terro, R., et al. 1987. Organism resembling *Neisseria gonorrhoeae* and *Neisseria meningitidis*. J. Clin. Microbiol. 25:1546.

10. Kellogg, D.S., Jr., Peacock, W.L., Jr., Deacon, W.E., et al. 1963. *Neisseria gonorrhoeae*: I. Virulence genetically linked to clonal variation. J. Bacteriol. 85:1274.

11. Knapp, J.S. 1988. Historical perspectives and identification of *Neisseria* and related species. Clin. Microbiol. Rev. 1:41.

12. Southern, P.M., Jr. and Kutscher, A.E. 1987. Bacteremia due to *Neisseria cinerea*: report of two cases. Diagn. Microbiol. Infect. Dis. 7:143.

BIBLIOGRAPHY

Morello, J.A., ed. 1989. Perspectives on pathogenic Neisseriae. Clin. Microbiol. Rev. Suppl. 2:S1-S149. (Entire issue devoted to Neisseriae.)

27 Enterobacteriaceae

Bacteria belonging to the family Enterobacteriaceae are the most commonly encountered organisms isolated from clinical specimens. They are gram-negative bacilli, able to grow readily on all supportive media (blood and chocolate agars), and they form distinctive colonies on selective agars depending on their metabolic capabilities and the components of the media, as discussed in Chapter 8. Some species are classical pathogens, assumed to be the etiologic agents of disease when they are encountered in clinical specimens, independent of the numbers of colony-forming units detected (such as *Salmonella*, *Shigella*, and *Yersinia pestis*). Other species can colonize humans without evoking any pathological response, such as those Enterobacteriaceae that colonize the human intestinal tract. These "commensal" organisms, if they are introduced into a susceptible site (peritoneal cavity, lung of an immunosuppressed host, cerebrospinal fluid, and so forth) are able to cause disease. Still others, such as *Escherichia coli*, are associated with certain syndromes based on the presence of virulence factors that are not possessed by all strains or even by the same strain at all times. Members of this ubiquitous family of similar organisms have been mentioned in association with each of the anatomic sites of infectious disease covered in previous chapters, including blood, cerebrospinal fluid, respiratory tract, gastrointestinal tract, urinary tract, soft tissue, sterile body fluids, and in a variety of loci in immunocompromised hosts. The only major category of infectious diseases with which Enterobacteriaceae have not yet been definitively associated is that of sexually transmitted disease.

Identification of the Enterobacteriaceae to species level is of importance epidemiologically as well as clinically. The susceptibility patterns of many species are predictable, allowing the clinician to choose therapy based on an isolate's identification. The presence of an epidemic or small outbreak, due to a particularly virulent strain of Enterobacteriaceae or due to a breakdown in technique among health care workers, is often first detected by microbiologists who have noticed a cluster of isolates of an unusual biotype. The discovery of an extremely rare biotype in a cluster of blood cultures led a Milwaukee microbiologist to discover the source of a nationwide outbreak of septicemia associated with contaminated intravenous fluids. The importance of species differentiation for epidemiologic purposes is discussed in Chapter 5.

Within the last several years, the number of recognized species of Enterobacteriaceae has grown from 26 to over 100 (approximately 80 species have been named), and more species are being validated monthly.[6] This rapid expansion is somewhat overwhelming to clinical microbiologists, who are not taxonomists and generally wish only to convey some meaningful information to clinicians concerning bacterial species isolated from clinical material. Most microbiology laboratories are able to identify the newly recognized species of Enterobacteriaceae, primarily because of the availability of commercially produced multibiochemical and enzymatic parameter test systems. This chapter will focus on the 13 genera of Enterobacteriaceae that are most likely to be encountered in clinical specimens. Although we advocate the definitive identification of isolates that can be causally related to disease, particularly from systemic sites of infection such as blood, cerebrospinal fluid, tissue, or other sterile body fluids, it is not practical for routine clinical laboratories to maintain all of the unusual, rarely used, or technically demanding media or test reagents necessary for thorough studies of rarely isolated organisms. Such isolates should be forwarded to a reference laboratory for further studies.

27.1. Epidemiology and Pathogenesis of Infections due to Enterobacteriaceae

Enterobacteriaceae are the predominant facultative flora in the human bowel, a site from which they can easily be disseminated. Lapses in personal hygiene, especially during periods of diarrheal disease, can contribute to the fecal-oral route of transmission of the agents of gastroenteritis and related diseases. Countries with poor sanitation systems are more likely to have environmental reservoirs of the Enterobacteriaceae, from which disease is maintained

in the population. Hospitalized patients quickly become colonized on the skin or in the respiratory tract with strains endemic to the hospital, allowing these organisms easy access to the host under any compromising situation.

In addition to their presence as normal human fecal flora, Enterobacteriaceae are found in natural habitats worldwide, including soil, water, plants of all types, fish, insects, and other animals. Their importance in human disease is at least equaled by their importance as causes of disease in poultry, domestic livestock, fish, and several vegetable and plant crops, with major economic consequences. Although the genera that have not been associated with human disease will be listed here (Table 27.1), they will not be discussed in detail. It is possible that any species of Enterobacteriaceae may be isolated from clinical specimens, especially as more immunocompromised patients survive long enough to become infected, technical proficiency among microbiologists is increasing, and commercial identification systems are expanding their data bases. Only by identifying unusual clinical isolates can microbiologists discover previously unrecognized agents of human disease.

27.1.a. Enterobacteriaceae associated with gastroenteritis and enteric fevers. Several Enterobacteriaceae have been associated with gastroenteritis and food-borne disease (also mentioned in Chapter 17). *Salmonella* species are the etiologic agents of most of the food-borne gastroenteritis in the United States. Over 50,000 cases were reported to the Centers for Disease Control (CDC) in 1987. For some reason, the incidence of salmonellosis increased steadily from 1955 to 1985, particularly among elderly patients. The organism is naturally found in poultry, but disease can be transmitted in a wide variety of foods. The most recent major outbreak occurred in Chicago in spring 1985, when contaminated milk infected a large number of individuals. Ultimately, more than 5000 individuals contracted *Salmonella* gastroenteritis, resulting in several fatalities. Because *Salmonella* are susceptible to gastric acid, a large inoculum (approximately 10^5 organisms) must be ingested.

Salmonella are able to invade the intestinal mucosa. Some strains produce an enterotoxin. *S. typhi*, the paratyphoid bacilli, and *S. cholerae-suis* are more likely to invade systemically, entering the bloodstream and causing serious febrile disease (typhoid or enteric fever). These strains are usually carried only in human hosts, passed among individ-

Table 27.1
Genera and Species of Enterobacteriaceae

GENUS	SPECIES	COMMENTS
Budvicia*	aquatica	Found in drinking and surface water. Isolated from human feces.
Buttiauxella	agrestis	Found in water, not associated with human disease.
Cedecea*	davisae lapagei neteri (others)	Isolated from humans, primarily respiratory tract and wounds.
Citrobacter*	amalonaticus diversus freundii (others)	Isolated from humans, wound infections, urine, sepsis; fecal flora. Also isolated from environment.
Edwardsiella*	hoshinae ictaluri tarda (others)	Isolated from humans and animals; associated with diarrhea, wound infections, sepsis.
Enterobacter	aerogenes* agglomerans* amnigenus* asburiae cloacae* dissolvens gergoviae* intermedium nimipressuralis sakazakii* taylorae* (others)	Very common, normal fecal flora; isolated from wounds, respiratory tract, urine, blood. *E. agglomerans* also in animals, others found in environment. *E. cloacae* most clinically significant. *E. agglomerans* and *E. sakazakii* yellow-pigmented.
Erwinia	amylovora (others)	Associated with diseases of plants.
Escherichia	blattae coli* fergusonii* hermannii* vulneris*	Isolated from humans and animals, *E. coli* most common human pathogen. *E. blattae* found only in cockroaches. *E. hermannii* and *E. vulneris* isolated from wounds. Others normal stool flora.
Ewingella*	americana	Isolated from humans, respiratory tract, blood. No environmental source known.
Hafnia*	alvei (others)	Isolated from humans, respiratory tract, other sources. No environmental source known.
Klebsiella	oxytoca* ozaenae* planticola* pneumoniae* rhinoscleromatis* terrigena	Normal stool flora, some strains found in environment. Isolated from respiratory tract, urine, wounds, blood. *K. terrigena* found only in water.
Kluyvera*	ascorbata cryocrescens	Probably normal stool flora. Isolated from human infections, respiratory tract, blood, urine.
Koserella*	trabulsii	Isolated from human feces, wounds, respiratory tract, knee joint. (Synonym for *Yokenella regensburgei*.)
Leclercia*	adecarboxylata	Isolated from humans, respiratory tract, blood, urine, wounds; also found in food and water.
Leminorella*	grimontii richardii	Isolated from human feces. H_2S-positive, not known to be pathogenic for humans.
Moellerella*	wisconsinsis	Isolated from human stool and natural water. Not known to be pathogenic for humans. Resistant to colistin.
Morganella*	morganii (others)	Normal stool flora. Isolated from human infections (urine, blood, others).

*Isolated from clinical specimens.

Continued.

Table 27.1

Genera and Species of Enterobacteriaceae—cont'd

GENUS	SPECIES	COMMENTS
Obesumbacterium	*proteus*	Isolated from brewery yeast. Not known to be pathogenic for humans.
Proteus	*mirabilis** *myxofaciens* *penneri** *vulgaris**	Most species normal fecal flora. Isolated from human infections, urine, wounds, blood, others, *P. myxofaciens* isolated from moths only. *P. penneri* resembles *P. vulgaris*, including spreading growth, but is indole-negative and chloramphenicol-resistant.
Providencia	*alcalifaciens** *heimbachae* *rettgeri** *rustigianii** *stuartii**	Most species are normal fecal flora. Isolated from human infections, urine, wounds, blood. *P. rustigianii* not known to be pathogenic for humans.
Rhanella*	*aquatilis*	Isolated from water. Only one human isolate reported. Not known to be pathogenic for humans.
Salmonella*	(*enterica*) >2000 serovars	Widely distributed in humans and animals. Cause of gastroenteritis and enteric fever. Genus *Arizona* now included in *Salmonella*. Nomenclature still undecided.
Serratia*	*ficaria* "*fonticola*" *liquefaciens* *marcescens* *odorifera* *plymuthica* *rubidaea* (others)	Isolated from humans, water, rarely animals. Some species important human pathogens. Isolated from respiratory tract, wounds, blood, urine, others. *S. ficaria, odorifera, plymuthica, rubidaea* not known to be human pathogens. *S. fonticola* probably not true member of *Serratia* genus.
Shigella*	*boydii* *dysenteriae* *flexneri* *sonnei*	Human reservoir only, not normal flora. Cause of gastroenteritis and bacterial dysentery. Genetically identical to *E. coli*.
Tatumella*	*ptyseos*	Isolated from humans, respiratory tract, urine, blood. Unlike other Enterobacteriaceae, *Tatumella* has polar flagella; susceptible to penicillin; poor grower, better at 25° C.
Xenorhabdus	*luminescens* *nematophilus*	Isolated from nematodes only. Grow only at 25° C, not at 35° C. No human isolates.
Yersinia*	*aldovae* *enterocolitica* *frederiksenii* *intermedia* *kristensenii* *pestis* *pseudotuber- culosis* *ruckeri*	Isolated from humans, animals, environment. Some important human pathogens. Agents of plague, gastroenteritis, other infections. Isolated from stool, blood, urine, wounds. *Y. ruckerii* not found in humans, cause of "red mouth" disease of fish. *Y. ruckeri* probably not true member of genus *Yersinia*.

uals by fecal contamination of food or water. Very young, very old, and other compromised hosts are most likely to become seriously ill. One third of all cases of salmonellosis reported in 1987 occurred in children less than 5 years old.

The incidence of typhoid fever in the United States is quite low (400 cases reported in 1987), and in approximately half of these the disease was acquired during foreign travel. Domestically acquired typhoid fever, however, is often transmitted by a chronic carrier of *S. typhi*. After recovering from typhoid fever, some individuals carry the bacterium asymptomatically for long periods of time. Another set of individuals will be asymptomatic carriers without ever suffering from disease. The silent carriers contribute to continued episodes of infections.

Shigella species are carried primarily by humans and are not disseminated in nature. The organism is able to resist gastric acidity, allowing a very small inoculum (as few as 10 organisms) to cause disease. Shigellosis also occurs primarily in children, although the incidence is not as high as that of salmonellosis. In 1987 approximately 24,000 cases of shigellosis were reported to the CDC. *Shigella* produce an enterotoxin, but it is not as important to virulence as is their invasiveness. The organisms invade the epithelial cells of the large bowel, causing a dysentery-like syndrome (Chapter 17). *Shigella* rarely invade systemically.

E. coli is also an important cause of gastrointestinal disease. It can be associated with nursery outbreaks of diarrhea as well as with travelers' diarrhea (turista, Delhi belly, and other amusing epithets), an important source of morbidity to Americans traveling to other countries. Virulence mechanisms of *E. coli* include production of an enterotoxin similar to that of *Vibrio cholerae*, invasiveness, production of cytotoxins, and adherence (Chapter 17). In previous years, nursery outbreaks of *E. coli*-associated gastroenteritis were associated with particular serotypes of the organism, called **enteropathogenic E. coli. (EPEC)** Serotypes may still be associated with epidemics or geographic regions, but the serotype is not the only significant factor; it does serve as a marker for a particular strain. Toxin production is carried on a plasmid, a transmissible genetic element that can be easily transferred from strain to strain among and between species. For this reason, serotyping of single isolates of *E. coli* from pediatric patients with diarrhea is not recommended. For epidemiologic reasons and when outbreaks are suspected, serotyping is still a valuable tool. Local health departments are better equipped to handle such situations than are most clinical laboratories.

Tests for toxin production and tests utilizing genetic probes to detect the toxin gene sequences (although not universally available) more accurately identify etiologic agents (**enterotoxigenic** *E. coli*; **[ETEC]**). A particle agglutination test for detection of heat-labile and heat-stable toxins of *E. coli* is available commercially but is not widely used in clinical laboratories. The gastrointestinal disease associated with invasive or traditional cytotoxic *E. coli* can resemble shigellosis, and the disease mediated by enterotoxigenic *E. coli* can resemble cholera. Additionally, serious hemorrhagic colitis and hemolytic uremic syndrome have been associated with infection with verotoxin (a specific cytotoxin)-producing

E. coli.[5] Other mechanisms of pathogenicity also occur in still other types of *E. coli*.

The fourth genus of Enterobacteriaceae containing organisms that are major etiologic agents of diarrheal disease is *Yersinia*, which also includes the etiologic agent of human plague. *Y. enterocolitica* and, less commonly, *Y. pseudotuberculosis* and *Y. intermedia*[1] have only recently been implicated as significant causes of gastroenteritis. The organisms possess the ability to invade the intestinal mucosa, as well as to produce a heat-stable enterotoxin similar to that of some strains of *E. coli*. Virulence factors shared among other members of *Yersinia* species, such as the ability to survive intracellularly, may also contribute to pathogenesis. Symptoms that accompany *Y. pseudotuberculosis*, and occasionally *Y. enterocolitica* infections may mimic those of appendicitis (although the symptoms are actually due to mesenteric lymphadenitis). The organisms can invade the epithelium to cause systemic disease. *Y. enterocolitica* has also been associated with exudative pharyngitis.

Although the incidence of diarrheal disease associated with *Yersinia* is much higher in Europe and Canada than in the United States, more isolations are occurring in the United States over time, aided by increased awareness of the organism and better laboratory techniques designed especially for its detection (Chapter 17). Certain serotypes (primarily 03 and 09) have been recovered from patients with diarrhea in Europe and Scandinavia. These serotypes are less common in the United States, where 08 predominates. The incidence of 03 isolations, however, seems to be increasing, at least in the New York area, with an accompanying greater risk of acquiring disease via human-to-human transmission.[2]

Gastroenteritis has also been associated with *Edwardsiella tarda*, a member of the Enterobacteriaceae that resembles salmonellae in its pathogenic mechanisms, as well as morphologically. The organism has also been known to invade through the intestinal epithelium, causing systemic disease. Reported cases of *Edwardsiella*-associated gastroenteritis are uncommon.

27.1.b. *Yersinia pestis*. The agent of human plague, *Y. pestis*, causes disease among many wild animal species, including prairie dogs, squirrels, rabbits, chipmunks, and others. The organism is transmitted among these animals by fleas and other ectoparasites, which also spread the organism to carnivores that prey upon the smaller rodents. Humans acquire the disease when bitten by an infected flea or by handling the carcass of an infected animal. Rarely, infection can be spread from person to person via infected aerosol droplets from respiratory secretions of patients who have plague pneumonia (the Black Death). Most cases occur among young individuals in the southwestern and western United States; Navajos are at higher risk because of intense rodent plague in areas of the reservation in Arizona. The incidence increased steadily beginning in 1965, with 19 cases reported in 1982 and 40 cases reported in the peak year of 1983. Cases dropped considerably after 1983, with only 12 cases reported in 1987. This probably reflects a natural cycle of plague within the wild rodent population.

Once the organisms penetrate the skin, through small breaks or via flea bites, or are breathed in, they are taken up by macrophages and polymorphonuclear neutrophils, within which they can multiply. During this first intracellular phase, the bacteria are stimulated by their immediate environment (lack of Ca^{++}, temperature, ionic concentration) to produce a protein and a lipoprotein antigen, called V and W antigens, that render the organism less susceptible to intracellular killing by other reticuloendothelial cells once they escape the original cell through lysis of that cell. The genetic determinants that code for these antigens are located on plasmids. *Y. pestis* also possesses an envelope antigen (F-1) that may contribute to resistance to phagocytosis. Virulent *Y. pestis* produces three factors, a bacteriocin called pesticin I, coagulase, and fibrinolysin. These three factors, produced together, are plasmid-mediated; coagulase and fibrinolysin contribute to virulence by promoting invasiveness. Other factors that are associated with virulence include the ability of virulent strains to absorb hemin and basic aromatic dyes to form colored colonies (related to iron transport and storage), the ability to synthesize purines, and production of a toxin.

Primary disease is usually of the "bubonic" variety, characterized by infected and swollen lymph nodes and fever. Sepsis and sometimes pneumonia follow within several days. Septicemic and pneumonic plague may also occur without the lymphadenopathy stage. Untreated human plague is 50% to 60% fatal. Streptomycin and tetracycline are the antimicrobial agents of choice. If meningitis develops, chloramphenicol should be added to the regimen.

27.1.c. Other infections associated with members of Enterobacteriaceae.

Enterobacteriaceae, particularly *E. coli*, are the most common cause of urinary tract infections. Urinary tract infections are the largest category of nosocomial infections (Chapter 23); they may lead to secondary sepsis, shock, and death. Nosocomial infections associated with Enterobacteriaceae also include pneumonia, surgical wound infections, and catheter-related sepsis. The species that are most likely to be recovered from urine of infected individuals are those that are able to adhere to urinary epithelium. Attachment-mediating, fingerlike projections composed of protein, called **fimbriae,** are often found on strains that are able to adhere, not only to urinary tract epithelial cells but also to many other human and animal epithelial cell types (Figure 16.1). Fimbriae are also found among gastroenteritis-producing strains, especially in animals. The ability to colonize the gastrointestinal tract, resisting the action of peristalsis and other factors, is mediated at least in part by fimbriae.

Most of the Enterobacteriaceae may be involved in bacterial pneumonia, but *Klebsiella pneumoniae* seems especially suited to this role. The copious polysaccharide capsular material produced by this species probably aids the organism to escape phagocytosis. Chapter 16 contains a discussion of those factors that contribute to the pathogenesis of pneumonia. Elderly patients and those compromised by influenza, alcoholism and other chronic diseases are most likely to contract community-acquired *Klebsiella* pneumonia. It is a significant cause of hospital-acquired pneumonia as well.

Neonatal meningitis has been associated with certain strains of *E. coli*, most of which possess the K1 capsular antigen (shared by group B streptococci, the other principal cause of neonatal meningitis). Capsular polysaccharide may also contribute to the pathogenesis of this disease. *Citrobacter* species, also encapsulated, have been associated with neonatal meningitis as well. It is postulated that the organisms can somehow invade through infant intestinal epithelium to cause systemic disease. *E. coli* is no more likely to be the etiologic agent of adult meningitis than are any other members of the Enterobacteriaceae. The role of capsular polysaccharide as a factor in the development of meningitis is mentioned in Chapter 15.

Serratia species are sometimes associated with especially severe hospital-acquired infections, including pneumonia and surgical wound infections.[8]

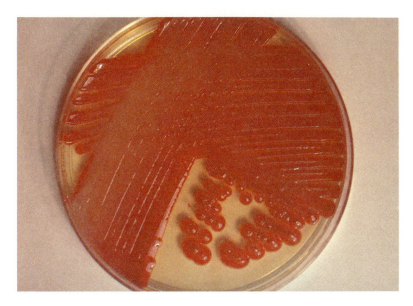

Figure 27.1
A pigmented *S. marcescens* species.

The organisms recovered from blood may be resistant to the bactericidal activity of serum and complement. Nosocomially derived *Serratia* strains are often resistant to multiple antibiotics. Rarely, strains of *S. marcescens* will display a red, non-water-soluble pigment (Figure 27.1). These pigmented strains are less likely to be resistant and are more likely to be community-acquired.

Most members of the Enterobacteriaceae have been associated with various infections, particularly among hospitalized and otherwise compromised hosts. The *Proteus*, *Providencia*, and *Morganella* species are most often recovered from urine of patients with urinary tract infections, although they can also be found associated with pneumonia, wound infections, and other syndromes. Those strains that are able to hydrolyze urea have been associated with the development of renal calculi in infected patients.

A virulence factor possessed by all Enterobacteriaceae (as well as all gram-negative bacteria) is the cell wall lipopolysaccharide, **endotoxin.** Biological activity of this component, released during growth and breakdown of gram-negative bacterial cells, was discussed in Chapter 14. The major pathological consequence of gram-negative septicemia, that of shock, is mediated by endotoxin. Patients may experience disseminated intravascular coagulopathy, respiratory tract problems, cellular and tissue injury, fever, and other debilitating problems. Multiple organ failure

may result. Although species of Enterobacteriaceae possess flagella, and species other than those mentioned possess polysaccharide capsules and fimbriae, the effect of these factors on the virulence of a particular strain has not been completely elucidated.

27.2. Taxonomy of Enterobacteriaceae

With increasing use of multifactorial biotyping systems routinely by clinical microbiology laboratories, unusual and rare biotypes of bacteria are being recognized and sent to reference centers such as the Centers for Disease Control (CDC) for collection and characterization. The application of deoxyribonucleic acid (DNA) homology technology to the study of the relatedness of two bacterial clones has been the major factor leading to the ability to assign definitively such morphologically or biochemically distinct strains of bacteria to species and occasionally to new genera. As described and illustrated in Chapter 10, the more closely related two strains of bacteria are, the greater the chromosomal homology shared between them, as demonstrated by the extent to which single strands of DNA from one strain will realign with single strands of DNA from the other strain under carefully controlled experimental conditions (called *stringent* conditions). The recombined DNA, possessing one strand from each of two test strains, is called a *hybrid,* and the analysis to determine relatedness is called *DNA-DNA hybrid-*

ization. Arbitrarily, clones of bacteria that share 70% or more of their chromosomal sequences are considered to belong to the same species. Definition of genera is not so easily determined. In addition to DNA-DNA hybridization studies, relatedness of bacteria can be determined by differences in the melting temperature of DNA, which is directly related to the number of guanine and cytosine bonds compared to the number of adenine and thymine bonds. The guanine and cytosine content ($\%G + C$) can be used to begin to characterize strains of bacteria, but DNA-DNA hybridization is the most definitive arbitrator. Ribonucleic acid typing (ribotyping) has also been used to determine relatedness among bacterial strains.

Table 27.1 lists the genera and species of Enterobacteriaceae that have been validly published as of this writing. With the exception of *Erwinia amylovora*, most previous *Erwinia* species have been renamed as *Enterobacter* species. A number of the newer species have not yet been isolated from humans, although in the future they may be found to be associated with human disease. The identification of these species is possible with many of the commercial identification systems (Chapter 9). Those laboratories that do not use such systems should refer to the publication by Farmer et al.(Bibliography) and subsequent descriptions of newly characterized species for biochemical tests used to identify these isolates, if they do not choose to send the isolates to a suitable reference laboratory. Recent publications are listed in the Bibliography of this chapter. Tests described in this chapter as well as in Chapter 9 will often be used to characterize the new species as well. The bulk of discussion in this chapter, however, will focus on the 13 genera most likely to be encountered in clinical specimens. The basic differential characteristics of the most commonly isolated Enterobacteriaceae are given in Table 27.2.

27.3. Laboratory Identification of Enterobacteriaceae

27.3.a. Isolation of Enterobacteriaceae from clinical material. Material from any site can harbor members of the family Enterobacteriaceae. Specimens of fecal material, in which these organisms are normal flora, are inoculated to selective and differential agars for detection of those organisms known to be the etiologic agents of gastroenteritis to the exclusion of the nonpathogenic commensal fecal Enterobacteriaceae. Strategies for cultivation of stool are dis-

cussed in Chapter 17, and an overview of culture media to inoculate initially is presented in Chapter 6. A screening agar for verotoxin-producing *E. coli*, such as MacConkey/sorbitol agar, will detect the most common serotype of verotoxin-producing strains, O157:H7. Other toxin-positive strains must be detected using Vero cells in a tissue culture cytotoxin assay, beyond the scope of most clinical laboratories.

Most other clinical specimens, including material from wounds, respiratory tract secretions, aspirations from abscesses, sterile body fluids, urines, tissues, and blood cultures, are inoculated to at least one supportive medium, such as blood or chocolate agar, that will allow the growth of all Enterobacteriaceae, as well as to one selective agar for gram-negative bacilli, usually MacConkey agar. Discussion of initial selection of media for isolation of etiologic agents of disease from each of these sites is found in the appropriate chapters of this text. Descriptions of colony morphologies of isolates on various selective and differential media commonly used for cultivation of Enterobacteriaceae are found in Chapter 8. Except for the most fastidious or biologically damaged strains, all Enterobacteriaceae will grow on MacConkey agar, yielding pink or reddish colonies if they are able to ferment lactose, and colorless, translucent colonies if they are slow- or non-lactose-fermenters (Figure 27.2). Growth on MacConkey agar is one of the first criteria used to establish the identification of an unknown gram-negative bacillus. Except for a few *Bacillus* species and tiny pinpoint colonies of enterococci, staphylococci, and an occasional yeast, gram-positive organisms do not grow on MacConkey agar.

27.3.b. General phenotypic features shared by all or most Enterobacteriaceae. The Enterobacteriaceae are straight-sided gram-negative bacilli that grow well on most laboratory media. The Enterobacteriaceae are facultative anaerobes—all will grow in air or anaerobically; CO_2 does not appreciably enhance growth. If they are motile, with the exception of *Tatumella ptyseos*, they possess peritrichous flagella. *T. ptyseos* has polar flagella. All species of *Klebsiella* and *Shigella* are nonmotile. Some species of *Escherichia*, *Salmonella*, and *Yersinia*, among clinically important Enterobacteriaceae, are nonmotile as well. Selected strains within other species may also be nonmotile.

All Enterobacteriaceae ferment glucose and are oxidase-negative, and almost all are able to reduce

Table 27.2

Identification of Clinically Important Enterobacteriaceae*

SPECIES	INDOLE PRODUCTION	METHYL RED	VOGES-PROSKAUER	CITRATE (SIMMONS')	HYDROGEN SULFIDE (TSI)	UREA HYDROLYSIS	PHENYLALANINE DEAMINASE	LYSINE DECARBOXYLASE	ARGININE DIHYDROLASE	ORNITHINE DECARBOXYLASE	MOTILITY (36°C)	GELATIN HYDROLYSIS (22°C)	D-GLUCOSE, GAS	LACTOSE FERMENTATION	SUCROSE FERMENTATION	D-MANNITOL FERMENTATION	DULCITOL FERMENTATION	ADONITOL FERMENTATION	D-SORBITOL FERMENTATION	L-ARABINOSE FERMENTATION	RAFFINOSE FERMENTATION	L-RHAMNOSE FERMENTATION	D-XYLOSE FERMENTATION	MELIBIOSE FERMENTATION	DNase, 25°C	ONPG†
Escherichia coli	98	99	0	1	1	1	0	90	17	65	95	0	95	95	50	98	60	5	94	99	50	80	95	75	0	95
Shigella serogroups A, B, and C	50	100	0	0	0	0	0	0	5	1	0	0	2	0	0	93	2	0	30	60	50	5	2	50	0	2
Shigella sonnei	0	100	0	0	0	0	0	0	2	98	0	0	0	2	1	99	0	0	2	95	3	75	2	25	0	90
Salmonella, most serotypes	1	100	0	95	95	1	0	98	70	97	95	0	96	1	1	100	96	0	95	99	2	95	97	95	2	2
Salmonella typhi	0	100	0	0	97	0	0	98	3	0	97	0	0	1	0	100	0	0	99	2	0	0	82	100	0	0
Salmonella paratyphi A	0	100	0	0	10	0	0	0	15	95	95	0	99	0	0	100	90	0	95	100	0	100	0	95	0	0
Citrobacter freundii	5	100	0	95	80	70	0	0	65	20	95	0	95	50	30	99	55	0	98	100	30	99	99	50	0	95
Citrobacter diversus	99	100	0	99	0	75	0	0	65	99	95	0	98	35	45	100	50	98	99	100	0	100	100	0	0	96
Edwardsiella tarda	99	100	0	1	100	0	0	100	0	100	98	0	100	0	0	0	0	0	0	9	0	0	0	0	0	0
Klebsiella pneumoniae	0	10	98	98	0	95	0	98	0	0	0	0	97	98	99	99	30	90	99	99	99	99	99	99	0	99
Klebsiella oxytoca	99	20	95	95	0	90	1	99	0	0	0	0	97	100	100	99	55	99	99	98	100	100	100	99	0	100
Enterobacter aerogenes	0	5	98	95	0	2	0	98	0	98	97	0	100	95	100	100	5	98	100	100	96	99	100	99	0	100
Enterobacter cloacae	0	5	100	100	0	65	0	0	97	96	95	0	100	93	97	100	15	25	95	100	97	92	99	90	0	99
Hafnia alvei	0	40	85	10	0	4	0	100	6	98	85	0	98	5	10	99	0	0	0	95	2	97	98	0	0	90
Serratia marcescens	1	20	98	98	0	15	0	99	0	99	97	90	55	2	99	99	0	40	99	0	2	1	7	0	98	95
Proteus mirabilis	2	97	50	65	98	98	98	0	0	99	95	90	96	2	15	0	0	0	0	0	1	1	98	0	50	0
Proteus vulgaris	98	95	0	15	95	95	99	0	0	0	95	91	85	2	97	0	0	0	0	0	1	5	95	0	80	5
Providencia rettgeri	99	93	0	95	0	98	98	0	0	0	94	0	10	5	15	0	0	100	1	0	5	70	10	5	10	5
Providencia stuartii	98	100	0	93	0	30	95	0	0	0	85	0	0	2	50	100	0	5	1	1	7	0	7	0	10	10
Providencia alcalifaciens	99	99	0	98	0	0	98	0	0	1	96	0	85	0	15	10	0	98	1	1	1	0	1	0	0	1
Morganella morganii	98	97	0	0	5	98	95	0	0	98	95	0	90	1	0	2	0	0	0	0	0	0	0	0	0	5
Yersinia enterocolitica	50	97	2	0	0	75	0	0	0	95	2	0	5	5	95	98	0	0	99	98	5	1	70	1	5	95
Yersinia pestis	0	80	0	0	0	5	0	0	0	0	0	0	0	0	0	97	0	0	50	100		1	90	20	0	50
Yersinia pseudotuberculosis	0	100	0	0	0	95	0	0	0	0	0	0	0	0	0	100	0	0	0	50	15	70	100	70	0	70

*Each number gives the percentage of positive reactions after 2 days of incubation at 36°C. The vast majority of these positive reactions occur within 24 h. Reactions that become positive after 2 days are not considered.

†ONPG, orthonitrophenyl-beta-D-galactopyranoside.

From Farmer, J.J. III, Davis, B.R., Hickman-Brenner, F.W., et al. 1985. Biochemical identification of the new species and biogroups of Enterobacteriaceae isolated from clinical specimens. J. Clin. Microbiol. 21:46.

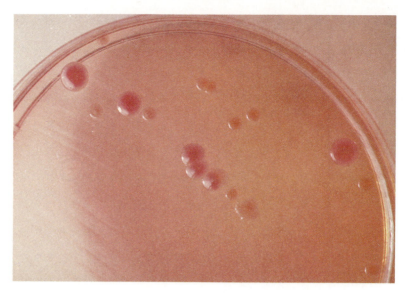

Figure 27.2
Colonies of lactose-fermenting (pink) and non-lactose-fermenting (colorless) gram-negative bacilli on MacConkey agar.

nitrates to nitrites. Performance of the nitrate test was outlined in Chapter 9. Except for one group of *Shigella* species and a species of *Xenorhabdus*, all Enterobacteriaceae are catalase-positive. An additional clue to the identification of an unknown organism as an Enterobacteriaceae is luxuriant growth on most routine media incubated at 35°C in air within 24 hours. Colonies on blood agar are usually gray, shiny, entire, convex, and opaque. Hemolysis may be present. Strains of some *Proteus* species display a recognizable "swarming" pattern that resembles waves of growth spreading from the original inoculum (Figure 27.3) due to their active motility. Most Enterobacteriaceae will yield large (at least 1 to 2-mm diameter after 24 hours) colonies on blood agar and MacConkey agar plates. A few strains of Enterobacteriaceae isolated from clinical specimens, however, may not grow well on MacConkey agar, especially if the organisms have been damaged previously by antibiotic treatment.

The first test that should be performed on a gram-negative bacillus isolated from clinical material is the oxidase test, as described in Chapter 9. The oxidase test must be performed with colonies growing on plates that do not contain dyes that may obscure the results. Plates yielding mixed cultures from clinical material may often contain colonies of more than one species of Enterobacteriaceae. If several colony mor-

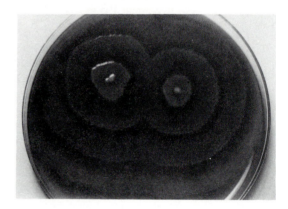

Figure 27.3
Appearance of swarming *Proteus* species on blood agar. Note successive waves of growth extending from a central inoculum.

phologies can be differentiated only on MacConkey agar, each morphotype should be subcultured to a portion of a blood agar plate for performance of an oxidase test. Oxidase negative, luxuriantly growing, facultatively anaerobic bacilli (initially isolated aerobically, in most cases) are likely to be members of the Enterobacteriaceae.

The ability to utilize glucose anaerobically with formation of acidic end products (fermentation) is tested by inoculating portions of a colony to a Kligler's iron agar (KIA) or triple sugar iron agar (TSIA)

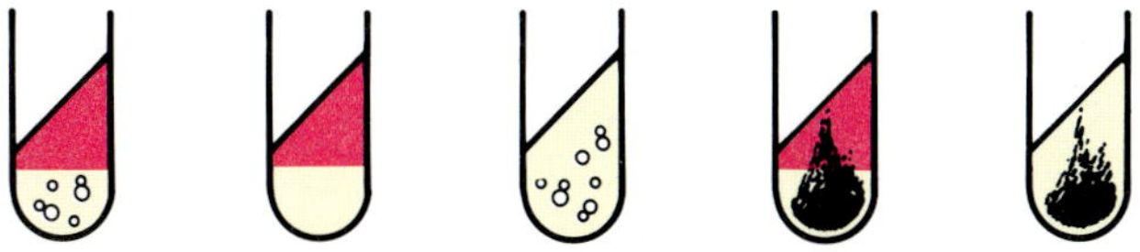

Alk/A gas	Alk/A no gas	A/A gas	Alk/A H₂S	A/A H₂S	Possible species
+	+	+	−	−	Escherichia coli Hafnia alvei
+	+	−	−	−	Morganella morganii Providencia alcalifaciens P. rettgeri P. stuartii Serratia sp.
+	−	+	−	−	Enterobacter aerogenes E. cloacae
+	−	+	+	+	Citrobacter sp.
+	+	−	+	−	Salmonella sp.
−	+	−	−	−	Shigella sp.
−	+	+	−	−	Yersinia sp.
−	−	+	−	−	Klebsiella sp.
−	−	−	+	+	Proteus mirabilis P. vulgaris
−	−	−	+	−	Edwardsiella tarda

*Some species show slight gas.

Figure 27.4
Chart showing basic reactions of Enterobacteriaceae on Kligler's iron agar.

slant (Chapter 9). These three preliminary tests will place the unknown organism into one of several categories, helping to determine which tests are necessary for further identification. Enterobacteriaceae are fermentative, oxidase-negative, MacConkey-positive bacilli. Those organisms that are grouped as nonfermentative gram-negative bacilli or other non-Enterobacteriaceae are further identified, as described in Chapters 28, 29, and 30. More rarely, isolates will fall into categories as described in Chapter 39. Initial reactions in KIA (or TSIA) agar can be used to guide identification of the 13 more commonly isolated genera of Enterobacteriaceae (Figure 27.4).

Many laboratories no longer rely on KIA for initial testing of gram-negative bacilli, but instead inoculate a commercial identification system (Chapter 9) with a suspension made from one isolated colony. Depending on the system, results are available within 4 hours or after overnight incubation, at which time the oxidase reaction can be correlated with the biochemical reactions for definitive identification. Because these systems usually include a larger number of differential parameters than can be utilized cost-effectively as individual components, the identifications that result are more specific. The immense data bases used by the commercial sys-

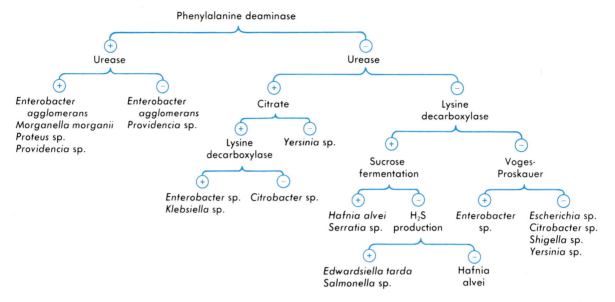

Figure 27.5

Flow chart for initial identification of Enterobacteriaceae based on basic biochemical reactions.

tems, as discussed in Chapter 9, contribute to the detection of unusual and new biotypes.

There are a few basic biochemical parameters, however, that have classically been employed by microbiologists to categorize the Enterobacteriaceae (and other bacteria) into species groups. Even if laboratories are using commercial identification systems, with the exception of the totally automated instruments (such as Vitek and Abbott MS-2 or Avantage, outlined in Chapter 11), technologists can still observe visual changes in indicators that correlate to individual biochemical reactions. Technologists are urged to try to identify isolates based on manually observed biochemical patterns before the organisms are identified by comparing the numerical code generated by the pattern of results with the company-furnished list of profile numbers and species identifications. Trying to identify species by recognizing their biochemical patterns is challenging and contributes to the continued maintenance of cognitive abilities.

Toward this end, the performance of some of the classical biochemical tests used to identify Enterobacteriaceae will be outlined in this chapter. These reactions are used not only to identify Enterobacteriaceae but also are often necessary for identification of more fastidious, unusual, or relatively metabolically inactive microorganisms (not only bacteria)

that cannot be identified with commercially available systems. A rudimentary flow chart that begins to differentiate commonly isolated Enterobacteriaceae on the basis of a few biochemical reactions is shown in Figure 27.5. Excellent commentaries on the biochemical bases of these tests and their performance are found in the ASM Manual of Clinical Microbiology, Washington's laboratory manual, and in the books by MacFaddin and by Howard and others (Bibliography). Media for performing these tests are all available from commercial suppliers, either already prepared or in dry powder form for in-house preparation. The results listed in Table 27.2 are based on conventional tests. Results of individual tests performed as part of a miniaturized or automated biochemical identification system cannot with complete reliability be compared with the results obtained with conventional methods. Identifications that result from miniature systems are based on patterns generated from the entire system and not on results of individual tests. Identifications are based on the "best fit."

27.3.c. **Urease test**. The ability of an organism to hydrolyze urea to ammonia and CO_2, as described in Chapter 9, is determined classically by heavily inoculating a urea-containing agar slant (Christensen urea agar, available commercially) or a urea-containing, buffered broth of the sort available commercially. (Rustigian and Stuart urea broth, which is highly buffered, described in Chapter 45 and also available commercially, yields reliable results.) Organisms should be well dispersed in broth for best results. The media are incubated at 37°C, preferably in a water bath or small incubator. Strongly urease-positive organisms will begin to produce alkaline products, which turn the phenol red indicator red to purple within minutes. The heavier the inoculum, the more rapid the positive result. Tubes or broths should be examined at 10 minutes, 30 minutes, 1 hour, and several hours after inoculation. Several suppliers (including Key Scientific Products, E-Y Laboratories, and Difco Laboratories) produce a rapid urease test reagent containing substrates impregnated on filter paper or in tablets, as mentioned in Chapter 9. Of particular utility for identification of *Proteus* and *Providencia* species are the filter paper disks produced by Remel Laboratories, which test for urease and phenylalanine deaminase. In addition to differentiation of Enterobacteriaceae, the classical urease test is also used to differentiate between certain *Brucella* species, to aid in identification of encapsulated yeasts, and as an additional test for identification of certain gram-negative coccobacilli.

27.3.d. Decarboxylation and dihydrolation of amino acids. Differentiation among many species of Enterobacteriaceae requires determining the ability of the organism to break down the amino acids lysine, arginine, and ornithine, forming an amine end product and CO_2. Lysine and ornithine are decarboxylated, whereas arginine is broken down first by dihydrolation and then by decarboxylation. The amine end product of these reactions is alkaline, causing a shift in the pH indicators bromcresol purple and cresol red to purple (also discussed in Chapter 9). The ability to decarboxylate lysine is a prominent feature of most species of *Salmonella*, *Klebsiella*, *Enterobacter aerogenes*, *Hafnia alvei*, and *Serratia marcescens*.

Definitive tests for lysine and ornithine decarboxylases and arginine dihydrolase are carried out in broth media developed by Moeller, called *Moeller's decarboxylase medium* (also discussed in Chapter 9). Performance of the test entails inoculation of Moeller's medium, which contains glucose, bromcresol purple, a nitrogen source, cresol red indicator, the enzyme activator pyridoxal, and the amino acid to be tested. In addition to tubes containing each amino acid, a control tube containing only the basal medium must be inoculated each time the test is performed, to ascertain that the organism does not form alkaline end products in the absence of an available amino acid.

The tubes are inoculated with a small amount of growth from isolated colonies, being certain that the inoculum is emulsified in the broth below its surface. All tubes are overlayed with sterile mineral oil or vaspar to a depth of 1 cm to prevent introduction of oxygen. Tubes are incubated at 35° to 37°C for up to 14 days, although results can usually be read in 4 days. A more rapid result is possible if the amount of broth is reduced and the inoculum is extremely turbid. A change in the color of the medium to purple indicates a positive test and the ability of the organism to utilize the amino acid to form alkaline end products (purple = positive). A yellow color indicates that only the glucose was utilized, with the formation of acid. The control tube, of course, should remain its original color (pale purple) or turn yellow if the organism is a glucose fermenter. A gray color may indicate reduction of the indicator, rather than alkaline end products. If the test is critical, the addition of more bromcresol purple solution (0.01% aqueous solution) to the broth below the seal may allow detection of a pH shift. Additional incubation of tubes displaying intermediate results after 4 days often allows interpretation of results later. Other bacteria in addition to those within the Enterobacteriaceae may be inoculated to Moeller's broths for detection of decarboxylase and dihydrolase enzymes. The test is particularly useful in the identification of viridans streptococci, *Aeromonas*, *Plesiomonas*, *Vibrio* species, and nonfermentative gram-negative bacilli.

Lysine iron agar (LIA) detects hydrogen sulfide (H_2S) formation, lysine decarboxylation, and phenylalanine deamination (positive for *Proteus*, *Providencia*, and *Morganella*) and is often used to differentiate H_2S-producing nonpathogens isolated on selective agar such as Hektoen and xylose-lysine-deoxycholate (Chapter 8) from etiologic agents of gastroenteritis. *Citrobacter* species, often confused with *Salmonella* on initial isolation, are lysine-negative. LIA contains glucose, lysine, ferric ammonium citrate, and sodium thiosulfate for H_2S detection, and bromcresol purple pH indicator. Organisms are inoculated in the same manner as for KIA, except that it is helpful to stab the butt of LIA several times to ensure an adequate inoculum. After 18 hours incubation at 35°C with a *loose cap*, the tube is examined. The formation of a black precipitate in the butt is indicative of H_2S production, although LIA is less sensitive than either TSI or KIA for detection of H_2S. Organisms that are able to decarboxylate lysine (a reaction that takes place anaerobically in the butt) will produce alkaline end products that result in a purple color. Those bacteria that do not decarboxylate lysine will ferment the small amount of glucose, yielding acid by-products and causing the bromcresol purple to turn the butt yellow. Even in the presence of a large amount of black precipitate, the yellow-colored butt can be seen by observing the tube with light behind it. Deamination of phenylalanine is detected by a change in the color of the slant from purple to reddish. LIA is often used as a basic preliminary screening medium to detect fecal pathogens because it incorporates several parameters into one medium. With the exception of *Salmonella paratyphi A*, most of the salmonellae and *Edwardsiella tarda* are lysine decarboxylase-positive.

27.3.e. **Methyl red and Voges-Proskauer tests.** Organisms that utilize glucose may do so by producing abundant acidic end products such as formate and acetate from the intermediate pyruvate metabolite, or they may metabolize the carbon compounds to acetoin and butanediol, which are more neutral in pH. The methyl red and Voges-Proskauer (MR and VP) tests detect the presence of the end products of these two divergent metabolic pathways. The same substrate broth, MR/VP broth, is used for both tests. Tubes of broth (5 ml per tube), containing peptones, glucose, and buffer, are available commercially or can be prepared in the laboratory from powder base. The organism is inoculated below the surface of the medium in the tube, and the tube is incubated with a loose cap at 35° to 37°C for at least 48 hours. A longer incubation period may be necessary, especially for the demonstration of a positive VP reaction. To perform the test, the substrate broth is divided into two equal aliquots, one of which is used for the MR test and the other for the VP test (Procedure 27.1). The subtle nature of this reaction demands that all reagents and substrates are controlled. As for all of the tests described in this section, the MR/VP test is sometimes used in the identification of organisms other than Enterobacteriaceae.

27.3.f. **Indole test.** The ability of an organism to degrade the amino acid tryptophan can be detected by testing for indole, the product of tryptophanase (tryptophan deamination of indolepyruvic acid). Reaction of indole with an aldehyde will result in a colored end product. The rapid indole test described in Chapter 9 is performed with dimethylaminocinnamaldehyde reagent, which turns blue or blue-green in the presence of indole. The classic test described here (Procedure 27.2) calls for *p*-dimethylaminobenzaldehyde as the indicator substrate. When the indole test described here is used to test bacteria other than Enterobacteriaceae, the more sensitive Ehrlich's reagent (described in Chapter 28) should be used to detect indole.

27.3.g. **Citrate utilization test.** Certain organisms are able to utilize a single substrate as a sole carbon source. The ability to use citrate can help to differentiate among members of the Enterobacteriaceae. The medium, Simmons' citrate agar, contains buffers, salts, cations, citrate, and bromthymol blue as the pH indicator. The medium can be purchased prepared or as dry powder. Since the reaction requires oxygen, the organism is inoculated to the surface of an agar slant of the medium. A very light inoculum (usually picked with a straight wire) is necessary to prevent false positive reactions due to carryover of substrates from previous media. The tube is incubated for 24 hours or up to 4 days at 35° to 37° C with a *loose cap*. Growth of the organism on the slant, with change of the color indicator from green to blue, or turquoise blue, is evidence of a positive test, indicating that the organism was able to grow and produce acetate and other alkaline carbonate end products. There may be a rare citrate-positive organism that can utilize the substrate without producing enough alkaline reaction to change the pH indicator. Luxuriant growth on the slant without a blue color may indicate a positive test, but the test should be repeated with a minimal inoculum.

27.3.h. **Motility test.** Another important differential test among Enterobacteriaceae and many other bacteria is motility. The fastest and most direct method for detection of motility is to examine microscopically (under oil immersion [$1,000 \times$]) a wet preparation of the organism from the initial isolation plates or broth incubated at room temperature for 2 to 4 hours, as described in Chapter 7. After the organisms have settled, the directed and purposeful movement of a single bacterium or several bacteria, as opposed to the flowing movement of all bacteria within a field, is indicative of motility. Motility must

PROCEDURE 27.1

Methyl Red and Voges-Proskauer Tests

Principle

The presence of certain metabolic enzymes can be used to differentiate organisms based on end products of glucose metabolism detected with various color indicator reagents. Acid products produced by enzymes of the mixed acid fermentation pathways are detected by development of a red color by the methyl red indicator (indicating pH <4.5). Acetoin and butanediol, products of the butanediol fermentation pathway, yield a pink or red color in the presence of α-naphthol in the relatively alkaline environment. Most Enterobacteriaceae demonstrate either one or the other metabolic pathway, but rarely both pathways.

Method

1. Prepare methyl red (MR) reagent as follows:

Methyl red (Mallinckrodt)	0.1 g
Ethyl alcohol (95%)	300 ml
Distilled water	200 ml

   Dissolve the methyl red in the alcohol before adding the distilled water. Store in a brown bottle in the refrigerator.

2. Prepare Voges-Proskauer (VP) reagent A as follows:

α-Naphthol (Sigma Chemical Co.)	5 g
Ethyl alcohol (absolute)	100 ml

   Dissolve the α-naphthol in a small amount of ethyl alcohol and bring the volume to 100 ml in a volumetric flask or cylinder. The alcohol should be almost colorless. Store in a brown bottle in the refrigerator.

3. Prepare (VP) reagent B as follows:

Potassium hydroxide (KOH)	40 g
Distilled water	100 ml

   Weigh out the KOH very quickly, as it is hygroscopic and will become caustic when moist. Add less than 100 ml water to the pellets in a flask in a cold water bath to prevent overheating. Bring the volume to 100 ml in a volumetric flask or cylinder. Store this reagent in the refrigerator in a polyethylene bottle or one that has been specially treated for storage of caustic chemicals.

4. From a tube of inoculated MR/VP broth base that has been incubated for at least 48 hours, remove 2.5 ml to another tube for the VP test.

5. To the 2.5 ml of organism suspension, add 0.6 ml (6 drops) of VP reagent A (α-naphthol). Then add 0.2 ml (2 drops) of VP reagent B (40% KOH). Gently shake the tube and allow it to sit for as long as 15 min.

6. Observe for the formation of a pink to red color, indicating the presence of acetoin (acetyl methyl carbinol). A pink color in the medium is indicative of a positive test. A negative test will appear colorless or yellow.

7. While the VP reaction is developing, the remaining 2.5 ml of substrate is tested for acidity by adding 0.5 ml (5 drops) of the methyl red reagent and observing the color. If the indicator remains red, the methyl red test result is positive. A change to yellow indicates that the pH of the medium is greater than 6.0, a negative MR test. If the reagent remains orange, the test must be repeated after a longer incubation period.

Quality control

E. coli ATCC 25922 and *Klebsiella pneumoniae* ATCC 13883 should be inoculated to MR-VP broths and tested.

Expected results

E. coli should be MR-positive and VP-negative, whereas *K. pneumoniae* is MR-negative and VP-positive.

Performance schedule

Quality control organisms must be used to test each batch of reagents and media prepared before they are used.

Modified from MacFaddin, J. 1980. Biochemical tests for identification of medical bacteria, ed. 2. Williams & Wilkins, Baltimore.

PROCEDURE 27.2

Indole Test

Principle

Tryptophanase enzymes degrade the tryptophan in peptones and other components of media to indole, skatole, and indoleacetic acid. When combined with certain aldehydes, indole yields a red-colored product. Organisms are grown in a medium rich in tryptophan and the medium is then tested for the presence of the indole end product. Either Kovacs' reagent (described here) or Ehrlich's reagent (Chapter 28) provides the aldehyde indicator.

Method

1. Prepare Kovacs' reagent as follows:

p-Dimethylaminobenzaldehyde (Sigma Chemical Co.)	10 g
Isoamyl or isobutyl alcohol (absolute)	150 ml
Concentrated hydrochloric acid	50 ml

   Dissolve the p-dimethylaminobenzaldehyde in the alcohol and slowly add the acid while constantly stirring the mixture. The reagent should be pale-colored and should be stored refrigerated in a brown bottle. If it turns brown or if quality control organisms fail to give correct reactions, discard the reagent and make a fresh lot. The aldehyde may require gentle heating in order to go into solution.

2. Inoculate the organism into a broth that contains tryptophan and incubate for at least 24 h. Most commercial peptone, pancreatic enzymatic casein hydrolysate, or tryptone (a pancreatic digest of casein) broths will contain enough tryptophan for use in this test. Note that acid hydrolysate of casein broths that do not contain tryptone are not suitable for the indole test.

3. To perform the test, remove 2 ml of the broth suspension to a second tube. Add 0.5 ml (5 drops) of Kovacs' reagent to the broth. Gently shake the tube and observe for a pink color in a ring around the interface between the broth and the alcoholic reagent, which rises to the surface (Figure 27.6).

4. If the test is negative, the remaining broth may be reincubated for an additional 24 h and the test may be repeated.

Quality control

Inoculate *E. coli* ATCC 25922 and *Enterobacter cloacae* ATCC 23355 as above.

Expected results

The *E. coli* is indole-positive and yields a red ring in the lower portion of the alcohol phase layer above the medium. The *E. cloacae* is indole-negative, showing either only a cloudy ring or a slight yellow-colored ring at the alcohol interface.

Performance schedule

Quality control strains should be tested with each new batch of media and reagents.

---

be distinguished from Brownian motion, which usually involves all visible organisms equally.

Motility can be encouraged by growing bacteria in semisolid media. Good commercial motility semisolid media are available from Difco Laboratories and BBL Microbiology Systems, as well as from other commercial media suppliers. The media are prepared as butt tubes with a depth of 5 cm or greater. The organism is inoculated by stabbing a straight wire carrying the inoculum once vertically into the center of the agar butt to a depth of approximately 2 cm. After overnight incubation, motility will be evident as a haze of growth extending into the agar from the stab line. It is not recommended to include a colored growth indicator in motility medium, such as tetrazolium salts, since it may be inhibitory to some bacteria. Because a much larger sample of a bacterial population can be tested with the semisolid motility agar than can be visualized microscopically, these media are probably

PROCEDURE 27.3

Phenylalanine Deaminase Test

Principle

Deamination of phenylalanine yields phenylpyruvic acid. Deamination of tryptophan yields indolepyruvic acid. These α-keto acids react with ferric chloride to form a green end product (phenylpyruvic acid) or an orange-brown end product (indolepyruvic acid).

Method

1. Prepare ferric chloride reagent as follows:

Ferric chloride ($FeCl_3$) (Sigma Chemical Co.)	12 g
Distilled water	94.6 ml
Concentrated HCl (37%)	5.4 ml

   Dissolve $FeCl_3$ in water and slowly add the hydrochloric acid while working under a fume hood. Store the reagent in a brown bottle in the refrigerator.
2. After overnight incubation of the test organism on an agar slant containing phenylalanine, add 0.5 ml (5 drops) of the reagent to the growth on the surface of the slant and gently rotate the tube so that the reagent covers the entire surface. Observe for an immediate development of a green color, indicating the presence of phenylpyruvic acid and a positive test result. Within 10 min the color will fade, so observation must take place immediately after the reagent has been added. Adding of additional reagent will usually regenerate the color. Certain species may deaminate phenylalanine so rapidly that the test will be positive within 4 h of incubation.

Quality control

Test *Proteus vulgaris* ATCC 33420 and *E. coli* ATCC 25922 as described.

Expected results

The *Proteus* will yield a positive test (green slant) and the *E. coli* slant will remain yellow after addition of the ferric chloride.

Performance schedule

Test quality control organisms with each new batch of media or reagents.

Modified from MacFaddin, J. 1980. Biochemical tests for identification of medical bacteria, ed. 2. Williams & Wilkins, Baltimore.

more sensitive for detection of motility. Solid and semisolid motility detection media are read after overnight incubation at the temperature preferred by the organism being tested. For example, *Y. enterocolitica* are motile at room temperature but not at 37° C. Organisms other than Enterobacteriaceae for which semisolid motility media are commonly used include *Listeria monocytogenes* and nonfermentative gram-negative bacilli. The nonfermentative bacteria show enhanced motility when nitrate is incorporated into the semisolid media due to their more active aerobic metabolism.

27.3.i. Phenylalanine deaminase test. Of the well-characterized Enterobacteriaceae, only *Enterobacter agglomerans* (20% of strains), *Enterobacter sakazakii* (50% of strains), *Morganella morganii, Proteus* species, *Providencia* species, *Rhanella aquatilis,* and *Tatumella ptyseos* are able to deaminate the amino acid phenylalanine. The organism to be tested is grown overnight on an agar slant containing phenylalanine, salts, yeast extract, and buffers. Phenylalanine agar is available prepared or in dry powder form. The product of phenylalanine deamination, phenylpyruvic acid, is detected by a colored end product that forms when phenylpyruvic acid combines with ferric chloride solution. Procedure 27.3 describes performance of the test.

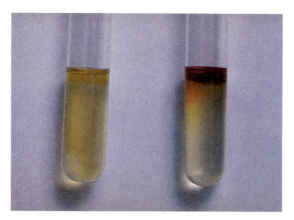

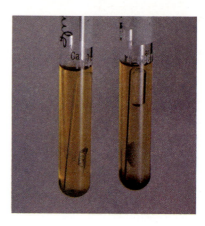

Figure 27.6
Indole test; positive result is visible as a red to pink ring around the top of the tube where the reagents float. A negative test is seen as no change in color of the reagents.

Figure 27.7
Fermentation of glucose with the production of gas, as seen by the bubble that has collected in the inverted Durham tube in the tube on the right. The organism in the tube on the left does not produce gas.

27.3.j. Substrate fermentation tests. A large proportion of the tests used to differentiate among members of the Enterobacteriaceae (as well as among other microorganisms) determines the ability of the organism to utilize a carbohydrate with the production of acid metabolic end products. In addition to detecting acid, carbohydrate fermentation media can be modified to detect the formation of gas by placing a very small, inverted glass tube (called a **"Durham tube"**) into the broth. If gas is produced during fermentation of the carbohydrate, it will be collected in the inverted tube and will be visible as a bubble (Figure 27.7). Most Enterobacteriaceae produce gas during glucose fermentation, but *Shigella*, *S. typhi*, *Providencia stuartii*, most *Yersinia* species, and certain *E. coli* species do not produce gas (called **anaerogenic**).

The carbohydrates are usually prepared as individual aqueous solutions and filter-sterilized to prevent their destruction by the heat of the autoclave. The heart infusion or other broth base containing a pH indicator, which may be 0.0018% (wt/vol) phenol red, 1% Andrade's acid fuchsin, or 0.0016% (wt/vol) bromcresol purple (originally dissolved in 95% ethanol, 1.6 g/100 ml ethanol), is made up, autoclaved, and allowed to cool before the sterile carbohydrate solutions are aseptically added to a final concentration of 1% carbohydrate. For most applications, bromcresol purple yields satisfactory and consistent results. A variety of sugars, including lactose, su-

crose, maltose, glucose, and others, and a variety of alcohols, including mannitol, erythritol, dulcitol, and others, can be added to carbohydrate broth base for fermentation tests. All generally used carbohydrate broths are available commercially from several media suppliers.

27.3.k. ONPG test. Enterobacteriaceae are preliminarily grouped according to their ability to ferment lactose, a β-galactoside. *Salmonella*, *Shigella*, *Proteus*, *Providencia*, and *Morganella* are usually considered to be non-lactose-fermenters. Other organisms, including certain *E. coli*, *Shigella sonnei*, *H. alvei*, *S. marcescens*, and some *Yersinia* species, may appear to be non-lactose-fermenters because they lack the enzyme (permease) that actively transports lactose across the cell membrane, making it available to intracellular β-galactosidase. True non-lactose-fermenters do not possess β-galactosidase. If β-galactosidase but not permease is produced by a species, strains will eventually be able to ferment lactose that slowly diffuses across the cell membrane, although this process may be too slow for detection with carbohydrate fermentation broths. A rapid test for the presence of β-galactosidase (determination of whether an organism has the capability of utilizing lactose) is the ONPG test (Procedure 27.4). Organisms other than Enterobacteriaceae, including *Neisseria* and streptococci, can also be differentiated with the ONPG test.

Because the reagents are difficult to prepare, we

PROCEDURE 27.4

*ONPG (o-Nitrophenyl-*β-D-Galactopyranoside*)* Test for β-Galactosidase

Principle

β-Galactosidase acts on the substrate **ONPG** in the same way as the enzyme hydrolyzes lactose to form galactose and glucose, although the end product of ONPG hydrolysis is a visible (yellow) product, orthonitrophenol.

Method

1. Prepare peptone water as follows:

Peptone (Difco)	1 g
NaCl	0.5 g
Distilled water	100 ml

   Autoclave at 121° C for 15 min.

2. Prepare sodium phosphate buffer as follows:

Na_2HPO_4	13.8 g
Distilled water	90 ml

   Add the sodium phosphate to the distilled water in a 100-ml volumetric flask. Dissolve it by warming at 37° C. Slowly add approximately 15 ml of 5 N NaOH (or approximately 6 g) until the pH stabilizes at 7.0. Bring the volume to 100 ml with distilled water. Because of its causticity, NaOH should be handled carefully, and manipulations should be performed in a fume hood.

3. Prepare ONPG solution as follows:

ONPG (Sigma)	0.6 g
Sodium phosphate buffer (step 2)	100 ml

   Add the ONPG to the buffer, sterilize this by filtration, and store solution in a sterile brown glass bottle, refrigerated at 4° to 10° C.

4. Prepare ONPG broth as follows:
   Aseptically add 25 ml of ONPG solution to 75 ml peptone water. Aseptically dispense this solution into sterile 13 × 100 mm plastic snap-capped tubes, 0.5 ml per tube. Store refrigerated for 1 month or frozen at −20° C for up to 6 months. If the solution appears yellow, discard it.

5. Inoculate one tube of ONPG broth with a heavy suspension of the organism to be tested (taken from a KIA or TSIA slant or from the surface of a fresh subculture plate). Incubate the tubes for a minimum of 1 h (preferably overnight) at 37° C.

6. Examine tubes for color change. A change to yellow indicates a positive result (presence of β-galactosidase), and no color change indicates a negative result (absence of the enzyme). If the test organism has not changed color after 1 h incubation, incubation should be continued for additional time up to the full 24 h. Tubes may be checked at hourly intervals. If the organism produces yellow pigment, the test cannot be performed, and the longer test for utilization of lactose must be substituted.

Quality control

Inoculate control organisms *E.coli* ATCC 25922 and *Proteus mirabilis* ATCC 29245 as in step 5.

Expected results

The *E. coli* should be positive (yellow), and the *Proteus* sp. should be negative (clear).

Performance schedule

Quality control strains should be tested each time new reagents are received and monthly thereafter.

Modified from MacFaddin, J. 1980. Biochemical tests for identification of medical bacteria, ed. 2. Williams & Wilkins, Baltimore; and from Hendrickson, D.A. 1985. Reagents and stains. In Lennette, E.H., Balows, A., Hausler, W.J., Jr., and Shadomy, H.J., editors. Manual of clinical microbiology, ed. 4. American Society for Microbiology, Washington, D.C.

recommend that laboratories purchase ONPG-impregnated filter paper disks from Difco Laboratories or Remel Laboratories or the tablets produced by Key Scientific Products. To perform the tests, an *extremely heavy* inoculum of the organism to be tested is suspended in a small volume of buffer and the reagents are eluted from the disk or tablet into the liquid. After several hours of incubation, a yellow color is indicative of hydrolysis of the substrate by β-galactosidase, or a positive test. The medium remains colorless when the test is negative. Manufacturers' recommendations and strict quality control practices should be followed.

27.3.l. Gelatin hydrolysis test. Enzymes that degrade proteins, often important virulence factors, are produced by relatively few members of the Enterobacteriaceae. *Serratia, Proteus, Xenorhabdus*, some *Yersinia*, and several of the unnamed groups produce proteinases. Gelatinase production can be detected by observing whether an organism can remove the gelatin coating from exposed x-ray film. A small piece of exposed but not developed x-ray film (obtained from the hospital radiology department) is dropped into a tube containing a very heavy suspension of the organism in trypticase soy or other nutrient broth. After 1 to 48 hours of incubation, the film is observed for removal of the gelatin layer, leaving behind the pale blue clear plastic film.

A commercially purchased gelatin broth medium may also be used. Duplicate tubes of media are inoculated with the culture. One tube is incubated at 37° C, and the other is incubated at room temperature. At the same time, an uninoculated tube is incubated at 37° C to serve as a control. All media will be liquid at incubator temperatures. After sufficient growth (which may take as long as 30 days) the tubes are placed in the refrigerator for 30 minutes, or until the uninoculated control tube resolidifies. If the test organism made gelatinase, either one or both of the inoculated tubes will remain liquid, indicating breakdown of the gelatin present in the medium. A positive control should always be tested with each assay. The gelatinase test is also used in identification schemes for many other organisms in addition to Enterobacteriaceae.

27.3.m. DNase test. Extracellular nucleases are produced primarily by the same species that produce the protease gelatinase. The detection of these enzymes is most sensitive at room temperature. Tests for DNase detection were outlined in Chapter 9.

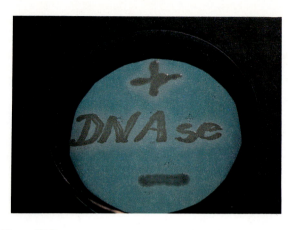

Figure 27.8
DNAse test agar containing methyl green indicator. Organisms that produce DNAse are identified by production of a clear zone (hydrolysis of DNA and subsequent breakdown of the indicator) surrounding growth of the organism after overnight incubation.

Commercially produced agars, either prepared as plates or as slants, are available from several sources, as are dry powder media (Figure 27.8).

27.3.n. Rapid catalase supplemental test. A recently described rapid catalase test may help to separate genera of Enterobacteriaceae that are morphologically difficult to differentiate. Chester and Moskowitz[3] observed the time for bubbles to appear after placing a single colony from a fresh agar culture into a drop of 3% hydrogen peroxide. Genera were divided into two groups. Those in which bubbles appeared *immediately* were *Cedecea, Hafnia, Morganella, Proteus, Providencia, Serratia*, and *Yersinia*. Those from which bubbles were delayed (usually 1 second or longer, but any slight delay was considered "delayed") included *Citrobacter, Edwardsiella, Escherichia, Enterobacter, Klebsiella, Kluyvera, Salmonella, Shigella*, and *Tatumella*. This test may be useful for differentiating similar-appearing strains of *Yersinia* from *E. coli* and *Shigella*, and *Serratia* from *Enterobacter* species.

27.4. Serologic Characterization of Enterobacteriaceae

27.4.a. General antigenic features. In addition to biochemical and morphologic features, the Enterobacteriaceae can also be differentiated serologically, based on their possession of at least three classes of antigenic determinants. The cell wall structure of a typical Enterobacteriaceae was illustrated in Chapter 14 (Figure 14.2). Not all species have been antigenically characterized yet, but those that have been intensely studied include *E. coli*, *Klebsiella*, *Shigella*, and most extensively, *Salmonella*. The first category of antigens is associated with the lipopolysaccharide, or endotoxin moiety of the cell wall, called "O" antigens or **somatic** (body) antigens. These antigens are heat-stabile.

Among *E. coli*, certain O antigens are associated with specific virulent phenotypes, such that *E. coli* O111 and O125, for example, are often found as etiologic agents of infantile diarrhea; *E. coli* O112 is often an invasive strain that causes a dysentery-like syndrome; and O157 has been associated with verocytotoxin production. Serotypes O1, O26, O91, O113, O121, O145, O157, and others have been isolated from cases of serious hemorrhagic colitis and hemolytic uremic syndromes caused by verotoxin-positive *E. coli*.

Shigella species have classically been grouped according to O serotypes. Since the *Shigella* have now been shown to be identical to *Escherichia* by DNA hybridization studies, no new serotypes will be added. For the convenience of clinicians and microbiologists, the name *Shigella* will continue to be used for those organisms that can be distinguished biochemically from the *E. coli* group (Table 27.2). Classically, the serotypes of *Shigella* correspond to species as follows: *S. dysenteriae*, serotype A; *S. flexneri*, serotype B; *S. boydii*, serotype C; and *S. sonnei*, serotype D.

The second category of antigens are the capsular polysaccharide antigens, called "K" antigens. These antigens are heat-labile, and they are known to be produced by organisms that include *Klebsiella*, *Salmonella*, and *E. coli*. The K antigens of some strains of *Salmonella* are called "Vi" antigens. Certain *Citrobacter* species may also possess Vi antigens, although they can be differentiated from the salmonellae biochemically. The presence of capsular antigens may inhibit the ability of antiserum to detect the underlying O antigen. By heating the organism suspension to boiling for 30 minutes or longer, technologists may be able to detect the masked O antigens. Nomenclature for *E. coli* antigens associated with virulence became confused when certain antigens, important to adherence of the organisms to intestinal epithelium, were named "K" antigens before their composition was known. These antigens, called K88 and K99, are now known to be protein,

analogous to fimbriae; they are not capsular polysaccharide and should not be called "K." Under new classification schemes, fimbriae-associated K antigens have been renamed as F antigens.

The third category of antigens possessed by Enterobacteriaceae are flagellar, or "H" antigens. These antigens are protein in nature and heat labile. *Salmonella* species often will produce two different antigenic types of flagella, or H antigens, called "phase 1" and "phase 2." Obviously, only motile strains will display H antigens, but certain salmonellae may express only one of their two phases of antigens at a given time. These strains can be encouraged to express the second phase of their H antigens by cultivation in special media.

27.4.b. Serological characterization of *Salmonella* species. *Salmonella* species are characterized according to their O and H antigens in a scheme called the Kauffmann-White scheme. There are many more than 2000 different serovars of *Salmonella*, based on the combined O, Vi, and H antigens that each serovar expresses. In addition to their α-numeric serovars, each serovar is named for the town in which it was first isolated or some other factor with which it is associated. For practical purposes, these organisms are treated as if the name is a species; e.g., *Salmonella* subgroup I 1,4,5,12:i:1,2, representing the O:phase 1:phase 2 antigens, is called *Salmonella typhimurium*. Serotyping of isolates of Enterobacteriaceae is important for epidemiologic purposes (Chapter 5). The unabridged list of all currently accepted serovars can be found in *Bergey's Manual of Systematic Bacteriology*. Clinical laboratories often perform a very abbreviated preliminary serologic grouping on isolates of *Salmonella*, using commercially available polyvalent antisera designated A, B, C_1, C_2, D, E, F, G, H, and Vi. Some of the more common etiologic agents of gastrointestinal disease and enteric fever can be classified by their agglutination in antisera belonging to one of the pools. For example, *S. paratyphi* A is agglutinated by antiserum A, *S. typhimurium* is agglutinated by antiserum B, and *S. typhi* is agglutinated by antiserum D, unless it is Vi-positive.

The slide agglutination test is performed as described in Chapter 12. A suspension of the organism in physiologic saline must be tested for autoagglutination before antiserum is added. Those biochemically suspicious organism isolates that fail to agglutinate in the polyvalent antisera should be boiled by placing a heavy suspension of the organisms, in 0.5 ml sterile physiologic saline in a small screw-capped glass tube, into a beaker of boiling water for 15 to 30 minutes. Some isolates may require prolonged (up to 1 hour) boiling. After cooling, the suspension is retested for specific agglutination. All isolates that biochemically resemble *Salmonella* but fail to agglutinate in any typing sera should be sent to a reference laboratory for definitive identification. The widespread use of commercial biotyping systems with many parameters (discussed in Chapter 9) has allowed almost every laboratory, no matter how small, to identify definitively (by biotype) isolates that resemble stool pathogens recovered from patients with gastroenteritis. It is important to notify both the physician caring for the patient and public health workers (or the hospital epidemiologist) so that the patient may be appropriately isolated if he or she is in the hospital, or so that the patient may be instructed as to hygienic practices if at home, to prevent spread of the disease.

DNA homology studies have shown all *Salmonella* to be genetically identical. It has been proposed that they be given a new species name, *Salmonella enterica*, and that microbiologists continue to call them by their serovar names as is current practice.[7] It remains to be seen whether the microbiological community will accept this proposal.

27.5. Treatment of Infections due to Enterobacteriaceae

The great diversity among species of Enterobacteriaceae, as well as their propensity to indiscriminately pass genetic elements containing resistance factors among each other, makes it difficult to make specific statements about antimicrobial resistance. Multiple resistance is common among hospital strains of Enterobacteriaceae, those most involved in serious nosocomial infections. A few generalizations can be made, however. Environmental strains of Enterobacteriaceae are usually susceptible to aminoglycosides, trimethoprim-sulfamethoxazole, imipenem, and third generation cephalosporins. A recent study examining new species of Enterobacteriaceae showed *Klebsiella terrigena*, *Klebsiella planticola*, *Enterobacter amnigenus*, *Enterobacter intermedium*, *Rahnella aquatilis*, *Serratia fonticola*, *Serratia plymuthica*, and *Buttiauxella agrestis* to be resistant to chloramphenicol (which is rarely used for treatment today).[4]

Several genera of Enterobacteriaceae display patterns of resistance that aid in their identification. Technologists can check the biochemically derived identification with the known susceptibility pattern as a form of quality assurance. *K. pneumoniae* and *Citrobacter diversus* are resistant to ampicillin and carbenicillin; most *Enterobacter* species and *Hafnia* are resistant to ampicillin and cephalothin, although newer cephalosporins are more active against *Enterobacter*. Swarming *Proteus* species are usually resistant to nitrofurantoin, and *Proteus*, *Morganella*, and *Serratia* are resistant to colistin. *Providencia* and *Serratia* are multiply resistant, and *E. coli* (particularly community-acquired strains), in contrast, are often susceptible to all antibiotics tested.

Treatment of nosocomial infections associated with any of the Enterobacteriaceae usually consists of an aminoglycoside, alone or, more commonly, in combination with another agent such as a β-lactam. Some of the newer agents, such as cefoperazone, ceftazidime, cefotaxime, or mezlocillin, may be effective against *Proteus*, *Citrobacter*, *E. coli*, and *Klebsiella*. For nosocomially acquired infections, the best policy is to start empiric therapy based on the prevailing susceptibility patterns for known isolates in the institution, changing therapy if results of in vitro susceptibility tests indicate the necessity for change. For this reason, it is very important that the laboratory have available statistics concerning the percentage of susceptible isolates, categorized by species and antimicrobial agent. These statistics should be distributed to all clinicians and updated regularly. In the case of seriously ill patients, the best agents should be used in combination until data are available regarding the specific susceptibility pattern of the etiologic agent in question.

Treatment of Enterobacteriaceae-associated gastroenteritis varies with the severity of disease. Many infections, particularly with *Salmonella*, are self-limiting and should not be treated. Treatment may encourage development of the carrier state. If treatment is warranted, ampicillin or trimethoprim-sulfamethoxazole is the drug of choice. Quinolones may also be effective. Chloramphenicol may be necessary for life-threatening illness. Susceptibility tests are important, however, since ampicillin and multiply-resistant strains of *Salmonella* are being reported more frequently. *Shigella* are usually ampicillin-resistant. Trimethoprim-sulfamethoxazole, the quinolones, and furazolidone may be useful agents for treatment of bacillary dysentery. *Yersinia* are susceptible to chloramphenicol, aminoglycosides, tetracycline, and trimethoprim-sulfamethoxazole. *Y. enterocolitica* and *Y. pseudotuberculosis* septicemia have high fatality rates despite therapy; these syndromes require aggressive treatment with an aminoglycoside, ampicillin, or both. As stated previously, streptomycin or tetracycline is the preferred agent for treatment of plague. For severe disease, chloramphenicol can be added.

REFERENCES

1. Agbonlahor, D.E. 1986. Characteristics of *Yersinia intermedia*-like bacteria isolated from patients with diarrhea in Nigeria. J. Clin. Microbiol. 23:891.

2. Bottone, E.J. 1981. *Yersinia enterocolitica*. CRC Press, Boca Raton, Fla.

3. Chester, B., and Moskowitz, L.B. 1987. Rapid catalase supplemental test for identification of members of the family Enterobacteriaceae. J. Clin. Microbiol. 25:439.

4. Freney, J., Husson, M.O., Gavini, F., et al. 1988. Susceptibilities to antibiotics and antiseptics of new species of the family Enterobacteriaceae. Antimicrob. Agents Chemother. 32:873.

5. Karmali, M.A. 1989. Infection by verocytotoxin-producing *Escherichia coli*. Rev. Infect. Dis. 2:15.

6. Miller, J.M., and Farmer, J.J. III 1987. Recent additions to the Enterobacteriaceae. Clin. Microbiol. Newsletter 9:173.

7. Minor, L.L., and Popoff, M.Y. 1987. Designation of *Salmonella enterica* sp. nov., nom. rev., as the type and only species of the genus *Salmonella*. Int. J. Syst. Bacteriol. 37:465.

8. Yannelli, B., Schoch, P.E., and Cunha, B.A. 1987. *Serratia marcescens*. Clin. Microbiol. Newsletter 9:157.

BIBLIOGRAPHY

Akhurst, R.J. 1986. *Xenorhabdus nematophilus* subsp. *beddingii* (*Enterobacteriaceae*): a new subspecies of bacteria mutualistically associated with entomopathogenic nematodes. Int. J. Syst. Bacteriol. 36:454.

Brenner, D.J. 1984. Enterobacteriaceae Rahn 1937. In Krieg, N.R., and Holt, J.G., editors: Bergey's manual of systematic bacteriology, vol. 1. Williams & Wilkins, Baltimore.

Brenner, D.J., McWhorter, A.C., Kai, A., et al. 1986. *Enterobacter asburiae* sp. nov., a new species found in clinical specimens, and reassignment of *Erwinia dissolvens* and *Erwinia nimipressuralis* to the genus *Enterobacter* as *Enterobacter dissolvens* comb. nov. and *Enterobacter nimipressuralis* comb. nov. J. Clin. Microbiol. 23:1114.

Brubaker, R.R. 1984. Molecular biology of the dread Black Death. ASM News 50:240.

Centers for Disease Control. 1988. Summary of notifiable diseases United States. M.M.W.R. 36:1.

Clarridge, J.E., and Weissfeld, A.S. 1987. Enterobacteriaceae infections. p. 233-296. In Wentworth, B.B., Baselski, V.S., Doern, G.V., et al., editors. Diagnostic procedures for bacterial infections, ed. 7. American Public Health Association, Washington, D.C.

Farmer, J.J. III, Davis, B.R., Hickman-Brenner, F.W., et al. 1985. Biochemical identification of new species and biogroups of *Enterobacteriaceae* isolated from clinical specimens. J. Clin. Microbiol. 21:46.

Gavini, F., Izard, D., Grimont, P.A., et al. 1986. Priority of *Klebsiella planticola* Bagley, Seidler, and Brenner 1982 over *Klebsiella trevisanii* Ferragut, Izard, Gavini, Kersters, DeLey, and Leclerc 1983. Int. J. Syst. Bacteriol. 36:486.

Hendrickson, D.A. 1985. Reagents and stains. In Lennette, E.H., Balows, A., Hausler, W.J., Jr., and Shadomy, H.J., editors. Manual of clinical microbiology, ed. 4. American Society for Microbiology, Washington, D.C.

Hickman-Brenner, F.W., Fanning, G.R., Müller, H.E., and Brenner, D.J. 1986. Priority of *Providencia rustigianii* Hickman-Brenner, Farmer, Steigerwalt, and Brenner 1983 over *Providencia friedericiana* Müller 1983. Int. J. Syst. Bacteriol. 36:565.

Hickman-Brenner, F.W., Huntley-Carter, G.P, Fanning, G.R., et al. 1985. *Koserella trabulsii*, a new genus and species of *Enterobacteriaceae* formerly known as Enteric group 45. J. Clin. Microbiol. 21:39.

Howard, B.J., Klaas, J. II, Rubin, S.J., et al., editors. 1987. Clinical and pathogenic microbiology. The C.V. Mosby Co., St. Louis.

Karmali, M.A. 1987. Laboratory diagnosis of verotoxin-producing *Escherichia coli* infections. Clin. Microbiol. Newsletter 9:65.

Kosako, Y., Sakazaki, R., Huntley-Carter, G.P., and Farmer, J.J. III. 1987. *Yokenella regensburgei* and *Koserella trabulsii* are subjective synonyms. Int. J. Syst. Bacteriol. 37:127.

Lennette, E.H., Balows, A., Hausler, W.J., Jr., and Shadomy, H.J., editors. 1985. Manual of clinical microbiology, ed. 4. American Society for Microbiology, Washington, D.C.

MacFaddin, J. 1980. Biochemical tests for identification of medical bacteria, ed. Williams & Wilkins, Baltimore.

Müller, H.E., O'Hara, M., Fanning, G.R., et al. 1986. *Providencia heimbachae*, a new species of *Enterobacteriaceae* isolated from animals. Int. J. Syst. Bacteriol. 36:252.

Owen, R.J., Ahmed, A.U., and Dawson, C.A. 1987. Guanine-plus-cytosine contents of type strains of the genus *Providencia*. Int. J. Syst. Bacteriol. 37:449.

Washington, J.A. II., editor. 1985. Laboratory procedures in clinical microbiology, ed. 2. Springer-Verlag, New York.

28

Nonfermentative Gram-Negative Bacilli and Coccobacilli

The nonfermentative gram-negative bacilli are found in nature as inhabitants of soil and water and as harmless parasites on the mucous membranes of humans and animals. These bacteria can cause disease by colonizing and subsequently infecting immunocompromised individuals or by gaining access to normally sterile body sites through trauma. Less than one fifth of all gram-negative bacilli isolated from clinical specimens received in a routine clinical microbiology laboratory are likely to be nonfermentative bacilli, and the predominant species among those strains is *Pseudomonas aeruginosa*. Although nonfermenters comprise a small percentage of the total isolates recovered, they generally require more effort for their identification and often require specialized tests.

Pseudomonas is the second most common etiologic agent of nosocomial infections (after *Escherichia coli*) in many hospitals. Former members of the genus have been placed in new genera recently; further taxonomic changes are likely in the future. The genera *Moraxella* and *Acinetobacter*, covered in this chapter, are included in the family Neisseriaceae. Another genus in that family, *Kingella*, will be discussed in Chapter 29, since it is able to ferment glucose. *Moraxella urethralis* has been removed from the genus *Moraxella* and the family Neisseriaceae and placed into a new genus, *Oligella*.[21] The genus *Achromobacter*, formerly a valid taxon, has not been included in the *Approved Lists of Bacterial Names*, published in 1980. Organisms that were called "*Achromobacter xylosoxidans*" are now called *Alcaligenes xylosoxidans*.[12] In addition to the named bacteria covered in this chapter, there are several unnamed species, including Centers for Disease Control (CDC) Groups IVc-2, EO-2, and others (often similar to *Alcaligenes* or *Pseudomonas*) that have been recovered from clinical specimens. The definitive identification of all of the various nonfermentative gram-negative bacilli that might be encountered in a clinical laboratory is beyond the scope of this text. Readers are referred to the excellent references by Gilardi,[6] Pickett and Greenwood,[18] and Clark et al.[3] for detailed information and identification schemes.

28.1. Epidemiology and Pathogenesis of Infections due to Nonfermenters

28.1.a. *Pseudomonas aeruginosa.* The most frequently isolated nonfermentative bacillus found in clinical specimens, *P. aeruginosa*, has one of the broadest ranges of infectivity among all pathogenic microorganisms. This species can cause disease in plants, insects, fish, amphibians, reptiles, birds, and mammals. It is a significant cause of burn wound infections and nosocomial infections, and an unusual mucoid variant is almost universally found to colonize the respiratory tract of patients with cystic fibrosis. Particularly destructive infections of the eye (keratitis and endophthalmitis) are associated with *P. aeruginosa*; contact lens wearers are one group at increased risk for such infections. *P. aeruginosa* is the third most frequently isolated etiologic agent in hospital-acquired pneumonia. The organisms are so well adapted to survival in harsh environments that they can exist on the minimal organic nutrients present in distilled water. Underchlorinated water used to fill hot tubs was thought to be the vehicle of a widespread epidemic of *P. aeruginosa*–associated folliculitis that initially appeared across the United States during the late 1970s. Strains of *P. aeruginosa* have even been isolated from the disinfectant soap solutions used by nurses and physicians to wash their hands. When hospital environments are sampled, *P. aeruginosa* is found in drains, water faucets, sinks, cleaning solutions, medicines, and other sites, including the flowers in patients' rooms.

Although *P. aeruginosa* possesses many possible virulence factors, it must be remembered that it is a significant human pathogen only in compromised patients. Those strains that cause pneumonia appear to possess fimbriae that mediate adherence to respiratory epithelial cells. The mucoid polysaccha-ride, particularly pronounced in strains isolated from patients with cystic fibrosis, seems to protect the bacteria from phagocytosis. The ability of *P. aeruginosa* strains to destroy tissue may be related to the production of a number of extracellular enzymes, including proteases, elastase, and pigments that may inhibit growth of other bacteria (called **pyocins**), and hemolysins. In addition, virulent strains produce an exotoxin, called "exotoxin A," which inhibits protein synthesis much as does the toxin of *Corynebacterium diphtheriae*. Exotoxin A also seems to promote tissue destruction and aggravate the host's inflammatory response, further contributing to tissue damage. As do all other nonanaerobic gram-negative bacteria, *P. aeruginosa* possesses endotoxin.

28.1.b. Other pseudomonads, *Shewanella (Alteromonas), Comamonas, Chryseomonas, Flavimonas*, and *Methylobacterium.* Other pseudomonads that have been isolated from human clinical sources include a number of species that are saprophytic inhabitants of the soil and water, infecting humans as opportunistic pathogens. The number of isolations of *P. cepacia* in association with *P. aeruginosa* in respiratory secretions from cystic fibrosis patients has recently increased dramatically. The presence of this organism seems to be associated with decreased pulmonary function. Many strains of *P. cepacia* produce protease and lipase, and a number of strains also produce biologically active endotoxin. Most of the other pseudomonads and many other nonfermenters are isolated more frequently from respiratory specimens from cystic fibrosis patients than from patients with other types of pneumonia. These patients are particularly at risk for pulmonary infection due to these agents.

There are at least 24 species of *Pseudomonas* that have been implicated as the etiologic agents of human disease. Many more species can be recovered from the environment, including soil, water, and plants. Most of these species probably do not possess any particular virulence properties but infect humans opportunistically.

Specific syndromes, however, can be attributed to *P. mallei*, the agent of "glanders," and *P. pseudomallei*, the agent of "melioidosis", both considered to be "true" pathogens. Glanders, a disease of horses and occasionally other animals such as goats, sheep, donkeys, and dogs, is transmitted to humans by contact with infected animals. The disease, rarely seen in the United States, may present as a systemic septicemic infection, a local suppurative infection with lymphadenopathy, acute pneumonia, or chronic disease. Melioidosis, found primarily among returning Vietnam veterans and Southeast Asian immigrants, is usually a pneumonia-like illness, although it may be a systemic, febrile illness or an acute or chronic suppurative infection. Although *P. pseudomallei* can be found in the soil, *P. mallei* has been isolated only from animals that are susceptible to infection with this agent. The etiologic *Pseudomonas* species can be recovered from blood, aspirated lesion material, or respiratory secretions from patients suffering from glanders or melioidosis. *P. pseudomallei* and *P. mallei* both produce extracellular toxins, and *P. mallei* has an endotoxin-like material that may contribute to pathogenesis.

The relatively new genera *Shewanella* (originally named "*Alteromonas*"), *Protomonas*, and *Comomonas* include former *Pseudomonas* species that were found to differ from *P. aeruginosa* (the type strain) by cell wall component structures and genetic composition.[22] They are opportunistic pathogens similar to the pseudomonads. The new genera *Chryseomonas* and *Flavimonas* produce a yellow pigment but unlike most pseudomonads (with the major exception of *P. maltophilia*) they are oxidase-negative.[11] Virulence factors have not been studied for these species, although they have been isolated from human clinical specimens.

28.1.c. *Acinetobacter, Agrobacterium, Alcaligenes, Flavobacterium, Sphingobacterium*, and *Weeksella* species. These nonfermenters are found in soil and water. They infect humans when they have been introduced into a traumatic wound or by opportunistic colonization and infection of compromised hosts. In addition, *Acinetobacter* species have been isolated as the etiologic agent of pneumonia in healthy individuals, although they are primarily found as nosocomial pathogens.[13] *Alcaligenes*, which has recently undergone taxonomic changes to include former *Achromobacter xylosoxidans* and the naming of a new species, "*Alcaligenes piechaudii*," is most commonly recovered from sputum, cerebrospinal fluid, and blood of hospitalized patients. Although no definite virulence factors have been elucidated for any of these organisms, *Flavobacterium* species, in particular *F. meningosepticum*, is associated with outbreaks and sporadic cases of neonatal meningitis and septicemia. These bacteria must possess some mechanism such as neurotropism that allows them to produce such a syndrome. The flavo-

bacteria also produce proteases and gelatinase, which may contribute to virulence.[7] *Sphingobacterium multivorum*, formerly known as *Flavobacterium multivorum* and CDC Group IIk, is rarely isolated from humans.[5] *Weeksella zoohelcum* has been isolated from human wounds, especially those resulting from dog bites.[10] *Agrobacterium radiobacter* (synonym *A. tumefaciens*) has been isolated from sputum, blood, mucous membrane sites, and wounds.

28.1.d. *Eikenella, Moraxella, Taylorella*, and *Oligella* species. These genera are normal inhabitants of human mucous membranes of the mouth, upper respiratory tract, and genitourinary tract. From these sites, they can cause disease in immunosuppressed hosts. As with the other nonfermenters, infection may follow deposition in normally sterile tissues. *Eikenella corrodens* is a commonly recovered etiologic agent of human bite wound infections and is an important pathogen in many other types of infection on occasion. *Oligella urethralis*, formerly *Moraxella urethralis*, is a commensal in the human genitourinary tract and is an uncommon pathogen.[21] The new species *O. ureolytica*, formerly CDC group IVe, is also isolated from urine.[21] Its pathogenicity has not been documented. *Taylorella equigenitalis* was previously called *Haemophilus equigenitalis*; it has been isolated only from horses as the etiologic agent of equine metritis and will not be discussed further. The virulence factors that contribute to pathogenesis of disease due to these nonfermentative bacteria are not well characterized.

28.2. Laboratory Identification

28.2.a. General considerations. Once it has been determined that a gram-negative bacillus isolated from clinical material is not a member of the Enterobacteriaceae by criteria listed in Chapter 27 (Enterobacteriaceae are oxidase-negative; able to ferment glucose, as detected by production of a yellow butt in triple sugar iron agar [TSIA] or Kligler's iron agar [KIA]; and grow well on MacConkey and other media) and that the isolate is not *P. aeruginosa* (as detailed in Section 28.2.b), a set of preliminary tests must be performed to categorize the isolate so that it can be identified by the most expedient method. These tests include determining the ability of the organism to grow on MacConkey agar, the oxidase reaction, and determining whether the organism is able to metabolize carbohydrates or the circumstances under which the organism produces acid from the carbohydrates glucose and maltose. The

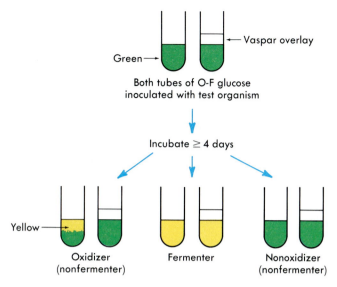

Figure 28.1
Interpretation of oxidative-fermentative (O-F) utilization of glucose test.

ability of an isolate to utilize carbohydrates and whether it does so oxidatively (in the presence of air) or fermentatively (in the absence of air) or both is one of the most important characteristics needed to separate the nonfermenters from Enterobacteriaceae.

It was first realized by Hugh and Leifson that organisms that were able to utilize carbohydrates only very minimally would produce tiny amounts of acid. In media containing large amounts of peptones and other protein sources, these organisms would utilize the peptones preferentially, producing enough alkaline end products to overshadow any pH indicator changes that might occur because of acid production. They developed a *low-peptone* medium, called "oxidative-fermentative" medium (O-F medium), that would allow detection of acid production by weak metabolizers. Preparation, inoculation, and interpretation of O-F medium test results are described in Procedure 28.1.

Oxidative-fermentative reactions are interpreted as shown in Figure 28.1. Fermentation takes place in the medium without oxygen (the overlaid tubes). Organisms that are able to ferment a carbohydrate are also able to oxidize it (the open tubes). These organisms are still called "fermenters." Organisms that produce acid products and yellow reactions only in open tubes are "oxidizers," and organisms that do not utilize glucose, either fermentatively or oxidatively, are called "nonoxidizers." Some nonoxidizers

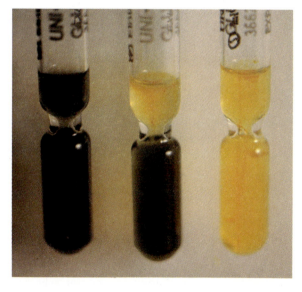

Figure 28.2
Commercially produced O-F media that incorporates both tests into one tube (Flow Diagnostics).

may actually produce such a large volume of alkaline end products that the indicator turns blue; this is called an "alkaline" O-F result. O-F media may be purchased from most media manufacturers. Flow Laboratories produces a single tube that can be inoculated for determination of both oxidative and fermentative glucose utilization (Figure 28.2).

Based on their reaction in oxidative-fermentative

PROCEDURE 28.1

Oxidative-Fermentative (O-F) Test For Carbohydrate Utilization

Principle

The small amount of acid produced by certain fermenters and oxidizers may be masked by larger amounts of alkaline products of protein metabolism. Carbohydrate fermentation reactions can thus be determined by testing such organisms in a medium with minimal proteins.

Method

1. Prepare O-F base medium as follows:

Peptone or tryptone	2 g
Sodium chloride	5 g
Agar	2.5 g
Dipotassium phosphate	0.3 g
Bromthymol blue	0.03 g
Distilled water	1000 ml

   Combine all ingredients, which are available from Difco Laboratories and standard chemical supply companies, or purchase O-F base from commercial suppliers of media (Appendix C). Adjust pH to 7.1 and divide the solution into several smaller flasks with known volume, one flask for each carbohydrate being prepared. For example, if O-F glucose, maltose, sucrose, lactose, and mannitol are to be made, divide the O-F base into five flasks containing 200 ml each. Autoclave the flasks at 121° C for 15 min.

2. Prepare 10% aqueous carbohydrate solutions by adding 2 g carbohydrate (glucose, lactose, etc.) to 20 ml distilled water. Immediately sterilize the carbohydrate solutions by passing them through a 0.2 μg membrane filter. Autoclave sterilization will destroy some of the carbohydrates. These solutions can be refrigerated for several months, although they may require redissolving before use.

3. When the O-F base has cooled to 55° C after autoclaving, aseptically add 20 ml of the sterile 10% carbohydrate solution to the 200 ml flask of O-F base, for a final concentration of 1% carbohydrate. The correctly prepared medium is green, but it appears somewhat bluish while it is still hot.

4. Dispense the 1% carbohydrate O-F media into 16 × 125 mm screw cap test tubes, 5 ml per tube. Allow the tubes to solidify upright (forming a semisoft butt), tighten caps, and refrigerate. The medium should be usable for several months. If desired, the base can be

(O-F) glucose, ability to grow on MacConkey agar, and oxidase reaction, all unusual non-Enterobacteriaceae may be placed preliminarily into a category requiring particular additional tests for identification (Figure 28.3). The ability of these organisms to utilize carbohydrates other than glucose is also usually tested in O-F medium; standard methods (Chapter 9) are used for performance of most of the other biochemical tests required to identify these organisms. Since indole production may be an important characteristic, a more sensitive method for extracting indole is often used for the nonfermenters (Procedure 28.2). The rapid spot indole test that uses *p*-dimethylaminocinnamaldehyde reagent (Chapter 9)

may also be satisfactory. Key differential characteristics of commonly recovered nonfermenters and related strains are shown in Table 28.1. Other clinically significant gram-negative bacilli that grow on conventional media, other than the nonfermenters mentioned in this chapter, are discussed in Chapters 29, 30, and 39.

In addition to biochemical metabolism, another important taxonomic feature of organisms classified as nonfermenters is the arrangement of their flagella. Performance of a flagella stain is not easy; it is an art that must be developed with experience. Flagella are fragile and tend to break off from the surface of bacteria during manipulation. Many individual bac-

dispensed without carbohydrates, which can then be added to melted and cooled tubes of base as needed (0.5 ml 10% carbohydrate to 5 ml base).

5. For testing the nature of glucose utilization, two tubes of 1% O-F glucose are inoculated. Material from isolated colonies is picked up with a straight wire and stabbed at least four times into each medium. Stabs should extend approximately 5 mm deep into the surface layer of the butt.

6. The medium in one of each of the two identical tubes is overlayed with sterile melted petrolatum or melted paraffin combined with an equal volume of petroleum jelly (called "vaspar") approximately 1 cm deep to prevent oxygen from reaching the inoculum. Sterile mineral oil is not recommended for overlaying the medium, because some lots are acidic and can contribute to false-positive results.

7. The tubes are incubated at 35° C for as long as 4 days and examined daily for production of acid, as indicated by a change in the bromthymol blue indicator from green to yellow.

Quality control

Test *P. aeruginosa* ATCC 27853 and *Alcaligenes faecalis* ATCC 8750 in O-F glucose and maltose.

Expected results

P. aeruginosa will be oxidative for glucose (yellow reaction in non-overlaid glucose and no color change in the overlaid tube) and non-fermentative, non-oxidative for maltose (will show no change in either of the maltose tubes). *A. faecalis* will show no change or a blue color indicating alkaline end products in the four tubes, as it is asaccharolytic.

Performance schedule

Test the quality control organisms each time a new batch of media is prepared and every 2 months thereafter.

teria within a culture will not produce flagella, and the stain sometimes fails to work. Procedure 28.3 outlines a flagella stain that should yield excellent results if all of the steps are followed carefully.

28.2.b. Identification of *P. aeruginosa.* As noted earlier, by far the most commonly encountered nonfermenter is *P. aeruginosa*. These organisms can grow on most routine laboratory media, including MacConkey agar. On 5% sheep blood agar, colonies are flat with a feathered edge, rough- or "ground glass"–appearing, and β-hemolytic (Figure 28.5). Colonies can grow to 3 to 5 mm in diameter within 48 hours incubation at 35°-37° C in air, and growth is equally good at room temperature. The mucoid (alginate-producing) strains isolated primarily from patients with cystic fibrosis may be blue-green or pale yellow-green, and they are extremely mucoid. This mucoid material may be produced in such quantities that it slides across the surface of the plate when the plate is tipped (Figure 28.6). *P. aeruginosa* exhibits a particularly striking characteristic odor, which resembles overripe grapes (or corn tortillas). Most strains of *P. aeruginosa* produce pyocyanin, a turquoise blue or blue water-soluble and chloroform-extractable pigment, visible on uncolored media, such as Mueller-Hinton agar (Figure 28.7), and especially visible on *Pseudomonas* P agar (Difco Laboratories) and Tech agar (BBL Microbiology Sys-

Table 28.1

Key Differential Characteristics of Commonly Recovered Nonfermenters and Related Strains

	CATALASE	OXIDASE	INDOLE	PIGMENT	UREASE
Acinetobacter	+	−	−	−	− / +
Agrobacterium	+	+	−	−	+ R
Alcaligenes	+	+	−	−	− / +
Bordetella	+	+	−	−	+ R
Chyrseomonas	+	−	−	Y	− / +
Comamonas	+	+	−	−	−
Eikenella	−	+	−	− / Y	−
Flavimonas	+	−	−	Y	− / +
Flavobacterium	+	+	− / +	Y	− / +
Kingella	−	+	− / +	− / Y	−
Methylobacterium	+	+	−	Pink	−
Moraxella	+	+	−	−	− / +
Ochrobactrum	+	+	−	−	+ R
Oligella	+	+	−	−	+ R / −
Pasteurella	+	+	+ / −	−	+ / −
Pseudomonas	+	+	−	+ / −	+ / −
Shewanella	+	+	−	+	− / +
Sphingobacterium	+	+	−	Y	+
Weeksella	+	+	+	Tan	+ R / −

+ = > 90% of strains positive; − = > 90% of strains negative; + / − = variable (most strains positive); − / + = variable (most strains negative); NM = nonmotile; N = none; P = peritrichous; Po = polar; PT = polar tuft; Y = yellow; R = rapid urease; ND = not done; O = oxidative; F = fermentative.
Modified from G. Gilardi (personal communication).

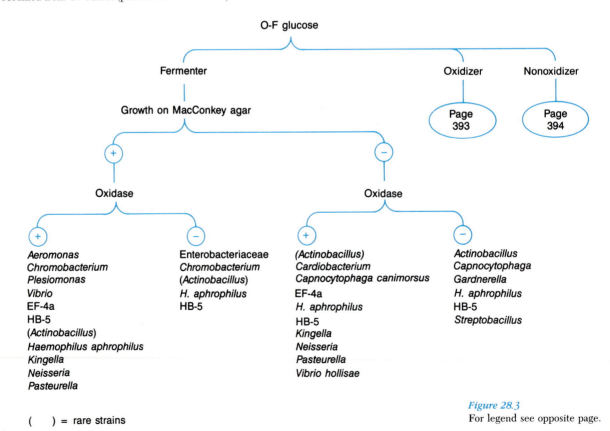

( ) = rare strains

Figure 28.3
For legend see opposite page.

H₂S IN TSI	SUSCEPTIBLE TO PENICILLIN	FLAGELLA	SUSCEPTIBLE TO POLYMYXIN	ARGININE DIHYDROLASE	OXIDATIVE/ FERMENTATIVE
−	−	N	+	−	O/ −
− / +	−	P	+	−	O
−	−	P	+	−	− / O
−	−	P	+	−	−
−	−	Po	+	+	O
−	−	PT	+	−	− / O
−	+	N	+	−	−
−	−	Po	+	−	O
−	−	NM	−	−	O/ −
−	+	N	+	ND	F
−	−	Po	− / +	−	O
−	+	N	+	−	−
−	−	P	+	−	O
−	+ / −	N/P	+	−	−
−	+	N	+	−	F
−	−	Po/P +	+ / −	+ / −	O/ −
+	−	Po	+	−	O
−	−	NM	−	−	O
−	+	NM	+ / −	−	−

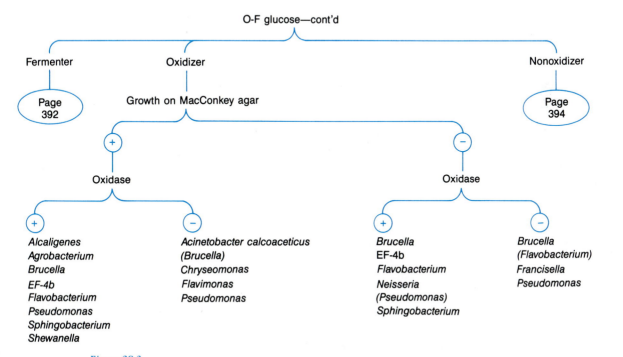

Figure 28.3
Initial characterization of gram-negative bacilli based on utilization of glucose in oxidative-fermentative (O-F) media, growth on MacConkey agar, and oxidase reaction.

Continued.

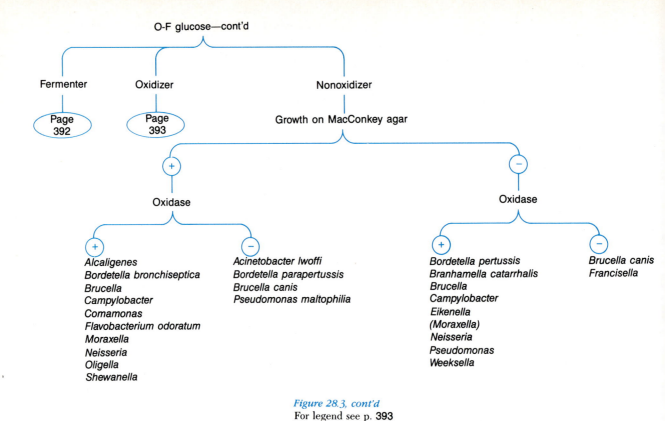

Figure 28.3, cont'd
For legend see p. **393**

PROCEDURE 28.2

Xylene Extraction For Demonstration of Indole Production

Principle

Small amounts of indole produced from the breakdown of tryptophan by tryptophanase must be extracted with xylene before they can be detected.

Method

1. Prepare Ehrlich's reagent as follows:

   Paradimethylaminobenzaldehyde
   (Sigma Chemical Co.)   2 g
   Ethyl alcohol (95%)   190 ml
   Hydrochloric acid
   (concentrated)   40 ml
   Store refrigerated in a brown bottle.

2. Add 1 ml of xylene to a 48 h culture of organisms in tryptone or trypticase broth or other appropriate medium. Shake the tube well, and allow it to stand for a few minutes until the solvent rises to the surface.

Modified from Bohme. 1906. Zentralbl. Bakt., Orig. 40:129.

3. Gently add about 0.5 ml of the reagent down the sides of the tube, so that it forms a ring between the medium and the solvent. If indole has been produced by the organisms, it will, being soluble in solvent, be concentrated in the solvent layer, and on addition of the reagent, a brilliant *red ring* will develop just below the solvent layer. If no indole is produced, no color will develop.

Quality control

Test *E. coli* ATCC 25922 and *Pseudomonas aeruginosa* ATCC 27853.

Expected results

The *E. coli* is strongly indole-positive (red ring) and the *Pseudomonas* is negative (no color or pale yellow ring).

Performance schedule

Test quality control organisms each time fresh reagents are made and monthly thereafter.

PROCEDURE 28.3

Flagella Stain

Principle

Tannic acid and fuchsin coat flagella, lending them enough thickness to be observed microscopically.

Method

1. Prepare solution A as follows:

   Basic fuchsin (certified for flagella stain;
     Aldrich Chemical Co.)   0.6 g
   Ethyl alcohol (95%)   50 ml
   Add the fuchsin to the alcohol and allow to stir overnight on a magnetic stirring plate to dissolve the fuchsin.

2. Prepare solution B as follows:

   Sodium chloride   0.37 g
   Tannic acid (Sigma Chemical Co.)   0.75 g
   Distilled water   50 ml

3. Combine solutions A and B and mix thoroughly. Adjust the pH to 5.0 with 1.0 N NaOH. Place the stain into a tightly capped brown bottle and let it remain for 3 days in the refrigerator (4° C) before using it, to allow it to cure. It is stable in the refrigerator for 1 month and in the freezer for at least 1 year. The stain deteriorates rapidly at room temperature. Use only the clear supernatant for the staining procedure; do not disturb the sediment that settles in the bottom of the bottle. Before performing each staining procedure, draw a small amount of the stain from the bottle and allow it to warm to room temperature. Discard the stain that is left over after the procedure.

4. Clean slides by soaking them in 3% concentrated hydrochloric acid in 95% ethanol for 4 days. Rinse thoroughly in tap water (by allowing tap water to run through the slides in a beaker for 10 min), and then rinse with several changes of distilled water. Lean the slides against an upright surface to drain and air dry.

5. Flame a clean slide in the blue flame portion of a gas burner. Do not allow carbon to be deposited on the slide. Enclose a rectangular area with a thick wax pencil line.

6. Place a large drop of distilled water at one end of the slide, within the wax-penciled area.

7. Pick up a small amount of growth from the tops of several young colonies on an agar plate or from a freshly inoculated slant on the end of an inoculating needle. Touch the needle to the drop of water on the slide in several places, allowing a small amount of the organism to disperse in the water. Tip the slide slightly to allow the drop of water to run toward the opposite end of the slide. Allow the suspension to air dry and do not heat fix before staining.

8. Apply 1 ml of the stain to the dry slide and observe the slide for the formation of a fine, metallic red precipitate (which will take 5-15 min). Each new batch of stain should be tested for optimal timing with a known flagella-producing organism.

9. Rinse the slide gently in tap water, holding the slide horizontally. Do not tilt to drain the water, and allow the slide to air dry.

10. Examine under oil immersion (1,000×) for flagella (Figure 28.4). It is possible that only a few of the bacteria in the suspension retained intact flagella; thorough examination is often required.

Quality control

Test a fresh culture of *P. aeruginosa* ATCC 27853.

Expected results

The organism should display polar flagella on at least 10% of cells seen.

Performance schedule

Test a quality control organism each time a flagella stain is performed.

Modified from Clark. 1976. J. Clin. Microbiol. 3-632.

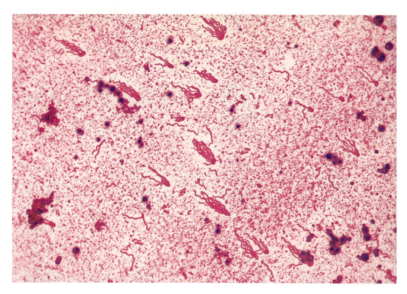

Figure 28.4
Bacteria stained with the flagella stain demonstrating peritrichous flagella.

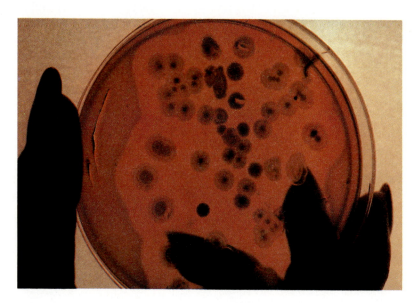

Figure 28.5
Strong β-hemolysis exhibited by most strains of *P. aeruginosa*.

tems). No other bacteria produce this pigment, so its detection is sufficient for identification of an isolate as *P. aeruginosa*. Some strains of *P. aeruginosa* produce other pigments, pyoverdins (yellow), pyorubrin (red), and pyomelanin (brown), which may mask the pyocyanin. Such strains, which appear yel-

low-green, blue-green, red, purple, or brown, must be further characterized. Occasional strains of *P. aeruginosa* fail to produce pyocyanin. These strains, however, are able to grow at 42° C, are able to dihydrolyze arginine, are motile by means of polar flagella, and are unable to produce acid in O-F lac-

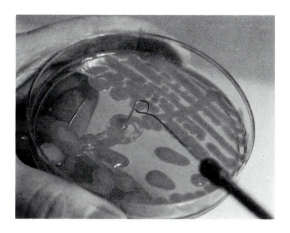

Figure 28.6
Abundant mucoid material produced by a strain of
P. aeruginosa isolated from a patient with cystic fibrosis.

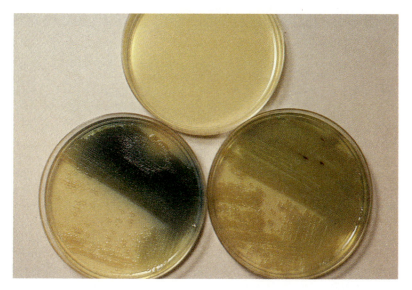

Figure 28.7
Two different pyocyanin-producing strains of *P. aeruginosa* and a control plate with no growth.

tose or sucrose. *P. aeruginosa* and other pseudo-monads isolated from humans often produce water-soluble fluorescent pigments; pyoverdin is also one of these. Fluorescent pigment–producing strains fluoresce under *short-wave* ultraviolet light (Figure 28.8). A standard Wood's lamp emits light at 365 nm; the fluorescence of pseudomonads is best observed at 254 nm.

Several selective agars have been developed for isolation of *P. aeruginosa* from "contaminated" spec-imens, such as stool. It has been shown that devel-opment of nosocomial infection with *P. aeruginosa* is often preceded by gastrointestinal colonization;

thus detection of colonized persons at risk of devel-oping *Pseudomonas* infection may aid in prevention of subsequent morbidity. Agar containing *cetrimide* (cetrimethylammonium bromide), available as Pseu-dosel agar (BBL Microbiology Systems); *irgasan* (2,2,2-trichloro-2-hydroxydiphenyl ether), available as irgasan agar (Difco Laboratories); and noncom-mercially available agar containing 30 µg/ml C-390 (9-chloro-9-[diethylaminophenyl]-10-pheny-lacridan), available from Norwich-Eaton Pharmaceu-ticals, have been used successfully.[19] Since C-390 inhibits the growth of all other bacteria, it may be used in an identification scheme. Isolates that grow

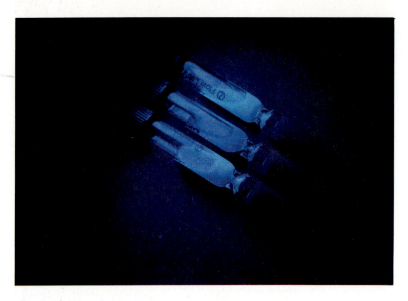

Figure 28.8
The two outer tubes were inoculated with fluorescing strains of pseudomonads; the central tube is the uninoculated control. Photograph taken under ultraviolet light.

on trypticase soy agar containing 30 μg/ml C-390 can be presumptively identified as *P. aeruginosa*.

For practical purposes, isolates on blood agar that exhibit the characteristic colonial morphology and odor, that are β-hemolytic, and that are oxidase-positive can be presumptively identified as *P. aeruginosa*. When the susceptibility pattern also agrees with that generally exhibited by *P. aeruginosa*, that of resistance to most antimicrobial agents except for aminoglycosides and colistin (polymyxin B), the identification is more certain. All *P. aeruginosa* strains are oxidase-positive, motile by means of polar flagella, able to oxidize glucose in O-F carbohydrate base, unable to oxidize maltose, unable to decarboxylate lysine or ornithine, and able to dihydrolyze arginine. As are all pseudomonads, they are catalase-positive. In addition to growth on C-390, all *P. aeruginosa* are able to grow at 42° C, an ability shared by several of the other *Pseudomonas* species but none of the other species that produce fluorescent pigment, such as *P. fluorescens* and *P. putida*. Fluorescent pigment may be enhanced by growth on *Pseudomonas* F agar (Difco Laboratories), GNF agar (Flow Laboratories), or Flo agar (BBL Microbiology Systems). In KIA or TSIA, *P. aeruginosa* yields an alkaline slant over a red or unchanged butt. Growth on the slant surface often appears metallic. Table 28.2 lists key characteristics used to differentiate

some more frequently isolated species of clinically important pseudomonads.

28.2.c. Identification of other *Pseudomonas* and similar species. *P. maltophilia* is second to *P. aeruginosa* in frequency of isolation. As the name implies, this species is able to oxidize maltose as well as glucose. Because *P. maltophilia* lacks certain key traits of the genus *Pseudomonas* (*P. maltophilia* possesses multitrichous polar flagella and is usually oxidase-negative), some workers have proposed moving it to the genus *Xanthomonas*, a group of yellow-pigment-producing plant pathogens. *Xanthomonas*, on the other hand, possesses a single polar flagellum, unlike *P. maltophilia*. The taxonomic status of *P. maltophilia* is uncertain at this time.

Colonies of *P. maltophilia* on blood agar are rough, lavender-green, and have an ammonia-like odor (Figure 28.9). They may be slightly α-hemolytic. The organism is oxidase-negative, arginine dihydrolase–negative, ornithine decarboxylase–negative, but lysine decarboxylase–positive (may be delayed). It does not produce pyoverdin, and most strains are unable to grow on cetrimide. *P. maltophilia*, rare strains of *P. cepacia* and *P. paucimobilis*, and some strains of *P. mallei* and *P. gladioli* (synonym *P. marginata*; very rarely isolated) are the only named oxidase-negative pseudomonads named (several unnamed strains are oxidase-negative).

Table 28.2
Some Characteristics of Commonly Encountered *Pseudomonas* and Related Species (Given as Percent Positive Reactions)

SPECIES (NUMBER OF STRAINS)	OXIDASE	GROWTH AT 42° C	GAS FROM NITRATE	ACID IN O-F† GLUCOSE	ACID IN O-F LACTOSE	ACID IN O-F FRUCTOSE	LYSINE DECARBOXYLASE	ARGININE DIHYDROLASE	ORNITHINE DECARBOXYLASE	GELATIN HYDROLYSIS
*P. aeruginosa** (91)	100	100	62	98	0	90	0	99	0	47
P. maltophilia (645)	2	50	0	100	86	99	99	0	0	100
P. cepacia (208)	93	60	0	100	99	100	91	0	66	74
P. fluorescens (217)	100	0	4	100	11	99	0	99	0	100
P. putida (310)	100	0	0	100	14	99	0	99	0	0
P. stutzeri (171)	100	90	100	100	0	94	0	0	0	0
P. putrefaciens (72)	100	76	0	97	0	53	0	0	99	94
P. paucimobilis (168)	90	0	0	100	100	100	0	0	0	0
Comamonas acidovorans (106)	100	9	0	0	0	100	0	0	0	2
P. alcaligenes (52)	100	54	0	0	0	0	0	8	0	2
Ochrobactrum anthropi (52)	100	10	96	98	0	98	0	40	0	0
Alteromonas putrefaciens (13)	100	0	0	100	15	100	0	0	92	100
Flavimonas oryzihabitans (101)	0	26	0	100	0	100	0	0	0	5
P. diminuta (44)	100	23	0	0	0	0	0	0	0	61
P. pickettii (56)	100	41	93	100	57	100	0	0	0	60
P. pseudoalcaligenes (76)	100	75	5	17	0	100	0	36	0	1
P. vesicularis (47)	100	0	0	58	0	0	0	0	0	38
Methylobacterium extorquens (22)	100	0	0	18	0	41	0	0	0	0

+ = > 90% of strains positive; − = > 90% of strains negative; +/− = variable (most strains positive); −/+ = variable (most strains negative).
*Apyocyanogenic strains.
†O-F, oxidative fermentative.
Data from Gilardi, G.L. 1984. Identification of glucose-nonfermenting gram-negative bacilli. Clin. Microbiol. Newsletter 6:111, 127; updated in January 1987 (personal communication).

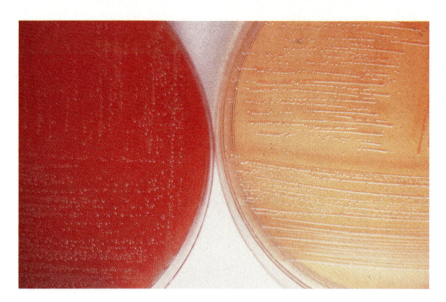

The pseudomallei group includes organisms that grow on a wide variety of organic compounds as single sources of carbon and energy. Several species in the group are not human pathogens, but *P. pseudomallei*, *P. mallei*, *P. cepacia*, *P. pickettii*, and *P. gladioli* have been isolated from clinical specimens. *P. pseudomallei* grows slowly on blood agar, forming colonies that may be wrinkled at first, becoming umbonate with time (Figure 28.10). Colonies exhibit varying degrees of hemolysis. Growth is characterized by a putrid odor followed by an aromatic, pungent odor. The organisms possess polar tufts of flagella and are able to grow at 42° C and on MacConkey agar. Of course, the clinical history of the patient is usually suggestive for melioidosis, which aids the microbiologist in identifying the etiologic agent.

P. mallei is the only nonmotile species in the genus *Pseudomonas*. This species, which may be suspected because of a clinical picture suggestive of glanders, is unable to grow at 42° C and may not grow on blood agar. Colonies on brain-heart infusion agar (with added glycerol) are grayish white and translucent after 48 hours incubation, later becoming yellowish and opaque. A Gram stain will reveal coccal forms and occasional filaments and pleomorphic forms that may branch. The CDC considers this organism to be too dangerous for routine laboratory study.[3]

The third species in the pseudomallei group is *P. cepacia*. Next to *P. aeruginosa*, *P. cepacia* is the pseudomonad most commonly isolated from cystic fibrosis patients and is an important nosocomial pathogen. *P. cepacia* may produce diffusible pigments, appearing as yellow or yellow-green, rough, serrate-edged colonies. It does not fluoresce. Strains are motile and able to oxidize glucose, lactose, maltose, and mannitol. It is resistant to polymyxin B.

In addition to *P. aeruginosa*, there are two other species that may produce fluorescent pigments, *P. fluorescens* and *P. putida*. Whereas *P. aeruginosa* has one polar flagellum, these two species have polar tufts of flagella. Many strains grow best at 30° C, and none grow at 42° C. Both species are resistant to carbenicillin. *P. stutzeri*, isolated from wounds, urogenital sources, and other sites, is distinguished by production of yellow to tan, flat, dry, and wrinkled colonies that resemble those of *P. pseudomallei* (Figure 28.11). *P. putrefaciens* (divided into two biovars based on oxidation of sucrose and maltose and requirement for Na[+]) is the only nonfermenter known to produce hydrogen sulfide (H_2S) in the butt of a TSIA or KIA slant. For this reason, an isolate may be mistaken for an H_2S-producing Enterobacteriaceae strain unless the oxidase result is checked. These strains are oxidase-positive. A number of other pseudomonads and similar organisms have been isolated from clinical material, including *Chryseomonas*

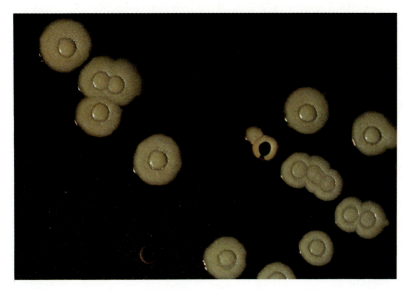

Figure 28.10
Colonies of *P. pseudomallei* after 96 hours of incubation on blood agar.

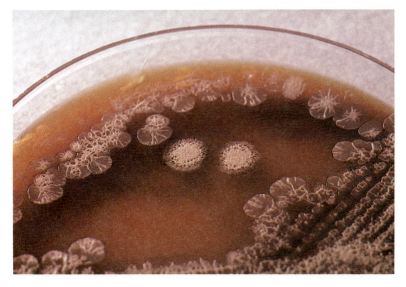

Figure 28.11
Dry, wrinkled colonies of *P. stutzeri* on blood agar after 48 hours of incubation.

luteola (formerly CDC group Ve-1), *Comamonas acidovorans, Comomonas. testosteroni, Flavimonas oryzihabitans* (formerly CDC group Ve-2), *Ochrobactrum anthropi* (formerly CDC group Vd), *Pseudomonas alcaligenes, P. diminuta, P. mendocina, P. mesophilica, P. paucimobilis, P. pickettii (P. tho-* *masii), P. pseudoalcaligenes, P. putida, Methylobacterium extorquens* (formerly *P. mesophilica* and *P. extorquens*, a pink-pigmented species), and *P. vesicularis*.[8,11,12,15-17] The reader is referred to references by Gilardi[6] and Clark et al.[3] for methods for definitive identification of these organisms. If a clin-

Table 28.3
Alcaligenes species

	NITRATE → NITRITE	NITRITE → GAS	ACID IN O-F XYLOSE
xylosoxidans subsp. *denitrificans*	+	+	−
xylosoxidans subsp. *xylosoxidans*	+	+	+
piechaudii	+	−	−
faecalis	−	+	−

+ = > 90% of strains positive; − = > 90% of strains negative; + / − = variable (most strains positive); − / + = variable (most strains negative).
Data from Clark et al.[3] and Kiredjian et al.[12]

ically significant isolate must be identified, it should be sent to an appropriate reference laboratory.

28.2.d. Genus *Alcaligenes* (including organisms formerly called *Achromobacter* species). The *Alcaligenes* species of clinical importance have been isolated from blood, respiratory secretions, infected wounds, urine, and several other sources. They are usually opportunistic pathogens, infecting patients with impaired host defenses. The genus *Alcaligenes* consists currently of four species, *A. faecalis* (also called "*A. odorans*" by CDC), *A. xylosoxidans* subsp. *xylosoxidans* (formerly called *Achromobacter xylosoxidans* and briefly known as *Alcaligenes denitrificans* subsp. *xylosoxidans*), *A. xylosoxidans* subsp. *denitrificans*, and the newly described *A. piechaudii* (Table 28.3).[12] *Alcaligenes* belong to the family *Alcaligenaceae*, which also includes *Bordetella* (Chapter 29) based on genetic similarity. All *Alcaligenes* are oxidase-positive and catalase-positive, possess peritrichous flagella (which distinguishes them from pseudomonads), asaccharolytic, and are able to utilize acetate as a sole source of carbon. On blood agar, the colonies are flat, spreading, and rough with a feathery edge. *Alcaligenes* does grow on MacConkey agar. *A. faecalis* is biochemically quite inert, whereas *A. xylosoxidans* species are able to reduce nitrate to nitrite. The strain of *A. faecalis* previously called *A. odorans* produces a distinctive sweet odor, reminiscent of fresh apple cider; colonies may be slightly α-hemolytic on sheep blood agar. *A. xylosoxidans* subsp. *xylosoxidans* oxidizes xylose and some strains may oxidize glucose weakly.

28.2.e. Genus *Acinetobacter*. Found as a major constituent of the flora of soil, water, and sewage and within the hospital environment, *Acinetobacter* is also found to colonize the skin of hospitalized patients. It may be involved in wound infections, par-

ticularly if there has been soil or water contamination of the wound. After *P. aeruginosa*, *A. calcoaceticus* is the most commonly isolated nonfermenter in clinical laboratories. It is possible that *Acinetobacter* species are actually normal flora of the skin and mucous membranes of humans. They have been implicated as etiologic agents of pneumonia (both community- and hospital acquired) and urinary tract infection. They may also be involved in sepsis and other infections.[13] The genus has recently been expanded to include species *A. baumannii*, *A. calcoaceticus*, *A. lwoffii*, *A. haemolyticus*, *A. johnsonii*, and *A. junii*, in addition to several unnamed species.[2]

Colonies on blood agar are convex, gray to white, 2 to 3 mm in diameter, and variably hemolytic (Figure 28.12). They are oxidase-negative and catalase-positive and may initially be confused with Enterobacteriaceae, since colonies resemble nonlactose-fermenting Enterobacteriaceae on MacConkey agar. *Acinetobacter* cannot, however, grow in the butt of a TSIA or KIA, and it cannot reduce nitrate. Differentiation from *P. maltophilia*, which is also oxidase-negative, may be based on the lysine decarboxylase reaction. *Acinetobacter* cannot utilize lysine in Moeller's decarboxylase media, whereas *P. maltophilia* is lysine decarboxylase–positive. *A. calcoaceticus* and *A. lwoffii* are clinically important. *A. calcoaceticus* (formerly known as *Herellea vaginicola*) is able to oxidize glucose, xylose, and some other sugars in oxidative-fermentative (O-F) carbohydrate base; whereas *A. lwoffi* (formerly known as *Mima polymorpha*) is inactive biochemically (Table 28.4). On Gram stain, the cells of *Acinetobacter* are very plump, almost coccoid rods that tend to resist alcohol decolorization; they may be mistaken for *Neisseria* sp. particularly when found intracellularly.

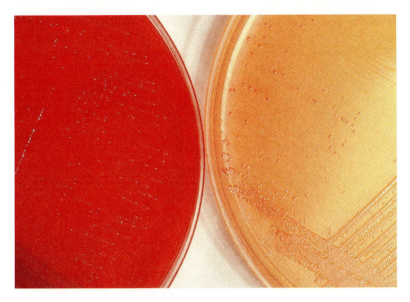

Figure 28.12
Colonies of *A. calcoaceticus* on blood and MacConkey agars.

Table 28.4
Acinetobacter,* Moraxella, and Oligella Species

	GROWTH AT 42° C	GELATIN HYDROLYSIS	UREASE	CITRATE	GROWTH AT 37° C	ACID IN O-F GLUCOSE	GROWTH IN 3% NaCl
Acinetobacter calcoaceticus	−	−	+ / −	+	+	+	NA
A. baumannii	+	−	NA	+	+	+	NA
A. haemolyticus	−	+	NA	+	+	+ / −	NA
A. junii	+	−	NA	+	+	−	NA
A. johnsonii	−	−	NA	+	−	−	NA
A. lwoffii	−	−	−	−	+	−	NA
Moraxella osloensis	−	−	−	−	+	−	−
M. lacunata	−	+ / −	−	−	+	−	+
M. phenylpyruvica	+ / −	−	+	−	+	−	+
Oligella urethralis	+	−	−	+ / −	+	−	+
O. ureolytica	−	−	+ †	− / +	+	−	+

+ = > 90% of strains positive; − = > 90% of strains negative; + / − = variable (most strains positive); − / + = variable (most strains negative); NA = not applicable.
*Only named species are listed.
†Rapid reaction.

Similar to most gram-negative bacilli but unlike other *Moraxella*-like organisms, *Acinetobacter* species are usually resistant to penicillin in vitro.

28.2.f. Genera *Moraxella* and *Oligella*. *Moraxella atlantae*, *M. lacunata*, *M. nonliquefaciens*, *M. osloensis*, and *M. phenylpyruvica* are important isolates from human clinical material. All are normal flora of the mucous membranes of humans and other animals. They have been isolated as the etiologic agents of nosocomial infections, wound infections, pneumonia, and other types of opportunistic infections. *Moraxella* species are gram-negative coccobacilli, and in the case of *Moraxella (Branhamella) catarrhalis*, the cells are true cocci. For this reason and because all *Moraxella* are oxidase-positive, *M. (B.) catarrhalis* will always be identified initially as a *Neisseria* species. The complete discussion of this organism has been included, therefore, in Chapter 26 with the *Neisseria* species, although *M. (B.) catarrhalis* is, by DNA homology studies, a true subgenus of the genus *Moraxella*.

Moraxella and *Oligella* are nonpigmented and are unable to utilize carbohydrates. Whereas *Moraxella* is nonmotile, *Oligella ureolytica* is usually motile. *Moraxella* and *Oligella urethralis*, but not *Oligella ureolytica*, are susceptible to penicillin. Most strains grow slowly on MacConkey agar, resembling non-lactose- fermenting Enterobacteriaceae. *M. lacunata*, isolated most frequently from eye infections, fails to grow on MacConkey agar but may produce pitting of blood agar. The organism is able to liquefy serum, so that depressions are formed on the surface of Loeffler's serum agar slants. Strains of *M. nonliquefaciens* may be very mucoid. *M. phenylpyruvica* is able to hydrolyze urea and deaminate phenylalanine. Other characteristics are shown in Table 28.4.

Oligella urethralis (formerly *Moraxella urethralis*) and *O. ureolytica*, newly named for species called CDC group IVe, are asaccharolytic, oxidase-positive, catalase-positive, small, coccoid bacilli. *O. ureolytica* is strongly urease-positive, with reactions detected within 30 minutes. *Bordetella* species also display such rapid urease reactions. Penicillin susceptibility will help differentiate *O. urethralis* from similar species.

28.2.g. Genus *Eikenella*. *E. corrodens*, the only species within the genus, is usually characterized by the ability to pit ("corrode") the agar. The organisms are found as normal flora in the human mouth and gastrointestinal tract, and they are common etiologic agents of human bite wounds and clenched fist wounds. They have also been isolated from cases of meningitis, endocarditis, aspiration pneumonia, osteomyelitis, brain and intra-abdominal abscess, and periodontitis. Because some isolates will initially grow only anaerobically, the organism was first thought to be an anaerobe and named "*Bacteroides corrodens*." An obligately anaerobic organism that greatly resembles *Eikenella* had been named *Bacteroides corrodens* and later *Bacteroides ureolyticus*. *Eikenella* is facultatively anaerobic and grows best in a humidified, capnophilic atmosphere.

E. corrodens is oxidase-positive but is unable to utilize carbohydrates. It is catalase-, urease-,

indole-, and arginine dihydrolase–negative, but lysine decarboxylase–and nitrate positive. Blood is required for growth, and chocolate agar is the most supportive medium. Colonies are yellowish, opaque, and consist of three distinct zones of growth: a moist, shiny central zone; a refractile circle of growth with a pearly sheen, resembling a mercury drop; and an outer flat, rougher spreading zone. The colonies are quite tiny, however, and because they often are sunk into small craters in the agar (pitting), they must be viewed under magnification. The colonies produce a bleachlike odor. In broth, the organisms grow in discrete granules, often adherent to the sides of the tube. Noncorroding colonies may also be seen, either as morphologic variants among the initial colonies of an isolate or as a homogeneous strain. Fresh isolates require hemin for growth. Gram stains reveal a small, even, straight-sided gram-negative bacillus. Because they are so resistant to clindamycin, a clindamycin-impregnated filter paper disk (5 μg clindamycin) may be used to help isolate the organism in mixed culture.

28.2.h. Genera *Flavobacterium*, *Sphingobacterium*, and *Weeksella*. So named because of their typical yellow pigment (Figure 28.13), the flavobacteria are ubiquitous inhabitants of soil and water, and they have been found in food as well as from sources within the hospital.[7] Although the flavobacteria grow best at 25° to 30° C, clinical isolates will grow at 35° C on initial isolation. The most clinically significant species is *F. meningosepticum*, an etiologic agent of neonatal meningitis and sepsis. Episodes of this syndrome are likely to occur as small epidemics, affecting a number of babies in the same nursery. Although many infants are asymptomatically colonized with the organism, mortality can be 50% among those who contract disease.

Other species, *F. breve*, *F. indologenes*, *F. odoratum*, and others, have only rarely been isolated from humans. *Sphingobacterium multivorum* and *S. spiritovorum*, former flavobacteria, were placed into a new genus based on cell wall structure. All species have been implicated as the etiologic agents of sepsis, wound infections, endocarditis, and pneumonia.[5] Flavobacteria, in addition to producing yellow pigmentation, usually grow on MacConkey agar (except for some unnamed strains), are catalase- and oxidase positive and nonmotile and (except for *F. odoratum*) are able to produce acid from glucose in O-F carbohydrate medium. *F. odoratum* produces a sweet,

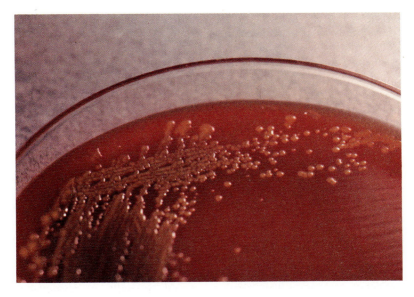

Figure 28.13
Yellow-pigmented colonies of *Flavobacterium* species on blood agar.

fruity odor similar to that of *A. odorans,* by which it can be recognized. All flavobacteria are resistant to penicillins and polymyxin. Because of extensive proteolytic enzyme production, colonies on blood agar are usually surrounded by a lavender-green discoloration. Gram stains of colonies reveal long, thin, filamentous gram-negative bacilli with occasional swollen ends. They are nonfermentative; some species are oxidizers. Indole, produced by many strains, must be detected using xylene extraction. Gelatinase is produced by most strains. The extracellular proteins and gelatinase may account in part for the virulence of some species.

Weeksella zoohelcum, formerly CDC group IIj, is nonsaccharolytic and nonmotile, unable to grow on MacConkey agar, and urease-positive. Growth on rabbit blood agar may yield sticky colonies.[3] This species is almost exclusively associated with animal bite wounds and scratches.

28.2.i. Genus *Agrobacterium.* Only one species of *Agrobacterium, A. tumefaciens,* formerly *A. radiobacter* (from the Greek *radius,* meaning "ray"; star-shaped aggregates of bacteria are observed occasionally), has been recovered from human clinical material. Normally an invasive plant pathogen, *A. tumefaciens,* has been isolated from wound infections, sputum, urine, and blood. Whether this organism is a true pathogen or only a saprophytic

contaminant has not been determined. *Agrobacterium* is oxidase variable (by Kovacs' method), rapidly urease positive, able to hydrolyze esculin, and motile by means of peritrichous flagella, unlike *Alcaligenes* and certain *Pseudomonas* species with which it may be confused.

28.3. Nonconventional Methods for Identification of Nonfermentative Bacilli

Numerous identification package systems, rapid methods, and automated methods are available for identification of nonfermenters. Because of the complexity and diversity of this group of organisms, no one system has proved to identify all nonfermenters accurately. New products are in developmental stages, so that eventually microbiologists will be able to obtain definitive identification more easily.

Several manufacturers produce miniature biochemical identification systems (Chapter 9). The Uni N/F Tek (Flow Laboratories), Oxi-ferm (Roche Diagnostics), Minitek (BBL Microbiology Systems), and two API systems, API Rapid NFT and the API 20E (Analytab Products), have all been used to identify nonfermenters. With those species that comprise the great majority of the isolates seen in routine clinical microbiology laboratories, each of the systems performs adequately. The unusual or rare species are identified with difficulty even in reference laboratories; the commercial systems should not be relied on for definitive identifications of such organisms. An example of the results of an early evaluation found that 72% of 229 clinical isolates were correctly identified by one commercial system.[14]

The makers of automated identification and identification/susceptibility testing systems have incorporated substrates and data bases for identification of nonfermenters. The AMS AutoMicrobic System (Vitek Systems, Inc.), the Avantage (Abbott Diagnostics), the Autobac IDX (General Diagnostics), and several manufacturers of MIC/ID systems in the microdilution tray format (Sceptor, BBL Microbiology Systems; MicroScan, American Scientific Products; and Fox, Micro-Media Systems) each include gram-negative nonfermenter identification capability. For all of these systems, approximately 90% of the clinically relevant nonfermenters tested will be identified accurately. Microbiologists should retain a slight skepticism, however, and correlate the results of the identification system of choice with the morphological characteristics, both cellular and colonial, growth characteristics, and other traits (smell, hemolysis, speed of growth) of the organism being examined. A novel approach for identification of oxidase-positive, glucose-negative, motile species of nonfermenters has been suggested by Pickett and Greenwood[18] to circumvent the arduous flagella stain. These tests use alkalinization of acetamide, arginine, histidine, saccharate, and urea to identify the bacteria. The media are available commercially.

Perhaps one of the most exciting prospects for identification of this complex group of organisms is the analysis of cell wall fatty acids by gas-liquid chromatography.[1,4] Available commercially as the MIS System (Microbial ID), this system uses extracts of cell wall components analyzed in a fused-silica capillary column in a GLC instrument (Hewlett-Packard) to arrive at species designations based on patterns of fatty acid methyl esters, unique for each species (Chapter 11). Preliminary results are very promising. Organisms are grown under standard conditions for 24 to 48 hours before extraction. The subsequent identification process requires approximately 4 hours.

28.4. Treatment of Infections Caused by Nonfermentative Gram-Negative Bacilli

Pseudomonads, particularly *P. aeruginosa*, are notoriously resistant to a large number of commonly used antimicrobial agents; they are usually susceptible to aminoglycosides, the drugs of choice. There is a tremendous amount of literature concerning treatment of *Pseudomonas* infections; treatment choices vary with the clinical situation and the site of infection. Certain medical centers experience a high rate of aminoglycoside-resistant *P. aeruginosa* isolates. New β-lactam antimicrobials, including cefsulodin, ceftazidime, imipenem, and others, have shown promise, although resistance can occur during a course of therapy. If the organism is susceptible, piperacillin, mezlocillin, carbenicillin, or moxalactam may be chosen. For serious infections, high dosage of the β-lactam drug and combination therapy (addition of an aminoglycoside) is recommended. It is beyond the scope of this text to discuss the many ramifications of therapy of *Pseudomonas* infections.

Most strains of *Alcaligenes* are susceptible to some aminoglycosides, carbenicillin, rifampin, piperacillin, cefoperazone, cefamandole, trimethoprim-sulfamethoxazole, and colistin. For *Alcaligenes* species, in vitro susceptibility test results should be used to guide therapy. *Acinetobacter* species are usually susceptible to trimethoprim-sulfamethoxazole, carbenicillin, cefotaxime, and ceftizoxime. Aminoglycosides and imipenem are also usually effective. The new quinolones are extremely active against *Acinetobacter* species.[20] For serious infections, combinations of an aminoglycoside and a β-lactam drug are recommended. *Moraxella* species are susceptible to penicillin, ampicillin, chloramphenicol, and aminoglycosides in vitro. *E. corrodens* has been successfully treated with penicillin, ampicillin, carbenicillin, and tetracycline. Newer agents such as moxalactam and third-generation cephalosporins, as well as the quinolones, are also effective against *Eikenella* in vitro.[9]

Flavobacteria are multiply resistant, although most isolates are susceptible to trimethoprim-sulfamethoxazole, rifampin, moxalactam, cefotaxime, and clindamycin. In vitro bactericidal susceptibility tests should be used to guide therapy of serious infections. Treatment with erythromycin has not been generally successful, although in vitro test results indicate susceptibility. Most strains are resistant to aminoglycosides, penicillins, and chloramphenicol. Limited susceptibility data available for *Agrobacterium* species indicate most strains tested were susceptible to carbenicillin, gentamicin, piperacillin, and tetracycline and resistant to penicillin, chloramphenicol, cephalosporins, amikacin and tobramycin.[6]

REFERENCES

1. Alexander, H. 1987. Gas-liquid chromatography as an aid in identification of glucose-nonfermenting gram-negative bacilli. Clin. Microbiol. Newsletter 9:25.
2. Bouvet, P.J.M., and Grimont, P.A.D. 1986. Taxonomy of the genus *Acinetobacter* with the recognition of *Acinetobacter baumannii* sp. nov., *Acinetobacter haemolyticus* sp. nov., *Acinetobacter johnsonii* sp. nov., and *Acinetobacter junii* sp. nov. and emended descriptions of *Acinetobacter calcoaceticus* and *Acinetobacter lwoffi*. Int. J. Syst. Bacteriol. 36:228.
3. Clark, W.A., Hollis, D.G., Weaver, R.E., et al. 1984. Identification of unusual pathogenic gram-negative aerobic and facultatively anaerobic bacteria, CDC. U.S. Department of Health and Human Services, Atlanta, Ga.
4. Dees, S.B., Moss, C.W., Hollis, D.G., et al. 1986. Chemical characterization of *Flavobacterium odoratum*, *Flavobacterium breve*, and *Flavobacterium*-like groups IIe, IIh, and IIf. J. Clin. Microbiol. 23:267.
5. Freney, J., Hansen, W., Ploton, C., et al. 1987. Septicemia caused by *Sphingobacterium multivorum*. J. Clin. Microbiol. 25:1126.
6. Gilardi, G.L. 1984. Identification of glucose-nonfermenting gram-negative bacilli. Clin. Microbiol. Newsletter 6:111. Updated periodically in the Newsletter and available from Dr. Gilardi, North General Hospital, 1919 Madison Ave., New York, NY 10035.
7. Gilardi, G.L. 1986. *Flavobacterium*. Clin. Microbiol. Newsletter 8:143.
8. Gilchrist, M.J.R., Kraft, J.A., Hammond, J.G., et al. 1986. Detection of *Pseudomonas mesophilica* as a source of nosocomial infections in a bone marrow transplant unit. J. Clin. Microbiol. 23:1052.
9. Goldstein, E.J.C., Citron, D.M., Vagvolgyi, A.E., et al. 1986. Susceptibility of *Eikenella corrodens* to newer and older quinolones. Antimicrob. Agents Chemother. 30:172.
10. Holmes, B., Steigerwalt, A.G., Weaver, R.E., et al. 1986. *Weeksella zoohelcum* sp. nov. (formerly group IIj), from human clinical specimens. System. Appl. Microbiol. 8:191.
11. Holmes, B., Steigerwalt, A.G., Weaver, R.E., et al. 1987. *Chryseomonas luteola* comb. nov. and *Flavimonas oryzihabitans* gen. nov., comb. nov., *Pseudomonas*-like species from human clinical specimens and formerly known, respectively, as groups Ve-1 and Ve-2. Int. J. Syst. Bacteriol. 37:245.
12. Kiredjian, M., Holmes, B., Kersters, K., et al. 1986. *Alcaligenes piechaudii*, a new species from human clinical specimens and the environment. Int. J. Syst. Bacteriol. 36:282.
13. Lyons, R.W. 1983. *Acinetobacter calcoaceticus*. Clin. Microbiol. Newsletter 5:87.
14. Martin, R., Siavoshi, F., and McDougal, D.L. 1986. Comparison of Rapid NFT System and conventional methods for identification of nonsaccharolytic gram-negative bacteria. J. Clin. Microbiol. 24:1089.
15. Morrison, A.J., and Shulman, J.A. 1986. Community-acquired bloodstream infection caused by *Pseudomonas paucimobilis*: case report and review of the literature. J. Clin. Microbiol. 24:853.
16. Morrison, A.J., Jr., and Boyce, K. IV. 1986. Peritonitis caused by *Alcaligenes denitrificans* subsp. *xylosoxydans*: case report and review of the literature. J. Clin. Microbiol. 24:879.
17. Peel, M.M., Hibberd, A.J., King, B.M., et al. 1988. *Alcaligenes piechaudii* from chronic ear discharge. J. Clin. Microbiol. 26:1580.
18. Pickett, M.J., and Greenwood, J.R. 1986. Identification of oxidase-positive, glucose-negative, motile species of nonfermentative bacteria. J. Clin. Microbiol. 23:920.
19. Robin, T., and Janda, J.M. 1984. Enhanced recovery of *Pseudomonas aeruginosa* from diverse clinical specimens on a new selective agar. Diagn. Microbiol. Infect. Dis. 2:207.
20. Rolston, K.V.I., and Bodey, G.P. 1986. In vitro susceptibility of *Acinetobacter* species to various antimicrobial agents. Antimicrob. Agents Chemother. 30:769.
21. Rossau, R., Kersters, K., Falsen, E., et al. 1987. *Oligella*, a new genus including *Oligella urethralis* comb. nov. (formerly *Moraxella urethralis*) and *Oligella ureolytica* sp. nov. (formerly CDC Group IVe): relationship to *Taylorella equigenitalis* and related taxa. Int. J. Syst. Bacteriol. 37:198.
22. Tamaoka, J., Ha, D.-M., and Komagata, K. 1987. Reclassification of *Pseudomonas acidovorans* den Dooren de Jong 1926 and *Pseudomonas testosteroni* Marcus and Talalay 1956 as *Comamonas acidovorans* comb. nov. and *Comamonas testosteroni* comb. nov., with an emended description of the genus *Comamonas*. Int. J. Syst. Bacteriol. 37:52.

BIBLIOGRAPHY

Hugh, R., and Gilardi, G.L. 1980. *Pseudomonas*. In Lennette, E.H., Balows, A., Hausler, W.J., Jr., and Truant, J.P., editors. Manual of clinical microbiology, ed. 3. American Society for Microbiology, Washington, D.C.

Palleroni, N.J. 1984. Genus *Pseudomonas Migula 1894*. In Krieg, N.R., and Holt, J.G., editors. Bergey's manual of systematic bacteriology, ed. 9. Williams & Wilkins, Baltimore.

Symposium on *Pseudomonas aeruginosa* infections. 1983. Rev. Infect. Dis. 5(suppl.5):δ833.

29

Gram-Negative Facultatively Anaerobic Bacilli and Aerobic Coccobacilli

Nine named genera and three unnamed species of gram-negative organisms are discussed in this chapter. Three genera, *Pasteurella*, *Brucella*, and *Francisella*, are primarily agents of zoonoses and infect humans only by accident, when the humans come into close contact with the preferred animal hosts, with insects that have acquired the organisms from the animals, or environmental contamination. *Capnocytophaga canimorsus* (formerly DF-2), named **dysgonic** fermenter by the Centers for Disease Control (CDC) because the organism grows poorly in standard microbiological media, is also carried by animals as normal oral flora, particularly in dogs and rarely in cats. DF-3 may also be normal flora of animals. Six other genera: *Haemophilus, Bordetella, Kingella, Cardiobacterium, Capnocytophaga,* and *Actinobacillus,* are found among the normal flora of the human respiratory tract and occasionally other mucosal surfaces. Organisms designated by the CDC as HB-5 seem to be normal flora of the human genitourinary mucosa. All of the organisms discussed in this chapter are morphologically **pleomorphic,** occurring as short bacilli, coccobacilli, or exhibiting chains or filamentous forms. *Cardiobacterium, Capnocytophaga, Pasteurella,* HB-5, *Kingella,* and *Actinobacillus* species will grow on routine laboratory media, but the other genera may require specialized growth factors.

29.1. Genus *Francisella*

29.1.a. Epidemiology and pathogenesis of *Francisella* infection. *Francisella* consists of *F. tularensis,* the agent of human and animal tularemia, and two other related species. *F. novicida,* a rare human pathogen that is genetically identical to *F. tularensis* (it has been proposed to reclassify this organism as a biogroup of *F. tularensis*), and the proposed species "*F. philomiragia.*" *F. novicida* was isolated from lymph nodes and blood, respectively, of two human patients whose disease resembled tularemia (R. E. Weaver, CDC), although *F. novicida* is primarily an animal pathogen. "*F. philomiragia*" has been isolated from several patients, many of whom were immunocompromised or were victims of near-drowning incidents. The organism is present in animals and ground water.

F. tularensis is carried by many species of wild rodents, rabbits, beavers, and muskrats in North America. Humans become infected by handling the carcasses or skin of infected animals, through insect vectors (chiefly deerflies and ticks in the United States), by being bitten by carnivores that have themselves eaten infected animals, or by inhalation. The capsule of *F. tularensis* may be a factor in virulence, allowing the organism to avoid immediate destruction by polymorphonuclear neutrophils. The organism is extremely invasive, being one of only a few infectious agents reported to penetrate intact skin, still a debatable property. In addition to invasiveness, the organisms are intracellular parasites, able to survive in the cells of the reticuloendothelial system, where they reside after a bacteremic phase.

Granulomatous lesions may develop in various organs. Patients experience high fevers, headache, lymphadenopathy, and an ulcerative lesion at the site of inoculation. Pneumonia and rhabdomyolysis (evidenced by elevated creatine phosphokinase levels and hemoglobinuria without red blood cells) are common complications. Pneumonia may be seen as a primary infection. Tularemia is primarily a disease of adult men who hunt since they have the most contact with wild animals and are most likely to be exposed to the insect vectors.

29.1.b. Laboratory identification. *F. tularensis* is a Biosafety level 2 pathogen, a designation that requires technologists to wear gloves and to work within a biological safety cabinet when handling material that potentially harbors this agent. Because tularemia is one of the most common laboratory-acquired infections, however, most microbiologists do not attempt to work with infectious material from suspected cases. We recommend that specimens be sent to reference laboratories or state or other public health laboratories that are equipped to handle *Francisella.* The CDC has fluorescent antibody stains available for direct detection of the organism in lesion smears, but such procedures are best performed by reference laboratories.

F. tularensis is strictly aerobic and requires enriched media (containing cysteine and cystine) for primary isolation. Commercial media for cultivation of the organism are available (glucose cystine agar, BBL Microbiology Systems, and cystine heart agar, Difco Laboratories); both require the addition of 5% sheep or rabbit blood. *F. tularensis* may also grow on chocolate agar and rarely on Thayer-Martin agar with prolonged incubation. It does not grow on MacConkey agar, and growth is not enhanced by carbon dioxide. The organisms, which grow slowly, requiring 2 to 4 days for maximum colony formation, are weakly catalase positive and oxidase-negative. Some strains may require up to 2 weeks to develop visible colonies. A recent report has documented isolation of *F. tularensis* in the Bactec 460 blood culture system (Johnston Laboratories) from blood of four patients.[16] Organisms did not show positive growth indices until a minimum of three days after inoculation.

Colonies are transparent, mucoid, and easily emulsified. Although carbohydrates are fermented, isolates should be identified serologically (by agglutination) or by a fluorescent antibody stain. Ideally they should be sent to a reference laboratory for characterization. Diagnosis of disease in patients is usually accomplished serologically by whole cell agglutination (febrile agglutinins, Chapter 12) or by newer enzyme-linked immunosorbent assay (ELISA) techniques.

F. novicida and "*F. philomiragia*" do not require cysteine or cystine for isolation, although they resemble *F. tularensis* by being small, coccobacillary rods that grow poorly or not at all on MacConkey agar. These two species differ from *F. tularensis* biochemically; *F. philomiragia* is oxidase-positive and most strains will produce H_2S in triple sugar iron agar medium, produce gelatinase, and grow in 6% NaCl (no strains of *F. tularensis* share either characteristic). *F. novicida* is oxidase-negative, may grow on MacConkey agar and in 6% NaCl, and all three strains tested are able to oxidize glucose and sucrose in oxidative-fermentative media.

29.1.c. Treatment of *Francisella* infections. The organism is susceptible to aminoglycosides, and streptomycin is the drug of choice. Gentamicin is a possible alternative; tetracycline and chloramphenicol have also been used, although the latter two agents have been associated with a higher rate of relapse following treatment.

29.2. Genus *Brucella*

29.2.a. Epidemiology and pathogenesis of *Brucella* infection. The agents of brucellosis, *Brucella* species, are normal flora of the genital and urinary tracts of many animals including goats, pigs, cows, and dogs. Most humans acquire disease through ingestion of contaminated milk or through occupational exposure; the disease is particularly common among abattoir workers. Farmers and veterinarians are also at increased risk. The primary virulence factor for *Brucella* seems to be the organism's ability to survive intracellularly. It is probably this characteristic, as well as granuloma and abscess formation, that accounts for the chronic and relapsing nature of the febrile disease. Patients often present with a gradual onset of nonspecific systemic symptoms, including fever, malaise, chills, sweats, fatigue, and mental changes. Localized lesions can occur in most any organ or bone; they may be granulomatous or suppurative and destructive. An infectious, mononucleosis like illness may occur. Pulmonary, cardiovascular, hepatic, skeletal, genitourinary, and central nervous system localization are also possible complications.

29.2.b. Collection and transport of specimens. *Brucella* species are usually isolated from blood cultures or bone marrow cultures during the acute illness. Organisms may also be recovered from joint fluid of patients with arthritis. Blood cultures may require prolonged incubation times, as mentioned in Chapter 14. Bone marrow cultures are handled as discussed in Chapter 21. Material from infected lymph nodes, other tissue, cerebrospinal fluid, and urine may also yield *Brucella*. The laboratory should be notified that brucellosis is suspected so that supplemented media that better support growth of the organism can be inoculated. Although most strains will grow on chocolate and blood agar and some strains will grow on MacConkey agar, *Brucella* agar (Gibco Laboratories and BBL) or some type of infusion base agar is recommended. The addition of 5% heated horse or rabbit serum will enhance growth on all media. Cultures should be incubated in 5% to 10% CO_2 in a humidified atmosphere, such as a candle extinction jar.

Blood cultures are held for 4 weeks, and inoculated plates are incubated for 3 weeks before being discarded as negative. It has been found that organisms may be present in blood culture broths without visible evidence and without an increase in the growth index as measured on the Bactec radiometric blood culture instrument. For this reason, weekly blind subcultures to *Brucella* broth are recommended for optimal recovery of *Brucella* species from blood cultures. The use of biphasic blood culture bottles (Castañeda type with an agar slant and broth) is a more cost-effective option, and the bottles are less likely to become contaminated during repeated subcultures. *Brucella* is also considered to be a type 2 biohazard and should be handled with all appropriate precautions. Many laboratory-acquired cases of brucellosis have been documented; it is one of the most prevalent laboratory-acquired infections.

29.2.c. Laboratory identification. Serologic tests are used for diagnosis more commonly than are cultures (*Brucella* is one of the "febrile agglutunins"), but culture results are more definitive. Both IgM and IgG are quantified initially; IgM is then inactivated by 2 mercaptoethanol to reveal rising antibody titers of IgG without IgM interference. Definitive serologic diagnosis should be performed by an experienced reference laboratory.

On culture, colonies appear small, convex, smooth, translucent, and slightly yellow and opales-

PROCEDURE 29.1

Special Tests for Species Differentiation Among Brucella

1. Urease activity is determined by inoculating a large loopful of growth from a broth suspension made from isolated colonies to the surface of a Christensen's urea agar slant (Chapter 9).

2. Examine the slant immediately and incubate the slant at 37° C, examining at 15 min, 1 h, 2 h, and 24 h.

3. Urease activity is evidenced by a change in color on the slant surface from yellow to pink to bright pinkish-purple.

4. Production of hydrogen sulfide is determined by placing a strip of lead acetate–impregnated filter paper (available from Remel Laboratories and other suppliers) suspended in the atmosphere above an agar slant culture (trypticase soy agar or serum-supplemented agar) of the organism being tested. The paper must not contact the agar or the sides of the tube. This can be accomplished by bending the paper over the edge of the tube mouth before lightly screwing on the cap, leaving a length of the strip inside the tube.

5. The tube is incubated at 37° C in air or CO_2, as required, and the paper strip is examined and changed daily. A complete blackening of the entire strip after the first day, or slight

blackening of the strip on subsequent days, is indicative of hydrogen sulfide production.

6. Growth on media containing aniline dyes is determined by incorporating the dyes thionine and basic fuchsin (available from National Aniline Division, Allied Chemical and Dye Co.) in tryptic soy agar plates. Dyes are prepared by boiling 0.1 g of each dye in 100 ml distilled water and adding 2 ml dye solution to 100 ml molten agar before pouring plates of 20 ml agar per plate to yield a final dye concentration of 1:50,000 (wt/vol). Different lots of dye may vary, so testing plates with quality control strains is necessary.

7. Equal quantities of the organisms are inoculated to plates without dyes and plates with each dye, and the inocula are streaked for isolation in four quadrants. The plates are incubated at 37° C in the appropriate atmosphere for up to 4 days and examined for growth. Growth in at least three quadrants is considered positive.

Quality control

Because strains of *Brucella* must be maintained and manipulated to assess the performance characteristics of these media adequately, we recommend that only reference laboratories with extensive experience with this genus perform the tests described above.

Modified from Corbel, M.J. and Brinley-Morgan, W.J. 1984. Genus *Brucella* (Meyer and Shaw 1920). In Krieg, N.R., and Holt, J.G., editors. Bergey's manual of systematic bacteriology, vol 1. Williams & Wilkins, Baltimore.

---

cent after at least 48 hours incubation. The colonies may become brownish with age. The organisms are catalase-positive and most strains are oxidase-positive. None of the *Brucella* species oxidize carbohydrates; other nonfermentative gram-negative coccobacilli that may be confused with *Brucella* are *Bordetella*, *Moraxella*, *Kingella*, *Acinetobacter* species, and others (Chapter 28). *Brucella*, however, is nonmotile, urease- and nitrate-positive, and strictly aerobic.

The most rapid test for presumptive identification of *Brucella* is the particle agglutination test with antismooth *Brucella* serum, available from Difco Lab-

oratories. Agglutination is carried out as described in Chapter 12. This test cannot be performed on rough colony variants. Six species of *Brucella* may be isolated from humans: *B. melitensis*, *B. abortus*, *B. suis*, *B. canis*, *B. ovis* (rare), and *B. neotomae* (also rare). The species are differentiated by the rapidity with which they hydrolyze urea, their relative ability to produce hydrogen sulfide (H_2S) gas, their requirements for CO_2, and their susceptibility to the aniline dyes thionine and basic fuchsin, as briefly described in Procedure 29.1. Performance of the urease and H_2S detection tests is also described in Procedure 29.1. Differential characteristics are

Table 29.1

Characteristics of *Brucella* Species

SPECIES	CO₂ REQUIRED FOR GROWTH	TIME TO POSITIVE UREASE	H₂S PRODUCED	GROWTH ON MEDIA CONTAINING	
				THIONINE*	FUCHSIN*
abortus	$+/-$	2 h (rare 24 h)	$+$ (most strains)	$+/-$	$+/-$ (most strains $+$)
melitensis	$-$	2 h (rare 24 h)	$-$	$+$	$+$
suis	$-$	15 min	$+/-$	$+$	$-$ (most)
ovis	$+$	≥ 7 days	$-$	$+$	$-$ (most)
neotomae	$-$	15 min	$+$	$-$	$-$
canis	$-$	15 min	$-$	$+$	$-$ (most)

$+$ = >90% of strains positive; $-$ = >90% of strains negative; $+/-$ = variable results.
*1:50,000 wt/vol, as described in text.

listed in Table 29.1. For determination of CO_2 requirement, identical plates of *Brucella* agar or brain heart infusion agar should be given equal inocula (with a calibrated loop, for example) of a broth suspension of the organism to be tested. One plate should be incubated in a candle jar and the other plate should be incubated in air, both in the same incubator. Most strains of *B. abortus* and all strains of *B. ovis* will not grow in air but will show growth in the candle jar. Isolates of *Brucella* should be sent to state or other reference laboratories for confirmation or definitive identification since most clinical laboratories lack the necessary media and containment facilities. The tests are variable enough to necessitate very stringent quality control measures employing known strains of *Brucella*. Because of the difficulty of isolating the organism, many cases of brucellosis are diagnosed serologically by the *Brucella* **febrile agglutinin** test. Titers of $\geq 1:80$ are always considered to be significant; a fourfold increase in titer between acute and convalescent sera is considered to be more definitive, however. An ELISA procedure has also been described.

29.2.d. Treatment of brucellosis. For initial therapy, tetracycline combined with an aminoglycoside, streptomycin or gentamicin, is probably best. Trimethoprim-sulfamethoxazole has also been effective for treatment of brucellosis in adults.

29.3. Genus *Bordetella*

29.3.a. Epidemiology and pathogenesis of *Bordetella* infection. *Bordetella* species are obligate parasites of animals and humans, residing on the mucous membranes of the respiratory tract. The organisms colonize the ciliated epithelial cells, adhering closely to the surface; the adherence may be mediated by fimbriae. Mechanisms of pathogenesis of etiologic agents of respiratory tract infections were discussed in Chapter 16. Bordetellae seem to be the only bacteria that adhere only to ciliated mucosal cells. Other virulence factors associated with Bordetellae, particularly *B. pertussis*, include a capsule that surrounds the cells of virulent strains, production of dermonecrotic toxins, production of a filamentous hemagglutinin, production of extracellular enzymes (adenylate cyclase), and production of other biologically active substances including endotoxin (Chapter 14), tracheal cytotoxin, and an exotoxin (pertussis toxin) that acts on various cells of the immune system and other tissues.[4]

There are four species, *B. pertussis*, *B. bronchiseptica*, *B. avium*, and *B. parapertussis*; *B. avium* is found in turkeys and *B. bronchiseptica* is found naturally in animals such as rabbits, dogs, swine, and many other wild and domestic animals. Except for *B. avium*, all species can cause respiratory disease in humans; although the disease associated with *B. pertussis*, "pertussis" or "whooping cough", is most severe. *B. bronchiseptica* has been isolated from infected wounds as well as from the respiratory tract of humans. Documented infections have occurred.[3,14] Incidence of whooping cough in the United States had steadily declined since 1950 when vaccine became widely used, leveling at approximately 1900 cases reported annually. An increase has been seen since 1981, however, and more than 2800

Figure 29.1
Colonies of *Bordetella pertussis* resembling mercury drops on Bordet-Gengou agar after 48 h incubation.

cases were reported in 1987 (>4000 cases in 1986). Fatalities still occur. Recent epidemiologic studies in New York and Wisconsin have shown recovery of *B. pertussis* from children and adults with respiratory tract disease that does not resemble classical whooping cough. The organism may be more prevalent than is currently assumed, since very few laboratories use methods that allow its detection unless requested by a clinician who suspects the disease.

29.3.b. Collection and transport of specimens. Specimens are collected either as nasopharyngeal washings or on a nasopharyngeal swab (calcium alginate on a wire handle). The swab is bent to conform to the nasal passage and held against the posterior aspect of the nasopharynx. If coughing does not occur, another swab is inserted into the other nostril to initiate the cough. The swab is left in place during the entire cough, removed, and immediately inoculated onto a selective medium such as Bordet-Gengou agar containing 20% sheep blood cells and 2.5 µg/ml methicillin instead of penicillin or the recently evaluated Jones-Kendrick charcoal agar containing 40 µg/ml cephalexin. Stauffer and others[19] have found cephalexin to be superior to methicillin for inhibition of normal respiratory flora and Jones-Kendrick agar to be acceptable for transport and cultivation of *Bordetella* species from respiratory tract specimens. This agar will remain effective even after 2 months storage in tightly wrapped plastic bags in the refrigerator. Other ce-

phalexin-containing media have also shown good yields.[1,21] Agar developed for isolation of *Legionella*, buffered-charcoal-yeast-extract, will also support growth of *Bordetella* sp. A recent study advocates Regan-Lowe media for best recovery of *B. pertussis* from nasopharyngeal swabs.[11] A fluid transport medium may be used for swabs (it must be held for less than 2 hours). Half-strength Regan-Lowe agar enhanced yields when used as a transport and enrichment medium.[10] Cold casein hydrolysate medium and casamino acid broth (available commercially) have been found to be an effective transport media, particularly for preparation of slides for direct fluorescent antibody staining.

29.3.c. Laboratory identification. Plates are incubated at 35° to 37° C in a humidified atmosphere; they do not require increased CO_2. If grown on Bordet-Gengou agar with 20% blood, colonies will show a diffuse zone of hemolysis. Colonies will grow within 7 days, appearing small, smooth, convex, with a pearly luster, resembling mercury drops (Figure 29.1). The colonies are mucoid and tenacious. A Gram stain of the organism will reveal minute, faintly staining coccobacilli singly or in pairs. The use of a 2 minute safranin O counterstain or a carbolfuchsin counterstain will enhance their visibility. *B. bronchiseptica* and *B. parapertussis* will grow on MacConkey agar; *B. pertussis* will not.

A direct fluorescent antibody stain is available for detection of *B. pertussis* in smears made from na-

PROCEDURE 29.2

Direct Fluorescent Antibody Stain for Bordetella pertussis

Principle

The presence of even one bacterium of *B. pertussis* is indicative of disease; therefore, direct visualization of the organism, specifically stained by an immunofluorescent reagent, is pathognomic.

Method

1. Prepare casamino acid transport and holding medium. Add 1 g casamino acids (commercially available) to 100 ml distilled water in acid-washed glassware. Adjust pH to 7.2 and dispense in 0.5 ml amounts in acid-washed screw capped 12 × 75 mm tubes. Tighten caps and autoclave 20 min. This medium can be stored for 1 year at refrigerator temperature.

2. Immediately after collection, insert nasopharyngeal swab or material obtained by aspiration into cool casamino acid medium. Incubate the specimen for 1 h at 35° C.

3. With a sterile capillary pipette, place a heaped drop of the well-mixed medium onto each of two circles of a clean glass slide suitable for fluorescent staining. Allow the smears to air dry and reapply material for a total of three applications. Heat fix the slide. Remove a

known positive and a known negative control slide (prepared from stock cultures) from the freezer at the same time, following an identical procedure for each slide.

4. Place a drop of fluorescein-conjugated anti–*B. pertussis* antibody to cover one of the smears completely and place a drop of fluorescein-conjugated normal rabbit serum over the second control smear. Incubate at room temperature in a humidified chamber in the dark (placing the slide on a broken wooden applicator stick in a Petri dish with a moist gauze pad works well) 30 min.

5. Rinse the slides two times in phosphate buffered saline, pH 7.5 (commercially available), allowing them to remain in the second buffer rinse for 10 min, and then rinse in distilled water.

6. Mount with glycerol buffered mounting fluid, pH 8.5 (commercially available), and examine under ultraviolet light for bright fluorescing coccobacilli with bright rims and darker centers. The patient control smear should show no fluorescence, and the known positive smear should yield brightly fluorescing short bacilli and coccobacilli.

Quality control

Obtain a *B. pertussis* culture (from your local health department or large university laboratory), pass it on the agar used for specimens, and prepare slides from suspensions of colonies. Stain one control slide each time a patient specimen is examined.

Modified from Anhalt, J. 1981. In Washington, J.A. Jr., editor: Laboratory procedures in clinical microbiology. Springer-Verlag, New York; and Parker and Linneman. 1980. In Lennette, E.H., Balows, A., Hausler, W.J. Jr., and Truant, J.P., editors: Manual of clinical microbiology, ed. 3. American Society for Microbiology, Washington, D.C.

---

sopharyngeal material. The procedure is described in Procedure 29.2. In experienced hands, this reagent has been very efficient for early diagnosis of cases of whooping cough.[20,21] Slides may be prepared, heat fixed, and mailed to a reference laboratory for evaluation. This reagent may also be used to identify presumptively organisms growing on

agar. The fluorescent antibody identification method is much faster than conventional biochemicals.

Whole cell agglutination reactions in specific antiserum may also be used for species identification (Chapter 12). Abbreviated biochemical reactions of the three known species of *Bordetella* are shown in Table 29.2. A fourth organism, designated *Borde-*

Table 29.2

Characteristics of *Bordetella* Species

SPECIES	GROWTH ON HEART INFUSION AGAR	UREASE	NITRATE REDUCTION	MOTILITY
pertussis	−	−	−	−
parapertussis	+	+ (18 h)	−	−
bronchiseptica	+	+ (4 h)	+	+

+ = All strains positive; − = all strains negative.

tella-like, has been isolated from domestic poultry but has not been well characterized.

An enzyme immunoassay for detection of antibody to *B. pertussis* was recently shown to be valuable in diagnosing culture-negative individuals.[20] Commercial variations of this test have recently become available (Labsystems-USA, Chicago, Ill). Preliminary trials have yielded promising results for early diagnosis of pertussis.

29.3.d. Treatment of pertussis. Adequate microbiological therapy may not alter the course of the disease. Erythromycin does eradicate organisms from the respiratory tract, however, and should be given to all patients with pertussis, as well as to contacts prophylactically.

29.4. Genus *Haemophilus*

The following three genera, *Haemophilus*, *Actinobacillus*, and *Pasteurella*, are all members of the family Pasteurellaceae, a group of organisms that are pleomorphic, gram-negative, nonmotile bacilli and coccobacilli that are able to reduce nitrates and utilize carbohydrates either fermentatively or with oxygen as the terminal electron acceptor. All three genera live on animals, including humans, primarily on mucosal surfaces. They may be differentiated by their requirements for nicotinamide adenine dinucleotide (NAD), as well as by other criteria. A proposal to move *Actinobacillus actinomycetemcomitans* to the genus *Haemophilus* was recently rejected.

29.4.a. Epidemiology and pathogenesis of *Haemophilus* infection. Carried in the normal respiratory tract (and occasionally genital tract) of humans, pigs, sheep, and most other vertebrates, the organisms cause upper respiratory tract infections, suppurative infections, primarily in areas adjacent to the respiratory tract, and systemic infections, particularly meningitis. In humans, *Haemophilus influen-*

zae is the most common etiologic agent of acute bacterial meningitis in young children. *H. influenzae*, the most important human pathogen among the species of *Haemophilus*, is also associated with acute, contagious conjunctivitis ("pinkeye" [biogroup aegyptius, formerly called *H. aegyptius*]), acute and chronic otitis media, epiglottitis, cellulitis, and other infections. *H. influenzae* has even been isolated from the urine of patients with urinary tract infections.[5] A recently recognized serious disease in children, Brazilian purpuric fever, preceded by conjunctivitis, has been associated with *H. influenzae* biogroup aegyptius.[2]

H. ducreyi, not found as part of normal genital flora of humans or known to be harbored by any animals, is the cause of chancroid, a widespread venereal disease, found most commonly in tropical parts of the world. Other species of *Haemophilus*, which include *H. parainfluenzae*, *H. haemolyticus*, *H. aphrophilus*, *H. paraphrophilus*, and *H. segnis*, are normal flora of humans only, occasionally causing upper and lower respiratory tract infections. These organisms may also occasionally enter the bloodstream from a mucosal focus, disseminating to cause systemic disease, including endocarditis, metastatic abscesses,[15] (especially brain abscess) septic arthritis, and osteomyelitis. They have also been known to infect tissue adjacent to the mucosa, causing jaw infections, dental abscesses, appendicitis,[22] and, when they are traumatically inoculated into healthy tissue, bite wound infections. *H. influenzae* and *H. parainfluenzae* are associated with invasive disease in humans more often than are the other species. *H. parainfluenzae* tends to grow in tangled clumps or strands of filamentous bacterial forms; these may easily break off the main colony. Particularly in cases of sepsis or endocarditis, there may be metastatic abscess formation.

The polysaccharide capsule is clearly a virulence

Table 29.3

Biotypes of *H. influenzae*

BIOTYPE	SYNDROME (SITE OF INFECTION)	INDOLE	UREASE	ORNITHINE
I	Sepsis, meningitis	+	+	+
II	Eye (United States), bacteremia, ear, lower respiratory tract	+	+	−
III	Eye (Europe), respiratory tract	−	+	−
IV	Ear (rare), respiratory tract	−	+	+
V	Ear, lower respiratory tract	+	−	+
VI	Upper respiratory tract (rare)	+	−	−

+ = > 90% of strains positive; − = > 90% of strains negative.

Modified from Kilian, M., and Biberstein, E.L. 1984. Genus *Haemophilus* (Winslow, Broadhurst, Buchanan, Krumwiede, Rogers and Smith) 1917. In Kreig, N.R., and Holt, J.G., editors. Bergey's manual of systematic bacteriology, vol. 1. Williams & Wilkins, Baltimore.

factor for *H. influenzae*, since anticapsular antibody is protective against acquisition of meningitis. A number of immunological reagents have been developed for the rapid identification of *H. influenzae* capsular polysaccharide type b (the most common pathogenic agent), as described in section 29.4.e and in Chapter 15. Unencapsulated strains, however, are often recovered from specimens taken from patients with infections other than meningitis, including pneumonia, cellulitis, otitis media, and soft tissue infections. Pathogenic mechanisms of the *Haemophilus* species are not well understood. Since the organisms enter the bloodstream so readily after colonization of the respiratory epithelium, they may possess some invasive properties. Their ability to multiply in host tissues and evoke an inflammatory response contributes to the pathology of pyogenic *Haemophilus* disease. The presence of a specific plasmid was significantly associated with severe disease among strains of *H. influenzae* biogroup aegyptius isolated from children with Brazilian purpuric fever.[2] The nature of a possible virulence factor on this plasmid, however, is not known.

Recent studies on identification of *H. influenzae* have shown that certain biotypes of that organism are more commonly associated with particular syndromes, as outlined in Table 29.3.[8,9] Biotyping can be easily accomplished, and microbiologists should routinely identify significant *H. influenzae* isolates to biotype. As more laboratories procure such definitive identifications, our understanding of the epidemiology and pathogenesis of infection with this prevalent microorganism will expand.

29.4.b. Collection and transport of specimens. Most any specimen may harbor *Haemophilus* species, and it is primarily for isolation of this organism that most clinical material received for routine culture in microbiology laboratories is inoculated to chocolate agar and incubated in 5% to 10% CO_2. Blood, cerebrospinal fluid, middle ear exudate collected by tympanocentesis, joint fluids, respiratory tract specimens, swabs from inflamed conjunctivae, and abscess drainage are a few of the many types of specimens that are likely to yield *Haemophilus* species.

Most swabs routinely used for collection of material for culture, including calcium alginate, cotton, and Dacron, are suitable for collection of specimens for detection of most species of *Haemophilus*. Modified Stuart's transport medium or Amie's charcoal transport medium will adequately maintain viability of the organism until the specimen is inoculated to growth media. For recovery of *H. ducreyi* from genital ulcers, however, special measures are necessary due to the fastidious nature of the bacterium. The ulcer should be cleansed with sterile gauze moistened with sterile saline. A physician uses a cotton swab premoistened with phosphate buffered saline to collect material from the ulcer base. This swab must be plated to media (described in Chapter 19 and mentioned in Section 29.4.c) within 10 minutes of collection for maximum yield. A gram stain of material from a chancroid lesion may display the characteristic "school of fish" arrangement, seen as numerous gram-negative coccobacilli in groups resembling fish (Figure 19.3).

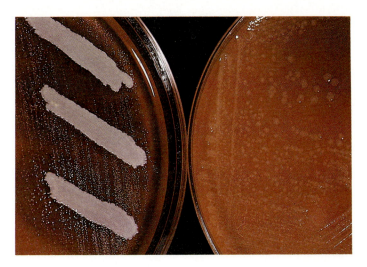

Figure 29.2
Satelliting colonies of *Haemophilus influenzae* surrounding the *Staphylococcus aureus* streaks on the right. The *Haemophilus* was streaked for confluent growth on the blood agar plate, but colonies appear only close to the *Staphylococcus* growth. Chocolate agar (plate on left) provides all nutrients necessary for growth of *H. influenzae*. (Photograph by Pete Rose.)

29.4.c. Media and incubation conditions for isolation of *Haemophilus* species. Chocolate agar supplies the factors necessary for growth of most *Haemophilus* species. These factors are *hemin* (called "X factor") and *nicotine adenine dinucleotide (NAD;* called "V factor"). *H. influenzae, H. haemolyticus,* and *H. ducreyi* require X factor, whereas *H. aphrophilus* requires X factor only for initial isolation. All clinically significant species except *H. aphrophilus* and *H. ducreyi* require V factor. Chocolate agar, horse blood agar, and rabbit blood agar all contain adequate quantities of both growth factors and support the growth of *Haemophilus* species that require both factors. Either rabbit blood or horse blood is used for visualization of hemolysis. Sheep blood that has not been chocolatized contains enough NADase (produced by the sheep blood cells) to destroy the NAD normally present, although sheep blood agar does contain adequate hemin for growth of *Haemophilus* that requires hemin. *Haemophilus* species that require both X and V factors can grow on sheep blood agar if the V factor is exogenously provided. Several other bacterial species produce V factor as a metabolic by-product. Therefore, tiny colonies of *Haemophilus* may be seen growing very close to colonies of bacteria on sheep blood agar that produces V factor. This phenomenon, known as "satelliting"

(Figure 29.2), often occurs around hemolytic staphylococci because they produce sufficient V factor. Pneumococci, neisseriae, and many other organisms also produce enough NAD to allow satellite colonies of *Haemophilus* species to form in their vicinity. With the exceptions of *H. aphrophilus* and *H. ducreyi,* all clinically significant *Haemophilus* species require V factor.

Media that adequately support growth of *H. ducreyi* are Mueller-Hinton base chocolate agar supplemented with 1% IsoVitaleX (BBL Microbiology Systems) and 3 µg/ml vancomycin, and heart infusion base agar with 10% fetal bovine serum and 3 µg/ml vancomycin. For best recovery, material from suspected chancroid lesions should be inoculated to two plates, one of each different agar formula, both of which are incubated in a candle jar at 35° to 37° C for a maximum of 7 days.

H. influenzae is a significant etiologic agent of lower respiratory tract infection, particularly among elderly patients and young individuals with cystic fibrosis. The number of isolates of *Haemophilus* species is increased when selective media such as horse blood–bacitracin developed by Klein and Blazevic (Chapter 45) are employed for recovery of these organisms. Such media are particularly important for isolating *Haemophilus* from respiratory secretions of

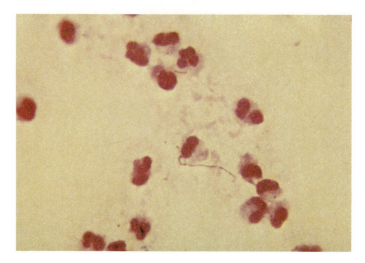

Figure 29.3
Gram stain of cerebrospinal fluid containing many polymorphonuclear leukocytes and *Haemophilus influenzae*. Note both coccobacilli and long filamentous forms.

patients with cystic fibrosis, where the organisms may be etiologic agents of disease, but they are overgrown and their presence obscured by the coexisting mucoid *Pseudomonas aeruginosa*.

Most strains of *Haemophilus* are able to grow aerobically and anaerobically. Growth is usually stimulated by 5% to 10% CO_2 (*H. paraphrohaemolyticus* requires CO_2) so that incubation in a candle extinction jar or carbon dioxide incubator is recommended. The organisms usually grow within 24 hours, but some strains, particularly *H. ducreyi*, may require as long as 7 days.

29.4.d. Laboratory identification of clinically significant *Haemophilus* species. *Haemophilus* species are often not visible in broth, especially in blood culture media, since they do not grow to turbidity. For this reason, blind subcultures to chocolate agar or examination of smears (acridine orange fluorescent stain is recommended), is necessary for their detection. *H. parainfluenzae* may appear as filamentous, intertwining strands of gram-negative bacilli, whereas the other species usually are seen as coccobacilli with long filamentous forms occasionally interspersed (Figure 29.3). Gram stains from colonies growing on solid agar are more typical, showing pleomorphic coccobacilli.

Colonies on chocolate agar are transparent, moist, smooth, convex, with a distinct odor, variously described as "mousy" or "bleachlike." X and

V factor requirements are carried out using the **porphyrin test** (Procedure 29.3). This test detects the presence of enzymes that convert δ-aminolevulinic acid (ALA) into porphyrins or protoporphyrins. The more traditional method for detection of X and V factor requirements, that of inoculating the organism to media without blood and placing X and V factor-impregnated filter paper strips on the plate, incubating overnight, and examining for growth around the appropriate strip, cannot be recommended. Many X factor–requiring organisms are able to carry over enough X factor from the primary medium to yield false negative tests with the filter paper method.

A commercial ALA reagent impregnated on a filter paper disk is available from Remel Laboratories. The test is performed in 4 hours. The technologist must be careful not to overmoisten the disk, as false negative results can occur due to dilution of the end product.[6]

In addition to the porphyrin test, *Haemophilus* isolates may be identified using biochemical parameters (Table 29.4). Although conventional media are acceptable for performance of these tests, several new rapid enzymatic biochemical systems have been developed for identification of *Haemophilus*, including the Minitek System (BBL Microbiology Systems), the RapID-NH (Innovative Diagnostics), HNID (American MicroScan), and others.

PROCEDURE 29.3

Porphyrin Test for X Factor Requirement

Principle

Non-hemin-requiring *Haemophilus* species can use delta-aminolevulinic acid (ALA) as a substrate for the synthesis of porphyrin (another name for hemin). Porphyrin will fluoresce reddish orange under ultraviolet light and can thus be detected.

Method

1. Prepare delta-aminolevulinic acid substrate as follows:

δ-Aminolevulinic acid (Sigma Chemical Co.) (2 mol/L)	0.34 g
MgSO4 (0.08 mol/L)	0.0096 g
Phosphate mol/L buffer (0.1 mol/L, pH 6.9)	1,000 ml

   The $MgSO_4$ may be prepared in a more concentrated solution and diluted to reach the desired final concentration. Mix thoroughly, dispense into small plastic snap top tubes (12 × 75 mm) 0.5 ml per tube, and freeze at −20° C until use.
2. Thaw the substrate and add a very heavy loopful of the organism to be tested, making a heavy suspension.
3. Incubate the tubes at 37° C for 4 h and then take the tubes into a darkroom and shine an ultraviolet light source of 360 nm wavelength (long wave) on the contents of the tube.
4. Presence of a brick red to orange fluorescence indicates that porphyrins were produced, and that the organism does not require hemin (X factor).

Quality control

Test *H. influenzae* ATCC 43065 and *H. parainfluenzae* ATCC 7901 in the same manner as test organisms.

Expected results

H. parainfluenzae, the positive control, will show red fluorescence in the tube; *H. influenzae*, the negative control, should display no fluorescence.

Performance schedule

Test fresh subcultures of the quality control strains each time the test is performed.

Modified from Kilian and Biberstein. 1984.[9]

Those species that require V factor have been grouped into biotypes but the biotypes have not yet been associated with particular clinical syndromes. *H. segnis* is the only oxidase- negative species among this group. *H. aphrophilus* can be confused with a closely related organism, *A. actinomycetemcomitans*. As discussed in section 29.5.b, *A. actinomycetemcomitans* is catalase-positive, does not require V factor, and cannot ferment lactose or sucrose. For these and other reasons, the genus name *Actinobacillus* has been retained. *H. aphrophilus* yields the opposite reactions in those tests. Colony morphology of *H. aphrophilus* on a clear medium can be used to aid in differentiating it from *A. actinomycetemcomitans*. The colony of *H. aphrophilus* is round and convex and displays an opaque zone near the center (Figure 29.4), whereas *A. actinomycetemcomitans* colonies appear to have a central star-shaped structure (Figure 29.5).

29.4.e. Rapid identification of *H. influenzae* type b. The clinical significance of *H. influenzae* type b has prompted workers to develop rapid immunological methods for detection of its capsular polysaccharide directly in clinical specimens, such as cerebrospinal fluid, serum, and urine. The organism, once isolated, can also be rapidly identified with the same reagents. Coagglutination reagents produced by Pharmacia Biotechnology and latex agglutination reagents (BBL Microbiology Systems, Wellcome Diagnostics, Wampole Laboratories) have been shown to be very sensitive and specific for detecting the presence of *H. influenzae* type b in cerebrospinal

Table 29.4

Characteristics of *Haemophilus* Species Isolated from Humans

SPECIES	REQUIRES V FACTOR FOR GROWTH	ALA→ PORPHYRINS	UREASE	INDOLE	ACID FROM GLUCOSE	LACTOSE	BETA HEMOLYTIC*	CATALASE
H. influenzae	+	–	+/–	+/–	+	–	–	+
H. parainfluenzae	+	+	+/–	–	+ (some gas)	–	–	+/– (slow)
H. haemolyticus	+	–	+	+/–	+ (some gas)	–	+	+
H. aphrophilus	–	+ (weak)	–	–	+ (gas)	+	–	–
H. paraphrophilus	+	+	–	–	+ (gas)	+	–	–
H. segnis	+	+	+	–	+ (weak)	–	–	+/– (slow)
H. influenzae subsp *aegyptius*	+	–	+	–	+	–	–	+
H. ducreyi	–	–	–	–	+/–	–	–	–
H. parahaemolyticus	+	+	+	–	+ (some gas)	–	+	+/–
H. paraphrohaemolyticus†	+	+	+	–	+	–	+	+/–

+ = >90% of strains positive; – = >90% of strains negative; +/– = variable results, some gas = some strains produce gas.

*Rabbit or horse blood agar.

†Requires CO_2 for growth.

Modified from Kilian, M., and Biberstein, E.L. 1984. *Genus Haemophilus* (Winslow, Broadhurst, Buchanan, Krumwiede, Rogers and Smith 1917). In Krieg, N.R., and Holt, J.G., editors. *Bergey's manual of systematic bacteriology*, vol. 1. Williams & Wilkins, Baltimore.

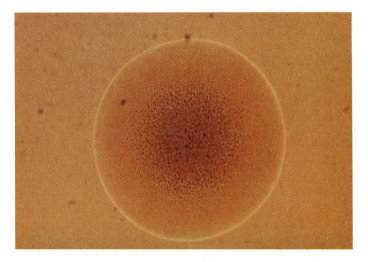

Figure 29.4
Colony of *Haemophilus aphrophilus* on heart infusion agar. Note opaque central area.

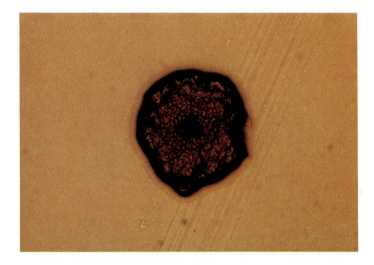

Figure 29.5
Colony of *Actinobacillus actinomycetemcomitans* on heart infusion agar. Note the central star-shaped structure.

fluid and slightly less sensitive when used with other body fluids (Chapter 15). Because of false-negative tests, however, and rare cross-reactive antigens, such tests should not be used as the sole diagnostic modality.

In addition to rapid detection and identification of the organism, the increasing incidence of ampicillin resistance necessitates that microbiologists perform a rapid test for detection of β-beta lactamase. Because of widespread chloramphenicol re-sistance found in other parts of the world (and occasional chloramphenicol-resistant isolates seen in the United States), microbiologists may wish to perform a rapid test for detection of chloramphenicol resistance as well. These tests, produced commercially as reagent-impregnated filter paper disks, are discussed fully in Chapter 13.

29.4.f. Treatment of *Haemophilus* infections. During meningitis, certain antimicrobial agents that would normally be unable to do so can penetrate the blood-brain barrier, allowing agents such as ampicillin to be used for treatment of this disease. However, because of the recent increase in resistance of *H. influenzae* to ampicillin and the possibility of chloramphenicol resistance, the current recommended initial therapy for meningitis is a combination of ampicillin and chloramphenicol pending the results of in vitro susceptibility tests. Chloramphenicol achieves excellent levels in most tissues, including bone, and is the drug of choice for serious infections caused by susceptible *Haemophilus* species, alone or in combination with ampicillin. Once an isolate has been shown to be susceptible to ampicillin, this agent may be used alone to continue treatment. Newer cephalosporins, such as cefotaxime and cefuroxime, are effective as single drug regimens for treatment of meningitis. Patients with less severe disease caused by *H. influenzae* being treated as outpatients are usually given oral amoxicillin-clavulanic acid, amoxicillin, ampicillin, or trimethoprim-sulfamethoxazole. Other species of *Haemophilus* may often be successfully treated with tetracycline in addition to the agents mentioned. Treatment for chancroid involves either oral erythromycin or trimethoprim-sulfamethoxazole. Rifampin is the antimicrobial agent of choice for prophylaxis of close contacts of a patient with *H. influenzae* meningitis. Capsular polysaccharide vaccines for use in children have recently been released. Their efficacy in all situations has not been verified. Clinical trials are ongoing.

29.5. Genus *Actinobacillus*.

29.5.a. Epidemiology and pathogenesis of *Actinobacillus* infection. *A. lignieresii*, *A. equuli*, *A. suis*, and *A. capsulatus* are found as pathogens and as part of the normal oral flora of many domestic animals, including cows, horses, sheep, and pigs. *A. actinomycetemcomitans* is normal flora of human oral mucosa and is not found in other animals. Humans are infected with the animal species through traumatic inoculation of the organism, such as via a bite wound or other wound.[18] Infections associated with *A. actinomycetemcomitans* are probably all of endogenous origin. This species is often isolated along with *Actinomyces* or *Arachnia* from actinomycotic lesions of the jaw or abscesses within the thoracic cavity. Failure to eradicate the *Actinobacillus* may account for persistence of actinomycosis, even after the *Actinomyces* or *Arachnia* has been cleared. *A.*

actinomycetemcomitans has recently been associated with a destructive periodontitis that occurs in adolescents. This species, as well as the closely related *H. aphrophilus*, is occasionally isolated as the etiologic agent of endocarditis.[7] The organism probably possesses very low virulence, acting as a pathogen only opportunistically.

29.5.b. Laboratory identification. *A. actinomycetemcomitans*, the clinically important species, grows on blood and chocolate agars; unlike the other species of *Actinobacillus*, it does not grow on MacConkey agar. Growth is enhanced in a candle jar or a CO_2 incubator, but colonies may require up to 7 days to achieve maximum size. Growth in broth media is often barely visible, with no turbidity produced. Microcolonies may be seen as tiny puffballs growing on the blood cell layer in blood culture bottles, or alternatively, growth may appear as a film or as tiny puffs on the sides of a bottle or tube. On blood agar, the medium surrounding the colonies exhibits a slight greenish tinge. The colonies themselves are rough and sticky. A characteristic finding is the presence of a four- to six-pointed starlike configuration in the center of a mature colony growing on clear medium (such as brain heart infusion agar); this star pattern can be easily visualized by examining the colony under low power (100 ×) with a standard microscope (Figure 29.5). On Gram stain, the organisms are gram-negative bacilli, often displaying coccoid forms. The coccoid shapes may be found at the end of bacilli, giving the overall appearance of the dots and dashes of Morse code. *Actinobacillus* species may resemble *Haemophilus* species and *Pasteurella* species; their differentiation is outlined in Table 29.5. Key characteristics of certain *Actinobacillus* species are shown in Table 29.6. Characteristics of *Pasteurella*-like species that are genetically more similar to *Actinobacillus* are shown in Table 29.7.

29.5.c. Treatment of *Actinobacillus* infections. All members of the genera are susceptible to tetracycline and chloramphenicol. Penicillin resistance has been reported, and the organisms are all resistant to aminoglycosides and clindamycin.

29.6. Genus *Pasteurella*

29.6.a. Epidemiology and pathogenesis of *Pasteurella* infection. *Pasteurella* species are normal flora of the respiratory and gastrointestinal tracts of many species of domestic and wild animals and birds.

Table 29.5
Differential Characteristics of Morphologically Similar Gram-Negative Bacilli and Coccobacilli

GENUS/SPECIES	OXIDASE	CATALASE	CELL SHAPE		INDOLE	NITRATE TO NITRITE	FERMENTATION OF		
			COCCOID	FUSIFORM			MALTOSE	SUCROSE	LACTOSE
Actinobacillus	+/-	+	+	-	-	+	+	-	-
Capnocytophaga (except DF-2)	-	-	-	+	-	+/-	+	+	+/-
Cardiobacterium	+	-	-	-	+	-	+	+*	-
DF-2 (now C. canimorsus)	+ (weak)	+	-	+	-	-	+	-	+
Eikenella	+	-	+/-	-	-	+	-	-	-
Haemophilus aphrophilus	-/+ (weak)	-	+/-	-	-	+	+	+	+
HB-5	+ (weak)	-	+/-	-	+ (weak)†	+	-	-	-
Kingella kingae	+	-	-	-	-	-	+	-	-
Pasteurella multocida	+	+	+/-	-	+	+	-	+	-

+ = >90% of strains positive within 2 days; − = >90% of strains negative; +/− = variable (most strains positive); −/+ = variable (most strains negative).
*Positive results may require extended incubation period.
†Xylene extraction required.

Table 29.6

Characteristics of *Actinobacillus* Species

				FERMENTATION OF		
SPECIES	**OXIDASE**	**UREASE**	**ESCULIN HYDROLYSIS**	**TREHALOSE**	**SALICIN**	**SODIUM HIPPURATE HYDROLYSIS**
A. actinomycetemcomitans	− / +	−	−	−	−	ND
A. lignieresii	+	+	−	−	−	−
A. equuli	+	+	−	+	−	+
A. suis	+	+	+	+	+	+

+ = >90% of strains positive; − = >90% of strains negative; − / + = variable results; ND = not done.

Table 29.7

Characteristics of *Pasteurella* and Related Species of Possible Clinical Significance

	β-HEMOLYSIS	GROWTH ON MacCONKEY AGAR	INDOLE	UREASE	ORNITHINE DECARBOXYLASE	GAS FROM GLUCOSE	FERMENTATION OF			
							MALTOSE	MANNITOL	SORBITOL	DULCITOL
P. multocida ss. multocida	−	−	+	−	+	−	−	+	+	−
P. multocida ss. gallicida	−	−	+	−	+	−	−	+	+	+
P. multocida ss. septica	−	−	+	−	+	−	−	+	−	−
P. dagmatis	−	−	+	+ / −	−	+ / −	+	−	−	−
P. canis	−	−	+ / −	−	+	−	−	−	−	−
P. (Actinobacillus) pneumotropica	−	+ / −	+	+	+	−	+	−	NA	NA
P. (Actinobacillus) urease	−	−	−	+	−	−	+	+	NA	NA
P. (Actinobacillus) haemolyticus	+	+	−	−	−	−	+	+ / −	NA	NA
P. (Actinobacillus) aerogenes	−	+	−	+	+ / −	+	+	−	NA	NA

+ = >90% of strains positive; − = >90% of strains negative; + / − = variable results.
Modified from Carter, G.R. 1984. Genus *Pasteurella* (Trevisan 1887). In Krieg, N.R., and Holt, J. G., editors. Bergey's manual of systematic bacteriology, vol. 1. Williams & Wilkins, Baltimore.

They are etiologic agents of hemorrhagic septicemia, gastrointestinal infections, and respiratory tract infections in many animals. Humans acquire *Pasteurella* primarily through animal exposure. The majority of human infections are associated with animal bites, but a large number of respiratory tract and intra-abdominal infections are associated with possible inhalation of the organism or with no known source of acquisition. *Pasteurella multocida* (which now includes three subspecies, subsp. *multocida*, subsp. *septica*, and subsp. *gallicida*), the most common human pathogen among the Pasteurellae, can be isolated from animal bite wounds, respiratory secretions from patients with pneumonia, cerebrospinal fluid, abscesses, biopsy specimens from patients with osteomyelitis, blood, joint fluid from septic arthritis, and many other sites. Other species of *Pasteurella*, *P. dagmatis*, *P. gallinarum*, *P. canis*, *P. stomatis*, *P. anatis*, *P. langaa*, *P. avium*, *P. volantium*, and several unnamed species, are more com-

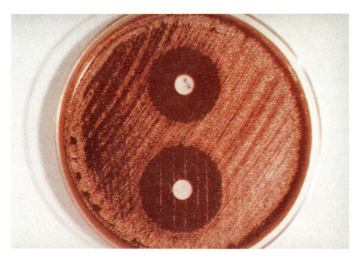

Figure 29.6
Susceptibility of *Pasteurella multocida* to a 2-unit penicillin disk.

monly associated with animal disease, although they have been reported from human cases of endocarditis, pneumonia, septicemia, and primarily from infected wounds, occasionally involving osteomyelitis.[12] Previously described species of *Pasteurella, haemolytica, ureae,* and *aerogenes,* have been shown to be significantly different from true Pasteurellae by DNA homology studies. *P. pneumotropica, P. ureae,* and *P. haemolytica* appear to be similar to the genus *Actinobacillus.*[12]

Virulence of *Pasteurella* is related to the polysaccharide capsule that allows the organism to resist phagocytosis. Although some strains produce a cytotoxin, its role in the pathogenesis of disease has not been elucidated. *P. multocida* appears to be the most virulent of the species. Virulence may be enhanced by the ability of the organism to utilize free iron, a factor in the pathogenicity of several bacterial strains.

29.6.b. Laboratory identification. Since *Pasteurella* species grow well on routinely inoculated laboratory media including blood agar, they are easily isolated from all sites in which they may be present. Growth is not appreciably enhanced by increased concentrations of CO_2. Colonies are small and translucent and may be smooth or rough. A brown discoloration of the medium may develop around colonies of *P. multocida.* The colonies on blood agar have a musty or "mushroom" sort of smell, which is recognizable to experienced microbiologists. All species should be oxidase-positive by the Kovacs' test;

several subcultures may be necessary to demonstrate this. They are nitrate- and catalase- positive, spot indole–positive, and glucose fermenters. A quick screening procedure used for presumptive identification of *Pasteurella* species takes advantage of their penicillin susceptibility, unusual for gram-negative bacteria. The surface of a Mueller-Hinton blood agar plate is inoculated with a suspension of the organism equal to a McFarland 0.5 turbidity, using a cotton swab and streaking in three directions, as for the disk-diffusion susceptibility test. A filter paper disk containing 2 U of penicillin (used for susceptibility testing) is placed in the center of the plate, which is then incubated overnight in air. A zone of inhibition around the disk is indicative of susceptibility; most other gram-negative bacilli are resistant to penicillin (Figure 29.6).

The organism is a small, coccoid or rod-shaped bacillus that often exhibits bipolar staining. All species are nonmotile. Differentiation among species can be achieved using biochemical parameters listed in Table 29.7. Only some strains of *P. dagmatis* produce gas from glucose. Isolates of this species (previously called "new species" or "gas") are often associated with dog and cat bites and may go on to cause systemic disease.

Most of the biochemical identification systems available commercially will identify *Pasteurella,* at least to genus. *Pasteurella* should be suspected when any isolate is associated with an animal bite. Again, it is important for clinicians to inform the laboratory of the source of a wound specimen and pertinent clinical information so that the microbiologist can perform the appropriate tests early in the identification protocol.

29.6.c. Treatment of Pasteurella infections. Penicillin is the antimicrobial agent of choice for all *Pasteurella* infections. Tetracycline and chloramphenicol are also effective, but aminoglycosides, erythromycin, and clindamycin are not recommended. Cephalothin has also been found to be effective for therapy of wound infections due to *Pasteurella*.

29.7. Genus *Kingella*

29.7.a. Epidemiology and pathogenesis of *Kingella* infection. The three species of *Kingella*, *K. kingae*, *K. denitrificans*, and *K. indologenes*, are normal oropharyngeal flora of humans. Although the pathogenicity of *K. denitrificans* is unknown, *K. indologenes* has been isolated (rarely) from eye infections. *K. kingae*, on the other hand, has been associated with infection more often. The organism has been found as the etiologic agent of bacteremia and skin lesions, and it seems to be particularly associated with septic arthritis.[17] Pathogenic mechanisms have not been well characterized.

29.7.b. Laboratory identification. Colonies of *K. kingae* on 5% sheep blood agar are small with a clear zone of hemolysis. Initial growth may require several days of incubation. Increased CO_2 seems to enhance growth. Colony morphology may vary; one morphotype pits the agar and assumes a "fried egg" appearance with a thin, spreading haze of growth surrounding the central colony. Gram stain reveals short, plump bacilli with squared-off ends that may form chains.

K. denitrificans produces nonhemolytic colonies resembling those of *K. kingae*. One distinguishing feature is the ability of *K. denitrificans* to grow on Thayer-Martin medium. Because it is also oxidase-positive and able to produce acid from glucose, *K. denitrificans* may be confused with *Neisseria gonorrhoeae*. Differential tests include nitrate reduction (*N. gonorrhoeae* is unable to reduce nitrate, whereas most *K. denitrificans* are nitrate-positive) and inhibition of growth of *N. gonorrhoeae* by amylase. All of 52 *K. denitrificans* isolates tested by Odugbemi and Arko[13] were not inhibited from growing up to a 13 mm diameter filter paper disk impregnated with 0.05 ml diluted human saliva or α-amylase (Sigma

Chemical Co.) when inoculated to the surface of plates made from GC agar base with IsoVitaleX (BBL Microbiology Systems).

All *Kingella* species are oxidase-positive and nonmotile and able to ferment glucose. Most *Kingella* species are catalase-negative, which helps to differentiate them from *Moraxella* species and *Neisseria* species. In contrast to the other two species, *K. indologenes* is indole-positive, as the name suggests. None of the species will produce acid in the butt of a triple sugar iron agar tube; they may not grow at all in that medium. Oxidative-fermentative carbohydrate media (Chapter 28) may need to be supplemented with 5% horse serum to allow sufficient growth.

29.7.c. Treatment of *Kingella* infections. Penicillin appears to be the drug of choice for treatment of infections due to *K. kingae*. The organism is also susceptible to gentamicin and chloramphenicol, both of which have been used successfully to treat septic arthritis. There is limited information on susceptibilities of the other two species.

29.8. Genus *Capnocytophaga* (Except the Former DF-2)

29.8.a. Epidemiology and pathogenesis of *Capnocytophaga* infection. The *Capnocytophaga* are **capnophilic** (carbon dioxide–loving) gram-negative bacilli, found as normal oral flora in humans. These organisms are often found in significantly larger numbers within the gingival pockets of patients with periodontal disease. The organisms produce proteases that are able to cleave secretory immunoglobulins, which are postulated to have a protective effect in preventing oral disease. An additional possible virulence factor is production by *Capnocytophaga* of a heat-stable factor that alters polymorphonuclear neutrophil chemotactic activity. Interestingly, young patients with severe periodontitis also often display a neutrophil dysfunction that may spontaneously revert with the effective treatment of their periodontitis. The role of the extracellular products of *Capnocytophaga* in virulence of the organism has not yet been fully elucidated.

In addition to periodontal disease, *Capnocytophaga* is associated with sepsis or systemic infection, usually in leukemic and/or granulocytopenic patients. However, there are several reports of osteomyelitis, septic arthritis, endocarditis, and soft tissue infections in normal hosts from which *Capnocyto-*

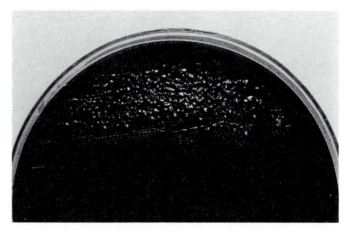

Figure 29.7
Colonies of *Capnocytophaga* growing on 5% sheep blood agar. Note haze of growth extending from
colonies, evidence of gliding motility of the bacteria.

phaga has been isolated. The portal of entry is thought to be the oral cavity. Many of the patients with predisposing immunosuppression had bleeding gums or oral mucosal erosion before they developed sepsis.

29.8.b. Laboratory identification of *Capnocytophaga*. The organism grows well on trypticase soy agar with 5% sheep blood, the standard blood agar plate used by most microbiology laboratories for routine cultures, as well as on chocolate or trypticase soy agar without blood. After 48 to 72 hours incubation at 37° C in 5% CO_2 or anaerobically, colonies are 1 to 5 mm in diameter, opaque, shiny, and nonhemolytic, with a pale beige or yellowish color. The color may be more apparent if growth is scraped from the surface with a loop and examined against a white background. The organism will not grow in air. Occasionally, gliding motility of the organism may be observed as outgrowths from the colonies or as a haze on the surface of the agar (Figure 29.7). The gliding motility is best observed on media containing 3% agar. The organism fails to grow on MacConkey agar.

Gram stain reveals gram-negative, fusiform shaped bacilli with one rounded end and one tapered end and occasional filamentous forms (Figure 29.8). The organisms may appear as aggregates. They are oxidase- and catalase-negative. A negative spot indole test is also helpful. There are three named species of *Capnocytophaga*, *C . ochracea*, *C . sputigena*, and *C . gingivalis*, and there is one unnamed group, that can be distinguished with difficulty biochemi-

cally (Table 29.8). Commercially available anaerobic identification systems, such as the RapID ANA (Innovative Diagnostics, Inc.), Minitek System (BBL Microbiology Systems), and API AnIdent (Analytab Products), and the multiparameter API ZYM enzymatic identification system can be used to differentiate *Capnocytophaga* species. For most situations, however, a presumptive identification to genus is as beneficial to clinicians as is definitive identification. In addition, all species share the traits of acid production from glucose and sucrose, negative urease, lysine and ornithine decarboxylases. The organism differs from morphologically similar organisms, such as *A . actinomycetemcomitans*, *H . aphrophilus*, *Eikenella corrodens*, *Gardnerella vaginalis*, and CDC Group HB-5. Table 29.5 outlines some of the major differential characteristics among these fastidious gram-negative organisms.

29.8.c. Treatment of *Capnocytophaga* infections. Sepsis caused by this organism is severe, especially in immunocompromised patients, and must be approached aggressively. Bactericidal activity has been shown for penicillin, carbenicillin, clindamycin, and erythromycin. All strains are resistant to aminoglycosides.

29.9. Genus *Cardiobacterium*

29.9.a. Epidemiology and pathogenesis of *Cardiobacterium* infection. *Cardiobacterium hominis*, the only species in the genus, is normal flora in the human mouth, and perhaps on other mucous membranes. It is noninvasive and has not been associated

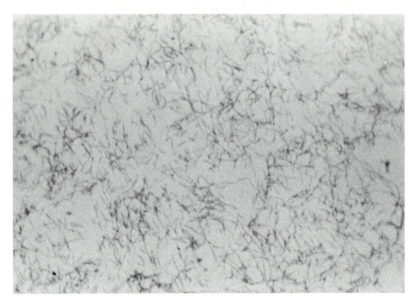

Figure 29.8
Gram stain of *Capnocytophaga*.

Table 29.8
Key Differential Characteristics Among Species of *Capnocytophaga**

TEST	C. OCHRACEA	C. SPUTIGENA	C. GINGIVALIS	GROUP IV
Fructose	100	46	0	0
Lactose	82	31	0	100
Maltose	93	100	0	100
Mannitol	79	0	0	0
Raffinose	75	0	0	0
Rhamnose	71	92	79	0
Trehalose	93	0	7	80
NO$_2$ to nitrogen	82	92	100	0

*Carbohydrate fermentations were performed in buffered single substrate medium. Results are given as a percentage of positive reactions observed from testing 60 strains.
Modified from Forlenza, S.W. 1985. *Capnocytophaga:* an opportunistic pathogen. Clin. Microbiol. Newsletter 7:17.

with any type of infection other than bacteremia or endocarditis. The incidence of *Cardiobacterium*-related bacteremia, however, is increasing. This may be because of the increased number of susceptible hosts, or, more likely, because of increased awareness among microbiologists as well as better blood culturing techniques. Only 34 cases of *C. hominis* infection had been reported until 1983. Most patients had prior cardiac valvular disease. No specific virulence factors have been delineated for this organism.

29.9.b. Laboratory identification of *C. hominis*. As an etiologic agent of disease, this organism has been isolated only from blood. It grows well in standard blood culture media and can be subcultured to 5% sheep blood agar, chocolate agar, and trypticase soy agar without blood. The organism does not grow on MacConkey agar. Incubation of blood agar subcultures at 37° C in 5% CO2 or in air with increased humidity (a candle jar probably provides the best atmosphere) for 48 hours yields colonies that are 1 to 2 mm in diameter, slightly α-hemolytic, smooth, round, glistening, and opaque. The organism will grow equally well at 30° and 37° C. Colonies grown on trypticase soy agar without blood should be observed microscopically under low power (100 ×) after 24 hours incubation for typical rough appearance with an internal serpentine pattern of bacilli, some of which stream from the edge of the colony toward adjacent colonies. This appearance is in contrast to the prominent starlike pattern seen in colonies of *A. actinomycetemcomitans*, with which *Cardiobacterium* may be confused. *Cardiobacterium* is a pleomorphic gram-negative bacillus that tends to form rosettelike arrangements.

The organism is oxidase-positive. *C. hominis* is able to utilize carbohydrates in media with sufficient nutritional factors. The addition of 10% horse serum to standard fermentation media will allow sufficient growth of the organism. A key biochemical parameter of *C. hominis* is the weak production of indole. The spot indole test (Chapter 9), performed on a colony grown on blood agar for 72 hours, may be positive even if the conventional test is negative. Alternatively, the more sensitive indole reagent described in Chapter 28, that of Ehrlich, combined with xylene extraction, may be required for demonstration of this property. *C. hominis* is urease-negative, catalase-negative, and nitrate-negative, as outlined in Table 29.5.

29.9.c. Treatment of *C. hominis* infections. The organism is susceptible in vitro to penicillin, ampicillin, cephalothin, chloramphenicol, aminoglycosides, and tetracycline. Penicillin is probably the drug of choice, although the organism's identity must be certain, as *A. actinomycetemcomitans* and *H. aphrophilus*, with which *C. hominis* may be confused, are often resistant to penicillin.

29.10. *Capnocytophaga canimorsus* (Formerly DF-2) and DF-3

C. canimorsus, probably normal oral flora in dogs and possibly cats, has been isolated from numerous cases of severe infection, often following a dog bite.[1a] Patients with underlying immunocompromising disorders are more likely to develop infection. The organism is usually isolated from blood or cerebrospinal fluid, but it may be missed in other specimens because of its fastidious nature and slow growth rate. After 4 days or longer of incubation at 37° C in 5% to 10% CO_2, pinpoint colonies appear on chocolate agar. Heart infusion agar with 5% rabbit blood may yield better growth. The organisms display a characteristic morphology of long, thin, pleomorphic gram-negative bacilli with occasional curved forms. Spindle- and cigar-shaped rods, some with tapered

ends, may also be seen. *C. canimorsus* (DF-2) is catalase- and oxidase-positive (other *Capnocytophaga* are catalase-negative) and indole-, nitrate-, and urease-negative. Some strains may hydrolyze esculin or produce arginine dihydrolase. The addition of 3% rabbit serum may be necessary for growth of the organism in carbohydrate broths. Alternatively, the rapid enzymatic carbohydrate tests described in Chapter 9 may be used. *C. canimorsus* is susceptible to penicillin, cephalothin, chloramphenicol, and carbenicillin but may be resistant to aminoglycosides. Resistance to colistin may help differentiate *C. canimorsus* from similar organisms, such as *P. multocida*, EF-4, *Kingella* sp., *Capnocytophaga*, *Eikenella*, and *C. hominis*, all of which are susceptible to colistin.

Other organisms resembling *C. canimorsus*, such as *C. cynodegmi* and DF-3, have been isolated from blood, wounds, and other sources, again associated with animal bites. DF-3 is catalase-negative, oxidase-negative, nitrate-negative, and may be indole-positive or negative. *C. cynodegmi* resembles *C. canimorsus* but is more active metabolically.

29.11. HB-5

HB-5 is isolated from the genitourinary tract of men and women. The organism has been associated with skin infections and abscesses. It is a gram-negative coccobacillus. Growth occurs as nonhemolytic colonies on blood agar after 24 hours of incubation at 37° C in 5% to 10% CO_2. Oxidase is variable and catalase is not produced. The organisms are nitrate-positive and weakly indole-positive. A triple sugar iron agar slant inoculated with HB-5 will be uniformly yellow after overnight incubation; glucose is fermented with the production of gas (unlike *Pasteurella*, *Cardiobacterium*, *Capnocytophaga*, and DF-3), but neither sucrose nor lactose is fermented.

REFERENCES

1. Aoyama, T., Murase, Y., Iwata, T., et al. 1986. Comparison of blood-free medium (cyclodextrin solid medium) with Bordet-Gengou medium for clinical isolation of *Bordetella pertussis*. J. Clin. Microbiol. 23:1046.

1a. Brenner, D.J., Hollis, D.G., Fanning, G.R., and Weaver, R.E. 1989. *C. canimorsus* sp. nov. (formerly CDC group DF-2), a cause of septicemia following dog bite, and *C. cynodegmi* sp. nov., a cause of localized wound infection following dog bite. J. Clin. Microbiol. 27:231.

2. Brenner, D.J., Mayer, L.W., Carlone, G.M., et al. 1988. Biochemical, genetic, and epidemiologic characterization of

Haemophilus influenzae biogroup Aegyptius (*Haemophilus aegyptius*) strains associated with Brazilian purpuric fever. J. Clin. Microbiol. 26:1524.

3. Ehrhardt, M.A., Lynch, K.M., Tyson, G.M., and Beckwith, D.G. 1986. Bordetella bronchiseptica: pathogen vs. commensal. Clin. Microbiol. Newsletter. 8:26.
4. Friedman, R.L. 1988. Pertussis: the disease and new diagnostic methods. Clin. Microbiol. Rev. 1:365.
5. Gabre-Kidan, T., Lipsky, B., and Plorde, J.J. 1984. *H. influenzae* as a cause of urinary tract infections in men. Arch. Intern. Med. 144:1623.
6. Gadberry, J.L. and Amos, M.A. 1986. Comparison of a new commercially prepared porphyrin test and the conventional satellite test for the identification of *Haemophilus* species that require X factor. J. Clin. Microbiol. 23:637-39.
7. Kaplan, A.H., Weber, D.J., Oddone, E.Z., and Perfect, J.R. 1989. Infection due to *Actinobacillus actinomycetemcomitans*: fifteen cases and review. Rev. Infect. Dis. 11:46.
8. Kilian, M. 1980. A taxonomic study of the genus *Haemophilus*, with the proposal of a new species. J. Gen. Microbiol. 93:9.
9. Kilian, M., and Biberstein, E.L. 1984. Genus *Haemophilus* Winslow, Broadhurst, Buchanan, Krumwiede, Rogers and Smith 1917. In Krieg, N.R., and Holt, J.G., editors. Bergey's manual of systematic bacteriology, ed. 9. Williams & Wilkins, Baltimore.
10. Kurzynski, T.A., Boehm, D.E., Rott-Petri, J.A., et al. 1988. Comparison of modified Bordet-Gengou and modified Regan-Lowe media for isolation of *Bordetella pertussis* and *Bordetella parapertussis*. J. Clin. Microbiol. 26:2661.
11. Morrill, W.E., Barbaree, J.M., Fields, B.S., et al. 1988. Effects of transport temperature and medium on recovery of *Bordetella pertussis* from nasopharyngeal swabs. J. Clin. Microbiol. 26:1814.
12. Mutters, R., Ihm, P., Pohl, S., et al. 1985. Reclassification of the genus *Pasteurella* Trevisan 1887 on the basis of deoxyribonucleic acid homology, with proposals for the new species *Pasteurella dagmatis*, *Pasteurella canis*, *Pasteurella stomatis*, *Pasteurella anatis*, and *Pasteurella langaa*. Int. J. Syst. Bact. 35:309.
13. Odugbemi, T., and Arko, R.J. 1983. Differentiation of *Kingella denitrificans* from *Neisseria gonorrhoeae* by growth on a semisolid medium and sensitivity to amylase. J. Clin. Microbiol. 17:389.

14. Papasian, C.J., Downs, N.J., Talley, R.L., et al. 1987. *Bordetella bronchiseptica* bronchitis. J. Clin. Microbiol. 25:575.
15. Papasian, C.J., Reintjes, S., Rengachary, S.S., et al. 1987. *Haemophilus paraphrophilus* brain abscess. Diagn. Microbiol. Infect. Dis. 7:205.
16. Provenza, J.M., Klotz, S.A., and Penn, R.L. 1986. Isolation of *Francisella tularensis* from blood. J. Clin. Microbiol. 24:453.
17. Raymond, J., Bergeret, M., Bargy, F., and Missenard, G. 1986. Isolation of two strains of *Kingella kingae* associated with septic arthritis. J. Clin. Microbiol. 24:1100.
18. Ruddy, A., Hughes, J., and Bourbeau, P. 1986. *Actinobacillus suis*: finger isolate following horse bite. Clin. Microbiol. Newsletter 8:187.
19. Stauffer, L.R., Brown, D.R., and Sandstrom, R.E. 1983. Cephalexin-supplemented Jones-Kendrick charcoal agar for selective isolation of *Bordetella pertussis*: comparison with previously described media. J. Clin. Microbiol. 17:60.
20. Steketee, R.W., Burstyn, D.G., Wassilak, S.G.F., et al. 1988. A comparison of laboratory and clinical methods for diagnosing pertussis in an outbreak in a facility for the developmentally disabled. J. Infect. Dis. 157:441.
21. Young, S.A., Anderson, G.L., Mitchell, P.D. 1987. Laboratory observations during an outbreak of pertussis. Clin. Microbiol. Newsletter 9:176.
22. Welch, W.D., Southern, P.M. Jr., and Schneider, N.R. 1986. Five cases of *Haemophilus segnis* appendicitis. J. Clin. Microbiol. 24:851.

BIBLIOGRAPHY

Corbel, M.J., and Brinkley-Morgan, W.J. 1984. Genus *Brucella* (Meyer and Shaw 1920). In Krieg, N.R., and Holt, J.G., editors. Bergey's manual of systematic bacteriology, ed. 9. Williams & Wilkins, Baltimore.

Friedman, R.L. 1988. Pertussis: the disease and new diagnostic methods. Clin. Microbiol. Rev. 1:365.

Hicklin, A., Verghese, A., and Alvarez, S. 1987. Dysgonic fermenter-2 septicemia. Rev. Infect. Dis. 9:884.

Weaver, R.E., Hollis, D.G., and Bottone, E.J. 1985. Gram-negative fermentative bacteria and *Francisella tularensis*. In Lennette, E.H., Balows, A., Hausler, W.J. Jr., and Shadomy, H.J., editors. Manual of clinical microbiology, ed. 4. American Society for Microbiology, Washington, D.C.

30 Vibrio and Related Species, Aeromonas, Plesiomonas, Campylobacter, and Others

Members of the genera *Vibrio*, *Campylobacter*, *Aeromonas*, and *Plesiomonas* have a few features in common: most of them are oxidase-positive gram-negative rods, some with curved cellular morphology, and some species from each genus are the etiologic agents of diarrheal disease in humans. Some species in all genera are motile by means of polar flagella, although the types of flagella and their arrangements vary. The Vibrionaceae family has classically included the genera *Vibrio*, *Plesiomonas*, and *Aeromonas*. It has been proposed that *Plesiomonas* be moved to the Enterobacteriaceae (it most resembles *Proteus* species).[3] Genera to remain in the family Vibrionaceae, "*Shewanella*" (includes former *Pseudomonas putrefaciens*; see Chapter 28), "*Photobacterium*," and "*Listonella*," have been proposed for some members of *Vibrio* species. Because they are more closely related to Enterobacteriaceae than Vibrionaceae, the new family "Aeromonadaceae" has been proposed for all *Aeromonas* species and some organisms previously classified as *Vibrio* species.[6] The Vibrionaceae are found in seawater and freshwater, where they are pathogenic for aquatic animals. Recovery of *Vibrio* species as the etiologic agents of diarrheal disease may require the use of special media, and for some *Campylobacter*, special atmosphere and temperature of incubation may be required as well.

Campylobacter species differ from vibrios by requiring a microaerophilic atmosphere. They display curved cellular morphology with occasional "seagull" forms representing two organisms end to end. Members of the genus are found in domestic animals, in soil and water, and in humans.

30.1. *Vibrio* Species

30.1.a. Epidemiology and pathogenesis of *Vibrio* infection. Members of the genus *Vibrio* are natural inhabitants of seawater. All organisms in this group are able to grow in media containing increased salt concentrations, and with the exception of *V. cholerae* and *V. mimicus* (the so-called "nonhalophilic" vibrios), they require sodium chloride for growth. The sodium ion–requiring members are called **halophilic** (based on the assumption that the chloride ion was required) vibrios. There are eleven species of potential clinical importance among the *Vibrio*. Table 30-1 lists the more common species.[19] *V. metschnikovii* and *V. cincinnatiensis* have been reported from rare human infections; they are not likely to be seen in a routine clinical laboratory.[2,8] *V. cholerae*, no longer rare in the United States, is usually acquired during foreign travel, although more than 40 cases of domestically acquired *V. cholerae* infection have been reported in the United States since 1973. In almost every case from which a *Vibrio* has been isolated from a domestically acquired infectious process, there has been some association with water or seafood. Although selective media are helpful for recovery of *Vibrio* from stool, the organisms grow well on routine bacteriologic media (sheep blood agar) and would not be overlooked when isolated from blood, wound cultures, or other sources as long as all gram-negative colonies are screened for oxidase production.

The enterotoxin of *V. cholerae* is one of the best characterized among bacteria (Chapter 17). The action of the toxin is to activate the adenylate cyclase of intestinal mucosal cells, which in turn raises the intracellular level of cyclic adenosine monophosphate (AMP), ultimately causing an active secretion of electrolytes into the intestinal lumen by altering ion transport across the cell membranes of the gastrointestinal mucosa epithelial cells. The outpouring of ions is followed by a release of water. Patients with cholera have been known to secrete fluid volumes equal to their body weight within 4 days. More importantly, the loss of water can dehydrate the patient so quickly that death occurs within 12 hours of onset of disease. In addition to the toxin, adherence to intestinal epithelium and motility are important factors in the pathogenicity of *V. cholerae*. Cholera-like toxin activity has also been observed in strains of *V. cholerae* non-O1 and *V. mimicus*. Other enterotoxins are produced by other vibrios.

Table 30.1

Clinically Significant *Vibrio* Species and Their Associated Infections (in Order of Relative Frequency)

TYPE OF INFECTION	ASSOCIATED SPECIES
Gastroenteritis	*cholerae* serotype 01
	cholerae non-01
	parahaemolyticus
	fluvialis
	mimicus
	furnissii
	hollisae
Wound infection	*alginolyticus*
	vulnificus
	*damsela**
Sepsis	*cholerae* non-01
	vulnificus
Ear infection	*alginolyticus*
	cholera non-01
	mimicus
	parahaemolyticus

*V. damsela proposed to be moved to new genus *"Listonella."*

Other species of *Vibrio* produce a number of extracellular cytolytic toxins or cytotoxins and enzymes that may contribute to their virulence. Pathogenicity of *V. vulnificus* and *V. damsela* is probably enhanced by cytolysin production. *V. fluvialis* has been shown to produce a cytotoxin. *V. parahaemolyticus* can produce disease that resembles dysentery. It appears that *V. parahaemolyticus* virulence may be associated with hemolysin production.

V. vulnificus, the lactose-positive halophilic *Vibrio*, appears to have a remarkable invasive potential, perhaps mediated by proteases. Primarily seen in patients with underlying hepatic or immunocompromising disease, but also in healthy patients, this organism produces a primary septicemia (with 50% mortality in patients with underlying disease). The organisms are assumed to enter the bloodstream via the gastrointestinal tract, usually within 24 to 48 hours after ingestion of raw shellfish, particularly oysters. Infections caused by *V. vulnificus* have been reported primarily from coastal states.

30.1.b. Isolation of *Vibrio* species from feces. Fecal specimens received in microbiology laboratories in the United States are not routinely inoculated to media selective for vibrios due to the low incidence of *Vibrio*-related gastroenteritis in the United States. If a patient with diarrheal disease has a history of

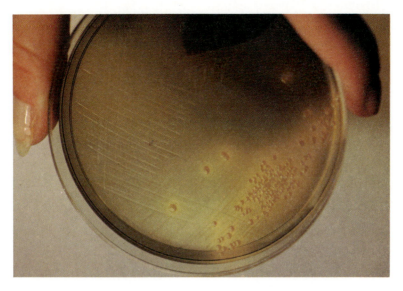

Figure 30.1
Colonies of *V. cholerae* on TCBS agar.

travel, of having consumed shellfish, or had other contact with seawater, vibrios should be considered. Recent foreign travel is the most important risk factor. Stool should be transported in Cary-Blair transport media if it cannot be plated to selective agar immediately. Plating onto 5% sheep blood agar will also adequately support the growth of *Vibrio* species. The most commonly used selective agar is thiosulfate citrate—bile salts—sucrose agar (TCBS; Appendix A), which can be heavily inoculated. Eiken (Japan) produces a highly regarded product (Michael Janda, personal communication). An evaluation of dry powder TCBS from four different commercial manufacturers showed media produced by Oxoid Ltd. in England to perform consistently better for isolation and typical colony morphology formation than three other media tested.[35] Conventional selective enteric agars (Chapter 8) should be inoculated, of course, for isolation of other possible etiologic agents. All vibrios will grow on nonselective media, but their colonies will not be distinctive enough to ensure their detection in mixed flora containing large numbers of other bacteria unless some screening procedure (such as oxidase) is used. In very dilute, typical "rice water" stools of cholera, vibrios are present in large numbers, often to the exclusion of much of the normal flora. An enrichment broth particularly

useful for detection of small numbers of *V. cholerae* is alkaline peptone water (pH 8.4, Appendix A). Janda and colleagues[19] recommend that alkaline peptone water be prepared in 20-ml amounts to retain proper pH. This broth should be subcultured to selective media (TCBS) as soon as possible after 5 hours' incubation (at 35° C) to prevent overgrowth of other bacteria. Longer incubation times are acceptable with lower incubation temperatures (room temperature). Supplementing media with NaCl is not necessary, since these organisms do grow in brain-heart infusion broth and on blood agar without added salt.

30.1.c. **Laboratory identification.** After 18 to 24 hours' incubation at 35° C in air, sucrose-fermenting vibrios (*V. cholerae, V. alginolyticus, V. cincinnatiensis V. fluvialis, V. furnissii, V. metschnikovii,* and some *V. vulnificus*) will appear as medium-sized, smooth, opaque, thin-edged yellow colonies on TCBS agar (Figure 30.1). The other clinically important vibrios do not ferment sucrose and will appear olive-green (Figure 30.2).

On Gram stain, vibrios are small gram-negative bacilli that may occasionally exhibit slightly curved forms (Figure 30.3). Morphology cannot reliably be used for identification. Oxidase-positive fermentative organisms isolated from wound cultures, blood,

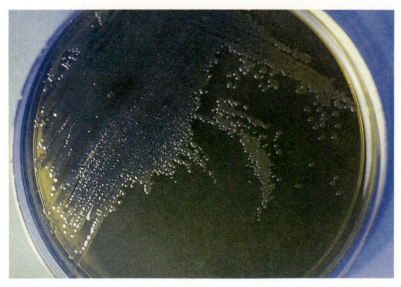

Figure 30.2
Colonies of *V. parahaemolyticus* on TCBS agar.

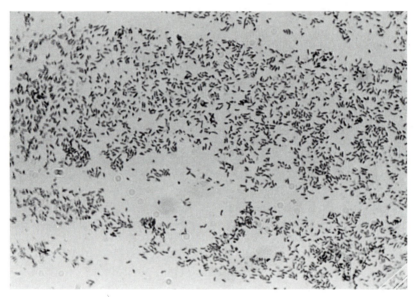

Figure 30.3
Gram stain of smear made from *Vibrio cholerae* colony on TCBS agar.

and other sources may be vibrios, and biochemical tests should be performed. The commercially produced biotyping systems may identify the most common *Vibrio* species; newly described and unusual species are less likely to be reliably identified by such kits. Except for *V. metschnikovii*, all vibrios are oxidase-positive. The halophilic vibrios may require the addition of NaCl (up to a total of 3%) to all identification media and prepackaged commercial systems in order to display proper reactions. Systems that utilize a saline suspension of the inoculum are likely to support the growth of some of the clinically important vibrios without added salt. Identification procedures are no different than those used for other gram-negative bacilli. Key differential characteristics of the more commonly isolated clinically relevant vibrios are listed in Table 30.2.

Vibrios have been divided into serogroups based on their somatic "O" antigens; thus all cholera-producing strains were assigned to serotype "O," subgroup 1 (O1). Other grouping systems identify more than 70 non-O1 serogroups.[19] Although there is no genetic basis for a division, *V. cholerae* have been divided by morphological difference into two biovars or biotypes: classical and eltor (formerly El Tor). The eltor biovar is Voges-Proskauer-positive, will agglutinate chicken red blood cells, and is resistant to a 50-U disk of polymyxin B, whereas the classical biovar yields the opposite reactions. Many recently isolated eltor biovars are nonhemolytic on sheep blood agar, in contrast to the typical β-hemolysis displayed by organisms of this biovar that were isolated several years ago.

V. cholerae of both serotypes, O1 and non-O1, cause cholera-like disease, although only serotype O1 is associated with epidemic disease. These two serotypes are biochemically identical but differ in their ability to agglutinate in *V. cholerae* O1 antiserum. Non-O1 vibrios have been associated with large outbreaks. In the United States the occasional isolate of *V. cholerae* is likely to be nonagglutinable in O1 typing serum.

Gastroenteritis-associated strains of *V. parahaemolyticus* are usually able to produce a hemolysin that hemolyzes human red blood cells in mannitol agar with a high salt content, called Kanagawa phenomenon. Environmental strains seem to lack this ability. It is interesting that strains of urease-positive *V. parahaemolyticus* are currently being isolated from patients with gastroenteritis in many countries and particularly in the United States, in contrast to the predominance of urease-negative strains recovered before 1980.[19]

Oxidase-positive organisms that may be confused with vibrios include *Aeromonas* species, *Plesiomonas* species, and *Pseudomonas* species. Key differential characteristics are outlined in Table 30.3. One important test for differentiation of vibrios from *Aeromonas* species (discussed below), which they closely resemble, is susceptibility to the vibriostatic agent 2,4-diamino-6,7-diisopropylpteridine phosphate (O/129). This agent, available in 10- and 150-µg disks (or as powder) from Oxoid USA inhibits the growth of all vibrios at a concentration of 150 µg/ml or greater. *Aeromonas*, Enterobacteriaceae, and

Pseudomonas species are resistant. Of organisms likely to be confused with vibrios, most *Plesiomonas* are susceptible to O/129 at 10 µg, and all are susceptible to O/129 at 150 µg. However, *Plesiomonas* will not grow on TCBS and fails to grow in 6% salt; all the vibrios (except for strains of *V. hollisae*) grow on TCBS, and all vibrios, with the exception of certain *V. mimicus* and *V. cholerae* strains, are able to grow in media containing 6% salt.

30.1.d. Treatment of *Vibrio* disease. Cholera is best treated with fluid and electrolyte replacement, although tetracycline or furazolidone will shorten the course of disease and may decrease bacterial excretion. In areas of the world where cholera is endemic, such as Bangladesh, tetracycline resistance is common. The decision of whether to treat a patient with antimicrobial agents depends on demographic, economic, and clinical factors, including the nutritional status of the patient. There have been ampicillin-trimethoprim-sulfamethoxazole- and tetracycline-resistant isolates reported from the developed world as well, so a susceptibility test should be performed. The agar disk diffusion test is adequate; Mueller-Hinton agar will support the growth of halophilic and nonhalophilic vibrios; salt should not be added, as it alters the activity of certain antimicrobial agents. Most strains of *V. parahaemolyticus*, *V. alginolyticus*, *V. damsela*, *V. vulnificus*, and *V. hollisae* are susceptible to gentamicin, tetracycline, and chloramphenicol. Resistance to ampicillin, cephalothin, and carbenicillin has been reported for *V. parahaemolyticus*, *V. alginolyticus*, and *V. furnissii*.

30.2. *Aeromonas* Species

30.2.a. Epidemiology and pathogenesis of *Aeromonas* infection. *Aeromonas* are ubiquitous inhabitants of natural waters, both fresh and salt, where they infect animals, including amphibians, reptiles, and fish. In humans, they are most commonly associated with infections of wounds acquired near or in water, or with diarrheal disease. The nonmotile species, *A. salmonicida* and *A. media*, and the motile species, *A. hydrophila* group (*A. hydrophila*, *A. caviae-punctata*, and *A. sobria*), *A. schubertii*,[13] and *A. veronii*,[14] have all been associated with human disease. The fish pathogen, *A. salmonicida*, because of its preferential growth temperature of 23° C, is least likely to cause human infections. *Aeromonas* species have been recovered from blood, cerebrospinal fluid, exudate from otitis media, urine, peritoneal fluid, necrotic muscle, infected heart valves, and

Table 30.2

Differential Characteristics of *Vibrio* Species Likely to be Recovered from Clinical Specimens

	GROWTH IN NaCl (%)					VOGES-PROSKAUER	LYSINE DECARBOXYLASE
	0	**3**	**6**	**8**	**10**		
alginolyticus	−	+	+	+	+	+	+
cholerae	+	+	+ / −	−	−	+ / −	+
cincinnatiensis	−	+	+	−	−	+	+
damsela *	−	+	+	−	−	+	+ / −
fluvialis	−	+	+	+ / −	+ / −	−	−
furnissii†	−	+	+	+ / −	−	−	−
hollisae	−	+	+	−	−	−	−
metschnikovii‡	+ / −	+	+	+ / −	−	+	+ / −
mimicus	+	+	+ / −	−	−	−	+
parahaemolyticus§	−	+	+	+	−	−	+
vulnificus	−	+	+	−	−	−	+

+ = ≥90% positive; − = ≥90% negative; ± = variable results; ND = test not done.
* Urease positive.
† Gas from glucose.
‡ Oxidase-negative and nitrate-negative.
§ Rare urease-positive strains.

Table 30.3

Key Characteristics of Oxidase-Positive Gram-Negative Bacilli

CHARACTERISTIC	AEROMONAS	PLESIOMONAS	VIBRIO	PSEUDOMONAS
Susceptible to 0/129				
10 µg	−	+ / −	+ / −	−
150 µg	−	+	+	−
Ferment glucose	+	+	+	−
Acid from				
Inositol	−	+	−	NA
Mannitol	+	−	+	NA
Gelatin liquefaction	+	−	+	+ / −
Growth on TCBS	−	−	+	−
Requires or stimulated by Na⁺	−	−	+	−

+ = most strains positive; − = most strains negative; + / − = variable results; NA = not applicable.

bone.[17] Gastroenteritis, however, is the most common infection associated with this organism.

Janda and Duffey[18] describe five diarrheal presentations for *Aeromonas*-related gastroenteritis: secretory (acute watery diarrhea, often with vomiting), dysenteric (accompanied by blood and mucus in the stool), chronic (lasting longer than 10 days), choleric ("rice-water" stools), and traveler's. Drinking untreated water is one risk factor for acquisition of *Aeromonas*-related gastroenteritis, an increasingly recognized syndrome. Other risk factors for acquisition of gastroenteritis by adults, including current gastrointestinal or liver disease, reduced stomach acidity, and recent antibiotic administration, were reported by George and others.[10] *A. hydrophila*, *A. sobria*, *A. caviae*, and *A. veronii* have been associated with gastrointestinal disease and *A. schubertii*, *A. veronii*, *A. hydrophila*, and *A. sobria* have been recovered from infected wounds and blood.[15,18,24] *A. caviae* is rarely isolated from blood, suggesting that it is less virulent.

It has been shown that *A. hydrophila* produces a heat-labile enterotoxin (synonymous with the β-hemolysin) and a heat stable cytotoxic enterotoxin. *Aeromonas* also produces a large number of extracellular enzymes, including protease, amylase, li-

ORNITHINE DECARBOXYLASE	ARGININE DIHYDROLASE	INDOLE	ACID FROM			SENSITIVITY TO O/129	
			LACTOSE	SUCROSE	ARABINOSE	10 μg	150 μg
+ / −	−	+ / −	−	+	−	−	+
+	−	+	−	+	−	+	+
−	−	−	−	+	+	−	+
−	+	−	−	−	+	+	+
−	+	+ / −	−	+	+	−	+
−	+	−	−	+	+	−	+
−	−	+	−	−	+	−	+
−	+	+ / −	+	+	−	+	+
+	−	+	−	−	−	+	+
+	−	+	−	−	+ / −	−	+
+ / −	−	+	+	−	−	+	+

pase, nuclease, and others. The role of these enzymes in the pathogenesis of *Aeromonas* infections, if any, has not been defined. Adherence may also serve as a virulence factor.

30.2.b. Laboratory identification. *Aeromonas* species grow on standard laboratory media, including blood agar and MacConkey agar. They would be identified as would any other gram-negative bacillus isolated from a source such as a sterile body fluid, tissue, or wound. On Gram stain, the cells are straight-sided, medium-sized, nonpleomorphic gram-negative bacilli. Recognition of *Aeromonas* species as etiologic agents of diarrhea, however, is more difficult, since many strains ferment lactose and sucrose and would not be distinctive enough to be recognized on MacConkey agar. The selective media commonly used to detect *Salmonella*, *Shigella*, and *Campylobacter* species are inhibitory to some *Aeromonas*. Many *Aeromonas* are β-hemolytic on 5% sheep blood agar, allowing one to choose colonies to screen for the presence of oxidase by Kovacs' method. Nonhemolytic colonies should be screened as well. All members of the Vibrionaceae family are oxidase-positive (except *V. metschnikovii*), and they can be differentiated from oxidase-positive pseudomonads by their ability to ferment glucose in triple sugar iron (TSI) agar and by the spot indole test (Chapter 9). *Pseudomonas* species are all indole-negative, whereas many Vibrionaceae are indole-positive. If a predominance of non-pseudomonas-appearing oxidase-positive colonies are found on the blood agar plate inoculated with diarrheal stool, the possibility of *Aeromonas* should be further explored. Trypticase soy agar with 5% sheep blood and 10 or 30 μg/ml ampicillin is also useful for selective isolation of *Aeromonas*.[9] A combination of ampicillin blood agar and CIN agar, used to select for *Yersinia enterocolitica*, showed best recovery of strains of *Aeromonas* from feces in one recent study.[21] Prilxylose-ampicillin agar has been used successfully for recovery of aeromonads from clinical specimens.[18,28]

Aeromonas are distinguished from the Enterobacteriaceae, which they closely resemble both morphologically and biochemically, by the oxidase test; Enterobacteriaceae are oxidase-negative. *Aeromonas* are differentiated from oxidase-positive vibrios by their resistance to the vibriostatic agent O/129 (Table 30.3). Table 30.4 outlines differentiation of the *Aeromonas* species pathogenic for humans, as well as the closely related *Plesiomonas shigelloides*. The commercial biochemical and enzymatic identification systems routinely used for characterization of Enterobacteriaceae will identify *Plesiomonas* and *Aeromonas*, at least to genus, with the addition of the oxidase test result to the profile number generated. At least one widely used system (API 20E, Analytab Products) does not distinguish between *Aeromonas* and certain *Vibrio* species, the performance of the O/129 test or growth on TCBS is, therefore, critical.

30.2.c. Treatment of *Aeromonas* infection. *Aeromonas*-associated diarrhea is usually self-limited and

Table 30.4
Key Differential Characteristics of *Aeromonas* Species (Isolated from Humans) and *Plesiomonas shigelloides*

SPECIES	ESCULIN HYDROLYSIS	VOGES-PROSKAUER*	LYSINE DECARBOX-YLASE	ARGININE DIHYDRO-LASE	ORNITHINE DECARBOX-YLASE	GAS FROM GLUCOSE	ACID FROM	
							MAN-NITOL	ARABI-NOSE
A. hydrophila	+	+	+	+	−	+	+	+
A. caviae	+	−	−	+	−	−	+	+
A. sobria	−	+	+	+	−	+	+	−
A. veronii	+	+	+	−	+	+	+	−
A. schubertii†	−	+	+	+	−		−	
P. shigelloides	−	−	+	+	+	−	−	−

+ = ≥90% positive; − = ≥90% negative.
* Plus 1% NaCl.
† Indole-negative.

normally does not require treatment. For protracted, bloody, or chronic diarrhea and for more severe infections, several antimicrobial agents are effective. The organisms are susceptible to quinolones, gentamicin, trimethoprim-sulfamethoxazole, third generation cephalosporins, and chloramphenicol. They are resistant to streptomycin, penicillins, and most first- and second-generation cephalosporins.

30.3. Plesiomonas

The one species of *Plesiomonas*, *P. shigelloides*, resembles *Aeromonas*, although it is not β-hemolytic. *Plesiomonas* also maintains a water habitat. Although primarily associated with gastroenteritis, the organism has been isolated as the etiologic agent of meningitis, bacteremia, septic arthritis, cholecystitis, and endophthalmitis.[3] The pathogenesis of diarrhea associated with *Plesiomonas* has not been conclusively established, although epidemiologic studies and other lines of evidence strongly suggest a causal relationship.[3,16] Disease is associated with eating raw shellfish and foreign travel. Virulence factors include enterotoxin,[22] possible invasiveness (using classical tests for this property), and adherence to intestinal epithelial cells.[3]

Gram-stained colonies may reveal long filamentous forms as well as regular bacilli. Although the colonies are not distinctive from Enterobacteriaceae on MacConkey agar, they are oxidase-positive and may be detected in the same manner as *Aeromonas* colonies. Both lactose-fermenting and non-lactose-fermenting strains exist, exhibiting different colony morphologies on MacConkey agar. *P. shigelloides* is identified biochemically, as outlined in Table 30.4.

As with *Aeromonas*, only patients with under-

lying disease or very severe infections should be treated. Patients treated with tetracycline or trimethoprim-sulfamethoxazole have recovered from *Plesiomonas* infection. Chloramphenicol, trimethoprim-sulfamethoxazole, cephalothin, and aminoglycosides are active against *Plesiomonas* in vitro. Most isolates have been resistant to penicillin, ampicillin, and carbenicillin.

30.4. Campylobacter Species

30.4.a. **Epidemiology and pathogenesis of *Campylobacter* infection.** *Campylobacter* species are microaerophilic inhabitants of the gastrointestinal tracts of a number of animals, including poultry, dogs, cats, sheep, and cattle, as well as the reproductive organs of several animal species (Table 30.5). When fecal samples from chicken carcasses chosen at random from butcher shops in the New York City area were tested for *Campylobacter*, 83% of the samples yielded over 10^6 colony-forming units per gram of feces. Species of *Campylobacter* produce two primary syndromes in humans: systemic disease characterized by fever and, most commonly, gastroenteritis. Extraintestinal disease, including meningitis, endocarditis, and septic arthritis, is being recognized increasingly, particularly in AIDS patients. The *Campylobacter* species associated with the most human infections (*jejuni* and *coli*) are usually transmitted via contaminated food, milk, or water. Outbreaks have been associated with contaminated drinking water and consumption of improperly pasteurized milk, among other sources. In contrast to other agents of foodborne gastroenteritis, including *Salmonella* and staphylococci, *Campylobacter* does not multiply in food.

Table 30.5

Campylobacter species and associated factors

SPECIES HUMANS	PREDOMINANT HOST(S)	INFECTION IN
"*cinaedi*"	Homosexual males	Enteritis
coli	Pigs	Enteritis
concisus	Humans	? Periodontal disease
cryaerophila	Cows, pigs	Diarrhea
"*fennelliae*"	Homosexual males	Enteritis
fetus subsp. *fetus*	Cows, sheep	Sepsis, meningitis, abscesses, other
fetus subsp. *venerealis*	Cows	None
hyointestinalis	Pigs	Proctitis, diarrhea
jejuni	Numerous animals, birds	Enteritis
jejuni subsp. *doylei*	Humans	? Diarrhea
laridis	Seagulls	Enteritis
mucosalis	Pigs	None
nitrofigilis	Salt marsh plant roots	None
pylori	Humans	Gastritis, peptic ulcer
sputorum	Cattle, sheep, humans	Unknown
"*upsaliensis*"	Dogs, humans	Gastroenteritis, sepsis

C. hyointestinalis, recently implicated in human disease, was isolated from patients who drank untreated water, were compromised in some way, or were returning from international travel.[7] The newest among named strains, *C. jejuni* subsp. *doylei*, was isolated from children with diarrhea and from gastric biopsies from adults.[29] As more laboratories differentiate among these species, their etiologic roles will be delineated. Among homosexual populations, *Campylobacter* is thought to be transmitted sexually, as are other agents of gastroenteritis. "*Campylobacter cinaedi*" and "*Campylobacter fennelliae*" have been proposed for new species isolated from stools of homosexuals with enteritis or proctitis. Although isolated from the human gingival crevice of patients with periodontal disease, the role of *C. concisus* in this syndrome is not clear. The taxonomy of *Campylobacter* has been reviewed recently.[27]

Recent studies have amassed evidence for the role of *C. pylori* as an etiologic agent of gastritis and probably peptic ulcer.[1,4,12] Pathogenic mechanisms have not yet been elucidated and studies are ongoing. Because of genetic differences, *C. pylori*, and perhaps *C. concisus* as well, is likely to be moved to a different genus. The genus name *Helicobacter* has been proposed.

Campylobacter species (usually *jejuni*) has been recognized as the most common etiologic agent of gastroenteritis in the United States. Ratios of recovery of *Campylobacter* vs *Salmonella* range from 2:1

to 46:1.[5] *Campylobacter* species seem to possess several virulence factors. The production of bloody diarrhea, characterized by the presence of numerous polymorphonuclear neutrophils in patients with gastroenteritis and the appearance of certain strains of *Campylobacter* in the blood of patients after ingestion of contaminated material, are indicative of the invasive capacity of the organism. *Campylobacter* species (*coli*, *jejuni*, and *laridis*) are known to produce a cytotoxin, a cytotonic factor, and an enterotoxin, which may account for those cases characterized by watery diarrhea.[20] The actual importance of toxin production in development of disease is still being investigated.[34]

Although 97% of patients with diarrhea due to *C. jejuni* cease excreting the organism within 4 to 7 weeks even without treatment, the remaining patients (now asymptomatic) continue to carry the organism for long periods of time (1 to several years). Carriers of *C. jejuni* are far more common in tropical countries than in the United States. Increased prevalence of infection in tropical countries results in an endemic level of mild disease, probably due to herd immunity.

30.4.b. Isolation of *Campylobacter* species from blood cultures. *C. fetus* subsp. *fetus*, *C. laridis*, *C. jejuni*, "*C. cinaedi*," and "*C. upsaliensis*" have been documented as agents of sepsis[26,27,30,32] and will grow in most blood culture media, although they may require as long as 2 weeks for growth to be detected.

Subcultures from broths must be incubated in a microaerophilic atmosphere or the organisms will not multiply. There is often no visible turbidity in blood culture media, therefore blind subcultures or visual examination using acridine orange stain is necessary. The presence of *Campylobacter* species in blood cultures is detected effectively by CO_2 monitoring (Bactec system). Isolation from sources other than blood or feces (extremely rare) is ideally accomplished by inoculating the material (macerated tissue, wound exudate) to a nonselective blood or chocolate agar plate and incubating the plate at 37° C in a CO_2-enriched, microaerophilic atmosphere. Selective agars containing a cephalosporin, rifampin, and polymyxin B may inhibit growth of some strains and should not be used for isolation from normally sterile sites.

30.4.c. Isolation of *Campylobacter* species from feces. The most common agents of gastroenteritis, *C. jejuni* and *C. coli*, are able to grow well at 42° C and are resistant to cephalosporin, characteristics useful for their initial isolation. There is not an increased number of colonies at this temperature, but the colonies are larger and the growth of most normal fecal flora is inhibited. Feces may be transported to the laboratory directly for inoculation onto media. If a delay of longer than 2 hours is anticipated, material should be placed either in Cary-Blair transport medium or in campy thio—a thioglycollate broth base with 0.16% agar and vancomycin (10 mg/L), trimethoprim (5 mg/L), cephalothin (15 mg/L), polymyxin B (2,500 U/L), and amphotericin B (2 mg/L). The same antimicrobial agents are incorporated into *Brucella* agar base with 10% sheep blood to produce campy-BAP, one of the selective agars that is useful for cultivation of these strains. A number of media manufacturers produce commercial plates for *Campylobacter* isolation. Since these *Campylobacter* are resistant to cold, refrigeration of fresh stools for as long as 24 hours before plating will probably not result in false-negative cultures. The stool should be plated onto a selective agar and incubated at 42° C in a microaerophilic atmosphere. The atmosphere can be generated in several ways, including commercially produced gas-generating envelopes meant to be used in conjunction with plastic bags or plastic jars. Evacuation and replacement in plastic bags or anaerobic jars with an atmosphere of 10% CO_2, 5% O_2, and the balance N_2 is the most cost-effective method, although it is somewhat labor-

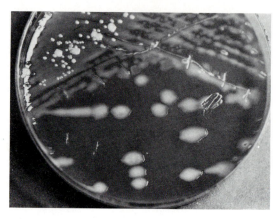

Figure 30.4
C. jejuni growing on a campy blood agar plate after 48 hours' incubation.

intensive.[31] Plates should be held for 72 hours before being discarded as negative.

Isolation of *C. fetus* subsp. *fetus*, *C. laridis*, *C. hyointestinalis*, *C. cryaerophila*, "*C. fennelliae*," "*C. cinaedi*," and "*C. upsaliensis*" from stool may be attempted by inoculating a selective medium without cephalosporins and incubating for up to 7 days at 37° C microaerophilically. Skirrow's medium, containing blood agar base, 5% lysed horse blood, vancomycin (10 mg/L), polymyxin (2,500 U/L) and trimethoprim (5 mg/L) would adequately support growth of the less common species.

Filtration of feces has been promoted as an alternative method for isolation of *Campylobacter* species from feces. Either a 0.65- or a 0.8-μm pore-size cellulose acetate filter can be used.[31] The stool is diluted if necessary, and several drops of filtrate are placed directly onto nonselective agar and incubated at 42° C in a microaerophilic atmosphere. In a modification, a filter is placed onto the agar surface, and a drop of stool is placed on the filter. The plate is incubated upright. After overnight incubation the filter is removed, and the plates are reincubated. *Campylobacter* species are able to move through the filter to produce colonies on the agar surface.

Plates should be examined at 24 and 48 hours for characteristic colonies, which are gray to pinkish or yellowish gray, slightly mucoid-looking colonies; some colonies may exhibit a tailing effect along the streak line (Figure 30.4). Other colony morphologies are also common.

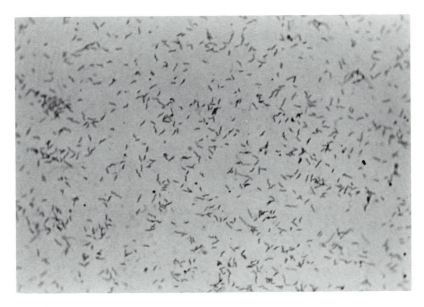

Figure 30.5
Gram stain appearance of *C. jejuni* smeared from primary isolation plate. Note seagull-shaped and curved forms.

30.4.d. Laboratory identification. Suspicious-looking colonies seen on selective media incubated at 42° C may be presumptively identified as *Campylobacter* species (usually *jejuni* or *coli*) with a few simple tests. A wet preparation of the organism may be examined under phase or darkfield microscopy for characteristic darting motility and curved forms. On Gram stain, the organisms are small, curved, or seagull-winged gram-negative rods (Figure 30.5). Most all of the pathogenic *Campylobacter* species are oxidase- and catalase-positive. For most laboratories, reporting of such isolates from feces as "*Campylobacter* species" should suffice.

Campylobacter species are asaccharolytic, able to grow in the presence of 1% glycine and 3.5% NaCl, and, with the exception of *C. cryaerophila*, are unable to grow in air. Susceptibility to nalidixic acid and cephalothin, an important differential characteristic among species (Table 30.6), is determined by inoculating a 5% sheep blood agar plate or a Mueller-Hinton agar plate with a McFarland 0.5 turbidity suspension of the organism as for agar disk diffusion susceptibility testing, placing 30-µg disks on the agar surface, and incubating microaerophilically at 37° C. Other tests useful for identifying these species are the rapid hippurate hydrolysis test (Chapter 9, Procedure 9.9), production of H$_2$S in TSI agar butts,

nitrate reduction,[29] and a promising new test, hydrolyis of indoxyl acetate (Procedure 30.1.).[23] The indoxyl acetate test, positive only for *C. jejuni, C. coli,* "*C. fennelliae,*" and *C. cryaerophila* and weakly positive for some strains of "*C. cinaedi,*" was reliable for colonies grown on any medium, although limited numbers of some species have been evaluated.[23] Definitive differentiation of *C. jejuni, C. coli,* and *C. pylori* is also accomplished by detecting C-19 cyclopropane fatty acid methyl ester as a component of the cell wall using gas-liquid chromatographic methods.[11] This method is not available to most clinical microbiology laboratories.

30.4.e. Detection of *C. pylori* in gastric specimens. Tissue biopsy material should be transported to the laboratory in a sterile container. It may be refrigerated for up to 5 hours before processing. Smears and cultures should be examined for presence of the organisms. Parsonnet and others[25] report good recovery using the following technique. Tissue is rinsed in dextrose phosphate broth, blotted onto a sterile gauze or filter paper to remove excess broth, and pressed onto the surface of a sterile glass slide. After the smear has been prepared, the tissue is ground in dextrose phosphate broth and inoculated to media. Nonselective agar media, including chocolate agar and brucella agar with 5% sheep blood,

Table 30.6
Differential Characteristics of Clinically Relevant *Campylobacter* Species

SPECIES	GROWTH AT		HIPPURATE HYDROLYSIS	CATALASE	H₂S IN TSI	INDOXYL ACETATE HYDROLYSIS	NITRATE TO NITRITE	SUSCEPTIBLE TO 30-µg DISK	
	25° C	42° C						CEPHALOTHIN	NALIDIXIC ACID
"cinaedi"	–	–/+	–	+	–	–/+	+	+/–	+
coli	–	+	–	+	–	+	+	–	+
concisus	–	+	–	–	+	ND	+	–	–
cryaerophila	+	–	–	+	–	+	+	–	+/–
"fennelliae"	–	–	–	+	–	+	–	+	+
fetus subsp. *fetus*	+	–/+	–	+	–	–	+	+	–
hyointestinalis	+/–	+	–	+	+	–	+	+	–
jejuni	–	+	+	+	–	+	+	–	+
jejuni subsp. *doylei*	–	+/–	+	+/– or weak +	–	ND	–	+	+
laridis	–	+	–	+	–	–	+	–	–
*pylori**	–	+	–	+	–	–	+/–	+	–
sputorum	–	+	–	–/+	+	–	+	+	–/+
"upsaliensis"	–	+	–	–/weak +	–	ND	+	+	+

+ = Most strains positive; – = most strains negative; +/– = variable results; ND = not done.
*Strong and rapid positive urease.

PROCEDURE 30.1

Hydrolysis of Indoxyl Acetate

Principle

Certain species of *Campylobacter* produce a bacterial esterase that hydrolyzes indoxyl acetate to produce a blue end product.

Method

1. Prepare indoxyl acetate disks as follows:
   a. Dissolve 1 g indoxyl acetate (Sigma Chemical) in 10 ml acetone.
   b. Place filter paper disks (0.25 inch [0.64 cm] diameter, available from Difco and BBL) on a dry surface and add 0.5 ml of the indoxyl acetate solution to each disk.
   c. Allow the disks to air dry and store desiccated in an amber bottle at 4° C. Disks are stable for at least 1 year.
2. To test an isolate, place several colonies on the surface of an indoxyl acetate disk and moisten the disk with a drop of sterile water. Observe for up to 10 min for a blue color, indicating hydrolysis of the substrate.

Quality control

Test a fresh subculture of *C. jejuni* (ATCC 29428) on one disk and simply add water to a second disk.

Expected results

The *C. jejuni,* as a positive control, should yield a blue color reaction within 10 min. The uninoculated disk should remain the original color, as a negative control.

Performance schedule

Perform a qualtiy control check when disks are first prepared and monthly thereafter.

Modified from Mills and Gherna.[23]

---

have been useful for isolation of *C. pylori* from gastric antral biopsy specimens. Selective agar, such as Skirrow's agar also support growth.[33] Modified Thayer-Martin medium (intended for gonococci) yielded the best recovery in at least one study.[25] Several agars must be evaluated before a laboratory determines that which is best in their circumstances.

Incubation up to 1 week in a humidified, microaerophilic atmosphere at 35 to 37° C may be required before growth is visible as small, translucent, circular colonies. *C. pylori* is identified presumptively by typical cellular morphology and by positive results for oxidase, catalase, and rapid urease tests.

Presumptive evidence of the presence of the organism in biopsy material may be obtained by placing a portion of crushed tissue biopsy material directly into urease broth. A positive test is considered indicative of the organism's presence. Problems of low sensitivity and the necessity for a 24 hour incubation have precluded universal acceptance of this test. Microbiologists and pathologists should decide whether to incorporate tests for *C. pylori* in their routine procedures based on input from the gastroenterologists served by a laboratory.

30.4.f. Treatment of *Campylobacter* infection. Erythromycin is the drug of choice for those patients with complicated gastroenteritis (hyperpyrexia, dehydration, or bacteremia). For patients with bacteremia, therapy is continued for 4 weeks. Gastroenteritis is usually treated for 10 days. Tetracycline is an alternative choice in the United States, although 15% to 20% of strains are resistant; children under 7 years should be given clindamycin. The gastroenteritis-associated *Campylobacter* species are susceptible to gentamicin, other aminoglycosides, chloramphenicol, cefotaxime, and ciprofloxacin.

C. pylori displays in vitro susceptibility to erythromycin, rifampin, tetracycline, and metronidazole and resistance to nalidixic acid and sulfonamides. Bismuth salts have activity against *C. pylori* and have been efficacious in treating some patients with gastritis, although controlled studies are rare. Evidence for efficacy of furazolidone and metronidazole in treatment of gastritis has been presented; final recommendations await further studies.[1]

REFERENCES

1. Blaser, M.J. 1987. Gastric *Campylobacter*-like organisms, gastritis, and peptic ulcer disease. Gastroenterology 93:371.

2. Brayton, P.R., Bode, R.B., Colwell, R.R., et al. 1986. *Vibrio cincinnatiensis* sp. nov., a new human pathogen. J. Clin. Microbiol. 23:104.

3. Brenden, R.A., Miller, M.A., and Janda, J.M. 1988. Clinical disease spectrum and pathogenic factors associated with *Plesiomonas shigelloides* infections in humans. Rev. Infect. Dis. 10:303.

4. Buck, G.E. 1987. *Campylobacter pylori (C. pyloridis)*: a new organism implicated as a cause of gastritis and peptic ulcers. Clin. Microbiol. Newsletter 9:141.

5. Centers for Disease Control. 1988. *Campylobacter* isolates in the United States, 1982-1986. M.M.W.R. 37(SS-2):1.

6. Colwell, R.R., MacDonell, M.T., and De Ley, J. 1986. Proposal to recognize the family *Aeromonadaceae* fam. nov. Int. J. Syst. Bacteriol. 36:473.

7. Edmonds, P., Patton, C.M., Griffin, P.M., et al. 1987. *Campylobacter hyointestinalis* associated with human gastrointestinal disease in the United States. J. Clin. Microbiol. 25:685.

8. Farmer, J.J. III, Hickman-Brenner, F.W., Fanning, G.R., et al. 1988. Characterization of *Vibrio metschnikovii* and *Vibrio gazogenes* by DNA-DNA hybridization and phenotype. J. Clin. Microbiol. 26:1993.

9. George, W.L. 1987. *Aeromonas*-associated diarrhea. Clin. Microbiol. Newsletter 9:121.

10. George, W.L., Nakata, M.M., Thompson, J., et al. 1985. *Aeromonas*-related diarrhea in adults. Arch. Intern. Med. 145:2207.

11. Goodwin, C.S., McCulloch, R.K., Armstrong, J.A., et al. 1985. Unusual cellular fatty acids and distinctive ultrastructure in a new spiral bacterium (*Campylobacter pyloridis*) from the human gastric mucosa. J. Med. Microbiol. 19:257.

12. Graham, D.Y., and Klein, P.D. 1987. *Campylobacter pyloridis* gastritis: the past, the present, and speculations about the future. Am. J. Gastroenterol. 82:283.

13. Hickman-Brenner, F.W., Fanning, G.R., Arduino, M.J., et al. 1988. *Aeromonas schubertii*, a new mannitol-negative species found in human clinical specimens. J. Clin. Microbiol. 26:1561.

14. Hickman-Brenner, F.W., MacDonald, K.L., Steigerwalt, A.G., et al. 1987. *Aeromonas veronii*, a new ornithine decarboxylase-positive species that may cause diarrhea. J. Clin. Microbiol. 25:900.

15. Holmberg, S.D., Schell, W.L., Fanning, G.R., et al. 1986. *Aeromonas* intestinal infections in the United States. Ann. Intern. Med. 105:683.

16. Holmberg, S.D., Wachsmuth, I.K., Hickman-Brenner, F.W., et al. 1986. *Plesiomonas* enteric infections in the United States. Ann. Intern. Med. 105:690.

17. Isaacs, R.D., Paviour, S.D., Bunker, D.E., et al. 1988. Wound infection with aerogenic *Aeromonas* strains: a review of twenty-seven cases. Eur. J. Clin. Microbiol. Infect. Dis. 7:355.

18. Janda, J.M., and Duffey, P.S. 1988. Mesophilic aeromonads in human disease: current taxonomy, laboratory identification, and infectious disease spectrum. Rev. Infect. Dis. 10:980.

19. Janda, J.M., Powers, C., Bryant, R.G., et al. 1988. Current perspectives on the epidemiology and pathogenesis of clinically significant *Vibrio* spp. Clin. Microbiol. Rev. 1:245.

20. Johnson, W.M., and Lior, H. 1986. Cytotoxic and cytotonic factors produced by *Campylobacter jejuni, Campylobacter coli*, and *Campylobacter laridis*. J. Clin. Microbiol. 24:275.

21. Kelly, M.T., Stroh, E.M.D., and Jessop, J. 1988. Comparison of blood agar, ampicillin blood agar, MacConkey-ampicillin-tween agar, and modified cefsulodin-irgasan-novobiocin agar for isolation of *Aeromonas* spp. from stool specimens. J. Clin. Microbiol. 26:1738.

22. Matthews, B.G., Douglas, H., and Guiney, D.G. 1988. Production of a heat stable enterotoxin by *Plesiomonas shigelloides*. Microb. Pathog. 5:207.

23. Mills, C.K., and Gherna, R.L. 1987. Hydrolysis of indoxyl acetate by *Campylobacter* species. J. Clin. Microbiol. 25:1560.

24. Moyer, N.P. 1987. Clinical significance of *Aeromonas* species isolated from patients with diarrhea. J. Clin. Microbiol. 25:2044.

25. Parsonnet, J., Welch, K., Compton, C., et al. 1988. Simple microbiologic detection of *Campylobacter pylori*. J. Clin. Microbiol. 26:948.

26. Patton, C.M., Shaffer, N., Edmonds, P., et al. 1989. Human disease associated with "*Campylobacter upsaliensis*" (catalase-negative or weakly positive *Campylobacter* species) in the United States. J. Clin. Microbiol. 27:66.

27. Penner, J.L. 1988. The genus *Campylobacter*: a decade of progress. Clin. Microbiol. Rev. 1:157.

28. Rogol, M., Sechter, I., Grinberg, L., et al. 1979. Pril-xylose-ampicillin agar, a new selective medium for the isolation of *Aeromonas hydrophila*. J. Med. Microbiol. 12:229.

29. Steele, T.W., and Owen, R.J. 1988. *Campylobacter jejuni* subsp. *doylei* subsp. nov., a subspecies of nitrate-negative campylobacters isolated from human clinical specimens. Int. J. Syst. Bacteriol. 38:316.

30. Tauxe, R.V., Patton, C.M., Edmonds, P., et al. 1985. Illness associated with *Campylobacter laridis*, a newly recognized *Campylobacter* species. J. Clin. Microbiol. 21:222.

31. Tenover, F.C., and Gebhart, C.J. 1988. Isolation and identification of *Campylobacter* species. Clin. Microbiol. Newsletter 10:81.

32. Totten, P.A., Fennell, C.L., Tenover, F.C., et al. 1985. *Campylobacter cinaedi* (sp. nov.) and *Campylobacter fennelliae* (sp. nov.); two new *Campylobacter* species associated with enteric disease in homosexual men. J. Infect. Dis. 151:131.

33. von Wulffen, H., Heesemann, J., Butzow, G.H., et al. 1986. Detection of *Campylobacter pyloridis* in patients with antrum gastritis and peptic ulcers by culture, complement fixation test, and immunoblot. J. Clin. Microbiol. 24:716.

34. Walker, R.I., Caldwell, M.B., Lee, E.C., et al. 1986. Pathophysiology of *Campylobacter* enteritis. Microbiol. Rev. 50:81.

35. West, P.A., Russek, E., Brayton, P.R., et al. 1982. Statistical evaluation of a quality control method for isolation of pathogenic *Vibrio* species on selected thiosulfate-citrate-bile-salts-sucrose agars. J. Clin. Microbiol. 16:1110.

31 Spirochetes and Other Spiral-shaped Organisms

The Spirochaetaceae family includes organisms that have been known to cause human disease since prehistoric times, such as *Treponema carateum*, the agent of pinta, as well as organisms that have been discovered and associated with disease as recently as 1975, such as *Borrelia burgdorferi*, the agent of Lyme disease. Most of the spirochetes multiply within a living host, having no natural reservoir in the inanimate environment. Treponemes pathogenic for humans are transmitted from person to person through direct contact, either sexual or otherwise. *Borrelia* species pass through an arthropod vector, and *Leptospira* species are contracted accidentally by humans who come into contact with water contaminated by animal urine or who are bitten by an infected animal. Although the spirochete *Treponema hyodysenteriae* has been unequivocally established as an agent of swine dysentery, the role of intestinal spirochetes in human gastroenteritis is still largely unknown. Intestinal spirochetosis will be briefly mentioned in this chapter.

31.1. Morphology

The spirochetes are all long, slender, helically curved gram-negative bacilli, with the unusual morphological features of axial fibrils and an outer coating, the sheath. These fibrils, or axial filaments, are flagellalike organelles that wrap around the cell wall of the bacteria, are enclosed within the outer sheath, and facilitate motility of the organisms. The fibrils are attached within the cell wall by platelike structures located near the ends of the cells, called insertion disks. The protoplasmic cylinder gyrates around the fibrils, causing bacterial movement to

Table 31.1

Spirochetes Pathogenic for Humans

GENUS	AXIAL FIBRILS	INSERTION DISKS
Treponema	6-10	1
Leptospira	2	3-5
Borrelia	30-40	2
*Brachyspira**	4	2

*Proposed name.

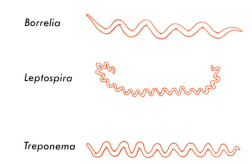

Figure 31.1

Species designation of spirochetes based on general morphology.

appear as a corkscrewlike winding. Differentiation of genera within the Spirochaetaceae is based on the number of axial fibrils, the number of insertion disks present (Table 31.1), as well as on biochemical and metabolic features. The spirochetes, in general, also fall into genera based loosely on their gross morphology (Figure 31.1). Treponemes are slender with tight coils; *Borrelia* are somewhat thicker with fewer and looser coils, and the *Leptospira* resemble the *Borrelia* except for their hooked ends.

31.2. Taxonomic Considerations

The genera that contain organisms pathogenic for humans are *Treponema*, including the causative agents of syphilis, pinta, yaws, and bejel; *Borrelia*, including vector-borne agents of relapsing fever and Lyme disease; *Leptospira*, which includes the agents of leptospirosis; and the newly proposed genus *Brachyspira*, the type species of which, *B. aalborgi*, may cause intestinal disease. *Leptospira* species, in contrast to the other spirochetes, contain diaminopimelic acid in their cell walls instead of ornithine. *Leptospira* organisms can be cultivated more easily in vitro than the other genera, but the *Borrelia* species associated with relapsing fever stain more readily and are thus more easily visualized microscopically. *Borrelia*, except for *B. burgdorferi*, are named primarily for the vector in which they are transmitted.

31.3. *Treponema* Species

Virulent strains of these spirochetes, the agents of syphilis and several other diseases, had not been cultivated in the laboratory except by animal passage in rabbit testicles or mouse footpads until 1981. At that time, Fieldsteel and others,[5,11] using a very complex tissue culture system of fibroblast cell monolayers, reported in vitro growth of *Treponema pallidum* biotype *pallidum*, the causative agent of syph-

ilis. The organisms were microaerophilic, in contrast to the anaerobic non-syphilis-associated treponemes that had been cultivated before. To cause disease, the spirochetes must attach to host cell membranes, penetrate, and multiply. Inflammatory responses by the host mediate pathology. Recent studies indicate that these organisms are able to escape host defenses by being antigenically rather inert.

31.3.a. Laboratory diagnosis of syphilis—serology and darkfield examination. Cultivation of this organism is still not possible for clinical laboratories, so for the most part the diagnosis of syphilis must rest on serologic methods and clinical acumen. Serologic diagnosis of syphilis is discussed in Chapters 12 and 19.

The microbiology laboratory can, however, examine the primary lesion of syphilis, the chancre, or secondary lesions for the presence of motile spirochetes under darkfield illumination. Although the darkfield examination is very much dependent on technical expertise and the numbers of organisms in the lesion, it can be highly specific when performed on genital lesions. Since the normal oral cavity contains spirochetes that are usually nonpathogenic but can mimic *T. pallidum* in appearance, one should not perform darkfield microscopy on material from lesions within the oral cavity.

The method for collection of the specimen is described in Chapter 19. Treponemes, if present in material from the lesion, will be long (5 to 20 μm), slender, tightly coiled spirochetes, moving very slowly (rarely spiraling) and perhaps bending in the middle (Figure 31.2). It is best to examine the darkfield preparation under the darkfield oil immersion lens (1000×) to substantiate the morphology. Since

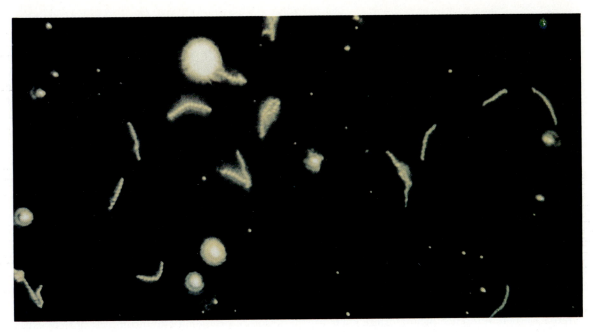

Figure 31.2
Appearance of *T. pallidum* in darkfield preparation.

positive lesions may be teeming with viable spiro-chetes that are highly infectious, all supplies and patient specimens must be handled with extreme caution and carefully discarded as required for con-taminated materials. Although a fluorescent anti-body reagent for *T. pallidum* is available, its use on exudate from lesions has not yielded consistently reliable results.

31.3.b. Other treponemes. The other species of treponemes associated with human disease include *T. pallidum* biotype *pertenue*, the agent of yaws; *T. pallidum* biotype *endemicus*, the agent of endemic syphilis (bejel); and *T. carateum*, the agent of pinta. These diseases are primarily found in tropical or sub-tropical regions and are usually spread by human contact. Poor personal hygiene plays a role in their transmission. The serologic tests and the microscopic morphologies of all of these organisms, including *T. pallidum* biotype *pallidum*, are indistinguishable from each other; only manifestations of the disease vary.

Another group of treponemes are normal inhab-itants of the oral cavity or the human genital tract; these include *T. vincentii*, *T. denticola*, *T. refrin-gens*, *T. macrodentium*, and *T. oralis*. These organ-isms are cultivable anaerobically on artificial media.

Patients with acute necrotizing ulcerative gingivitis (also known as Vincent's gingivitis), a destructive lesion of the gums, show combinations of morpho-logical types of bacteria on methylene blue–stained material from the lesions, which include spirochetes and fusiforms. It appears that oral spirochetes, par-ticularly an unusually large one, may be important in this disease, along with other anaerobes. Further discussion of oral infections is found in Chapter 22. Penicillin G (or tetracycline in penicillin-allergic pa-tients) is effective in all treponematoses.

31.4. *Borrelia* Species

31.4.a. Relapsing fever. Human relapsing fever is caused by more than 15 species of *Borrelia* and is transmitted to humans by the bite of a louse or a tick. Those carried by lice are called *B. recurrentis*. All others that cause disease in the United States are transmitted via tick bites and are named after the species of tick (usually of the genus *Ornithodoros*) from which they are recovered. Common species in the United States include *B. hermsii*, *B. turicatae*, *B. parkeri*, and *B. bergmanni*.

Although the organisms can be cultured in nu-tritionally rich media under microaerophilic condi-tions, the procedures are cumbersome and unreliable and are used primarily as research tools. Clinical laboratories rely on direct observation of the organism in peripheral blood from patients for diagnosis. Organisms can be found in 70% of cases when blood specimens from febrile patients are examined. The organisms can be seen either directly in wet preparations of peripheral blood (mixed with equal parts of sterile nonbacteriostatic saline) under darkfield illumination, in which the spirochetes move rapidly, often pushing the red blood cells around, or by staining thick and thin films with Wright's or Giemsa stains, by procedures similar to those used to detect malaria.

Serologic tests for *Borrelia*-caused relapsing fever have not proved reliable for diagnosis because of the many antigenic shifts undergone by the *Borrelia* organisms during the course of disease. Patients may exhibit increased titers to *Proteus* OX K antigens (up to 1:80), but other cross-reacting antibodies are rare. Certain reference laboratories, such as those at the Centers for Disease Control in Atlanta, may perform special serologic procedures on sera from selected cases. Several antibiotics, including tetracycline, are effective therapeutically.

31.4.b. Lyme disease. Lyme disease, named after its discovery as the cause of an epidemic of "pseudojuvenile rheumatoid arthritis" among young boys living in Lyme, Connecticut, is the most prevalent tick-borne disease in the United States. It is characterized by three stages, not all of which occur in any given patient. The first stage, erythema chronicum migrans, is the characteristic red, annular skin lesion with central clearing that first appears at the site of the tick bite but may develop at distant sites as well. Patients may experience headache, fever, muscle and joint pain, and malaise during this stage. The second stage, beginning weeks to months after infection, may include arthritis, but the most important features are neurologic disorders (meningitis, neurologic deficits) and carditis. The third stage is usually characterized by chronic arthritis and may continue for years.

The agent of Lyme disease is *B. burgdorferi*. The spirochete has been recovered from the blood, cerebrospinal fluid, and skin lesions (erythema chronicum migrans) of patients, and rarely from joint fluid.[13] The bacteria are transmitted by the bite of a tick. Several genera of ticks act as vectors in the United States, including *Ixodes pacificus* in California and in other areas *I. dammini*. The ticks' natural hosts are deer and rodents, although they will attach to pets as well as humans; all stages of tick can harbor the spirochete and transmit disease. The nymphal form of the tick is most likely to transmit disease because it is active in the spring and summer when people are dressed lightly and present in the woods habitat. This stage of the tick is very tiny (pinhead size); thus the initial tick bite may be overlooked. Ticks require a lengthy period of attachment, a minimum of 24 hours, before they transmit disease. The use of insect repellent and careful inspection for ticks daily during outdoor activity in high-risk areas are the best preventive strategies. Endemic areas of disease have been identified in 14 states (including Massachusetts, Connecticut, Maryland, Wisconsin, Minnesota, Oregon, and California), as well as in Europe, Russia, Japan, and Australia.

Culture of the spirochete may be attempted, although the yield is low. The periphery of the annular lesion of erythema chronicum migrans, blood, and cerebrospinal fluid provide the best specimens for culture. The resuspended plasma from blood, spinal fluid sediment, or macerated tissue biopsy is inoculated into a tube of modified Kelly's medium (BSK II; described in Appendix A) and incubated tightly capped at 33° C for 1 month. Blind subcultures (0.1 ml) are performed weekly from the lower portion of the broth to fresh media, and the cultures are examined by darkfield microscopy for the presence of spirochetes.

The organism may also be visualized in tissue sections stained with Warthin-Starry silver stain and in blood and cerebrospinal fluid stained with acridine orange, specific fluorescent stain, or Giemsa.[3]

Serologic diagnosis is the best routine test available for clinical laboratory performance today. Several commercial products are available. Patients show a rise in titer of IgM against the spirochete within 2 to 3 weeks of onset of symptoms and a concomitant rise in IgG very early in the disease. These antibodies both last for at least several years. Due to antigenic similarity, however, antibodies produced by patients with Lyme disease often cross-react with other spirochetal antigens, leading to false-positive and false-negative tests.[10] Patients with syphilis may harbor antibodies that cross-react with antigens of *B. burgdorferi*. Problematic, also, are the more than 15% of patients with Lyme disease who fail to develop antibody.[4,6] Western blot tests and tests for antigen in urine are being developed.

Phenoxymethyl penicillin or erythromycin is a first choice drug for therapy. Broad-spectrum cephalosporins, particularly ceftriaxone, and chloramphenicol have been successful with patients who fail initial treatment.[3] Treatment, however, may result in lack of antibody response in the patient, and treatment failures, particularly in patients with chronic disease, have been reported.

31.5. Leptospirosis

The leptospires include both free-living and parasitic forms. Pathogenic species are called *Leptospira interrogans*, and most saprophytic leptospires are called *L. biflexa*. The pathogens include over 180 different serologically defined types, which used to be designated as species and are now known as serovars or serotypes of *L. interrogans*. Physiologically, the saprophytes can be differentiated from pathogens by their ability to grow at 10° C and lower, or at least 5° C lower than the growth temperature of pathogenic leptospires.[8]

The organisms are too small to be seen in wet preparations made from fresh blood, and they do not push the erythrocytes around as the *Borrelia* do. Currently, the most reliable method for laboratory diagnosis of leptospirosis is to culture the organisms from blood or cerebrospinal fluid during the first week of illness or from urine thereafter for several months. A few drops of heparinized or sodium-oxalate anticoagulated blood are inoculated into tubes of Fletcher's or Ellinghausen, McCullough, Johnson, and Harris (EMJH) media (both described in Appendix A). Urine should be inoculated soon after collection, as acidity (diluted out in the broth medium) may harm the spirochetes. One or two drops of undiluted and a 1:10 dilution of urine are added to 5 ml medium. The addition of 200 μg/ml of 5-fluorouracil (an anticancer drug) may prevent contamination by other bacteria without harming the leptospires. Tissue specimens (especially liver and kidney) may be aseptically triturated (macerated) and inoculated in dilutions of 1:1, 1:10, and 1:100 as for urine cultures.

All cultures are incubated at room temperature or 30° C in the dark for up to 6 weeks. The organisms grow below the surface. Material collected from a few centimeters below the surface of broth cultures should be examined weekly for the presence of growth using a direct wet preparation under darkfield illumination. Leptospires will exhibit cork-screwlike motility. A more complete discussion of these methods can be found in Alexander.[1] A new species of *Leptospira*, "*L. inadai*" serovar *lyme*, was recovered recently from a skin biopsy of a patient with Lyme disease.[12] The spirochete displayed typical morphology, failed to agglutinate in antisera against any known strains, and showed low DNA homology with other species and serovars of leptospires. Based on growth at low temperature and low antibody titers in the patient from whom it was recovered, it was thought to be nonpathogenic.

Serologic diagnosis of leptospirosis is best performed using pools of bacterial antigens containing many serotypes in each pool. Positive results are visualized by examining for the presence of agglutination under darkfield examination. A macroscopic agglutination procedure is more readily accessible to routine clinical laboratories. Reagents are available commercially. Indirect hemagglutination and an enzyme-linked immunosorbent assay (ELISA) test for IgM antibody are also available. Penicillin or tetracycline may modify the course of the illness, but only if started not later than the fourth day of illness.

31.6. Miscellaneous Spiral-shaped Organisms

The normal gastrointestinal tract of humans is colonized with spirochetes, most of which cause no harm to the host. Since 1981, however, several groups have reported patients with diarrhea, inflammatory cellular responses, and numerous spirochetes found to be invading the intestinal epithelium (into the lamina propria), as well as within macrophages. Many of these patients also suffered from other illnesses such as Crohn's disease. Hovind-Hougen and others were able to culture the spirochetes from five patients in vitro and found that they differed from other known genera morphologically.[2,7] Since growth characteristics and morphology differed from previously named spirochetes, they designated this organism *Brachyspira aalborgi*. Jones and others[9] recovered spirochetes from diarrheal stool from homosexual males. Some of the isolates resembled *B. aalborgi* and others showed different colony morphologies and biochemical characteristics. The role, if any, of these organisms in the etiology of the patients' diarrhea is not known.

Whether intestinal spirochetosis is a real entity and a more common syndrome than has been appreciated until now remains to be elucidated.

Spirillum minus, the other agent of rat-bite fever

(in addition to *Streptobacillus moniliformis*, Chapter 39), is a short, helical organism with only a few spirals that resembles *Campylobacter* more than spirochetes. Its taxonomic position is unclear at this time; it may be reassigned to a new genus. It is mentioned again in Chapter 40.

REFERENCES

1. Alexander, A.D. 1980. *Leptospira*. In Lennette, E.H., Balows, A., Hausler, W.J., Jr., and Truant, J.P., editors. Manual of clinical microbiology, ed. 3. American Society for Microbiology. Washington, D.C.

2. Antonakopoulos, G., Newman, J., and Wilkinson, M. 1982. Intestinal spirochetosis; an electron microscopic study of an unusual case. Histopathology 6:477.

3. Barbour, A.G. 1988. Laboratory aspects of Lyme borreliosis. Clin. Microbiol. Rev. 1:399.

4. Dattwyler, R.J., Volkman, D.J., Luft, B.J., et al. 1988. Seronegative Lyme disease: discussion of specific T- and B-lymphocyte responses to *Borrelia burgdorferi*. N. Engl. J. Med. 319:1441.

5. Fieldsteel, A.H., Cox, D.L., and Moeckii, R.A. 1981. Cultivation of virulent *Treponema pallidum* in tissue culture. Infect. Immun. 32:908.

6. Grodzicki, R.L., and Steere, A.C. 1988. Comparison of immunoblotting and indirect enzyme-linked immunosorbent assay using different antigen preparations for diagnosing early Lyme disease. J. Infect. Dis. 157:790.

7. Hovind-Hougen, K., Birch-Anderson, A., Henrik-Nielsen, R., et al. 1982. Intestinal spirochetosis: morphological characterization and cultivation of the spirochete *Brachyspira aalborgi* gen. nov., sp. nov. J. Clin. Microbiol. 16:1127.

8. Johnson, R.C., and Harris, V.G. 1967. Differentiation of pathogenic and saprophytic leptospires. I. Growth at low temperatures. J. Bacteriol. 94:27.

9. Jones, M.J., Miller, J.N., and George, W.L. 1986. Microbiological and biochemical characterization of spirochetes isolated from the feces of homosexual men. J. Clin. Microbiol. 24:1071.

10. Magnarelli, L.A., Anderson, J.F., and Johnson, R.C. 1987. Cross-reactivity in serologic tests for Lyme disease and other spirochetal infections. J. Infect. Dis. 156:183.

11. Norris, S.J. 1982. In vitro cultivation of *Treponema pallidum*; independent confirmation. Infect. Immun. 36:437.

12. Schmid, G.P., Steere, A.C., Kornblatt, A.N., et al. 1986. Newly recognized *Leptospira* species ("*Leptospira inadai*" serovar *lyme*) isolated from human skin. J. Clin. Microbiol. 24:484.

13. Steere, A.C., Grodzicki, R.L., Craft, J.E., et al. 1984. Recovery of Lyme disease spirochetes from patients. Yale J. Biol. Med. 57:557.

BIBLIOGRAPHY

Alexander, A.D. 1980. Serological diagnosis of leptospirosis. In Rose, N.R., and Friedman, J., editors. Manual of clinical immunology, ed. 2. American Society for Microbiology, Washington, D.C.

Benach, J.L., and Bosler, E.M., editors. 1988. Lyme disease and related disorders. Ann. N.Y. Acad. Sci. 539:1-513. (Entire book devoted to Lyme disease.)

Burgdorfer, W. 1985. Spirochetes. In Lennette, E.H., Balows, A., Hausler, W.J., Jr., and Shadomy, H.J., editors. Manual of clinical microbiology, ed. 4. American Society for Microbiology, Washington, D.C.

Coleman, J.L., and Benach, J.L. 1987. Isolation of antigenic components from the Lyme disease spirochete: their role in early diagnosis. J. Infect. Dis. 155:756.

Steere, A.C., Grodzicki, R.L., Kornblatt, A.N., et al. 1983. The spirochetal etiology of Lyme disease. N. Engl. J. Med. 308:733.

32

Aerobic or Facultative Spore-Forming Rods (*Bacillus* Species)

The genus *Bacillus* contains a large number of species that are aerobic or facultative, usually gram-positive and spore-forming; several of these species have been involved in clinically significant infections of a variety of types. *Bacillus* species are widely distributed in nature and are therefore frequent contaminants in laboratory cultures from clinical specimens. Contamination of radiometric blood culture apparatus and of alcohol swabs has also led to clusters of pseudobacteremia. Species identification within the genus is not important for clinical purposes, but identification of *Bacillus anthracis* (the agent of anthrax) is a major exception. Reference laboratories may be used for this purpose.

32.1. Morphology and General Characteristics

Bacillus species are able to grow on most nonselective laboratory media; they may or may not grow on eosin–methylene blue (EMB) agar. Those with typical Gram stain appearance (Figure 32.1) are easily identified as *Bacillus* species. Because atypical strains may vary in Gram stain, oxidase, and other reactions and spores may not be evident, they may resemble nonfermentative gram-negative bacilli. When identification is attempted using gram-negative schemes, these organisms cannot be classified in any known gram-negative species or Centers for Disease Control (CDC) taxon. *Bacillus* strains that are strict aerobes may appear as nonfermentative gram-negative bacilli on Kligler's or triple sugar iron (TSI) agar as well. Most do not grow on enteric agars, but some show limited growth. However, several

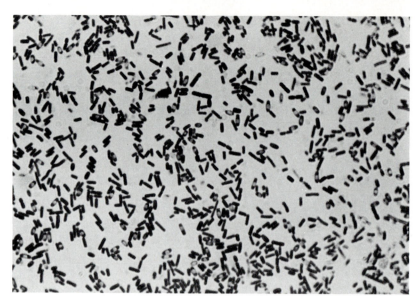

Figure 32.1
Gram stain of *Bacillus* species visualized under oil immersion (1000 ×) showing the clear intracellular (subterminal) spores that fail to pick up the stain.

gram-negative nonfermenters also fail to grow on such media.

The colonial morphology of the *Bacillus* strains that simulate gram-negative rods is not typical of the usual *Bacillus* species (which exhibit large, flat colonies and frequent β-hemolysis). Some of these strains even have minute colonies. Spore formation often fails to occur within the time required to report a clinical isolate. Sporulation may be stimulated by subculture onto esculin agar and may be facilitated on acidified media such as TSI agar. Two other tests may be useful. One is susceptibility to vancomycin; with the exception of *Flavobacterium* species, no gram-negative nonfermenter is known to be susceptible to vancomycin (30-μg disk), whereas most *Bacillus* species are susceptible. However, there are strains of *Bacillus* species that are vancomycin-resistant, so only vancomycin susceptibility can be used diagnostically. The second procedure that may be helpful is the KOH test (described in Chapter 7) in which gram-negative organisms show a viscous thread. Some *Bacillus* strains, particularly from older cultures that have also lost their gram-positive characteristic, may give a "gram-negative" reaction by this test. Accordingly, the test is of value for

identification of *Bacillus* species only if no viscous thread is formed.

Treatment of specimens or mixed cultures that may contain *Bacillus* species with 50% ethanol for 1 hour is effective for selecting *Bacillus* species, just as it is for selecting spore-forming anaerobes (Chapter 34).

32.2. Differentiation of *Bacillus* Species

Species differentiation within the genus *Bacillus* is based on cell morphology, whether the organism is obligately aerobic or facultative, action on xylose and arabinose, starch hydrolysis, indole production, nitrite production from nitrate, presence of protein bodies, susceptibility to gamma phage, capsule production, the "string of pearls" test (see Section 32.3.b below), and animal pathogenicity. Table 32.1 shows differential characteristics of a number of species likely to be encountered in clinical specimens. The three groups are based on size of cell and whether the spore swells the cell wall (group I cells are 0.9 μm wide; group II cells are smaller than group I; and group III spores cause swelling of the cell wall). Identification of a sporadic isolate, past verifying that the organism is not *B. anthracis*, is not warranted in most circumstances.

Table 32-1

Identification of *Bacillus* species*

	USUAL CELL DIAMETER (μm)	PENICILLIN (10 U)	MOTILITY	WIDE ZONE LECITHINASE	β-HEMOLYSIS	SPORES SWELL CELLS	VOGES-PROSKAUER	NITRATE REDUCTION	STARCH	DISTINGUISHING CHARACTERISTICS
Group I										
B. anthracis	≥0.9	S	0	27	−	−	85	100		Produces capsule
B. cereus	≥0.9	R	99	100	+	−	84	89		
B. mycoides	≥0.9	R	63	100	−	−	50	100		Rhizoid colony
B. megaterium	≥0.9	V	42	0	−	−	0	10		
B. thuringiensis	≥0.9	R	+	+	+	−	V	+		Insect pathogen that produces toxin crystals
Group II										
B. subtilis	<0.9	S	84	−	V	−	71	89	80	
B. pumilus	<0.9	S	100	−	V	−	78	0	6	
B. licheniformis	<0.9	S	80	−	+	−	83	100	100	
B. firmus	<0.9	S	90	−	V	−	0	70	50	
B. coagulans	<0.9	S	+	−	V	−	V	0		Grows at 55° and 35° C
Group III										
B. circulans	<0.9		+	−	−	+	6	76		Colonies may migrate on agar
B. sphaericus	<0.9		+	−	−	+	0	26		Produces spherical spores
B. laterosporus	<0.9		+	V	−	+	0	90		Produces canoe-shaped spores
B. brevis	<0.9		+	−	−	+	−	26		
B. polymyxa	<0.9		+	−	−	+	100	0		
B. alvei (H₂S + Bacillus)	<0.9		+	−	V	+	V	+		
B. stearothermophilus	<0.9		+	−	−	+	V	0		Grows at 65° C, no growth at 35° C

+ = >90% positive; − = <10% positive; V = 10% to 90% positive.

*Percentages are given when available.

From Howard, B.J., Klaas, J.J. II, Rubin, S.J., et al. 1987. Clinical and pathogenic microbiology. The C.V. Mosby Co., St. Louis.

32.3. *Bacillus anthracis*

B. anthracis is the primary human pathogen in the genus. Anthrax is a rare disease in the United States, so the organism is seldom encountered in the average hospital or public health laboratory. Cases in the United States are most often related to handling of imported wool or goat hair, animal hides, shaving brushes, and so forth, originating principally in Asia, the Middle East, and Africa. Cases may also result from contact with diseased animals, primarily cattle, swine, and horses, and from inadvertent self-inoculation of veterinary anthrax vaccine. During the last decade there has been an average of 2.5 cases of anthrax per year in the United States.

Anthrax is manifested in humans in three forms:

1. *Cutaneous anthrax* (malignant pustule) is the most common form in the United States. Infection is initiated by the entrance of bacilli through an abrasion of the skin. A pustule usually appears on the hands or forearms. The bacilli are readily recognized in the serosanguineous discharge.

2. *Pulmonary anthrax* is also known as woolsorter's disease. The bacilli may be found in large numbers in the sputum. Spores are inhaled during shearing, sorting, or handling of animal hair. If not properly treated, this form progresses to fatal septicemia.

3. *Gastrointestinal anthrax* is the most severe and

rarest form of anthrax. The bacilli or spores are swallowed, thus initiating intestinal infection. The organisms may be isolated from the patient's stools. This form is also usually fatal if not treated.

32.3.a. **Structure, extracellular products.** The organism is a facultative, large, square-ended, nonmotile rod, with an ellipsoidal to cylindrical centrally located spore. The sporangium is not swollen as a rule. The cells frequently occur in long chains, giving a bamboo appearance, especially on primary isolation from infected tissue or discharge. The chains of virulent forms are usually surrounded by a capsule. Encapsulation occurs also in enriched media and when grown on sodium bicarbonate agar under 5% CO_2. Avirulent forms are usually unencapsulated. Sporulation occurs in the soil and on culture media, but not in living tissue.

The colonies of *B. anthracis* are normally large (4 to 5 mm), opaque, raised, and irregular, with a curled margin. When the margin of the colony is pushed inward and then lifted gently with an inoculating needle, the disturbed portion of the colony stands up like beaten egg whites. Comma-shaped colony outgrowths are common. On sheep blood agar, the colonies are invariably nonhemolytic. Smooth and rough colony forms may be observed, and both of these may be virulent. In broth, the bacillus produces a heavy pellicle, with little if any subsurface growth.

Two potent exotoxins are produced. Both toxin molecules are dependent on a third protein, called protective antigen (PA), for their biological activity. The two exotoxins are known as lethal factor (LF) and edema factor (EF). It appears that PA is essential for the toxins to enter into the target cells. The combination of EF and PA increases host susceptibility to infection by suppressing polymorphonuclear neutrophil function.

32.3.b. **Identification methods.** When working with suspected *B. anthracis*, one should use extreme caution, work in a bacteriologic safety hood, avoid creating aerosols, and decontaminate all areas thoroughly with a sporicidal germicide such as Alcide.

The optimal growth temperature for the organism is 35° C; when grown at 42° or 43° C, it becomes attenuated or avirulent. This is because of the loss of the capsule. Biochemically, the organism is characterized as follows:

- Carbohydrate fermentation: glucose, fructose, maltose, sucrose, and trehalose are fermented with acid only; arabinose, xylose, galactose, lactose, mannose, raffinose, rhamnose, adonitol, dulcitol, inositol, inulin, mannitol, and sorbitol are not fermented.
- Gelatin: inverted pine tree growth; slow liquefaction.
- Nitrates: reduced to nitrites.
- Starch: hydrolyzed.
- Voges-Proskauer: positive.

A simple presumptive test for identification of *B. anthracis* has been proposed. It is a modification of the string of pearls test, which reflects the susceptibility of a strain to penicillin. Single streaks of the suspect organism, as well as positive and negative controls, are made on a Mueller-Hinton agar plate. Ten-unit penicillin disks are placed on each streak, and a coverslip is placed over the streak. After incubation for 3 to 6 hours at 37° C, growth beneath the coverslip is examined microscopically for the presence of strings of spherical cellular forms of the organism. The presence of such cells resembling strings of pearls is considered a positive test. Specific identification may be made by use of a gamma bacteriophage (at CDC or state health department laboratories).

The pathogenicity of *B. anthracis* may be determined by injecting each of 10 white mice (2 to 3 weeks of age) subcutaneously with 0.2 ml of a saline suspension of the organism. Rabbits or guinea pigs may also be used. Animals usually die 2 to 5 days after inoculation from septicemia; the organism is readily recovered from the heart, blood, spleen, liver, and lungs of the animal. Animal inoculation is not generally done in clinical laboratories.

32.3.c. **Susceptibility to antimicrobial agents.** Penicillin is the drug of choice for treatment. Alternative drugs for the penicillin-sensitive patient are tetracycline, erythromycin, and chloramphenicol.

32.3.d. **Noncultural methods of identification.** Encapsulated strains may be used for fluorescent antibody staining; this is available through CDC. Both the cell wall and the capsule fluoresce simultaneously. This test would presumably work well directly on clinical specimens, if it were feasible to perform the test promptly.

Antibodies to the organism may be detected by an indirect hemagglutination or enzyme-linked immunosorbent test (using the PA component of the toxin as the capture antigen). These tests are available through state health department laboratories.

32.4. *Bacillus cereus*

This organism is the cause of serious infections of various types, usually, but not always, in immunocompromised hosts. Other patient background factors include surgery and other trauma, burns, intravenous drug abuse, implantation of catheters and various prosthetic devices (including heart valves), and use of hemodialysis and peritoneal dialysis. Types of infections described include septicemia, endocarditis, necrotizing pneumonia with or without empyema, meningitis, rapidly destructive ophthalmitis, peritonitis, wound infection, myonecrosis, and osteomyelitis. Myonecrosis has followed surgery and trauma and may simulate clostridial myonecrosis (gas gangrene). Injection of *B. cereus* exotoxin into the skin of rabbits causes increased vascular permeability and necrosis; production of this toxin seems to correlate with the severity of clinical infection. Rabbit skin necrosis is attributed to two factors, an enterotoxin and a hemolysin. Phospholipase C (lecithinase) is produced by almost all strains of *B. cereus*; its pathogenic role is doubtful. The toxin can also be demonstrated to cause fluid accumulation in the rabbit ileal loop model. *B. cereus* produces β-lactamase.

B. cereus has long been known as an important cause of food poisoning. The short incubation type of food poisoning due to *B. cereus* is most often associated with fried rice that has been cooked and held warm for extended periods; it is due to preformed toxin. Long incubation food poisoning due to *B. cereus* is frequently associated with meat or vegetable dishes; in these cases, toxin is formed in vivo. These entities are discussed in greater detail in Chapter 17.

32.4.a. Laboratory identification. *B. cereus* colonies vary from small, shiny, and compact to the large, feathery, spreading type. A lavender colony with β-hemolysis is seen on sheep blood agar.

Unlike *B. anthracis*, *B. cereus* is resistant to gamma phage, is usually resistant to penicillin, does not encapsulate on bicarbonate agar, and on fluorescent antibody–stained smears does not exhibit fluorescence of both cell wall and capsule. Lecithinase and hemolysin production are very useful in the provisional identification of *B. cereus*.

32.4.b. Susceptibility to antimicrobial agents. Because of β-lactamase production, *B. cereus* is usually not susceptible to penicillin and many other β-lactam antimicrobial agents. It is also resistant to trimethoprim. It is susceptible to gentamicin, clindamycin, erythromycin, vancomycin, and probably to chloramphenicol. Most strains are inhibited by sulfonamides and tetracycline.

32.5. Other *Bacillus* Species

Several other of the 60 or so species in this genus have been encountered in significant infections, especially *B. subtilis* and *B. licheniformis*. The latter two species have been implicated in food poisoning and in a number of infections, including septicemia, panophthalmitis, pneumonia, wound infection, and peritonitis. Ocular infection has been produced by a biological insecticide made up of *Bacillus thuringiensis*; the material was inadvertently splashed into the patient's eye. Other *Bacillus* species incriminated in infection of one type or another on at least one occasion include *B. brevis*, *B. circulans*, *B. coagulans*, *B. macerans*, *B. megaterium*, *B. pumilus*, and *B. sphaericus*. Allergic reactions in workers manufacturing laundry detergent containing derivatives of *B. subtilis* have been described. Also, hypersensitivity pneumonitis related to exposure to wood dust contaminated with *B. subtilis* has been described.

32.5.a. Morphology and extracellular products. *B. subtilis* colonies are usually large, flat, and dull, with a ground glass appearance (Figure 32.2). Several species produce collagenases. *B. megaterium* produces a filterable hemolysin, and *B. mycoides* produces potent toxins that can be lethal to experimental animals.

32.5.b. Susceptibility to antimicrobial agents. Susceptibility to penicillin G and other older β-lactam antibiotics is variable and may be species-related, tending to be high for *B. subtilis* and intermediate for *B. pumilus*. Although clindamycin is generally considered to be an effective drug for treating *Bacillus* infections, there is a report of one strain of *B. licheniformis* that was resistant to clindamycin and susceptible to penicillin. Vancomycin should be one of the more dependable drugs for therapy of serious infections due to *Bacillus* species. Obviously, the type and the location of the infection will influence the choice of therapy.

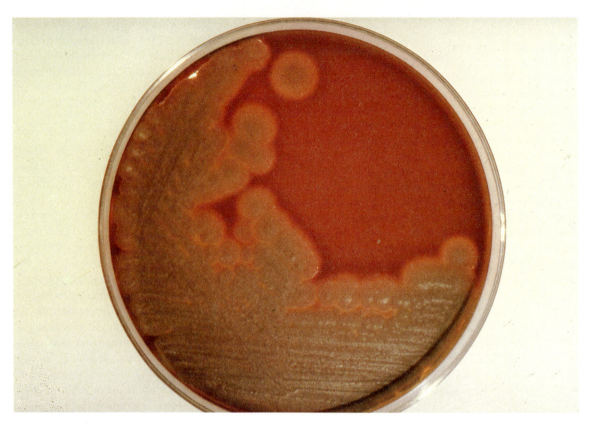

Figure 32.2
B. subtilis on BAP.

BIBLIOGRAPHY

Bekemeyer, W.B., and Zimmerman, G.A. 1985. Life-threatening complications associated with *Bacillus cereus* pneumonia. Am. Rev. Respir. Dis. 131:466.

Blachman, U., Gilardi, G.L., Pickett, M.J., et al. 1980. *Bacillus* spp. strains posing as nonfermentative gram-negative rods. Clin. Microbiol. Newsletter 2:8.

Brachman, P.S. 1983. Anthrax. In Hoeprich, P.D., editor. Infectious diseases, ed. 3., Harper & Row, Publishers, Philadelphia.

Clarridge, J.E. 1987. Gram-positive bacilli. In Howard, B.J., Klass, J. II, Rubin, S.J., et al., editors. 1987. Clinical and pathogenic microbiology. The C.V. Mosby Co., St. Louis.

Editorial. 1983. *Bacillus cereus* as a systemic pathogen. Lancet 2:1469.

Parry, J.M., Turnbull, P.C.B., and Gibson, J.R. 1983. A colour atlas of *Bacillus* species. Wolfe Medical Atlases—19. Wolfe Medical Publications, Ltd., Ipswich, England.

Pennington, J.E., Gibbons, N.D., Strobeck, J.E., et al. 1976. *Bacillus* species infection in patients with hematologic neoplasia. J.A.M.A. 235:1473.

Tuazon, C.V., Murray, H.W., Levy, C., et al. 1979. Serious infections from *Bacillus* sp. J.A.M.A. 241:1137.

Turnbull, P.C.B., and Kramer, J.M. 1983. Non-gastrointestinal *Bacillus cereus* infections: an analysis of exotoxin production by strains isolated over a two-year period. J. Clin. Pathol. 36:1091.

33

Aerobic, Non-Spore-Forming, Gram-Positive Bacilli

Aerobic, gram-positive, non-spore-forming bacilli are taxonomically diverse and are ubiquitous inhabitants of the natural environment. The group comprises a large number of genera (see box on p. 460). For purposes of this chapter the discussion will be limited to the aerobic *Actinomyces, Arcanobacterium, Corynebacterium, Erysipelothrix, Kurthia, Lactobacillus, Listeria, Nocardia, Oerskovia, Rothia,* and *Rhodococcus*. The remaining genera will not be discussed either because they are rarely, if ever, isolated in the clinical laboratory or because they are covered in other chapters.

With the exception of *Corynebacterium diphtheriae,* the aerobic, gram-positive, non-spore-forming bacilli are of low pathogenicity and generally require a major break in the immunological defenses of the host to cause significant infection. However, because they constitute a large portion of the normal bacterial flora of patients and the environment they are frequently isolated in the clinical laboratory. Given their widespread distribution and the fact that some of these organisms may be highly antibiotic-resistant, it is not surprising that both epidemic and sporadic infections with certain of these organisms are becoming increasingly recognized.

Most of the bacteria in this group are pleomorphic, exhibiting various morphologies that include branching, clubbing, coccoid forms, and palisading. These organisms all grow well on commonly used nonselective media, including 5% sheep blood agar. As outlined by Clarridge and Weissfeld[7] and Hollis and Weaver,[14] the organisms may be divided into groups on the basis of the catalase test. Figure 33.1 illustrates a basic strategy for preliminary identification of aerobic, gram-positive, non-spore-forming bacilli.

Aerobic, Gram-Positive, Non-Spore-Forming Bacilli	
Actinomyces	Erysipelothrix
Agromyces	Gardnerella
Arcanobacterium	Kurthia
Arthrobacter	Lactobacillus
Aureobacterium	Listeria
Arachnia	Microbacterium
Brevibacterium	Mycobacterium
Brochothrix	Nocardia
Caryophanon	Nocardiopsis
Caseobacter	Oerskovia
Cellulomonas	Propionibacterium
Corynebacterium	Rothia
Curtobacterium	Rhodococcus
Dermatophilus	Renibacterium
Streptomyces	

33.1. *Listeria* Species

33.1.a Epidemiology and pathogenesis of listeriosis. The genus *Listeria* contains eight species: *monocytogenes, denitrificans, grayi, innocua, ivanovii, murrayi, seeligeri,* and *welshimeri.* Although both *L. ivanovii* and *L. monocytogenes* have been associated with human disease, only *L. monocytogenes* is commonly encountered in clinical laboratories. *L. monocytogenes* is ubiquitous in the environment and has been isolated from soil and decaying vegetation as well as from a number of wild and domestic animals. Stool-carriage studies have also documented asymptomatic intestinal carriage of *L. monocytogenes* in 1% to 5% of humans. *L. monocytogenes* is a well-known cause of spontaneous abortions in animals as well as the cause of basilar meningitis or "circling disease" in sheep.

Human listeriosis has been a reportable disease since 1986, and although our knowledge of the epidemiology remains incomplete, recent analysis of both epidemic and sporadic disease has provided considerable insight into the epidemiology and transmission of *L. monocytogenes.* Four major epidemics of listeriosis have occurred in North America and one in Switzerland since 1981. The total number of cases ranged from 36 to 142, with case fatality rates between 27% and 44%. The cases were linked to the ingestion of contaminated dairy products in three of the epidemics, contaminated cabbage in one, and no source could be implicated in the fifth outbreak. Studies of dairy products, raw vegetables, and sausages have documented the presence of *L. monocytogenes* in low numbers, suggesting that this organism may be a common contaminant of both processed and unprocessed foods of plant and animal origin. Because the organism can survive and multiply at refrigerator temperatures, even a small amount of contamination may be significant.[5]

Most human cases are sporadic, and the source of the infection is usually unknown. Active surveillance conducted by the Centers for Disease Control (CDC) in six areas of the United States has provided estimates of at least 1700 serious infections, 450 deaths, and 100 stillbirths due to listeriosis annually in the United States. Listeriosis is seen almost exclusively in neonates, pregnant women, and immunocompromised individuals. The clinical presentation ranges from sepsis and meningitis in neonates and immunocompromised patients to a nonspecific febrile illness in pregnant women. Transplacental infection is common, possibly due to deficiencies in local immunoregulation at the placenta, and results in premature labor, septic abortion, and neonatal listeriosis. The case fatality rate ranges from 3% to 50% with perinatal disease and is estimated at 35% in nonperinatal cases.

Outside of the perinatal period, the most common presentation of listeriosis is meningitis. In persons with meningitis the cerebrospinal fluid (CSF) is purulent and the CSF protein is usually elevated; however, the CSF glucose level is normal and the Gram stain is negative in greater than 60% of cases. Cultures of blood and CSF are positive in 60% to 75% of cases and remain the most reliable means of diagnosis. The pathogenesis of listeriosis is related to several factors, including host immunity, inoculum size, and possibly strain-specific virulence factors. *L. monocytogenes* is commonly cited as a classic example of an intracellular pathogen, and the importance of T cell–mediated immunity to this organism is well established. The available data support the alimentary tract as the major portal of entry of *L. monocytogenes*; however, it is unclear whether disruption of the mucosal barrier is necessary for the organism to cause systemic disease. Although β-hemolysis on blood agar distinguishes *L. mono-*

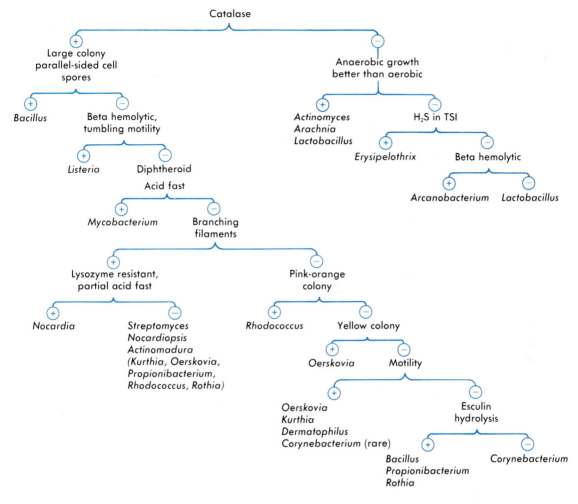

Figure 33.1
Flow chart for preliminary identification of aerobic, gram-positive non-spore-forming bacilli.

cytogenes from the nonpathogenic species of *Listeria*, additional virulence factors have been difficult to demonstrate. Currently it appears that virulence is mediated by action of at least three components: a phospholipase, a hemolysin, and a lipopolysaccharide.

33.1.b Laboratory identification. On Gram stain *L. monocytogenes* appears as a pleomorphic, non-spore-forming, gram-positive bacillus. It is somewhat smaller than most gram-positive bacilli, with cells ranging from 0.4 to 0.5 μm × 1 to 2 μm. The cells may be coccobacillary and occur in pairs and short chains suggestive of *S. pneumoniae* or other species of streptococci. The organisms may palisade and thus resemble diphtheroids or may be confused with *Haemophilus* species on overdecolorized preparations.

L. monocytogenes grows well on most laboratory media, yielding small, smooth, translucent gray colonies with a narrow zone of β-hemolysis (Figure 33.2). The colony morphology closely resembles that of group B β-hemolytic streptococci, with which it is often confused. *L. monocytogenes* also hydrolyzes sodium hippurate and yields a positive reaction in the CAMP test (used for Group B streptococci); however, it can readily be distinguished from *Streptococcus agalactiae* by positive tests for catalase and esculin hydrolysis (*S. agalactiae* is negative in both). Colonies grown on clear media, such as nutrient agar, will display a blue-green color when they are

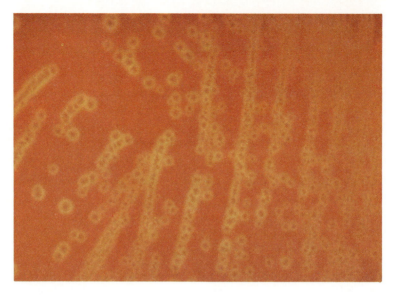

Figure 33.2
Colonies of *L. monocytogenes* on sheep blood agar after 48-hour incubation, showing the diffuse zone of β-hemolysis surrounding the colonies.

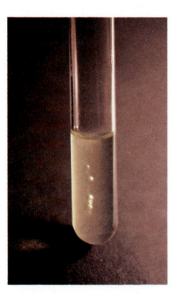

Figure 33.3
Characteristic umbrella-shaped motility pattern exhibited by colonies of *L. monocytogenes* after overnight incubation.

observed with an oblique (45-degree angle) light source. *Listeria* can also be presumptively identified by observation of motility under direct wet preparation. *Listeria* exhibits a characteristic end-over-end tumbling motility when incubated in nutrient broth for 1 to 2 hours at room temperature. An identical broth culture incubated at 37°C will show very little, if any, motility. This motility pattern will also be illustrated by the "umbrella-shaped" pattern that develops after overnight incubation at room temperature of a culture that has been stabbed into a tube of semisolid agar (Figure 33.3). Table 33.1 summarizes the basic biochemical and enzymatic tests used to differentiate *L. monocytogenes* from organisms with which it might be confused.

Although *L. monocytogenes* grows readily from cerebrospinal fluid, blood, and most other specimens, it may be difficult to isolate from placenta and other tissue. Placing the specimen at 4°C for several weeks to months and subculturing at frequent intervals may serve to enhance recovery. This procedure, called *cold enrichment*, is particularly useful for epidemiologic studies when specimens are contaminated with other flora. A procedure for handling tissue suspected of containing *Listeria* is given in Chapter 21.

Table 33.1

Differentiation of *L. monocytogenes* from Other Bacteria it Resembles

ORGANISM	CATALASE	ESCULIN	MOTILITY	β-HEMOLYSIS	H₂S/TSI
L. monocytogenes	+	+	+	+	−
Corynebacterium sp.	+	−	− / +	− / +	−
Propionibacterium sp.	+	+ / −	−	+ / −	−
E. rhusiopathiae	−	−	−	−	+
Lactobacillus sp.	−	−	−	−	−
S. agalactiae	−	−	−	+	−
Enterococci	−	+	−	− / +	−

+ = 90% of strains positive; − = >90% of strains negative; + / − = variable (most strains positive); − / + = variable (most strains negative).

33.1.c. Therapy. *L. monocytogenes* is susceptible to a wide variety of antimicrobial agents in vitro, including penicillin, ampicillin, tetracyclines, erythromycin, chloramphenicol, rifampin, sulfamethoxazole and trimethoprim, and the aminoglycosides. Of these, only sulfamethoxazole and trimethoprim (the combination) and the aminoglycosides are bactericidal.

The optimal therapy for listeriosis is controversial and has not been established in controlled clinical trials. Ampicillin is generally considered to be more active than penicillin, and the combination of ampicillin plus an aminoglycoside results in synergistic bactericidal activity in vitro. The current therapy of choice for listeriosis is a combination of ampicillin plus gentamicin. Clinical failures have been observed with chloramphenicol, and little or no data exist evaluating the efficacy of agents such as rifampin. The combination of sulfamethoxazole and trimethoprim may be useful in treatment of patients who are allergic to penicillin. This regimen is bactericidal, achieves adequate levels in serum and CSF, and has documented clinical efficacy.

33.2. *Erysipelothrix rhusiopathiae*

33.2.a. Epidemiology and pathogenesis. *E. rhusiopathiae* is the only species in the genus and is a well-known veterinary pathogen of considerable economic importance. *E. rhusiopathiae* is ubiquitous in nature and has been isolated from a variety of environmental sources, including soil, food, and water. Contamination of the environment is thought to occur secondary to excretion of the organism by infected or colonized animals. Human infection is usually related to occupational exposure (veterinarians,

farmers) and occurs most commonly in those who have direct contact with animals or with organic matter in which the organism is commonly found. The most common form of human disease is a spreading, cellulitis-like lesion of the hands and fingers known as *erysipeloid*. Rarely a septic form may be observed that presents with bacteremia and skin involvement and is almost always associated with endocarditis. A total of 49 cases of sepsis and endocarditis due to *E. rhusiopathiae* have been reported since 1912, and 89% occurred in patients with an occupational risk for cutaneous infection with *Erysipelothrix*. The crude mortality in these patients was 38%, almost twice as high as that for other causes of bacterial endocarditis. Although pathogenicity of *E. rhusiopathiae* for swine has been related to neuraminidase production, surface antigen structure, endothelial adherence, and fibrin deposition on synovial membrane during bacteremia, little is known about the pathogenesis of infection due to this organism in humans.

33.2.b. Laboratory identification. *E. rhusiopathiae* is a facultatively anaerobic, nonmotile, nonsporulating gram-positive rod. The organism grows well on blood agar, showing α-hemolysis after prolonged incubation. Older colonies may show a tendency to become gram-negative. Aspirated material or biopsy specimens of skin lesions should be inoculated into brain-heart infusion broth with 1% dextrose and incubated in air or CO_2 at 35° C for initial isolation. Subcultures of this broth to blood agar are made at 24-hour intervals.

On primary isolation, the organism may yield two or more different morphological colony types, each containing bacteria with different cellular morphol-

Table 33.2

Corynebacteria Associated with Human Infection

SPECIES	INFECTION(S)
C. diphtheriae	Pharyngeal, nasal, cutaneous*
C. jeikeium (group JK)	Systemic, catheter, cutaneous, endocarditis, pneumonia
Group D2	Cystitis, systemic, cutaneous, catheter
C. pseudotuberculosis	Lymphadenitis, pneumonia
C. minutissimum	*Associated with erythrasma, bacteremia (rare)*
Leprosy-derived	*Associated with leprosy*
C. haemolyticum	Pharyngitis, rash
C. aquaticum	Meningitis, peritonitis (rare)
Rhodococcus equi	Systemic, pneumonia, osteomyelitis
Arcanobacterium haemolyticum	Wound, pharyngitis, abscess, cutaneous
Actinomyces pyogenes	Cutaneous, endocarditis (rare)

*Although the infection is localized, the effects of the toxin are systemic.

ogies, mimicking a polymicrobic infection. *E. rhusiopathiae* smeared from large, rough colonies is a slender, filamentous gram-positive bacillus with a tendency to overdecolorize and become gram-negative. A Gram stain made from the smaller, smooth, translucent colony yields small, slender bacilli. *E. rhusiopathiae* may be distinguished from other gram-positive rods, such as *Listeria*, lactobacilli, and *Corynebacterium* species, by type of hemolysis, presence or absence of motility, and catalase production; however, its primary distinguishing characteristic is that it is the only catalase-negative, gram-positive, aerobic bacillus that produces H_2S when inoculated into triple sugar iron or Kligler's iron agar slant tubes. The important biochemical characteristics for the identification of *E. rhusiopathiae* are listed in Table 33.1.

33.2.c. Therapy. Clinical isolates of *E. rhusiopathiae* are usually highly susceptible to penicillins, cephalosporins, erythromycin, and clindamycin. Most notably, this organism is usually resistant to vancomycin as well as sulfonamides, trimethoprim-sulfamethoxazole, and the aminoglycosides. Variable susceptibility is reported for tetracycline and chloramphenicol. The treatment of choice is penicillin. Addition of an aminoglycoside does not appear to be warranted. Given the resistance of *Erysipelothrix* to

vancomycin, prompt identification and antimicrobial susceptibility testing of gram-positive bacilli isolated from blood or skin lesions should be performed in order to minimize the risk of complications due to inappropriate therapy.

33.3. *Corynebacterium* and Related Species, Including *Rhodococcus, Arcanobacterium*, and *Actinomyces pyogenes*

33.3.a. General considerations, epidemiology, and pathogenesis. The corynebacteria are pleomorphic, primarily nonmotile, aerobic, or facultative, gram-positive bacilli. Preferential synthesis of cell wall components at one end of the cell often results in clubbing and uneven division during binary fission, seen as "Chinese letter forms" (Figure 33.4). The *Corynebacterium* species and related genera most likely to be encountered in the clinical laboratory include *C. diphtheriae, C. ulcerans, C. aquaticum, C. pseudodiphtheriticum, C. xerosis, C. renale, C. pseudotuberculosis, C. bovis, C. minutissimum, C. jeikeium* (formerly CDC group JK),[15] *C. matruchotii* (formerly *Bacterionema matruchotii*), CDC groups D2, A4, and G2, *Arcanobacterium haemolyticum* (formerly *C. haemolyticum*), and *Actinomyces pyogenes* (formerly *C. equi*).

These organisms are found throughout nature, acting as pathogens and parasites of plants and animals. Although most species are harmless saprophytes and many are part of the normal human skin and mucous membrane flora, *C. diphtheriae*, the agent of diphtheria, and *C. jeikeium* (group JK)[15] and group D2, both relatively common causes of infection in compromised hosts, are major pathogens of humans.[25] Species other than *C. diphtheriae, C. jeikeium* (group JK), and group D2 have also been associated with human infection, however, as outlined in Table 33.2.* Certain strains have been placed in new genera that were formerly within *Corynebacterium*, such as *Rhodococcus equi* (formerly *C. equi*), *Arcanobacterium haemolyticum* (formerly *C. haemolyticum*), and *Actinomyces pyogenes* (formerly *C. pyogenes*). *C. xerosis, C. pseudodiphtheriticum, C. minutissimum, C. ulcerans, C. bovis* and others have also been reported to cause human disease, but rarely.[6,9,12,14] *C. aquaticum*, recently associated with serious disease in immunocompromised

*References 1, 3, 4, 6, 9, 14, 17, 19.

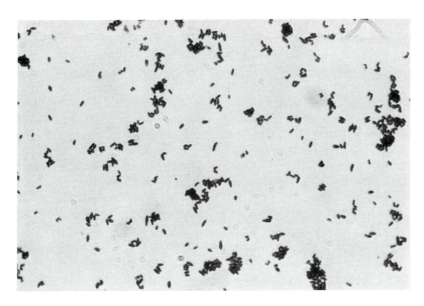

Figure 33.4
Pleomorphic forms of *Corynebacterium* species seen on Gram stain.

patients, may initially be confused with *L. monocytogenes* because of its similar motility.[3,4] A newly described group of corynebacteria, closely related to each other genetically and closely related immunologically to *Mycobacterium leprae*, are the leprosy-derived corynebacteria, reviewed by Cocito and Delville.[8] These organisms can be cultivated from lesions of leprosy and may contribute synergistically with *M. leprae* in development of disease.

Diphtheria is a well known toxin-mediated infectious disease caused by *C. diphtheriae*. The disease is an acute, contagious, febrile illness characterized by local oropharyngeal inflammation and pseudomembrane formation and damage to the heart and peripheral nerves caused by the exotoxin produced by the organisms. The exotoxin of *C. diphtheriae* is one of the most well-studied bacterial toxins and acts to inhibit protein synthesis, particularly in the heart muscle and neural cells. The gene for toxin production is carried into the bacteria by a bacteriophage, which then produces a nonlytic infection within the bacteria, replicating with the bacterial genome. Such an infection that does not lyse the host cell is called *lysogenic*. Although *C. diphtheriae* that are not infected with toxin-producing phage can cause diphtheria-like disease, the disease is usually not as severe. Diphtheria may occur in both endemic and epidemic forms; however, the an-

nual incidence has declined from 200 cases per 100,000 population in 1920 to approximately 0.001 per 100,000 in the 1980s, largely because of vaccination efforts in the United States. Recent endemic foci include skid row inhabitants of Seattle, who suffered from wound infections with *C. diphtheriae*. The toxin can be elaborated from wound colonization as well as from pharyngeal sites of infection.

C. jeikeium (group JK) and group D2 are of particular interest among the nondiphtheriae species of *Corynebacterium*. Both of these organisms are resistant to a wide range of antimicrobial agents such as penicillins, cephalosporins, and aminoglycosides. In addition, both organisms have been recognized as the etiologic agent in an increasing number of serious infections among hospitalized and immunocompromised individuals.

C. jeikeium (group JK) causes a variety of infections, including septicemia, meningitis, and peritonitis; however, the most frequent type of infection with this agent is bacteremia or foreign body infection (for example, intravascular device or cerebrospinal fluid shunts).[15] Most commonly, the infections are nosocomial, occurring in patients with compromised host defenses, exposure to broad-spectrum antimicrobials, and with an extended hospital stay.[25] Nosocomial transmission of *C. jeikeium* has been well documented; bacteremia due to this organism can be prevented by the introduction of control measures such as reduction of catheter manipulation and wearing of sterile gloves.

Corynebacterium group D2 has also been reported as a cause of nosocomial bacteremia and pneumonia, but most commonly it is found to cause cystitis, bacteriuria, and pyelonephritis. *Corynebacterium* group D2 is a urea-splitting organism, and as is the case with many other urea-splitting organisms, the urease produced seems to play an important role in its pathogenicity. Infection with this organism produces an alkaline urine and promotes the formation of struvite (ammonium magnesium phosphate) stones in the bladder. Most patients infected with *Corynebacterium* group D2 are elderly and have a history of urologic abnormalities, instrumentation, and exposure to broad-spectrum antimicrobial therapy.

Colonization of hospitalized patients with *C. jeikeium* or *Corynebacterium* group D2 is common; however, only a few patients are colonized by both organisms simultaneously. The sites most frequently colonized are the groin and rectum, with *C. jeikeium* isolated more frequently from males and group D2 isolated more frequently from females.[25]

33.3.b. Isolation of *C. diphtheriae* from suspected cases of diphtheria. Although the cornyebacteria will grow well on most routinely used laboratory media, selective and differential media for *C. diphtheriae* should be used if diphtheria is suspected. Cystine tellurite blood agar (Appendix A) will reliably support growth of *C. diphtheriae*. The colonies appear black, or gray with a characteristic garliclike odor, usually after 24 hours' incubation in air. Colony morphology differences on cystine tellurite agar have been used to differentiate the three subspecies of *C. diphtheriae: mitis, intermedius,* and *gravis.* They may occasionally require 48 hours' incubation for initial isolation. Modified Tinsdale agar (Appendix A) has been used for isolation of *C. diphtheriae*; colonies are black with dark brown halos. The halos develop particularly around colonies that have grown into stabbed areas of the agar. This medium must be used within 4 days of preparation and does not support growth of many strains. When small numbers of organisms must be isolated, primary inoculation to a Loeffler slant and overnight incubation at 35°C in air before subculturing to cystine tellurite blood agar may improve recovery. Gram-stained colonies that exhibit coryneform morphology should be

streaked to a sheep blood agar plate for purity before biochemical tests are performed. Identification of subspecies of diphtheria isolates is best accomplished biochemically.

33.4.c. Laboratory identification of corynebacteria. *Corynebacterium* species grow well on most commonly used media and usually appear as opaque, white, or gray colonies. They may, however, resemble nonhemolytic or α-hemolytic streptococci, yeast, staphylococci, and commensal *Neisseria* species. Gram-stain morphology is typical of the genus, and no true branching should be observed. Most corynebacteria are catalase-negative.

As described by Thompson et al.,[29] rapid biochemical tests are reliable for identification of several groups of corynebacteria. In addition, two supplementary tests, that of pyrazinamidase activity[27] and production of the enzyme phospholipase D,[2] can be used to differentiate among corynebacteria. Performance of these tests is described in Procedures 33.1 to 33.3. Selected biochemical reactions of some clinically relevant species are shown in Table 33.3. Additionally, definitive schemes for species identification within *Corynebacterium* and related genera are available.[6,9]

Several investigators have reported on the usefulness of various commercial biochemical kits in the identification of *C. jeikeium, Corynebacterium* group D2, and other species of *Corynebacterium*. The API 20S (Analytab Products, Inc.; developed for identification of streptococci) reliably identified multiply antibiotic-resistant strains of group JK (*C. jeikeium*) and D2, often with the addition of urease and nitrate tests.[16,30] The Minitek system (BBL Microbiology Systems) was found to identify correctly 20 different species of *Corynebacterium*, including 44 isolates of group JK, from a test population of 90 clinical and stock isolates of corynebacteria.[24] Similarly, Grasmick and Bruckner used the Rapid Identification Method (RIM series; Austin Biological Laboratories, Inc.) tests for carbohydrate utilization, nitrate reduction, and urease activity in combination with conventional overnight tests to differentiate group JK isolates from other species of *Corynebacterium*.[11]

33.3.d. In vitro toxigenicity test. Definitive identification of a strain of *C. diphtheriae* as a true pathogen requires demonstration of toxin production. A patient may be infected with several strains at once,

Text continued on p. 471.

PROCEDURE 33.1

Pyrazinamidase Test for Corynebacteria

Principle

The enzyme pyrazine-carboxylamidase (pyrazin-amidase), which hydrolyzes pyrazinamide to free pyrazinoic acid, is present in most corynebacteria but absent in three species.

Method

1. Prepare substrate medium as follows:

Agar (Bacto agar, Difco Laboratories)	2 g
Pyrazinamide (Sigma Chemical Co.)	0.1 g
Pyruvic acid, sodium salt (Sigma)	2 g
Distilled water	1000 ml

   Mix thoroughly, heat to dissolve, and dispense in 5-ml amounts in 16 × 125 mm screw-cap test tubes. Autoclave for 15 min at 121° C. Allow the medium to harden upright to form a butt. Medium will keep 6 months at 4° C.
2. Inoculate a *heavy* suspension of the test organism into the top half of the substrate medium tube by scraping up growth from a 24 to 72-hour culture on blood or chocolate agar with a cotton swab and gently rotating the swab in the medium. The suspension should be milky.

Modified from Coyle, M.B. Harborview Medical Center, Seattle, Wash., and from Sulea I.T., et al.[17]

3. Incubate the tubes for 2 h at 37° C in a water bath or a dry bath.
4. To the tube of each test organism, add 1 ml of freshly prepared 1% ferrous ammonium sulfate (0.1 g ferrous ammonium sulfate [Sigma] in 10 ml sterile distilled water).
5. Examine tubes after 1-5 min at room temperature for a rusty pink band in the agar, indicating hydrolysis of pyrazinamide and presence of pyrazinamidase. An additional incubation of 4 h in the refrigerator may enhance color formation.
6. Only *C. diphtheriae, C. ulcerans,* and *C. pseudotuberculosis* lack pyrazinamidase.

Quality control

Inoculate identical tubes of medium with a negative control *(C. ulcerans)* and a positive control *(C. xerosis).* Stock organisms should be used; specific quality control strains have not been designated for this test.

Expected results

C. xerosis will show a rusty pink band in the agar, indicating free pyrazinoic acid. The *C. ulcerans* will show no color.

Performance schedule

Test quality control organisms each time the test is performed.

PROCEDURE 33.2

Detection of Phospholipase D by Inhibition of CAMP Test

Principle

The enzyme phospholipase D acts to prevent the enhanced hemolysis seen when the hemolysins of *S. aureus* and *S. agalactiae* interact synergistically (CAMP test, Chapter 25).

Method

1. Fresh cultures of each organism needed for performance of the test are incubated overnight on blood agar plates
   a. *S. aureus*, β-toxin-positive strain
   b. *S. agalactiae*, known to be positive in the CAMP test (Chapter 25)
   c. *C. ulcerans* as positive control
   d. Unknown strain of *Corynebacterium* to be tested

Modified from Barksdale et al. 1981.[2]

2. A 5% sheep blood agar plate is inoculated with the test organisms by swabbing the colonies with a cotton-tipped swab and rubbing the swab on the surface of the test plate in the pattern shown in Figure 33.5.
3. The plate is incubated 48 h at 37° C. Inhibition of the enhanced zone of hemolysis formed at the junction of the staphylococcal hemolysin and the streptococcal hemolysin is caused by phospholipase D.

Quality control

The quality control organisms are included in the test as described. Standard *C. ulcerans* have not been designated for this test.

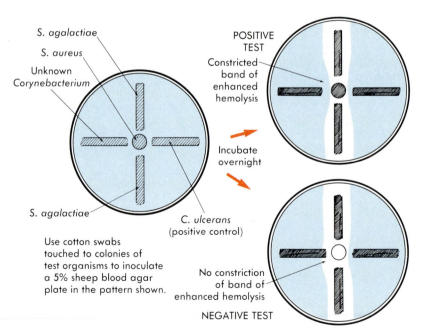

Figure 33.5
Pattern of inoculation of plate for test for phospholipase D (inhibition of **CAMP** test).

PROCEDURE 33.3

Rapid Biochemical Tests for Identification of Corynebacterium *Species*

Principle

Corynebacteria can be identified biochemically if large inocula are used with buffered substrates.

Method

1. Prepare biochemicals as follows:

   Biochemical medium base

Casamino acids (Difco Laboratories)	20 g
L-cysteine HCl (Sigma Chemical Co.)	0.3 g
Sodium sulfate (J. T. Baker Chemical Co.)	0.3 g
Neopeptone (Difco Laboratories)	25 g
Phenol red (Difco Laboratories)	0.1 g
Distilled water	1 L

   Dispense in 50-ml quantities into six 100 ml screw-cap flasks.
   To one flask, add:

   Starch (Difco Laboratories) 1 g

   To another flask, add:

   Glycogen (Difco Laboratories) 1 g

   Autoclave all of the flasks for 10 min at 121° C. Prepare 20% carbohydrate solutions of dextrose, maltose, sucrose, and trehalose in distilled water (4 g carbohydrate in 20 ml distilled water). Filter sterilize through a 0.45 μm membrane filter. Add 5 ml of each carbohydrate solution to one each of the four remaining flasks of autoclaved broth base.
   Also prepare nitrate broth and urea broth (Appendix A) or purchase such media commercially (Appendix C).
   Store all media in sterile dropper bottles.

   Modified from Thompson, J.S., et al.[29]

2. Just before use, dispense 1 drop (approximately 0.025 ml) of each medium into a sterile microtube (6 × 50 mm borosilicate disposable glass, Kimble Division of Owens-Illinois) held upright in a microdilution plate.
3. Inoculate each medium with one third of a large loopful of a colony from overnight growth on blood agar. Be certain that the inoculum is very evenly dispersed in the medium. Complete emulsification is required for rapid reactions.
4. Overlay the inoculated urea tube with mineral oil.
5. Incubate the tubes for 1 h in a shallow water bath at 37° C. Results are interpreted as for conventional tests: positive carbohydrate utilization is shown by yellow; negative is red; urea hydrolysis turns the indicator pink, and the nitrate test requires addition of standard reagents (Chapter 9), after which a positive test is red.

Quality control

Enterobacteriaceae can be chosen to determine that the carbohydrate reactions are acceptable and for a positive nitrate control. *Proteus vulgaris* can be used as a positive control for the urease test (pink color). An asaccharolytic organism, such as an inactive *C. jeikeium*, should be tested as a negative control.

Performance schedule

Control organisms should be tested each time the test is performed.

Table 33.3
Differentiation of *Corynebacterium* Species

SPECIES	CATALASE	NITRATE	UREASE	DEXTROSE	MALTOSE	SUCROSE	STARCH	TRE-HALOSE	GLYCOGEN	PYRAZIN-AMIDASE	PHOSPHO-LIPASE
C. diphtheriae (*mitis*)	+	+*	−	+	+	−	−	−	−	−	−
C. diphtheriae (*gravis*)	+	+	−	+	+	−	+	−	+	−	−
C. diphtheriae (*intermedius*)	+	+	−	+	+	−	−	−	−	−	−
C. ulcerans	+	−	+	+	+	−	+	+	−/+	−	+
C. pseudodiphtheriticum	+	+	+	−	−	−	−	−	−	+	−
C. pseudotuberculosis	+	+/−	+	+	+	−	−	−	−	−	+
C. xerosis	+	+	−	+	+/−	+	−	−	−	+	−
C. jeikeium (group JK)	+	−	−	+/−	+/−	−	+/−	+/−	+/−	+	−
Group D2	+	−	+	−	−	−	−	−	−	NT	NT
Actinomyces pyogenes	−	−	−	+	+	+/−	+/−	+/−	NT	+	+
Arcanobacterium haemolyticum	−	−	−	+	+	+/−	+/−	+/−	NT	+	+

+ = >90% of strains positive; − = >90% of strains negative; +/− = variable (most strains positive); −/+ = variable (most strains negative); NT = not tested.
C. diphtheriae (*mitis*, belfanti strain) is nitrate-negative.
Compiled from material presented by Coyle, M.B., Harborview Medical Center, Seattle, Wash., and from Thompson, J.S., Gates-Davis, D.R., and Young, D.C. 1983. Rapid microbiochemical identification of *Corynebacterium diphtheriae* and other medically important corynebacteria. J. Clin. Microbiol. 18:926.

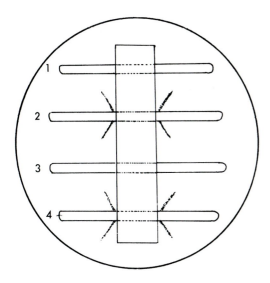

Figure 33.6
Diagram of an Elek plate for demonstration of toxin production by *C. diphtheriae*.

so that testing a pooled inoculum will enhance chances of detecting toxin activity. The most useful test is that described originally by Elek, the in vitro toxigenicity test, or *Elek plate*.[10] The test should be performed only in reference laboratories today, since the incidence of diphtheria is quite low and the test poses numerous technical problems because of variability of reagents. Briefly, a filter paper strip impregnated with diphtheria antitoxin is buried just below the surface of a special agar plate before the agar hardens. Strains to be tested and known positive and negative toxigenic strains are streaked on the surface of the agar in a line across the plate, at a right angle to the antitoxin paper strip (Figure 33.6). After 24 hours' incubation at 37° C, plates are examined with transmitted light for the presence of fine precipitin lines at a 45-degree angle to the streaks. The presence of precipitin lines indicates that the strain produced toxin that reacted with the homologous antitoxin. Under some circumstances, precipitin lines may take up to 72 hours to develop.

33.3.e. Therapy of infections caused by corynebacteria. *C. diphtheriae* are usually susceptible to penicillin, erythromycin, and most other antimicrobial agents useful against gram-positive bacteria. In all cases of diphtheria, antibiotic therapy should be initiated. Antitoxin therapy is given to patients from whom toxigenic strains are isolated or if the clinical picture dictates such therapy. The isolates should be tested for susceptibility, however, since erythromycin and tetracycline resistance has been observed. The other corynebacteria are variable in susceptibility. All corynebacteria are resistant to oxacillin, methicillin, and nafcillin. *C. jeikeium* and group D2, additionally, commonly exhibit multiple resistance, usually being susceptible only to vancomycin, which is the drug of choice for treatment of infections with those strains. Although some of the newer antimicrobial agents, such as teichoplanin and the quinolones, are also active against *C. jeikeium* and group D2 and although synergy between aminoglycosides and such agents has been demonstrated, it is not clear what role these agents will have in the prevention and therapy of infections due to the *Corynebacterium* species.[26]

33.4. *Nocardia* Species

33.4.a. General considerations, epidemiology, and pathogenesis. *Nocardia* organisms are members of the group of aerobic actinomycetes, which include *Streptomyces, Nocardiopsis, Actinomadura, Dermatophilus*, and other genera that rarely cause human infection. Some of these organisms are discussed briefly in Section 33.5. *Dermatophilus* is discussed in Chapter 39. *Nocardia* are inhabitants of the soil and water. They infect humans after inhalation of the organisms and primary establishment of growth in the lungs or by inoculation through breaks in the skin. The infection is usually chronic, but occasionally is fulminant, and is usually seen in immunosuppressed patients. The clinical syndrome of a chronic disease with both respiratory and central nervous system components, particularly if abscess formation is apparent, is suggestive of nocardiosis.

Nocardiosis is most commonly caused by *N. asteroides* (over 90% of cases) and rarely by *N. brasiliensis, N. caviae*, or other species. Infections due to *N. asteroides* occur most frequently in immunocompromised individuals, particularly following renal or cardiac transplantation. Infections caused by *Nocardia* are primarily suppurative, with necrosis and abscess formation. The incidence is higher in males than in females. Although pneumonic processes are often seen, a lymphocutaneous infection resembling sporotrichosis (Chapter 43) can occur. Spread to other tissues from the primary pulmonary lesions occurs by advancing growth (to produce empyema, chest wall involvement, and draining sinuses) or hematogenously. Hematogenous dissemi-

PROCEDURE 33.4

Partial Acid-Fast Stain for Identification of Nocardia

Principle

The nocardiae, because of unusual long-chain fatty acids in their cell walls, can retain carbolfuchsin dye during mild acid decolorization, whereas other aerobic branching bacilli cannot.

Method

1. Emulsify a very small amount of the organisms to be stained in a drop of distilled water on the slide. A known positive control and a negative control should be stained along with the unknown strain.
2. Allow to air dry and heat fix.
3. Flood the stain with Kinyoun's carbolfuchsin (Appendix B) and allow the stain to remain on the slide 3 min.
4. Rinse with tap water, shake off excess water, and decolorize briefly with 3% acid alcohol (940 ml of 95% ethanol and 60 ml of concentrated HCl) until no more red color rinses off the slides.
5. Counterstain with Kinyoun's methylene blue (Appendix B) for 30 s.
6. Rinse again with tap water. Allow the slide to air dry and examine the unknown strain compared with the controls. Partially acid-fast organisms show reddish to purple filaments, compared with non-acid-fast organisms, which are blue only.

Quality control

A known partially acid-fast organism, *N. asteroides*, and a known negative control, *Actinomadura madurai*, should be subcultured onto the same medium as the organism to be tested and incubated concurrently. The *Nocardia* should exhibit reddish and purple filaments with occasional areas of blue, whereas the *Actinomadura* will stain only blue. No designated strains have been reserved for quality control.

Performance schedule

Quality control strains should be tested each time the stain is performed.

---

nation involving the central nervous system, resulting in single or multiple brain abscesses, is particularly common, occurring in approximately 30% of patients. Osteomyelitis is also being recognized more commonly.[22] The organism seems to be able to resist phagocytosis and therefore persists in the host. Definitive determinants of pathogenicity are not known, but the filamentous stage of growth seems to be more virulent than the stationary coccoid phase.

33.4.b. **Laboratory identification.** Cells of *Nocardia* are pleomorphic, exhibiting branching and coccoid forms. The most distinguishing characteristic of *Nocardia* is its tendency to retain carbol-fuchsin stain with mild acid decolorization, called *partial acid-fastness*. The characteristic may be difficult to demonstrate. Growing the organism to be tested, along with a fresh subculture of a known positive control

(*Nocardia asteroides*) and a known negative control (*Actinomadura madurae*), for approximately 4 days on Middlebrook 7H11 agar (Appendix A) or in litmus milk broth (Appendix A) will enhance the acid fast nature of an isolate. The partial acid fast stain is performed as outlined in Procedure 33.4.

Nocardia may be first suspected when long, thin, branching gram-positive bacilli are seen in smears of lesion material or sputum. The organism also stains with Gomori methenamine silver stain (Figure 33.7). Since it grows slowly, *Nocardia* is often overgrown by normal flora and other bacteria on routine microbiological media. Insertion of a glass rod dipped in paraffin to a liquid culture of a contaminated specimen (sputum, for example) diluted 1:1 in buffered saline has been shown to enhance recovery of *Nocardia*, which can utilize paraffin as a sole carbon source.[21,23] Material from specimens

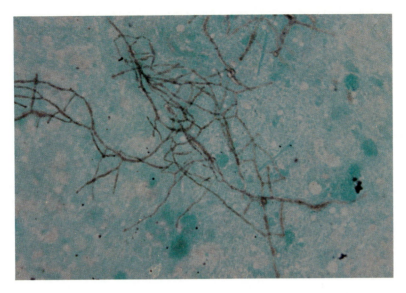

Figure 33.7
Nocardia in lesion of lower leg, stained with Gomori–methenamine silver stain.

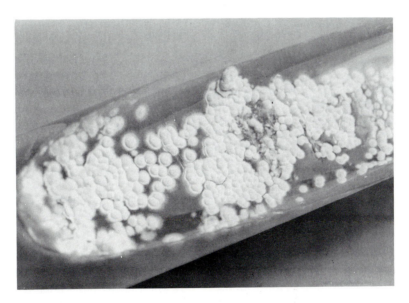

Figure 33.8
Colony of *N. asteroides* after 10 days of incubation.

that contain no other flora, such as tissue and abscess drainage, may be inoculated to brain-heart infusion agar, which supports growth of *Nocardia*. The organism grows well on Sabouraud dextrose agar but is inhibited by chloramphenicol. Occasional isolates will first be seen on mycobacterial culture media, since *Nocardia* can survive the usual decontamination procedures. Incubating at least one primary isolation medium at 45°C may enhance recovery of *N. asteroides*. *Nocardia* species grow better in 10% CO_2.

Colonies are visible from 3 to 30 days after inoculation, appearing as waxy, bumpy, or velvety rugose forms, usually with yellow to orange pigment (Figure 33.8). The presence of branching filaments and partial acid fastness differentiates these isolates

PROCEDURE 33.5

Lysozyme Resistance for Differentiating Nocardia *from* Streptomyces

Principle

The enzyme lysozyme, present in human tears and other secretions, can break down cell walls of certain microorganisms. Susceptibility to the action of lysozyme can differentiate among certain morphologically similar genera and species.

Method

1. Prepare basal broth as follows:

Peptone (Difco Laboratories)	5 g
Beef extract (Difco)	3 g
Glycerol (Difco)	70 ml
Distilled water	1000 ml

Dispense 500 ml of this solution into 16 × 125 mm screw-cap glass test tubes, 5 ml per tube. Autoclave the test tubes and the remaining solution for 15 min at 121° C. Tighten caps and store the tubes in the refrigerator for a maximum of 2 months.

2. Prepare lysozyme solution as follows:

Lysozyme (Sigma Chemical Co.)	100 mg
HCl (0.01 N)	100 ml
Filter-sterilize through a 0.45 μm membrane filter.	

3. Add 5-ml lysozyme solution to 95 ml basal broth, mix gently, avoiding bubbles, and aseptically dispense in 5 ml amounts to sterile, screw-cap tubes as in step 1. Store refrigerated for a maximum of 2 weeks.
4. Place several bits of the colony of the isolate to be tested into a tube of the basal glycerol broth without lysozyme (control) and into a tube of broth containing lysozyme.
5. Incubate at room temperature for up to 7 days. Observe for growth in the control tube. An organism that grows well in the control tube but not in the lysozyme tube is considered to be susceptible to lysozyme.

Quality control

Test a known negative control (*Streptomyces griseus*) and a known positive control (*N. asteroides*) in the same way. No specific strains have been designated for quality control.

Performance schedule

Test quality control organisms each time the test is performed.

Modified from McGinnis, et al. 1982.[18]

from mycobacteria. Differentiation from *Streptomyces* species is more difficult. Aerial hyphae of *Nocardia*, *Streptomyces*, *Nocardiopsis*, and *Actinomadura* are best displayed on the slightly acid Sabouraud dextrose agar made from Difco Laboratories' dry powder, according to Leonore Haley of the CDC. Mishra et al.[20] have developed a taxonomic scheme that divides these genera on the basis of biochemical characteristics. There are numerous species of *Nocardia*, not all of which have been recovered from clinical specimens. A simplified scheme for identification of the most commonly isolated species, developed by McGinnis, D'Amato,

and Land,[18] is shown in Table 33.5. Readers are referred to the publication by those authors for instructions on preparation of the media used to identify these organisms.

Nocardia are resistant to the action of lysozyme, while almost all *Streptomyces* are susceptible. Lysozyme resistance is tested according to Procedure 33.5. This test is subject to variation, however, and occasionally does not yield useful results. Another helpful test for differentiating *Nocardia*, *Nocardiopsis*, and *Streptomyces* from the other aerobic actinomycetes is ONPG (*o*-nitrophenyl-β-D-galactopyranoside), the test for β-galactosidase. The reagents

Table 33.4

Differentiation of Selected Aerobic Actinomycetes

ORGANISM	ACID FROM CELLOBIOSE	HYDROLYSIS OF					LYSOZYME RESISTANCE
		CASEIN	HYPOXANTHINE	TYROSINE	UREA	XANTHINE	
Actinomadura madurae	+	+	+	+	−	−	−
A. pelletieri	−	+	+/−	+	−	−	−
Nocardia asteroides	−	−	−	−	+	−	+
N. brasiliensis	−	+	+	+	+	−	+
N. caviae	−	−	+	+/−	+	+	+
Nocardiopsis dassonvillei	+	+	+	+	+/−	+	−
Streptomyces griseus	+	+	+	+	+	+	−
S. somaliensis	−	+	−	+	−	−	−
Streptomyces species (other)	+/−	+	+	+	+/−	+/−	+/−

+ = ≥90% of strains positive; − = ≥90% of strains negative; +/− = variable results.
Modified from McGinnis et al. 1982. Pictorial handbook of medically important fungi and aerobic actinomycetes. Praeger Publishers, New York.

are available commercially since they are usually used for identification of Enterobacteriaceae. The three genera mentioned are positive (able to utilize lactose), while other genera of actinomycetes are negative. In cases where definitive identification of a *Nocardia*-like organism is required, the isolate should be sent to a reference laboratory where cell wall analysis by gas-liquid chromatography (GLC) can be performed.

33.4.c. Therapy. Sulfonamides still appear to be the antimicrobial agents of choice for treatment of nocardiosis. Trimethoprim-sulfamethoxazole has not been shown to be as active as sulfonamides alone against *Nocardia*. Minocycline seems to be a good alternative for sulfonamide-allergic patients, and newer aminoglycosides such as amikacin are very promising. In vitro susceptibility tests can be performed by reference laboratories, and they should be attempted with isolates from cases that appear resistant to treatment.

33.5. Miscellaneous Other Aerobic Actinomycetes

Human infections with strains of the genera *Nocardiopsis*, *Actinomadura*, *Dermatophilus*, and *Streptomyces* are usually chronic, granulomatous lesions of the skin and subcutaneous tissue, acquired by inoculation. *Mycetoma*, a chronic lesion of the ex-

tremities (usually the feet), characterized by swollen tissue and draining sinus tracts, is usually associated with fungal infection, although it can be caused by members of the actinomycetes. The infection is then called *actinomycetoma*. These organisms are becoming more common as causes of infection in immunocompromised hosts. All of the aerobic actinomycetes are soil saprophytes.

With the exception of rare strains of *Streptomyces*, aerobic actinomycetes are susceptible to the action of lysozyme. Because the biochemical reactions that are used to identify these organisms are difficult to perform and because cell wall analysis is usually needed for ultimate species identification, clinically significant strains should be sent to a reference laboratory for testing. Table 33.4 illustrates a simplified scheme for differentiation among some medically important species.

Another group of actinomycetes, the thermophilic actinomycetes, are responsible for hypersensitivity pneumonitis. Clinical laboratories are rarely asked to diagnose such disease, which occurs in farmers, factory workers, and others who are exposed occupationally to spores or fungal elements from which they develop allergy. The species involved, *Thermoactinomyces*, *Saccharomonospora*, and *Micropolyspora*, grow readily on trypticase soy agar with 1% yeast extract or on one-half strength nutrient agar. A practical scheme for identification of the most common etiologic agents has been presented by Hollick.[13] Because there is no effective therapy, patients must prevent disease by altering life-style to avoid exposure to these sensitizing agents.

33.6. Other Aerobic Non-Spore-Forming Bacilli: *Rothia, Kurthia, Oerskovia,* and *Lactobacillus*

33.6.a. *Rothia dentocariosa*. The genus *Rothia* was created in 1967 to accommodate an organism that resembled *Actinomyces* (but grew well aerobically) and resembled *Nocardia* (but did not contain the same cell wall constituents). The only species, *R. dentocariosa*, has caused abscesses and endocarditis and is part of normal human oral flora. It has also been recovered from gingival crevices of patients with periodontal disease and can cause periodontitis in germ-free rats. Unlike other filamentous, gram-positive organisms, *Rothia* contains fructose as a component of the cell wall. The organism grows well on nutrient agar, producing smooth colonies at 48 hours that become rough or globose on prolonged incubation. Microscopically, the cells are coccoid, only becoming branched after several days of incubation in broth. The organism is catalase-positive, lactose-negative, and produces acetoin from glucose (exhibits a positive Voges-Proskauer test). *Rothia* is susceptible to most antimicrobial agents, including penicillin, erythromycin, aminoglycosides, and cephalosporins.

33.6.b. *Kurthia* and *Oerskovia* species. Both of these genera are soil saprophytes, being only rarely implicated in human infection. *Kurthia bessonii* has been isolated from endocarditis. The organism resembles *Bacillus cereus* by forming irregular colonies and by its cellular morphology (large, straight-sided, motile gram-positive bacilli). *Kurthia*, however, does not form spores and is strictly aerobic and nonsaccharolytic.

At least two species of *Oerskovia*, *O. turbata* and *O. xanthineolytica*, can cause human infection. Isolates have been recovered from infected heart valves, blood, wounds, and other sites. Most strains of *Oerskovia* produce a yellow pigment. Microscopically, the organisms are branching, filamentous bacilli that fragment into coccoid forms after prolonged incubation. Differentiation from *Corynebacterium* species is extremely difficult. The ability of *Oerskovia* to hydrolyze esculin and motility may be helpful.

Only very rare strains of corynebacteria (*C. aquaticum* and a few CDC groups) are motile.

33.6.c. *Lactobacillus* species. The lactobacilli are common inhabitants of the oral cavity, gastrointestinal tract, and female genital tract of humans. They have only rarely been reported to cause serious human infection. Lactobacilli have been isolated from blood, cerebrospinal fluid, abscess material, amniotic fluid, and pleural fluid. One series of endocarditis cases has been reported.[28] The organism is a facultative or strict anaerobe, usually preferring to grow microaerophilically; strains are usually identified using anaerobic media and methods (Chapters 34 and 35). The presence of large numbers of lactobacilli in the culture or Gram stain of vaginal contents is indicative of a healthy vagina. When the organism gains access to an unnatural site, it is able to cause suppurative infection. Large amounts of lactic acid are produced as by-products of metabolism, which helps to maintain the acid pH that lactobacilli thrive in. It is possible that endocervical lactobacilli play a role in protecting human females from gonococcal infection and bacterial vaginosis.

The colonies can assume any morphology on blood agar, ranging from pinpoint, α-hemolytic colonies resembling streptococci to large, rough, gray colonies. The microscopic morphology is highly variable as well, with the existence of forms similar to *Bacillus* species, possibly chaining, as well as coccobacilli, spiral forms, and others. All species are catalase-negative. Differentiation from streptococci may be difficult, but the formation of chains of rods in thioglycollate broth and moderate vancomycin resistance (unusual for any gram-positive organism) help to characterize isolates as lactobacilli. Using prereduced, anaerobically sterilized carbohydrate media (Chapter 34), microbiologists can identify some species of lactobacilli. Minimal characteristics of four of the more commonly isolated species that are able to grow aerobically are shown in Table 33.5.

Penicillin, ampicillin, clindamycin, and cephalothin are able to inhibit growth of lactobacilli, but bactericidal activity is not commonly seen. It is possible that the acid environment produced by the organisms contributes to the decreased activity of certain antimicrobial agents against lactobacilli. Strains of lactobacilli that are resistant to vancomycin have been isolated from colonized, but not infected, hospitalized individuals; however, these isolates remain susceptible to penicillin. For treatment of en-

Table 33.5

Selected Key Features of Lactobacilli most Commonly Isolated from Clinical Specimens

SPECIES	ARGININE TO AMMONIA	GROWTH AT 45° C	ACID FROM	
			MANNITOL	RAFFINOSE
Lactobacillus acidophilus	−	−	−	+ / −
L. casei	−	+	+	−
L. leichmannii	+	−	−	+ / −
L. plantarum	−	+ / −	+ / −	+

+ = ≥90% of strains positive; − = ≥90% of strains negative; + / − = variable results.

docarditis, it is recommended that combinations of penicillin and aminoglycosides be used, perhaps with addition of rifampin for increased bactericidal activity.[28]

REFERENCES

1. Banck, G., and Nyman, M. 1986. Tonsillitis and rash associated with *Corynebacterium haemolyticum*. J. Infect. Dis. 154:1037.

2. Barksdale, L., Lindr, R., Sulea, I.T., and Pollice, M. 1981. Phospholipase D activity of *Corynebacterium pseudotuberculosis* (*Corynebacterium ovis*) and *Corynebacterium ulcerans*, a distinctive marker within the genus *Corynebacterium*. J. Clin. Microbiol. 13:335.

3. Beckwith, D.G., Jahre, J.A., and Haggerty, S. 1986. Isolation of *Corynebacterium aquaticum* from spinal fluid of an infant with meningitis. J. Clin. Microbiol. 23:375.

4. Casella, P., Bosoni, M.A., and Tommasi, A. 1988. Recurrent *Corynebacterium aquaticum* peritonitis in a patient undergoing continuous ambulatory peritoneal dialysis. Clin. Microbiol. Newsletter 10: 62.

5. Ciesielski, C.A., and Swaminathan, B. 1987. *Listeria monocytogenes*—a foodborne pathogen. Clin. Microbiol. Newsletter 9:149.

6. Clarridge, J.E. 1986. When, why, and how far should coryneforms be identified? Clin. Microbiol. Newsletter 8:32.

7. Clarridge, J.E., and Weissfeld, A.S. 1984. Aerobic asporogenous gram-positive bacilli. Clin. Microbiol. Newsletter 6:115.

8. Cocito, C., and Delville, J. 1983. Properties of microorganisms isolated from human leprosy lesions. Rev. Infect. Dis. 4:649.

9. Coyle, M.B., Hollis, D.G., and Groman, N.B. 1985. *Coryhnebacterium* spp. and other coryneform organisms. In Lennette, E.H., Balows, A., Hausler, W.J., Jr., and Shadomy, H.J., editors. Manual of clinical microbiology, ed. American society for Microbiology, Washington, D.C.

10. Elek, S.D. 1949. The plate virulence test for diphtheria. J. Clin. Pathol. 2:250.

11. Grasmick, A.E., and Bruckner, D.A. 1987. Comparison of rapid identification method and conventional substrates for identification of *Corynebacterium* group JK isolates. J. Clin. Microbiol. 25:1111.

12. Guarderas, J., Karnad, A., Alvarez, S., and Berk, S.L. 1986. *Corynebacterium minitissimum* bacteremia in a patient with chronic myeloid leukemia in blast crisis. Diagn. Microbiol. Infect. Dis. 5:327.

13. Hollick, G.E. 1986. Isolation and identification of thermophilic actinomycetes associated with hypersensitivity pneumonitis. Clin. Microbiol. Newsletter 8:29.

14. Hollis, D.G., and Weaver, R.E. 1981. Gram-positive organisms: a guide to identification. Centers for Disease Control, Atlanta, May 1981.

15. Jackman, P.J.H., Pitcher, D.G., Pelcynska, S., and Borman, P. 1987. Classification of corynebacteria associated with endocarditis (group JK) as *Corynebacterium jeikeium* sp. nov. System. Appl. Microbiol. 9:83.

16. Kelly, M.C., Smith, I.D., Anstey, R.J., et al. 1984. Rapid identification of antibitoic-resistant corynebacteria with the API 20S system. J. Clin. Microbiol. 19:245.

17. Kunke, P.J. 1987. Serious infection in an AIDS patient due to *Rhodococcus equi*. Clin. Microbiol. Newsletter 9:163.

18. McGinnis, M.R., D'Amato, R.F., and Land, G.A. 1982. Pictorial handbook of medically important fungi and aerobic actinomycetes. Praeger Publishers, New York.

19. Miller, R.A., Brancato, F., and Holmes, K.K. 1986. *Corynebacterium hemolyticum* as a cause of pharyngitis and scarlatiniform rash in young adults. Ann. Intern. Med. 105:867.

20. Mishra, S.K., Gordon, R.E., and Barnett, D.A. 1980. Identification of nocardiae and streptomycetes of medical importance. J. Clin. Microbiol. 11:728.

21. Mishra, S.K., and Randhawa, H.S. 1969. Application of paraffin bait technique to the isolation of *Nocardia asteroides* from clinical specimens. Appl. Microbiol. 18:686.

22. Schwartz, J.G., and Tio, F.O. 1987. Nocardial osteomyelitis: a case report and review of the literature. Diagn. Microbiol. Infect. Dis. 8:37.

23. Singh, M., Sandhu, R.S., and Randhawa, H.S. 1987. Comparison of paraffin baiting and conventional culture techniques for isolation of *Nocardia asteroides* from sputum. J. Clin. Microbiol. 25:176.

24. Slifkin, M., Gil, G.M., and Engwall, C. 1986. Rapid identification of group JK and other corynebacteria with the Minitek system. J. Clin. Microbiol. 24:177.

25. Soriano, F., Rodriguez-Tudela, J.L., Fernandez-Roblas, R., et al. 1988. Skin colonization by *Corynebacterium* groups D2 and JK in hospitalized patients. J. Clin. Microbiol. 26:1878.

26. Spitzer, P.G., Eliopoulos, G.M., Karchmer, A.W., and Moellering, R.C., Jr. 1988. Synergistic activity between vancomycin or teichoplanin and gentamicin or tobramycin against pathogenic diphtheroids. Antimicrob. Agents Chemother. 32:434.

27. Sulea, I.T., Pollice, M.C., and Barksdale, L. 1980. Pyrazine carboxylamidase activity in *Corynebacterium*. J. Clin. Microbiol. 30:466.

28. Sussman, J.I., Baron, E.J., Goldberg, S.M., et al. 1986. Clinical manifestations and therapy of *Lactobacillus* endocarditis: report of a case and review of the literature. Rev. Infect. Dis. 8:771.

29. Thompson, J.S., Gates-Davis, D.R., and Yong, D.C. 1983. Rapid microbiochemical identification of *Corynebacterium diphtheriae* and other medically important corynebacteria. J. Clin. Microbiol. 18:926.

30. Tillotson, G., Arora, M., Robbins, M., and Holton, J. 1988. Identification of *Corynebacterium jeikeium* and *Corynebacterium* CDC group D2 with the API 20 Strep system. Eur. J. Clin. Microbiol. Infect. Dis. 7:675.

BIBLIOGRAPHY

Ciesielski, C.A., Hightower, A.W., Parsons, S.K., and Broome, C.V. 1988. Listeriosis in the United States: 1980-1982. Arch. Intern. Med. 148:1416.

Curry, W.A. 1980. Human nocardiosis: a clinical review with selected case reports. Arch. Intern. Med. 140:819.

Fagnant, J.E., Sanders, C.C., and Sanders, W.E., Jr. 1982. Development of and evaluation of a biochemical scheme for identification of endocervical lactobacilli. J. Clin. Microbiol. 16:926.

Gellin, B.G., and Broome, C.V. 1989. Listeriosis. J. Am. Med. Assoc. 261:1313.

Goodfellow, M., Alderson, G., and Lacey, J. 1979. Numerical taxonomy of *Actinomadura* and related organisms. J. Gen. Microbiol. 112:95.

Gorby, G.L., and Peacock, J.E. Jr. 1988. *Erysipelothrix rhusiopathiae* endocarditis: microbiologic, epidemiologic, and clinical features of an occupational disease. Rev. Infect. Dis. 10:317.

Haley, L.D., and Calloway, C.S. 1978. Isolation and identification of some aerobic actinomycetes. In Laboratory methods in medical mycology, ed. U.S. Department of Health, Education, and Welfare Publication CDC 78-8361. Washington, D.C.

Kerry-Williams, S.M., and Noble, W.C. 1987. Group JK coryneform bacteria. J. Hosp. Infect. 9:4.

Lipsky, B.A., Goldberger, A.C., Tompkins, L.S., and Plorde, J.J. 1982. Infections caused by nondiphtheria corynebacteria. Rev. Infect. Dis. 4:1220.

McGowan, J.E. 1988. JK coryneforms: a continuing problem for hospital infection control. J. Hosp. Infect. 11(Suppl. A):358.

Middlebrook, J.L., and Dorland, R.B. 1984. Bacterial toxins: cellular mechanisms of action. Microbiol. Rev. 48:199.

Philip, A., and Roberts, G.D. 1984. *Nocardiopsis dassonvillei* cellulitis of the arm. Clin. Microbiol. Newsletter 6:14.

Prauser, H., editor. 1970. The actinomycetales. VEB Gastov Fischer Verlag, Jena.

Schwartz, B., Hexter, D., Broome, C.V., et al. 1989. Investigation of an outbreak of listeriosis: new hypotheses for the etiology of epidemic *Listeria monocytogenes* infections. J. Infect. Dis. 159:680.

Slack, J.M., and Gerencser, M. 1975. Actinomyces, filamentous bacteria: biology and pathogenicity. Burgess Publishing Co., Minneapolis.

Smego, R.A., Jr., and Gallis, H.A. 1984. The clinical spectrum of *Nocardia brasiliensis* infection in the United States. Rev. Infect. Dis. 6:164.

Soriano, F., and Fernandez-Roblas, R. 1988. Infections caused by antibiotic-resistant *Corynebacterium* group D2. Eur. J. Clin. Microbiol. Infect. Dis. 7:337.

Tisdall, P.A., and Roberts, G.D. 1979. Aerobic actinomycetes and the clinical laboratory. Clin. Microbiol. Newsletter 1:1.

Van Etta, L.L., Filice, G.A., Ferguson, R.M., and Gerding, D.N. 1983. *Corynebacterium equi*: a review of 12 cases of human infection. Rev. Infect. Dis. 5:1012.

34

Processing Clinical Specimens for Anaerobic Bacteria: Isolation and Identification Procedures

Martha A.C. Edelstein

34.1. Initial Processing Procedure

Properly collected and transported specimens for anaerobic culture may be processed on the bench, in an anaerobic chamber, or with the roll tube system (Chapters 6 and 8). Initial processing includes a direct examination and inoculation of the specimen onto appropriate media as represented in Figure 34.1.

34.1.a. Direct examination. Direct examination involves a macro- and microscopic examination of the clinical material and may include end product analysis by gas-liquid chromatography (GLC), dark-field examination, or fluorescent antibody screening techniques. Direct examination provides immediate semiquantitative information about the types of organisms present. This could be important for initial therapy, since culture results may not be available for several days.

The specimen is inspected for characteristics that strongly indicate the presence of anaerobes such as (1) foul odor; (2) brick-red fluorescence upon exposure to long-wave ultraviolet (UV) light (wavelength, 366 nm), suggesting dark pigmented *Bacteroides* or *Porphyromonas* sp.; and (3) sulfur granules (see Figures 35-13 and 35-14) associated with *Actinomyces* sp., *Propionibacterium propionicum* (formerly *Arachnia*), or *Eubacterium nodatum*. The presence of blood, purulence, or other distinguishing characteristics of the specimen are also noted.

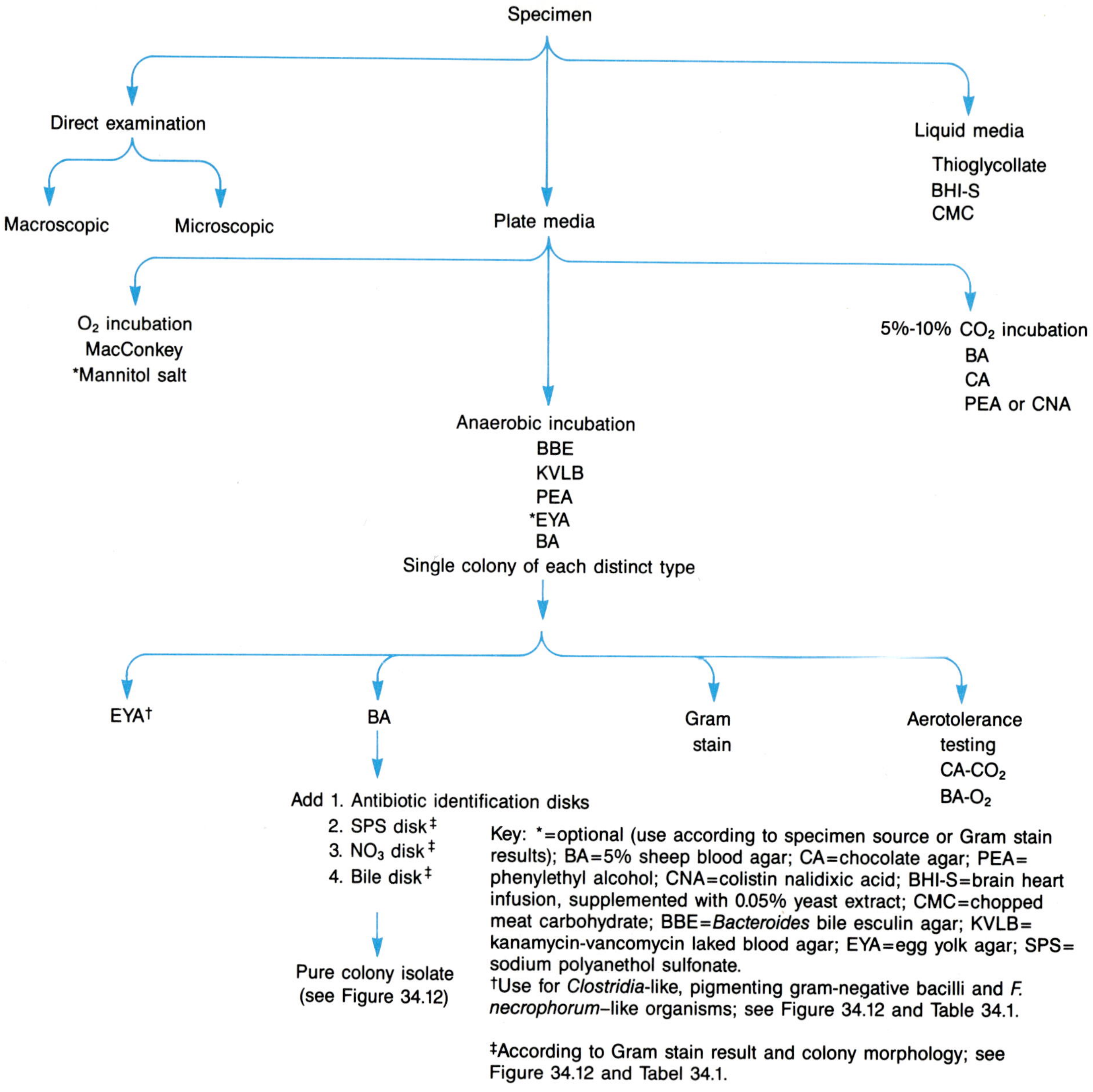

Specimen

Direct examination

Macroscopic   Microscopic

Plate media

Liquid media
Thioglycollate
BHI-S
CMC

O_2 incubation
MacConkey
*Mannitol salt

5%-10% CO_2 incubation
BA
CA
PEA or CNA

Anaerobic incubation
BBE
KVLB
PEA
***EYA**
BA
Single colony of each distinct type

EYA†   BA   Gram
stain   Aerotolerance
testing
CA-CO_2
BA-O_2

Add 1. Antibiotic identification disks
2. SPS disk‡
3. NO_3 disk‡
4. Bile disk‡

Key: *=optional (use according to specimen source or Gram stain
results); BA=5% sheep blood agar; CA=chocolate agar; PEA=
phenylethyl alcohol; CNA=colistin nalidixic acid; BHI-S=brain heart
infusion, supplemented with 0.05% yeast extract; CMC=chopped
meat carbohydrate; BBE=*Bacteroides* bile esculin agar; KVLB=
kanamycin-vancomycin laked blood agar; EYA=egg yolk agar; SPS=
sodium polyanethol sulfonate.
†Use for *Clostridia*-like, pigmenting gram-negative bacilli and *F.
necrophorum*–like organisms; see Figure 34.12 and Table 34.1.

Pure colony isolate
(see Figure 34.12)

‡According to Gram stain result and colony morphology; see
Figure 34.12 and Tabel 34.1.

Figure 34.1
Initial specimen processing scheme with suggested choices from which to select media. (From Sutter,
V.L., Citron, D.M., Edelstein, M.A.C., and Finegold, S.M. 1985. Wadsworth anaerobic bacteriology
manual, ed. 4 Star Publishing Co., Belmont, Calif.)

The microscopic examination always includes a
Gram stain (Chapter 7). The Gram stain reveals the
types and relative numbers of microorganisms and
host cells present and serves as a quality control
measure for the adequacy of anaerobic techniques.
Results of the Gram stain may also indicate the need

for additional media such as egg yolk agar for clostridia. Some anaerobes have characteristic cell morphology on Gram stain (for example, boxcar-shaped
cells of *Clostridium perfringens* (Figure 34.2) or
thin, pointed-ends cells of *Fusobacterium nucleatum*
(Figure 34.3), which is important presumptive evi-

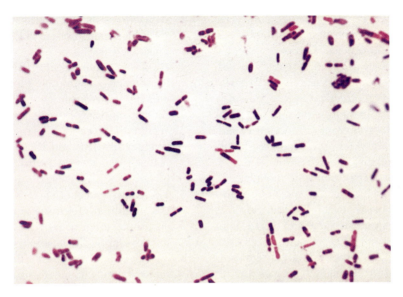

Figure 34.2
C. perfringens. Boxcar-shaped cells. (From Sutter, V.L., Citron, D.M., Edelstein, M.A.C., and Finegold, S.M. 1985. Wadsworth anaerobic bacteriology manual, ed. 4 Star Publishing Co., Belmont, Calif.)

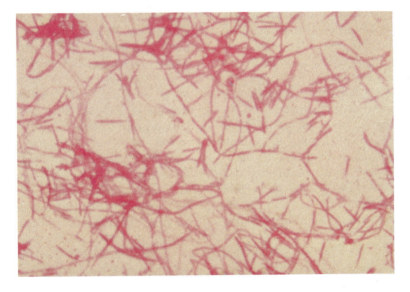

Figure 34.3
F. nucleatum. Thin bacillus with pointed ends.

dence for the presence of anaerobes. However, isolation and aerotolerance testing are required to confirm the presumptive results. It is also useful to correlate the source of the specimen with the gram-stain result to make an educated guess as to the presumptive identity of bacteria present. For example, a tangled mass of branching or clubbing gram-positive bacilli observed on a gram-stain smear from a jaw is good presumptive evidence for actinomycosis. A positive Gram stain with a negative culture may indicate (1) poor collection or transport methods, (2) poor processing procedures, (3) poor anaerobic atmosphere, (4) poor or inadequate types of media, or (5) nonviable cells due to antibiotic use or presence of other bactericidal factors.

Darkfield or phase-contrast microscopy may aid in detecting poorly staining organisms and spores and in observing motility directly, but it is generally not useful. A 2-hour direct fluorescent antibody stain (FA) for *Bacteroides fragilis* group (Fluoretec-F) and some pigmented *Bacteroides* sp. (Fluoretec-M) is available (Organon-Teknika). (See Section 34.6.)

34.1.b. Specimen preparation and inoculation. After direct visual examination, the specimen is inoculated onto appropriate anaerobic and aerobic plating media, into a liquid medium, and onto a slide for Gram stain. In preparation for culture, grossly purulent material is vortex-mixed in a gas-tight anaerobe transport vial or an anaerobic chamber, to ensure even distribution of the bacteria and their viability. Specimens transported in a syringe are injected into an anaerobic tube for vortexing. Pieces of tissue or bone fragments are homogenized with approximately 1 ml of liquid medium using a tissue grinder to make a thick mixture. Grinding should be done in an anaerobic chamber to minimize aeration. If a chamber is not available, process the specimen as rapidly as possible. Swab specimens are "wrung out" in about 0.5 ml of broth and treated as a liquid specimen. Using a Pasteur pipette, transfer the prepared specimen as follows:

- 1 drop per plate for purulent material
- 2 to 3 drops per plate for nonpurulent material
- 0.5 to 1 ml to middle or bottom of liquid medium
- 1 drop evenly spread onto a slide.

If the swab specimen is inoculated directly onto the media, inoculate the nonselective plates first (both aerobic and anaerobic plates) and then the selective and differential plates. The plates are then streaked for isolation.

The direct smear is fixed in methanol for 30 seconds, rather than heat-fixed, in order to preserve red and white cell morphology. Standard Gram stain procedures and reagents are used, except that the counterstain is dilute basic fuchsin (Appendix B), or Kopeloff's method can be followed (see Holdeman et al. 1977).

Enriched and selective media are required for optimum recovery of anaerobes, because anaerobes are fastidious and most anaerobic infections are mixed with aerobes and other anaerobes. The following media are used for the primary isolation of obligately anaerobic bacteria:

1. *Brucella* 5% sheep blood agar supplemented with vitamin K_1 and hemin (BA) for the isolation of most bacteria.
2. *Bacteroides* bile esculin (BBE) agar for the selection and presumptive identification of *B. fragilis* group organisms.
3. Kanamycin-vancomycin–laked blood (KVLB) agar for the selection of pigmented and other *Bacteroides* sp. BBE and KVLB are available as biplates from several prepared media manufacturers.
4. Phenylethyl alcohol sheep blood agar (PEA) for the inhibition of enteric and certain other nonanaerobic gram-negative bacilli that otherwise may overgrow the anaerobes.
5. Thioglycollate medium (BBL 135C), supplemented with vitamin K_1 (0.1 μg/ml) and hemin (5 μg/ml), and a marble chip or sodium bicarbonate (1 mg/ml, added prior to use). This medium must be boiled or steamed to drive off residual oxygen and is used on the day of steaming. After inoculation and tightening of the cap, the tube may be incubated aerobically.

Primary plates should be reduced in an anaerobic atmosphere for at least 24 hours before use, unless they have been freshly prepared *no more than 4 hours previously*. Prereduced anaerobically sterilized (PRAS) plate media are available (Anaerobe Systems). BA plates used for subculture usually do not need to be reduced. Freshness of media is an important consideration except for prepackaged PRAS media.

Blood agar media may also be prepared with Columbia, Schaedler, or brain-heart infusion base medium *supplemented with 0.5% yeast extract*. Unsupplemented trypticase soy and heart infusion or brain-heart infusion agar plates should not be used, because these do not adequately support the growth of all anaerobes. The following supplements are added to the basal medium:

- 5% sheep, horse, or rabbit blood for enrichment and for detecting hemolysis and pigment production (rabbit blood is best for the latter)
- Vitamin K_1 (final concentration, 10 μg/ml for solid media and 0.1 μg/ml for liquid media) for growth of some pigmented *Bacteroides* and *Porphyromonas*
- Hemin (final concentration 5 μg/ml) for growth enhancement of the *B. fragilis* group and other *Bacteroides* sp.

BBE agar is useful for the rapid isolation and

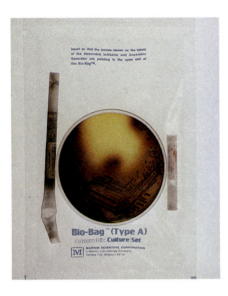

Figure 34.4
B. fragilis growing on *Bacteroides* bile esculin agar (positive esculin reaction) in Bio-Bag.

presumptive identification of the *B. fragilis* group (Figure 34.4). Rapid presumptive evidence of the *B. fragilis* group is important as it is the most commonly isolated pathogenic anaerobe and is often more resistant to some antibiotics than are other anaerobes. The medium contains 100 μg/ml of gentamicin, which inhibits most aerobic organisms; 20% bile, which inhibits most anaerobes except for the *B. fragilis* group and a few other species; and esculin, which differentiates esculin-positive and esculin-negative *B. fragilis* group (most are esculin-positive). Other non–*B. fragilis* group organisms that may rarely grow on this medium are *Fusobacterium mortiferum*, *Klebsiella pneumoniae*, enterococci, and yeast. However, unlike the *B. fragilis* group, their colony size is usually less than 1 mm in diameter, and their colony morphology is unlike the *B. fragilis* group.

KVLB agar is useful for the rapid isolation of *Bacteroides* sp. The medium contains 75 μg/ml kanamycin, which inhibits most aerobic, facultative, and anaerobic gram-negative rods except for *Bacteroides*, and 7.5 μg/ml vancomycin, which inhibits most gram-positive organisms. The laked blood allows earlier pigmentation by the pigmented anaerobic gram-negative bacteria. However, *Porphyromonas* sp. (formerly *Bacteroides asaccharolyticus* group) will not grow on this medium because of their

susceptibility to vancomycin. Yeast and other kanamycin-resistant organisms sometimes grow on this medium; therefore, one should prepare a Gram stain and check the aerotolerance of all isolates.

PEA agar inhibits nonanaerobic gram-negative rods. It prevents *Proteus* sp. from swarming and other enterics from overgrowing the anaerobes. Most gram-positive and gram-negative anaerobes will grow on the primary PEA plates, especially in mixed culture. Colony morphology on PEA is similar to that on the blood agar, but it may take an additional 48 hours' incubation to detect the more slowly growing and pigmenting anaerobes.

Thioglycollate broth serves only as a backup source of culture material, which may be needed in the event of a jar failure or growth inhibition on plates due to antibiotic or bacteriostatic factors in the specimen; these factors will be diluted in the broth. PRAS broths such as chopped meat carbohydrate, chopped meat and supplemented brain-heart may substitute for the thioglycollate described in no. 5 above. The PRAS tubes must be gassed with anaerobic gas after inoculating or incubated with the cap loosened in an anaerobic atmosphere.

If clostridia are suspected (because of the clinical picture, or if spores or large gram-positive rods are seen on the initial Gram stain), an egg yolk agar (EYA) plate is inoculated to check for the production of lecithinase and lipase. If boxcar-shaped cells resembling *C. perfringens* are seen on Gram stain (Figure 34.2), a direct Nagler test (Procedure 34.6) can also be set up along with the primary plates.

34.2. Incubation of Cultures

Inoculated plates are immediately placed into an anaerobic environment (jars, chamber, GasPak pouch [BBL], or a Bio-Bag type A [Becton, Dickinson]), as described in Chapter 8, and are incubated at 35° C for 48 hours. In general, cultures must not be exposed to oxygen until after 48 hours of incubation, since anaerobes are most sensitive to oxygen during their log phase of growth, and colony morphology often changes dramatically between 24 and 48 hours. Plates incubated in a chamber or anaerobic bag can be observed at 24 hours or earlier without oxygen exposure. At 24 hours, check for the presence of *B. fragilis* group on the BBE plate and *Clostridium*-like organisms on the BA or EYA plates. Isolates from the BBE and EYA plates may be further characterized when good growth is evident. Large colonies on the BA plate resembling *Clostridium* sp. can be

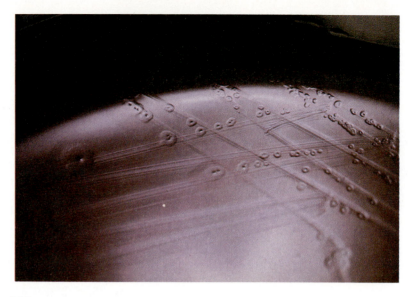

Figure 34.5
B. ureolyticus. Pitting colonies on blood agar. (From Sutter, V.L., Citron, D.M., Edelstein, M.A.C., and Finegold, S.M. 1985. Wadsworth anaerobic bacteriology manual, ed. 4. Star Publishing Co., Belmont, Calif.)

subcultured at 24 hours in a chamber. Plates showing no growth are incubated anaerobically for 7 days before discarding.

The thioglycollate broth culture associated with plates showing no growth is inspected daily for 7 days and, when turbid or on day 7, subcultured to a BA plate (anaerobic incubation) and a chocolate agar plate (CO_2 incubation). A 24-hour inspection for growth in the broth is important in the case of no growth on the primary aerobic plates. Growth in the broth, especially in the lower half of the tube, suggests the presence of anaerobes. A final report of a negative culture should be issued at 7 days, although the liquid medium is held for at least 1 more week before a final visual examination and discarding of the broth.

34.3. Examination of Primary Plates

Anaerobes are usually present in mixed culture with other anaerobes or with facultative bacteria; the combination of enrichment and selective agar plates yields information that will suggest the presence and perhaps the type of anaerobe(s). Primary anaerobic plates should be examined with a hand lens (× 8) or, preferably, a stereoscopic microscope. Colonies are described from the various media and semi-quantitated.

The *B. fragilis* group grows selectively on BBE; therefore only colonies greater than 1 mm in diameter should be described, enumerated, and subcultured. At 48 hours, *B. fragilis* group colonies are greater than 1 mm in diameter, circular, entire, and raised, with three distinct morphotypes:

1. Low convex, dark gray, friable, and surrounded by a dark gray zone (esculin hydrolysis) and a precipitate (bile)
2. Glistening, convex, light to dark gray, and surrounded by a gray zone
3. Similar to the second morphotype, but with no gray zone (esculin not hydrolyzed)

Growth on the KVLB plate suggests the presence of *Bacteroides* sp. Check carefully for pigment (this may take more than 48 hours to appear) and brick-red fluorescence, which is detected with a long-wave UV light (Wood's lamp), since these may indicate the presence of pigmented *Bacteroides* sp. or of *Porphyromonas*. All colony types, however, should be subcultured to purity plates and for an aerotolerance test.

All colony morphotypes from the nonselective BA plate are characterized, since facultative and obligately anaerobic bacteria sometimes have similar colony appearances. Nevertheless, the distinct colony morphology of certain anaerobes is highly suggestive

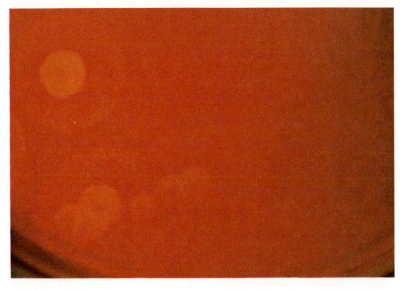

Figure 34.6
C. perfringens. Double zone of β-hemolysis on blood agar. (From Sutter, V.L., Citron, D.M., Edelstein, M.A.C., and Finegold S.M. 1985. Wadsworth anaerobic bacteriology manual, ed. 4 Star Publishing Co., Belmont, Calif.)

of their presence in a culture. Pitting colonies present on the anaerobic but not on the CO_2 plate are suggestive of the *Bacteroides ureolyticus*–like group, (Figure 34.5). Large colonies with a double zone of β-hemolysis (Figure 34.6), made up of large gram-positive bacilli, are presumptively *C. perfringens*. These colonies may be subcultured additionally to an egg yolk agar plate for the Nagler test. Slender fusiform gram-negative bacilli (see Figure 34.3) from breadcrumb-like or speckled colonies showing greening of the agar around the colonies suggest *F. nucleatum*. Dark, pigmented (Figure 34.7) or brick-red fluorescent colonies (Figure 34.8) that are gram-negative coccobacilli are pigmented *Bacteroides* sp. or *Porphyromonas*. A molar tooth colony (Figure 34.9) of gram-positive branching rods (Figure 34.10) may be *Actinomyces israelii*.

Colonies on the PEA plate are processed further only if they are different from ones growing on the BA plate or if colonies on the BA plate are impossible to subculture because of overgrowth by clostridia, swarming *Proteus*, or other organisms.

34.4. Subculture of Isolates

A single colony of each distinct type described is examined microscopically using a Gram stain and is subcultured to the following (Figure 34.1):

• BA plate to be incubated anaerobically for isolation of the organism and subsequent testing (purity plate)
• Chocolate agar plate to be incubated in CO_2 for aerotolerance testing
• EYA plate for suspected lipase and lecithinase producers (*Clostridium* sp., *Fusobacterium necrophorum, Bacteroides intermedius*)—optional
• Rabbit blood (preferably laked) agar for gram-negative bacilli to better detect pigment production

Use a sterile wooden applicator stick to subculture colonies; enough cells can usually be picked up to inoculate numerous plates, a broth, and a slide for Gram stain.

Inoculum from the same colony subcultured to the purity plate is used for aerotolerance testing and the Gram stain. If the original colony is not large enough to determine atmospheric requirements directly, use growth from the purity plate for aerotolerance testing. Four to six isolates can be inoculated onto a single chocolate agar plate. An additional BA plate incubated in air will further define the atmospheric requirements of facultative organisms (for example, microaerophilic streptococci). The Centers for Disease Control (CDC) Anaerobe Laboratory recommends using five different atmospheres, al-

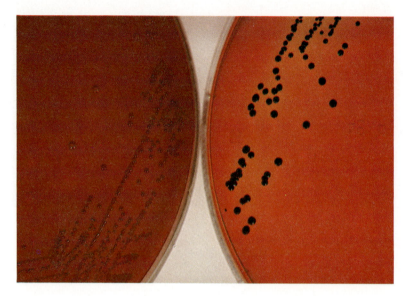

Figure 34.7
B. intermedius. Black pigmentation on sheep blood agar (*left*) vs rabbit blood agar (*right*). (From Sutter, V.L.,Citron, D.M., Edelstein, M.A.C., and Finegold, S.M. 1985. Wadsworth anaerobic bacteriology manual, ed. 4. Star Publishing Co., Belmont, Calif.)

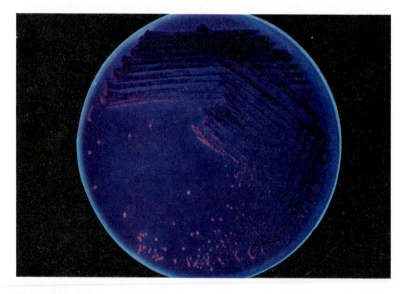

Figure 34.8
Pigmented *Bacteroides* sp. Red fluorescence under ultraviolet light (366 nm).

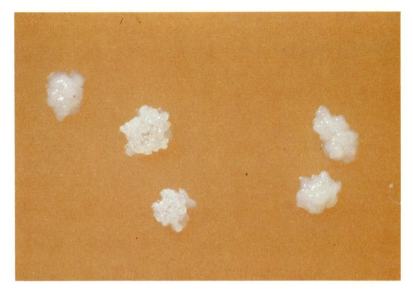

Figure 34.9
Actinomyces israelii. "Molar tooth" colonies.

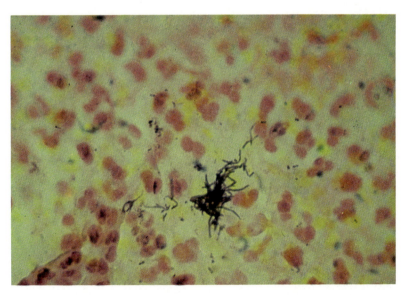

Figure 34.10
A. israelii. Sulfur granule demonstrating gram-positive branching bacilli on microscopic examination.

though this is usually not necessary for routine identification. An assay for pyruvate oxidase or resistance to a 5-μg metronidazole disk may also aid in determining atmospheric requirements of the organism. These may be helpful for those aerobic bacteria that may require an anaerobic, or reduced oxygen, environment for initial or good growth.

The following antibiotic identification disks are placed on the first quadrant of the purity BA plate (Procedure 34.1): kanamycin, 1 mg (BBL or Anaerobe Systems): colistin, 10 μg; and vancomycin, 5 μg (Figure 34.11) These disks aid in preliminary grouping of anaerobes and serve as a Gram stain check but *do not* imply susceptibility of an organism for antibiotic therapy.

PROCEDURE 34.1

Antibiotic Identification Disks

Principle

Most anaerobes have a characteristic susceptibility pattern to colistin (10 μg), vancomycin (5 μg), and kanamycin (1 mg) disks. The pattern generated will usually confirm a dubious Gram-stain reaction (with few exceptions, most gram-negative anaerobes are resistant to vancomycin) and aid in subdividing the anaerobic gram-negative bacilli into groups (see Table 34.2 and Section 34.5.c).

Method

1. Reagents
   a. Vancomycin 5-μg disk (Va)
   b. Kanamycin 1-mg disk (K)
   c. Colistin 10-μg disk (Co)
   d. Brucella blood agar plate (BA)
2. Procedure
   a. Allow the three disks to equilibrate to room temperature. A small supply of disks is stored desiccated at 2° to 8° C, and a larger supply at −20° C.
   b. Transfer a portion of one colony to a BA plate. Streak the first quadrant several times to produce a heavy lawn of growth and then streak the other quadrants for isolation.
   c. Place the Co, K, and Va disks in the first quadrant, well separated from each other (Figure 34.11).
   d. Incubate the plates anaerobically for 48 h at 35° C.
3. Reading and interpretation: Observe for a zone of inhibition of growth. A zone of 10 mm or less indicates resistance, and a zone greater than 10 mm indicates susceptibility. *Do not* use the zone-size interpretation as an indicator of the susceptibility of the organism for clinical treatment purpose.

Quality control

Test *F. necrophorum*, *B. fragilis*, and *C. perfringens* as described under Method. Two isolates can be inoculated per plate.

Expected results

The disks meet performance standards when the following patterns are obtained:
1. *F. necrophorum* is susceptible to K and Co and resistant to Va.
2. *B. fragilis* is resistant to all three antibiotics.
3. *C. perfringens* is sensitive to Va and K and resistant to Co.

Performance schedule

Test each new lot of disks and weekly thereafter.

Three other disks can be added to the BA at this time. A sodium polyanethol-sulfonate (SPS) disk can be placed near the colistin disk for rapid presumptive identification of *Peptostreptococcus anaerobius*. A nitrate disk may be placed on the second quadrant for subsequent determination of nitrate reduction. A bile disk is added to the second quadrant to detect bile inhibition.

If processing is performed on the open bench, all plates should promptly be incubated anaerobically, since some clinical isolates (for example, *F. necrophorum* and pigmented *Bacteroides* sp.) may die after relatively short exposure to oxygen. The primary plates are reincubated along with the purity plates for an additional 48 hours and are again inspected for new morphotypes of slow growers and pigmenters.

34.5. Identification of Isolates

Pure culture isolates are processed for identification as shown in Figure 34.12. As in mycobacteriology, the extent of identification and susceptibility testing of anaerobes will vary according to the laboratories' interests and resources. Three laboratory levels can be defined. All laboratories should be able to identify colonies presumptively from primary plates as belonging to major groups of anaerobes and to isolate and maintain an anaerobe in pure culture so that it

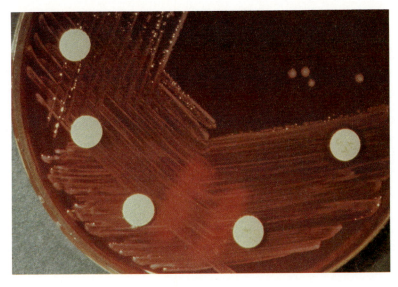

Figure 34.11
B. fragilis. Special potency antibiotic disks, bile resistance, and spot indole test.

can be sent to a reference laboratory if needed (level I). Most laboratories should be able to use simple tests for further grouping of the anaerobes and to identify certain ones to species level (level II). Reference laboratories or laboratories with a special interest in anaerobes should be able to identify most isolates definitively using a variety of techniques (level III). These methods may include prereduced anaerobically sterilized (PRAS) biochemicals, miniaturized biochemical systems (for example, API and Minitek; also described in Chapter 9), rapid-enzyme detection panels (for example, RapID-ANA, AnIDENT) or individual tests (Rosco ID Disks, H.B. Company), gas-liquid chromatography (GLC) (Chapter 11), toxin assays, and so on.

34.5.a. Level I identification. As described in Section 34.3, information from the primary plates in conjunction with the atmospheric requirements, Gram stain, and colony morphology of a pure isolate provides presumptive identification of many anaerobic organisms. Table 34.1 summarizes the extent to which isolates can be identified using this information. It is also useful to correlate specimen source and expected organisms from that site to aid in presumptive identification.

34.5.b. Level II identification tests. Preliminary grouping of anaerobes and identification of some are based on colony and cell morphology, Gram reac-

tion, susceptibility to antibiotic identification disks, nitrate reduction (disk test), indole and catalase production, plus several other simple tests. The following characteristics are noted and tests are performed from the purity BA plate on all isolates as depicted schematically in Figure 34.12:

Colony morphology. Colony features of the isolate are described from a 48-hour pure BA culture and include the shape, edge, elevation, opacity, color, and any other distinguishing characteristics (for example, irregular, smooth, convex, opaque, white, speckling).

Hemolysis. Transmitted light is used to look for hemolysis, especially a double zone of hemolysis (clear zone of hemolysis extending just beyond the colony edge and a zone of partial hemolysis extending well beyond the colony edge) (see Figure 34.6), and greening of the agar, which is more apparent after exposure to air.

Pigment. Few anaerobes produce pigment, but colors common among those that do vary from light tan to black (for example, pigmented *Bacteroides* sp. or *Porphyromonas*) or pink to red (for example, *Actinomyces odontolyticus*). Whole or hemolyzed laked rabbit blood is best for detecting pigment, and it is helpful to pick up several colonies on a white cotton swab to increase the contrast.

Fluorescence. Long-wave UV light (366 nm) is used

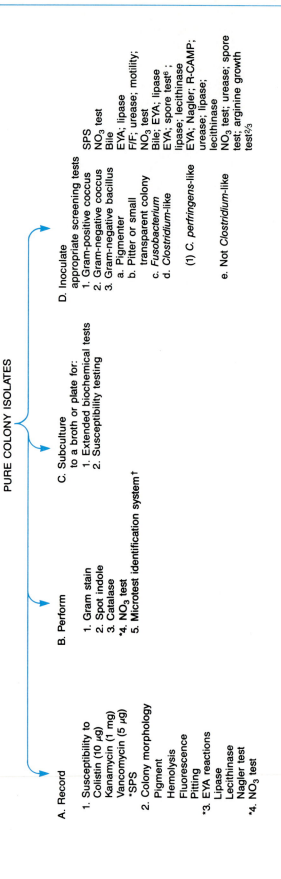

PURE COLONY ISOLATES

A. Record
1. Susceptibility to
   Colistin (10 µg)
   Kanamycin (1 mg)
   Vancomycin (5 µg)
   *SPS
2. Colony morphology
   Pigment
   Hemolysis
   Fluorescence
   Pitting
*3. EYA reactions
   Lipase
   Lecithinase
   Nagler test
*4. NO_3 test

B. Perform
1. Gram stain
2. Spot indole
3. Catalase
*4. NO_3 test
5. Microtest identification system†

C. Subculture
   to a broth or plate for:
1. Extended biochemical tests
2. Susceptibility testing

D. Inoculate
   appropriate screening tests
1. Gram-positive coccus — SPS
2. Gram-negative coccus — NO_3 test
3. Gram-negative bacillus — Bile
   a. Pigmenter — EYA; lipase
   b. Pitter or small transparent colony — F/F; urease; motility; NO_3 test
   c. *Fusobacterium* — Bile; EYA; lipase
   d. *Clostridium*-like — EYA; spore test[6]; lipase; lecithinase
      (1) *C. perfringens*-like — EYA; Nagler; R-CAMP; urease; lipase; lecithinase
   e. Not *Clostridium*-like — NO_3 test; urease; spore test; arginine growth test[2/3]

Key: *=if available at this time; SPS=sodium polyanethol
sulfonate;EYA=egg yolk agar; F/F=formate-fumarate growth test;
R-CAMP=reverse CAMP test
† Use test systems selectively and with appropriate
organisms. See Section 34.5.g for guidance.
‡ Perform when spores are not detected on Gram stain.
§ Perform on tiny gram-positive rod.

Figure 34.12
Pure culture isolate processing scheme. (From Sutter, V.L., Citron, D.M., Edelstein, M.A.C., and Finegold, S.M. 1985. Wadsworth anaerobic bacteriology manual, ed. 4 Star Publishing Co., Belmont, Calif.)

Table 34.1

Level I Identification

ORGANISM	GRAM REACTION	CELL SHAPE	COMMENTS	AERO-TOLER-ANCE	DISTINGUISHING CHARACTERISTICS	USUAL SOURCE; COMMENTS
B. fragilis group	−	B	Can be pleomorphic with safety pin feature	−	Grows on BBE; >1 mm in diameter; ± esculin	Infections below the waist; blood; β-lactamase + (usually)
Pigmenter	−	B, CB	Can be very coccoid or *Haemophilus*-like	−	Foul odor; black or brown pigment; some fluoresce brick-red	Head-neck; dental; bite wounds; TTA; many β-lactamase +
B. ureolyticus–like	−	B	Thin; some are curved	−	May pit agar or spread; transparent colony	Head-neck; dental
F. nucleatum	−	B	Slender cell with pointed ends	−	Foul odor; 3 colony types: breadcrumb, speckling, or smooth	Infections above the waist: brain abscess, head-neck, dental, bites, lung
Gram-negative bacillus	−	B		−		Any type infection
Gram-negative coccus	−	C	*Veillonella* cells are tiny	−		Head-neck; dental; bite wounds; TTA; pleural fluids
Gram-positive coccus	+	C, CB	Variable size	−		Any type infection
C. perfringens (presumptive)	+	B	Large boxcar shape; no spores observed; may appear gram-negative	−	Double zone β-hemolysis	Intra-abdominal; blood; gangrene
Clostridium sp.	+	B	Spores observed; may appear gram-negative	−		Infections below the waist
Gram-positive bacillus	+	B, CB	No spores observed; no boxcar cells	− +		
Actinomyces-like	+	B	Branching cells	− +	Sulfur granules on direct examination; molar-tooth colony	Head-neck; brain; lung

− = negative; + = positive; − + = some strains positive; B = bacillus; C = coccus; CB = coccobacillus; BBE = *Bacteroides* bile esculin agar; TTA = transtracheal aspirate.
Data from Sutter, V.L., Citron, D.M., Edelstein, M.A.C., and Finegold, S.M. 1985. Wadsworth anaerobic bacteriology manual, ed. 4. Star Publishing Co., Belmont, Calif., and Edelstein, M.A.C. Laboratory diagnosis of anaerobic infections in humans. In Finegold, S.M., and George, W.L., editors. 1989. Anaerobic infections in humans, Academic Press, Orlando, Fla.

to detect fluorescing colonies. A variety of colors may be seen, including brick red, pink, orange, and chartreuse (see Figure 34.8). Certain pigmented *Bacteroides* sp. and *Porphyromonas* fluoresce yellow-green, brick red, or not at all. Fluorescence often disappears or is masked as pigmentation of the pigmented *Bacteroides* sp. and *Porphyromonas* deepens. A few other *Bacteroides* sp. fluoresce yellow-green or coral. Many of the fusobacteria fluoresce yellow-green. *Veillonella* fluoresces red, but this property is medium-dependent and dissipates rapidly upon exposure to air. Certain clostridia strains fluoresce yellow-green, red, coral, and orange.

Pitting. The top of the colony usually appears just above the level of a craterlike depression in the agar; this depression has been created by an agarase en-

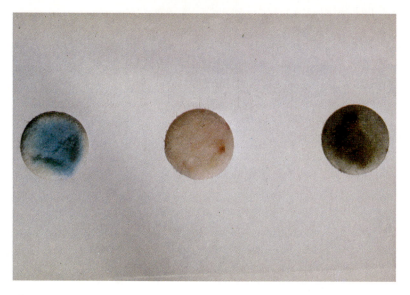

Figure 34.13

Spot indole test using *p*-dimethylaminocinnamaldehyde. Blue = positive; colorless or other than blue = negative. (From Sutter, V.L., Citron, D.M., Edelstein, M.A.C., and Finegold, S.M. 1985. Wadsworth anaerobic bacteriology manual, ed. 4. Star Publishing Co., Belmont, Calif.)

zyme produced by the organism. Hold the BA plate at an angle to the light source to observe this phenomenon better. This characteristic may be easier to detect after 4 days of incubation (see Figure 34.5).

Catalase. See Section 9.2.a. and Procedure 9.1. Use 15% hydrogen peroxide in place of 3% hydrogen peroxide. Most anaerobes are catalase-negative; some of the exceptions include several species in the *B. fragilis* group, a few anaerobic cocci, several *Propionibacterium* sp., and *Actinomyces viscosus*.

Spot indole. See Section 9.2.d. and Procedure 9.4. (Figure 34.13). The reagent is *p*-dimethylaminocinnamaldehyde.

Antibiotic identification disks (Procedure 34.1) (Table 34.2). Anaerobes vary in their susceptibility to colistin (10 μg), vancomycin (5 μg), and kanamycin (1 mg), and the reaction patterns aid in interpreting the Gram reaction, in separating *Bacteroides* sp. and *Fusobacterium* sp., and in subdividing the *Bacteroides* (see Tables 34.2 to 34.4). Generally, grampositive organisms are resistant to colistin and sensitive to vancomycin, whereas the gram-negative organisms are resistant to vancomycin. An accurate interpretation of the Gram stain reaction is important because the result is often used for selection of subsequent tests. Young cultures of pigmenting *Bacteroides* and clostridia may appear gram-variable and

Table 34.2

Grouping of Anaerobes Using the Antibiotic Identification Disks Pattern

GROUP	VANCOMYCIN (5 μg)	KANAMYCIN (1 mg)	COLISTIN (10 μg)
Gram-positive	S	V	R
Gram-negative	R	R[s]	S*
B. fragilis group	R	R	R
Other *Bacteroides*	R	R	V
Pigmented *Porphyromonas* sp.†	S	R	R
Fusobacterium	R	S	S
B. ureolyticus group	R	S	S

S = sensitive; R = resistant; R[s] = some stains sensitive; V = variable.

*Unusual gram-negative anaerobes may be resistant (see *Porphyromonas*).

†*Porphyromonas* is one of the exceptions; it is a gram-negative bacillus with a gram-positive disk pattern.

some clostridia consistently stain gram-negative; the *Clostridium* would be sensitive to vancomycin and the pigmenter would be resistant. A few exceptions do occur, such as the pigmenting *Porphyromonas* sp. (formerly *B. asaccharolyticus* group), which are

PROCEDURE 34.2

Twenty-Percent-Bile Tube Test

Principle

Anaerobic bacteria vary in their ability to grow in the presence of 20% bile (equivalent to 2% oxgall). Bile tolerance is most helpful in separating the *B. fragilis* group from other *Bacteroides* sp. and in separating *Fusobacterium mortiferum-varium* from most other clinically significant fusobacteria.

Method

1. Reagents
   a. Oxgall (Difco Laboratories): Prepare a solution of 40% oxgall (Difco Laboratories). Sterilize by autoclaving and store at 2° to 8° C.
   b. Thioglycollate broth (thio)
2. Procedure
   a. Add 0.5 ml of 40% oxgall to a 10-ml tube of freshly steamed or boiled thio or to any broth supporting good growth of the organism. This yields a concentration of 2% oxgall, equivalent to 20% bile. Add the bile to a warm tube, since this facilitates mixing of the bile and thio.
   b. Inoculate both the thio-bile tube and an unsupplemented thio control tube with 1 to 2 colonies from a pure BA plate or broth culture of the organism. Do not vigorously mix the thio tubes, since this will introduce too much air into the system.
   c. Incubate the thio tubes aerobically 24 to 48 h with the caps tightened. If the tubes have been aerated or another broth is used, loosen the caps and incubate anaerobically.
3. Reading and interpretation: Compare the growth in the bile-supplemented tube to the growth in the plain tube. Record as "bile inhibited" when there is no growth or significantly less growth in the bile tube. Record as "bile tolerant" when there is good growth in both tubes.

Quality control

Test *B. fragilis* (bile tolerant) and any bile-sensitive organism (e.g., *B. oralis* or *B. melaninogenicus*) by inoculating each into bile-supplemented and unsupplemented thio broth tubes as described in the Method.

Expected results

B. fragilis is bile tolerant and will therefore grow to the same turbidity in broth containing 20% bile as in non-bile-containing broth. *B. oralis* is inhibited by bile, so it grows poorly if at all in the presence of bile.

Performance schedule

Test each new lot of oxgall and each batch of the 40% oxgall solution.

---

resistant to colistin and sensitive to vancomycin. *Fusobacterium* sp. are susceptible to both kanamycin and colistin, and the *Bacteroides* are usually resistant to kanamycin but variable in susceptibility to colistin. The *B. ureolyticus* group is an exception, as its pattern is the same as that of *Fusobacterium*. Some of the unusual or less frequently isolated anaerobic gram-negative bacilli may not conform to these generalizations. In that case, a motility test, a flagellar stain, and GLC may be required to place the organism in the correct genus.

As with any disk diffusion test, many variables affect zone sizes. It is important to inoculate and streak the plate so that a heavy lawn is produced.

The organism may appear susceptible if the inoculum is too light. The disks must be placed well apart, as a large zone around one disk may interfere with interpretation of an adjacent disk. The elapsed time between inoculation, streaking, disk application, and incubation should be kept to a minimum. It may be necessary to inoculate the plates in batched groups of 5 to 10 plates.

With the addition of some of the following tests, further grouping or definitive identification of several selected anaerobes may be possible.

Bile test (Procedure 34.2) (Figure 34.11). The ability to grow in 20% bile is a key for separating the bile-resistant *B. fragilis* group from other *Bacter-*

PROCEDURE 34.3

Formate-fumarate (F/F) Growth Stimulation Test

Principle

In broth culture, *Bacteroides ureolyticus*, *B. gracilis*, and *Wolinella* sp. derive energy (ATP) during the transfer of electrons from formate to fumarate via a formate dehydrogenase-sulfur molybdenum protein complex and fumarate reductase. Other anaerobes do not require this metabolic pathway for energy production.

Method

1. Reagents
   a. Prepare a solution of formate-fumarate:

Sodium formate (Fisher Scientific Co.)	3 g
Fumaric acid (Fisher Scientific Co.)	3 g
Distilled water	50 ml
Sodium hydroxide	18 pellets

   (1) Combine ingredients, stirring until pellets are dissolved and fumaric acid is in solution.
   (2) Adjust pH to 7.0 with 4 N sodium hydroxide.
   (3) Sterilize by filtration through a 0.2-μm membrane filter. Store at 2° to 8° C.
   b. Thioglycollate broth (thio)
2. Procedure
   a. Add 0.5 ml F/F to a 10-ml freshly steamed or boiled thio tube.
   b. Inoculate both an F/F-supplemented thio and an unsupplemented thio with several colonies from a 48- to 72-h BA plate culture.
   c. Incubate aerobically with the caps tightened for 24 to 72 h at 35° C.
3. Reading and interpretation: Compare the growth in the F/F-supplemented tube to that in the plain tubes. Record as "F/F stimulated" when there is growth in the supplemented tube and poor to no growth in the plain tube.

Quality control

Test *B. ureolyticus* (requires F/F for growth in thio broth) and *B. fragilis* (doesn't require F/F for growth in thio broth) by inoculating both into F/F supplemented and unsupplemented thio as described under Method.

Expected results

Performance standards are met when *B. ureolyticus* grows only in the F/F-supplemented broth and *B. fragilis* grows in both the F/F-supplemented and unsupplemented broth.

Performance schedule

Test each new lot of reagents and each new batch of working solutions.

---

oides sp. and for differentiating *F. mortiferum-varium* from most of the other fusobacteria. The test can be performed using bile-containing agar, a bile tube test, or bile-impregnated disks (Remel, Oxoid, or Anaerobe Systems). The disk test is performed as with the antibiotic identification disks test, and appearance of any zone denotes susceptibility, whereas growth up to the disk shows resistance.

Nitrate disk test. The principle, reagents, and reactions are the same as those discussed in Section 9.3.e, Chapter 9. Test tiny indole-negative gram-positive rods (*Eubacterium lentum*–like), curved or straight gram-negative bacilli that form small transparent colonies or pit the agar (*B. ureolyticus*–like), and gram-negative cocci.

Formate and fumarate (F/F) growth stimulation test (Procedure 34.3). The *B. ureolyticus*–like organisms grow poorly if at all in broth medium that is not supplemented with formate and fumarate. These organisms require formate or hydrogen as an electron donor and fumarate or nitrate as an electron acceptor in their metabolic processes. A simple test method is to supplement a thioglycollate broth or comparable medium with formate and fumarate and compare growth in that tube with growth in an unsupplemented broth culture. Test all gram-negative rods

PROCEDURE 34.4

Ethanol Spore Test

Principle

Alcohols, such as ethanol, kill vegetative cells in a hydrated environment by coagulating proteins. Spores are not readily hydrated and are usually resistant to ethanol. This test will separate spore-formers (*Clostridium* and *Bacillus* sp.) from non-spore-formers.

Method

1. Reagents
   a. 95% ethanol
   b. Chopped meat carbohydrate (CMC) (Carr Scarborough) or thioglycollate (thio) broth
   c. Brucella blood agar plate (BA)
2. Procedure
   a. Inoculate 1 to 2 colonies of the isolate into a CMC or thio tube. Incubate 48 h at 37° C and then incubate an additional 1 to 2 days at room temperature.
   b. Add 1 ml of the broth culture to 1 ml of 95% ethanol.
   c. Gently mix and allow to stand for 30 to 45 min.
   d. Dip a swab into the alcohol mixture and spread onto a BA plate.
   e. Dip a second swab into the original broth culture; spread this onto a BA; and streak for isolation. This plate serves as a control for purity and viability of the organism.
   f. Incubate both plates in an anaerobic environment at 35° C for 48 h.
3. Reading and interpretation: Observe for growth. If growth occurs only on the control plate, then the organism is considered a non-spore-former. If growth occurs on both plates, then the organism is considered a spore-former. If there is no growth on the control plate, then the test is inconclusive. Be certain that the colony morphology on all the plates is the same as the original colony (that is, the growth is not due to a contaminant). Also, *C. perfringens*, *C. clostridioforme*, and a few other *Clostridium* sp. may not survive exposure to ethanol, so their identification is based on other characteristics (see Chapter 35).

Quality control

The control plate serves as an internal quality control. The media used must have already met quality control performance standards.

---

that form small transparent colonies or pit the agar.

Urease test. This test is useful for differentiating between the two indole-positive, Nagler-positive clostridia (*C. sordellii* and *C. bifermentans*), among the *B. ureolyticus*–like group, and among the *Actinomyces* sp. A broth and disk (Difco) test is available. See Section 9.2.g. for the principle and reagents. This test is incubated aerobically at 37° C. A positive, bright pink to red color often occurs within 5 to 30 minutes of incubation if a heavy inoculum is prepared.

Motility. Motility is occasionally helpful for identification of anaerobes isolated from human infections, primarily for the gram-negative bacilli. Almost all the clinically isolated gram-negative bacilli belong to the genera *Bacteroides*, *Porphyromonas*, or *Fusobacterium*, all of which are nonmotile; however,

do test the *B. ureolyticus*–like group, because it includes *Wolinella* and *Campylobacter* species, which are motile. Test any other gram-negative bacillus that does not key out otherwise according to Table 36.3. Motility is optimally performed on young broth or plate cultures.

SPS susceptibility test. *P. anaerobius* is susceptible to a 1-mg SPS disk, whereas the other anaerobic gram-positive cocci are resistant. Follow the procedure used for the antibiotic identification disks. A zone size greater than or equal to 12 mm is considered susceptible. Test all anaerobic gram-positive cocci that resemble *P. anaerobius* (large colony, sweetish foul odor, large cocci in chains).

Ethanol spore test (Procedure 34.4). Spores are resistant to the effect of alcohol, whereas vegetative cells are killed. Test gram-positive bacilli to separate

PROCEDURE 34.5

Lecithinase Test

Principle

Bacterial lecithinase splits lecithin (a normal component of egg yolk) to insoluble diglycerides, resulting in an opaque halo surrounding a colony growing on egg-yolk-containing medium.

Method

1. Reagents: Commercially prepared egg yolk agar (EYA) plates are available from many sources. If preparing the medium in house, egg yolk emulsion is available from Difco Laboratories, Hana Biologics, and Oxoid USA. Store the plates at 2° to 8° C. Reducing the plates prior to use is not usually necessary.
2. Procedure
   a. Transfer one colony of a 24- to 72-h plate culture or 2 to 3 drops of a broth culture of the test organism to an EYA plate.
   b. Incubate anaerobically at 35° C for at least 24 h. If negative, reincubate the plate for an additional 24 to 48 h.
3. Reading and interpretation: Examine for a white opacity in the medium that surrounds the colony and extends beyond the edge of

growth; this is a positive lecithinase test. Some organisms require extended incubation to demonstrate a positive test; however, this is not practical in a clinical laboratory, so 72 h is chosen as an arbitrary maximum incubation time.

Quality control

Test *C. perfringens* (lecithinase positive) and *C. difficile* (lecithinase negative) by streaking each onto one half of an EYA plate as described under Method.

Expected results

Performance standards are met when both organisms grow on the medium. *C. perfringens* produces a white opaque zone in the medium extending beyond the colony edge (lecithinase positive), and *C. difficile* produces no opaque zone in the medium (lecithinase negative).

Performance schedule

Test each new lot of egg yolk agar plates.

Clostridium sp. from other gram-positive bacilli if spores are not seen on a gram-stain smear.

Lecithinase test (Procedure 34.5). The compound lecithin, a normal component of egg yolk, is split by the enzyme lecithinase to release insoluble diglycerides. This results in an opaque halo in egg-yolk-containing medium that extends beyond the edge of colony growth (Figure 34.14). It is important to test all clostridia and clostridia-like organisms.

Lipase reaction. Free fats present in egg yolk are broken down by the enzyme lipase to produce glycerol and fatty acids. The fatty acids appear either as a surface "oil-on-water" layer that covers the colony and may extend beyond the colony edge or as a zone of opacity directly beneath the colony (Figure 34.15). All clostridia, pigmented *Bacteroides* sp., and fusobacteria are tested for lipase production.

When testing anaerobic gram-negative bacilli, use an egg yolk agar plate that does not contain antibiotics and is supplemented with vitamin K_1 and hemin. Inoculate and incubate the egg yolk agar plate as described in the lecithinase test (Procedure 34.5). Hold the plate at an angle to the light source to detect the "oil-on-water" phenomenon more easily. It may be necessary to reincubate the plate for up to 2 weeks to detect slow lipase producers.

Nagler test (Procedure 34.6) (Figure 34.16). *C. perfringens, Clostridium baratii, C. bifermentans,* and *C. sordellii* produce an α-lecithinase that is detected by a neutralization test using type-A *C. perfringens* antitoxin. One should test *C. perfringens*–like and other lecithinase-positive clostridia.

Reverse CAMP test (Figure 34.17). This test is similar to the CAMP test for identifying group B β-

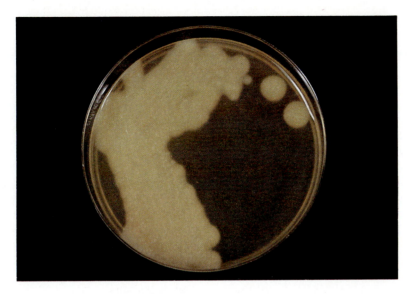

Figure 34.14
C. perfringens. Lecithinase reaction. (From Sutter, V.L., Citron, D.M., Edelstein, M.A.C., and Finegold, S.M. 1985. Wadsworth anaerobic bacteriology manual, ed. 4. Star Publishing Co., Belmont, Calif.)

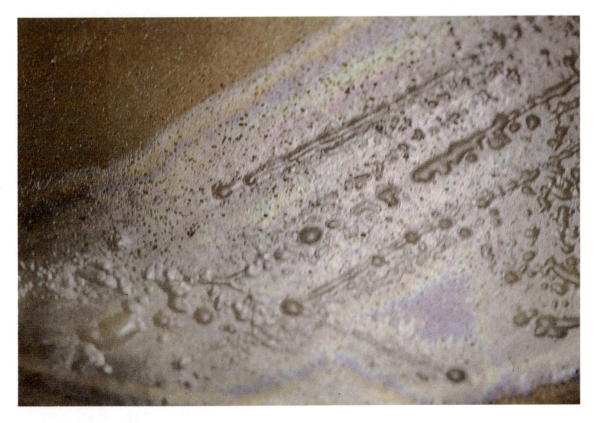

Figure 34.15
Clostridium. Positive lipase reaction on egg yolk agar.

PROCEDURE 34.6

Nagler Test

Principle

α-Lecithinase-producing clostridia (*C. perfringens, C. baratii, C. bifermentans*, and *C. sordellii*) are detected by inhibition of the lecithinase reaction by an α-lecithinase antitoxin. This results in a drastic reduction or complete disappearance of the white opaque zone produced by the splitting of lecithin to insoluble diglycerides (positive lecithinase reaction).

Method

1. Reagents
   a. Egg yolk plate
   b. *Clostridium welchii (perfringens)* type A antitoxin (Cooper Animal Health)
2. Procedure
   a. Swab one-half of an egg yolk agar plate with antitoxin.
   b. Allow the liquid to dry.
   c. Inoculate the test organism on the antitoxin-free half and then streak once across to the antitoxin side of the plate.
   d. Incubate anaerobically 24 to 48 h at 37° C.
3. Reading and interpretation: Examine for the disappearance or dramatic reduction of the opacity on the antitoxin half of the plate. This

denotes neutralization of the type-A lecithinase and is a positive Nagler test (Figure 34.16).

Quality control

Test *C. perfringens* (α-lecithinase producer) and a lecithinase positive (but not α) *C. subterminale. C. haemolyticum* and *C. novyi* type B are also lecithinase producers not of the alpha type, but they are oxygen sensitive and may be difficult to maintain.

Expected results

Performance standards are met when both organisms grow on the egg-yolk-containing agar; both organisms produce a white, opaque halo in the medium; the opacity in the medium is dramatically decreased or obliterated in the presence of α-lecithinase antitoxin with *C. perfringens;* and the opacity remains in the presence of the antitoxin with *C. subterminale.*

Performance schedule

Test each new lot of antitoxin and each time the test is performed.

---

hemolytic streptococci (Chapter 25), except that the putative *Clostridium* sp. replaces *Staphylococcus aureus* and a known group B β-hemolytic streptococcus is used. Although group B streptococci may exhibit some enhanced hemolysis with other clostridia, it is only with *C. perfringens* that the characteristic arrowhead form is demonstrated. Test all *C. perfringens*–like gram-positive bacilli with this test. Only the typical arrowhead of synergistic β-hemolysis (Figure 34-17) indicates a positive test.

Arginine growth stimulation test. Eubacterium lentum is one of the few anaerobic gram-positive rods whose growth is enhanced by arginine; therefore, test all small gram-positive bacilli that do not resemble diphtheroids. This test is performed in a manner

similar to the formate-fumarate growth test, but uses arginine hydrochloride in a final concentration of 0.5% (wt/vol).

• • •

A few of the preceding tests are incorporated in the Lombard-Dowell (LD) Presumpto 1 plate, which is available from many sources, including Remel Laboratories. The more fastidious organisms (certain pigmenters, cocci, *Fusobacterium*) do not grow well on the LD basal medium, and some manufacturers supplement it. Good growth on the basal medium is required to interpret results accurately.

34.5.c. Level II group identification: gram-negative organisms. The gram-negative organisms are di-

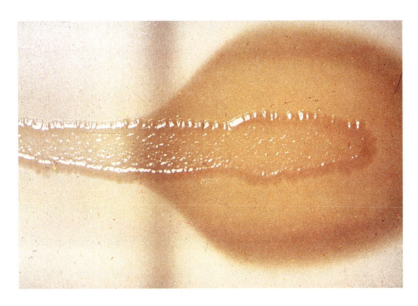

Figure 34.16
C. perfringens. Positive Nagler test on egg yolk agar. Inhibition of lecithinase reaction by antitoxin (*left*).

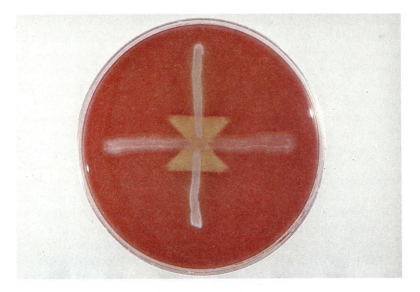

Figure 34.17
C. perfringens. Reverse CAMP test with group B β-hemolytic *Streptococcus* (vertical) and *C. perfringens* (horizontal). (From Sutter, V.L., Citron, D.M., Edelstein, M.A.C., and Finegold, S.M. 1985. Wadsworth anaerobic bacteriology manual, ed. 4. Star Publishing Co., Belmont, Calif.)

vided into the following major categories based on microscopic morphology, antibiotic identification disks pattern, or a few other simple tests.

B. fragilis *group.* These gram-negative bacilli grow in 20% bile and are almost always resistant to all three special potency antibiotic disks.

Pigmented Bacteroides *sp. and* Porphyromonas *sp.* Colonies that fluoresce brick red or produce brown-to-black pigment are placed in this group. Some species are coccobacillary.

B. ureolyticus–*like group.* Members of this group reduce nitrate and require formate and fumarate for growth in broth culture. Their disk pattern is the same as the fusobacteria; however, colony morphology is different. *B. ureolyticus, Bacteroides gracilis, Wolinella,* and *Campylobacter concisus* form small translucent to transparent colonies that may corrode the agar, whereas the *Fusobacterium* colony is generally larger and more opaque.

Other Bacteroides *sp.* This term is applied to gram-negative bacilli that do not fit the preceding categories or the *Fusobacterium* sp.

Fusobacterium *sp.* Gram-negative bacilli are placed in this group by their characteristic antibiotic identification disks pattern (sensitive to colistin and kanamycin and resistant to vancomycin) and colony and microscopic morphology.

Anaerobic gram-negative cocci. This category is based solely on Gram stain morphology and includes *Veillonella, Megasphaera,* and *Acidaminococcus.*

34.5.d. Level II group identification: gram-positive organisms. The gram-positive organisms are divided into three major categories based on microscopic morphology and the presence of spores.

Anaerobic gram-positive cocci. The genera of clinical importance are *Peptostreptococcus* and *Streptococcus.* If a coccus is resistant to metronidazole, it probably is a *Streptococcus* or *Staphylococcus saccharolyticus.*

Clostridium *sp.* These are the endospore-forming, anaerobic, gram-positive bacilli. If spores are not present on Gram stain, the ethanol or heat-spore test will separate this group from the non-spore-forming anaerobic bacilli. *C. perfringens, C. ramosum,* and *C. clostridioforme* may not produce spores or survive a spore test procedure, so it is important to recognize these organisms using other characteristics. Again, a few clostridia grow aerobically, but they produce quantitatively fewer spores aerobically.

Anaerobic non-spore-forming bacilli. This group includes the genera *Actinomyces, Bifidobacterium, Eubacterium,* anaerobic *Lactobacillus,* and *Propionibacterium.* It is impossible to differentiate this group accurately to the genus level without end product analysis, except for *Propionibacterium acnes* and *E. lentum.* They can be identified with a few additional tests, as discussed in the next section.

34.5.e. Level II final identification. Those anaerobes that can be definitively identified using simple tests are shown in Tables 34.3 and 34.4. The results of characteristics in bold type are keys to identification. It is necessary that all stated characteristics be present to identify them definitively. If a characteristic is not present, only a group name can be applied, unless further biochemical testing is carried out.

The *B. fragilis* group and other *Bacteroides* require further biochemical tests for definitive identification. Two species of pigmented *Bacteroides* sp. can be identified readily. An indole-positive and lipase-positive gram-negative coccobacillus that forms dark pigmented colonies or fluoresces brick red may be identified as *B. intermedius.* Lipase-negative strains must be identified using other biochemical tests. A lipase-positive, indole-negative pigmented *Bacteroides* is identified as *B. loescheii;* however, lipase-positive strains of *B. loescheii* are encountered infrequently.

The *B. ureolyticus* group includes *B. ureolyticus, B. gracilis, C. concisus,* and *Wolinella* sp. Transfer of this group to the *Campylobacter* genus has been proposed. These organisms are thin gram-negative rods with round ends and are susceptible to colistin and kanamycin. The colonies are small, translucent or transparent, and may produce greening of the agar. Three colony morphotypes exist: smooth and convex, pitting, and spreading. All three can occur in the same culture. The organisms are asaccharolytic, nitrate- or nitrite-positive, and require formate and fumarate for growth in broth culture. The organisms can use nitrate and hydrogen in place of formate and fumarate. The *Wolinella* sp. and *C. concisus* are motile; oxidase may be useful in differentiating between them. *B. ureolyticus* and *B. gracilis* are nonmotile, although *B. gracilis* may demonstrate "twitching" in a wet preparation and "gliding" on agar. *B. ureolyticus* is urease-positive, whereas *B. gracilis* is urease-negative.

Table 34.3
Level II Identification of Gram-Negative Anaerobes

	CELL CURVED	CELL SHAPE	SLENDER CELLS WITH POINTED ENDS	KANAMYCIN (1 mg)	VANCOMYCIN (5 µg)	COLISTIN (10 µg)	GROWTH IN BILE	INDOLE	CATALASE	PIGMENTED COLONY	BRICK-RED FLUORESCENCE	LIPASE	PITS THE AGAR	REQUIRES FORMATE-FUMARATE	NITRATE REDUCTION	UREASE	MOTILE	STRONG OXIDASE
B. fragilis group	−	B	−	R	R	R	+	V	V	−	−	−	−	−	−	−		
Pigmented *Bacteroides* sp.	−	B, CB	−	R	R	V	−	V	−	+*	V	V	−	−	−	−		
B. intermedius	−	B, CB	−	R	R	S	−	+	−	+	+	+	−	−	−	−		
B. loescheii	−	B, CB	−	R	R	R^s	−	−	−	+−*	−+	+	−	−	−	−		
Porphyromonas sp.	−	B, CB	−	R	S	R	−	+	−	+	+−‡	−	−	−	−	−		
Other *Bacteroides* sp.	−	B, CB	−	V	R	V	−	V	−	−†	−	−	−	−	−	−		
B. ureolyticus–like	V	B	−	S	R	S	−	−	−	−	−	−	V	+	+	V	V	V
B. ureolyticus			−	S	R	S	−	−	−	−	−	−	+−	+	+	+	−	
B. gracilis	−	B	−	S	R	S	−	−	−	−	−	−	V	+	+	−	−§	
Wolinella	V	B	−	S	R	S	−	−	−	−	−	−	V	+	+	−	+	−
Campylobacter concisus	V	B	−	S	R	S	−	−	−	−	−	−	V	+	+	−	+	+
Fusobacterium sp.	+−	B	V	S	R	S	V	V	−	−	−	V	−	−	−	−		
F. nucleatum	−	B	+	S	R	S	−	+	−	−	−	−	−	−	−	−		
F. necrophorum	−	B	−	S	R	S	−+	+	−	−	−	+−	−	−	−	−		
F. mortiferum-varium	−	B	−	S	R	S	+	V	−	−	−	−	−	−	−	−		
Gram-negative cocci	−	C	−	S	R	S	−	−	V	−	V	−	−	−	V	−	−	
Veillonella	−	C	−	S	R	S	−	−	V	−	−+	−	−	−	+	−	−	

Reactions in **bold type** are key tests; B = bacillus; CB = coccobacillus; R = resistant; S = sensitive; V = variable; + = positive; − = negative; superscripts indicate reactions of occasional strains.

*B. melaninogenicus group often requires prolonged incubation before pigment is observed.

†B. bivius produces pigment on prolonged incubation.

‡P. gingivalis does not fluoresce.

§B. gracilis displays a "twitching" motion.

Modified from Sutter, V.L., Citron, D.M., Edelstein, M.A.C., and Finegold, S.M. 1985. Wadsworth anaerobic bacteriology manual, ed. 4. Star Publishing Co., Belmont, Calif.

Two *Fusobacterium* sp. can be identified with a few simple tests. *F. nucleatum* is an indole-positive thin bacillus with pointed ends. The colony fluoresces chartreuse and produces greening of the agar upon exposure to air. There are three colony morphotypes of *F. nucleatum*: speckled, breadcrumb-like, and smooth. The colony size varies from less than 0.5 to 2 mm in diameter. The breadcrumb colony is white, whereas the speckled and smooth types are gray to gray-white. A lipase-positive *Fusobac-*terium is *F. necrophorum*. It is a pleomorphic rod with rounded ends and sometimes forms bizarre shapes. It is indole-positive, fluoresces chartreuse, and produces greening of the agar. The colonies are umbonate and range in size from 0.5 to 2 mm in diameter. Lipase-positive strains are often β-hemolytic. Lipase-negative strains require further biochemical tests for identification. A bile-resistant *Fusobacterium* may be identified tentatively as *F. mortiferum-varium* group. Other species of *Fuso-*

Table 34.4
Level II Identification of Gram-positive Anaerobes

Organism	CELL SHAPE	SPORES OBSERVED	BOXCAR-SHAPED CELLS	DOUBLE ZONE β-HEMOLYSIS	KANAMYCIN (1 mg)	VANCOMYCIN (5 µg)	COLISTIN (10 µg)	INDOLE	SPS	CATALASE	SURVIVES ETHANOL SPORE TEST	LECITHINASE	NAGLER TEST	STRONG R-CAMP TEST	ARGININE STIMULATION	UREASE	NITRATE REDUCTION	GROUND GLASS YELLOW COLONIES ON CCFA MEDIUM	COMMENTS
Gram-positive cocci	C, CB	–	–	–	V	S	R	V	V	V	–	–	–		–		$-^{+}$	–	Sweet, putrid odor; may chain
P. anaerobius	C, CB	–	–	–	R^{s}	S	R	–	S	–	–	–	–		–		–	–	
P. asaccharolyticus	C	–	–	–	S	S	R	+	R	V	–	–	–		–	–	–	–	
Clostridium sp.	B	$+^{-}$	$-^{+}$	–	V	S	R	V		V	$+^{-}$	V	–		–	V	$-^{+}$	V	"Indole" odor
Nagler-positive																			
C. perfringens	B	–	+	$+^{-}$	S	S	R	–		–	$-^{+}$	+	+	+	–	–	$+^{-}$	–	
C. baratii	B	+	–	–	S	S	R	–		–	+	+	$+^{w}$	–	–	–	V	–	
C. sordellii	B	+	–	–	S	S	R	+		–	+	+	$+^{w}$	–	–	$+^{-}$	–	–	
C. bifermentans	B	+	–	–	S	S	R	+		–	+	+	$+^{w}$	–	–	–	–	–	
Nagler-negative Presumptive																			
C. difficile	B	$+^{-}$	–	–	S	S	R	–		–	+	–	–	–	–	–	–	+	"Horse stable" odor; fluoresces charteuse
Non-spore-forming	B, CB	–	–	–	V	S	R	V		V	–	V	–		V	V	V	–	
P. acnes	B, CB	–	–	–	S	S	R	$+^{-}$		$+^{-}$	–	–	–		–	V	$+^{-}$	–	May branch; diphtheroid
E. lentum	B	–	–	–	S	S	R	–		–	–	–	–		+	–	+	–	Small bacillus

Reactions in **bold type** are key tests; B = bacillus; CB = coccobacillus; C = coccus; R = resistant; S = sensitive; V = variable; + = positive; – = negative; w = weak; superscripts indicate reactions of occasional strains.

Modified from Sutter, V.L., Citron, D.M., Edelstein, M.A.C., and Finegold, S.M. 1985. Wadsworth anaerobic bacteriology manual, ed. 4. Star Publishing Co., Belmont, Calif.

bacterium (e.g., *F. necrophorum*) may grow in 20% bile; therefore further testing is required to confirm the presumptive identification.

A gram-negative coccus less than 0.5 mm in diameter that reduces nitrate or nitrite is *Veillonella* sp. The other gram-negative cocci do not reduce nitrate. Catalase is variable. The colonies are small and nearly transparent.

A gram-positive coccus sensitive to sodium polyanetholsulfonate (SPS) is *P. anaerobius*. It is a large coccobacillus and often occurs in chains. The colonies vary in size from 0.5 to 2 mm in diameter (usually larger than most anaerobic cocci) and are gray-white and opaque. A sweet, fetid odor is associated with this organism. An indole-positive, gram-positive coccus is *Peptostreptococcus asaccharolyticus*. *Peptostreptococcus indolicus*, another indole-positive coccus, is rarely isolated from clinical specimens and, unlike *P. asaccharolyticus*, converts lactate to propionate and is usually nitrate-positive and coagulase-positive.

Four *Clostridium sp.* are fairly simple to identify, because they are all Nagler-positive. *C. perfringens* is readily recognizable by its microscopic and colony morphology. It is a boxcar-shaped gram-positive rod with a typical double zone of β-hemolysis surrounding the colony (see Figure 34.6). It is reverse CAMP test–positive, whereas other clostridia have been reported to be negative. The reverse CAMP-negative strains are identified with other biochemical tests. *C. sordellii* and *C. bifermentans* are indole-positive. *C. sordellii* is usually urease-positive, and *C. bifermentans* is urease-negative.

Propionibacterium acnes is an indole-positive, catalase-positive, small pleomorphic (diphtheroid-like) gram-positive bacillus. It usually reduces nitrate. The colonies are initially small and white and become larger and more yellowish tan with age. Indole- or catalase-negative strains are identified with more extensive biochemical tests.

E. lentum is a nitrate-positive, small, gram-positive bacillus whose growth in broth is stimulated by arginine. It forms small, gray, translucent colonies.

34.5.f. Level III identification. In addition to tests performed at level II, species identification of most anaerobes requires additional biochemical tests and often metabolic end product analysis by GLC. Differentiation of genera of anaerobes is shown in tables in Chapters 35 to 37. For level III identification tables and flow diagrams, fermentation reactions are

based on use of prereduced anaerobically sterilized (PRAS) liquid media, and preformed enzyme reactions are based on test kits and individual tube tests. Thioglycollate-based media with bromthymol blue indicator (*CDC Laboratory Manual*) give similar results for fermentation reactions, whereas results obtained in other systems may not agree with these tables. Gas chromatographic analysis may be performed from any carbohydrate-containing medium that supports good growth of the organism.

34.5.g. Level III identification systems. Several identification systems are available, including macrotube and microtube, agar plate, and enzyme substrate types. The PRAS system (macrotube) is still the standard method, but other chemical and biochemical tests may be required. Table 34.5 compares features of some of these systems.

Macrotube systems. Macrotube systems rely on the metabolic breakdown of substrates and production of specific end products during growth of the organism. The substrates are incorporated into prereduced anaerobically sterilized (PRAS) peptone yeast (refer to the VPI Anaerobe Manual or Wadsworth Anaerobic Bacteriology Manual) or thioglycollate broth (refer to the *CDC Anaerobe Manual*). A wide variety of biochemicals is available. End products of metabolism are determined using GLC. Identification is determined by comparing reaction patterns of the unknown to tables of reaction patterns of specific organisms. The PRAS II system (Scott) uses a computer program for interpretation of reaction patterns. However, less than 100% agreement with expected results (see Table 34.6) occurs with this system. The macrotube system, including GLC, is required for the identification of most gram-positive non-spore-forming bacilli, most *Clostridium* sp., some anaerobic cocci, and unusual or less frequently isolated gram-negative bacilli. Additional non-PRAS tests may be required for some organisms. For example, *B. oris* and *B. buccae* have the same PRAS and GLC patterns; α-fucosidase (available in preformed enzyme kits) and colistin disk susceptibility are used to separate them.

PRAS biochemicals are inoculated by either the open or the closed technique. The open technique uses a special apparatus that allows for a continuous flow of anaerobic gas into the tube during manipulations, whereas the closed technique uses a needle and syringe to inject the inoculum into the tube through a rubber stopper (Carr-Scarborough) or a diaphragm in a Hungate type screw cap (PRAS II, Scott Laboratories). Appropriate biochemicals are processed for GLC. See the *Wadsworth Anaerobic Bacteriology Manual* or *Virginia Polytechnic Institute (VPI) Anaerobe Manual* for details.

The PRAS system is expensive, labor-intensive, and not problem-free. The major problem is uninterpretable biochemical results that may be due to (1) an inadequate, nonviable, or mixed inoculum, (2) partial oxidation of tubes, or (3) contamination. Repeat testing is required about 10% to 20% of the time. Because proper interpretation requires good growth, incubation may need to be for as long as 1 week. Careful anaerobic technique is required to maintain an anaerobic atmosphere during manipulations.

Microtube systems. The microtube systems also require growth of the organism for substrate degradation. The API 20A strip contains 16 carbohydrates and tests for indole, urea, gelatin, esculin, and catalase. The indicator is bromcresol purple, which turns yellow at a pH of 6.8. The Minitek system offers a wide choice of biochemical tests using microtray plates and disks saturated with various substrates. The indicator is phenol red, which turns yellow at pH 5.2. A 24- to 48-hour plate culture of the test organism is harvested and suspended in inoculating fluid (Lombard Dowell) to a density equal to a No. 3 MacFarland turbidity standard for API 20A and No. 5 for Minitek. After a 24- to 48-hour anaerobic incubation period, the required reagents are added and the tests are read. The code number generated is matched to a code number representing a specific organism. A codebook or a more extensive computer data bank is available.

The color reactions in both these systems are not always clear-cut (shades of brown [API] and yellow-orange [Minitek]) and make interpretation of test results difficult. In this situation neither system should be relied upon for identification. Of the few current reports, the percent agreement of final identification between PRAS plus GLC and these microtube systems demonstrates that neither system is adequate for identification of many anaerobes without GLC and other tests.

Agar plate system. The agar plate system developed by the CDC Anaerobe Laboratory also requires growth of the organism for substrate degradation. The substrates in the Presumpto I, II, and III four-quadrant plates are incorporated into Lombard-Dowell agar base medium. GLC, motility, and other tests are required for identification.

Preformed enzyme. Several rapid identification systems are available that do not require growth of the organism but instead rely on chromogenic and conventional substrate breakdown by preformed enzymes. Most kits use two chromogens, ortho-, pare-, or beta-naphthylamides and ortho- or para-nitrophenyls. When the colorless chromogen-substrate complex is split, the chromogen is detected directly (yellow nitrophenyl) or after the addition of a "developer" (usually cinnamaldehyde) that complexes with β-naphthylamides to produce a red to pink color. The chromogenic and conventional substrates of the various kits are similar. Some of the substrates may become available as individual tests, so a battery of selected tests can be used; these individual substrates require further evaluation and FDA approval (Rosco disks distributed by ProLab, Inc.).

A pure culture of the organism grown on an individual nonselective agar plate medium is harvested and suspended in inoculating fluid to the appropriate turbidity (see Table 34.5). The panels are inoculated following manufacturer's instructions and incubated aerobically at 35° to 37° C for 4 hours. It is important to adhere strictly to the manufacturer's instructions as culture plate medium, inoculum density, correct filling of wells, and incubation time and atmosphere can affect results.

The IDS and API products have been on the market the longest and are the most commonly used 4-hour systems. The RapID-ANA has 10 test wells, 8 of which are bifunctional (that is, 2 tests per well), for a total of 18 tests. The developer is added to the first set of reactions after they have been read. The AnIDENT panel is a series of 20 substrate wells with a total of 25 tests. The developer is added to 9 of the wells.

Austin Biological Laboratories (ABL), MicroScan, and Vitek also produce 4-hour rapid enzyme test kits. These are similar to IDS and API, except the ABL kit requires separate inoculation of four conventional substrates. A codebook or computer access or both are available, except that ABL uses charts. There are very few reports regarding correlation of these systems to PRAS and GLC identification. The API Zym system has nearly 40 tests, but there is no data base available for anaerobes.

Some of the advantages and disadvantages of these rapid systems are listed in the box on p. 504.

Table 34.5
Comparison of Anaerobic Identification Systems

| PARAMETER | PRAS BIO-CHEMICALS | 4 H PREFORMED ENZYME KITS | | | | MICROTUBE KITS | |
		AnIDENT	RapID-ANA	MICROSCAN	VITEK	MINITEK	API 20A
Inoculum							
Source	Broth*	Plate†	Plate‡	Plate†	Plate	Plate	Plate†
Age	24-48 h	24 h	24-72 h	24-48 h	24-48 h	Not specified	Fresh
Diluent	None	Sterile distilled H$_2$O	Available	Sterile deionized H$_2$O	Sterile saline	Provided (Lombard-Dowell)	Provided (Lombard-Dowell)
Turbidity§							
Size	>2+ in 10 ml 2-10 drops per tube	No. 5 in 3 ml About 85 µl per cupule	No. 3 in 1 ml About 0.1 ml per well	No. 3 in 3 ml 50 µl per well	No. 3 Semiautomatic filling	No. 5 in 1.5 ml 0.05 ml per well	≥ No. 3 in 5 ml —
Tests							
Number	5-30	20	18	24	28	20	21
Type	Variable	Fixed	Fixed	Fixed	Fixed	Variable	Fixed
Incubation							
Time	24 h to 1 wk	4 h	4 h	4 h	4 h	48 h	24 h
Atmosphere	Anaerobic	Aerobic	Aerobic	Aerobic	Aerobic	Anaerobic	Anaerobic
Data base	Charts	Codebook Computer-assist	Codebook Computer-assist	Codebook Computer-assist	Computer program	Codebook Computer-assist	Codebook Computer-assist
Cost ($)/tube or panel||	0.50/tube	3.08	4.50	4.75	4.50	4.50	4.58

*Peptone yeast glucose, thioglycollate, or any broth that supports the growth of the isolate can be used. If a supplement is required, add the supplement to each tube to be inoculated.

†The inoculum is prepared from growth on a nonselective medium. Read the package insert for specific media.

‡Selective media may be used, except for those that detect esculin with a ferric ion (for example, BBE agar). Read the package insert for specific media.

§Expressed in terms of McFarland turbidimetric standard, except for PRAS, which is a subjective estimate of turbidity.

\|\|Based on the list price of the panel; it does not include the cost of the codebook or any other required materials. Except for Minitek and API 20A, it does not include the cost of the diluent.

Modified from handout material from Anaerobe Systems (Santa Clara, Calif.) Anaerobe Workshop Lecture Series and product package inserts.

Advantages and Disadvantages of Rapid Identification Systems

Advantages	Disadvantages
· Aerobic incubation · Short incubation time · Direct inoculum from a plate · Easy handling of kits · Minimal storage space · Expanded computer service · Updated data banks · Amenability to taxonomic changes	· Considerable training time and materials required for familiarity with test reactions · Interpretation somewhat difficult because of gradations in color reactions (color charts are provided by some manufacturers to decrease the problem) · Kits available designed only for common clinical isolates from human sources · Misidentifications possible for organisms not listed in the data base · Additional testing including GLC sometimes required · Accuracy of kits better for some anaerobes than for others

---

Table 34.6 is a compilation of several studies showing the agreement of identification between various systems without the use of additional tests and PRAS plus GLC. It is important to know the percent agreement of identification at the species level, as this is an indicator of accuracy. There are several other studies, but few used PRAS and GLC as the reference method and most did not present their data in a standard format, so interpretation for all categories is not possible. Wide ranges of percent agreement for some categories may be due to differences in the types and numbers of anaerobes tested, the general expertise in identifying anaerobes, the preliminary tests used (for example, Gram stain, antibiotic disk identification pattern, indole, catalase), previous experience in using the test kits, the number of times the test was repeated, the method and criteria of calculating percent agreement, or inclusion or exclusion of isolates that did not have an interpretation for a code number. The RapID-ANA and API AnIDENT are probably adequate for identifying members of the *B. fragilis* group, anaerobic gram-positive cocci, *C. perfringens*, *Clostridium septicum*, and some but not all of the bile-sensitive gram-negative bacilli (for example, high agreement with *B. bivius* and *B. disiens*) (see Dellinger and Moore, 1986, and Tanner et al., 1985). The kits are rarely helpful for identifying other *Clos-*

tridium sp., gram-positive non-spore-forming bacilli (except *P. acnes*), and most gram-negative cocci. In most instances one should not use the kits to identify those anaerobes that can be identified with a few simple tests (for example, *P. anaerobius*), unless warranted by the clinical setting. In all cases, use preliminary test results to confirm the kit-generated identification. For example, the bile reaction is necessary, because *B. fragilis* could be identified as *Bacteroides oralis* and vice versa. There are few reports of the efficacy of the kits for the identification of nonhuman strains. Adney and Jones found the RapID-ANA system to be promising, but suggested that further evaluation was required.

34.6. Other Identification methods

Serology, GLC of both volatile fatty acid end products and cellular fatty acids, and DNA probes offer other techniques for the identification of anaerobes.

34.6.a. **Serology.** Serologic methods have been used to detect either bacterial cell wall antigens or extracellular toxins. Agglutination, immunodiffusion, immunofluorescence, immunoperoxidase, and enzyme immunosorbent assays have been developed for a myriad of bacteria, including the pigmented anaerobic gram-negative bacilli (especially of the oral cavity), *B. fragilis* group and its individual members, and the toxins of *C. perfringens*, *Clostridium bot-*

Table 34.6

Agreement of Identification Systems with PRAS and GLC

	AGREEMENT FOR DEFINITIVE IDENTIFICATION (%)				
	RapID-ANA	AnIDENT	VITEK	API20A	MINITEK
Gram-negative bacilli	43-94 (5)*	74-76 (2)	74 (1)	53-91 (3)	74-80 (2)
Bacteroides	33-88 (4)	81 (1)	77 (1)	67-88 (4)	83 (1)
B. fragilis group	29-87 (3)	79 (1)	83 (1)	68-84 (2)	90 (1)
Pigmented	—	—	58 (1)	—	—
Other *Bacteroides*	89 (1)	89 (1)	65 (1)	67 (1)	—
Fusobacterium	60-100 (4)	58 (1)	27 (1)	0-100 (4)	8 (1)
Gram-positive cocci	64-96 (5)	77-86 (2)	66 (1)	29-80 (3)	55-67 (2)
Gram-positive bacilli					
Clostridium	38-100 (5)	59-63 (2)	64 (1)	66-80 (3)	72-74 (2)
C. perfringens	100 (3)	100 (1)	100 (1)	82-100 (2)	88 (1)
C. difficile	100 (5)	9-78 (3)	64 (1)	96 (1)	69-91 (2)
Non-spore-forming	64-100 (5)	44-77 (2)	62 (1)	61-80 (3)	79-80 (2)
Overall					
Species	53-92 (5)	67-94 (2)	71 (1)	57-85 (3)	70-76 (2)
Genus	94-97 (2)	90 (1)	77 (1)	69-76 (3)	—

*Number in parenthesis is the number of studies used to determine percent agreement.

Data from Applebaum et al., 1983 and 1985; Bate, 1986; Gulletta et al., 1985; Karachewski et al., 1985; Murray et al., 1985; Schreckenberger et al., 1988; Stenson et al., 1986; Tanner et al., 1985.

ulinum, and *Clostridium difficile*. Although there are distinct serologic differences between the genera of anaerobic gram-positive cocci, no test has been developed commercially. A latex test for *C. difficile* is commercially available; its usefulness in predicting disease is controversial (See Chapter 17, Section 17.6). The other serologic tool commercially available is an immunofluorescence kit for certain members of the *B. fragilis* group and some species of the pigmented anaerobic gram-negative bacilli (Fluoretec-F and Fluoretec-M, Organon-Teknika). For the organisms tested, the sensitivity and specificity were near 90%. False-negative results are seen with *B. ovatus*, *B. vulgatus*, and *B. distasonis*. Cross-reactions have been reported with both kits, and certain pigmented anaerobic gram-negative bacilli could not be detected. The CDC has antiserum for *Actinomyces* sp.; they accept slides *only* after prior approval. With the development of monoclonal antibodies for some *B. fragilis* group species and *B. gingivalis*, perhaps more specific kits will be developed for anaerobes of clinical importance.

34.6.b. Gas-liquid chromatography (GLC). As with serology, GLC is not a new tool in anaerobic microbiology. Some of the newer techniques increase the sensitivity for detecting certain metabolic end products (for example, use of electron-capture and headspace chromatography to detect characteristic products of *C. difficile* in stool specimens). Their major drawback has been specificity. GLC has also been used to detect changes in a series of chemically defined media, and the pattern obtained is compared with patterns of known strains of bacteria (that is, GLC used to detect preformed enzyme reactions). Taxonomists use GLC to determine cell wall fatty acid composition, and this application has been developed for species-specific identification by Hewlett-Packard (Microbial Identification System). After a series of multistep procedures, including processing, saponification, methylation, and extraction and washing, the sample is injected into a flame ionization detector GLC fitted with a glass capillary column. The chromatogram produced is automatically matched to a best-fit chromatogram in a computer library. This system is currently under evaluation at several centers and should be regarded as a research tool until these evaluations show good specificity.

34.6.c. Nucleic acid probes. DNA probes for the *Bacteroides fragilis* group, *B. fragilis*, *B. thetaiotaomicron*, and a multiprobe for *Bacteroides* sp.–*F. nucleatum*–*F. necrophorum* complex have been developed but are not commercially available. The major problem with these techniques is relatively low sensitivity.

BIBLIOGRAPHY

Adney, W.S., and Jones, R.L. 1985. Evaluation of the RapID-ANA system for identification of anaerobic bacteria of veterinary origin. J. Clin. Microbiol. 22:980.

Applebaum, P.C., Kaufmann, C.S., and Depenbusch, J. 1985. Accuracy and reproducibility of a four-hour method for anaerobe identification. J. Clin. Microbiol. 21:894.

Applebaum, P.C., Kaufmann, C.S., Keifer, J.C., and Venbrux, H.J. 1983. Comparison of three methods for anaerobe identification. J. Clin. Microbiol. 18:614.

Bartholomew, B.A., Stringer, M.F., Watson, G.N., and Gilbert, R.J. 1985. Development and application of an enzyme linked immunosorbent assay for *Clostridium perfringens* type A enterotoxin. J. Clin. Pathol. 38:222.

Bate, G. 1986. Comparison of Minitek Anaerobe II, API An-Ident, and RapID-ANA systems for identification of *Clostridium difficile*. Am. J. Clin. Pathol. 85:716.

Beaucage, C.M., and Onderdonk, A.B. 1982. Evaluation of prereduced anaerobically sterilized medium (PRAS II) system for identification of anaerobic microorganisms. J. Clin. Microbiol. 16:570.

Cooper, S.W., Szymczak, E.G., Jacobus, N.V., and Tally, F.P. 1984. Differentiation of *Bacteroides ovatus* and *Bacteroides thetaiotaomicron* by means of bacteriophage. J. Clin. Microbiol. 20:1122.

Dellinger, C.A., and Moore, L.V.H. 1986. Use of the RapID-ANA system to screen for enzyme activities that differ among species of bile-inhibited *Bacteroides*. J. Clin. Microbiol. 23:289.

Dezfulian, M., and Bartlett, J.G. 1984. Detection of *Clostridium botulinum* type A toxin by enzyme-linked immunosorbent assay with antibodies produced in immunologically tolerant animals. J. Clin. Microbiol. 19:645.

Dowell, V.R., Jr., and Hawkins, T.M. 1974. Laboratory methods in anaerobic bacteriology. In CDC laboratory manual, DHEW Publication No. (CDC) 74-8272, U.S. Government Printing Office, Washington, D.C.

Dowell, V.R., Jr., and Lombard, G.L. 1981. Reactions of anaerobic bacteria in differential agar media. U.S. Department of Health and Human Services, Public Health Service, Centers for Disease Control. Atlanta, Ga.

Ebersole, J.L., Frey, D.E., Taubman, M.A., et al. 1984. Serological identification of oral *Bacteroides* spp. by enzyme-linked immunosorbent assay. J. Clin. Microbiol. 19:639.

Edelstein, M.A.C. 1989. Laboratory diagnosis of anaerobic infections in humans. In Finegold, S.M., and George, W.L., editors. Anaerobic infections in humans. Academic Press, Orlando, Fla., pp. 111-135.

Finegold, S.M., and Edelstein, M.A.C. 1988. Coping with anaerobes in the 80s. In Hardie, J.M., and Borriello, S.P., editors. Anaerobes today. John Wiley & Sons, London, pp. 1-10.

Gulletta, E., Amato, G., Nani, E., and Covelli, I. 1985. Comparison of two systems for identification of anaerobic bacteria. Eur. J. Clin. Microbiol. 4:282.

Harpold, D.J., and Wasilauskas, B.L. 1987. Rapid identification of obligately anaerobic gram-positive cocci using high-performance liquid chromatography. J. Clin. Microbiol. 25:996.

Head, C.B., and Ratnam, S. 1988. Comparison of API ZYM system with API An-Ident, API 20A, Minitek Anaerobe II, and RapID-ANA systems for identification of *Clostridium difficile*. J. Clin. Microbiol. 26:144.

Holdeman, L.V., Cato, E.P., and Moore, W.E.C. 1977. Anaerobe laboratory manual, ed. 4. VPI Laboratory, Virgina Polytechnic Institute and State University, Blacksburg, Va.

Holmberg, K., and Forsum, U. 1973. Identification of *Actinomyces, Arachnia, Bacterionema, Rothia*, and *Propionibacterium* species by defined immunofluorescence. Appl. Microbiol. 25:834.

Hoopes, W.L., Rissing, J.P., Smith, J.W., and White, A.C. 1980. Radioimmunoassay for *Bacteroides fragilis* infections. J. Clin. Microbiol. 12:205.

Hsu, P.C., Minshew, B.H., Williams, B.L., and Lennard, E.S. 1979. Use of an immunoperoxidase method for identification of *Bacteroides fragilis*. J. Clin. Microbiol. 10:285.

Hussain, Z., Lannigan, R., Schieven, B.C., et al. 1987. Comparison of RapID-ANA and Minitek with a conventional method for biochemical identification of anaerobes. Diagn. Microbiol. Infect. Dis. 6:69.

Karachewski, N.O., Busch, E.L., and Wells, C.L. 1985. Comparison of PRAS II, RapID-ANA and API 20A systems for identification of anaerobic bacteria. J. Clin. Microbiol. 21:122.

Kasper, D.L., Fiddian, A.P., and Tabaqchali, S. 1979. Rapid diagnosis of *Bacteroides* infections by indirect immunofluorescence assay of clinical specimens. Lancet 1:239.

Kuritza, A.P., Getty, C.E., Shaughnessy, P., et al. 1986. DNA probes for identification of clinically important *Bacteroides* species. J. Clin. Microbiol. 23:343.

Lambert, M.A., and Moss, C.W. 1980. Production of *p*-hydroxyhydrocinnamic acid from tyrosine by *Peptostreptococcus anaerobius*. J. Clin. Microbiol. 12:291.

Livingston, S.J., Kominos, S.D., and Yee, R.B. 1978. New medium for selection and presumptive identification of the *Bacteroides fragilis* group. J. Clin. Microbiol. 7:448.

Marler, L., Allen, S., and Siders, J. 1984. Rapid enzymatic characterization of clinically encountered anaerobic bacteria with the API ZYM system. Eur. J. Clin. Microbiol. 3:294.

Millar, S.J., Chen, P.B., Haussman, E. 1987. Monoclonal antibody for identification of *Bacteroides gingivalis* lipopolysaccharide. J. Clin. Microbiol. 25:2437.

Mills, C.K., Grimes, B.Y., and Gherna, R.L. 1987. Three rapid methods compared with a conventional detection of urease production in anaerobic bacteria. J. Clin. Microbiol. 25:2209.

Moss, C.W., Lambert, M.A., and Lombard, G.L. 1977. Cellular fatty acids of *Peptococcus variabilis* and *Peptostreptococcus anaerobius*. J. Clin. Microbiol. 5:665.

Murray, P.R., Weber, C.J., and Niles, A.C. 1985. Comparative evaluation of three identification systems for anaerobes. J. Clin. Microbiol. 22:52.

Narikawa, S., and Nakamura, M. 1987. Differentiation of obligate anaerobes by assay of pyruvate: ferredoxin oxidoreductase activity. Eur. J. Clin. Microbiol. 6:74.

Okuda, K., Ohta, K., Kato, T., et al. 1986. Antigenic characteristics and serological identification of 10 black-pigmented *Bacteroides* species. J. Clin. Microbiol. 24:89.

Salyers, A.A., Lynn, S.P., and Gardner, J.F. 1983. Use of randomly cloned DNA fragments for identification of *Bacteroides thetaiotaomicron*. J. Bacteriol. 154:287.

Schreckenberger, P.C., Celig, D.H., and Janda, W.M. 1988.

Clinical evaluation of the Vitek ANI card for identification of anaerobic bacteria. J. Clin. Microbiol. 26:225.

Senne, J.E., and McCarthy, L.R. 1982. Evaluation of a metronidazole disk test for the presumptive identification of anaerobes. Am. J. Med. Tech. 48:613.

Stenson, M.J., Lee, D.T., Rosenblatt, J.E., Contezac, J.M. 1986. Evaluation of the AnIdent system for the identification of anaerobic bacteria. Diagn. Microbiol. Infect. Dis. 5:9.

Sutter, V.L., Citron, D.M., Edelstein, M.A.C., and Finegold, S.M. 1985. Wadsworth anaerobic bacteriology manual, ed. 4. Star Publishing Co., Belmont, Calif.

Tanner, A.C.R., Strzempko, M.N., Belsky, C.A., and McKinley, G.A. 1985. API-ZYM and API An-Ident reactions of fastidious oral gram-negative species. J. Clin. Microbiol. 22:333.

Viljanen, M.K., Linko, L., and Lehtonen, O. 1988. Detection of *Bacteroides fragilis, Bacteroides thetaiotaomicron,* and *Bacteroides ovatus* in clinical specimens by immunofluorescence with a monoclonal antibody to *B. fragilis* lipopolysaccharide. J. Clin. Microbiol. 26:448.

Weissfeld, A.S., and Sonnenwirth, A.C. 1981. Rapid detection and identification of *Bacteroides fragilis* and *Bacteroides melaninogenicus* by immunofluorescence. J. Clin. Microbiol. 13:798.

Wong, M., Catena, A., and Hadley, W.K. 1980. Antigenic relationships and rapid identification of *Peptostreptococcus* species. J. Clin. Microbiol. 11:515.

35

Anaerobic Gram-Positive Bacilli

Martha A.C. Edelstein

The anaerobic gram-positive bacilli of human clinical significance consist of one genus of endospore-formers, *Clostridium*, and five genera of non-spore-formers, *Actinomyces*, *Bifidobacterium*, *Eubacterium*, *Lactobacillus*, and *Propionibacterium*. These anaerobic bacilli are ubiquitous and are part of the normal flora of the oral cavity, gastrointestinal and genitourinary tracts, and skin. The *Clostridium* species can cause acute severe or chronic infections, while the non-spore-formers usually cause chronic disease. Some *Clostridium* species are resistant to antimicrobials, and many of the non-spore-formers are resistant to metronidazole.

Although members of this group are by definition obligate anaerobes, many of the non-spore-formers and a few species of clostridia are aerotolerant. Because they grow in air or a CO_2-enriched atmosphere, they may be difficult to distinguish from aerobic bacilli. Generally, colonies of the aerotolerant anaerobic gram-positive bacilli are larger, or the spore-formers produce many more spores anaerobically than aerobically.

Differentiation of genera of gram-positive bacilli is represented in Table 35.1. They are initially separated into spore-formers and non-spore-formers; however, some *Clostridium* species rarely form spores and may not demonstrate spores with various spore tests. The non-spore-formers are differentiated by their metabolic end products.

SPORE-FORMING BACILLI
35.1. *Clostridium* Species

There are more than eighty described species in the genus *Clostridium*. Some are highly pathogenic or

Table 35.1

Differentiation of Genera of Anaerobic, Gram-Positive Bacilli

CHARACTERISTICS	GENERA
Spore-forming	*Clostridium*
Non-spore-forming	
1. Produces propionic and acetic acids with or without succinic acid	*Propionibacterium*
2. No major propionic acid produced	
a. Produces acetic and lactic acid (A > L)	*Bifidobacterium*
b. Produces lactic acid as sole major end product	*Lactobacillus*
c. Produces major succinic acid and moderate acetic acid with or without lactic acid	*Actinomyces*
d. Other: Butyric ± others, acetic, or no major acids	*Eubacterium*

Data from Sutter et al., 1985; Holdeman et al., 1977; Schal, 1986.

Table 35.2

Taxonomic Changes of Anaerobic, Gram-Positive Bacilli

NEW	OLD
Actinomyces pyogenes	*Corynebacterium pyogenes*
Bifidobacterium dentium	*B. eriksonii*
Clostridium	
C. argentinense	*C. botulinum* type G and some strains of *C. hastiforme* and *C. subterminale*
C. baratii	*C. barati, C. perenne,* and *C. paraperfringens*
C. clostridioforme	*C. clostridiiforme*
C. spiroforme	sp. nov.
C. symbiosum	*Fusobacterium symbiosum*
Eubacterium	
E. brachy	sp. nov.
E. nodatum	sp. nov.
E. plautii	*Fusobacterium plautii*
E. timidum	sp. nov.
E. yurii	sp. nov.
E. yurii ssp. *yurii*	sp. nov.
E. yurii ssp. *margaretiae*	sp. nov.
Lactobacillus oris	sp. nov.
Propionibacterium propionicus	*Arachnia propionica*

Data from Sutter et al., 1985; Moore et al., 1988; Charfreitag et al., 1988; and Suen et al., 1988.

toxigenic, such as *C. tetani*, while others are rarely pathogenic. Most clostridia are obligate anaerobes, but some can grow on an enriched medium in air. These aerotolerant clostridia can be confused with *Bacillus* species. In general, the *Clostridium* species produce larger colonies and quantitatively more spores in an anaerobic than aerobic atmosphere, and the clostridia are usually catalase-negative. *C. perfringens, C. ramosum,* and *C. clostridioforme* do not readily sporulate in vitro and could be confused with non-spore-formers; however, these clostridia are usually easy to recognize by a characteristic Gram stain or colony morphology.

Several new species have been described, but few have been isolated from human clinical material. All *C. botulinum* type G and a few strains of *C. hastiforme* and *C. subterminale* have been named *C. argentinense. C. perenne* and *C. paraperfringens* are now *C. baratii* (Table 35.2).

35.1.a. Normal flora and infections. Clostridia are widely distributed in soil, dust, and water and are common inhabitants of the intestinal tract and, to a much lesser extent, the genital tract. They are often found in unclean wounds and wound infections. Most infections are mixed with other anaerobes and aerobes, and they are either endogenous (that is, spread from a normal flora site to a contiguous area) or exogenous (that is, originate from outside the body).

Clostridial disease syndromes of exogenous origin include tetanus and sometimes gas gangrene (clostridial myonecrosis); intoxications include tetanus, botulism, and *C. perfringens* food poisoning. Some clostridia participate in either endogenous or exogenous types of infections. The pathogenic species can be placed in five categories by virtue of the disease syndromes or intoxications they produce, with some species occurring in more than one category. *C. perfringens* and *C. ramosum* are by far the most commonly isolated clostridia.

35.1.b. Disease syndromes and intoxications.

Group I: Gas gangrene. C. perfringens (type A), *C. septicum, C. novyi* type A, *C. bifermentans, C. histolyticum, C. sordellii, C. sporogenes,* and a few other clostridia can cause gas gangrene; the first three species are the most important. Infection can be either of endogenous or exogenous origin. Bacteremia occurs in about 15% of the patients with clostridial myonecrosis. *C. septicum* is associated

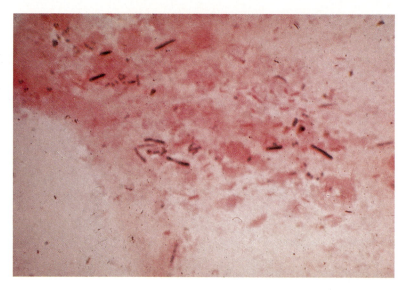

Figure 35.1
Perineal gas gangrene. *C. perfringens* (large, broad gram-positive rods), coliforms, and white blood
cells badly distorted by toxin of *C. perfringens*.

with cancer of the cecum and other organs and is
isolated from blood. The gram stain may be helpful
in substantiating the clinical diagnosis of gas gangrene (Figures 35.1 to 35.3). The two findings of
note are absence or distortion of white blood cells
and other host cells in the stained smear of exudate
or aspirated material and the presence of large, relatively short, fat, gram-positive rods with blunt ends
and without evidence of spores. The changes in the
host cells are due to the α-toxin produced by *C.
perfringens*. Isolation and identification of the organism is required to confirm the presence of *Clostridium* species.

Group II: Tetanus. *C. tetani* is the etiologic agent
of tetanus. The bacterium and its spores of exogenous origin (usually a soil-contaminated sharp object)
are usually inoculated in a puncture wound. When
the proper conditions exist, the toxin (tetanospasmin) is produced, and disease may follow.

Group III: Botulism. The primary agent of botulism
is *C. botulinum;* however, there are reports of rare
cases due to *C. butyricum* and *C. baratii* that can
produce types E and F botulinal neurotoxins. The
three manifestations of disease are food, wound, and
infant botulism. Food botulism occurs with the
ingestion of preformed toxin in contaminated food
and wound botulism occurs with the introduction of
spores or bacteria into a wound. With infant botu-

lism, the bacterium colonizes the gastrointestinal
tract of the infant (presumably because the infant's
own flora is not yet fully developed) and produces
toxin within the gastrointestinal tract; the toxin is
then absorbed to produce the disease (Chapter 17).
It is speculated that in vivo toxin production and
absorption may be a mechanism in certain cases of
adult botulism as well. Cultivation of *C. botulinum*
should be attempted only by reference laboratories;
personnel involved should be immunized. Determination of toxigenicity, where indicated, should be
done by reference laboratories.

*Group IV: Antibiotic-associated pseudomembranous
colitis.* The primary etiologic agent is *C. difficile*.
Rare cases may be due to *C. perfringens* type C and
other clostridia, as well as to *Staphylococcus aureus*.
C. difficile may also be involved in pseudomembranous colitis not related to the use of antimicrobial
therapy, in disease following the use of methotrexate
and other cytotoxic agents, in exacerbations of inflammatory bowel disease (at least partly related to
therapy), and in complications of bowel obstruction.
Most strains of *C. difficile* produce at least two toxins;
one is cytopathic for most tissue culture cell lines
and the other is an enterotoxin. Diarrhea without
colitis following antimicrobial therapy may involve
C. difficile on occasion. There is evidence to implicate type A *C. perfringens* in some of these cases as

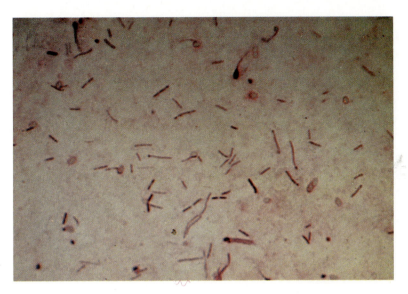

Figure 35.2
C . septicum, microscopic. Note free spores.

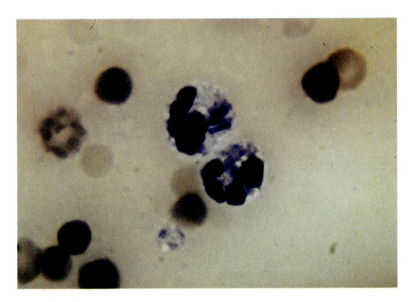

Figure 35.3
Intracellular *C . perfringens* in peripheral blood smear.

well. Details on examination of specimens for *C . difficile* and its cytopathic toxin are presented in Chapter 17.

Group V. Miscellaneous. These infections are more commonly encountered than those in Groups I to IV. *C . perfringens* and a number of other species of clostridia are more commonly isolated from an as-

sortment of infections throughout the body, similar to those caused by the non-spore-forming anaerobes rather than the other four groups. However, clostridia are found in such infections only about one-tenth as often as non-spore-formers. Miscellaneous infections include brain abscess, aspiration pneumonia, thoracic empyema, intra-abdominal infec-

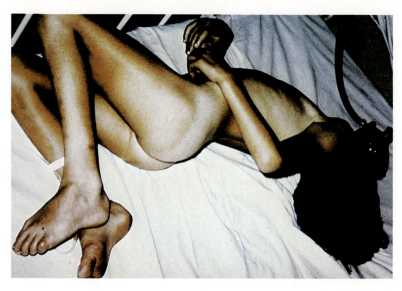

Figure 35.4
Tetanus. Patient exhibits opisthotonos (head and legs bent backward toward each other).

tion, postoperative wound infection, infections related to gynecologic disease or surgery, and soft tissue infections. The classic infections involving *C. perfringens*, aside from gas gangrene, are gangrenous cholecystitis (with or without visceral gas gangrene) and postabortal sepsis with intravascular hemolysis. Bacteremia is seen occasionally with *C. perfringens* and rarely with other clostridia. The isolation of clostridia from blood in the absence of clinical signs of disease may be a transient event and not necessarily related to disease, except as noted for *C. septicum*.

35.1.c. Virulence factors. The clostridia produce many virulence factors such as spores, toxins of numerous types, and other extracellular products such as collagenase and proteases. The spores of some pathogenic species may survive in impro perly home-canned produce (in which they can develop vegetatively under normal domestic conditions) (*Clostridium botulinum*), in insufficiently sterilized surgical dressings and bandages, in plaster of Paris for casts, and on the clothing and skin of humans (primarily *C. perfringens* in the latter three examples).

The toxins of *C. difficile* have already been mentioned. The exotoxins of *Clostridium tetani* and *C. botulinum* are among the most potent poisons known to man (estimated to be one million times as potent as rattlesnake poison). The toxin produced by *C.*

tetani, tetanospasmin, becomes bound to gangliosides within the central nervous system; like strychnine, it suppresses the central inhibitory balancing influences on motor neuron activity, thus leading to intensified reflex response to afferent stimuli and to spasticity and convulsions (Figure 35.4). It also acts on the sympathetic nervous system and on the neurocirculatory and neuroendocrine systems. Botulinal toxin attaches to individual motor nerve terminals, preventing acetylcholine release at the nerve endings. *C. perfringens* produces at least ten toxins, including hemolysins, proteases, RNase, collagenase, hyaluronidase, neuraminidase, and an enterotoxin with activity similar to *Vibrio cholerae*. The β-toxin of type C (and B) *C. perfringens* is the key factor in necrotizing enterocolitis ("Darmbrand," pig-bel). A number of other clostridia produce toxins, some of which are important. The interested reader is referred to Smith's and Willis' excellent books cited in the bibliography.

35.1.d. Morphology and general characteristics. The clostridia possess no one typical cell shape or size. Some are very large rods, whereas others are slender and short or long and sometimes even coiled. Most strains are gram-positive, but a few always appear gram-negative (for example, *C. clostridioforme*) and others gram-variable depending on growth medium and age of the culture. Sporangia are often characteristically swollen, showing spindle, drum-

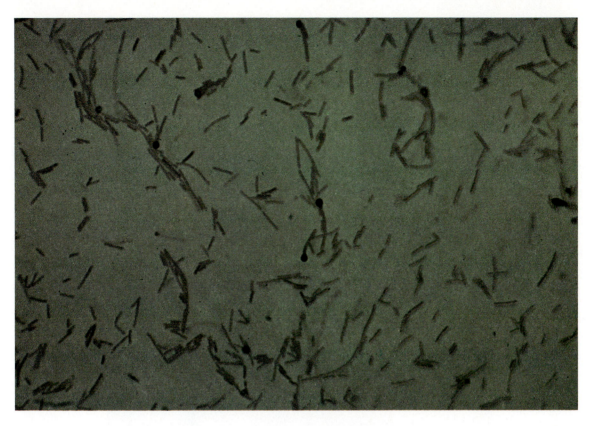

Figure 35.5
C. tetani, microscopic. Note round terminal spores, the "drumstick" appearance.

stick (*C. tetani*) (Figure 35.5), and "tennis racket" (*C. botulinum*) forms and containing central, subterminal or terminal spores. Spores may be apparent on Gram's stain or a wet preparation using phase-contrast or darkfield microscopy. It is difficult to detect spores of *C. perfringens*, *C. ramosum*, and *C. clostridioforme*. *C. perfringens* and *C. clostridioforme* are usually differentiated from non-spore-formers by their cell morphology; *C. perfringens* is boxcar-shaped (Figure 35.3); *C. clostridioforme* has an elongated football shape with cells often in pairs, and it stains gram-negative. *C. ramosum* cells are slender and usually longer than *C. perfringens* cells; other tests are required to differentiate *C. ramosum* from non-spore-formers.

As with cell morphology, the clostridia possess no one typical colony morphology, although generally a large colony (>2 mm) with irregular edges or swarming growth (occurring only on the anaerobic plate) is probably a *Clostridium* (Figures 35.6 to

35.8). Some *Clostridium* sp., however, form small, convex nonhemolytic colonies with an entire edge, such as *C. ramosum* and *C. clostridioforme*. Many clostridia produce several different-looking colony types at one time, so the culture often looks mixed. A subculture of a single colony that yields the same pleomorphism should be considered pure. A few *Clostridium* species have distinct colony characteristics. *C. perfringens* usually produces a double zone of hemolysis (see Figure 34.6). The inner zone (which may be only immediately beneath the colony) shows complete hemolysis and the outer zone shows discoloration and incomplete hemolysis. *C. septicum* produces a "medusa-head" colony in a few hours that spreads over the entire plate in less than 24 hours (Figure 35.6). *C. tetani* and *C. sporogenes* may also swarm. *C. difficile* produces a yellow ground-glass colony on the selective medium cycloserine-cefoxitin egg yolk fructose agar (Figure 35.9); relatively few organisms other than *C. difficile* grow on the CCFA

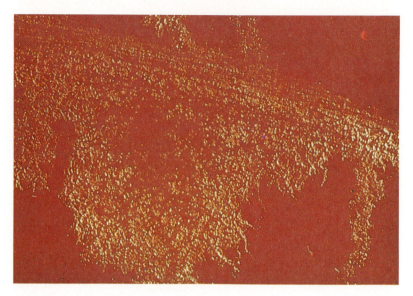

Figure 35.6
C. septicum. "Medusa head" colony on BA.

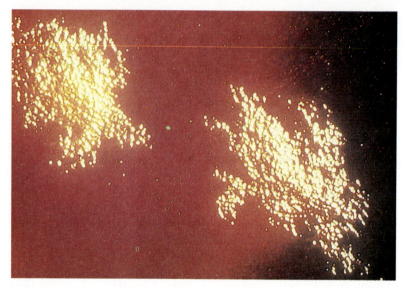

Figure 35.7
C. tetani on BA. Note irregular edge.

medium, and their colonies are unlike those of *C. difficile*. *C. difficile* colonies on blood agar are usually 2 mm or more in diameter after 24 hours of incubation (Figure 35.10), fluoresce yellow-green, and emit a horse stable odor. Such colonies, which on Gram stain show typical gram-positive rods, constitute good presumptive evidence of the presence of *C. difficile*. Most clostridia grow well in broth, with some strains producing abundant gas (for example, *C. perfringens* and *C. septicum*) and foul odor.

35.1.e. **Identification: isolation techniques.** Although most clostridia are mixed with other anaerobes or facultative aerobes in infections, their iso-

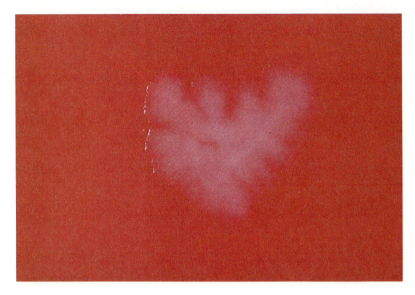

Figure 35.8
C. sordellii on BAP.

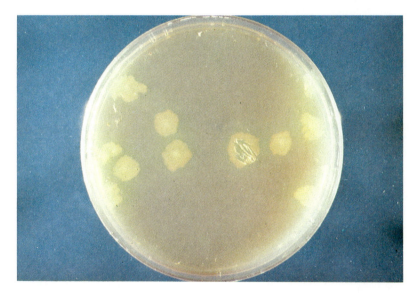

Figure 35.9
C. difficile on cycloserine cefoxitin fructose agar.

lation is not usually difficult when the selective agar phenylethyl alcohol (PEA) or colistin nalidixic acid (CNA) agar is included as one of the primary culture media. In the event these media do not adequately isolate the clostridia, heat shock, ethanol exposure, or other selective agars are alternative isolation methods (see Procedure 35.1). Always split the spec-imen, so that part is treated and the other is pro-cessed in the usual manner. If the specimen amount is too small, use the backup broth culture or cell paste from a sweep of the primary BA plate as the inoculum for the test. If *C. perfringens* is expected (typical Gram stain or clinical condition), set up a Nagler test directly with a portion of the specimen.

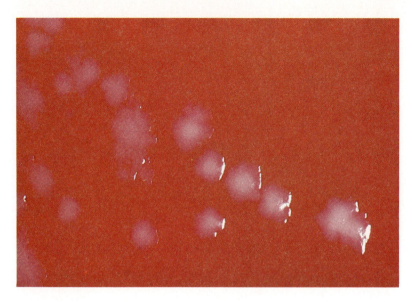

Figure 35.10
C. difficile on BAP.

Table 35.3

Characteristics of Nagler-Positive *Clostridum* Species

	INDOLE PRODUCTION	GELATING HYDROLYSIS	UREASE	GROWTH ENHANCED BY 1% MANNOSE	GLUTAMIC ACID DECARBOXYLASE	REVERSE CAMP TEST	MOTILITY
C. perfringens	−	+	−		+	**+**	−
C. baratii	−	−	−		+	−	+
C. bifermentans	**+**	+	−	**+**	−*	−	+
C. sordellii	**+**	+	+⁻	−	+	−	+

Reactions: Results in **bold type** are key reactions; + = positive; − = negative; +⁻ = rare strain negative.
*Only a few strains have been tested.
Data from Sutter et al., 1985; Banks et al., 1989; Cato et al., 1986; Jilly et al., 1984.

Media with 5% agar may be useful to minimize swarming of some species. Neomycin (100 μg/ml; McClung-Toabe agar) or cycloserine (500 μg/ml)-containing blood agar or egg yolk agar are good selective media. If the plates are being prepared in house, neomycin can be added before autoclaving, but filter-sterilized cycloserine is added after autoclaving. Nonselective media should always be inoculated in parallel with selective media.

35.1.f. Grouping and definitive identification. The *Clostridium* species can be divided into the following three groups using aerotolerance, lecithinase production, and the Nagler reaction: (1) aerotolerant, (2) Nagler-positive, and (3) Nagler-negative obligate anaerobes. Table 35.3, Table 35.4, and Figure 35.11 show tests that are useful for definitive identification. Results in **bold type** are key reactions. Use the flow diagram as a guide, because atypical strains may give variable reactions.

Isolating Clostridia from Mixed Culture

Heat shock

Principle

Most *Clostridium* sp. produce spores resistant to heating at 80° C for 10 min, whereas vegetative cells are usually killed. *Bacillus* sp. also produce heat-resistant spores, so all isolates must be further processed (see Chapter 34). A few clostridia produce spores sensitive to exposure to 80° C.

Method

1. Original specimen or liquid backup culture source
   a. Remove an aliquot of liquid specimen or an aliquot of the original broth culture and transfer it to a sterile screw-cap glass tube.
   b. Place the tube in an 80° C water bath for 10 min. Be certain the water level is above the liquid level in the tube.
   c. Transfer 1 to 2 drops of the heated samples onto enriched *Brucella* 5% sheep blood and egg yolk agar (EYA) plates. Streak for isolation.
   d. Incubate plates anaerobically for 24 to 48 h.
   e. Process colonies for identification as described in Chapters 34 and 35.
2. Plate source
   a. If the patient specimen has been inoculated onto agar plates and no broth culture is available or spores were observed on a Gram-stain smear of the original plates, a sweep of the first quandrant of growth can be used for the spore test.
   b. Sweep across the first quadrant with a loop and inoculate into a freshly steamed tube of thioglycollate or a PRAS starch broth tube.
   c. Heat immediately at 80° C for 10 min.
   d. Incubate the broth tube 24 to 48 h.
   e. If growth occurs, subculture 2 to 3 drops of the heat-treated broth to a blood agar and an egg yolk agar plate.
   f. Incubate plates 24 to 48 h and process colonies for identification as described in Chapters 34 and 35.

Quality control

A specific quality control procedure for clinical material is difficult and not required. The best assurance that spore-formers will be recovered is to determine that equipment, reagents, and media are performing properly. Failure to recover spore-formers observed on a Gram-stain smear may be due to killing of the spores at 80° C or to a failure in the system. If possible, repeat the test at a lower temperature or perform the ethanol spore test.

Ethanol Treatment

Principle

To significantly reduce non-spore-forming organisms and enhance recovery of spore-formers, a portion of the patient's sample is exposed to ethanol, because ethanol (or other alcohols) kills vegetative cells but not most spores.

Method

1. The specimen source may be an aliquot of the patient's specimen or the original backup broth culture, or a sweep of the first quadrant of the primary culture plate.
2. Add 1 ml of liquid culture to 1 ml of 95% ethanol or a loopful of bacterial cell paste from a plate culture to 1 ml of 50% ethanol.
3. Gently mix and allow mixture to stand for 35 to 45 min.
4. Dip a swab into the alcohol mixture and spread onto the first quadrant of a BA and an EYA plate. Streak the other quadrants for isolation.
5. Incubate the plates anaerobically at 37° C for 48 h.
6. Process colonies for identification as described in Chapters 34 and 35.

Quality control

A specific quality control procedure for clinical material is difficult and not required. The best assurance that spore-formers will be recovered is to determine that equipment, reagents, and media are performing adequately. Repeat the test if spores are observed on a Gram-stain smear of material, but spore-formers are not recovered.

Table 35.4
Characteristics of Clostridium Species

| | AEROBIC GROWTH | GELATIN HYDROLYSIS | LECITHINASE | LIPASE | INDOLE PRODUCTION | UREASE | BUTYRIC ACID PRODUCED IN PYG | ISOACIDS PRODUCED IN PYG | FERMENTATION OF | | | | | SPORE SHAPE AND LOCATION | FATTY ACID END PRODUCTS FROM PYG |
									GLUCOSE	LACTOSE	MALTOSE	FRUCTOSE	XYLOSE		
Aerotolerant															
C. histolyticum	+[-]	+	-	-	-		-	-	-	-	-	-	-	OS	A (l s)
C. tertium	+	-	-	-	-		+	-	+	+	+	+	+[-]	OT	A B L (s)
Nagler-positive*															
C. perfringens†	-	+	+	-	-		+	-	+	+	+	+	-	OST†	A B L (p s)
C. baratii	-	-	+	-	-	-	+	-	+	+[w]	+[w]	+	-	R/OS/T	A B L (p s)
C. bifermentans	-	+	+	-	+	-	+	-	+	-	w[-]	V	-	OS/T	A B L
C. sordellii	-	+	+	-	+	+[-]	+[-]	+[-]	+	-	w[+]	V	-	OS/T	A (p ib b iv ic l)
Nagler-negative															
Saccharolytic; proteolytic															
C. botulinum‡	-	V	-	+[-]	-		+	+[-]	+	-	V	V	-	OS	A B (P ib iv v ic l s)
C. novyi type A	-	+	+	+	-		+	-	+	-	V	-[w]	-	OS	A P B
C. sporogenes§	-	+	-	+	-		+	+[-]	+	-	-[w]	-[w]	-	OS	A B ib iv (p v l s)
C. cadaveris	-	+	-	-	+		+	+[-]	+	-	-	V	-	OT	A b
C. septicum	-	+	-	-	-		+	-	+	+	+	+	-	OS	A B (p)
C. difficile	-	+[w]	-	-	-		+	+	+	-	-	+	-[w]	OS	A ib B iv ic (v)
C. putrificum	-	+	-	-	-		+	+	+	-	-[w]	-[w]	-	O/RT/S	A ib B iv (p v l s)
Saccharolytic; nonproteolytic															
C. butyricum	-	-	-	-	-		**+**	-	+	+	+	+	-	OS	A B (l s)
C. innocuum	-	-	-	-	-		**+**	-	+	-	-	+	-	OT	A B L (s)
C. ramosum†,‖	-	-	-	-	-				+	+	+	+	-[w]	R/OT	a L (s)
C. clostridioforme†,‖	-	-	-	-	-[+]	-			+	+[-]	+[w]	+	+	OS	l (s)
Asaccharolytic; proteolytic															
C. tetani	-	+	-	-	+[-]		+	-	-	-	-	-	-	RT	A B (l s)
C. hastiforme	-	+	-	-	-		+	+	-	-	-	-	-	OT	A B iv ib (p ic)
C. subterminale	-	+	-	-[+]	-		+	+	-	-	-	-	-	OS	A B ib IV (p ic l s)

Reactions: Results in **bold type** are key reactions; superscripts represent rare strain reactions; − = negative; + = positive; w = weakly positive; V = variable.

PRAS carbohydrates: + = pH < 5.5; W = pH 5.5-5.7; − = pH > 5.7.

Spore shape and location: O = oval; R = round; S = subterminal; T = terminal.

Fatty acids: A = acetic; P = propionic; IB = isobutyric; B = butyric; IV = isovaleric; V = valeric; IC = isocaproic; L = lactic; S = succinic. NOTE: (1) Capital letters indicate major metabolic products. (2) Small letters indicate minor products. (3) Parentheses indicate a variable reaction. (4) Isoacids are primarily from carbohydrate-free media (such as PY) in the case of saccharolytic organisms.

*Refer to Table 35.3.

†Spores almost never observed.

‡*C. botulinum* types vary in proteolytic, +saccharolytic, and lipase reactions. Send suspected isolates or *C. botulinum*–containing material to the appropriate local or state agency.

§*C. sporogenes* and *C. botulinum* types A, B, and F behave biochemically the same; these two clostridia can be differentiated only by toxin neutralization studies.

‖Cell morphology useful differential feature; see Section 35.1.d. *C. clostridioforme* often appears gram-negative.

Data from Sutter et al., 1985; Cato et al., 1986; Holdeman et al., 1977; Willis, 1977.

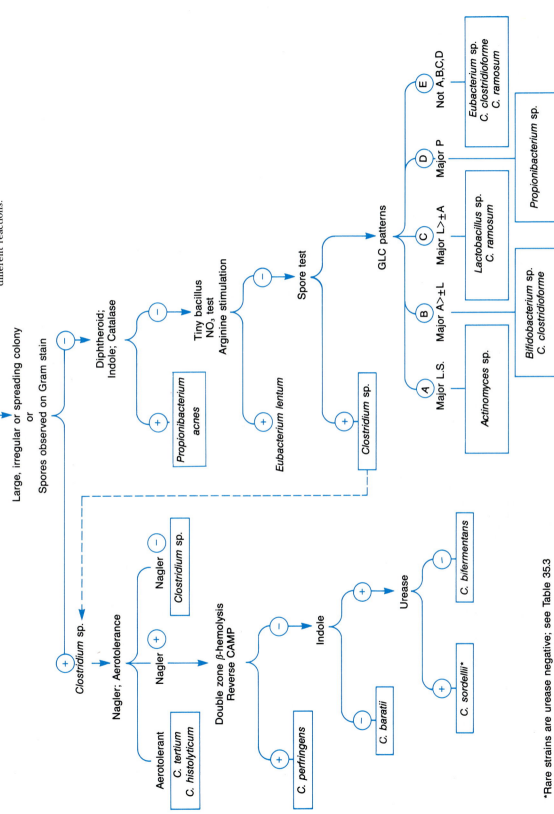

Figure 35.11
Flow diagram for identification of gram-positive anaerobic bacilli. Use only as a guide, as atypical strains may have different reactions.

*Rare strains are urease negative; see Table 35.3

C. tertium and *C. histolyticum* are the more frequently encountered aerotolerant clostridia. Growth can be very good in air, but a Gram stain of growth from an aerobic plate will show fewer spores than the anaerobic plate.

Identification of the four Nagler-positive *Clostridium* species (*C. perfringens*, *C. baratii*, *C. sordellii*, and *C. bifermentans*) is presented in Chapter 34 and Table 35.3. Briefly, *C. perfringens* demonstrates the most complete neutralization of the α-lecithinase in the Nagler test. It is readily differentiated from the other Nagler-positive bacteria by displaying double-zone hemolysis, boxcar-shaped cells, and a positive reverse-CAMP test. It is also nonmotile. *C. baratii* is infrequently isolated from clinical material. *C. sordellii* is indole-positive and almost always urease-positive, whereas *C. bifermentans* is indole-positive and urease-negative.

There are a myriad of obligately anaerobic, Nagler-negative *Clostridium* sp. Overall, these organisms are infrequently isolated. Of this group, *C. ramosum*, *C. septicum*, and *C. clostridioforme* are the most frequently isolated. *C. difficile* is infrequently isolated from nonstool specimens. Lipase-positive *C. botulinum* strains and *C. sporogenes* are phenotypically similar, so that differentiation traditionally relies on animal toxicity studies; these studies should be performed by a reference laboratory. As with *C. difficile*, detection of the toxin is probably more important for diagnosis than isolation of the bacterium. Production of lecithinase and lipase (egg yolk agar reactions), hydrolysis of gelatin, and fermentation of glucose are useful for subdividing this diverse group. *C. novyi* type A is the only *Clostridium* that consistently produces both lecithinase and lipase. Definitive identification relies on end product analysis using gas-liquid chromatography (GLC), carbohydrate fermentation patterns, and various other tests. Characteristics of some *Clostridium* species are included in Table 35.4.

35.1.g. Susceptibility to antimicrobials. Overall, penicillin is the drug of choice to treat clostridial infections, but minimal inhibitory concentrations of *C. ramosum* are as high as 8 U/ml. Occasional strains of *C. perfringens* and other clostridia are resistant to penicillin G. *C. ramosum* is not as virulent as *C. perfringens*, but about 15% of strains are highly resistant to clindamycin, and many strains are resistant to tetracycline and erythromycin. Some 20% to 30% of certain clostridial species other than *C. perfrin-*

gens are also resistant to clindamycin. One third of clostridia other than *C. perfringens* are resistant to cefoxitin. Chloramphenicol and metronidazole are essentially active against all clostridia. Surgical debridement and drainage are the essential part of the therapeutic approach to clostridial infections. Oral vancomycin or metronidazole is the drug of choice for the treatment of *C. difficile* colitis, and oral bacitracin is equally effective.

NON-SPORE-FORMING BACILLI

The genera of anaerobic non-spore-forming bacilli encountered in human clinical material are *Actinomyces*, *Bifidobacterium*, *Eubacterium*, *Lactobacillus*, and *Propionibacterium*. The genus *Arachnia* has been essentially eliminated, and *A. propionica* has been transferred to the genus *Propionibacterium* as *P. propionicus*. Several new species of *Eubacterium* sp. associated with the oral flora have been described. See Table 35.2 for some other taxonomic changes.

These organisms are found as normal flora in the upper respiratory tract and oral cavity, the bowel, the vagina, and, in the case of *Propionibacterium*, on the skin. The anaerobic gram-positive non-spore-forming bacilli are considered nonpathogenic, except for the *Actinomyces* sp. and a few others (e.g., *Eubacterium brachy*). They are rarely isolated in pure culture. They are usually isolated with a mixture of many other types of organisms and may at times represent contamination of the specimen with normal flora.

35.2. Differentiation of genera

With rare exceptions, differentiation of this group is by variation in the pattern of volatile and nonvolatile fatty acids produced during carbohydrate fermentation or peptone degradation (Table 35.1). However, a few generalizations can be made based on a few simple tests (Table 35.5):

1. A catalase-positive non-spore-former is probable *Propionibacterium* species or *A. viscosus*.
2. A nitrate-positive bacterium is probably *not* a *Lactobacillus* or *Bifidobacterium* species.
3. An aerotolerant strain is *not* a *Eubacterium* species.
4. A straight bacillus with parallel sides is probably *not* an *Actinomyces*, *Bifidobacterium*, or *Propionibacterium* species.

Usually, morphologic features are not adequate

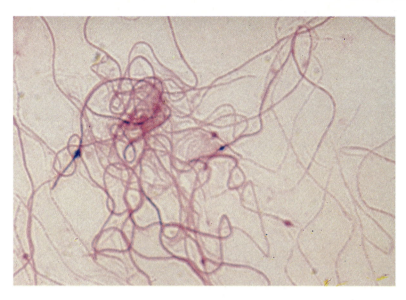

Figure 35.12
Eubacterium species. Gram's stain. Anaerobes may be overdecolorized easily or they may lose their gram positivity.

Table 35.5

Simple Tests for Presumptive Differentiation of Non-Spore-Forming Bacilli*

GENERA	AEROBIC GROWTH	CATALASE	NITRATE REDUCTION	CELLS WITH PARALLEL SIDES
Actinomyces	+ −	− +	+ −	−
Bifidobacterium	− +	−	−	−
Eubacterium	−	−	+ −	+ −
Lactobacillus	+ −	−	− +	+ −
Propionibacterium	+ −	+ −	+ −	− +

Reactions: Superscripts represent reactions of rare strains; + = positive; − = negative.
*Also, see Table 35.2 for fatty acid metabolic end products.
Data from Sutter et al., 1985; Schal, 1986.

for distinguishing between different gram-positive, non-spore-forming, anaerobic bacilli. Moreover, there may be problems distinguishing this group of organisms from others, since they may look coccoid at times, may destain (Figure 35.12) and appear gram-negative, and may be confused with clostridia that do not demonstrate spores. Use of antibiotic identification disks may help resolve gram-stain problems, and the use of egg yolk agar (EYA) can be helpful in differentiating clostridia from these organisms. On EYA, none of the non-spore-forming bacilli produce lecithinase and only a few produce lipase. *Nocardia* can be differentiated from *Actinomyces* and *P. propionicus* by the modified acid-fast

stain described in Chapter 33; *Nocardia* are weakly acid-fast.

Other methods that may be useful for differentiation of the genera of gram-positive non-spore-forming bacilli include ultrastructural features of the cell wall and cell wall fatty acid analysis, neither of which is currently available for routine use.

35.3. *Actinomyces* Species

35.3.a. Normal flora, infections, and virulence factors. *Actinomyces* are residents of the mouth, including tonsillar crypts and dental plaque, and the female genital tract. They produce infection primarily as endogenous opportunists. The etiologic

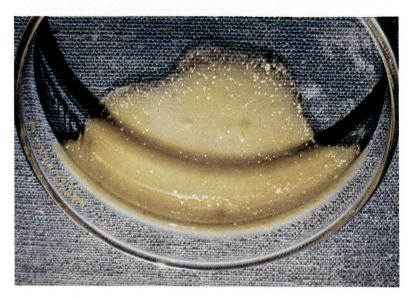

Figure 35.13
Sulfur granules in thoracic empyema fluid. Actinomycosis. (Photograph courtesy Charles V. Sanders.)

agents of human actinomycosis within the *Actinomyces* species include the most common and important organism, *A. israelii,* and several other species: *A. naeslundii, A. odontolyticus, A. viscosus,* and *A. meyeri.* Actinomycosis is typically a mixed infection with *Actinomyces* or one of the other etiologic agents plus pigmented anaerobic gram-negative bacilli, *Bacteroides* species, other anaerobes, and perhaps *Actinobacillus (Haemophilus) actinomycetemcomitans.* A large number of cases of pelvic actinomycosis caused by *Actinomyces* or *Eubacterium* have been described in association with the use of intrauterine contraceptive devices (IUDs). The *Actinomyces* are also associated with periodontal disease.

Actinomyces species, particularly *A. israelii,* produce phosphatases and capsular material.

35.3.b. Morphology and general characteristics. Except for *A. meyeri* whose rods are usually small and nonbranching, *Actinomyces* cells are often branching and beaded. Diphtheroid and coccal forms are also seen. The microscopic morphology of a Gram stain of "sulfur granules" (Figure 35.13) from actinomycotic pus shows a tangled mass of long filamentous forms displaying a similar morphology (Figure 35.14). Two *Actinomyces* have characteristic colony morphology. *A. israelii* typically produces a characteristic white, heaped, rough, lobate colony

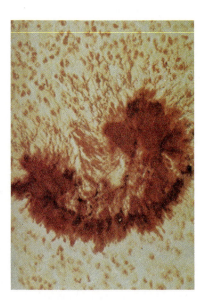

Figure 35.14
Sulfur granule, microscopic. Actinomycosis. Note aggregate of filamentous bacilli and other debris.

resembling a molar tooth (see Figure 34.9) but may also produce a breadcrumblike, raspberry, or smooth colony; *A. odontolyticus* colonies usually turn red on blood agar after several days' incubation. Colonies of the other *Actinomyces* generally are smooth, flat to convex, gray-white, and translucent, with entire margins. *A. pyogenes* and sometimes *A. odontolyticus* produce β-hemolysis. The *Actinomyces* are generally slow growers, so agar plates should be incubated for a minimum of 7 days. Many require CO_2 for growth. Some of the *Actinomyces* produce tight aggregates (balls) in broth (Figure 35.15). Growth in broth may be enhanced with Tween 80 supplementation. Most of the *Actinomyces* are microaerophilic, although many grow better anaerobically. *A. meyeri* is an obligate anaerobe.

35.3.c. Identification. With rare strain variation, the *Actinomyces* produce major succinic and lactic acid. There are several selective media for *Actinomyces*, but no one medium will isolate all species. A metronidazole–cadmium sulfate–containing medium effectively isolates and presumptively identifies *A. viscosus* and *A. naeslundii* from dental specimens. A metronidazole disk added to a PEA plate may help select for *Actinomyces* and other aerotolerant, anaerobic, gram-positive bacilli.

Most *Actinomyces* are nitrate-positive and all are indole-negative (Figure 35.16). Other useful simple tests for identification are urease, catalase, and gelatin hydrolysis. *A. naeslundii* is urease-positive, while the others are urease-negative, except for *A. viscosus*, which is rarely urease-positive. *A. viscosus* is catalase-positive. It is often overlooked, because it is assumed to be a *Propionibacterium* or diphtheroid and therefore less likely to be important. Unlike *P. acnes*, it grows equally well aerobically and anaerobically, usually hydrolyzes esculin, does not produce indole, is nonproteolytic, does not produce a pink sediment in thioglycollate broth, and is more fermentative. Definitive identification of *Actinomyces* sp. requires further biochemical tests (see Table 35.6). Some workers have found the microcolony (the colony at a very young age) morphology on supplemented brain-heart infusion agar to be helpful in differentiating species.

35.3.d. Susceptibility to antimicrobials. Penicillin G remains the drug of choice in the treatment of actinomycosis. Tetracycline, clindamycin, and erythromycin also demonstrate activity against these organisms. Metronidazole is relatively poor in activity against *Actinomyces*, in sharp contrast to its excellent activity against virtually all other clinically important anaerobes (other non-spore-forming, anaerobic, gram-positive rods also tend to be resistant to metronidazole). Clindamycin treatment failures are probably due to the presence of clindamycin-resis-

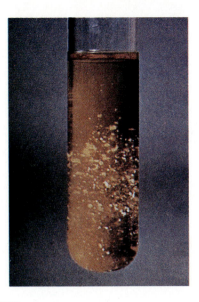

Figure 35.15
A. israelii in thioglycollate broth showing no growth near the surface and tight aggregates of growth.

tant bacteria, such as *Actinobacillus (Haemophilus) actinomycetemcomitans*.

34.4. *Bifidobacterium* Species

35.4.a. Normal flora and infections. *Bifidobacterium* species are part of the normal flora in the gastrointestinal tract and may play a protective role in preventing ingrowth of pathogens. They may reside as normal flora in the oral cavity. These organisms are rarely isolated from clinical material, although *B. dentium* (formerly *B. eriksonii*) has been isolated from mixed flora pulmonary infections, some of which may be severe.

35.4.b. Morphology and general characteristics. The most conspicuous feature of bifidobacteria cells is their various shapes, with pronounced clubbing or bifurcated ends. Diphtheroidal and branching forms may also be observed, but the cells are usually thicker than *Actinomyces*. *B. dentium* produces a white, convex, shiny colony with an irregular edge and has diffuse growth in broth (unlike most *Actinomyces* species). Like *Lactobacillus* species, they are acidophilic and grow best on low pH agar (for example, tomato juice agar). Some bifidobacteria grow aerobically in the presence of CO_2.

35.4.c. Identification. *Bifidobacterium* species produce major amounts of acetic and lactic acids in peptone yeast glucose broth, with acetic acid in

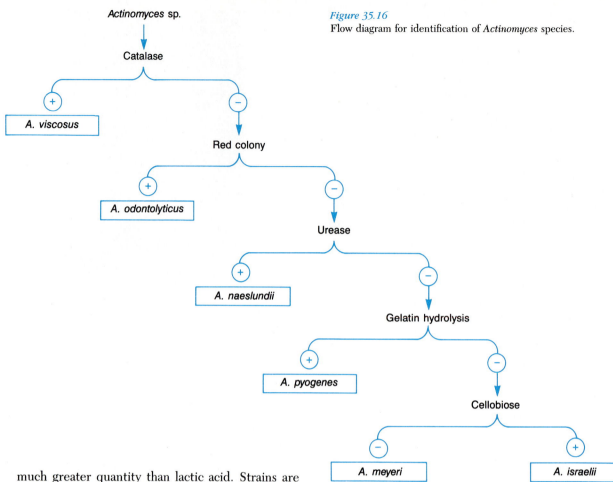

Figure 35.16
Flow diagram for identification of *Actinomyces* species.

much greater quantity than lactic acid. Strains are generally indole-, nitrate-, and catalase-negative, with a rare catalase-positive strain. The bifidobacteria are saccharolytic and produce a low pH in carbohydrate media. Definitive identification requires many biochemical tests (Table 35.6).

35.5. *Eubacterium* Species

35.5.a. Normal flora and infections. *Eubacterium* species reside in the gastrointestinal tract and are usually part of the indigenous oral flora as well. *Eubacterium* species are usually not particularly pathogenic. In rare cases, they have caused endocarditis. These bacteria have been isolated from blood, abscesses, dental infections, and wounds, but always with other anaerobes or facultative bacteria. *E. nodatum* has been isolated from actinomycosis of the jaw and IUD-associated genital tract infections.

35.5.b. Morphology and general characteristics. The Gram-stain appearance of *Eubacterium* species varies greatly. They often appear as pleomorphic

rods to coccobacilli occurring in pairs or short chains, but also as straight uniform or curved rods. *E. alactolyticum* has a sea-gull-wing shape. *E. nodatum* may appear the same as *Actinomyces*—beading, filamentous, branching. *E. lentum* is a small, straight rod with rounded ends. Colonies of *Eubacterium* tend to be fairly nondescript—raised to convex and transparent to translucent. The colony apearance of *E. nodatum*, however, may be similar to *A. israelii* (heaped, raspberry, or molar tooth–like).

35.5.c. Identification. By default, any anaerobic gram-positive bacillus that does not fit any of the other described genera is classified as *Eubacterium* species. All members are obligate anaerobes and catalase-negative, and most are nonmotile. This genus can be divided into three groups based on volatile and nonvolatile fatty acid patterns: (1) butyric acid

Table 35.6
Characteristics of Gram-Positive Non-Spore-Forming Bacilli

Organism	INDOLE PRODUCTION	CATALASE	UREASE	NITRATE REDUCTION	RED COLONY	STRONG GELATIN HYDROLYSIS	ESCULIN HYDROLYSIS	OXYGEN TOLERANCE	FERMENTATION OF: AMYGDALIN	CELLOBIOSE	GLUCOSE	MALTOSE	MANNITOL	SUCROSE	FATTY ACIDS FROM PYG BROTH
Actinomyces															
A. israelii	−	−	−	$+^-$	−	−	+	AM	+	+	+	+	+	+	A L S
A. odontolyticus	−	−	−	+	+	−	V	AM	−	+	+	$+^-$	+	$+^-$	A S
A. meyeri	−	−	−	−	−	+	−	A	$+^-$	−	+	+	−	+	A S
A. pyogenes	−	−	$+^-$	−	−	−	−	AF	$+^-$	−	+	$+^-$	−	−	A L S
A. naeslundii	−	+	+	$+^-$	−	−	V	MF	$+^-$	$+^-$	+	$+^-$	−	+	A L S
A. viscosus	−	+	V	+	−	−	V	AMF	V	V	+	+	$-^+$	+	A L [A > L]
Bifidobacterium	−	−	V	−	−	−	+	AM	V	V	+	+	$-^+$	V	A L [A > L]
B. dentium	−	−		−	−	−	+	A	+	V	+	V	$-^+$	+	A L [A > L]
Eubacterium															
E. lentum	V	−	−	$+^-$	−	−	−	A	+	−	−	−	−	−	(a l s)
Lactobacillus	−	−	−	$-^+$	−	−	V	AM	V	V	$+^-$	$+^-$	V	$+^-$	A L [L > A]
Propionibacterium															
P. acnes	$+^-$	$+^-$	−	$+^-$	−	+	−	AM	−	−	+	+	$-^+$	−	A P (iv L s)
P. avidum	−	+	−	−	−	+	+	AMF	−	−	+	+	$-^+$	+	A P (iv s)
P. granulosum	−	+	−	−	−	$-^+$	−	AM	$-^+$	−	+	$+^-$	$+^-$	+	A P (iv s)
P. propionicus	−	−	−	+	−	$+^-$	+	AF	V	−	+	+	+	+	A P S (L)

Reactions: Results in **bold type** are key reactions; superscripts represent rare strain reactions; − = negative; + = positive; V = variable.

PRAS carbohydrates: + = pH <5.5; W = pH 5.5 to 5.7; − = pH >5.7.

Fatty acids: A = acetic; P = propionic; IV = isovaleric; L = lactic; S = succinic. NOTE: (1) Capital letters indicate major (2) Small letters indicate minor products. (3) Parentheses indicate a variable reaction. (4) Isoacids are primarily from carbohydrate-free media (such as PY in the case of saccharolytic organisms.

Oxygen tolerance: A = anaerobic; M = microaerophilic; F = facultative.

Data from Sutter et al., 1985; Cummins and Johnson, 1986; Hill et al., 1987; Holdeman et al., 1977; Schal, 1986.

producers, (2) nonbutyric acid producers, and (3) little or no fermentation acids. As described in Chapter 34, *E. lentum* can be presumptively identified on the basis of arginine stimulation in broth culture, nitrate reduction, and typical microscopic morphology.

35.6. *Lactobacillus* Species

35.6.a. Normal flora and infections. Lactobacilli are prominent as normal flora in the vagina and colon, and are found in smaller numbers in the mouth. They are only occasionally involved in human infections, usually pleuropulmonary infections or dental caries, and almost always as part of a mixed bacterial flora. They have been isolated, but rarely, from urinary tract infection, bacteremia, endocarditis, local suppurative infections, and chorioamnionitis.

35.6.b. Morphology and general characteristics. Generally, lactobacilli cells are straight and uniform with rounded ends, and they may form chains. Some are short and so coccobacillary as to be confused with streptococci. The organisms are microaerophilic, but usually form larger colonies in an anaerobic atmosphere. Colonies on sheep blood or chocolate agar grown in an enriched CO_2 atmosphere are usually small, and sometimes greening is observed. As with the bifidobacteria, they grow best on a low pH medium.

35.6.c. Identification. *Lactobacillus* species produce major amounts of lactic acid with or without smaller amounts of acetic acid. With rare exception, they are nonmotile and indole-, catalase-, and nitrate-negative. Definitive identification requires a battery of chemical and biochemical tests.

35.6.d. Susceptibility to antimicrobials. Most strains are susceptible to penicillin, but higher doses of the drug may be required for refractory cases.

35.7. *Propionibacterium* Species

35.7.a. Normal flora and infections. *Propionibacterium* species are part of the normal flora of the skin but are also recovered from the gastrointestinal tract, upper respiratory tract (especially the anterior nares), and the urogenital tract. Because of their presence on skin, propionibacteria are often contaminants. *P. acnes* is frequently a contaminant of blood cultures and other sterile body fluids. *P. granulosum* and *P. avidum* may also represent contaminants from the skin. Accordingly, particular care must be exercised in the preparation of the skin before veni-

puncture, lumbar puncture, aspiration of pus from an abscess, and so on, as described in Chapters 6 and 14. Recovery of the same organism on repeat cultures or from serial blood culture bottles is suggestive that the organism is a pathogen. Various *Propionibacterium* species, particularly *P. acnes*, have been implicated in infections related to heart valves and prosthetic devices, such as artificial joints and ventricular shunts. These infections may lead to osteomyelitis, bacteremia, endocarditis, and meningitis. Most of these infections are chronic in nature. *P. acnes* plays a role in acne. *P. avidum* and *P. granulosum* are rarely isolated from clinical material. *P. propionicus* (formerly *Arachnia propionica*) is a cause of actinomycosis.

P. acnes produces several enzymes, including hyaluronidase, chondroitin sulfatase, neuraminidase, acylneuraminic acid, lyase, and a lipase that hydrolyzes triglycerides but not phospholipids, cholesterol, linolenate or the lipids in egg yolk. The lipase frees long-chain fatty acids in the skin that may be irritating enough to contribute to formation of acne pustules, although other factors are certainly of importance as well. Many strains of anaerobic propionibacteria enhance cellular and humoral immunity in certain animals and in humans, under certain conditions.

35.7.b. Morphology and general characteristics. *Propionibacterium* species are often referred to as the anaerobic diphtheroids, because the bacilli are irregular, pleomorphic, and often club-shaped, with one end round and the other tapered. At times, short branching and beading forms can be observed. Young colonies of *P. acnes* are small and white to gray-white, and older colonies are often yellow. They are sometimes β-hemolytic. As with other anaerobic non-spore-forming bacilli, many *Propionibacterium* species are aerotolerant but demonstrate better growth anaerobically. *Propionibacterium* species generally grow well in broth, especially in the presence of Tween 80.

35.7.c. Identification. When grown in peptone yeast glucose broth, *Propionibacterium* species produce a major amount of propionic and acetic acids with a lesser amount of lactic, succinic, and isovaleric acids. Except for *P. propionica* and a few other strains, the propionibacteria are catalase-positive. When an anaerobic diphtheroid is nitrate- and indole-positive, it can be identified as *P. acnes* (Fig-

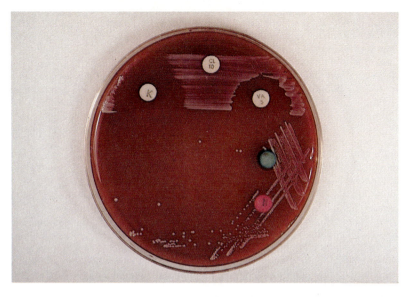

Figure 35.17
P. acnes. Disk identification tests: indole- and nitrate-positive. (From Sutter, V.L., Citron, D.M., Edelstein, M.A.C., and Finegold, S.M. 1985. Wadsworth anaerobic bacteriology manual, ed. 4. Star Publishing Co., Belmont, Calif.)

ure 35.17). A few strains of *P. acnes* are negative for one or all of the tests.

35.7.d. Susceptibility to antimicrobials. *P. acnes* is very sensitive to penicillin and most other antibiotics, except for the aminoglycosides. As with most other aerotolerant anaerobic gram-positive bacilli, these bacteria are resistant to metronidazole.

BIBLIOGRAPHY

Aureli, P., Fenicia, L., Pasolini, B., et al., 1986. Two cases of type E infant botulism caused by neurotoxigenic *Clostridium butyricum* in Italy. J. Infect. Dis. 154:207.

Banks, E.R., Allen, S.D., Siders, J.A., and O'Bryan, N.A. 1989. Characterization of anaerobic bacteria by using a commercially available rapid tube test for glutamic acid decarboxylase. J. Clin. Microbiol. 27:361.

Bartlett, J.G., Chang, T.W., Gurwith, M., et al., 1978. Antibiotic-associated pseudomembranous colitis due to toxin-producing clostridia. N. Engl. J. Med. 298:531.

Branger, C., Bruneau, B., and Goullet, P. 1987. Septicemia caused by *Propionibacterium granulosum* in a compromised patient. J. Clin. Microbiol. 25:2405.

Brazier, J.S. 1984. Ultra-violet fluorescence of *Clostridium perfringens*. Microbios letters 25:89.

Brock, D.W., Georg, L.K., Brown, J.M., and Hicklin, M.D. 1973. Actinomycosis caused by *Arachnia propionica:* report of 11 cases. Am. J. Clin. Pathol. 59:66.

Buchanan, A.G. 1982. Clinical laboratory evaluation of a reverse CAMP test for presumptive identification of *Clostridium perfringens*. J. Clin. Microbiol. 16:761.

Cato, E.P., George, W.L., and Finegold, S.M. 1986. Genus *Clostridium* Prazmowski 1880. In Sneath, P.H.A., Mair, N.S., Sharpe, M.E., and Holt, J.G., editors: Bergey's manual of systematic bacteriology, vol. 2, pp. 1141-1200. Williams & Wilkins, Baltimore.

Charfreitag, O., Collins, M.D., and Stackebrandt, E. 1988. Reclassification of *Arachnia propionica* as *Propionibacterium propionicus* comb. nov. Int. J. Syst. Bacteriol. 38:354.

Coleman, R.M., Georg, L.K., and Rozzell, A.R. 1969. *Actinomyces naeslundii* as an agent of human actinomycosis. Appl. Microbiol. 18:420.

Cummins, C.S., and Johnson, J.J. 1986. Genus I. *Propionibacterium* Orla-Jensen 1909. In Sneath, P.H.A., Mair, N.S., Sharpe, M.E., and Holt, J.G., editors: Bergey's manual of systematic bacteriology, vol. 2, pp. 1346-1353. Williams & Wilkins, Baltimore.

Dowell, V.R., Jr., and Hawkins, T.M. 1968. Detection of clostridial toxins, toxin neutralization tests, and pathogenicity tests. Centers for Disease Control, Atlanta, Ga.

Dunne, W.M., Jr., Kurschenbaum, H.A., Deshur, W.R., et al. 1986. *Propionibacterium avidum* as the etiologic agent of splenic abscess. Diagn. Microbiol. Infect. Dis. 4:87.

Finegold, S.M. 1977. Anaerobic bacteria in human disease. Academic Press, New York.

George, W.L. 1984. Antimicrobial agent–associated colitis and diarrhea: historical background and clinical aspects. Rev. Infect. Dis 6(Suppl.):S208.

George, W.L., Sutter, V.L., Citron, D., and Finegold, S.M. 1979. Selective and differential medium for isolation of *Clostridium difficile*. J. Clin. Microbiol. 9:214.

Gerencser, M.A., and Slack, J.M. 1969. Identification of human strains of *Actinomyces viscosus*. Appl. Microbiol. 18:80.

Gorbach, S.L., and Thadepalli, H. 1975. Isolation of *Clostridium* in human infections: evaluation of 114 cases. J. Infect. Dis. 131(Suppl.):S81.

Hill, G.B., Ayers, O.M., and Kohan, A.P. 1987. Characteristics and sites of infection of *Eubacterium nodatum, Eubacterium timidum, Eubacterium brachy,* and other asaccharolytic eubacteria. J. Clin. Microbiol. 25:1540.

Holdeman, L.V., Cato, E.P., and Moore, W.E.C. 1977. Anaerobe laboratory manual, ed. 4. Virginia Polytechnic Institute and State University, Blacksburg, Va.

Jilly, B.J., Schreckenberger, P.C., and LeBeau, L.J. 1984. Rapid glutamic acid decarboxylase test for identification of *Bacteroides* and *Clostridium* spp. J. Clin. Microbiol. 19:592.

Kornman, K.S., and Loesche, W.J. 1978. New medium for isolation of *Actinomyces viscosus* and *Actinomyces naeslundii* from dental plaque. J. Clin. Microbiol. 7:514.

Lambert, R.F., Jr., Brown, J.M., and Georg, L.K. 1967. Identification of *Actinomyces israelii* and *Actinomyces naeslundii* by fluorescent antibody and agar-gel diffusion techniques. J. Bacteriol. 94:1287.

McCroskey, L.M., Hatheway, C.L., Fenicia, L., et al. 1986. Characterization of an organism that produces type E botulinal toxin, but which resembles *Clostridium butyricum* from the feces of an infant with type E botulism. J. Clin. Microbiol. 23:201.

Midura, T.F., and Arnon, S.S. 1976. Infant botulism: identification of *C. botulinum* and its toxin in faeces. Lancet 2:934.

Moore, L.V.H., Cato, E.P., and Moore, W.E.C. 1987 and 1988. VPI Anaerobe laboratory manual update, supplement to the VPI anaerobe laboratory manual, ed. 4. 1977. Virginia Polytechnic Institute and State University, Blacksburg, Va.

Noble, R.C., and Overman, S.B. 1987. *Propionibacterium acnes* osteomyelitis: case report and review of the literature. J. Clin. Microbiol. 25:251.

Pine, L., Malcolm, G.B., Curtis, E.M., and Brown, J.M. 1981. Demonstration of *Actinomyces* and *Arachnia* species in cervicovaginal smears by direct staining with species-specific fluorescent-antibody conjugate. J. Clin. Microbiol. 13:15.

Rochford, J.C. 1980. Pleuropulmonary infection associated with *Eubacterium brachy*, a new species of *Eubacterium*. J. Clin. Microbiol. 12:722.

Schal, K.P. 1986. Genus *Actinomyces* Harz 1877 and Genus *Arachnia* Pine and Georg 1969. In Sneath, P.H.A., Mair, N.S., Sharpe, M.E., and Holt, J.G., editors: Bergey's manual of systematic bacteriology, vol. 2, pp. 1332-1342; 1383-1418. Williams & Wilkins, Baltimore.

Smith, L.DS. 1975. The pathogenic anaerobic bacteria, ed. 2. Charles C Thomas, Publisher, Springfield, Ill.

Suen, J.C., Hatheway, C.L., Steigerwalt, A.G., and Brenner, D.J. 1988. *Clostridium argentinense* sp. nov.: a genetically homogeneous group composed of all strains of *Clostridium botulinum* toxin type G and some nontoxigenic strains previously identified as *Clostridium subterminale* or *Clostridium hastiforme*. Int. J. Syst. Bacteriol. 38:375.

Sussman, J.I., Baron, E.J., Goldberg, S.M., et al. 1986. Clinical manifestations and therapy of lactobacillus endocarditis: report of a case and review of the literature. Rev. Infect. Dis. 8:771.

Sutter, V.L., Citron, D.M., Edelstein, M.A.C., and Finegold, S.M. 1985. Wadsworth anaerobic bacteriology manual, ed. 4. Star Publishing Co., Belmont, Calif.

Wang, W.L.L., Everett, E.D., Johnson, M., and Dean, E. 1977. Susceptibility of *Propionibacterium acnes* to seventeen antibiotics. Antimicrob. Agents Chemother. 11:171.

Willis, A.T. 1977. Anaerobic bacteriology: clinical and laboratory practice. Butterworth & Co. (Publishers), London.

Willis, A.T. 1969. Clostridia of wound infection. Butterworth & Co. (Publishers), London.

36 Anaerobic Gram-Negative Bacilli

Martha A.C. Edelstein

36.1. Bacteroidaceae

The anaerobic gram-negative rods belong to the family Bacteroidaceae (see Table 36.1 and box). They are obligately anaerobic, non-spore-forming bacilli that are straight, curved, or helical and either motile or nonmotile. They metabolize carbohydrates, peptones, or metabolic intermediates; most species produce organic acids. Although not a member of the Bacteroidaceae, the anaerobic bacterium *Campylobacter concisus* is included because it is similar to some *Bacteroides* and *Wolinella*.

The Bacteroidaceae are prevalent among the indigenous flora of humans and animals, primarily on mucosal surfaces. In many locations they are the dominant members of the normal flora.

Of the anaerobes, the gram-negative rods are those most commonly involved in infections and constitute one third of the total anaerobic isolates from clinical specimens. Anaerobic or mixed infections may develop by disruption of a mucosal surface or introduction of anaerobes into a normally sterile site through, for example, surgical manipulations, trauma, disease, aspiration of oropharyngeal secretions, or seeding of an organism in the course of bacteremia. Infection with gram-negative anaerobic bacilli, as with anaerobic infection generally, is characterized by abscess formation and tissue destruction. The most common infections in which gram-negative anaerobic rods participate are pleuropulmonary, intraabdominal, and female genital tract infections, but infections of any type anywhere in the body may involve these organisms (Figure 36.1). Most of the gram-negative bacilli isolated from

Table 36.1

Differentiation of Genera of Anaerobic Gram-Negative Bacilli

I. Nonmotile	
A. Major end product: butyric without isoacids	*Fusobacterium*
B. Major end product: lactic acid	*Leptotrichia*
C. Major end product: acetic; H_2S produced	*Desulfomonas*
D. Major end product: not as above (A, B, or C)	
1. Pigmented and nonfermentative	*Porphyromonas*
2. Other than D.1	
a. Common clinical isolate	*Bacteroides*
b. Rare clinical isolate	
(1) Strongly fermentative	*Mitsuokella*
(2) Weakly fermentative	*Anaerorhabdus*
II. Motile	
A. Fermentative	
1. Major end product: butyric acid	*Butyrivibrio*
2. Major end product: succinic acid	
a. Single, polar flagellum	
(1) Spiral-shaped cell	*Succinivibrio*
(2) Straight ovoid cell	*Succinimonas*
b. Bipolar tufts of flagella	*Anaerobiospirillum*
3. Major end product: propionic acid	
a. Single polar flagellum	*Anaerovibrio*
b. Tufts of flagella	
(1) Near center concave side	*Selenomonas*
(2) Lateral spiral arrangement	*Centipeda*
B. Nonfermentative	
1. Single polar flagellum	
a. Usually oxidase strongly positive	*Campylobacter*
b. Oxidase weak positive to negative	*Wolinella*
2. Tufts of flagella	*Mobiluncus*
3. Peritrichous flagellation	*Tissierella*

Data from Sutter et al., 1985; Holdeman et al., 1984.

human infections belong to the genera *Bacteroides,* *Porphyromonas,* or *Fusobacterium.*

Many of these organisms produce enzymes that may play a role in pathogenesis. For example, *Bacteroides, Porphyromonas,* and *Fusobacterium* produce collagenase, neuraminidase, DNase, heparinase, and proteinases. Several gram-negative anaerobic rods inhibit phagocytic uptake and killing of aerobes.

Specimen collection and transport are of utmost importance in documenting the role of gram-negative anaerobic rods in an infectious process (see Chapter 6). Since these organisms are so prevalent on mucosal surfaces, it is important to avoid contaminating the specimen with normal flora when collecting a specimen. Transport must be carried out in an oxygen-free atmosphere.

36.1.a. Morphology and general characteristics. Cell morphology varies greatly within the family

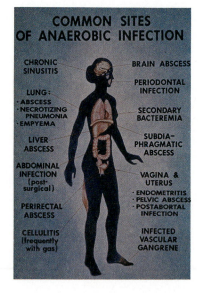

Figure 36.1

Common sites of anaerobic infection.

Family Bacteroidaceae

Bacteroides fragilis group (Table 36.3)

    B. fragilis
    B. vulgatus
    B. distasonis
    B. caccae
    B. merdae
    B. thetaiotaomicron
    B. uniformis
    B. ovatus
    B. stercoris

Pigmenting organisms (Table 36.4)

    Pigmenting *Bacteroides*
      B. intermedius
      B. corporis
      B. bivius
      B. melaninogenicus
      B. loescheii
      B. denticola
    Porphyromonas
      P. asaccharolyticus
      P. endodontalis
      P. gingivalis

Nonpigmenting, bile-sensitive organisms (Table 36.5)

    B. oralis group
      B. oralis
      B. veroralis
      B. buccalis
      B. oulorum
    Ferment pentoses
      B. oris
      B. buccae
      B. heparinolyticus
      B. zoogleoformans
    Other *Bacteroides*
      B. bivius
      B. disiens
    Require formate and fumarate
      B. ureolyticus
      B. gracilis
      Wolinella sp.
      "Campylobacter concisus"

Fusobacterium (Table 36.6)

    F. nucleatum
    F. necrophorum
    Bile-resistant
      F. mortiferum
      F. varium
      Other *Fusobacterium* sp.
    Other *Fusobacterium* sp.

Bacteroidaceae. Some cells may be filamentous, pleomorphic, vacuolated, or stain irregularly, and motile ones may be peritrichous or have polar or bipolar flagella. Cell morphology is a useful differential factor for some genera and species (see Table 36.1). For example, *Fusobacterium nucleatum* is a thin bacillus with pointed ends, whereas most other fusobacteria have rounded ends.

There is no one typical colony morphology for the Bacteroidaceae, and they cannot be easily differentiated from obligately aerobic or facultative anaerobic gram-negative bacilli without an aerotolerance test. Some species or groups within each genus have a characteristic morphology. For example, the pigmented *Bacteroides* sp. and *Porphyromonas* produce pigment, and the *B. ureolyticus* group produces an agarase that pits the agar around the colony. Some gram-negative anaerobic rods are encapsulated and some are surrounded by less well-defined polysaccharide material.

36.1.b. Differentiation of anaerobic gram-negative rods. Classically, the Bacteroidaceae are identified by motility and location of flagella in motile forms, metabolic end products, and cell shape (Table 36.1). Practically, few tests are needed for recognizing *Bacteroides*, *Porphyromonas*, and *Fusobacterium*. These tests are detailed in Chapter 34 and later in this chapter. A motility test is not routinely required, because most gram-negative anaerobic bacilli isolated from clinical material are nonmotile. However, a motility test and flagellar stain should be performed on curved or helical bacilli, ones with unusual cell or colony morphology, urease-negative formate- and fumarate-requiring rods, or when the organism cannot be identified by usual tests. Tests for the presence of malate and glutamate dehydrogenase, respiratory quinones, glucose-6-phosphate and 6-phosphogluconate dehydrogenase, and the guanine plus cytosine percent will likely supersede or augment current tests for determining genus identification.

36.2. *Bacteroides* and *Porphyromonas*

The anaerobic gram-negative bacilli *Bacteroides* and *Porphyromonas* are nonmotile straight rods with rounded ends and produce a variety of metabolic end products, usually including succinic acid.

36.2.a. **Taxonomic changes.** Some taxonomic changes in the *Bacteroides* are due to new chemotaxonomic approaches to categorizing bacteria and others to investigations into the bacterial flora of primarily healthy and diseased sites, particularly dental structures. Table 36.2 lists many of these taxonomic changes. It has recently been proposed to limit the genus *Bacteroides* to the *Bacteroides fragilis* group. Three previously unnamed members of the *B. fragilis* group have acquired species names: *B. caccae*, *B. stercoris*, and *B. merdae*. *B. caccae* (formerly "3452 A") has been isolated from clinical infections. So far the other two have been isolated only as part of the normal bowel flora. The asaccharolytic pigmented *Bacteroides* sp. now belong to the genus *Porphyromonas*. Several new species from animal sources have been described and these may be important in animal bite wounds. *B. ureolyticus* and *B. gracilis*, along with *Wolinella* sp., may be transferred in whole or in part to *Campylobacter*.

36.2.b. **Normal flora, infections, and virulence factors.** The *Bacteroides* and *Porphyromonas* are found as part of the indigenous flora of the oropharynx, gastrointestinal tract, and genitourinary tract. The *B. fragilis* group forms the largest part of the gut flora. The pigmented *Bacteroides* sp. reside in the oropharynx, upper respiratory tract, genitourinary and gastrointestinal tracts, and *Porphyromonas* is primarily isolated from dental structures.

In general, the *B. fragilis* group predominantly causes infections occurring below the diaphragm,

Table 36.2

Taxonomic Changes in Anaerobic Gram-Negative Bacilli

NEW	OLD
Bacteroides	
B. buccae	*B. ruminicola* subsp. *brevis* biotype 3
B. buccalis	Part of *B. oralis*
B. caccae	"3452A"
B. corporis	*B. melaninogenicus* ss. *intermedius*, in part
B. denticola	Part of *B. melaninogenicus*
B. forsythus	sp. nov.
B. gracilis	sp. nov.
B. heparinolyticus	sp. nov.
B. intermedius	*B. melaninogenicus* ss. *intermedius*, in part
B. loescheii	Part of *B. melaninogenicus*
B. melaninogenicus	*B. melaninogenicus* ss. *melaninogenicus*, in part
B. merdae	*B. fragilis* group "T4-1"
B. oris	Part of *B. ruminicola* subsp. *brevis* biotype 3
B. oulorum	sp. nov.
B. stercoris	*B. fragilis* group "subspecies a"
B. veroralis	Part of *B. oralis*
Fusobacterium	
F. alocis	sp. nov.
F. periodonticum	sp. nov.
F. sulci	sp. nov.
F. ulcerans	sp. nov.
Porphyromonas	genus nov.
P. asaccharolyticus	*B. asaccharolyticus*
P. endodontalis	*B. endodontalis*
P. gingivalis	*B. gingivalis*
Anaerorhabdus	genus nov.
A. furcosus	*B. furcosus*
Centipeda periodontii	genus nov., sp. nov.
Mitsuokella	genus nov.
M. dentalis	sp. nov.
M. multiacida	*B. multiacidus*
Selenomonas	
S. artemidis	sp. nov.
S. dianae	sp. nov.
S. flueggei	sp. nov.
S. infelix	sp. nov.
S. noxia	sp. nov.
Tissierella praeacuta	*B. praeacutus*
Wolinella	genus nov.
W. curva	sp. nov.
W. recta	sp. nov.
W. succinogenes	*Vibrio succinogenes*

such as intra-abdominal abscess, including liver abscess, and decubitus ulcers, but may cause any type of infection, including bacteremia. They have been isolated infrequently from pleuropulmonary infection or brain abscess. *B. fragilis* is the most commonly encountered pathogen of all the anaerobic bacteria. Other members of the *B. fragilis* group isolated from infected material include *B. thetaiotaomicron*, *B. distasonis*, *B. caccae*, *B. uniformis*, and *B. vulgatus*.

Pigmented anaerobic gram-negative bacteria, which include pigmenting *Bacteroides* and *Porphyromonas*, are not isolated as frequently as the *B. fragilis* group; however, some species play a major role in gingivitis and periodontitis, and some are commonly isolated from head and neck infection, aspiration pneumonia, and lung abscess. Pigmenters have been isolated from female genital tract infections, but not as frequently as some of the other *Bacteroides* sp. (especially *B. bivius* and *B. disiens*). These "other" *Bacteroides* sp. (non–*B. fragilis* group and nonpigmenters) have been isolated from a wide variety of infections, but much less frequently than the *B. fragilis* group.

Capsules are produced by several species, including *B. fragilis*, *P. asaccharolyticus*, and probably *B. melaninogenicus*, *B. intermedius*, *B. oralis*, *B. oris*, and *B. buccae*. The *B. fragilis* capsule can be demonstrated by ruthenium red staining, India ink staining, and electron microscopy. The endotoxin of *B. fragilis* differs from that of other gram-negative bacilli by structure and weaker biologic activity. Nonetheless, it is clear that the capsule is a virulence factor for *B. fragilis*. *B. bivius*, in contrast to *B. fragilis*, has a potent endotoxin. *B. fragilis* also produces many enzymes such as neuraminidase, DNase, hyaluronidase, gelatinase, fibrinolysin, superoxide dismutase, and heparinase. Certain pigmented *Bacteroides* produce phospholipase A, collagenase, hyaluronidase, and fibrinolysin. Heparinase is produced by *B. heparinolyticus*.

36.2.c. Differentiation and grouping. *Bacteroides* sp. and *Porphyromonas* sp. are readily divided into three major groups based on bile susceptibility, pigment production, and antibiotic disk identification patterns. The *B. fragilis* group is nonpigmented, and bile-resistant, and resistant to all three antibiotic identification disks; the pigmented *Bacteroides* sp. and *Porphyromonas* typically produce pigment and are bile-sensitive; and the "other" *Bacteroides* sp.

are nonpigmented and bile-sensitive. *Porphyromonas* has a unique antibiotic disk identification pattern; it is resistant to colistin and sensitive to vancomycin. See Chapter 34 for more details. Figure 36.2 illustrates the major means for differentiating between various groups of *Bacteroides* and between certain *Bacteroides*, *Porphyromonas*, and *Fusobacterium* groups.

36.2.d. Bile-resistant *Bacteroides*. This group of *Bacteroides* includes the *B. fragilis* group and two other bile-resistant species not commonly encountered—*B. eggerthii* and *B. splanchnicus*.

36.2.d.1. Morphology and general characteristics. Microscopically, the members of the *B. fragilis* group are pale-staining gram-negative bacilli with rounded ends. The cells are fairly uniform, although pleomorphism and irregularity of staining are common in direct smears of clinical material or from broth cultures (Figure 36.3). Cells of *B. ovatus* are usually more ovoid. *B. fragilis* group strains produce 1 to 3 mm in diameter, smooth, white to gray, nonhemolytic, translucent colonies on blood agar (Figure 36.4). *B. thetaiotaomicron* may appear whiter than colonies of *B. fragilis*. Colonies of *B. ovatus* are often mucoid.

36.2.d.2. Identification. The *B. fragilis* group is distinguished from the other two bile-resistant *Bacteroides* species by its ability to ferment sucrose (Table 36.3). Indole and catalase and perhaps esculin are good tests for initially separating the *B. fragilis* group into smaller categories. Further tests for differentiation of species within the *B. fragilis* group and the other bile-resistant *Bacteroides* are noted in Table 36.3. A discussion of preliminary grouping and identification procedures for the various anaerobes appears in Chapter 34.

36.2.d.3. Susceptibility to antimicrobial agents. *B. fragilis* is among the most resistant of the anaerobes. This resistance applies primarily to β-lactam drugs (such as penicillins and cephalosporins) and is mediated by production of β-lactamases which, although primarily cephalosporinases, also show significant ability to hydrolyze penicillins. Certain β-lactam agents such as broad-spectrum penicillins (e.g., ticarcillin, piperacillin, and related drugs), cefoxitin, and imipenem are largely resistant to these β-lactamases and thus retain activity against *B. fragilis*. However, resistance to the preceding drugs, except for imipenem, is seen in up to 5% of strains and a few strains have demonstrated resistance to

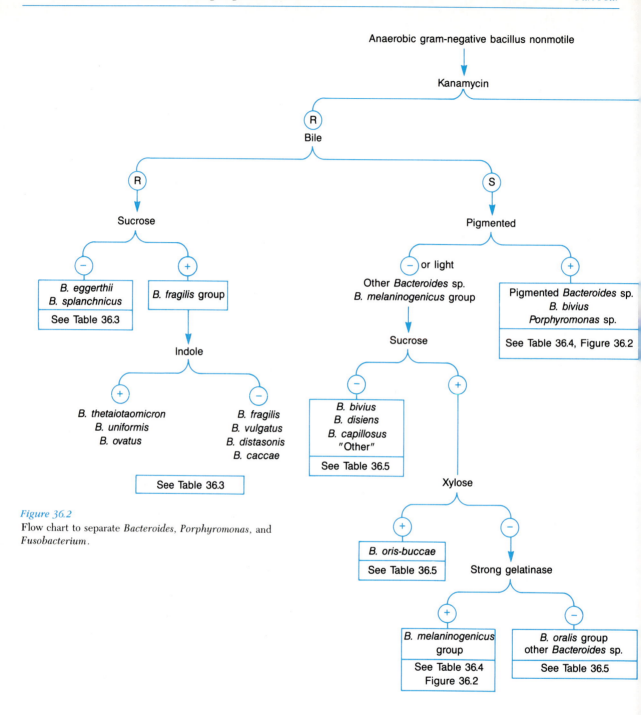

Figure 36.2
Flow chart to separate *Bacteroides, Porphyromonas,* and *Fusobacterium.*

imipenem. Resistance to tetracycline is common, and 5% to 25% of strains of *B. fragilis* are resistant to clindamycin in a number of centers. Metronidazole and chloramphenicol are active against essentially all strains of the *B. fragilis* group. Other mem-

bers of the *B. fragilis* group, notably *B. thetaiotaomicron, B. caccae,* and *B. distasonis,* may be much more resistant to antimicrobial agents.

36.2.e. **Pigmented** *Bacteroides* **and** *Porphyromonas.* Nine of the at least twelve species in this

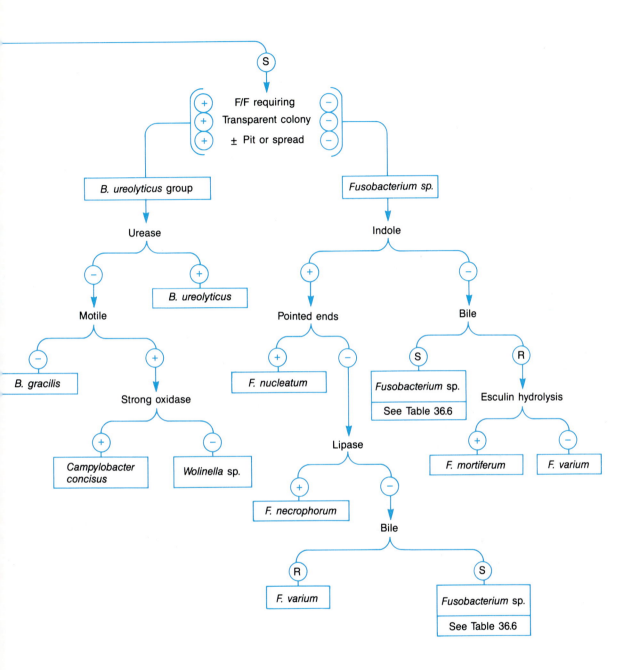

group have been isolated from human clinical material; the others are associated with animals. Those most commonly encountered are *P. asaccharolyticus*, *P. gingivalis*, *B. intermedius*, and *B. melaninogenicus*. *B. bivius* may be included here, because

it may produce pigment upon prolonged incubation.

36.2.e.1. Morphology and general characteristics. These organisms are usually seen as pale-staining coccobacilli (Figure 36.5) but may also appear as pleomorphic bacilli. Young cultures may appear

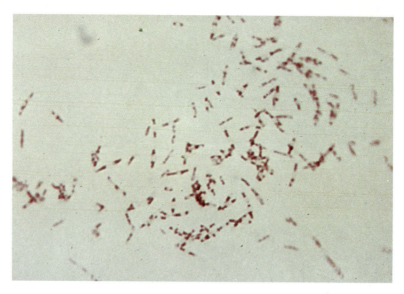

Figure 36.3
B. fragilis. Irregular staining and pleomorphism.

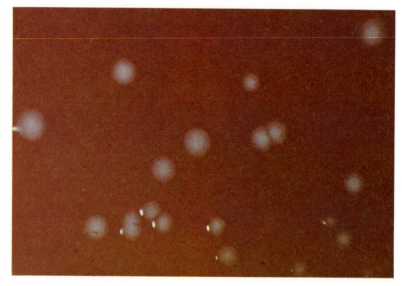

Figure 36.4
B. fragilis. Gray, shiny colony on BA.

gram-positive to gram-variable. The organisms produce a variety of colony types with varying amounts of pigment, and this may be helpful in subdividing the group. Generally, *B. intermedius* and *B. corporis* produce dark brown to black dry colonies; *Porphyromonas* colonies are usually more mucoid and dark brown to black; and the *B. melaninogenicus* group produces light tan or buff smooth colonies. Pigment production may not always be readily detected and may require prolonged incubation (greater than 2 weeks), especially with the *B. melaninogenicus* group. The use of *laked* rabbit blood agar allows the earliest and most reliable pigment production (see Figure 34.7). Colonies may fluoresce (see Figure

Table 36.3
Characteristics of Bile-Resistant *Bacteroides* Species

	GROWTH IN 20% BILE	INDOLE	CATALASE	ESCULIN HYDROLYSIS	FERMENTATION OF SUCROSE	MALTOSE	ARABINOSE	CELLOBIOSE	RHAMNOSE	SALICIN	TREHALOSE	XYLAN	α-FUCOSIDASE	FATTY ACIDS FROM PEPTONE YEAST GLUCOSE BROTH
B. fragilis group														
B. fragilis	+	–	**+**	+	+	+	–	$-^w$	–	–	–	–		A p S pa
B. vulgatus	+	–	**+**$^-$	$-^+$	+	+	+	–	+	–	–	V		A p S
B. distasonis	+	–	**+**$^-$	+	+	+	$-^+$	+	V	+	+	–		A p S (ib iv l pa)
B. merdae*	+	–	$-^+$	+	+	+	$-^+$	$-^+$	+	+	–	–		A S (p ib iv)
B. caccae	+	–	–	+	+	+	+	$-^+$	$+^-$	V	+	–	+	A S (p iv)
B. thetaiotaomicron	+	+	**+**	+	+	+	+	+	+	$-^+$	+	–		A p S pa
B. uniformis	w^+	+	$-^+$	+	+	+	+	$+^w$	$-^+$	$+^-$	–			a p l S (ib iv)
B. ovatus	+	+	$-^+$	+	+	+	+	+	$-^+$	+	+	+		A p S pa (ib iv l)
B. stercoris*	+	+	–	+	+	+	$-^+$	–	+	–	–	V	V	A p S (ib iv)
Other														
B. eggerthii*	+	+		+	–	+	+	$-^w$	w^-	–	–			A p S (ib iv l)
B. splanchnicus*	w^+	+	–	+	–	–	+	–	–	–	–			A P ib b iv S (l)

Reactions: Results in **bold type** are key characteristics; #, negative; $-^+$, rare strains positive; +, most strains positive; $+^-$, rare strain negative, $-^w$, rare strain weak positive; V, variable; w, weak positive.

PRAS carbohydrates: +, pH <5.5; 2, pH 5.5-5.7; –, pH >5.7.

Fatty acids: A, acetic; P, propionic; IB, isobuotryic; IV, isovleric; L, lactic; S, succinic; PA, phenylacetic. NOTE: (1) Capital letters indicate major metabolic products. (2) Small letters indicate minor products. (3) Parentheses indicate a variable reaction. (4) Isoacids are primarily from carbohydrate-free media (such as PY) in the case of saccharolytic organisms.

*Rarely isolated; part of the normal bowel flora.

Data from Sutter et al., 1985; Holdeman et al., 1984; Johnson et al., 1986; Moore et al., 1988.

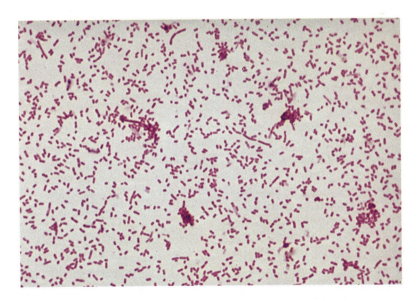

Figure 36.5
Pigmented *Bacteroides* sp. or *Porphyromonas*. Many coccobacillary forms as well as rods. (From Sutter et al. 1985)

Table 36.4

Characteristics of Pigmented Anaerobic Gram-Negative Bacilli

| | VANCOMYCIN (5 μg) | COLISTIN (10 μg) | INDOLE | LIPASE | FERMENTATION OF | | | | ESCULIN HYDROLYSIS | GROWTH 3% SALT | α-FUCOSIDASE | ARGININE DIHYDROLASE | FATTY ACIDS FROM PEPTONE YEAST GLUCOSE BROTH | PHENYLACETIC ACID |
					GLUCOSE	LACTOSE	CELLOBIOSE	SUCROSE						
Saccharolytic														
B. melaninogenicus	R	R^s	−	−	+	+	−	+	−$^+$		+	+	A S (ib iv 1)	−
B. denticola	R	R^s	−	−	+	+	−	+	+		−	−	A S (ib iv 1)	−
B. loescheii	R	R^s	−	−^{w}	+	+	+	+$^-$	−		+	−	a S (1)	−
Partially saccharolytic														
B. bivius	R	S	−	−	+	+	−	−	−		+	V	A iv S (ib)	−
B. corporis	R	S	−	−	+	−	−	−	−		−	−	A ib iv S (b)	−
B. intermedius	R	S	+	+$^-$	+	−	−	+	−		+	+	A iv S (p ib)	−
Asaccharolytic														
P. asaccharolyticus	S	R	+	−	−	−	−	−	−	G	+	+	A p ib B iv S	−
P. endodontalis	S	R	+	−	−	−	−	−	−	NG	−	−	a p ib b iv	−
P. gingivalis	S	R	+	−	−	−	−	−	−	NG	−	−	a p ib B IV s	+

Reactions: Results in **bold type** are key characteristics; R, resistant; R^s, some strains sensitive; S, sensitive; −, negative; −$^+$, rare strains positive; +, most strains positive; +$^-$, rare strain negative; −^{w}, rare strain weak positive; V, variable; G, growth; NG, no growth. *PRAS carbohydrates:* +, pH <5.5; w, pH 5.5-5.7; −, pH >5.7.
Fatty acids: A, acetic; P, propionic; IB, isobutyric; B, butyric; IV, isovaleric; L, lactic; S, succinic; PA, phenylacetic. NOTE: (1) Capital letters indicate major metabolic products. (2) Small letters indicate minor products. (3) Parentheses indicate a variable reaction. (4) Isoacids are primarily from carbohydrate-free media (such as PY) in the case of saccharolytic organisms.
Data from Sutter et al., 1985; Holdeman et al., 1984; Mayrand et al., 1984; Moore et al., 1988; Shah and Collins, 1988; van Winkelhoff et al., 1985 and 1986.

34.8) brick red, yellow-green, coral, or not at all under ultraviolet light. After pigment is produced, the fluorescence may not be detectable. Most *Porphyromonas* are difficult to grow in broth and on some selective agars containing vancomycin (for example, KVLB). Additional bicarbonate, serum, or hemin may enhance growth in broth.

36.2.e.2. Identification. The pigmenting anaerobic gram-negative bacilli are all sensitive to bile and form three groups using the antimicrobial disk identification pattern, indole reaction, and colony morphology (Table 36.4 and Figure 36.6): (1) *B. intermedius-corporis* are resistant to vancomycin and kanamycin and susceptible to colistin, their colonies are typically dry and black, and *B. intermedius* is indole-positive; (2) the *B. melaninogenicus* group (*B. loescheii, B. denticola,* and *B. melaninogenicus*) are indole-negative, often resistant to all antibiotic identification disks (colistin, kanamycin, and vancomy-

cin), and their colonies do not develop deep pigmentation; (3) *Porphyromonas* sp. are indole-positive, sensitive to vancomycin and kanamycin and resistant to colistin, and their colonies are often mucoid, shiny, smooth, and dark brown to black. Some key reactions for differentiation of species are production of indole, lipase, and phenylacetic acid; esculin hydrolysis; fermentation of glucose, lactose, and cellobiose; and salt tolerance. α-Fucosidase and arginine dihydrolase are also useful. As noted in Chapter 34, *B. intermedius* and *B. loescheii* are easy to identify when the lipase reaction is positive; *B. intermedius* is indole-positive and *B. loescheii* indole-negative.

36.2.e.3. Susceptibility to antimicrobial agents. Many of the pigmenting organisms produce β-lactamase. However, this does not always correlate with in vitro susceptibility or clinical outcome. Nonetheless, for seriously ill patients with aspiration pneu-

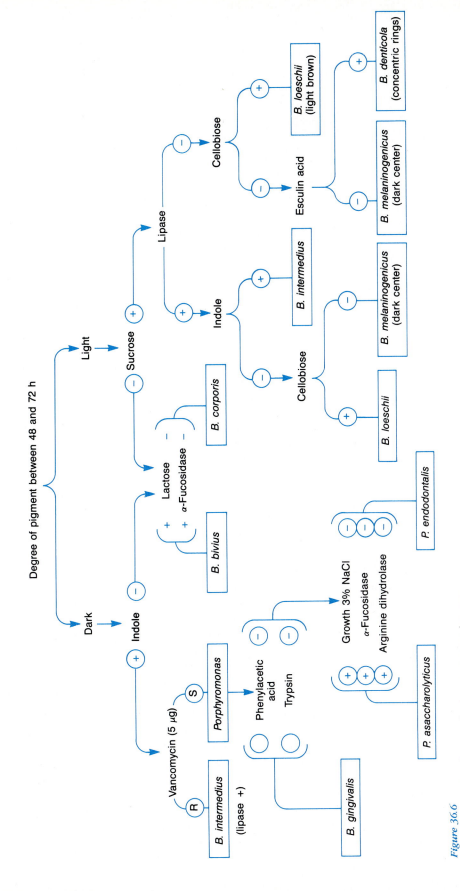

Figure 36.6
Flow chart for identification of pigmenting anaerobic gram-negative bacilli.

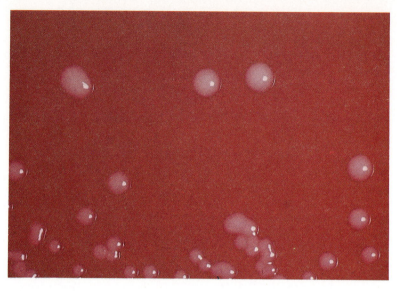

Figure 36.7
Bacteroides oris-buccae on BA. Colonies somewhat mucoid.

monia, penicillin G can no longer be considered the drug of choice for anaerobic coverage, because of the high probability of recovering a pigmenter or other resistant anaerobe from that infection. Metronidazole and chloramphenicol are universally active against these organisms; clindamycin is also usually effective. The broad-spectrum penicillins related to carbenicillin are active against about 95% of strains in this group, as is cefoxitin.

36.2.f. Bile-sensitive, nonpigmented *Bacteroides*. This remaining group of *Bacteroides* is very diverse and contains a number of organisms encountered with some frequency in various infections, but almost always as part of a mixed bacterial flora. The more frequently isolated members of this group are *B. oris* and *B. buccae* (Figure 36.7), *B. oralis*, *B. disiens*, *B. ureolyticus* (see Figures 34.5 and 36.8), and *B. gracilis*. These organisms are found as normal flora in the oral cavity, gastrointestinal tract, and genitourinary tract. They cause various infections, most commonly those of the lower respiratory and female genital tracts. *Bacteroides gracilis* may be found in serious, deep-seated infections, although its pathogenic role is not fully established.

36.2.f.1. Morphology and general characteristics. For the most part, the organisms in this group are not particularly distinctive morphologically. However, cells of *B. gracilis* and *B. ureolyticus* are usually thinner and less pleomorphic than some of the other

Bacteroides. *Wolinella* sp. and *C. concisus* may be curved rods. In addition, the colonies of these four are small and transparent and may pit the agar (see Figure 34.5) or spread (Figure 36.8). The pitting and spreading characteristics are not consistent. In broth, *B. zoogleoformans* forms a zoogleal mass (that is, the organisms are embedded in a jellylike matrix). *B. heparinolyticus* also produces a viscous mass.

36.2.f.2. Identification. This group can be subdivided into five groups (Table 36.5) based on proteolytic and fermentation activity and a requirement for formate and fumarate for growth: (1) saccharolytic pentose fermenters; (2) saccharolytic pentose nonfermenters (*B. oralis* group); (3) saccharolytic and proteolytic; (4) nonsaccharolytic or weakly saccharolytic fermenters; and (5) nonsaccharolytic formate- and fumarate-requiring. Further differentiation requires a combination of conventional biochemical tests and tests for preformed enzymes (available in rapid 4-hour identification test kits). *B. ureolyticus* and *B. gracilis* are readily differentiated from each other (*B. ureolyticus* is urease-positive) and from the motile *Wolinella* sp. and *C. concisus* (darting motility). *B. gracilis* may display a twitching motion.

36.2.f.3. Antimicrobial susceptibility. As with the pigmented *Bacteroides* and *Porphyromonas*, some resistance to β-lactam drugs has been observed, primarily with those strains producing β-lactamases.

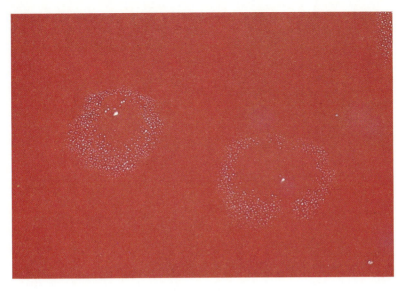

Figure 36.8
B. ureolyticus on BA. Note spreading and near transparency.

Most other antimicrobials are effective, except that 25% to 35% of *B. gracilis* strains exhibit significant resistance to clindamycin, cefoxitin, penicillin G, and piperacillin, and a very small percent of strains appear resistant to metronidazole and imipenem.

36.3. *Fusobacterium*

36.3.a. Introduction and taxonomic changes. Fusobacteria are anaerobic gram-negative bacilli that produce major butyric acid without isoacids and are nonmotile, straight, or slightly curved bacilli with pointed or rounded ends. With the exception of four newly described species—*F. alocis, F. sulcus, F. periodonticum,* and *F. ulcerans*—there have been few taxonomic changes within this genus (Table 36.2).

36.3.b. Normal flora, infections, and virulence factors. The fusobacteria are found as indigenous flora in the upper respiratory tract, in particular, but may also be found in the gastrointestinal and genitourinary tracts.

They may be implicated in infection throughout the body, but with some predilection for the lower respiratory tract, head and neck, periodontium, gingivae, and central nervous system. Of the seven fusobacteria most commonly encountered in human infections, *F. nucleatum* and *F. necrophorum* are isolated most often. *F. nucleatum* is encountered the most often by far and is clearly an important pathogen, particularly in head and neck and lower respiratory infections, but *F. necrophorum* is much more virulent. *F. necrophorum* invades the bloodstream with some frequency, particularly as part of a syndrome that begins with membranous tonsillitis, going on to septicemia and widespread metastatic infection that often includes lung abscess, empyema, liver abscess, osteomyelitis, and purulent arthritis. Other species of fusobacteria (Table 36.6) are isolated infrequently.

The lipopolysaccharide of *Fusobacterium* strains resembles that of nonanaerobic gram-negative rods in structure. With most strains, biological activity is strong. *F. necrophorum* produces a leukocidin and hemolyzes red blood cells of humans and a number of animal species. Phospholipase A and lysophospholipase are produced by *F. necrophorum*.

36.3.c. Morphology and general characteristics. The fusobacteria are pale-staining gram-negative bacilli with a diversity of cell shapes and colony morphology. *F. nucleatum* typically is a long, slender rod with tapered ends; the cells are often in pairs end-to-end (see Figure 34.3). *F. mortiferum* shows a bizarre pleomorphism, with spheroid swellings along irregularly stained filaments and free round bodies (Figure 36.9). *F. necrophorum* may occasionally resemble *F. mortiferum* or appear as a slightly pleomorphic bacillus with rounded ends. Colonies on blood agar are generally nonhemolytic

Table 36.5
Characteristics of Non-Pigmented Bile-Sensitive Anaerobic Gram-Negative Bacilli

Organism	KANAMYCIN (1 mg)	COLISTIN (10 μg)	GLUCOSE	XYLOSE (PENTOSE)	SUCROSE	LACTOSE	SALICIN	XYLAN	STRONG GELATIN HYDROLYSIS	INDOLE	ESCULIN HYDROLYSIS	α-FUCOSIDASE	NAG	ZOOGLEAL MASS	REQUIRES FORMATE-FUMARATE FOR GROWTH	NITRATE REDUCTION	MOTILE	UREASE	STRONG OXIDASE	PITS THE AGAR	FATTY ACIDS FROM PEPTONE YEAST GLUCOSE BROTH
B. oralis group																					
B. buccalis	R		+	−	+	+	−	−	−	−	+	+	+							−	a iv S
B. oulorum	R		+	−	+	+	+	−	−	−	+	+	+							−	a S
B. oralis	R		+	−	+	+	−	−	−	−	+	+	+							−	A S (1)
B. veroralis	R		+	−	+	+	−	+	−	−	+	+	+							−	a S
Pentose-fermenting																					
B. buccae	R	**S**	+	+	+	+	+	$+^-$	−	−	+	−	−							−	A S (p ib b iv 1)
B. oris	R	**R**	+	+	+	+	+	−	−	+	+	+	+							−	A S (p ib iv)
B. heparinolyticus*	R		+	+	+	+	V	−	−	−	+	+	+	$+^-$						−	S (a p iv)
B. zoogleoformans	R		+	+	+	+	−	−	−	−	+			+						−	A P S (ib iv)
Saccharolytic and proteolytic																					
B. bivius	R		+	−	−	+	−	−	+	−	−	+	+							−	A iv S (ib)
B. disiens	R		+	−	−	−	−	−	+	−	−	−	−							−	A S (p ib iv)
Weak or nonfermentative																					
B. capillosus	R		w^-	−	−	−	−	−	+	−	+									−	a s (p 1)
B. putredenis	R		−	−	−	−	−	−	+	+	−									−	a P ib b IV S (1)
Formate-fumarate-requiring																					
B. gracilis	S		−	−	−	−	−	−	−	−	−				+	+	−	−	−	$+^-$	a S (1)
B. ureolyticus	S		−	−	−	−	−	−	−	−	−				+	+	−	+	V	$+^-$	a S
Wolinella sp.	S		−	−	−	−	−	−	−	−	−				+	+	+	−	−	$-^+$	S
C. concisus	S		−	−	−	−	−	−	−	−	−				+	+	+	−	+	$-^+$	S

Reactions: Results in **bold type** are key characteristics; R, resistant; S, sensitive; −, negative; $-^+$, rare strains positive; +, most strains positive; $+^-$, rare strain negative; w^-, most strains weak, rare strains negative; V, variable. NAG, N-acetyl-glucosaminidase.

PRAS carbohydrates: +, pH <5.5; w, pH 5.5-5.7; −, pH >5.7.

Fatty acids: A, acetic; P, propionic; IB, isobutyric; B, butyric; IV, isovaleric; L, lactic; S, succinic. NOTE: (1) Capital letters indicate major metabolic products. (2) Small letters indicate minor products. (3) Parentheses indicate a variable reaction. (4) Isoacids are primarily from carbohydrate-free media (such as PY) in the case of saccharolytic organisms.

*Produces heparinase.

Data from Sutter et al., 1985; Holdeman et al., 1984; Moore et al., 1988.

Table 36.6

Characteristics of *Fusobacterium* Species

| | MICROSCOPIC FEATURES | INDOLE | GROWTH IN 20% BILE | LIPASE | GAS IN GLUCOSE AGAR | FERMENTATION OF | | | ESCULIN HYDROLYSIS | CONVERTS LACTATE TO PROPIONATE | CONVERTS THREONINE TO PROPIONATE | FATTY ACIDS FROM PEPTONE YEAST GLUCOSE BROTH |
						GLUCOSE	FRUCTOSE	MANNOSE				
F. nucleatum	**Slender pointed ends**	+	−	−	−²	−ʷ	−ʷ	−	−	−	+	a p B (L s)
F. gonidiaformans	Gonidia forms	+	−	−	4²	−	−	−	−	−	+	A p B (l s)
F. necrophorum	Round ends	+	−⁺	+⁻	4²	−ʷ	−ʷ	−	−	+	+	a p B (l s)
F. naviforme	**Boat shape**	+	−	−	−	Wˉ	−	−	−	−	−	a B L (p s)
F. varium	Small, round ends	+⁻	+	−	4	+ʷ	+ʷ	+ʷ	−	−	+	a p B L (s)
F. mortiferum	**Bizarre, round bodies**	−	+	−	4	+ʷ	+ʷ	+ʷ	+	−	+	a p B (v l a)
F. russii	Round ends	−	−	−	2ˉ	−	−	−	−	−	−	a B L

Reactions: Results in **bold type** are key characteristics; −, negative; −⁺, rare strains positive; +, most strains positive; +⁻, rare strain negative; −ʷ, rare strain weak positive; wˉ, most strains weak, rare strain.

PRAS carbohydrates: +, pH <5.5; w, pH 5.5-5.7; −, pH >5.7.

Gas in PYG agar deep: −, no gas detected; 2, splits agar horizontally; 3, agar displaced halfway to top of the tube; 4, agar displaced to top of the tube.

Fatty acids: A, acetic; P, propionic; B, butyric; V, valeric; L, lactic; S, succinic. NOTE: (1) Capital letters indicate major metabolic products. (2) Small letters indicate minor products. (3) Parentheses indicate a variable reaction. (4) Isoacids are primarily from carbohydrate-free media (such as PY) in the case of saccharolytic organisms.

Data from Sutter el al., 1985; Holdeman et al., 1977 and 1984.

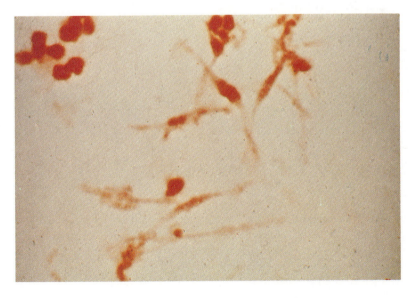

Figure 36.9

F. mortiferum. Very pleomorphic with round swellings. (From Sutter et al. 1985)

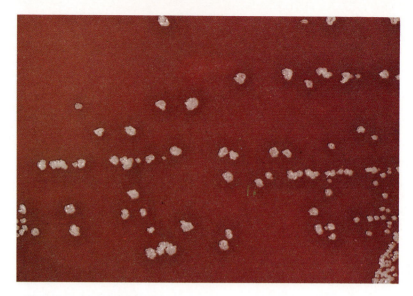

Figure 36.10
F. nucleatum. Breadcrumblike colonies and greening of agar.

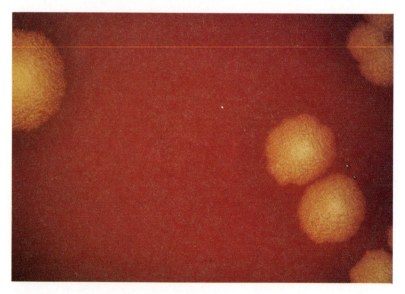

Figure 36.11
F. nucleatum. Note internal speckling in colonies.

but often show greening of the agar around the colonies after exposure to air. White breadcrumblike colonies (Figure 36.10) or convex, glistening α-hemolytic colonies with a flecked internal structure (Figure 36.11) are characteristic of *F. nucleatum*. *F. mortiferum* produces a colony with an opaque center and translucent, irregular margin (that is, "fried-

egg"), while *F. necrophorum* produces an umbonate colony (Fig. 36.12). *F. nucleatum* and sometimes *F. necrophorum* grow in balls in broth culture (Figure 36.13).

36.3.d. **Identification methods.** Besides the production of large amounts of butyric acid as a metabolic end product, the antibiotic disk identification

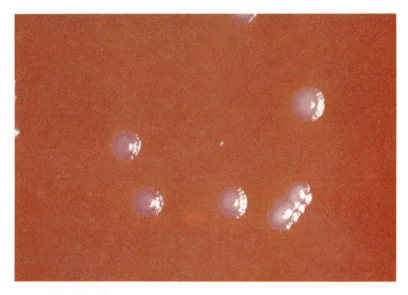

Figure 36.12
F. necrophorum on BA.

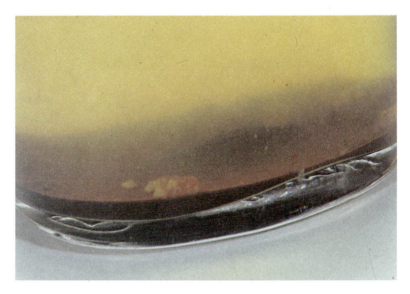

Figure 36.13
Positive blood culture. Note fluffy colonies at bottom of bottle *(F. necrophorum)*.

pattern is characteristic for fusobacteria; they are resistant to vancomycin and susceptible to kanamycin and colistin (see Chapter 34). This is the same pattern as the *B. ureolyticus* group, but the colony and growth characteristics usually distinguish them. There is some evidence that constitutive β-glucosidase may be used to differentiate between *Fuso-*

bacterium and *Bacteroides*. *F. nucleatum* is readily identified by microscopic and colony morphology and indole reaction (See Chapter 34). *F. necrophorum* is readily identified when the indole and lipase tests are both positive. Bile is inhibitory for most fusobacteria isolated from human clinical material except *F. mortiferum* and *F. varium* and some

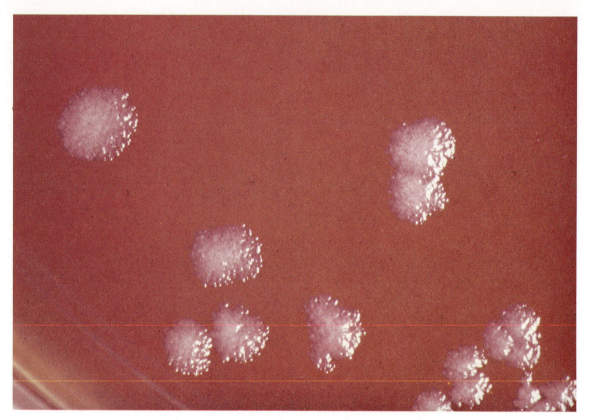

Figure 36.14
L. buccalis on BA.

strains of *F. necrophorum*. *F. mortiferum* is indole-negative and hydrolyzes esculin, whereas most strains of *F. varium* produce indole but do not hydrolyze esculin. Other characteristics useful in identifying the pathogenic species of *Fusobacterium* are indicated in Table 36.6.

36.3.e. Antimicrobial susceptibility. In general, fusobacteria are more susceptible to antimicrobial agents than are the *Bacteroides*. Unfortunately, resistance is beginning to appear in certain species of *Fusobacterium*. Some strains of *F. nucleatum* and of *F. varium* and *F. mortiferum* produce β-lactamase and, as a result, are manifesting some resistance. Imipenem and some quinolones are not as active against fusobacteria as with other anaerobes. Another phenomenon of interest with regard to fusobacteria is their ready production of L-form colonies upon exposure to cell wall–active antimicrobial agents, and the subsequent difficulty in interpreting susceptibility results.

36.4. Miscellaneous Bacteroidaceae

There are several genera of the family Bacteroidaceae other than *Bacteroides*, *Porphyromonas*, and *Fusobacterium*, and these have not been studied as closely. Those genera isolated from human clinical material are listed, along with key differential characteristics, in Table 36.1. Motility and cell shape provide an initial means of subdividing the group. Aside from those species associated with dental infections and vaginosis, most are infrequently isolated and then primarily from immunocompromised hosts. Several taxonomic changes have occurred within this family. Some *Bacteroides* sp. have been assigned to a new genus and many new species have been described (see Table 36.2). Several new species of *Selenomonas* associated with periodontitis have been described. The taxonomic status of *Mobiluncus* is unclear, because it has a gram-positive cell wall, but stains gram-variable to gram-negative.

36.4.a. Nonmotile rods. *Leptotrichia* and *Mitsuo-*

kella are nonmotile. *Leptotrichia buccalis* is part of the normal flora of the oral cavity and has been found, on occasion, in the intestine and the vagina. It has been recovered from dental infections, osteomyelitis of the mandible, bite wound infections, infections of the head and neck, and from the blood of a patient with a lung abscess. It is a long, plump, straight, or slightly curved gram-negative bacillus that grows end-to-end in pairs or chains. The ends that abut are flattened, whereas the other ends are often pointed. The colonies are 2 to 3 mm in diameter with a characteristic convoluted appearance (Figure 36.14). It is unique in producing lactic acid as its sole metabolic end product. *L. buccalis* is susceptible to virtually all antibacterial agents useful against anaerobes. *Mitsuokella dentalis* has been isolated from dental root canals. The bacterium produces a characteristic "water-drop" colony and grows poorly.

36.4.b. Motile or curved rods. The various anaerobic vibrios and curved rods are rarely recovered from clinical material; they have been involved in infections such as bacteremia, central nervous system infection, pulmonary infection, intra-abdominal infection, soft tissue infection, and endophthalmitis. Some have been isolated from dental infections. *Wolinella* sp. have been isolated from empyema fluid, decubitus and foot ulcers, and jaw abscesses. Both *Wolinella* and *C. concisus* have been isolated from significant dental infections. *Mobiluncus* is associated with vaginosis, but its pathogenic role is not clear. *Anaerobiospirillum succiniciproducens* bacteremia has been reviewed recently; this may be an underreported cause of bacteremia. Definitive identification within the group of anaerobic vibrios and curved rods is often time-consuming and difficult with the exception of *Wolinella* sp. and *C. concisus*. *Wolinella* sp. and *C. concisus* are similar to *B. ureolyticus* and *B. gracilis* in their requirement for formate and fumarate for growth, reduction of nitrate, and similar colony morphology. Oxidase may be useful for differentiating between *Wolinella* sp. and *C. concisus*.

BIBLIOGRAPHY

Adriaans, B., and Shah, H. 1988. *Fusobacterium ulcerans* sp. nov. from tropical ulcers. Int. J. Syst. Bacteriol. 38:447.

Cato, E.P., Moore, L.V.H., and Moore, W.E.C. 1985. *Fusobacterium alocis* sp. nov. and *Fusobacterium sulci* sp. nov. from the human gingival sulcus. J. Clin. Microbiol. 35:475.

Collins, M.D., and Shah, H.N. 1986. Reclassification of *Bacte-*
roides praeacutus Tissier (Holdeman and Moore) in a new genus, Tissierella, as *Tissierella praeacuta* comb. nov. Int. J. Syst. Bacteriol. 36:461.

Cooper, S.W., Pfeiffer, D.G., and Tally, F.P. 1985. Evaluation of xylan fermentation for the identification of *Bacteroides ovatus* and *Bacteroides thetaiotaomicron*. J. Clin. Microbiol. 22:125.

Edberg, S.C., and Bell, S.R. 1985. Lack of constitutive β-glucosidase (esculinase) in the genus *Fusobacterium*. J. Clin. Microbiol. 22:435.

Felner, J.M., and Dowell, V.R., Jr. 1971. "Bacteroides" bacteremia. Am. J. Med. 50:787.

Finegold, S.M. 1977. Anaerobic bacteria in human disease. Academic Press, New York.

George, W.L., Kirby, B.D., Sutter, V.L., et al. 1981. Gram-negative anaerobic bacilli: their role in infection and patterns of susceptibility to antimicrobial agents. II. Little-known *Fusobacterium* species and miscellaneous genera. Rev. Infect. Dis. 3:599.

Haapasalo, M., Ranta, H., Shah, H., et al. 1986. *Mitsuokella dentalis* sp. nov. from dental root canals. Int. J. Syst. Bacteriol. 35:566.

Holdeman, L.V., Cato, E.P., and Moore, W.E.C. 1977. Anaerobe laboratory manual, ed. 4. VPI Anaerobe Laboratory and Virginia Polytechnic Institute and State University, Blacksburg, Va.

Holdeman, L.V., Kelley, R.W., and Moore, W.E.C. 1984. Family I Bacteroidaceae Pribram, 1933. In Sneath, P.H.A, Mair, N.S., Sharpe, M.E., and Holt, J.G., editors: Bergey's Manual of Systematic Bacteriology, vol. 1, pp 602-637. Williams & Wilkins, Baltimore.

Johnson, C.C., and Finegold, S.M. 1987. Uncommonly encountered, motile anaerobic gram-negative bacilli associated with infection. Rev. Infect. Dis. 9:1150.

Johnson, C.C., Reinhardt, J.F., Edelstein, M.A.C., et al. 1985. *Bacteroides gracilis*, an important anaerobic bacterial pathogen. J. Clin. Microbiol. 22:799.

Johnson, J.L., Moore, W.E.C., and Moore, L.V.H. 1986. *Bacteroides caccae* sp. nov., *Bacteroides merdae* sp. nov., and *Bacteroides stercoris* sp. nov. isolated from human feces. Int. J. Syst. Bacteriol. 36:499.

Kirby, B.D., George, W.L., Sutter, V.L., et al. 1980. Gram-negative anaerobic bacilli: their role in infection and patterns of susceptibility to antimicrobial agents. I. Little-known *Bacteroides* species. Rev. Infect. Dis. 2:914.

Mayrand, D., Bourgeau, G., Grenier, D., and LaCroix, J-M. 1984. Properties of oral asaccharolytic black-pigmented *Bacteroides*. Can. J. Microbiol. 30:1133.

McCarthy, L.R., and Carlson, J.R. 1981. *Selenomonas sputigena* septicemia. J. Clin. Microbiol. 14:684.

McNeil, M.M., Martone, W.J., and Dowell, V.R., Jr. 1987. Bacteremia with *Anaerobiospirillum succiniciproducens*. Rev. Infect. Dis. 9:737.

Moore, L.V.H., Cato, E.P., and Moore, W.E.C. 1988. Anaerobe Lab Manual Update. Published as a supplement to the VPI Anaerobe Laboratory Manual, ed. 4. 1977. Virginia Polytechnic Institute, Blacksburg, Va.

Moore, L.V.H., Johnson, J.L., and Moore, W.E.C. 1987. *Selenomonas noxia* sp. nov., *Selenomonas flueggei*, sp. nov., *Selenomonas infelix*, sp. nov., *Selenomonas dianae*, sp. nov., and

Selenomonas artemidis, sp. nov. from the human gingival crevice. Int. J. Syst. Bacteriol. 36:271.

Paster, B.J., and Dewhirst, F.E. 1988. Phylogeny of Campylobacters, Wolinellas, *Bacteroides gracilis*, and *Bacteroides ureolyticus* by 16S ribosomal ribonucleic acid sequencing. Int. J. Syst. Bacteriol. 38:56.

Rotstein, O.D., Pruett, T.L., and Simmons, R.L. 1985. Mechanisms of microbial synergy in polymicrobial surgical infections. Rev. Infect Dis 7:151.

Shah, H.N., and Collins, M.D. 1988. Proposal for reclassification of *Bacteroides asaccharolyticus*, *Bacteroides gingivalis*, and *Bacteroides endodontalis* in a new genus, *Porphyromonas*. Int. J. Syst. Bacteriol. 38:128.

Shah, H.N., and Collins, M.D. 1989. Proposal to restrict the genus *Bacteroides* (Castellani and Chalmers) to *Bacteroides fragilis* and closely related species. Int. J. Syst. Bacteriol. 39:85.

Slots, J., Potts, T.V., and Mashimo, P.A. 1983. *Fusobacterium periodonticum*, a new species from the human oral cavity. J. Dent. Res. 62:960.

Slots, J., and Reynolds, H.S. 1982. Long wave UV light fluorescence for identification of black-pigmented *Bacteroides* spp. J. Clin. Microbiol. 16:1148.

Sutter, V.L., Citron, D.M., Edelstein, M.A.C., and Finegold, S.M. 1985. Wadsworth anaerobic bacteriology manual, ed. 4. Star Publishing Co., Belmont, Calif.

Tarnvik, A., Sundqvist, G., Gothefors, L., Gustafsson, H. 1986. Meningitis caused by *Fusobacterium necrophorum*. Eur. J. Clin. Microbiol. 5:353.

Truant, A.L., Menge, S., Milliorn, K., et al. 1983. *Fusobacterium nucleatum* pericarditis. J. Clin. Microbiol. 17:349.

van Winkelhoff, A.J., van Steenbergen, T.J.M., Kippuw, N., and deGraaff, J. 1986. Enzymatic characterization of oral and non-oral black-pigmented *Bacteroides* sp. Antonie Van Leeuwenhoek 52:163.

van Winkelhoff, A.J., van Steenbergen, T.J.M., Kippuw, N., and deGraaff, J. 1985. Further characterization of *Bacteroides endodontalis*, an asaccharolytic black-pigmented *Bacteroides* species from the oral cavity. J. Clin. Microbiol. 22:75.

37 Anaerobic Cocci

Martha A. C. Edelstein

The anaerobic cocci form a diverse group with many genera but no family affiliation (Table 37.1). The anaerobic gram-negative cocci belong to the genera *Veillonella, Acidaminococcus,* or *Megasphaera.* The gram-positive cocci belong to the genera *Peptococcus, Peptostreptococcus, Streptococcus, Ruminococcus,* or *Coprococcus.* Anaerobic cocci have been isolated from human clinical material with some frequency. Included with the anaerobic cocci are a few streptococci and *Staphylococcus saccharolyticus* (formerly *Peptococcus saccharolyticus*), because they usually require good anaerobic transport and culture techniques for isolation and identification.

37.1. Taxonomic Changes

As with other groups of anaerobes, the taxonomy of the anaerobic cocci has undergone and is undergoing many changes. All the pathogenic strains of *Peptococcus* sp. have been transferred to *Peptostreptococcus,* except for *Peptococcus niger.* *P. tetradius* is the new name for the old *Gaffkya.* The coccobacillary-shaped *P. anaerobius* appears to be more closely related to *Eubacterium* species or *Clostridium* species and may be transferred out of the genus *Peptostreptococcus.* The taxonomic status of several of the anaerobic streptococci is uncertain. *S. hansenii* is an obligate anaerobe and appears to be more closely related to clostridia. Of the microaerophilic streptococci, *S. morbillorum* is reclassified with *Gemella,* and *S. constellatus* and *S. intermedius* may be the same as *S. anginosus.*

Table 37.1
Anaerobic Cocci

Gram-negative cocci	
I. Produce propionic and acetic acids	*Veillonella*
II. Produce butyric and acetic acids	*Acidaminococcus*
III. Produce isobutyric, butyric, isovaleric, valeric, and caproic acids	*Megasphaera*
Gram-positive cocci	
I. Require a fermentable carbohydrate	
A. Produce butyric acid (plus other acids)	*Coprococcus*
B. Do not produce butyric acid	*Ruminococcus*
II. Do not require a fermentable carbohydrate	
A. Lactic acid sole major product	*Streptococcus, Gemella*
B. Not as above	*Peptostreptococcus* or *Peptococcus*

Modified from Sutter, V.L., Citron, D.M., Edelstein, M.A.C., and Finegold, S.M. 1985. Wadsworth anaerobic bacteriology manual, ed. 4. Star Publishing Co., Belmont, Calif.

37.2. Normal Flora, Infections, and Virulence Factors

The anaerobic cocci are numerically important members of the indigenous flora in the bowel, female genital tract, and oral cavity and are found in other locations as well, including the skin. Next to the anaerobic gram-negative bacilli, the anaerobic gram-positive cocci are the anaerobes most commonly encountered in clinically significant infections. Reflecting differences in their location as normal flora, the gram-positive anaerobic cocci are relatively more prevalent in respiratory tract and related infections. They are isolated commonly in female genital tract infections; they are less often encountered in intra-abdominal processes than are the gram-negative anaerobic rods. Nevertheless, gram-positive anaerobic cocci may be found in virtually all types of infection. *Ruminococcus* and *Coprococcus* are found in the normal flora of the colon but are nonpathogenic and rarely are isolated from clinical material. The anaerobic gram-positive cocci most commonly encountered in infection are *Peptostreptococcus magnus, P. asaccharolyticus, P. prevotii, P. micros,* and *P. anaerobius*. The anaerobic gram-negative cocci are isolated less frequently than the anaerobic gram-

positive cocci and appear to be much less pathogenic. *Veillonella* is encountered with some frequency in clinical specimens, whereas *Acidaminococcus* and *Megasphaera* are rarely isolated. At the Mayo Clinic, anaerobic cocci have been recovered from 31% of all anaerobic cultures that yielded growth. Virulence factors of anaerobic cocci have not been studied as extensively as for clostridia and anaerobic gram-negative rods; however, lipopolysaccharides, hyaluronidase, collagenase, and capsules have been described for the anaerobic cocci.

37.3. Differentiation of Anaerobic Cocci

Differentiation between genera of anaerobic cocci is based on gram-stain reaction and cell wall characteristics, metabolic end products, and on whether a fermentable carbohydrate is required for growth (see Table 37.1).

37.4. Anaerobic Gram-Positive Cocci

This group includes one species of *Peptococcus, P. niger*, which is rarely encountered in clinical infection, two anaerobic species in the genus *Streptococcus (S. intermedius, S. constellatus), Gemella morbillorum*, and the genus *Peptostreptococcus*, seven species of which may be encountered in infection. *Coprococcus* and *Ruminococcus* are excluded from this discussion because they are part of the normal bowel flora and rarely are isolated from clinical specimens.

37.4.a. **Morphology and general characteristics.** Microscopically, the anaerobic cocci are not as varied as the gram-negative anaerobic rods, but there are some notable differences in size and arrangement. Some anaerobic cocci form chains; this is best observed in broth culture. *P. anaerobius* (Figure 37.1) and *P. productus* are large coccobacilli often found in chains. *P. tetradius* may occur in packets. *P. magnus* cells are greater than 0.7 μm in diameter and are found singly or in masses; they may look like staphylococcal cells (Figure 37.2). Other peptostreptococci may also be mistaken for staphylococci on the basis of microscopic appearance. Indeed, such an appearance on direct Gram stain, with no staphylococci recovered on aerobic culture after 18 to 24 hours, should suggest the possibility of *Peptostreptococcus*. *P. micros* cells are less than 0.7 μm in diameter and often form short chains (Figure 37.3); Difference in cell size has been used as a key to distinguish between *P. micros* and *P. magnus*, but this difference in cell diameter now seems less re-

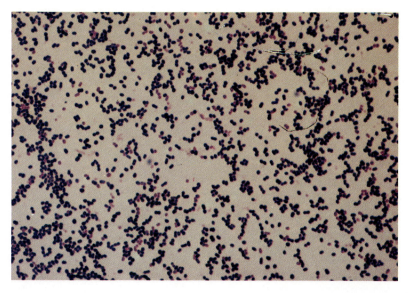

Figure 37.1
P. anaerobius. Large coccobacillary cells in chains, pairs, and singles. From Sutter, V.L., Citron, D.M., Edelstein, M.A.C., and Finegold, S.M. 1985. Wadsworth anaerobic bacteriology manual, ed. 4. Star Publishing Co., Belmont, Calif.

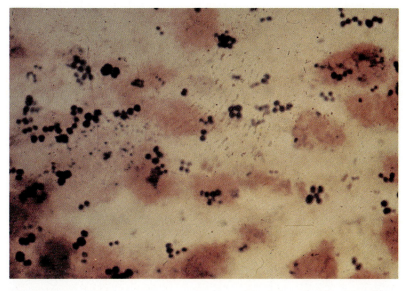

Figure 37.2
Peptostreptococcus magnus in pus (appearance identical to that of staphylococci). From Sutter, V.L., Citron, D.M., Edelstein, M.A.C., and Finegold, S.M. 1985. Wadsworth anaerobic bacteriology manual, ed. 4. Star Publishing Co., Belmont, Calif.

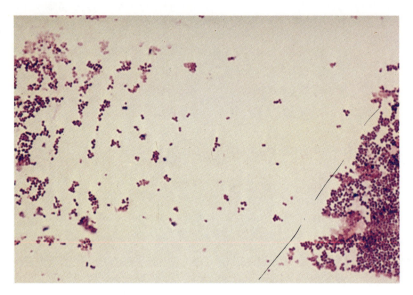

Figure 37.3
P. micros. Small cells, often form short chains. From Sutter, V.L. Citron, D.M., Edelstein, M.A.C., and Finegold, S.M. 1985. Wadsworth anaerobic bacteriology manual, ed. 4. Star Publishing Co., Belmont, Calif.

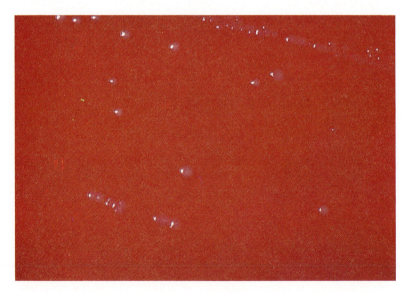

Figure 37.4
Typical colony morphology of anaerobic gram-positive coccus on blood agar *(P. asaccharolyticus)*.

liable. The anaerobic streptococci vary in size and occur in chains, pairs, or singly. Gram-positive anaerobic cocci produce minute to small, convex colonies that are gray to white and translucent to opaque (Figure 37.4). The edges are entire, and the colony surface may appear stippled or pock-marked. Colony size is usually <0.5 to 2 mm in diameter. There may be a halo of discoloration surrounding colonies of *P. micros*. *Peptococcus niger*, an organism that is rarely encountered, produces black-pigmented colonies. *P. anaerobius* typically produces larger and more opaque colonies than other anaerobic cocci (Figure 37.5); it also has a sweet, fetid odor. Growth of anaerobic cocci in broth is typically slow and results in balls, clumps, or aggregates of growth rather than diffuse turbidity. Tween 80 often enhances growth in broth culture.

37.4.b. Identification. Preliminary grouping and identification procedures for the anaerobic gram-positive cocci appear in Chapter 34. Tables 37.1 and 37.2 and Figure 37.6 list characteristics that aid in differentiation of the anaerobic gram-positive cocci. Results in bold type in the tables are key differential tests.

A few cocci can be identified with relatively simple tests. *P. anaerobius* is resistant to sodium polyanethol sulfonate (Figure 37.5) and produces isocaproic acid as an end product of metabolism. It is also one of the few cocci that degrades tyrosine crystals. *P. asaccharolyticus* and *P. indolicus* are indole-positive, but *P. indolicus* is rarely isolated from human clinical samples; it produces coagulase and reduces nitrate. There is evidence that some strains of *P. asaccharolyticus* are indole-negative.

Definitive identification requires end product analysis by gas-liquid chromotography (GLC); indole, alkaline phosphatase, and urease production; nitrate reduction; and carbohydrate fermentation. Alkaline phosphatase and catalase production and gelatin hydrolysis aid in differentiating *P. magnus* and *P. micros*. As mentioned in Chapter 34, the rapid 4-hour preformed enzyme kits identify the anaerobic gram-positive cocci fairly well without the use of GLC, except that there may be problems accurately separating *P. tetradius* and *P. prevotii*.

37.4.c. Susceptibility to antimicrobial agents. The drug of choice for anaerobic gram-positive coccal infections has generally been considered to be penicillin G. However, some strains require as much as 8 μg/ml for inhibition and rare strains may require as much as 32 μg/ml. Infection with the latter strains would best be treated with another, more active

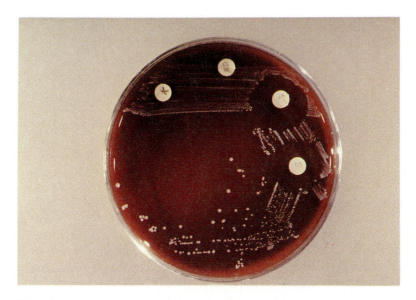

Figure 37.5
P. anaerobius. Compare colony morphology to Figure 37.4. Note disk identification tests: resistant to kanamycin and colistin, sensitive to vancomycin and sodium polyanethol sulfonate (SPS) (S disk).

Table 37.2
Characteristics of Anaerobic Gram-Positive Cocci

	ISOCAPROIC ACID	BUTYRIC ACID	LACTIC ACID	SPS	INDOLE	NITRATE	CATALASE	ALKALINE PHOSPHATASE	UREASE	CELLS <0.7 μm IN DIAMETER	GELATIN HYDROLYSIS	FERMENTATION OF GLUCOSE	MALTOSE	SUCROSE	FATTY ACIDS FROM PEPTONE YEAST GLUCOSE BROTH
Peptostreptococcus															
P. anaerobius	+	V	−	S	−	−	−	−	−		−ʷ	wˉ	wˉ	−ʷ	A IC (ib b iv)
P. asaccharolyticus	−	+	−	R	+ˉ	−	V	−	−		−	−	−	−	B (A l p)
P. indolicus	−	+	−	R	+	+ˉ					−	−	−	−	A B (p s)
P. prevotii	−	+	−	R	−	−	V	+	−⁺		−	w	wˉ	−ʷ	B (A L p)
P. tetradius	−	+	−	**R**	−	−	V	−	+		−	+	+	+	B L (a p)
P. magnus	−	−	−	R	−	−	+ˉ	−*	−	−	+ˉ	−	−	−	A
P micros	−	−	−	R	−	−	+	−	+		−	−	−	−	A (s)
P. productus	−	−	−	R	−	−	−		V*		−	+	+	+	A l (s)
Staphylococcus															
saccharolyticus	−	−	−	R	−	+	V				−	+	−	−	A (s)
"Anaerobic"															
streptococci	−	−	+	R	−	−	−				−	+	+	+	L (a s)

Reactions: Results in **bold type** are key differential tests; − = negative for majority of strains; + = positive for majority of strains; V = variable; w = most strains weakly positive; superscripts indicate reactions of occasional strains.
PRAS carbohydrates: + = pH <5.5; w = pH 5.5-5.7; − = pH >5.7.
Fatty acids: A = acetic; P = propionic; IB = isobutyric; B = butyric; IV = isovaleric; V = valeric; IC = isocaproic; C = caproic; L = lactic; S = succinic. NOTE: (1) Capital letters indicate major metabolic products. (2) Small letters indicate minor products. (3) Parentheses indicate a variable reaction. (4) Isoacids are primarily from carbohydrate-free media (such as PY) in the case of saccharolytic organisms.
*Varies with reporting laboratories.
Data from Sutter et al., 1985; Holdeman et al., 1977; Moore et al., 1986; Murdoch et al., 1988.

agent. Chloramphenicol, the carboxypenicillins and ureidopenicillins, and cefoxitin are active against all strains, although some strains require 16 μg/ml of cefoxitin for inhibition. Metronidazole is active against all but a few strains of obligately anaerobic gram-positive cocci and the "anaerobic" streptococci. Clindamycin is not active at achievable serum levels against about 10% of strains of cocci formerly classified in the genus *Peptococcus*. Cephalothin is quite active against all anaerobic gram-positive cocci. Occasional strains are resistant to cefamandole and ceftazidime; other cephalosporins are active against all strains, as is imipenem. Erythromycin is inactive at achievable levels against 20% to 30% of strains for-

merly classified in the genus *Peptococcus*. Tetracycline has poor activity against anaerobic gram-positive cocci; doxycycline is somewhat better but should not be used unless susceptibility of a given strain from an infection has been documented.

37.5. Anaerobic Gram-Negative Cocci

Only three of at least seven species of *Veillonella* are commonly found in human clinical infections. *Megasphaera* and *Acidaminococcus* are rarely encountered.

37.5.a. **Morphology and general characteristics.** *Veillonella* are tiny (less than 0.5 μm in diameter) gram-negative cocci that occur in masses or as dip-

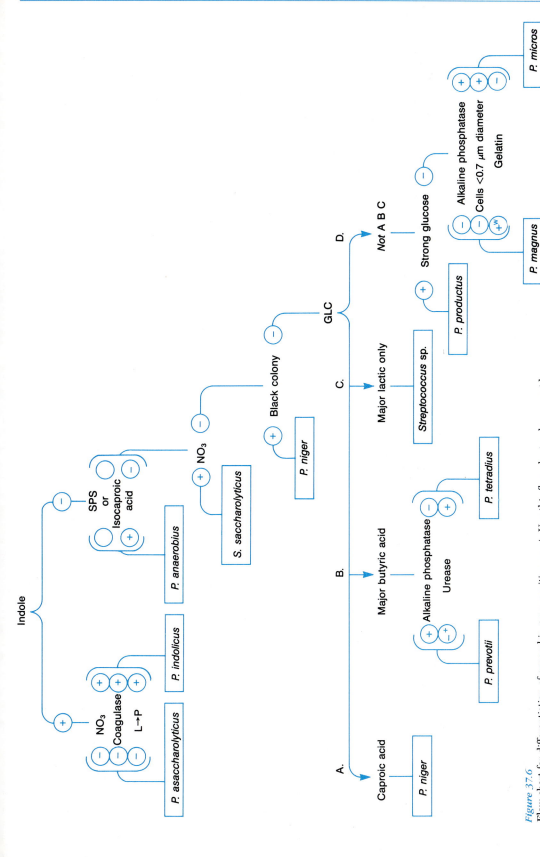

Figure 37.6

Flow chart for differentiation of anaerobic gram-positive cocci. Use this flow chart only as a guide; unusual strain variations may give anomalous results. *Reactions:* + = positive; − = negative; L→P = converts lactic acid to propionic acid (detected by GLC); SPS = sodium polyanethol sulfonate; S = sensitive; R = resistant; +ᵛ = most strains positive, some strains negative; GLC = results of end product analysis by GLC.

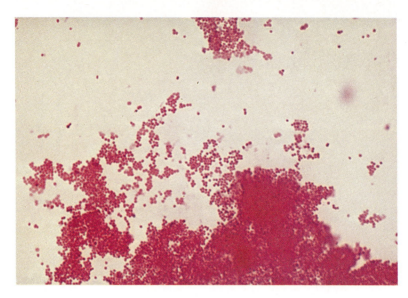

Figure 37.7
Veillonella. Small, gram-negative coccus. From Sutter, V.L., Citron, D.M., Edelstein, M.A.C., and Finegold, S.M. 1985. Wadsworth anaerobic bacteriology manual, ed. 4. Star Publishing Co., Belmont, Calif.

Table 37.3
Characteristics of Anaerobic Gram-Negative Cocci

	NITRATE REDUCTION	CATALASE	GLUCOSE	FATTY ACIDS FROM PEPTONE YEAST GLUCOSE BROTH
Veillonella sp.	+	V	−	A p
Acidaminococcus fermentans	−	−	−	A B
Megasphaera elsdenii	−	−	+	a ib b iv v C

Reactions: See Table 37.2.
PRAS carbohydrates: See Table 37.2.
Fatty acids: See Table 37.2.
Data from Sutter et al., 1985.

lococci (Figure 37.7). Negative staining of *Veillonella* cells reveals a convoluted surface. Unusually large cocci, especially when found in groups or packets, may suggest *Megasphaera*. *Megasphaera* commonly stains gram-positive but is really gram-negative on the basis of cell wall composition; it could initially be confused with *P. tetradius* by gram-stain morphology. *Veillonella* produce small, convex, translucent to transparent colonies with an entire edge. These colonies may show red fluorescence under long-wave ultraviolet light, but fluorescence is lost rapidly after exposure of colonies to air. *Veillonella*

grow poorly in broth and produce a very fine granular turbidity. Supplementation of broth with pyruvate may enhance growth for some strains.

37.5.b. Identification. Fatty acid end products are the key means for differentiation among the three genera of anaerobic gram-negative cocci (Table 37.1), but, as noted in Table 37.3, nitrate reduction, catalase production, and glucose fermentation are also useful in characterizing strains.

37.5.c. Susceptibility to antimicrobial agents. *Veillonella* is seldom a significant pathogen, and *Acidaminococcus* and *Megasphaera* are rarely encountered in infection, so that specific therapy directed against the anaerobic gram-negative cocci is seldom indicated. Penicillin G is quite active against these organisms, but other penicillins, including the carboxypenicillins and ureidopenicillins, are not active against all strains. Metronidazole, chloramphenicol, clindamycin, and cefoxitin are all active against the gram-negative coccal anaerobes, as are cephalothin, the newer cephalosporins, and imipenem.

BIBLIOGRAPHY

Babcock, J.B. 1979. Tyrosine degradation in presumptive identification of *Peptostreptococcus anaerobius*. J. Clin. Microbiol. 9:358.

Bourgault, A.-M., Rosenblatt, J.E., and Fitzgerald, R.H. 1980. *Peptococcus magnus:* a significant human pathogen. Ann. Intern. Med. 93:244.

Brazier, J.S., and Riley, T.V. 1988. UV red fluorescence of *Veillonella* sp. J. Clin. Microbiol. 26:383.

Coykendall, A.L., Wesbecher, P.M., and Gustafson, K.B. 1987. "*Streptococcus milleri*," *Streptococcus constellatus*, and *Streptococcus intermedius* are later synonyms of *Streptococcus anginosus*. Int. J. Syst. Bacteriol. 37:222.

Ezaki, T., Yamamoto, N., Ninomiya, K., et al. 1983. Transfer of *Peptococcus indolicus, Peptococcus asaccharolyticus, Peptococcus prevotii*, and *Peptococcus magnus* to the genus *Peptostreptococcus* and proposal of *Peptostreptococcus tetradius* sp. nov. Int. J. Syst. Bacteriol. 33:683.

Finegold, S.M. 1977. Anaerobic bacteria in human disease. Academic Press, New York.

Holdeman, L.V., Cato, E.P., and Moore, W.E.C. 1977. Anaerobe laboratory manual, ed. 4. VPI Laboratory, Virginia Polytechnic Institute and State University, Blacksburg, Va.

Huss, V.A.R., Festl, H., and Schleifer, K.H. 1984. Deoxyribonucleic acid hybridization studies and deoxynucleic acid base compositions of anaerobic, gram-positive cocci. Int. J. Syst. Bacteriol. 34:95.

Kilpper-Balz, R., and Schleifer, K.H. 1988. Transfer of *Streptococcus morbillorum* to the genus *Gemella* as *Gemella morbillorum* comb. nov. Int. J. Syst. Bacteriol. 38:442.

Knight, R.G., and Shlaes, D.M. 1988. Physiological characteristics and deoxyribonucleic acid relatedness of *Streptococcus intermedius* strains. Int. J. Syst. Bacteriol. 38:19.

Mays, T.D., Holdeman, L.V., Moore, W.E.C., et al. 1982. Taxonomy of the genus *Veillonella* Prevot. Int. J. Syst. Bacteriol. 32:28.

Moore, L.V.H., Johnson, J.J., and Moore, W.E.C. 1986. Genus *Peptococcus;* Genus *Peptostreptococcus*. In Sneath, P.H.A., Mair, N.S., Sharpe, M.E., and Holt, J.G., editors: Bergey's manual of systematic bacteriology, pp. 1082-1092. Williams & Wilkins, Baltimore.

Murdoch, D.A., Mitchelmore, I.J., Nash, R.A., et al. 1988. Preformed enzyme profiles of reference strains of gram-positive anaerobic cocci. J. Med. Microbiol. 27:65.

Pien, F.D., Thompson, R.L., and Martin, W.J. 1972. Clinical and bacteriologic studies of anaerobic gram-positive cocci. Mayo Clin. Proc. 47:251.

Rolfe, R.D., and Finegold, S.M. 1981. Comparative in vitro activity of new beta-lactam antibiotics against anaerobic bacteria. Antimicrob. Agents Chemother. 20:600.

Sutter, V.L., Citron, D.M., Edelstein, M.A.C., and Finegold, S.M. 1985. Wadsworth anaerobic bacteriology manual, ed. 4. Star Publishing Co., Belmont, Calif.

Sutter, V.L., and Finegold, S.M. 1976. Susceptibility of anaerobic bacteria to 23 antimicrobial agents. Antimicrob. Agents Chemother. 10:736.

Thomas, C.G.A., and Hare, R. 1954. The classification of anaerobic cocci and their isolation in normal human beings and pathological processes. J. Clin. Pathol. 7:300.

Weizenegger, W.L., Kilpper-Balz, R., and Schleifer, K.H. 1988. Phylogenetic relationships of anaerobic streptococci. Int. J. Syst. Bacteriol. 38:15.

Yatabe, J.H., Baldwin, K.L., and Martin, W.J. 1977. Isolation of an obligately anaerobic *Streptococcus pneumoniae* from blood culture. J. Clin. Microbiol. 6:181.

38 *Chlamydia, Mycoplasma,* and *Rickettsia*

Organisms of the genera *Chlamydia, Mycoplasma,* and *Rickettsia* are prokaryotes that differ from most other bacteria in their very small size, their unusual cell wall structure, or, in the case of *Rickettsia* and *Chlamydia,* their obligate intracellular parasitism. *Chlamydia* and *Mycoplasma* genera each include species that cause pneumonia and species that cause venereal disease. The fastidious nature of both of these organisms is at least one reason for the parallel development of similar disease syndromes; the organisms must adhere to and multiply within a protective environment, and the mucous membranes of the respiratory tract and the genitourinary tract provide favorable conditions at the first site at which the pathogen impinges on a hospitable host. Isolation of pathogenic chlamydiae and mycoplasma is possible for hospital clinical laboratories, but rickettsiae are extremely difficult to cultivate and too hazardous to work with for routine isolation attempts. These three genera will be treated separately in this chapter.

38.1. Chlamydiae

Members of the family Chlamydiaceae (order Chlamydiales) are obligate intracellular bacteria that were once regarded as viruses. *Chlamydia* are divided currently into two distinct species: *C. trachomatis* and *C. psittaci.* A third group of chlamydiae, the TWAR strain, has recently been described; TWAR shares less than 10% genetic homology with *C. trachomatis* and *C. psittaci* (which likewise share less than 10% homology between themselves).[2] The TWAR strain shares the *Chlamydia* genus-specific antigen but is otherwise serologically distinct. Based

Table 38.1
Differentiation Among *Chlamydia* Species

PROPERTY	C. TRACHOMATIS	C. PSITTACI	TWAR
Host range	Humans, mice	Birds, humans, lower mammals	Humans
Elementary body morphology	Round	Round	Pear-shaped
Inclusion morphology	Round, vacuolar	Variable, dense	Round, dense
Glycogen in inclusions	Yes	No	No
Susceptibility to sulfonamides	Yes	No	No
DNA homology	10%	10%	10%
Plasmid DNA	Yes	Yes	No

on these results, a third species, "*C. pneumoniae*," has been proposed to encompass TWAR strains.

C. psittaci is the agent of pneumonia and systemic disease associated with contact with birds; the disease is variously known as **psittacosis** or **ornithosis**. Although many species variants occur, they have not been separated further. The TWAR strain has also been implicated as a cause of lower respiratory tract infections.[5]

C. trachomatis is associated with four primary syndromes:

1. Endemic trachoma (repetitive conjunctival infection ultimately leading to blindness)
2. Sexually transmitted chlamydial disease (including nongonococcal urethritis and cervicitis)
3. Inclusion conjunctivitis (caused by the sexually transmitted strains and not leading to blindness)
4. Lymphogranuloma venereum (**LGV**).

C. trachomatis in some cases may infect the entire genital tract and may cause pneumonia in infants. Table 38.1 outlines some biological differences among these groups of organisms.

Although the chlamydiae possess a cell wall similar to that of gram-negative bacteria, their cell wall is distinctive in lacking a peptidoglycan layer. They do produce an endotoxin-like lipopolysaccharide antigen. Unlike any other bacteria, chlamydiae undergo an unusual developmental cycle (Figure 38.1). The infectious particles, rigid-enveloped structures approximately 0.3 μm in diameter called **elementary bodies,** attach to the surface of a susceptible host cell. They induce endocytosis and are enclosed within a cytoplasmic vesicle, a "phagosome." The organisms are able to prevent lysosomal fusion. After the initial stage, elementary bodies reorganize to a

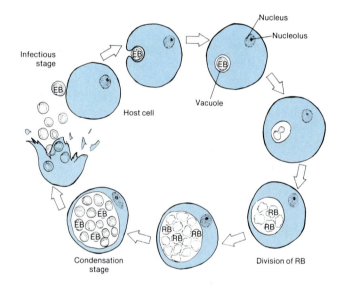

Figure 38.1
Life cycle of *Chlamydia*. *EB*, Elementary body. *RB*, Reticulate body. (From Boyd, R.F. 1984. General microbiology. The C.V. Mosby Co., St. Louis.

more metabolically active form, the **reticulate body.** Reticulate bodies multiply by binary fission until approximately 18 to 24 hours after infection, at which point many of the reticulate bodies reorganize again into infectious elementary bodies. Newly formed reticulate and elementary bodies are still enclosed within the phagosomic intracellular vesicle, which is visible microscopically as an **inclusion** after it has been highlighted with a special stain. The inclusions of *C. trachomatis* can be stained with iodine, since they consist primarily of glycogen and exist in a rather compact form, in contrast to the diffuse, Giemsa-staining inclusions of *C. psittaci*. At 48 to

72 hours after initial attachment, the cell ruptures to release a large number of infectious elementary bodies. The diseases caused by each of the species and the laboratory diagnosis of those diseases differ in several important ways. Each entity, *C. psittaci*, *C. trachomatis*, and the TWAR strain, will be discussed separately.

Tetracycline, erythromycin, sulfonamides, and broad-spectrum cephalosporins are usually effective for therapy of chlamydial infections.

38.1.a. Psittacosis. *C. psittaci* is an endemic pathogen of birds of all species. Psittacine birds (such as parrots and parakeets) are the major reservoir for human disease, but outbreaks have occurred among turkey processing workers and pigeon aficionados. The birds may show diarrheal illness or may be asymptomatic. Humans acquire the disease by inhalation of aerosols. The organisms are deposited in the alveoli, from which some are ingested by alveolar macrophages and carried to regional lymph nodes. From there, they are disseminated systemically, growing within cells of the reticuloendothelial system. Findings include pneumonia, severe headache, changes in mentation, and hepatosplenomegaly.

Diagnosis of psittacosis is almost always by serologic means. Because of hazards associated with working with the agent, only laboratories with type III biohazard containment facilities can safely culture *C. psittaci*. State health departments take an active role in consulting with clinicians about possible cases. Complement fixation has been most commonly used to detect psittacosis infection. A more recent test, microindirect immunofluorescence, seems to be more sensitive but is difficult to perform. For this test, various strains of *C. psittaci* are grown in hens' egg yolk sac cultures. The cultures, rich with elementary bodies, are diluted and vigorously dispersed in buffer. The tester uses a small pipette or pen and places a dot of each antigen in a geometric array on the surface of a glass slide. Several identical arrays, each containing a dot of every antigen, are prepared on a single slide. These slides are fixed and frozen until use. At the time of the test, serial dilutions of patients' serum are placed over the antigen arrays. After incubation and washing steps, fluorescein-conjugated antihuman immunoglobulin (either IgG or IgM) is overlayed on the slide. The slide is finally read for fluorescence of particular antigen dots with an ultraviolet microscope. Either a fourfold rise in titer between acute and convalescent serum sam-

ples or a single IgM titer of 1:32 in a patient with clinically suspicious illness is diagnostic.

38.1.b. Lymphogranuloma venereum. Lymphogranuloma venereum (LGV) is a sexually transmitted disease that is unusual in Europe and North America but not uncommon in Africa, Asia, and South America. The disease is characterized by a primary genital lesion of short duration at the site of initial infection. This lesion is often small and may be unrecognized, especially by female patients. The second stage, that of acute lymphadenitis, often involves the inguinal lymph nodes, causing them to enlarge, forming buboes. During this stage, infection may spread systemically to cause fever or locally to cause granulomatous proctitis. In a small number of cases (more women than men) the disease progresses to the third stage, that of a chronic inflammatory response that contributes to the development of genital hyperplasia, rectal fistulas, rectal stricture, draining sinuses, and other manifestations. Occasionally, chronic ulcerative or infiltrative lesions of the penis and scrotum may develop.

Diagnosis of LGV is established by the isolation of an LGV serotype strain from a bubo or other infected site. However, recovery rates of only 24% to 30% have been reported. A skin test that entails intradermal injections of LGV antigen, the Frei test, suffers from lack of sensitivity in early LGV and lack of specificity, since the Frei antigen is a genus-specific antigen. Moreover, the Frei test can remain positive for many years, limiting its usefulness. Again because a genus-specific antigen is used, antibody detection by complement fixation is also nonspecific. Despite its shortcomings, a complement fixation titer of 1:16 is presumptive evidence of infection. Other serologic tests, such as microimmunofluorescence and neutralization, are performed only in specialized laboratories.

38.1.c. *Chlamydia trachomatis* as a cause of non-LGV disease. Chlamydial infections have surpassed gonococcal infections as the most prevalent sexually transmitted disease in the United States. In addition to causing a spectrum of disease similar to that of gonococci, including urethritis, cervicitis, bartholinitis, proctitis, salpingitis, inclusion conjunctivitis (ophthalmia neonatorum), perihepatitis (Fitz-Hugh-Curtis syndrome), epididymitis, and endocarditis, chlamydiae are a significant cause of pneumonia in neonates. Chlamydiae have been found as one cause of the acute urethral syndrome in women, characterized by symptoms of a urinary tract infection with pyuria but few or no conventional bacteria.[16] Both chlamydiae and gonococci are major causes of pelvic inflammatory disease (PID), contributing significantly to the rising rate of infertility and ectopic pregnancies in young women. After only one episode of PID, as many as 10% of women may become infertile because of tubal occlusion. The risk increases dramatically with each additional episode of PID. Chlamydial salpingitis leading to infertility may be asymptomatic. Chlamydial infection can be transmitted to an infant from an infected mother during delivery. Approximately 0.5% of live births are complicated by neonatal chlamydial inclusion conjunctivitis or pneumonia.

Many genital chlamydial infections in people of either sex are asymptomatic. It is estimated that as many as 22% of women and 7% of men in some populations are asymptomatic carriers. The highest risk group is patients with gonococcal infection; 20% to 35% of men with gonorrhea and 50% of women with gonorrhea are likely to harbor *C. trachomatis* concomitantly. Furthermore, in the United States, 60% of cases of nongonococcal urethritis (NGU) are caused by chlamydiae. The incidence of this disease is even higher in Scandinavian countries. With the recently developed diagnostic tests outlined below, we expect that a much clearer epidemiologic picture and ultimately better control of this widespread disease are attainable goals for the near future.

Diagnosis of *C. trachomatis* can be achieved by cytology, culture, direct antigen detection in clinical specimens, and serologic testing. The organism can be recovered from infected epithelial cells from the urethra, cervix, conjunctiva, nasopharynx, rectum, and aspirates from fallopian tubes and epididymis.

Cytological examination of cell scrapings for the presence of inclusions was the first method used for diagnosis of *C. trachomatis*; it is still used occasionally for rapid diagnosis of inclusion conjunctivitis in newborns. However, this method is insensitive when compared with culture or direct immunofluorescence, the methods of choice today.[15]

Isolation of *C. trachomatis* in cell culture remains the most sensitive and specific diagnostic method. Cycloheximide-treated McCoy cells have been shown to produce consistently higher inclusion counts than other cell lines. Centrifugation of the specimen onto the cell monolayer (usually growing on a coverslip in the bottom of a vial, the "shell-vial") presumably facilitates adherence of elementary bodies. After 48 to 72 hours' incubation, monolayers are stained with iodine or an immunofluorescent stain and examined microscopically for inclusions. Procedure 38.1 is a method for isolation of chlamydiae. Despite the high sensitivity of culture, a number of technical problems adversely affect the recovery of *C. trachomatis* and relatively few laboratories perform cell culture isolation.

To circumvent the shortcoming of cell culture, antigen detection methods have been developed and are commercially available. Direct fluorescent antibody (**DFA**) staining methods employ fluorescein-isothiocyanate-conjugated monoclonal antibodies to either outer membrane proteins or lipopolysaccharides of *C. trachomatis* for the detection of elementary bodies in smears prepared from clinical material (Figure 38.2). The MicroTrak DFA (Syva Co.) is the most widely evaluated commercial system. DFAs achieved greater than or equal to 90% sensitivity compared with culture in evaluations in symptomatic men and high-risk women (sex partners of *Chlamydia*-positive men or women attending STD clinics).[9] In populations with asymptomatic infections, the sensitivity of DFA decreased, presumably because a lower number of inclusion-forming units were present.[1,19]

Chlamydial antigen has also been detected in clinical specimens by enzyme-linked immunosorbent assay (ELISA). A number of commercially available kits are marketed but only the Chlamydiazyme assay (Abbott Laboratories) has been extensively evaluated to date. The median sensitivity of this ELISA was approximately 79% in men with urethritis and 90% in high-risk women. However, only 50% sensitivity has been seen in asymptomatic men; in women with intermediate prevalence of disease (6% to 12%), sensitivity is approximately 85%.[6,7,18,20] A new direct antigen-detection method using an RNA-directed DNA probe conjugated to a chemiluminescent marker (PACE, Gen-Probe) has recently been introduced. Early studies are promising. In low-prevalence populations (<5%), however, culture remains the test of choice.

Serologic testing has limited value for diagnosis of urogenital infections in adults. Most adults with chlamydial infection have had a previous exposure to *C. trachomatis* and are seropositive. Antibodies to a genus-specific antigen can be detected by complement fixation. For type-specific antibodies of *C*.

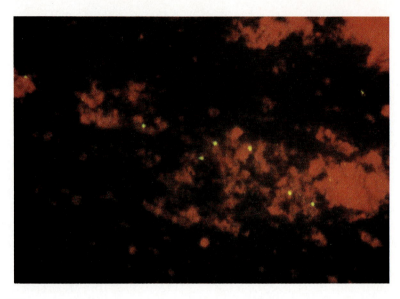

Figure 38.2
Appearance of fluorescein-conjugated monoclonal antibody–stained elementary bodies in direct smear
of urethral cell scraping from patient with chlamydial urethritis.

PROCEDURE 38.1

Cell Culture Method for Isolation of Chlamydiae

Method

1. Swab or tissue is collected in sucrose transport medium containing antibiotics and 2 to 4 sterile glass beads (Chapter 19). Specimens should be kept refrigerated at all times prior to transport to the laboratory. If the culture is not inoculated within 24 hours of collection, the specimen should be frozen at −70° C.

2. Vortex the specimen vigorously and remove the swab. The glass beads cause rupture of infected cells and release of elementary bodies. Tissue should be ground or minced and ground into a cell suspension using transport medium as a diluent.

3. Use aseptic technique and aspirate the cell culture medium above the McCoy cell monolayer in the shell vial (commercially available) and add 0.2 ml of the patient specimen to the vial.

4. Centrifuge the vial for at least 1 h at 2500 to 3000 × *g* at ambient temperature in a temperature-controlled centrifuge. Do not allow the temperature to increase past 40° C.

5. Aseptically remove the inoculum and add 1 ml fresh maintenance medium containing 1 μg/ml cycloheximide.

6. Recap the vials tightly and incubate at 35 to 37° C for 48 to 72 h.

7. Remove medium from the vials, fix with methanol or ethanol (according to manufacturer's instructions), and stain with iodine or fluorescein-conjugated chlamydial antibody.

8. Examine slides at 200 to 400 × magnification for dark brown (iodine stain; Figure 38.3) or apple green (fluorescent stain) intracytoplasmic inclusions (Figure 38.4).

Quality control

Laboratories performing chlamydial culture should subscribe to a commercial proficiency testing service to verify their procedures.

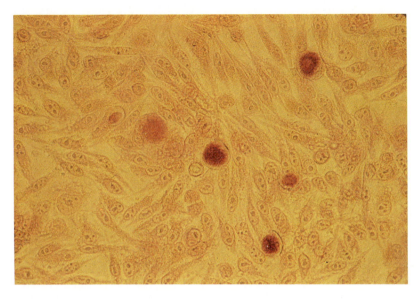

Figure 38.3
Iodine-stained inclusions in McCoy cell monolayer infected with *C. trachomatis*. (Courtesy Dr. Ellena Peterson, University of California, Irvine.)

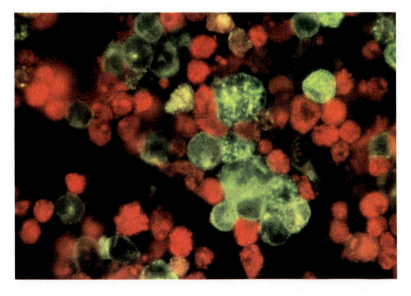

Figure 38.4
Fluorescent-antibody-stained inclusions in McCoy cell monolayer infected with *C. trachomatis*. (Courtesy Dr. Ellena Peterson, University of California, Irvine.)

trachomatis, the microimmunofluorescence assay, a tedious and difficult test, is used. A high titer of IgM (≥128) is suggestive of a recent infection; however, not all patients produce IgM.[10] Negative serologies can reliably exclude chlamydial infection. Detection of *C. trachomatis*–specific IgM is useful in diagnosis of neonatal infections.

38.1.d. TWAR (*"Chlamydia pneumoniae"*). The TWAR strain of *Chlamydia* was first isolated from the conjunctiva of a child in Taiwan. It was initially considered to be a psittacosis strain because the inclusions produced in cell culture resembled those of *C. psittaci*. Subsequently, the Taiwan isolate (TW-183) was shown to be serologically related to a pharyngeal isolate (AR-39), and thus the new strain was called "TWAR," an acronym for TW and AR (acute respiratory). Only one serotype of the proposed new species, *"C. pneumoniae,"* has been identified.

TWAR has been associated with pneumonia, bronchitis, pharyngitis, sinusitis, and a flulike illness. Infection in young adults is usually mild to moderate; the differential diagnosis primarily includes mycoplasmal pneumonia. Severe pneumonia is not uncommon in elderly or respiratory-compromised patients. Treatment with tetracycline and erythromycin has been successful.

Diagnosis of TWAR infection can be achieved by cell culture isolation and serology. A cell culture procedure similar to that used for *C. trachomatis* but substituting the more sensitive HeLa cell line for McCoy cells has been used. Complement fixation using a genus-specific antigen has been used, but it is not specific for TWAR. A microimmunofluorescence test using TWAR elementary bodies as antigen is more reliable but available only in specialized laboratories. A fourfold rise in either IgG or IgM is diagnostic, and a single IgM titer of ≥16 or an IgG titer of ≥512 is suggestive of recent infection.

38.2. Mycoplasmas

Members of the class Mollicutes, these organisms are found throughout the animal and plant kingdom as free-living saprophytes and parasites. First recognized from a case of pleuropneumonia in a cow, the organism was designated "pleuropneumonia-like" organism or PPLO. That term is still used today, particularly for certain mycoplasma media. The smallest organisms able to survive extracellularly, they are highly pleomorphic because they lack a cell wall, which also renders them completely resistant to β-lactam and other cell wall–active drugs. Although some species are normal human respiratory tract flora, *M. pneumoniae* is a major cause of respiratory disease (primary atypical pneumonia, sometimes called "walking pneumonia"). *M. pneumoniae* seldom causes invasive disease.

M. hominis, *M. genitalium*, and *Ureaplasma urealyticum* are important colonizers (and possibly pathogens) of the human genital tract. *M. hominis* has been associated with sepsis (particularly postpartum), arthritis, and recently with sternal wound infections.[4,17] A role for *U. urealyticum* in contributing to perinatal disorders and spontaneous abortion has been proposed; its association with acute urethral syndrome in women is fairly strong.[8,16] None of the other species, shown in Table 38.2, are definitely pathogenic for humans. These organisms colonize the mucosa of the respiratory and genital tracts of humans, growing extracellularly. By an unknown mechanism, infection with mycoplasma causes injury to mucosal cells. The tissue damage leads to impairment of ciliary function.

38.2.a. *Mycoplasma pneumoniae*. It is estimated that *M. pneumoniae* may cause as many as 50% of all community-acquired pneumonias during noninfluenza periods. The disease is primarily one of children and young adults, spreading from person to person via respiratory tract secretions. The most common syndrome produced is tracheobronchitis, but pneumonia, pharyngitis, rhinitis, ear infection (including bullous myringitis), meningitis, myocarditis, and pericarditis also occur.

Very few laboratories perform mycoplasma cultures. Accurate, rapid diagnosis is highly desirable, since penicillin and other β-lactam agents are ineffective treatment; erythromycin and tetracycline are the antibiotics of choice. Laboratory diagnosis is usually made serologically. Nonspecific production of cold agglutinins occurs in approximately half of patients with atypical pneumonia. The most widely used serologic tests today are complement fixation (CF) and ELISA. Although a fourfold rise in titer from acute to convalescent serum is better evidence, CF titers in single serum specimens ≥1:128 suggest recent infection. The RNA-directed DNA probe test (Gen-Probe) has been evaluated for detection of *M. pneumoniae* genes in sputum specimens with sensitivities similar to culture. Whether culture should be the "gold standard" has not been determined.

Table 38.2

Mycoplasmas Recovered from Humans

GENUS AND SPECIES	HEMADSORPTION	H₂O₂ PRODUCED	GLUCOSE-FERMENTED	HYDROLYSIS OF ARGININE	HYDROLYSIS OF UREA
Mycoplasma					
pneumoniae	+	+	+	−	−
salivarium	−	−	−	+	−
orale	−	−	−	+	−
buccale	−	−	−	+	−
faucium	−	−	−	+	−
lipophilum	−	−	−	+	−
primatum	−	−	−	+	−
fermentans	−	−	+	+	−
hominis	−	−	−	+	−
genitalium	+	+	+	−	−
Ureaplasma					
urealyticum	+ / −		−	−	+
Acholeplasma					
laidlawii	−		+	−	−

Collection and transport of respiratory tract specimens, including nasopharyngeal and throat swabs and washings, tracheal aspirates, sputa, and lung biopsy specimens, are detailed in Chapters 16 and 21. Procedure 38.2 is a method for isolation of *M. pneumoniae*.

Other methods are available for identifying *Mycoplasma* colonies isolated by Procedure 38.2, including hemadsorption, immunofluorescent stain of colonies, and inhibition by specific antisera impregnated onto filter paper disks.

38.2.b. Genital mycoplasmas. Of the species of mycoplasma found in the human genital tract, only *U. urealyticum* and *M. hominis* are suspected pathogens. Under what circumstances they are pathogenic is still unclear, as a large number of adults are asymptomatically colonized with both species. Ureaplasmas are a cause of nongonococcal urethritis in males, but they also colonize sexually active males without urethritis. Further studies are needed to elucidate the role of this organism in disease in males.[12] In females, ureaplasmas do not seem to cause disease, but they may possibly contribute to low birth weight of newborns born to colonized mothers. *M. hominis* does not seem to cause disease commonly in males, but it is a cause of postpartum fevers in women. Additionally, strains of the organism can be isolated significantly more often from patients with pelvic inflammatory disease than from controls.

Specimens are collected on swabs, as described in Chapter 19. Transport media such as modified Stuart's, 2-SP (used for chlamydiae), or trypticase soy broth (BBL Microbiology Systems) with 0.5% albumin and 400 U/ml penicillin will preserve viability for up to 24 hours at refrigerator temperatures. Specimens that must be held longer should be frozen at −70° C in a medium containing protein. Culture media may also be used for transport. Culture methods described here (Procedures 38.3 and 38.4) are modified from Mårdh[11] and from Clyde, Kenny, and Schachter.[3] Shepard's A7-B agar, a satisfactory medium for cultivation of genital mycoplasmas, is available from several commercial sources; a biphasic medium is also available (Hana Biologics).[14] Calcium chloride and urea incorporated into these media impart a dark brown color to *Ureaplasma* colonies (Figure 38.7) and remove the need to stain the colonies with magnesium chloride–urea reagent, described in Procedure 38.3.

Although serologic tests such as indirect hemagglutination and metabolism inhibition for genital mycoplasmas are available, they are rarely used. It is possible that ELISA tests for mycoplasmal antigen or RNA-directed DNA probes (PACE system, Gen-Probe) of sufficient specificity for diagnosis may be available in the future. Nucleic acid dot-blot hybridization methods have been used for detection of *M. genitalium*, which is difficult to isolate in culture.

Isolation of M. pneumoniae

1. Place 0.1 to 0.2 ml of liquid specimen or dip and twirl a specimen received on a swab in a vial of SP-4 culture medium (Appendix B). After expressing as much fluid as possible from the swab by "wringing" it at the mouth of the vial, remove the swab to prevent contamination.
2. Seal the vial tightly and incubate in air at 37° C for up to 3 weeks.
3. Inspect the vial daily. During the first 5 days a change in pH, indicated by a color shift from orange to yellow or violet, or increased turbidity is a sign that the culture is contaminated and should be discarded.
4. If either a slight acid pH shift (yellow color) with no increase in turbidity or no change occurs after 7 days' incubation, subculture several drops of the broth culture to Edward-Hayflick agar (Appendix B). Continue to incubate the original broth.
5. If broth that exhibited no changes at 7 days shows a slight acid pH shift at any time, subculture to agar as above. Broths that show no change at 3 weeks are blindly subcultured again, to agar.

6. Incubate the agar plates in a very moist atmosphere with 5% CO_2 at 37° C for 7 days.
7. Observe the agar surface under 40× magnification after 5 days for colonies, which appear as spherical, grainy, yellowish forms, embedded in the agar, with a thin outer layer ("fried egg," Figure 38.5).
8. Definitive identification of *M. pneumoniae* is accomplished by overlaying Edward-Hayflick agar plates showing suspicious colonies with 5% sheep or guinea pig erythrocytes in 1% agar made in physiologic saline (0.85% NaCl) instead of water. The 1% agar is melted and cooled to 50° C, the blood cells are added, and a thin layer is poured over the original agar surface.
9. Reincubate the plate for 24 h and observe for β-hemolysis around colonies of *M. pneumoniae* caused by production of hydrogen peroxide (Figure 38.6). Additional incubation at room temperature overnight will enhance the hemolysis. No other species of mycoplasma produces this reaction.

Modified from Clyde, Kenney, and Schachter.[3]

Isolation of U. urealyticum

1. Inoculate one *Ureaplasma* agar plate and one *Ureaplasma* broth (Appendix B) each with 0.1 ml specimen from transport medium.
2. Incubate broth in tightly sealed test tubes for 5 days. Observe twice daily for a color change in the broth to red with no increase in turbidity. If color change occurs, transfer one loopful to a *Ureaplasma* agar plate and streak for isolated colonies.
3. Agar plates are incubated in a candle jar or, optimally, in an anaerobic jar at 37° C. Colonies will appear on agar within 48 h. Plates

are inspected in the same way as described for *M. pneumoniae* (Procedure 38.2). *Ureaplasma* colonies will appear as small, granular, yellowish spheres that simulate the yolk of the "fried egg."
4. To definitively identify colonies on *Ureaplasma* agar after 48 h incubation, pour a solution of 1% urea and 0.8% $MnCl_2$ in distilled water over the agar surface. *U. urealyticum* will stain dark brown because of production of urease (Figure 38.8).

Figure 38.5
Colony of *Mycoplasma hominis* on A7 agar.

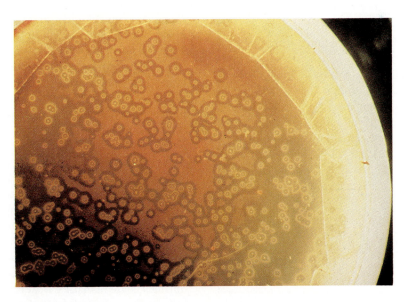

Figure 38.6
Mycoplasma pneumoniae colonies with sheep red blood cell overlay.

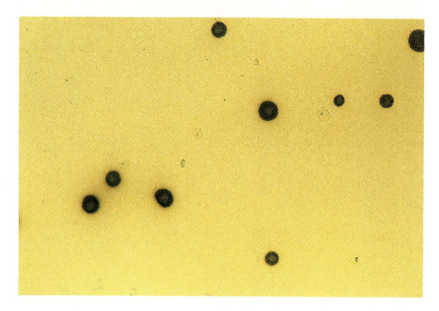

Figure 38.7
Colonies of *U. urealyticum* growing on Shephard A-7B agar visualized under 100× magnification.

PROCEDURE 38.4

Isolation of M. hominis

1. Inoculate one *M. hominis* agar plate and two *M. hominis* broth tubes (Chapter 45), one broth containing phenol red indicator and one without the possibly inhibitory phenol red, each with 0.1 ml specimen from transport media.
2. Incubate broths in tightly sealed test tubes for 5 days. If the phenol red–containing broth changes color to red or violet, both broths are subcultured to *M. hominis* agar. After 48 h incubation, transfer 0.1 ml or a loopful of broth from tubes that exhibited no change or only a slight increase in turbidity to *M. hominis* agar and streak for isolated colonies.
3. *M. hominis* agar plates are incubated in the same manner as *Ureaplasma* cultures. Plates should be observed daily for up to 5 days for colonies.

38.3. *Rickettsia, Coxiella,* and *Ehrlichia*

The Rickettsiaceae are a group of organisms that infect wild animals, with humans acting as accidental hosts in most cases. Most of these organisms are passed between animals by an insect vector. Since 1986, human infection due to *Ehrlichia canis* and *E. sennetsu, Rickettsia*-like organisms previously thought to infect only animals, has been recognized.[13] All rickettsiae multiply only intracellularly. *Coxiella burnetii,* which is similar to but distinct from the rickettsiae, can survive extracellularly. The rickettsiae cannot even survive outside of their animal hosts or insect vectors. The diseases caused in humans are usually characterized by fever, headache, and rash. With the exception of Q fever, caused by *C. burnetii,* the rickettsiae multiply in the endothelial cells of blood vessels, causing cell injury and death. Damage to cells results in vascular changes and the influx of inflammatory cells that serve to magnify the host's immune response and increase overall morbidity.

Rickettsiae are pleomorphic gram-negative coccobacilli. The organisms multiply by binary fission in the cytoplasm of host cells, which are finally lysed during release of mature rickettsiae. The rickettsiae, but not *C. burnetii,* infect humans following the bite of an infected arthropod vector. The agents, their

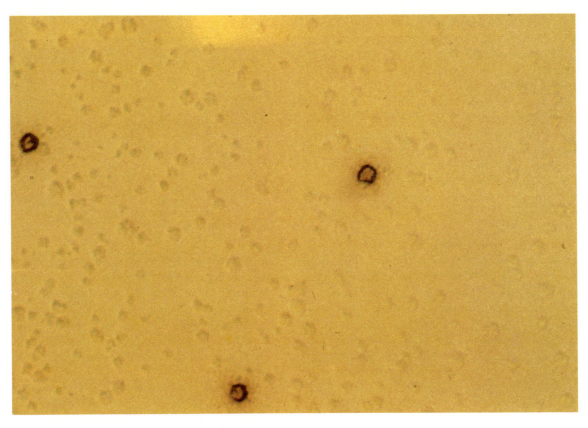

Figure 38.8
Colonies of *U. urealyticum* after 48 hour incubation, overlaid with urea-manganese chloride reagent.

vectors, and diseases are shown in Table 38.3. *C. burnetii* is more hardy than the others, resisting desiccation and sunlight. They infect humans by the aerosol route. In contrast to rickettsiae, *Coxiella* is passively phagocytized by host cells and multiplies within vacuoles. The other agents, after being deposited directly into the bloodstream through the bite of a louse, ixodid tick, flea, or mite, induce host cells to engulf them, after which they quickly escape the vacuole to become free in the cytoplasm. *Coxiella* is inhaled into the alveoli, picked up by macrophages, and carried to lymph nodes, from which it disseminates into the bloodstream. Granulomatous hepatitis and endocarditis are common sequelae.

Early diagnosis is usually made on clinical grounds based on the symptoms of fever, rash, and exposure to ticks. The characteristic spread of the rash from the extremities to the trunk helps to dis-

Table 38.3

Vectors of Selected Diseases Caused by *Rickettsia,* *Coxiella,* and *Ehrlichia*

AGENT	DISEASE	VECTOR
Rickettsia akari	Rickettsialpox	Mites
R. conorii	Boutonneuse fever	Ticks
R. prowazekii	Epidemic typhus Brill-Zinsser disease	Lice
R. rickettsii	Rocky Mountain spotted fever	Ticks
R. tsutsugamushi	Scrub typhus	Mites
R. typhi	Murine (endemic) typhus	Fleas
Rochalimaea quintana	Trench fever	Lice
Coxiella burnetii	Q fever	Ticks, aerosols
Ehrlichia canis	Ehrlichiosis	Ticks
E. sennetsu	Ehrlichiosis	Ticks

tinguish Rocky Mountain spotted fever (RMSF) from meningococcemia. Ehrlichiosis resembles "rashless" RMSF, since only 20% of patients infected with *Ehrlichia* develop rash, whereas almost 90% of RMSF patients exhibit a rash.

38.3.a. Laboratory identification. Biopsy specimens of skin tissue from the rash of RMSF can be stained directly with a specific immunofluorescent reagent. This test, available at certain state health laboratories and the Centers for Disease Control (CDC), can provide a diagnosis as early as 3 to 4 days after symptoms have appeared. The Giménez stain (Appendix C) is also used for examination of clinical material.

Although the rickettsiae can be cultured in embryonated eggs and in tissue culture, the risk of laboratory-acquired infection is extremely high, limiting culture techniques to a few specialized laboratories. Diagnosis of rickettsial disease and ehrlichiosis is primarily accomplished serologically. The least specific but most widely used test in the United States is the Weil-Felix reaction, the fortuitous agglutination of certain strains of *Proteus vulgaris* by serum from patients with rickettsial disease. Table 38.4 outlines the positive reactions associated with each disease. Commercial suppliers produce kits that contain all necessary antigens and human antirickettsial control antisera for performance of the Weil-Felix test. This test is only presumptive, however, and a more specific serologic test, such as complement fixation or direct immunofluorescence, must be used for confirmation of disease. These tests are performed primarily by reference laboratories, and kits are obtainable from CDC for performing tests for IgG antibody.

The microimmunofluorescent dot test, described previously for diagnosis of psittacosis, has shown excellent sensitivity for detecting antibodies to rickettsiae. By overlaying the antigen dots on the slide with fluorescein-conjugated antihuman IgM after the patient's serum has been allowed to form complexes, early diagnosis of RMSF can be achieved (within 7 to 10 days after onset of symptoms). Both immunofluorescent and a recently developed latex agglutination test method have shown good sensitivity for diagnosis of RMSF within the first week. Neither Q fever, ehrlichiosis, nor rickettsialpox induces Weil-Felix antibody in infected patients. Especially in those cases, specific immunofluorescent tests are valuable.

Table 38.4

Reactions of *Proteus* Strains in Weil-Felix Test

DISEASE	OX-19	OX-2	OX-K
Brill-Zinsser	V	V	−
Epidemic typhus	+	V	−
Murine typhus	+	V	−
Rickettsialpox	−	−	−
Rocky Mountain spotted fever	+	+	−
Scrub typhus	−	−	V
Q fever	−	−	−
Ehrlichiosis	−	−	−

+ = >90% positive agglutination; − = >90% negative agglutination; V = variable results.

C. burnetii undergoes an antigenic phase variation during infection. The organisms exist in phase II during initial infection, and humans produce antibody to phase II early in disease. If infection progresses to chronic disease, such as endocarditis or hepatitis, antibodies to phase I are present and can be measured by complement fixation or immunofluorescence.

Except for latex agglutination, immunofluorescence, and direct fluorescent antibody testing for diagnosing RMSF, none of the serologic tests is useful for diagnosing disease in time to influence therapy, since antibodies to rickettsiae other than *R. rickettsii* often cannot be detected until at least 2 weeks after the patient has become ill. With newer immunological reagents being developed, we can hope that more easily performed, sensitive, and specific tests for all rickettsial diseases will soon be available.

REFERENCES

1. Baselski, V.S., McNeeley, S.G., Ryan, G., and Robison, M.A. 1987. A comparison of nonculture-dependent methods for detection of *Chlamydia trachomatis* infections in pregnant women. Obstet. Gynecol. 70:47.
2. Campbell, L.A., Kuo, C.-C., and Grayston, J.T. 1987. Characterization of the new *Chlamydia* agent, TWAR, as a unique organism by restriction endonuclease analysis and DNA-DNA hybridization. J. Clin. Microbiol. 25:1911.
3. Clyde, W.A., Jr., Kenny, G.E., and Schachter, J. 1984. Cumitech 19: laboratory diagnosis of chlamydial and mycoplasmal infections. Drew, W.L., coordinating editor. American Society for Microbiology, Washington, D.C.
4. Gibbs, R.S., Cassell, G.H., Davis, J.K., et al. 1986. Further studies on genital mycoplasms in intra-amniotic infection: blood cultures and serologic response. Am. J. Obstet. Gynecol. 154:717.

5. Grayston, J.T., Kuo, C.-C., Wang, S.-P., and Altman, J. 1986. A new *Chlamydia psittaci* strain, TWAR, isolated in acute respiratory tract infections. N. Engl. J. Med. 315:161.

6. Hammerschlag, M.R., Roblin, P.M., Cummings, C., et al. 1987. Comparison of enzyme immunoassay and culture for diagnosis of chlamydial conjunctivitis and respiratory infections in infants. J. Clin. Microbiol. 25:2306.

7. Hipp, S.S., Yangsook, H., and Murphy, D. 1987. Assessment of enzyme immunoassay and immunofluorescence test for detection of *Chlamydia trachomatis.* J. Clin. Microbiol. 25:1938.

8. Kundsin, R.B., Driscoll, S.G., and Pelletier, P.A. 1980. *Ureaplasma urealyticum* incriminated in perinatal morbidity and mortality. Science 213:474.

9. Lipkin, E.S., Moncada, J.V., Shafer, M.A., et al. 1986. Comparison of monoclonal antibody staining and culture in diagnosing cervical chlamydial infection. J. Clin. Microbiol. 23:114.

10. Mahony, J.B., Chernesky, M.A., Bromberg, K., and Schachter, J. 1986. Accuracy of immunoglobulin M immunoassay for diagnosis of chlamydial infections in infants and adults. J. Clin. Microbiol. 24:731.

11. Mårdh, P.-A. 1984. Laboratory diagnosis of sexually transmitted diseases. In Holmes, K.K., Mårdh, P.-A., Sparling, P.F., and Wiesner, P.J., editors. Sexually transmitted diseases. McGraw-Hill Book Co., New York.

12. Oriel, J.D. 1983. Role of genital mycoplasmas in nongonococcal urethritis and prostatitis. Sex. Transm. Dis. 10 (Suppl.):263.

13. Peterson, L.R., Sawyer, L.A., Fishbein, D.B., et al. 1989. An outbreak of ehrlichiosis in members of an army reserve unit exposed to ticks. J. Infect. Dis. 159:562.

14. Phillips, L.E., Goodrich, K.H., Turner, R.M., and Faro, S. 1986. Isolation of *Mycoplasma* species and *Ureaplasma urealyticum* from obstetrical and gynecological patients by using commercially available medium formulations. J. Clin. Microbiol. 24:377.

15. Smith, J.W., Rogers, R.E., Katz, B.P., et al. 1987. Diagnosis of chlamydial infection in women attending antenatal and gynecologic clinics. J. Clin. Microbiol. 25:868.

16. Stamm, W.E., Running, K., Hale, J., and Holmes, K.K. 1983. Etiologic role of *Mycoplasma hominis* and *Ureaplasma urealyticum* in women with acute urethral syndrome. Sex. Transm. Dis. 10 (Suppl.):318.

17. Steffenson, D.O., Dummer, J.S., Granick, M.S., et al. 1987. Sternotomy infections with *Mycoplasma hominis.* Ann. Intern. Med. 106:204.

18. Taylor-Robinson, D., Thomas, B.J., and Osborn, M.F. 1987. Evaluation of enzyme immunoassay (Chlamydiazyme) for detecting *C. trachomatis* in genital tract specimens. J. Clin. Pathol. 40:194.

19. Tilton, R.C., Judson, F.N., Barnes, R.C., et al. 1988. Multicenter comparative evaluation of two rapid microscopic methods and culture for detection of *Chlamydia trachomatis* in patient specimens. J. Clin. Microbiol. 26:167.

20. Tjiam, K.H., van Heijst, B.Y., van Zuuren, A., et al. 1986. Evaluation of an enzyme immunoassay for the diagnosis of chlamydial infections in urogenital specimens. J. Clin. Microbiol. 23:752.

BIBLIOGRAPHY

Anonymous. 1983. International symposium on *Mycoplasma hominis*—a human pathogen. Sex. Transm. Dis. 10(suppl.). Entire issue devoted to human mycoplasmas.

Baca, O.G., and Paretsky, D. 1983. Q fever and *Coxiella burnetii:* a model for host-parasite interactions. Microbiol. Rev. 47:127.

Barnes, R.C. 1989. Laboratory diagnosis of human chlamydial infections. Clin. Microbiol. Rev. 2:119.

Batteiger, B.E., and Jones, R.B. 1987. Chlamydial infections. Infect. Dis. Clin. North Am. 1:55.

Cassel, G.H., and Cole, B.C. 1981. Mycoplasma as agents of human disease. N. Engl. J. Med. 304:80.

Centers for Disease Control. 1985. *Chlamydia trachomatis* infections: policy guidelines for prevention and control. M.M.W.R. 34 (Suppl.):53.

Couch, R.C. 1984. Mycoplasma diseases. In Holmes, K.K., Mårdh, P.-A., Sparling, P.F., and Wiesner, P.J., editors. Sexually transmitted diseases. McGraw-Hill Book Co., New York.

de Girolami, P.C., Drew, W.L., Gleaves, C.A., et al. 1988. Procedure manual for the detection of CMV and HSV in shell-vial cultures. Syva MicroTak Monograph. Syva Co., Palo Alto, Calif.

Hechemy, K.E. 1980. Rocky Mountain spotted fever: the clinical and immunoserologic picture. Clin. Immunol. Newsletter 1(10):1.

LaScolea, L.J., Jr. 1986. Chlamydial infections: the mother-infant connection. Clin. Microbiol. Newsletter 8:77.

Oriel, D., Ridgway, G., Schachter, J., et al., editors. 1986. Chlamydial infections. Cambridge University Press, Cambridge, England. (Entire book devoted to chlamydial topics.)

Philip, R.N., Casper, E.A., Ormsbee, R.A., et al. 1976. Microimmunofluorescence test for the serological study of Rocky Mountain spotted fever and typhus. J. Clin. Microbiol. 3:51.

Saah, A.J., and Hornick, R.B. 1985. *Coxiella burnetii* (Q fever). In Mandell, G.L., Douglas, R.G., Jr., and Bennett, J.E., editors. Principles and practice of infectious diseases, ed. 2. John Wiley & Sons, New York. (NOTE: Several other chapters by the same authors contain valuable information.)

Salgo, M.P., Telzak, E.E., Currie, B., et al. 1988. A focus of Rocky Mountain Spotted Fever within New York City. N. Engl. J. Med. 318:1346.

Schachter, J. 1984. Biology of *Chlamydia trachomatis.* In Holmes, K.K., Mårdh, P.-A., Sparling, P.F., and Wiesner, P.J., editors. Sexually transmitted diseases. McGraw-Hill Book Co., New York.

Stamm, W.E. 1988. Diagnosis of *Chlamydia trachomatis* genitourinary infections. Ann. Intern. Med. 108:710.

Weissfeld, A.S. 1983. Genital mycoplasma. Clin. Microbiol. Newsletter 5:65.

Woodward, W.E., and Hornick, R.B. 1985. *Rickettsia rickettsii* (Rocky Mountain spotted fever). In Mandell, G.L., Douglas, R.G., Jr., and Bennett, J.E., editors. Principles and practice of infectious diseases, ed. 2. John Wiley & Sons, New York.

Wyrick, P.B., Gutman, L.T., and Hodinka, R.L. 1988. Chlamydiae. In Joklik, W.K., Willett, H.P., Amos, D.B., and Wilfert, C.M., editors: Zinsser's Microbiology, ed. 19. Appleton & Lange, Norwalk, Conn.

The microorganisms discussed in this chapter were not placed in any of the previous chapters, either because they are unusual enough not to fit into existing classifications, or because they are isolated rarely or only in association with a defined syndrome. Although they are able to grow on media easily available to most clinical laboratories, several of the organisms discussed here require specific isolation techniques for their cultivation, necessitating that the physician communicate with the laboratory the need for special procedures.

39.1. Genus *Bartonella*

39.1.a. Epidemiology and pathogenesis of *Bartonella* infection.

Bartonella bacilliformis, the only species in the genus *Bartonella*, is closely related to *Chlamydia*, differing in the site of infection in the vertebrate host and in the requirement for intracellular multiplication. Although *Chlamydia* parasitize the epithelial cells of the respiratory and genital mucous membranes, *Bartonella* grow within and on the surface of erythrocytes and occasionally in vascular endothelium. In contrast to *Chlamydia*, *Bartonella* can be cultivated in vitro on nonliving media.

The disease bartonellosis is confined to the Andes region of Peru, Ecuador, and Colombia, where the arthropod vector, the sand fly, *Phlebotomus*, and susceptible humans both exist. Humans acquire the disease from the bite of the fly and humans serve as a reservoir for the organism in the region. Two forms of the disease are common, a febrile, systemic disease characterized by anemia, called "Oroya fever," and a chronic, cutaneous disease characterized by tumorlike lesions of the skin and mucous membranes, called "verruga peruana." Verruga peruana usually follows an episode of Oroya fever. The bacteria on the surface of and within erythrocytes seem to contribute to the anemia. Patients with partial immunity develop verruga peruana. It is not known exactly how the organisms damage the red blood cells. Patients with Oroya fever appear to be at increased risk for contracting *Salmonella* infection.

39.1.b. Laboratory diagnosis of bartonellosis.

The organisms can be isolated from blood and from material aspirated from lymph nodes or cutaneous lesions. Organisms grow best at room temperature and do not require increased CO_2 in the atmosphere. Brain-heart infusion agar, modified to contain 0.4% agar, with the addition of 5% human, rabbit, or horse blood, should support growth of *B. bacilliformis*. The organisms stain gram-negative and are visualized best with the carbol-fuchsin counterstain. They are curved or coccoid, with mixtures of rods and granules, which tend to grow in aggregates. In vitro, cells produce a polar tuft of flagella. Biochemically, *B. bacilliformis* is quite inert.

The organisms may also be visualized in blood films from infected patients.[16] They stain red-violet with Giemsa stain, appearing as cocci or bacilli, with occasional curved or ringlike forms. The cells may show polar enlargements (appearing only at one end).

39.1.c. Therapy of bartonellosis.

The disease seems to respond rapidly to therapy with penicillin, chloramphenicol, tetracycline, or streptomycin.

39.2. Genus *Chromobacterium*

39.2.a. Epidemiology and pathogenesis of *Chromobacterium* infection.

Chromobacterium violaceum, instantly recognizable by its purple pigment, is the etiologic agent of a particularly devastating and virulent bacteremia, usually acquired in the southeastern United States, particularly in Florida. The organism has been recovered from soil and water in tropical countries. Patients usually acquire the organism from puncture wounds or wounds that come into contact with soil or contaminated water. One patient, however, presumably acquired the infection by swallowing large amounts of water during a near-drowning accident. Since at least three of twelve patients were known to have chronic granulomatous disease and the status of several other patients is unknown, it has been suggested that an underlying neutrophil dysfunction places patients at increased risk for developing fulminant *C. violaceum* infections.[11]

The organism is extremely virulent; there is an overall mortality rate of 57% in patients with infection acquired in the United States. The infection often presents as a febrile illness, and skin lesions are common. Liver abscess and pulmonary involvement are also prominent features. Virulence factors have not been well studied, but extracellular proteases are produced by species of *C. violaceum*.

39.2.b. Laboratory identification of *Chromobacterium violaceum*.

The organisms are usually recognized by their violet pigment (Figure 39.1), produced on media containing tryptophan, such as 5% sheep blood agar. Although the organisms grow best at 25° C, they will grow at 37° C. *C. violaceum* is facultatively anaerobic. Cultures may smell of ammonium cyanide, since the organisms produce HCN. *C. violaceum* is resistant to penicillin and to the vibriostatic agent 0/129. Although it is usually oxidase-positive, the purple color may mask the reaction. It is catalase-, Voges-Proskauer, and esculin-negative. The rarely encountered pigment-negative strains may be confused with *Vibrio* species or *Aeromonas* species, but since they have not been implicated in human disease, they should not pose a problem. Resistance to 0/129 will distinguish *Chromobacterium* from vibrios, which are suscep-

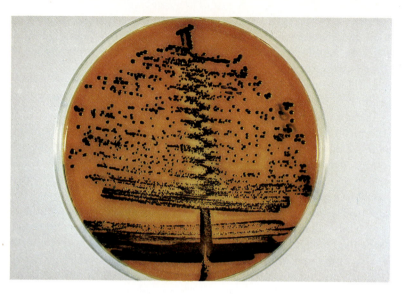

Figure 39.1
Colonies of violet-pigmented. *C. violaceum* on blood agar.

tible, and lack of indole production will differentiate *Chromobacterium* from *Aeromonas* and *Plesiomonas*, many of which are indole-positive. Unlike many of the other unusual gram-negative bacilli, *C. violaceum* grows well on MacConkey agar.

The organisms are always motile, as demonstrated by wet preparation. On Gram stain, they are medium to long bacilli with rounded ends; the bacilli are occasionally slightly curved. *Chromobacterium* possesses the unusual flagellar arrangement of both a single polar flagellum and lateral flagella. The other species of *Chromobacterium*, *C. fluviatile*, has not been associated with human infection. A former additional nonpathogenic species, *C. lividum*, has now been transferred to the genus *Janthinobacterium*.

39.2.c. Treatment of infections due to *C. violaceum.* Most isolates are susceptible in vitro to chloramphenicol, erythromycin, tetracycline, and trimethoprim-sulfamethoxazole. Resistance to ampicillin, cephalothin, carbenicillin, and penicillins has been reported. Those patients who recovered from septicemia in the series reported by Macher et al.[11] were treated with gentamicin, with or without chloramphenicol. Long-term therapy may be necessary to eradicate all foci of the infection.

39.3. Genus *Dermatophilus*

39.3.a. Epidemiology and pathogenesis of *Dermatophilus* infection. Within the same family as the *Actinomyces* species, and therefore classified as a bacterium, *Dermatophilus congolensis* is the etiologic agent of dermatophilosis (also called strawberry foot rot, lumpy wool, mycotic dermatitis, and streptotrichosis), a disease of the skin that is characterized by acute or chronic development of an exudative, scabbing dermatitis. The disease occurs worldwide in domestic animals, including cattle, sheep, goats, horses, other mammals, and humans. Manifestations of the disease are more severe in tropical regions. The organism has been isolated from both patients and wild animals in New York. Recently, a *Dermatophilus* infection of the tongue of a patient with human immunodeficiency virus (HIV) infection was reported; the lesions resembled those of Epstein-Barr-associated "hairy" leukoplakia.[2] As with the fungi, pathogenesis is probably related to the large size of the organism and its ability to resist cell-mediated killing. Extracellular enzymes may contribute to pathogenesis.

39.3.b. Laboratory identification of *Dermatophilus.* Biopsy material and touch preparations of the underside of scabs should be stained by Giemsa or methenamine silver. Typical organisms displaying septate hyphallike forms, tapering and dividing transversely, with production of packets of coccoid spores as a final morphotype, are visible, particularly around hair follicles. The organism is gram-positive, but fine structure is not visible with the Gram stain.

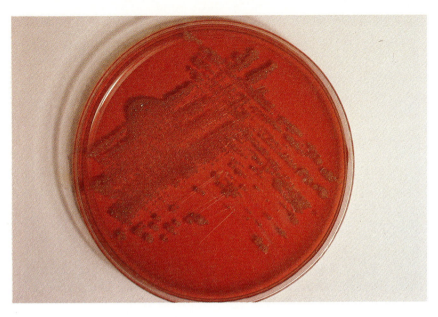

Figure 39.2
Colonies of *D. congolensis* on 5% sheep blood agar. (Organisms courtesy Dr. Morris Gordon.)

As described by Gordon,[7] biopsy specimens and tissue scrapings from skin lesions, as well as exudate aspirated from unopened pustules, should be streaked to blood agar, which is incubated in air at 37° C. Brain-heart infusion agar with 5% sheep blood, recommended for primary inoculation of all specimens for isolation of fungi, will also support growth of *D. congolensis*. Colonies develop to a diameter of approximately 5 mm after 2 to 4 days' growth. Colonies are grayish and usually become orange after several days, heaped, rough, glabrous, and adherent to the agar; pitting may be observed with early growth (Figure 39.2). In heavy areas, the colonies are β-hemolytic and in later stages they may become mucoid. The organisms will also grow in brain-heart infusion-peptone broth, but they do not grow on Sabouraud's dextrose agar. A direct wet preparation from a colony will show branching filaments from 0.5 to 5 μm in width; branches are at right angles. The filaments divide longitudinally and transversely, finally becoming aggregates of motile coccoid-shaped spores (Figure 39.3). If only coccoid forms are seen on wet preparation from a colony, a younger subculture should be examined for filaments. Because the Gram stain tends to obscure details, a plain methylene blue stain (such as Loeffler's methylene blue, Appendix B) should be used.

Although cellular morphology is characteristic, biochemical reactions may help confirm the identification. The organism is catalase- and urease-positive. *D. congolensis* produces extracellular enzymes, such as protease and gelatinase. All strains are indole-, nitrate-, and Voges-Proskauer-negative.

39.3.c. Treatment of infections caused by *Dermatophilus congolensis*. The organism is susceptible in vitro to penicillin, streptomycin, chloramphenicol, tetracycline, erythromycin, and sulfonamides. It is resistant to the antidermatophyte griseofulvin. The treatment of choice appears to be a penicillin in combination with an aminoglycoside.

39.4. Genus *Gardnerella*

39.4.a. Epidemiology and pathogenesis of *Gardnerella* infection. *Gardnerella vaginalis* is found in the genital and urinary tract of humans, where it may play a role in **bacterial vaginosis,** a possibly sexually transmitted disease of women characterized by copious, malodorous discharge. Although male partners of women with bacterial vaginosis can be found to harbor the organism in the genital tract, it does not seem to cause symptoms in males in that site. In addition to women with the characteristic discharge, approximately two thirds of asymptomatic normal controls also harbor the organism, although

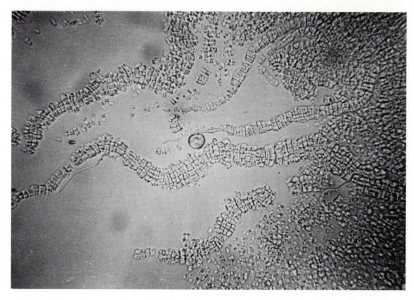

Figure 39.3
Methylene blue–stained organisms of *D. congolensis* from colony on blood agar plate. (Courtesy of Dr. Morris Gordon.)

the number of colony-forming units is often lower in asymptomatic females.

Bacterial vaginosis, formerly called "nonspecific vaginitis," is one of the most common complaints of postpubescent women visiting their gynecologists. The vaginal discharge of this syndrome is usually homogeneous, unaccompanied by pain or itching. Unlike the purulent discharge of gonococcal urethritis, *Trichomonas* vaginitis, and most yeast infections, there is a paucity of neutrophils in the discharge of patients suffering from bacterial vaginosis. For this reason, the term "vaginosis," rather than "vaginitis," was coined. Studies have implicated anaerobic bacteria in the etiology of bacterial vaginosis.[18] It is likely that *G. vaginalis* is an indicator organism for this syndrome; whether it is a true pathogen is not known. The organism does display some virulence for humans in addition to its role in vaginosis; a number of reports of postpartum sepsis, both in mothers and neonates, and of *G. vaginalis* as an agent of urinary tract infections in males and females have been published. The difficulty in cultivating the organism from blood has probably led to a lack of recognition of its role in postpartum bacteremia and fever.

39.4.b. Laboratory identification of *Gardnerella vaginalis*. Specimens most likely to be sent to the microbiology laboratory for cultivation of *G. vaginalis* include cervical, urethral, and vaginal swabs from patients with discharge, as well as urethral cultures from male sexual partners. Women suffering from postpartum fever, and neonates showing signs of sepsis may be infected with *G. vaginalis*, which may be isolated from blood. The sodium polyanethol sulfonate (SPS) currently used as an anticoagulant in most commercial blood culture media has been found to inhibit growth of *Gardnerella*, however, and these media are not suitable for culture. Good results have been achieved by direct plating of blood onto agar. Although there have been no studies, it seems likely that the lysis-centrifugation blood culture method would allow growth of *G. vaginalis* plated onto chocolate or other supportive agar, such as Columbia agar with colistin and nalidixic acid.

Most specimens of genital origin are contaminated with other flora. The fastidious nature of *G. vaginalis*, therefore, requires the use of a semiselective medium. The best selective and differential medium for detection of *G. vaginalis*, particularly from normal controls in which the number of organisms is small, is HBT (human blood tween) agar (Appendix A).[20] This medium consists of a base layer of Columbia agar base overlaid with a layer of the same base containing 5% human blood. HBT medium is

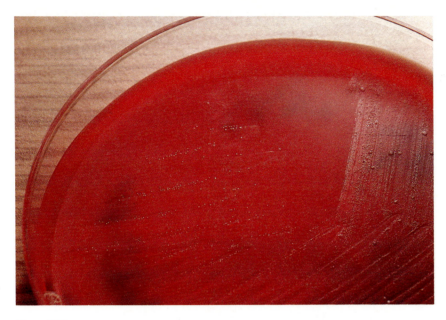

Figure 39.4
Culture of vaginal discharge after 48 hours incubation. Colonies of *G. vaginalis* growing in large numbers on CNA agar that also supports the growth of some normal flora.

available commercially. Material from genital discharge is inoculated within 4 to 6 hours of collection onto this medium and the plates are incubated in 5% to 10% CO_2 or in a candle jar for 48 hours. The organism has been shown to survive poorly in commonly used transport media. Colonies of *G. vaginalis* on HBT agar are convex, opaque, and gray, surrounded by a diffuse zone of β-hemolysis. On sheep blood agar these organisms are not hemolytic and are barely visible. They grow well on CNA agar, without yielding any hemolysis (Figure 39.4). The ability of the organism to hemolyze human erythrocytes forms the basis for the differential nature of the HBT agar. *G. vaginalis* will not grow on MacConkey agar.

The organisms are small, pleomorphic, gram-variable or gram-negative coccobacilli and short rods (Figure 39.5). They possess an unusual laminated cell wall structure with a possible glycocalyx, which may aid adherence to vaginal epithelium.[8] The organism is oxidase- and catalase-negative. Presumptive identification based on colonial morphology and hemolysis on HBT, cellular morphology, and the rapid enzyme tests mentioned here are adequate for isolates from female genital sources. *Gardnerella*

will hydrolyze sodium hippurate and ferment starch and raffinose.[22] The RIM system (Austin Biological Laboratories) can accurately identify *Gardnerella* biochemically, if such identification is clinically necessary.[10]

Presumptive diagnosis of bacterial vaginosis can be made without performing cultures, as described in Chapter 19. Aside from the distinctive clinical picture, a direct wet mount of vaginal discharge material will usually show "clue cells," squamous epithelial cells covered with tiny bacilli, especially around the periphery, giving the cell a stippled appearance. Discharge material will have a characteristic fishy odor, particularly after addition of 10% KOH (the sniff test), and the pH of the material will be greater than 4.5.

39.4.c. Treatment of *G. vaginalis* vaginosis. Although in vitro susceptibility of *G. vaginalis* to metronidazole is variable, metronidazole has consistently yielded the best cure of bacterial vaginosis. Since metronidazole is effective primarily against anaerobic bacteria, the ability of metronidazole to affect this syndrome speaks against a primary causative role for *Gardnerella*. All strains have been susceptible in vitro to ampicillin, carbenicillin, oxacillin, penicillin,

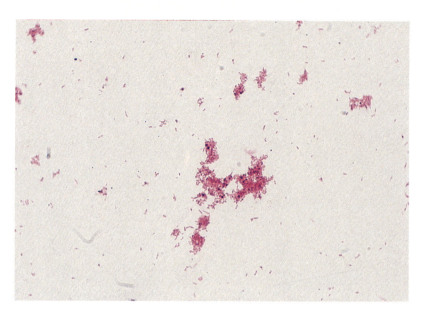

Figure 39.5
Gram stain of *G. vaginalis* from growth on CNA agar.

and vancomycin. Susceptibility to the latter three agents is usually a characteristic of gram-positive organisms, another enigmatic finding for *Gardnerella*.

39.5. Genus *Legionella*

39.5.a. **Epidemiology and pathogenesis of *Legionella* infection.** Species of *Legionella*, the only genus in the newly described family Legionellaceae, are distributed worldwide in surface water, soil, mud, lakes, and streams. The organisms are not known to have an animal reservoir, although they are maintained intracellularly in protozoa that function as their natural host. *Legionella* is the causative agent of Legionnaires' disease, a febrile and pneumonic illness with numerous clinical presentations. *Legionella* was discovered in 1976 by scientists at the Centers for Disease Control (CDC), who were investigating an epidemic of pneumonia among Pennsylvania state American Legion members attending a convention in Philadelphia. There is retrospective serologic evidence of *Legionella* infection as far back as 1947. Most of the studies to date have centered around *Legionella pneumophila*, the type species of the genus and the most prevalent etiologic agent of Legionnaires' disease. Many other species of *Legionella* have now been characterized, isolated from sporadic cases of pneumonia and from other

outbreaks, as well as from environmental sources. A recent outbreak of prosthetic-valve endocarditis due to *L. pneumophila* and *L. dumoffii* has been reported.[19] Many of the reported cases of non–*L. pneumophila* pneumonia have been nosocomial in nature.

Legionella species live in natural waters and can be found in air conditioning cooling tower water, air conditioning condensate, and reservoir waters, often in association with blue-green algae and free-living protozoa. The organisms can also multiply in relatively hot water and can be found in shower heads, whirlpool baths, and institutional potable water systems. They are able to grow at temperatures from 25° to 43° C on artificial media, and at even higher temperatures in nature. Patients usually acquire the organism by breathing in aerosols; no person-to-person transmission occurs. Eradication of *Legionella* from institutional water systems requires increased heat (hot water tanks must be heated to >70° C for 72 hours) or increased chlorination (to 2 parts per million of free chlorine). Surgical patients, those who are immunosuppressed (particularly those on corticosteroids), and persons who smoke are at increased risk for acquiring Legionnaires' disease.

The disease occurs sporadically, at low levels endemically, or as epidemics among susceptible hosts. It is not a rare infection (it is estimated that 25,000 to 50,000 cases occur annually in the United States); there is usually a seasonal peak during late summer. The disease involves multiple organ systems, but it is manifested primarily as severe, consolidated pneumonia. Bacteremia is probably not uncommon, especially in the immunosuppressed patient. Another manifestation of disease caused by *Legionella pneumophila* and occasionally by *L. anisa, L. feeleii*, and *L. micdadei*) is Pontiac fever, a multisystem disease with respiratory symptoms, fever, myalgia, and headache, but without pneumonia. Pontiac fever is a mild self-limited disease with no mortality, in contrast to Legionnaires' disease, which has a significant mortality. The clinical manifestations exhibited by infection with a particular species primarily are due to differences in the immune response of the host and perhaps to inoculum size; the same *Legionella* species gives rise to different expressions of disease in different individuals. Schlanger et al.[17] have reported a patient with sinusitis and no presenting pneumonia caused by *L. pneumophila*. The cellular immunodeficiency of this patient no doubt contributed to his acquisition of the infection.

Pathogenesis of *Legionella* infection has been studied quite extensively. Although the organisms produce several extracellular enzymes, including a phosphatase, a lipase, and nucleases, these have not been shown to contribute significantly to virulence. An extracellular toxin, however, may contribute to intracellular survival of the organisms by impairing the ability of phagocytic cells to utilize oxygen, and thus carry out oxidative bactericidal activities. The primary virulence mechanism of *Legionella* is its ability to survive within phagocytic host cells. Cell-mediated immune responses are necessary for the host to overcome disease. Serologic evidence exists for the presence of asymptomatic disease, since many healthy people surveyed possess antibodies to *Legionella* species, and in a recent hospital outbreak (VA Wadsworth Medical Center) there was a significant incidence of asymptomatic seroconversion.

39.5.b. Laboratory diagnosis of Legionnaires' disease by culture. The general isolation and direct detection of *Legionella* can be done effectively by all laboratories that possess a class II biological safety cabinet. Specimens from which *Legionella* can be isolated include respiratory tract secretions of all types, including sputum and pleural fluid; other sterile body fluids such as blood; and lung, transbronchial, or other biopsy material. Sputum specimens

are preferable to bronchial washings, which are likely to contain small amounts of inhibitory local anesthetic and are diluted by saline. Sputum from patients with Legionnaires' disease is usually nonpurulent and may appear bloody or watery. Therefore the grading system used for screening sputum for routine cultures is not applicable. Patients with Legionnaires' disease usually have detectable numbers of organisms in their respiratory secretions, even for quite some time after antibiotic therapy has been initiated. If the disease is present, the initial specimen is often likely to be positive. However, additional specimens should be processed if suspicion of the disease persists. Pleural fluid has not yielded many positive cultures in studies performed in several laboratories, but it may contain organisms. Specimens should be transported without holding media, buffers, or saline, which may be inhibitory to growth of *Legionella*. The organisms are actually very hardy and are best preserved by maintaining specimens in a small, tightly closed container to prevent desiccation and transporting them to the laboratory within 30 minutes of collection. If longer delay is anticipated, specimens should be refrigerated. If specimens cannot be assured of remaining moist, a small amount (1 ml) of sterile broth may be added.

Material should be inoculated to culture plates and applied to slides for direct fluorescent antibody testing (as described below) as soon as it is received in the laboratory. Technologists should work in a biological safety cabinet. As described in Chapter 16, sputum can best be picked from upper respiratory secretions with a wooden applicator stick, to which the mucus and pus cells will adhere. Sputum specimens that may contain contaminating bacteria should be diluted 1:10 in trypticase soy broth, the suspension should be vortexed with sterile glass beads, and plates should be inoculated with several drops of the diluted specimen. Lesser dilutions are recommended for aspirates. An acid-wash method may enhance recovery (Procedure 39.1).[6]

Sputum and respiratory secretions for direct fluorescent antibody tests are applied to slides without dilution. As described in Chapter 21, tissues are homogenized before smears and cultures are performed and clear sterile body fluids are centrifuged for 30 minutes at 4000 $\times$ g. The sediment is then vortexed and used for culture and smear preparation. Blood for culture of *Legionella* should probably be

PROCEDURE 39.1

Acid-wash Treatment of Contaminated Specimens for Recovery of Legionella *Species*

Principle

Acid washing may reduce contaminating organisms and increase the yield of *Legionella* organisms.

Method

1. Prepare stock solutions before preparing working solution and discard excess stock solutions

0.2 N HCl	50 ml
0.2 N KCl	50 ml

2. Add 5.3 ml HCl stock solution and 25 ml KCl stock solution to 100 ml distilled water.
3. Adjust pH to 2.2 by adding KCl or HCl.
4. Filter-sterilize working solution and dispense, 0.9 ml per tube plus sterile glass beads, into small screw-cap tubes.
5. Store refrigerated; stable for 6 months.
6. Add 0.1 ml specimen to 0.9 ml acid-wash solution.
7. Vortex vigorously and allow to sit on bench 4 min.
8. Revortex and plate 3 drops per plate to BCYE and BCYE-selective agar.

processed with the lysis-centrifugation tube system and plated directly to buffered charcoal yeast extract agar (BCYE). A biphasic culture medium containing BCYE agar and yeast extract broth, designed for isolation of *Legionella* from blood, is available from Remel Laboratories.

Specimens should be inoculated to two agar plates for recovery of *Legionella*, at least one of which is buffered charcoal yeast extract agar (BCYE) without inhibitory agents. This medium, developed at the CDC, contains charcoal to detoxify the medium, remove carbon dioxide, and modify the surface tension to allow the organisms to proliferate more easily. BCYE is also prepared with ACES buffer, and

growth supplements cysteine (required by *Legionella*), yeast extract, α-ketoglutarate, and iron. A second medium, BCYE base with polymyxin B, anisomycin (to inhibit fungi), and cefamandole, is recommended for specimens such as sputum that are likely to be contaminated with other flora. These media are commercially available from Remel Laboratories. Mueller-Hinton agar with 1% hemoglobin and 1% IsoVitaleX, first developed for susceptibility testing of *Haemophilus influenzae,* also will support the growth of most legionellae. Several other media, including a selective agar containing vancomycin and a differential agar containing bromthymol blue and bromcresol purple, are also available from Remel and others. Specimens obtained from sterile body sites may be plated to two media without selective agents, and perhaps also inoculated into the special blood culture broth without SPS. Of course, specimens should always be plated to standard media for recovery of pathogens other than *Legionella* that may be responsible for the disease.

Plates should be incubated in air or in a candle jar at 35° to 37° C in a humid atmosphere. Only growth of *L. gormanii* is stimulated by increased CO_2, so air incubation is preferable to 5% to 10% CO_2, which may inhibit some legionellae. Within 3 to 4 days, colonies should be visible. Plates should be held for a maximum of 2 weeks before discarding. Blood cultures in biphasic media should be held for 1 month. At 5 days, colonies are 3 to 4 mm in diameter, gray-white to blue-green, glistening, convex, circular, and may exhibit a cut-glass sort of internal granular speckling (Figure 39.6). A Giménez stain reveals small, coccobacillary organisms with occasional filamentous forms (Figure 39.7). A Gram stain yields thin, gram-negative bacilli.

All *Legionella* species are weakly catalase-positive (strongly catalase-positive organisms are less likely to be legionellae). Oxidase test results are variable. Another rapid differential screening test is the production of fluorescent pigment, visible under long-wave fluorescent light (long-wave light is generated at 365 nm; a Wood's light generates light of wavelength near 250 nm). *L. pneumophila, L. micdadei, L. jordanis, L. wadsworthii, L. oakridgensis,* and *L. longbeachae* fluoresce pale yellow-green; whereas *L. gormanii, L. dumoffii, L. bozemanii,* and *L. morrisii* fluoresce blue-white. All *Legionella* species described so far are able to liquefy gelatin.

The currently recognized species of legionellae

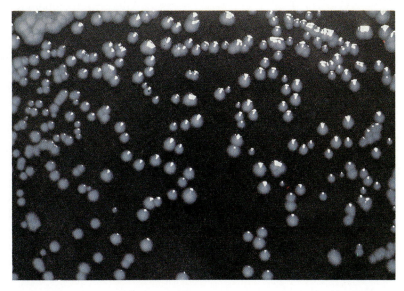

Figure 39.6
Colonies of *L. pneumophila* on BCYE agar. (Organism courtesy Dr. Clifford Mintz.)

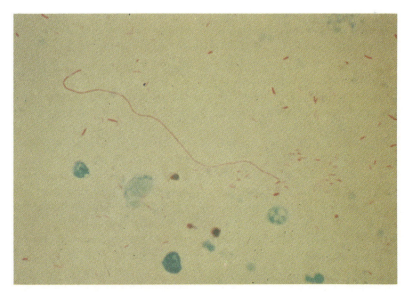

Figure 39.7
Giménez stain of *L. pneumophila* from a colony grown on BCYE.

Currently Recognized Species of Legionella

L. anisa	L. longbeachae*
L. birminghamensis	L. maceachernii*
L. bozemanii*	L. micdadei*
L. brunensis	L. moravica
L. cherrii	L. oakridgensis
L. cincinnatiensis	L. parisiensis
L. dumoffii*	L. pneumophila*
L. erythra	L. rubrilucens
L. feeleii*	L. sainthelensis
L. gormanii*	L. santicrucis
L. hackeliae*	L. spiritensis
I. israelensis	L. steigerwaltii
L. jamestowniensis	L. tucsonensis*
L. jordanis*	L. wadsworthii*

*Isolated from patient specimens.

---

are listed in the box. Most cases of Legionnaires' disease are associated with *L. pneumophila*. Definitive identification requires the facilities of a specialized reference laboratory. Identification of *L. pneumophila* species can be achieved, however, by a monoclonal immunofluorescent stain (Genetic Systems). Emulsions of organisms from isolated colonies are made in 10% neutral formalin, diluted 1:100 (to produce a very thin suspension), and placed on slides for fluorescent antibody staining, as described in Section 39.5.c. Clinical laboratories can probably perform sufficient service to clinicians by indicating the presence of *Legionella* species in a specimen. If further identification is necessary, the isolate should be forwarded to an appropriate reference laboratory. There are presently 28 named species, several of which have more than one serotype, and *L. pneumophila*, which has 14 serotypes.

39.5.c. Direct detection of *Legionella* in infected clinical material. The most rapid means of diagnosing Legionnaires' disease is direct detection of the presence of the bacilli in clinical specimens. Although *Pseudomonas* species and other contaminating material may occasionally cause cross-reactive and nonspecific fluorescence, direct fluorescent antibody (DFA) tests should be performed on specimens received in the laboratory for *Legionella* detection.

Antisera conjugated with fluorescein are available from several commercial suppliers (BioDx, Biological Products Division of Centers for Disease Control, Litton Bionetics, Genetic Systems, MarDx, Zeus Technologies, and others). Specimens are first tested with pools of antisera containing antibodies to several species or serotypes of *L. pneumophila*. Those that exhibit positive results are then reexamined with specific conjugated antisera. The Genetic Systems reagent is a monoclonal antibody directed against a cell wall protein common to *L. pneumophila*. Manufacturers' directions should be followed explicitly and material from commercial systems should never be divided and used separately. Laboratories should decide which serotypes to routinely test for based on the prevalence of isolates in their geographic area.

Briefly, material from the specimen is applied directly to two marked circles on an alcohol-cleaned microscope slide. Tissue is applied to the slide by touch preparation with adequate pressure to express bacteria from spaces. The slide is allowed to air dry, is heat-fixed, and then fixed by overlaying the slide with 10% buffered (pH 7.0) formalin for 10 minutes. The formalin is rinsed from the slide with sterile distilled water and the slide is allowed to air dry. If it cannot be stained immediately (delay is not acceptable for clinical specimens from living patients), the slide may be frozen at $-20°$ C in the dark for several weeks. One of the two specimen areas is tested against pooled antisera, and the other is tested against specific antiserum in the event of a positive result. The sensitivity of the DFA test is low, since 10^4 to 10^5 bacteria per milliliter of specimen are required for detection. Slides should be examined for 15 to 20 minutes before being declared negative, especially by technologists who rarely perform the test. The organisms appear as brightly fluorescent rods, with a velvety texture (Figure 39.8). Silver stains or even Giemsa stain may reveal organisms in tissue, and *L. micdadei* will stain acid-fast in tissue sections. Culture of specimens must always be performed as well, as it will detect those organisms that are not included within the usual battery of serotypes and because culture is more sensitive than DFA.

Two recently developed immunologic tests for Legionnaires' disease have shown great promise. Detection of *L. pneumophila* antigen in urine by means of a radioimmunoassay (RIA) (DuPont Co.)[1] or enzyme-linked immunosorbent assay (ELISA) test has yielded very specific and sensitive results.

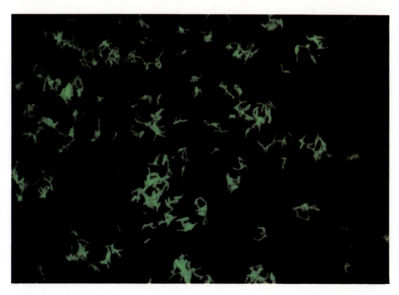

Figure 39.8
Fluorescent-antibody stained *L. pneumophila* from a positive control slide.

ELISA methods are also being used to detect circulating antigens in serum with good results. A nucleic acid probe that specifically detects genetic material of *L. pneumophila* in clinical specimens (Gen-Probe) is available as a diagnostic reagent. Early studies have revealed moderate sensitivity and specificity, similar to yields from direct fluorescent antibody stain.[5] The reagent is being modified to yield more reliable results.

39.5.d. Serologic and immunologic diagnosis of Legionnaires' disease. Most cases of legionellosis have been diagnosed retrospectively by detection of a fourfold rise in anti-*Legionella* antibody with an indirect fluorescent antibody test. Serum specimens no closer than 2 weeks apart should be tested. Confirmation of disease is accomplished by a fourfold rise in titer to >128, or, for unusual cases, a single serum with a titer of >256 and a characteristic clinical picture. However, as many as 12% of healthy persons will yield titers as high as 1:256, and unfortunately, individuals with Legionnaires' disease may not exhibit serologic titers until as long as 8 weeks after the primary illness or may never display significant antibody titer rises. Commercially prepared antigen-impregnated slides are available from numerous suppliers.

39.5.e. Treatment of Legionnaires' disease. Erythromycin, 4g per day intravenously in adults,

is the drug of choice for treatment of disease caused by *Legionella*. Penicillins, cephalosporins of all generations, and aminoglycosides are not effective and should not be used. In vitro susceptibility studies are not predictive of clinical response and should not be performed for individual isolates. High dose trimethoprim-sulfamethoxazole and tetracyclines have been effective in some cases. The concomitant administration of rifampin along with erythromycin may prove beneficial, especially in severe cases. For patients who cannot take erythromycin, doxycycline (plus rifampin for moderately and severely ill patients) is recommended. Clinical response usually follows the introduction of effective therapy within 48 hours.

39.6. Genus *Prototheca*

39.6.a. Epidemiology and pathogenesis of *Prototheca* infection. *Prototheca* are algae without chlorophyll that morphologically resemble green algae. The organisms are worldwide in distribution, found in water and soil. They enter the body through breaks in the skin, usually associated with minor trauma. The primary syndrome is a chronic, nodular skin lesion, although the organism can cause joint infection, wound infection, and rare disseminated disease in humans. The presence of the organism, which is resistant to killing by phagocytes, results in

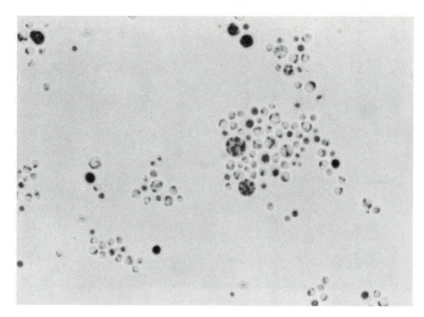

Figure 39.9
Prototheca organisms seen in wet mount stained with lactophenol cotton blue.

a granulomatous response. Spontaneous recovery does not occur.

39.6.b. Laboratory identification of *Prototheca*. There are two species of *Prototheca* associated with human disease, *P. wickerhamii* and *P. zopfii*. The organisms grow very well on Sabouraud's dextrose agar, and presumably on any other agar that will support the growth of yeast, such as brain heart infusion agar and Sabouraud's dextrose with heart infusion. Colonies are opaque, white to tan, smooth, heaped, moist, and resemble those of yeast. Examination under wet mount, however, reveals the characteristic structure of *Prototheca* (Figure 39.9). Cells are spherical, varying in size from tiny (1.5 μg diameter) to large (three times the size of a red blood cell). Within the cells (called sporangia), endospores can be seen developing.

For most laboratories, identification of *Prototheca* to genus by observation of typical cellular morphology is sufficient. If definitive identification is required, the API 20C system (Analytab Products, Inc.), a multiwell identification system for yeasts, will accurately determine the assimilation pattern and other biochemical parameters of *Prototheca* species within 4 days.[12]

39.6.c. Treatment of *Prototheca* infections. The infections caused by this organism must be treated or surgically excised. Most patients respond to am-

photericin B, although ketoconazole has been used successfully in at least one patient. *Prototheca* species are resistant to flucytosine.

39.7. Genus *Simonsiella*

39.7.a. Epidemiology and pathogenesis of *Simonsiella* infection. These strangely shaped gram-negative organisms are normal oral flora in mammals and other warm-blooded animals. They resemble fat caterpillars. Although isolated from gastric aspirate of a neonate, the species was not assumed to be pathogenic in one reported case.[21]

39.7.b. Laboratory identification of *Simonsiella*. *Simonsiella* grows well on blood agar aerobically. Colonies are translucent, gray, and 2 mm in diameter after overnight incubation. The isolate reported was oxidase- and catalase-positive.[21] Identification can be made on the basis of Gram stain morphology alone. The cells are arrayed side-by-side, tightly packed, to form a large structure approximately 3 μm wide by 10 to 20 μm long (Figure 39.10). Recognition of this organism may result in better definition of its role (if any) in infection.

39.8 Genus *Stomatococcus*

39.8.a. Epidemiology and pathogenesis of *Stomatococcus* infection. *Stomatococcus mucilaginosus*, a member of the family Micrococcaceae, is nor-

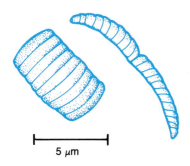

Figure 39.10
Diagram of structure of *Simonsiella* species.

mal oral flora in humans. It has been reported as an agent of endocarditis (primarily in intravenous drug abusers), bacteremia, and chronic ambulatory dialysis-associated peritonitis.[4,13,15]

39.8.b. Laboratory identification of *Stomatococcus*. *Stomatococcus* is differentiated from other micrococcaceae by its negative or weak catalase reaction. The organism does not grow in the presence of 5% NaCl. It hydrolyzes esculin and exhibits a positive PYR test. *Stomatococcus* has been characterized as "sticky staphylococci" when it is recognized among normal oral flora on culture. Important isolates should be sent to a reference laboratory for definitive identification.

39.8.c. Treatment of *Stomatococcus mucilaginosus* infections. Isolates have been reported susceptible to most antimicrobial agents, including penicillin and cephalosporins. Penicillin is the drug of choice. One strain, isolated from the blood of a drug abuser with endocarditis, was described as relatively resistant to penicillin.[13]

39.9. Genus *Streptobacillus*

39.9.a. Epidemiology and pathogenesis of *Streptobacillus* infection. *Streptobacillus moniliformis*, the only species within the genus, is one of the etiologic agents of "rat-bite fever." Humans acquire the infection via the bite of an infected rat (including laboratory rats) or less commonly via contaminated milk, food, or water. When the organism is acquired by ingestion, the disease is called "Haverhill fever." The organism is normal oral flora of wild and laboratory rats, although it is also associated with respiratory disease and fatal systemic disease in laboratory animals. Virulence factors have not been defined. The organism is known to spontaneously develop L forms (without cell walls), which may allow persistence of the organism in some sites.

Patients develop acute onset of chills, fever, headache, and severe joint pains. Within the first 2 days, patients exhibit a maculopapular, petechial, or morbilliform rash on the palms, soles of the feet, and extremities. Complications include endocarditis, septic arthritis, and pneumonia.[3,9]

39.9.b. Laboratory identification of *Streptobacillus*. Organisms may be cultured from blood, material aspirated from infected joints or lymph nodes, or aspirated from the pus within lesions. The organism requires the presence of blood, ascitic fluid, or serum for growth. Growth will occur on blood agar, incubated in a very moist environment with 5% to 10% CO_2, after 48 hours incubation at 37° C. Colonies are not hemolytic. Addition of 10% to 30% ascitic fluid (available commercially from some media suppliers, such as Difco Laboratories) or 20% horse serum should facilitate recovery of the organism. The organism grows as "fluff balls" or "breadcrumbs" near the bottom of the tube of broth or on the surface of the sedimented red blood cell layer in blood culture media. The sodium-polyanethol sulfonate present in most blood culture media is inhibitory.[3] Colonies grown on brain-heart infusion agar supplemented with 20% horse serum are small, smooth, glistening, colorless or grayish, with irregular edges.

Colonies may also exhibit a "fried egg" appearance, with a dark center and a flattened, lacy edge. These colonies have undergone the spontaneous transformation to the L form. Stains of L form colonies will yield coccobacillary or bipolar staining coccoid forms; usually a special stain, such as the Dienes stain (performed by pathologists) is required. Acridine orange stain will also reveal the bacteria when Gram stain fails because of lack of cell wall constituents.

Gram-stained organisms from standard colonies will show extreme pleomorphism, with long filamentous forms, chains, and swollen cells. The carbolfuchsin counterstain or the Giemsa stain may be necessary for visualization (Figure 39.11). With the same stains, organisms may be visualized directly in clinical material for rapid diagnosis.

S. moniliformis does not produce indole and is catalase-, oxidase-, and nitrate-negative, in contrast to organisms with which *Streptobacillus* may be confused, including *Actinobacillus*, *Haemophilus aprophilus*, and *Cardiobacterium*. In addition, the clinical history of a rat bite is usually elicited.

The other agent of rat-bite fever, *Spirillum minus*

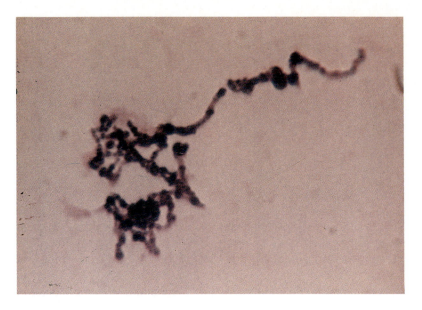

Figure 39.11
S. moniliformis smear made from a standard colony. Stained with Giemsa and visualized under oil immersion magnification (× 1000).

(Chapter 40), cannot be grown in vitro. Serologic diagnosis of rat-bite fever is also useful; most patients develop agglutinating titers to the causative organism. The specialized serologic tests are performed only at national reference laboratories, since the disease is extremely rare in the United States.

39.9.c. Treatment of *Streptobacillus moniliformis* infections. The organism is susceptible to penicillin and streptomycin. Therapy with a combined regimen of a penicillin and an aminoglycoside is probably most effective. The organism is only weakly susceptible to tetracycline in vitro. *S. moniliformis* is resistant to sulfonamides.

39.10. Thermophilic Bacteria

A new group of bacteria have been implicated as etiologic agents of human disease.[14] Isolated from specimens such as cerebrospinal fluid, blood, and heart valves, these organisms are able to grow at increased temperatures. Called "thermophilic" bacteria, most isolates grew better at 42° to 50° C than they did at 37° C, the temperature at which they were first isolated. All species were grown on tryptone-glucose-yeast extract agar. None were able to grow at room temperature. No strains were fermentative, and only a few strains were able to utilize glucose or maltose oxidatively in O-F media (Chap-

ter 28). No organisms grew on MacConkey agar and none grew on TSIA or KIA agar slants. All strains were oxidase-positive; none were indole-positive. There are probably several species among this group, but further studies are needed to delineate them. It is certain that at least several isolates were etiologic agents of disease in humans who had no predisposing conditions. They were all susceptible to penicillin and cephalosporins, and most were susceptible to aminoglycosides. Since the isolates grew poorly at normal incubator temperatures, they might be dismissed by microbiologists unless there is an index of suspicion. Other thermophilic microorganisms, such as certain actinomycetes (also mentioned in Chapter 33) and *Cytophaga* species, found in environmental sources, have been implicated as etiologic agents of human allergic pneumonitis, although they do not grow within the human body.

39.11. Unnamed Bacteria

A number of unnamed bacterial groups, morphologically similar but not yet definitively characterized, have been implicated as etiologic agents of human disease. Because the CDC is the national reference laboratory, most clinically significant isolates that cannot be identified by other laboratories in the United States are ultimately sent to CDC. Such organisms, designated by letters that reflect their characteristics (EF stands for eugonic fermenter, which means good-growing fermenter; DF stands for dysgonic fermenter, which means poor-growing fermenter; EO stands for eugonic oxidizer), or other letters (such as Ve-1, IVc-2, and HB), so that they can be categorized by microbiologists, may be isolated from clinical specimens. Although most of the individual groups are not discussed in this text, they may be listed in some tables and charts because they resemble organisms being discussed. Identification tables published by the CDC and the *Manual of Clinical Microbiology,* published by the American Society for Microbiology, should be consulted for further details concerning these organisms.

REFERENCES

1. Aguero-Rosenfeld, M., and Edelstein, P.H. 1988. Retrospective evaluation of the DuPont radioimmunoassay kit for detection of *Legionella pneumophila* serogroup I antigenuria in humans. J. Clin. Microbiol. 26:1775.
2. Bunker, M.L., Chewning, L., Wang, S.E., and Gordon, M.A. 1988. *Dermatophilus congolensis* and "hairy" leukoplakia. Am. J. Clin. Pathol. 89:683.
3. Clausen, C. 1987. Septic arthritis due to *Streptobacillus moniliformis*. Clin. Microbiol. Newsletter 9:123.
4. Coudron, P.E., Markowitz, S.M., Mohanty, L.B., et al. 1987. Isolation of *Stomatococcus mucilaginosus* from drug user with endocarditis. J. Clin. Microbiol. 25:1359.
5. Edelstein, P.H. 1986. Evaluation of the Gen-Probe DNA probe for the detection of legionellae in culture. J. Clin. Microbiol. 23:481.
6. Edelstein, P.H. 1984. Legionnaire's disease laboratory manual. National Technical Information Service. Publ. No. PB84-156827, U.S. Department of Commerce, Springfield, Va.
7. Gordon, M.A. 1985. Aerobic pathogenic Actinomycetaceae. In Lennette, E.H., Balows, A., Hausler, W.J., Jr., and Shadomy, H.J., editors. Manual of clinical microbiology, ed. 4. American Society for Microbiology, Washington, D.C.
8. Greenwood, J.R. 1983. Current taxonomic status of *Gardnerella vaginalis*. Scand. J. Infect. Dis. Suppl. 40:11.
9. Jenkins, S.G. 1988. Rat-bite fever. Clin. Microbiol. Newsletter 10:57.
10. Lien, E.A., and Hillier, S. 1989. Evaluation of the enhanced Rapid Identification Method for *Gardnerella vaginalis*. J. Clin. Microbiol. 27:566.
11. Macher, A.M., Casale, T.B., and Fauci, A.S. 1982. Chronic granulomatous disease of childhood and *Chromobacterium violaceum* infections in the southeastern United States. Ann. Intern. Med. 97:51.
12. Padhye, A.A., Baker, J.G., and D'Amato, R.F. 1979. Rapid identification of *Prototheca* species by the API 20C system. J. Clin. Microbiol. 10:579.
13. Pinsky, R.L., Piscitelli, V., and Patterson, J.E. 1989. Endocarditis caused by relatively penicillin-resistant *Stomatococcus mucilaginosus*. J. Clin. Microbiol. 27:215.
14. Rabkin, C.S., Galaid, E.I., Hollis, D.G., et al. 1985. Thermophilic bacteria: a new cause of human disease. J. Clin. Microbiol. 21:553.
15. Relman, D.A., Ruoff, K., and Ferraro, M.J. 1987. *Stomatococcus mucilaginosus* endocarditis in an intravenous drug abuser. J. Infect. Dis. 155:1080.
16. Ristic, M., and Kreier, J.P. 1984. Bartonellaceae Gieszczykiewicz 1939. In Krieg, N.R., and Holt, J.G., editors. Bergey's manual of systematic bacteriology, vol. 1. Williams & Wilkins, Baltimore.
17. Schlanger, G., Lutwick, L.I., Kurzman, M., et al. 1984. Sinusitis caused by *Legionella pneumophila* in a patient with the acquired immune deficiency syndrome. Am. J. Med. 77:957.
18. Spiegel, C.A., Amsel, R., Eschenbach, D., et al. 1980. Anaerobic bacteria in nonspecific vaginitis. N. Engl. J. Med. 303:601.
19. Tompkins, L.S., Roessler, B.J., Redd, S.C., et al. 1988. *Legionella* prosthetic-valve endocarditis. N. Engl. J. Med. 318:530.
20. Totten, P.A., Amsel, R., Hale, J., et al. 1982. Selective differential human blood bilayer media for isolation of *Gardnerella (Haemophilus) vaginalis*. J. Clin. Microbiol. 15:141.
21. Whitehouse, R.L.S., Jackson, H., Jackson, M.C., and Ramji, M.M. 1987. Isolation of *Simonsiella* sp. from a neonate. J. Clin. Microbiol. 25:522.
22. Yong, D.C.T., and Thompson, J.S. 1982. Rapid microbiochemical method for identification of *Gardnerella (Haemophilus) vaginalis*. J. Clin. Microbiol. 16:30.

BIBLIOGRAPHY

Csango, P.-A., Holmes, K.K., Jerve, F., Mårdh, P.-A., and Piot, P., editors. 1983. First international conference on vaginosis. Scand. J. Infect. Dis. Suppl. 40.

Fung, J.C., and Baron, E.J. 1985. *Gardnerella vaginalis* vaginitis. In Sun, T., editor. Sexually related infectious disease: laboratory and clinical aspects. Field and Rich Associates, New York.

Greenwood, J.R., and Pickett, M.J. 1984. Genus *Gardnerella Greenwood and Pickett 1980*. In Krieg, N.R., and Holt, J.G., editors. Bergey's manual of systematic bacteriology, vol. 1. Williams & Wilkins, Baltimore.

Lee, T.S., and Wright, B.D. 1981. Fulminating chromobacterial septicaemia presenting as respiratory distress syndrome. Thorax 36:557.

Sneath, P.H.A. 1984. Genus *Chromobacterium Bergonzini 1881*. In Krieg, N.R., and Holt, J.G., editors. Bergey's manual of systematic bacteriology, vol. 1. Williams & Wilkins, Baltimore.

Starr, A.J., Cribbett, L.S., Poklepovic, J., et al. 1981. *Chromobacterium violaceum* presenting as a surgical emergency. South. Med. J. 74:1137.

Winn, W.C. Jr. 1988. Legionnaires disease: historical perspective. Clin. Microbiol. Rev. 1:60.

40

New, Controversial, Difficult-to-Cultivate, or Noncultivatable Etiologic Agents of Disease

In addition to those diseases caused by agents that cannot be grown in culture using existing methods, there are a number of diseases that appear to be caused by an infectious agent, although such an agent has not been identified. Reasons for which an infectious agent might be considered to be associated with a disease include an epidemiologic pattern suggestive of dissemination by an agent or a clinical presentation that is similar to that produced by known etiologic agents. Once the suggestion of infectious etiology is advanced, tools of science can be used to investigate the problem. Within the last several years, a number of diseases, either newly recognized or described long ago, have been definitely traced to an etiologic agent for the first time. For example, *Borrelia burgdorferi* has been named recently as the agent responsible for Lyme disease, a multifaceted syndrome that had previously escaped proper diagnosis. More recently, *Helicobacter (Campylobacter) pylori* has been strongly associated with gastritis, a disease not thought to be infectious in nature. The diseases mentioned in this chapter are either syndromes in which the etiologic agent is difficult to isolate or demonstrate; well-described syndromes for which no etiologic agent has been found, although the diseases appear to be of an infectious nature; or diseases with which a newly described agent is associated. The agents mentioned in this chapter are usually not routinely sought by clinical microbiology laboratories at this time.

40.1. Diseases Associated with an Etiologic Agent

There are, of course, a number of infectious diseases for which the agent is well known but cannot be cultivated easily, if at all, such as syphilis, leprosy, hepatitis, warts (papillomavirus), and the slow virus diseases of progressive multifocal leukoencephalopathy (JC virus) and subacute sclerosing panencephalitis (measleslike paramyxovirus). Recently a new mycobacterium has been isolated from tissue biopsy material from the intestinal mucosa of patients with Crohn's disease (Chapter 41), although it is not established as a cause. Only with great difficulty can this agent be cultivated in the laboratory. Other intestinal organisms, including spirochetes, have been cultivated but not yet firmly associated with disease.[10,11,17]

40.1.a. *Spirillum minus*, an agent of rat-bite fever. *Spirillum minus* (formerly called *S. minor*, an incorrect Latin usage), an agent of rat-bite fever, has never been grown in culture. The organism has been visualized in Giemsa- or Wright-stained blood films and can be seen under darkfield microscopy. *S. minus* is a thick, spiral, gram-negative organism with two or three coils and polytrichous polar flagella. Infection can be transmitted by the bite or scratch of an infected animal. The bite wound heals spontaneously, but 1 to 4 weeks later reulcerates to form a granulomatous lesion at the same time that the patient develops constitutional symptoms of fever, headache, and a generalized, blotchy purplish maculopapular rash. Although it is rare that the organism can be seen in blood, it may be visualized in darkfield preparations made from the lesion.

Diagnosis is definitively made by injection of lesion material or blood into (experimental) white mice or guinea pigs, which then develop the disease. Differentiation between rat-bite fever caused by *S. minus* ("Sodoku") and that caused by *Streptobacillus moniliformis* (Haverhill fever; Chapter 39) is usually accomplished based on clinical presentations of the two infections and the isolation of the latter organism in culture. The incubation period for *S. minus* is much longer than that of streptobacillary rat-bite fever, which has occurred within 12 hours of the initial bite.

40.1.b. Cat-scratch disease. Cat-scratch disease was first recognized by Robert Debre in Paris during the 1930s. The disease is not uncommon, with over 750 reported cases and probably more than 100 cases occurring annually in the United States. Patients are usually children (80%), and the primary sites of lesions are the hands, arms and legs, and face and neck. Most cases are acquired following the scratch, bite, or lick of a cat or kitten, usually newly arrived to the household. Patients exhibit regional tender lymphadenopathy, anorexia, fatigue, fever, and headache, usually beginning 2 weeks after the cat scratch or contact. They may display a rash, generalized lymphadenopathy, seizures, and other systemic findings. The disease is usually self-limited; complications such as a suppurative lymph node or encephalitis have been reported. Cat-scratch disease has been recently seen in AIDS patients presenting as a proliferative endothelial cell lesion resembling Kaposi's sarcoma. Until 1983, clinical diagnosis required that a patient fulfill three of the following four criteria:

1. History of animal contact plus a site of primary inoculation
2. Negative laboratory studies for other causes of lymphadenopathy
3. Characteristic histopathology of the lesion or lymph node
4. A positive skin test.

The skin test antigen is prepared from heat-treated pus taken from another patient's lesion. Injection of 0.1 ml of this material intradermally elicits a wheal or papule within 72 hours, although the reaction can be the result of previous infection. Approximately 5% of patients will have false-negative skin test results, and 5% will have false-positive results.

In 1983, Wear and others[18] reported visualization of organisms in the lesions of cat-scratch disease. The organisms are gram-negative, 0.3 to 0.5 µm in diameter, and 0.5 to 1.0 µm in length. They are best visualized with the Warthin-Starry silver stain, such as that of Luna[14] (Procedure 40.1), usually used for spirochetes (Figure 40.1). The bacilli are not acid-fast and may not stain with the Gomori methenamine silver stain. They appear to be intracellular pathogens; the delayed-type hypersensitivity response to skin test antigen would appear consistent with an intracellular pathogen. Electron micrographs further support the findings of these scientists.[4,8]

Evidence that the gram-negative organism does cause the disease, however, is based on the fact that patients produce antibodies that, when coupled with immunoperoxidase or fluorescein, can be seen to bind to the organisms in lymph node material taken

PROCEDURE 40.1

Warthin-Starry Stain

Principle

Silver ions precipitate on the cell wall of bacteria and other structures; the black color enhances visibility of the organisms.

Method

1. Make solutions as follows:

   a. Acidulated water

Triple distilled water	1000 ml
1% aqueous citric acid	enough to bring triple distilled water to pH 4.0

   b. 1% silver nitrate solution

Silver nitrate, crystalline	1 g
Acidulated water	100 ml

   c. 2% silver nitrate solution

Silver nitrate, crystalline	2 g
Acidulated water	100 ml

   d. 5% gelatin solution

Sheet gelatin, high grade	10 g
Acidulated water	200 ml

   e. 0.15% hydroquinone solution

Hydroquinone crystals, photographic quality	0.15 g
Acidulated water	100 ml

   All chemicals should be available from a standard chemical supply company, such as Sigma Chemical Co. or E. Merck Darmstadt.

2. Fix tissue sections in buffered neutral formalin. Avoid chromate fixatives. This fixative is standard for most pathology laboratories. The tissue is embedded in paraffin; sections are cut at a thickness of 6 µm.

3. Warm the 2% silver nitrate, the 5% gelatin, and the 0.15% hydroquinone in 50 ml beakers in a water bath heated to 54° C.

4. Deparaffinize the (patient's) tissue slide and a known positive control slide through a series of xylene changes with increasing concentrations of water, until the slide is finally placed into triple distilled water for final hydration. These procedures are standard histologic methods. Place the slides into a Coplin jar containing the 1% silver nitrate solution, preheated in a 43° C water bath. Allow the silver to impregnate the slides for 30 min at 43° C in the water bath.

5. While the slides are being impregnated, prepare the developer as follows:

Silver nitrate solution (2%)	1.5 ml
Gelatin solution (5%)	3.75 ml
Hydroquinone solution (0.15%)	2 ml

   Prepare this developer, immediately before it is used, in a small beaker or flask.

6. Move the slides from the impregnator, lay them flat across a slide holder, and immediately flood them with the warm developer solution. Allow the sections to develop until they are light brown or yellow. Check the known control periodically, which should show black spirochetes or bacteria against a yellow or light brown background. When handling the slides, use paraffin-coated or plastic forceps.

7. Wash quickly and thoroughly in hot tap water, approximately 50° C. Rinse in distilled water.

8. Dehydrate in 95% alcohol, then absolute alcohol, and clear in xylene by placing the slides in two jars of each solution for 5 min each jar.

9. Mount with Permount or Histoclad (available from Baxter/American Scientific Products). Observe for characteristic black organisms against a light brown or yellow background.

Quality control

Stain a known positive control slide concurrently with each specimen staining procedure. Although most bacteria will stain black with Warthin-Starry, a thin, spiral organism will best control the procedure.

Modified from Luna.[14]

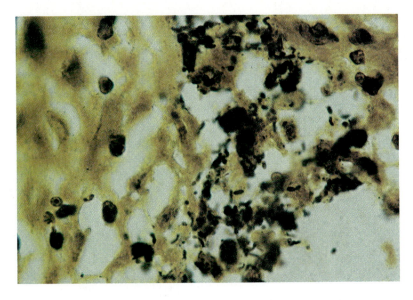

Figure 40.1
Cat-scratch disease bacillus in lymph node tissue (Warthin-Starry silver stain). (Photograph courtesy
Dr. Ellen Kahn, North Shore University Hospital, Manhasset, N.Y.)

from newly diagnosed patients. No specific reactions have occurred between these sera and preparations of any other infectious agents, and bacteria in lesion tissue sections do not react with immune sera made against any other morphologically similar bacteria. A gram-positive organism was cultured from a lymph node from a patient with cat-scratch disease, but whether it was the etiologic agent was controversial.[6] English and coworkers[4] recently isolated a cell-wall defective gram-negative bacillus from lymph nodes of patients with cat-scratch disease and were able to stimulate development of nodules in an armadillo injected with the organism. Although this isolate is likely to be the agent of cat-scratch disease, other laboratories have not confirmed these findings.

Treatment with antibiotics is not recommended, and one episode of disease probably imparts lifelong immunity. Once the etiologic agent has been unequivocally grown in culture, specific serologic reagents for diagnosis can be prepared and the need for lymph node biopsy will disappear. An excellent general discussion of this disease is found in the article by Hadfield, Schlagel, and Margileth.[9]

40.1.c. Granuloma inguinale. *Calymmatobacterium granulomatis* is the etiologic agent of "granuloma inguinale," or "donovanosis," a venereally transmitted disease characterized by subcutaneous nodules that enlarge and evolve to form beefy, erythematous, granulomatous, painless lesions that bleed easily. The lesions, which usually occur on the genitalia, have been mistaken for neoplasms. Patients often have inguinal lymphadenopathy. The organism has been isolated only from human lesions and the disease is confined primarily to the tropics, although it has been reported in the United States. Infectivity of this bacillus must be low, since sexual partners of infected patients often do not themselves become infected.

The organism can be visualized in scrapings of lesions stained with Wright's or Giemsa stain. Subsurface infected cells must be present; surface epithelium is not an adequate specimen. Groups of organisms are seen within mononuclear endothelial cells; this pathognomonic entity is known as a "Donovan body," named after the physician who first visualized the organism in such a lesion. The organism stains as a blue rod with prominent polar granules, giving rise to a "safety pin" appearance, surrounded by a large, pink capsule. The capsular polysaccharide shares several cross-reactive antigens with *Klebsiella* species, fueling speculation that *Calymmatobacterium* is closely related to *Klebsiella*.

Cultivation in vitro is very difficult, but it can be done using media containing some of the growth

PROCEDURE 40.2

Cultivation of C. **granulomatis**

1. Prepare medium as follows:

Peptone (Difco Laboratories)	10 g
Tryptone (Difco Laboratories)	3 g
Glucose	3 g
Commercial sea salts (any chemical supplier)	2 g
Agar (Bacto agar, Difco Laboratories)	1.2 g
Distilled water	1000 ml

Dissolve all ingredients by heating gently. Adjust pH to 7.3. Autoclave at 121° C for 15 min and cool to 45° C. Soak fresh eggs in 70% alcohol for 10 min before aseptically removing egg yolks. Dilute egg yolks with equal volume of sterile saline (0.85% NaCl) and mix with equal parts of the basal medium. Dispense the medium in sterile 16 × 125 mm tubes, 20 ml per tube. (Commercially available egg yolk [Difco Laboratories] may be suitable as a substitute for fresh egg yolks.)

2. A physician aspirates lymph node material or obtains material from the lesion with a sterile scalpel. The lesion is cleansed by carefully swabbing its surface with a sterile gauze pad soaked in sterile saline to remove surface contamination. A small slice near the edge of the lesion will allow removal of subsurface material. The best material is obtained from under the surface of the lesion near the edge.

3. Inoculate the medium well below the surface with the scraping or aspirated material. Incubate for at least 72 hours at 37° C. Incubating the tubes in a candle jar may help to retain the low oxygen concentration of the medium. Gram stain the broth, using a carbolfuchsin counterstain. *C. granulomatis* is gram-negative.

Modified from Dienst and Brownell.[3]

---

factors found in egg yolk (Procedure 40.2).[7] A medium described by Dienst has been used to culture *Calymmatobacterium* from aspirated bubo material, as described by Dienst and Brownell.[3]

Although gentamicin and chloramphenicol are effective for the therapy of granuloma inguinale, tetracycline or ampicillin is usually the drug of first choice. Trimethoprim-sulfamethoxazole or erythromycin has also been shown to be effective treatment for granuloma inguinale.

40.1.d. Hepatitis associated with hepatitis B virus, delta agent, and non-A, non-B hepatitis. The viruses of hepatitis A and B have been identified and characterized, but only hepatitis A virus has been grown in culture. The infectious particle of hepatitis B virus, the Dane particle, is present in the blood and hepatocytes of patients and can be visualized by electron microscopy. Several different antigenic constituents are released during infection. Diagnosis is based on detection of either antibodies to the constituents or the antigens themselves. Newer methods for detecting the surface antigen (HBsAg), an early protein antigen (HBeAg), and antibodies to HBsAg, HBeAg, and hepatitis core antigen (HBc) include radioimmunoassay (Chapter 11) and enzyme-linked immunosorbent assay (ELISA) (Chapter 10). Microbiology laboratories usually do not perform these tests.

Coinfection of patients with hepatitis B virus and a defective mutant virus, the "delta agent," is responsible for some proportion of the most severe cases of hepatitis. The delta agent requires coinfection with hepatitis B in the delta-infected cell for damage to occur. Persons at risk of acquiring delta agent hepatitis are those with chronic asymptomatic hepatitis B infection. Serologic tests for delta antigen and antibody are available in ELISA and RIA formats.

Non-A, non-B hepatitis is the most common transfusion-associated hepatitis. Researchers have recently cloned genetic material from a small, enveloped virus that transmitted non-A, non-B hepatitis to chimpanzees (called hepatitis C virus).[2] This clone reacted with antiserum from patients who had recovered from non-A, non-B hepatitis. The virus, characterized as a single-stranded RNA virus, appears to be similar to togaviruses (such as rubella virus, dengue virus, St. Louis encephalitis virus, and so forth). The virus itself has not been isolated or cultivated in vitro. It has been postulated that more than one etiologic agent is responsible for this type of hepatitis, although hepatitis C probably accounts for most transfusion-associated cases of non-A, non-B hepatitis. An ELISA test is available.

40.1.e. Rhinosporidiosis. Rhinosporidiosis is a chronic, celluloproliferative infection of the mucous membranes of the face and other areas, usually in the nose and less often in the conjunctiva, caused by a fungus that produces a spherule-like body similar to that of *Coccidioides immitis*. The disease is much more common in men than in women. The lesions ultimately develop into pedunculated polyps. Most prevalent in India, the infection has been described in the United States. A similar disease occurs in horses, cattle, and other animals. The agent, seen macroscopically in the polyp as tiny white dots, consists of large, thick-walled cysts or sporangia containing many endospores. The endospores, each about the size of a red blood cell, are released through a pore in the wall of the sporangium once it has matured to its full size of 200 to 300 μm. The agent of rhinosporidiosis, called *Rhinosporidium seeberi*, has recently been cultured in mammalian epithelial cell tissue culture, which may be a requirement for growth.[12] The fungus induced cellular proliferation in vitro. The cyst can be stained in biopsy material with mucicarmine; histologic studies are probably the best diagnostic tool available currently, although it may now be possible for laboratories to cultivate the agent from tissue biopsy material if appropriate tissue culture methods are used.

40.1.f. Lobomycosis. Lobomycosis is a presumed fungal infection from which an etiologic agent has not been cultured. Found in adult males, primarily living in the Amazon River basin, and in bottle-nose dolphins off the coast of Florida, the disease is characterized by chronic, progressive, subcutaneous nodules, usually on the face or extremities. The lesions can become verrucous or ulcerative. The organism, *Loboa loboi*, can be seen in scrapings and histological sections from the lesions as a large, thick-walled, spheroidal or oval yeast. The yeasts possess multiple buds and often appear in short chains. The buds are the same size as the mother cells, unlike the multiple buds of *Paracoccidioides brasiliensis*. The yeasts can be visualized with 10% KOH and stain with methenamine silver or periodic acid–Schiff (PAS). Diagnosis is made histologically.

40.1.g. Kuru and Creutzfeldt-Jakob disease. Kuru, a progressively fatal dementing disease of head-hunting tribes of New Guinea, was first thought to be of sex-linked genetic origin, since female adults were involved more often than males, and children were universally affected. When it was realized that the histologic lesions in the brains of patients with kuru resembled those found in sheep with a naturally occurring neurologic disease with similar symptoms, scrapie, the search began in earnest for an etiologic agent. Scrapie was known to be transmissible. In 1965, kurulike disease was transmitted to monkeys after intracerebral injection of material from the brains of humans who died from kuru. Brains of humans, monkeys, and sheep suffering from the disease show a characteristic spongiform degeneration of tissue (abnormal spaces in the tissue), with vacuoles in the neurons and extensive glial cell proliferation with almost no inflammatory changes. A similar histological and clinical picture was characteristic of another rare human disease, Creutzfeldt-Jakob disease (CJD). This disease, found in humans throughout the world, consists of a very slowly progressive first stage of intellectual deterioration and behavioral abnormalities, followed by a shorter, rapidly progressive terminal stage characterized by myoclonic contractions of various muscle groups. Patients suffer from ataxia, dementia, and delirium that progresses to stupor, coma, and death. There is no treatment for any of these diseases. Another histological feature of the brain of patients and laboratory animals with CJD, shared by patients with Alzheimer's disease (another progressive dementing disease of humans), is the presence of characteristically staining areas called amyloid plaques.

The putative agent of CJD and kuru was first purified by workers led by S. Prusiner in 1982.[16] The agent consisted primarily of a single protein of approximately 27 to 30 kilodaltons molecular weight, designated PrP 27-30. This structural component was called a **prion** (proteinaceous infectious agent) by Prusiner. Antibodies to PrP 27-30 react with the "amyloid" plaques found in brains of patients with CJD and with the same structures found in the brains of scrapie-infected experimental animals, all of which were found to be crystalline arrays of prion protein. The gene encoding this protein has been identified in human chromosome 20 and cloned.[13] This finding may negate the theory that prions are infectious agents and suggests that prion protein is an altered product of a normal gene. Although Alzheimer's disease also demonstrates similar-appearing amyloid plaques, the existence of this gene and differences in plaque morphology at the electron microscopic structural level argue against a direct association between prions and Alzheimer's syndrome.

The prion genes of humans and hamsters share 89% homology and there is no homology between this protein and other known proteins. The nature of the infectious process is still not understood. Perhaps another, yet unknown agent induces the prion gene to produce a modified protein that aggregates to cause symptoms of CJD and kuru. Until the pathogenesis of these and similar diseases are known, the tissues from patients with these syndromes must be handled as though they were infectious.

Prions are extremely resistant to denaturation by proteases, nucleases, heat, ultraviolet light, and chemicals. Phenolic compounds, active against most other infectious agents, have no effect on prions. Dilute chlorine bleach (1:10) is effective with increased exposure (more than 1 minute). Dilute (1 N) NaOH will also effectively render the prion noninfectious.[1] It is not known how or even whether they reproduce.

The pathogenesis of disease is still largely unknown; however, cases of CJD have been diagnosed in several individuals who ate the brains of wild or domestic animals. Ingestion of brains, even well cooked, cannot be recommended, since cooking practices would be entirely unable to reduce infectivity of an agent such as a prion. Direct inoculation of infectious material has been known to transmit disease, as has transplantation of corneas, cadaveric dura mater grafts, and administration of growth hormone from infected humans. Organs and tissues from any patients with degenerative neurologic diseases should not be used for transplantation.

Laboratory workers who must handle tissue from the brains of patients with CJD should take extra precautions. Double gloves, masks, and gowns should be worn, and all manipulations should take place within a biological laminar flow safety cabinet. A solution of 1 N NaOH should be used to soak all instruments, and even the hands of technologists can be soaked briefly in this alkali if accidental exposure occurs. Dilute chlorine bleach is another effective decontaminating agent.

40.1.h. Whipple's disease. Whipple's disease, found primarily in middle-aged men, is characterized by the presence of PAS-staining macrophages (indicating mucopolysaccharide or glycoprotein) in almost every organ system. Patients develop diarrhea, weight loss, arthralgia, lymphadenopathy, hyperpigmentation, often a long history of joint pain, and a distended and tender abdomen. Neurologic and sensory changes often occur.[5] It has been suggested that a cellular immune defect is involved in pathogenesis of this disease. Patients usually respond well to long-term therapy with antibacterial agents, including trimethoprim-sulfamethoxazole, tetracycline, and penicillin; tetracycline has been associated with serious relapses, however.[5] Without treatment the disease is uniformly fatal.

Bacterial forms can be seen within the macrophages and within numerous other cells of involved tissue. These bacteria are 0.25 μm in diameter and as long as 2.5 μm. Their cell wall stains gram variably, but there appears to be a trilaminar structure to the plasma membrane on electron microscopy, which is more characteristic of gram-negative organisms. An outer trilaminar cell membrane superficially resembles that found on the surface of *Gardnerella vaginalis*. The organisms are antigenically similar to certain streptococci. Electron microscopy is the most definitive diagnostic tool, since the organism has not been cultivated in vitro or passed to laboratory animals, although the bacteria can be seen with certain stains.

40.1.i. Erythema infectiosum (fifth disease) and aplastic crisis. Parvovirus B-19, the agent of the relatively mild febrile exanthematous disease called "fifth disease" (because it was the fifth childhood exanthem, after the four others: rubella, measles, scarlet fever, and roseola), has recently been associated with aplastic crisis, adult arthritis, and congenital infection. The rash of fifth disease begins on the cheeks, causing them to resemble slapped cheeks. The rash then moves to the extremities, where it may disappear and recur several times. Headache and fever may be associated with the rash in one fourth of patients. The more serious syndrome of aplastic crisis, characterized by a sudden and significant decrease in red blood cell production, is most common in children with congenital anemias, particularly sickle cell disease. A potentially important cause of birth defects, the virus has been shown to infect the fetus of infected pregnant women. At this time, most infected fetuses spontaneously abort. Arthritis, especially in children suffering from fifth disease and family contacts, has been described.

The parvoviruses are among the smallest DNA viruses, infecting a number of animals. Parvovirus B-19 has not been grown in culture, thus diagnosis is still difficult. The only source of antigen for creating ELISA tests, the most widely used diagnostic technique, is serum from an infected human. Obviously this reagent is scarce. Further attempts to isolate the virus are in progress.

40.2. Diseases for Which No Etiologic Agent Has Been Demonstrated

40.2.a. Kawasaki disease. Kawasaki disease occurs in children, usually less than 8 years old, primarily in Japan, but many cases have been reported in the United States. The symptoms include fever that lasts at least 5 days, congestion of the conjunctivae, dry, red lips and red, fissured or "strawberry" tongue, reddening of the palms of hands and soles of feet with ultimate desquamation, a rash over the trunk and face, and cervical lymphadenopathy. The disease has also been called "mucocutaneous lymph node syndrome." Patients are usually ill for 1 month, with the convalescent phase lasting 6 to 10 weeks. The most important sequela of the disease is cardiopathy, which occurs in 20% of patients. Diagnosis of Kawasaki disease can be made in patients in whom other etiologies are excluded and who meet five of the six criteria, providing also that antibiotic treatment does not ameliorate the fever. The rash and subsequent desquamation resemble that caused by staphylococci, particularly toxic shock syndrome staphylococci, but efforts to isolate an organism from patients with Kawasaki disease have been unsuccessful. Several studies have verified the efficacy of treating Kawasaki patients with intravenous gamma globulin plus aspirin, which dramatically reduced the incidence of the serious sequelae, coronary artery abnormalities.[15]

40.2.b. Other diseases. The childhood exanthem *roseola* is thought to have a viral cause, although no agent has been implicated. Like fifth disease, the illness is mild and self-limited and appears to be somewhat contagious. The rash of roseola occurs within 48 hours after the febrile period, which usually lasts 3 to 5 days. No infectious agent has been clearly associated with this infectious syndrome.

It seems reasonable to mention multiple sclerosis in this section. Epidemiologic studies point to an infectious agent, and the pattern of pathologic findings in the neural tissue resembles that found in a progressive multifocal leukoencephalopathy, a slow virus infection. No definite virus particles have been seen in electron microscopic studies of brain tissue from patients with multiple sclerosis, but these patients do exhibit high levels of serum antibodies against a number of known viruses. The pathogenesis of this relatively common demyelinating disease is unknown, but an infectious agent has not been ruled out.

REFERENCES

1. Brown, P., Rohwer, R.G., and Gajdusek, D.C. 1984. Sodium hydroxide decontamination of Creutzfeldt-Jakob disease virus. N. Engl. J. Med. 310:727.
2. Choo, Q.-L., Kuo, G., Weiner, A.J., et al. 1989. Isolation of a cDNA clone derived from a blood-borne non-A, non-B viral hepatitis genome. Science 244:359.
3. Dienst, R.B., and Brownell, G.H. 1984. Genus *Calymmatobacterium Aragao and Vianna 1913*. In Krieg, N.R., and Holt, J.G., editors. Bergey's manual of systematic bacteriology, vol. 1. Williams & Wilkins, Baltimore.
4. English, C.K., Wear, D.J., Margileth, A.M., et al. 1988. Cat-scratch disease: isolation and culture of the bacterial agent. J.A.M.A. 259:1347.
5. Fleming, J.L., Wiesner, R.H., and Shorter, R.G. 1988. Whipple's disease: clinical, biochemical, and histopathologic features and assessment of treatment in 29 patients. Mayo Clin. Proc. 63:539.
6. Gerber, M.A., MacAlister, T.J., Ballow, M., et al. 1985. The aetiological agent of cat scratch disease. Lancet 1:1236.
7. Goldberg, J. 1959. Studies on granuloma inguinale. IV. Growth requirements of *Donovania granulomatis* and its relationship to the natural habitat of the organism. Br. J. Ven. Dis. 35:266.
8. Hadfield, T.L., Malaty, R.H., Van Dellen, A., et al. 1985. Electron microscopy of the bacillus causing cat-scratch disease. J. Infect. Dis. 152:643.
9. Hadfield, T.L., Schlagel, C., and Margileth, A. 1985. Stalking the cause of cat-scratch disease. Diagn. Med. 8:23.
10. Henrik-Nielsen, R., Lundbeck, F.A., Teglbjaerg, P.S., et al. 1985. Intestinal spirochetosis of the vermiform appendix. Gastroenterology 88:971.
11. Jones, M.J., Miller, J.N., and George, W.L. 1986. Microbiological and biochemical characterization of spirochetes isolated from the feces of homosexual men. J. Clin. Microbiol. 24:1071.
12. Levy, M.G., Meuten, D.J., and Breitschwerdt, E.B. 1986. Cultivation of *Rhinosporidium seeberi* in vitro: interaction with epithelial cells. Science 234:474.
13. Liao, Y.-C.J., Lebo, R.V., Clawson, G.A., and Smuckler, E.A. 1986. Human prion protein cDNA: molecular cloning, chromosomal mapping, and biological implications. Science 233:364.
14. Luna, L.G. 1968. Warthin-Starry method for spirochetes and Donovan bodies. In Manual of histologic staining methods of the Armed Forces Institute of Pathology. McGraw-Hill Book Co., New York.

15. Newburger, J.W., Takahashi, M., Burns, J.C., et al. 1986. The treatment of Kawasaki syndrome with intravenous gamma globulin. N. Engl. J. Med. 315:341.

16. Prusiner, S.B. 1982. Novel proteinaceous infectious particles cause scrapie. Science 216:136.

17. Surawicz, C.M., Roberts, P.L., Rompalo, A., et al. 1987. Intestinal spirochetosis in homosexual men. Am. J. Med. 82:587.

18. Wear, D.J., Margileth, A.M., Hadfield, T.L., et al. 1983. Cat scratch disease: a bacterial infection. Science 221:1403.

BIBLIOGRAPHY

Bockman, J.M., Kingsbury, D.T., McKinley, M.P., et al. 1985. Creutzfeldt-Jakob disease prion proteins in human brains. N. Engl. J. Med. 312:73.

Cormier, D.P., and Mayo, D.R. 1988. Parvovirus B-19 infections. Clin. Microbiol. Newsletter 10:49.

Dobbins, W.O. III. 1985. Whipple's disease. In Mandell, G.L., Douglas, R.G., Jr., and Bennett, J.E., editors. Principles and practice of infectious diseases, ed. 2. John Wiley & Sons, New York.

Gajdusek, D.C., Gibbs, C.J., Asher, D.M., et al. 1977. Precautions in medical care of, and in handling materials from, patients with transmissible virus dementia (Creutzfeldt-Jakob disease). N. Engl. J. Med. 297:1253.

Gutman, L.T. 1988. *Campylobacter* and *Spirillum*. pp. 572-577. In Joklik, W.K., Willett, H.P., Amos, D.B., and Wilfert, C.M. editors. Zinsser's Microbiology, ed. 19. Appleton & Lange, Norwalk, Conn.

Lohr, J.A. 1985. Kawasaki disease (mucocutaneous lymph node syndrome). In Mandell, G.L., Douglas, R.G., Jr., and Bennett, J.E., editors. Principles and practice of infectious diseases, ed. 2. John Wiley & Sons, New York.

Melish, M.E., Hicks, R.V., and Reddy, V. 1982. Kawasaki syndrome: an update. Hosp. Pract. 17:99.

Murray, H.W., 1985. *Spirillum minor* (rat-bite fever). In Mandell, G.L., Douglas, R.G., Jr., and Bennett, J.E., editors. Principles and practice of infectious diseases, ed. 2. John Wiley & Sons, New York.

Taylor, A.F., Stephenson, T.G., Giese, H.A., and Petterson, G.R. 1984. Rat-bite fever in a college student. Calif. Morbid., No. 13. Department of Health Services, Sacramento, Calif.

41 Mycobacteria

O. George W. Berlin

Mycobacteria caused disease in humans long before recorded history, with evidence of disease found in the bones of prehistoric humans and animals. It continued into the eighteenth and nineteenth centuries as the white plague, decimating the populations of Europe. According to the World Health Organization, tuberculosis still kills 3 million people yearly in underdeveloped countries.

Mycobacterium tuberculosis, the cause of tuberculosis, is one of 54 recognized species of mycobacteria. Of these, 14 are known to cause disease in humans (Table 41.1).[10] For the first time since 1953, the United States experienced a 1.1% increase in new active cases of tuberculosis in 1986; it is thought that this increase is related to the acquired immune deficiency syndrome (AIDS) epidemic.[25] A remarkable increase in infections due to *M. avium* complex can also be attributed to AIDS patients.[43]

College of American Pathologists Extents of Service for Participation in Mycobacterial Interlaboratory Comparison Surveys

1. No mycobacterial procedures performed
2. Acid-fast stain of exudates, effusions, and body fluids, etc., with inoculation and referral of cultures to reference laboratories for further identification
3. Isolation of mycobacteria; identification of *M. tuberculosis* and preliminary identification of the atypical forms such as photochromogens, scotochromogens, nonphotochromogens, and rapid growers; drug susceptibility testing may or may not be performed
4. Definitive identification of mycobacteria isolated to the extent required to establish a correct clinical diagnosis and to aid in the selection of safe and effective therapy; drug susceptibility testing may or may not be performed

---

The physician is totally dependent on the microbiology laboratory for information that will help him or her to (1) make a definitive diagnosis of tuberculosis or other mycobacterial disease by isolation and identification of the etiologic agent, (2) treat the patient effectively by determining susceptibility of the isolated organisms, and (3) monitor the chemotherapeutic response of the patient by periodic examination of specimens for evidence of a decrease in numbers of organisms by smear and colony count in culture. The laboratory must determine what "level of service" it can provide most effectively. "Levels of Service" has been outlined by the American Society of Clinical Pathologists (box). At whatever level the laboratory chooses to operate, it must be prepared to offer exemplary service.[19]

41.1. Epidemiology and Pathogenesis of Mycobacterial Infections

Species of mycobacteria produce a spectrum of infections in humans and animals ranging from localized lesions to dissemination. While some species cause only human infections, others have been isolated from a wide variety of animals. Many of the species are also found in water and soil. A tentative classification is proposed based on pathogenesis and natural history. Species include: (1) obligate pathogens that cause exclusively human infections; (2) facultative pathogens that are found primarily in animals or the environment but produce documented human infections; (3) potentially "opportunistic" pathogenic species that are found in the environment but produce documented human infections; and (4) saprophytic species found in the environment that do not cause human infection (Table 41.1).

41.1.a. *Mycobacterium tuberculosis*. Tuberculosis still accounts for a large number of deaths and great morbidity worldwide. The disease is most common in parts of the developing nations of the world. Infection is spread from person to person by inhalation of airborne **droplet nuclei**, 1 to 5 μm in diameter. They are small enough to avoid being trapped by nasal turbinates or mucociliary membranes and may reach and impinge on the alveolar walls and be taken up by alveolar macrophages.[41] The pathogenesis of tuberculosis was discussed in Chapter 16.

Almost all tuberculosis acquired in the United States today is by aerosol inhalation. With the exception of leprosy, no other mycobacterial diseases are presumed contagious. Patients with cavitary disease are the primary reservoir for dissemination of *M. tuberculosis*. Although the disease incidence among Caucasians is falling, increasing numbers of cases are being discovered among Latin American and Southeast Asian immigrants and refugees. These patients, often infected with antibiotic-resistant strains of *M. tuberculosis*, pose new problems for public health officials and represent new foci for spread of the disease in certain locations, notably larger cities. Elderly patients, alcoholics, and non-Caucasians are more likely to develop disease. In addition, there is a resurgence of *M. tuberculosis* and other mycobacterial diseases in major metropolitan areas due to the advent of AIDS.

It has been shown that inhalation of a single viable organism can lead to infection, although close contact is usually necessary for acquisition of infection. Of persons who become infected, 15% to 20% go on to develop disease. Disease usually occurs some years after the initial infection, when the patient's immune system breaks down for some reason other than the presence of tuberculosis bacilli within the lung. In a small percentage of infected hosts, the disease becomes systemic, affecting such organs as the kidneys,

Table 41.1

Currently Recognized Species of the Genus *Mycobacterium* Isolated from Humans

GROUP	OBLIGATORY	FACULTATIVE	POTENTIAL	SAPROPHYTE	
Strict pathogens	*M. africanum* *M. leprae* *M. tuberculosis* *M. ulcerans*	*M. bovis*			
Photochromogens		*M. asiaticum* *M. kansasii* *M. marinum* *M. simiae*			
Scotochromogens		*M. scrofulaceum* *M. szulgai* *M. xenopi*	*M. gordonae* *M. flavescens*		
Nonchromogens*		*M. avium* *M. haemophilum* *M. intracellulare* *M. malmoense* *M. shimoidei*	*M. gastri* *M. nonchromogenicum* *M. terrae* *M. triviale*		
Rapid growers		*M. chelonae* *M. fortuitum*	*M. fallax* *M. smegmatis*	*M. agri* *M. aichiense* *M. austroafricanum* *M. aurum* *M. chitae* *M. chubuense* *M. diernhoferi* *M. duvalii* *M. gadium* *M. gilvum* *M. komossense*	*M. neoaurum* *M. parafortuitum* *M. obuense* *M. phei* *M. pulveris* *M. rhodesiae* *M. sphagni* *M. thermoresistible* *M. tokaiense* *M. vaccae*
Strict animal pathogens	*M. farcinogens* *M. lepraemu-* *rium* *M. porcinum*	*M. microti* *M. paratuberculosis* *M. senegalense*			

*Some strains of *M. avium* and *M. intracellulare* are pigmented.

Reproduced with permission from Good, R.C. 1985. Opportunistic pathogens in the genus *Mycobacterium*. Annu. Rev. Microbiol. 39:347. © 1985 by Annual Reviews Inc.

spleen, bone marrow, central nervous system, and intestinal tract. In most patients, however, the disease is restricted to the lungs, with granuloma formation, caseous necrosis, and ultimately cavitary disease (Chapter 16). A definitive diagnosis is made by isolating and identifying the etiologic agent, *M. tuberculosis*.

41.1.b. Other cultivatable mycobacteria. *M. bovis*, the agent of bovine tuberculosis, is an uncommon cause of disease in the United States today, although it used to be one of the primary agents of human intestinal tuberculosis, acquired through ingestion of contaminated milk. An attenuated strain of *M. bovis*, **bacille Calmette-Guérin (BCG),** has been used extensively in many parts of the world to immunize susceptible individuals against tuberculosis. BCG has recently been used as part of a controversial protocol to boost the nonspecific cellular immune response of certain immunologically deficient patients, particularly those with malignancies. Because mycobacteria are the classic examples of intracellular pathogens, and the body's response to BCG hinges on cell-mediated immunoreactivity, immunized individuals are expected to react more aggressively against all antigens that elicit cell mediated immunity. Rarely, the unfortunate individual's immune system will be so compromised that it cannot handle the BCG, and systemic BCG infection may develop.

Respiratory infection in immunocompetent hosts

is usually caused by *M. tuberculosis*, but *M. kansasii* and *M. avium-intracellulare* complex also cause tuberculosis-like disease. Other mycobacteria cause pulmonary disease, as well. *M. avium* complex is the most commonly isolated mycobacterial species in the United States today because of its high prevalence in patients suffering from AIDS (see Chapter 23).[11] In homosexual patients with AIDS the mode of acquisition of *M. avium* complex is believed to be through the gastrointestinal tract.[3,42] The first symptom of mycobacterial disease in many of these patients is protracted diarrhea. Acid-fast stains of feces or intestinal biopsy specimens reveal huge numbers of acid-fast bacilli. The infection usually disseminates in AIDS patients, with organisms being recovered from multiple sites, including blood, sputum, feces, semen, lymph nodes, and internal organs.

Isolation of *M. tuberculosis* or *M. bovis* is always indicative of disease, whereas isolation of other mycobacteria may or may not be clinically significant. *M. gordonae*, for example, one of the more common mycobacteria isolated from clinical specimens, is a normal inhabitant of tap water and rarely causes disease in humans. Table 41.1 lists the "mycobacteria other than tuberculosis (**MOTT**)" that have been implicated as etiologic agents of human disease.

41.1.c. Crohn's disease—associated *Mycobacterium*. Isolation of a new species of *Mycobacterium* that resembles the animal pathogen *M. paratuberculosis* from the bowel mucosa of patients with Crohn's disease has been reported by Chiodini and co-workers (see Bibliography). This news is particularly interesting, since the etiology of Crohn's disease, a chronic inflammatory bowel disease, previously had not been considered to be infectious. The organism is extremely fastidious, seems to require a growth factor, mycobactin, produced by other species of mycobacteria, such as *M. phlei*, a saprophytic strain, and may take as long as 6 to 18 months for primary isolation. Whether these mycobacteria actually contribute to development of Crohn's disease or are simply colonizing an environmental niche in the bowel of these patients remains to be elucidated.

41.1.d. *Mycobacterium leprae*. Possibly second to *M. tuberculosis* in worldwide importance is *M. leprae*, the agent of leprosy (also called Hansen's disease). The organism has not yet been cultivated in vitro. Leprosy is a chronic disease of the skin, mucous membranes, and nerve tissue, with a strong immunologic component to the pathology. Understanding of the pathogenesis and epidemiology of the disease is hampered by our inability to grow the organism in culture. In tropical countries, where the disease is most prevalent, it may be acquired from infected humans; however, infectivity is very low. Prolonged close contact and host immunologic status play a role in infectivity.

However leprosy is acquired, it passes through many stages in the host, characterized by various clinical and histopathological features. Although there are many intermediate stages, the primary stages include a silent phase, during which leprosy bacilli multiply in the skin within macrophages, and an indeterminate phase, in which the bacilli multiply in peripheral nerves and begin to cause sensory impairment. More severe disease states that may follow are called "tuberculoid," in which granulomas and hyperactive tissue are evident in the skin, and "lepromatous," in which the patient's immune response is virtually absent and the bacilli multiply rapidly, often within many organs of the body and the reticuloendothelial system. A patient may recover spontaneously at any stage, and there are several borderline stages defined by subtle differences in the host response to infection. Berlin and Martin[2] have summarized current knowledge about leprosy.

Diagnosis is usually made through histopathological examination of material taken from a skin lesion or from the earlobe of a suspected patient. While acid-fast bacilli are not seen during the early stages, they are later visualized in large numbers by the Fite stain or by routine Ziehl-Neelsen stain. Other sites from which positive smears may be seen include lymph nodes, bone marrow, and human milk. The stages of leprosy can be additionally pinpointed by a patient's response to "lepromin," a crude suspension of material taken from excised nodules of patients with Hansen's disease. Treatment consists of dapsone or DDS (4,4′-diaminodiphenyl sulfone), often given in combination with rifampin. Excellent results have also been seen with clofazimine, which requires several months to build up active concentrations within the patient's tissues.[32]

41.2. Laboratory Safety and Quality Control

Tuberculosis ranks high among laboratory-acquired infections. It is therefore mandatory that laboratory and hospital administrators provide laboratory personnel with facilities, equipment, and supplies that will reduce this risk to a minimum. All tuberculin-negative personnel should be skin-tested every 3 to

4 months. Tuberculin-positive persons should have a chest x-ray annually.

41.2.a. Facilities and equipment; safety measures

Facilities and equipment

1. A "hot room" devoted only to diagnostic mycobacteriology, maintained under negative air exhaust to adjacent corridors and work areas
2. Laminar flow biological safety cabinets, type 2B, which draw a minimum of 75 linear feet of air per minute across the front opening and exhaust 100% of the air to the outside
3. High-speed, refrigerated ultracentrifuges equipped with bucket covers and safety domes

Safety measures

1. Masks, gowns, and gloves must be worn when working in the "hot room."
2. Manipulations resulting in formation of aerosols must be kept to a minimum.
3. Hands should be scrubbed thoroughly before leaving the laboratory.
4. The increasing use of syringes and needles for BACTEC system inoculations requires extreme precaution to avoid finger sticks. Work slowly and deliberately and do not take your eyes off the needle.
5. Substitute egg and agar media in 1 ounce prescription bottles for media in test tubes. Bottles seldom break when dropped, whereas test tubes will always break. Bottles are easier to stack, store, and handle during incubation and examination.
6. In case of accident with formation of aerosols, hold your breath, make certain biological safety cabinets are on, centrifuges are turned off, and leave the room. Return in 30 minutes to cover the spill with 3% Amphyl and paper towels. Allow the Amphyl to stand for 30 minutes. Change clothing and shower if necessary. Return to the accident area for a final cleanup. Skin-test all tuberculin-negative personnel at 3 and 6 months after the accident.

41.2.b. Quality control. Quality control in diagnostic mycobacteriology requires the same attention to equipment, media, reagents, stains, and antimycobacterial susceptibility testing procedures as do other areas of the laboratory. Quality control of the decontamination and concentration procedures should be of particular concern, as the accuracy and reliability of these procedures determine whether mycobacteria are isolated from specimens. The slow rate of growth of mycobacteria interferes with prompt detection of deficiencies. Procedure 41.1 detects lethal effects of the decontaminating agents employed; it also detects deficiencies in media quality. However, two to three weeks will have elapsed before such deficiencies are noted. Therefore, routine monitoring with this procedure should help alert the laboratory to impending problems.

41.3. Specimen Collection

Acid-fast bacilli may infect almost any tissue or organ of the body (Table 41.3). The successful isolation of the organism depends on the quality of the specimen obtained and the appropriate processing and culture techniques employed by the mycobacteriology laboratory. In suspected mycobacterial disease, as in all other infectious diseases, the diagnostic procedure begins at the patient's bedside. Collection of proper clinical specimens requires careful attention to detail by the attending physician, nurse, or other ward personnel. An essential prerequisite of good specimen collection is the use of sturdy, sterile, leakproof containers, placed into bags to contain leakage should it occur.

41.3.a. Pulmonary specimens. Pulmonary secretions may be obtained by any one of the following methods: spontaneously produced or induced sputum, gastric lavage, transtracheal aspiration, bronchoscopy, and laryngeal swabbing. Sputum, aerosol induced sputum, bronchoscopic aspirations, and gastric lavage comprise the majority of specimens submitted for examination. Spontaneously produced sputum is the specimen of choice. In order to raise sputum, patients *must* be instructed to take a deep breath, hold it momentarily, and then cough deeply and vigorously. Patients must also be instructed to cover their mouths carefully while coughing and to discard tissues in an appropriate receptacle. Saliva and nasal secretions are not to be collected nor is the patient to use oral antiseptics during the period of collection. Sputum specimens must be free of food particles, residues, and other extraneous matter.

The aerosol induction procedure can best be done on ambulatory patients who are able to follow instructions. Aerosol-induced sputums have been collected from children as young as 5 years. The procedure should be avoided for patients with asthma or other respiratory difficulties. The patient must be questioned closely; if the patient admits to difficulty, the physician should confirm that the patient can be

PROCEDURE 41.1

Quality Control for Mycobacteriology

Reagents

1. Media: Routine media used for cultivation of mycobacteria
2. Quality control organism: A recent isolate of *M. tuberculosis* or *M. tuberculosis* strain H37Rv
3. Other materials:

   Autoclaved sputum (AFB-negative)
   7H9 liquid medium containing 15% glycerol
   Sterile buffer, pH 7.0
   50-ml plastic, conical centrifuge tubes

Procedure

1. Suspend several colonies of H37Rv in a tube containing 3 ml of 7H9 liquid medium and several plastic or glass beads. Mix vigorously on a test tube mixer; then allow large particles to settle for 15 min.
2. Prepare a dilution of approximately 10^6 organisms per milliliter by adding the above cell suspension drop-by-drop to 1 ml of buffer until a barely turbid suspension occurs. Transfer 0.5 ml of the 10^6 cells per milliliter dilution to 4.5 ml of glycerol broth to give a suspension of 10^5 cells per milliliter. Repeat the procedure to make a 10^4/ml and a 10^3/ml suspension.
3. Label fifteen 3-dram vials for each suspension (10^5, 10^4, and 10^3). Transfer 0.3 ml of the appropriate suspension to each vial. Store the vials at $-70°$ C to use for future quality control testing.
4. Thaw one vial of each of the three dilutions each time the quality control procedure is performed.
5. Add 2.7 ml autoclaved sputum to each cell suspension to effect a tenfold dilution and in-

oculate three sets of the media used for primary isolation with each of the three dilutions of sputum. Inoculate 0.1 ml of sputum per bottle.
6. Decontaminate and concentrate the remainder as you do with sputum specimens. Reconstitute the sediments with sterile buffer to 2.6 ml, resuspend vigorously, and inoculate a second set of media with 0.1 ml of each of the concentrated and resuspended samples.
7. Incubate at $37°$ C in 5%-10% CO_2 for 21 days.

Interpreting and recording results

The bottle of egg media should have been inoculated with approximately 10^4, 10^3, and 10^2 organisms, respectively. The first dilution should produce semiconfluent growth and the second and third dilutions should produce countable colonies in each bottle. Because of the retrospective nature of these determinations, close comparisons must be made between current and previous results to note trends or developing deficiencies. Failures may be due to faulty media, lethal effects of decontamination and concentration procedures, improperly prepared reagents, or overexposure of specimens to these reagents (Table 41.2). Should deficiencies become evident, techniques should be reviewed and attempts made to determine the source of the problem. New batches of media must be substituted for deficient media and the latter rechecked to verify deficiencies. Personnel should be included in all discussions of problems and corrective measures. All deficiencies and corrective actions should be recorded in the appropriate section of the Quality Control records.

safely induced. A physician should be present or close by when asthmatics are being induced. Aerosol induction can be done at any time during the day, but preferably approximately 2 hours after meals to avoid nausea and dizziness. The patient should be told that the procedure is being performed to induce coughing to raise sputum that the patient cannot

raise spontaneously and that the salt solution is irritating. The patient should be instructed to inhale slowly and deeply through the mouth and to cough at will, vigorously and deeply. The patient should be instructed to cover his or her mouth with tissues while coughing and to expectorate into a collection tube. The procedure should be discontinued if the

Table 41.2
Sample Results for Interpreting Quality Control Test of Decontamination and Concentration Procedure

SPUTUM SAMPLE	SPUTUM						INTERPRETATION
	UNPROCESSED			PROCESSED			
	10^4	10^3	10^2	10^4	10^3	10^2	
1	3+	2+	50-100 Col	2+	1+2+	Approx. 10	Media and D/C procedures are acceptable
2	3+	2+	50-100 Col	1+	0	0	Media acceptable; procedure too toxic
3	2+ or 1+	2+ or 1+	0	1+ or 0	1+ or 0	0	One or more of the media being used is not supporting growth of AFB adequately

Table 41.3
Types of Specimens and Species of Mycobacteria Likely to Be Recovered from Them

OCULAR	G.I. TRACT	CUTANEOUS	PULMONARY	GENITAL	VASCULAR (LYMPHATICS)	NERVOUS
M. fortuitum	M. bovis	M. leprae	M. tuberculosis	M. leprae	M. tuberculosis	M. leprae
M. chelonae	M. avium	M. marinum	M. africanum	M. tuberculosis	M. avium	M. tuberculosis
	M. intracellulare	M. haemophilum	M. kansasii	M. avium	M. intracellulare	
	M. sp. ("linda")	M. fortuitum	M. simiae	M. intracellulare	M. kansasii	
		M. chelonae	M. asiaticum	M. xenopi	M. leprae	
		M. ulcerans	M. scrofulaceum		M. scrofulaceum	
		M. smegmatis	M. szulgai		M. fortuitum	
			M. xenopi		M. chelonae	
			M. avium			
			M. intracellulare			
			M. malmoense			
			M. fortuitum			
			M. chelonae			

patient fails to raise sputum after 10 minutes or feels any discomfort. Ten milliliters of sputum should be collected in a 50-ml conical centrifuge tube; if the patient continues to raise sputum, a second specimen should be collected and submitted. Specimens should be delivered promptly to the laboratory and refrigerated if processing is delayed.

When the procedure is completed, the nebulizer should be thoroughly rinsed with filtered distilled water and allowed to soak in 2% acetic acid for 10 minutes. The nebulizer should then be rinsed with sterile filtered distilled water and air dried. The effluent should be collected weekly for bacteriological monitoring. Swabs of the transducer may be submitted as an alternative culture.

Gastric lavage is used to collect sputum from patients who may have swallowed their sputum during the night. The procedure is limited to senile, non-ambulatory patients, children less than 3 years old, and patients who fail to produce sputum by aerosol induction. The most desirable gastric lavage is collected at the patient's bedside before the patient arises and before exertion empties the stomach. *Gastric lavage cannot be performed as an office or clinic procedure.* A series of three specimens should be collected within 3 days. The patient should be told that the procedure is being performed to collect sputum that has been swallowed. If the patient appears unable to tolerate the procedure, gastric lavage should not be attempted.

The collector should wear a cap, gown, and mask and stand beside (not in front of) the patient, who should sit up on the edge of the bed or in a chair, if possible. The Levine collection tube is inserted through a nostril and the patient is instructed to swallow the tube. Small sips of filtered water and deep breaths may aid this process. When the tube is fully inserted, a syringe is attached to the end of the tube, and 5 ml of filtered distilled water is inserted through the tube. The syringe is then used to withdraw 20 to 25 ml gastric secretions. The fluid should be expelled slowly down the sides of the 50-ml conical collecting tube. Do not pump the syringe or otherwise create aerosols. The syringe is reattached to the Levine tube while the tube is slowly withdrawn, avoiding motion of the free end. Excess fluid is expelled into the collection tube, and the collection equipment and clothing are bagged in the appropriate hazardous waste containers. The top of the collection tube is screwed on tightly and the tube is held upright during *prompt* delivery to the laboratory. Bronchial lavages, washings, and brushings are collected and submitted by medical personnel. These are the specimens of choice for detecting nontuberculous mycobacteria and other opportunistic pathogens in patients with immune dysfunctions.

41.3.b. Urine specimens. In contrast to the overall decline in new cases of pulmonary tuberculosis, urogenital infections show little evidence of decreasing. It is presumed that there is a relatively long incubation period between the initial infection and later urinary tract manifestations. While 2% to 3% of patients with pulmonary tuberculosis exhibit urinary tract involvement, 30% to 40% of patients with genitourinary disease have tuberculosis at some other site. The clinical manifestations of urinary tuberculosis are variable, including frequency of urination (most common), dysuria, hematuria, and flank pain. Definitive diagnosis requires recovery of acid-fast bacilli from the urine.

Early morning voided urine specimens in sterile containers should be submitted daily for at least 3 days. Because of excessive dilution, higher contamination, and difficulty in concentrating, 24-hour urine specimens are undesirable.

41.3.c. Genital specimens. A variety of species of mycobacteria have been isolated from semen, seminal vesicles, prostate gland, and testes specimens; numerous isolations have been made from AIDS patients. Diagnosis requires biopsy of the suspected site for histological examination and culture.

41.3.d. Fecal specimens. Until recently, fecal specimens were rarely examined for acid-fast bacilli. However, the frequent isolation of *M. avium* complex from feces of AIDS patients has significantly increased the number of specimens submitted for this purpose. Feces should be submitted in a clean, dry container without preservative or diluent. Contamination with urine should be avoided.

41.3.e. Tissue specimens. Pus and exudates may be submitted on swabs or on small pieces of bandage, placed in sterile, leakproof containers. Swabs should be placed in a neutral transport medium to avoid desiccation. Tissue biopsy specimens should be submitted in large-mouth tubes or in petri dishes, bagged to prevent leakage.

41.3.f. Other specimens. Tuberculous meningitis is uncommon but still occurs in both immunocompetent and immunosuppressed patients. Most critical for isolation of acid-fast bacilli from cerebrospinal fluid is that the quantity of specimen be sufficient. There may be very few organisms in the spinal fluid, which makes their detection difficult. At least 10 ml of cerebrospinal fluid is recommended for recovery of mycobacteria.

The discovery of circulating mycobacteria in the blood of patients with AIDS has led to increased requests for such cultures. Best recovery can be achieved by collecting the blood in a lysis-centrifugation system. If the blood is allowed to remain in the lysing solution for approximately 1 hour, lysis of phagocytic cells may occur, allowing release and enhanced recovery of intracellular mycobacteria. In patients with AIDS, quantitation of such organisms can be used to monitor therapy and determine prognosis. For this purpose the 1.5 ml Pediatric Isolator tubes can be used, since the entire contents are plated and colony-forming units can be determined per milliliter of initial specimen. Other traditional methods have been described for isolation of mycobacteria from blood, including biphasic blood culture media, but the lysis-centrifugation system is the most practical so far. Automated radiometric detection of mycobacteria in blood is another alternative for such cultures. Use of this system is discussed in Section 41.5.b.

41.4. Specimen Processing for the Recovery of Acid-fast Organisms

Specimen processing for the recovery of acid-fast bacilli from clinical specimens involves a number of complex procedures, each of which must be carried out with precision. Specimens from sterile sites can be inoculated directly to media (small volume) or concentrated to reduce volume. Other specimens require decontamination and concentration. A

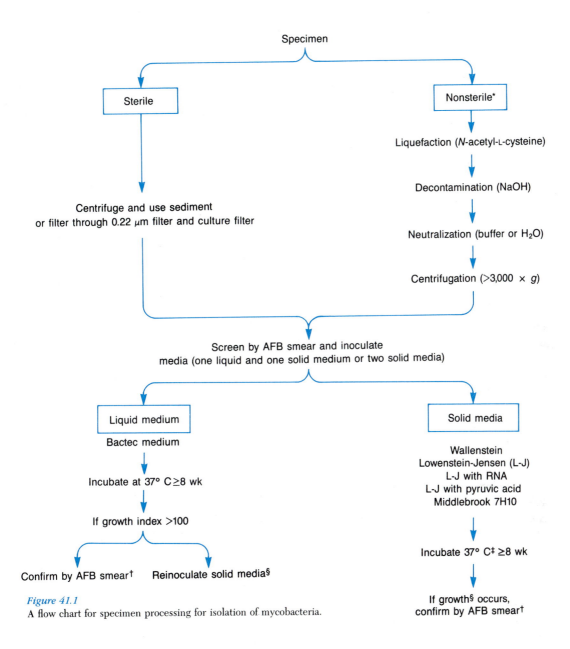

Figure 41.1
A flow chart for specimen processing for isolation of mycobacteria.

scheme for initial processing is depicted in Figure 41.1. The procedures will be explored in detail in the following sections.

41.4.a. Decontamination and concentration procedures. Many techniques for decontaminating and concentrating sputum and other specimens have been discarded because of a failure to fulfill some practical requirement, such as low toxicity to acid-fast bacilli, effective inhibition of contaminants, or

ability to completely liquefy mucoid sputum in a reasonable time period. The procedures outlined here, while still suffering some of these disadvantages, yield acceptable numbers of positive cultures *if properly performed*. Because of toxicity of the reagents toward acid-fast bacilli, it is mandatory that procedures be carried out within the stated time limits.

The *N*-acetyl-L cysteine–sodium hydroxide

N-Acetyl-L Cysteine–Sodium Hydroxide Method for Liquefaction and Decontamination of Specimens

Principle

Sodium hydroxide, an extremely toxic decontaminating agent, also acts as an emulsifier. The addition of a mucolytic agent, *N*-acetyl-L-cysteine (NALC), makes it possible to reduce the concentration of sodium hydroxide used and also shortens the time required for decontamination, thus aiding the optimal recovery of acid-fast bacilli.

Method

1. NALC–sodium hydroxide preparation
   For each day's cultures, add up the total volume of specimens to be treated and prepare an equal volume of the digestant-decontamination mixture, as follows:

1 N (4%) NaOH	50 ml
0.1 M (2.94%) trisodium citrate · 3H$_2$O	50 ml
N-Acetyl-L-cysteine (NALC) powder	0.5 g

   It is useful to use sterile distilled water for preparation of solutions to minimize chances of inadvertently adding acid-fast tap water contaminants to the specimens. Mix, sterilize, and store the NaOH and the citrate in sterile, screw-capped flasks for later use. This solution should be used within 24 h after the NALC is added.

2. 0.676 (1/15) M phosphate buffer preparation

   Solution A

Sodium monohydrogen phosphate (anhydrous)	9.47 g
Distilled water	1000 ml

   Solution B

Potassium dihydrophosphate	9.07 g
Distilled water	1000 ml

   Add 50 ml of solution B to 50 ml of solution A and adjust pH to 6.8.

3. Work within a biological safety cabinet and wear gloves. Transfer a maximum of 10 ml of sputum, urine, or other fluid to be processed to a sterile, disposable plastic 50-ml conical centrifuge tube with a leakproof and aerosol-free plastic screw-cap. Tubes with easily visible volume indicator marks are best.

4. Add an equal volume of freshly prepared digestant to the tube, being very careful when pouring digestant not to touch the lip of the specimen container, which might inadvertently transfer positive material to a negative specimen. Tighten the cap completely.

5. Vortex the specimen for approximately a slow count of 15, or for a maximum of 30 seconds, being certain to create a vortex in the liquid and not to merely agitate the material. Check for homogeneity by inverting the tube. If clumps remain, vortex the specimen intermittently while the rest of the specimens are being digested. An extra pinch of NALC crystals may be necessary to liquefy really mucoid sputa.

6. Start a 15-min timer as the first specimen is finished being vortexed. Continue digesting the other specimens, noting the amount of time that the entire run takes. The digestant should remain on the specimens for a maximum exposure of 20 min.

7. After 15 min of digestion, add enough phosphate buffer to reach within 1 cm of the top, screw the cap tightly closed, and invert the tube to mix the solutions and stop the digestion process. Addition of this solution also reduces the specific gravity of the specimen, aiding sedimentation of the bacilli during centrifugation.

8. Centrifuge all tubes at 3600 × g for 15 min.

9. Carefully pour off the supernatant into a splash-proof container (Figure 41.2). The lip of the tube may be wiped with an amphyl- or phenol-soaked gauze to absorb drips. Be careful not to touch the lip of any tube to another container. It is helpful to watch the sediment carefully as the supernatant is being decanted, since sometimes a very mucoid sediment can be loose and may pour right out with the supernatant. The technologist who sees the sediment beginning to slip can then stop decanting and use a sterile capillary pipette to remove the supernatant without losing the sediment.

10. Resuspend the sediment in 1 to 2 ml sterile water or buffer.

11. Inoculate the sediment to culture media and prepare slides.

Quality control

See Procedure 41.1.

PROCEDURE 41.3

Benzalkonium Chloride (Zephiran)—Trisodium Phosphate Method for Digestion and Decontamination

Principle

A milder decontaminating solution allows a longer time period for decontamination to occur.

Method

1. Prepare Zephiran–trisodium phosphate digestant as follows:

Trisodium phosphate ($Na_3PO_4 \cdot 2H_2O$)	500 g
Hot, sterile distilled water	2000 ml

   Add 3.25 ml of Zephiran concentrate (17% benzalkonium chloride, Winthrop laboratories). Mix. Store at room temperature.
2. Mix equal parts of the specimen and digestant, exactly as detailed in Procedure 41.2. Vortex for 30 s.
3. Allow the mixtures to stand without agitation for an additional 15 min.
4. Centrifuge as in Procedure 41.2 for 30 min.
5. Decant supernatant as in Procedure 41.2
6. Resuspend the supernatant in 20 ml of neutralizing buffer (obtained from Difco Laboratories). Although the 1/15 M phosphate buffer described in Procedure 41.3 may be used, the commercial buffer contains components to specifically neutralize the Zephiran.
7. Centrifuge the tubes as above for 20 min.
8. Decant supernatant fluids as above and retain the sediments for smears and cultures.

Quality control

See Procedure 41.1.

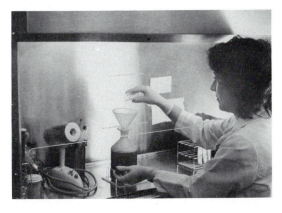

Figure 41.2
Supernatant from acid-fast specimen concentrates is carefully decanted into a splash-proof container that can be autoclaved and reused.

method (Procedure 41.2) is the most widely used decontamination and concentration procedure and may be considered the "gold standard."[18]

An alternative method for decontamination and concentration, the Zephiran–trisodium phosphate method (Procedure 41.3), permits a longer exposure of specimens to the decontaminating agents without affecting the recovery of acid-fast bacilli. A modification of this procedure (Procedure 41.4), which reduces the concentrations of the toxic reagents and requires a second wash of the sediment, further enhances survival of these organisms.

A decontaminating procedure utilizing oxalic acid is very useful for treating specimens known to harbor gram-negative rods, particularly *Pseudomonas* and *Proteus*, which are extremely troublesome contaminants (Procedure 41.5). Excellent discussions of decontamination and concentration procedures can be found elsewhere.[13,18,34]

Many other specimens that contain normal flora require decontamination and concentration; handling procedures for such specimens are described briefly here. Aerosol-induced sputums should be treated as sputums. Gastric lavages should be processed immediately or neutralized with 10% sodium carbonate (check with pH paper to determine that the specimen is at neutral pH) and refrigerated until processed as for sputum. If more than 10 ml of watery-appearing aspirate was obtained, the specimen can be centrifuged at 3600 × g for 30 minutes, the supernatant decanted, and the sediment processed as for sputum.

PROCEDURE 41.4

Modified Zephiran–Trisodium Phosphate (TSP) Method

Principle

By reducing the concentration of reagents and adding a second wash, survival of acid-fast bacilli is enhanced.

Method

Note: *All reagents should be prepared with filter-sterilized distilled water.*

1. Prepare Zephiran–trisodium phosphate (1:5000 Zephiran in 15% TSP) as follows:

Trisodium phosphate $Na_3PO_4 \cdot 2H_2O$)	150 g
Hot, sterile distilled water	1000 ml
Concentrated Zephiran chloride (17%)	1.1 ml
Bromthymol blue, 0.1% aqueous solution	10.0 ml

2. Prepare 1/15 M sterile phosphate buffer, pH 6.6, as follows:

   Stock solution A

Na_2HPO_4	9.47 g
Distilled water	1000 ml

   Stock solution B

KH_2PO_4	9.07 g
Distilled water	1000 ml

   Add 37.5 ml of solution A to 62.5 ml of solution B. Filter-sterilize through a 0.47-μm pore size nitrocellulose filter and autoclave for 15 min at 121° C. Aseptically add 15 U/ml penicillin G when the solution reaches room temperature.

3. To liquefy the specimen, add an equal volume of filtered distilled water to a maximum of 10-ml sputum in a 50-ml conical centrifuge tube. Sputolysin (Calbiochem, Inc.) may be used to liquefy thick, mucoid specimens. Vortex until the sputum is thoroughly homogenized; allow to stand 15 min.

   Note: *Sputolysin is a concentrated sterile solution of dithiothreitol (Cleland's reagent), used to liquefy sputum. Prepare a 1:10 dilution with sterile distilled water and use within 24 h.*

4. Add an equal volume of Zephiran-TSP to the diluted specimen (maximum of 10 ml to 10 ml sputum). Vortex thoroughly for approximately 30 s and allow the specimen to stand for 20 min.

5. Add 30 ml buffer. Vortex. Centrifuge at 1800 to 2400 × g for 20 min.

6. Decant to dryness, add 40 ml buffer, and vortex for 30 s to resuspend the sediment.

7. Centrifuge for 15 min as above, decant the supernatant, and add 1 to 2 ml phosphate buffer to the sediment. Resuspend by vortexing.

8. Prepare slides and inoculate media.

Quality control

See Procedure 41.1.

Urine specimens should be divided into a maximum of four 50 ml centrifuge tubes and centrifuged at 3600 × g for 30 minutes. The supernatant should be decanted, leaving approximately 2 ml of sediment in each tube. The tubes are vortexed to suspend the sediments and sediments are combined. If necessary, distilled water can be added to make the volume up to 10 ml. This urine concentrate is then treated as for sputum or with the sputolysin–oxalic acid method.

Feces are usually submitted for isolation of *M. avium* complex. One or two grams of formed stool or 5 ml of liquid stool is transferred to a 50-ml centrifuge tube and sterile, filtered distilled water is added to make the volume up to 10 ml. The suspension is vortexed thoroughly. The specimen is then filtered through gauze to remove particles. Add 10 ml NALC-NaOH to the suspension and allow to stand at room temperature for 45 to 60 minutes. Then add 25 ml phosphate buffer, mix thoroughly, and centrifuge for 20 minutes. The supernatant should be decanted and the sediment used to prepare slides and inoculate media.

Swabs and small pieces of bandage from pus and

PROCEDURE 41.5

Sputolysin–Oxalic Acid Method for Decontamination and Concentration

Principle

Oxalic acid provides an acid environment that is inhibitory to certain gram-negative rods, such as *Pseudomonas* and *Proteus*, which are difficult to remove from specimens without affecting recovery of mycobacteria.

Method

1. Prepare reagents as follows:

Sputolysin (Calbiochem)	1:10 dilution in distilled water
Oxalic acid	2.5% aqueous solution
Phosphate buffer (pH 7.0)	

2. Add an equal volume of Sputolysin to a maximum of 10 ml of sputum in a 50-ml conical centrifuge tube. Tighten the screw-cap and vortex thoroughly for 30 s. Allow to stand for 5 min.
3. Add an equal volume of 2.5% oxalic acid. Vortex thoroughly and allow to stand for 20 min.
4. Centrifuge at 3600 × g for 20 min and decant to dryness.
5. Add 40 ml phosphate buffer, resuspend the sediment, and centrifuge again for 15 min.
6. Decant the supernatant, add 1 to 2 ml phosphate buffer to the sediment, and vortex to thoroughly resuspend the sediment.
7. Prepare slides and inoculate media.

Quality control

See Procedure 41.1.

---

wound aspirates should be transferred to a sterile 50-ml centrifuge tube with 10 ml sterile, filtered distilled water. The specimen should be vortexed vigorously and allowed to stand for 20 minutes. The swab or bandage is removed and the resulting suspension is processed as for sputum.

Large pieces of tissue thought to be contaminated should be finely minced using a sterile scalpel and scissors. This material is transferred to a mortar and pestle for grinding or to a 50-ml centrifuge tube containing 6 to 8 glass beads. The tube is vortexed vigorously and allowed to stand for 20 to 30 minutes to permit the aerosol to settle. Alternatively, a Stomacher instrument can be used to homogenize tissue. Homogenate is poured through sterile gauze into a 50-ml centrifuge tube. An equal volume of NALC-NaOH is added; the tube is mixed vigorously and allowed to stand for 20 minutes. Then 25 ml phosphate buffer is added; the tube is mixed thoroughly and centrifuged at 3600 × g for 20 minutes. The supernatant is decanted and the sediment is suspended in 1 to 2 ml buffer and used to prepare slides and inoculate media. If the tissue is collected aseptically and not thought to be contaminated, it may be processed without treatment with NALC-NaOH.

Tissue specimens too small to be homogenized should be vortexed in 2 ml of buffer in a 50 ml centrifuge tube with 6 to 8 glass beads. The suspension should stand until aerosol settles after mixing. The volume is brought up to 10 ml with sterile, filtered distilled water and the decontamination process is continued as described for sputum.

41.4.b. Specimens that do not require decontamination. Processing a variety of clinical specimens that do not routinely require decontamination for acid-fast culture is described here. However, should such a specimen initially appear contaminated because of color, cloudiness, or foul odor, perform a Gram stain or acid-fast stain to detect bacteria other than acid-fast bacilli. Specimens found to be contaminated should be processed as in Section 41.4.a.

Cerebrospinal fluid should be handled aseptically and centrifuged for 30 minutes at 3600 × g to concentrate the bacteria. The supernatant is decanted and the sediment is vortexed thoroughly before preparing the smear and inoculating media. If insufficient quantity of spinal fluid is received, the specimen should be used directly for smear and culture. Because recovery of acid-fast bacilli from cerebrospinal fluid is difficult, additional solid and liquid media should be inoculated if material is available.

Pleural fluid should be collected in sterile anticoagulant (1 mg/ml ethylenediaminetetraacetic acid [EDTA] or 0.1 mg/ml heparin). If the fluid becomes clotted, it should be liquefied with an equal volume of Sputolysin and vigorous mixing. To lower the specific gravity and density of pleural fluid, transfer 20 ml to a sterile 50 ml centrifuge tube and dilute the specimen by filling the tube with distilled water. Invert several times to mix the suspension and centrifuge at 3600 $\times$ *g* for 30 minutes. The supernatant should be removed and the sediment should be resuspended for smear and culture.

Joint fluid and other sterile exudates can be handled aseptically and inoculated directly to media. Bone marrow aspirates may be injected into DuPont Pediatric Isolator tubes, which help to prevent clotting, and the specimen can be removed with a needle and syringe for preparation of smears and cultures. Alternatively, these specimens are either inoculated directly to media or, if clotted, treated with Sputolysin or glass beads and distilled water before concentration.

Several media have been described for recovery of acid-fast bacilli from blood, including trypticase soy broth, brain-heart infusion broth (fungal medium), 7H11-brain heart infusion biphasic medium, Ficoll-Hypaque isolation of white cell component, and the lysis-centrifugation system. In all patients with AIDS and other immune deficiencies, blood is the specimen of choice for detection of *M. avium* complex.[4,12,42]

41.5. Culture Media and Inoculation Methods

41.5.a. Conventional culture media. The following solid media are recommended because of the development of characteristic, reproducible colonial morphology, good growth from small inocula, and a low rate of contamination. Media in one ounce prescription bottles are preferred to screw-cap tubes for safety reasons described in Section 41.2.a. They also provide a larger surface area for examination of growth and contamination. A minimum of three bottles of at least two different media should be used for each specimen (media are all available from commercial sources). In addition, all aseptically collected specimens from normally sterile sites should be inoculated into 7H9 broth. If the Bactec system is being used (described in Section 41.5.b), one bottle of egg medium may be deleted. All specimens must be processed appropriately prior to inoculation. It is imperative to inoculate test organisms to commercially available products for quality control.

Wallenstein's medium, composed of egg yolk, 2.5% glycerin, malachite green, and water, is an excellent medium for the recovery of MOTT, par-

ticularly *M. avium* complex. Löwenstein-Jensen (L-J) medium supplemented with ribonucleic acid and L-J medium supplemented with pyruvic acid are two other preferred media (see box). The high rate of contamination and poor recovery of *M. tuberculosis* negate the value of 7H10 or 7H11 as a primary isolation medium. It has no equal, however, for the study of colony morphology, as a selective medium with antibiotics, or as a medium for susceptibility testing.

Cultures are incubated at 35° C in the dark in an atmosphere of 5% to 10% CO_2 and high humidity. A second set of cultures of material from skin lesions suspected of harboring *M. marinum* are incubated at room temperature (or at 30° C if such an incubator is available). Bottle caps should be slightly loose during the first 2 to 3 weeks to allow for evaporation of excess fluids and the entry of CO_2. Caps should be tightened when the surface of the medium is dry, but should be loosened and tightened weekly to allow for gas exchange.

Cultures are examined weekly for growth. Contaminated cultures are discarded and reported as "contaminated, unable to detect presence of mycobacteria," and repeat specimens are requested. If sediment is still available, it may be recultured after

---

Suggested Media for Cultivation of Mycobacteria from Clinical Specimens*

Solid

Agar-based
1. Middlebrook 7H10
2. Middlebrook 7H11
3. Mitchison's selective 7H11

Egg-based
1. Wallenstein
2. Löwenstein-Jensen (L-J) with RNA
3. L-J with pyruvic acid

Liquid

1. Bactec 12B medium
2. Middlebrook 7H9 Broth

*For optimal recovery of mycobacteria, a combination of liquid medium (Bactec) and a minimum of two solid media is recommended.

enhanced decontamination or by inoculating the sediment to a more selective medium. Most isolates will appear between 3 and 6 weeks; a few isolates will appear after 7 or 8 weeks of incubation. When growth appears, the rate of growth, pigmentation, and colony morphology are recorded. After 8 weeks of incubation, negative cultures (those showing no growth) from smear-negative specimens are reported, and the cultures are discarded.

41.5.b. Radiometric culture system. The Bactec system, a recent development for the rapid detection of mycobacteria based on radiometric monitoring, has added a new dimension to diagnostic mycobacteriology. It has reduced the turnaround time for isolation of acid-fast bacilli to approximately 10 days, compared with 17 days for conventional media.[23,29]

The Bactec system is based on the principle that the organisms multiply in the broth and metabolize ^{14}C-containing palmitic acid, producing radioactively labeled $^{14}CO_2$ in the atmosphere that collects above the broth in the bottle. The Bactec instrument withdraws this CO_2-containing atmosphere and measures the amount of radioactivity present. Those bottles that yield a radioactive index, called a "growth index," greater than 10 are considered to be positive.

The Bactec culture process may be described briefly as follows: after the specimen has been digested and decontaminated using NALC and NaOH, the sediment is resuspended in sterile phosphate buffer to a total volume of approximately 2 ml. A small quantity (0.4 to 0.5 ml) of this suspension is injected into a Bactec bottle containing 7H12 medium with added antimicrobial agents. The rest of the sediment is used for conventional smear and culture. Cultures are incubated as above and Bactec bottles are incubated in air at 37° C. The bottles are tested for $^{14}CO_2$ production three times weekly for 6 weeks. Bottles that register a growth index greater than 10 are subcultured to media and smeared for acid fast stain. Broth from bottles registering a growth index greater than 50 are split into two samples, each of which is injected into a fresh bottle of medium. A 5-µg quantity of p-nitro-α-acetylamino-β-hydroxypropiophenone (NAP) is added to one of the bottles, and they are both reincubated. These two bottles are then tested on the Bactec daily for 4 days. An increase in the growth index in the unaltered control bottle without a corresponding increase of the growth index in the bottle containing NAP indicates the presence of *M. tuberculosis* or

M. bovis, both of which are susceptible to NAP. NAP does not inhibit growth of MOTT. An additional medium containing TCH (thiophene-2-carboxylate hydrazide), to which only *M. bovis* is susceptible, can be used to separate *M. tuberculosis* and *M. bovis*. Definitive identification of mycobacteria other than the tuberculosis complex requires biochemical testing of isolated colonies, of course.

The Bactec system has also been adapted for performance of mycobacterial susceptibility testing. Sediments from acid-fast, smear-positive specimens are inoculated into Bactec bottles containing special Middlebrook 7H12 with antimicrobial agents and a control broth without antimicrobial agents. The bottles are incubated for a maximum of 2 weeks, and the growth index readings from the antibiotic-containing bottles are compared with those of the control. Once the growth index in the control bottle reaches 20, the test can be reported. A change in the growth index in the antibiotic media that is equal to or greater than that in the control medium indicates resistance, and a greater change in the control indicates susceptibility. Results of trials of this method compared with the conventional direct susceptibility testing method indicate that the Bactec agreed very well with conventional results, especially when large numbers of organisms were present in the sediment. The radiometric mycobacterial culturing and susceptibility testing systems are continuously improving. At this time, conventional media should be inoculated in addition to Bactec media for detection and isolation of mycobacteria.

41.6. Microscopic Examination

The mycobacteria possess cell walls that contain mycolic acids, long-chain multiply cross-linked fatty acids. These long-chain mycolic acids probably serve to complex basic dyes, contributing to the characteristic of "acid-fastness" that distinguishes them from other bacteria. Mycobacteria are not the only group with this unique feature. Species of *Nocardia* and *Rhodococcus* are also partially acid-fast; *Legionella micdadei*, the causative agent of Pittsburgh pneumonia, is partially acid-fast in tissue. Cysts of the genera *Cryptosporidium* and *Isospora* are distinctly acid-fast. The mycolic acids and lipids in the mycobacterial cell wall probably account for the unusual resistance of these organisms to the effects of drying and harsh decontaminating agents, as well as for acid-fastness.

PROCEDURE 41.6

Preparation of Smears for Acid-fast Stain from Direct or Concentrated Specimens

Method

1. Vortex concentrated sediment, unconcentrated sputum, other purulent material, or stool. Aspirate 0.1 to 0.2 ml into a Pasteur pipette and place 2 to 3 drops on the slide. Place the end of the pipette or a sterile applicator stick parallel to the slide and slowly spread the liquid uniformly to make a thin smear.

2. For cerebrospinal fluid sediment, vortex thoroughly and apply to the slide in heaped drops. A heaped drop is allowed to air dry, and a second application of sediment is placed on the same spot and allowed to dry. A minimum of three layers, applied to the same 1-cm diameter circle, should facilitate detection of small numbers of bacilli.

3. Fix the smear at 80° C for 15 min on an electric hot plate.
   Note: *Survival of mycobacteria at this temperature has been reported; handle all specimens with proper precautions.*

4. Stain slides by Ziehl-Neelsen or fluorochrome stain.

Modified from Allen, J. 1981. J. Clin. Pathol. 34:719.

When Gram-stained, mycobacteria usually appear as slender, poorly stained, beaded gram-positive bacilli; sometimes they appear as "gram-neutral" or "gram-ghosts" by failing to take up either crystal violet or safranin. It has been shown that acid-fastness is affected by age of colonies, media on which growth occurs, and ultraviolet light. Rapid-growing species appear to be acid-fast-variable. Three types of staining procedures are used in the laboratory for rapid detection and confirmation of acid-fast bacilli; fluorochrome, Ziehl-Neelsen, and Kinyoun. Smears for all methods are prepared in the same way (Procedure 41.6).

The visualization of acid-fast bacilli in sputum or other clinical material should be considered only presumptive evidence of tuberculosis, since stain does not specifically identify *M. tuberculosis*. The report form should indicate this. For example, *M. gordonae*, a nonpathogenic scotochromogen commonly found in tap water, has been a problem when tap water or deionized water has been used in the preparation of smears or even when patients have rinsed their mouths with tap water prior to the use of aerosolized saline solution for inducing sputum. However, the incidence of false-positive smears is very low when good quality control is maintained.

41.6.a. Fluorochrome stain. This is the screening procedure recommended for those laboratories that possess a fluorescent (ultraviolet) microscope (Procedure 41.7). This stain is more sensitive than the conventional carbolfuchsin stains because the fluorescent bacilli stand out brightly against the background; the smear can be initially examined at lower magnifications (250× to 400×), and therefore more fields can be visualized in a short period of time.[5] In addition, a positive fluorescent smear may be restained by the conventional Ziehl-Neelsen or Kinyoun procedure, thereby saving the time needed to make a fresh smear. Screening of specimens with rhodamine or rhodamine-auramine will result in a higher yield of positive smears and will substantially reduce the amount of time needed for examining smears. One drawback associated with the fluorochrome stains is that most strains of rapid growers may not appear fluorescent with these reagents. It is recommended that all negative fluorescent smears be confirmed with Ziehl-Neelsen stain; at least 100 fields should be examined before being reported as negative. It is important to wipe the immersion oil from the objective lens after examining a positive smear, since stained bacilli can float off the slide into the oil and may possibly contribute to a false-positive reading for the next smear examined.

41.6.b. Ziehl-Neelsen stain. This classic carbolfuchsin stain requires heating the slide for better penetration of stain within the mycobacterial cell wall; hence it is also known as the "hot stain" procedure (Procedure 41.8).[6] At least 100 oil immersion fields should be examined before reporting the smear as negative.

41.6.c. Kinyoun stain. Procedure 41.9 is the method of choice for small laboratories. The method is similar to the Ziehl-Neelsen stain but without heat; hence the term "cold stain."[15]

41.6.d. Interpretation and reporting of the smear. Smears should be examined carefully by scanning at least 100 fields before reporting a smear as "nega-

PROCEDURE 41.7

Auramine-Rhodamine Fluorochrome Stain

Principle

The fluorochrome dyes used in this stain complex to the mycolic acids in acid-fast cell walls. Detection of fluorescing cells is enhanced by the brightness against a dark background.

Method

1. Heat-fix slides at 80° C for at least 15 min.
2. Flood slides with auramine-rhodamine reagent (Appendix B) and allow to stain for 15 to 20 min at room temperature.
3. Rinse with deionized water and tilt slide to drain.
4. Decolorize with acid alcohol (70% ethanol and 0.5% hydrochloric acid) for 2 to 3 min.
5. Rinse with deionized water and tilt slide to drain.
6. Flood slides with 0.5% potassium permanganate for 2 to 4 min.
7. Rinse with deionized water and air dry.
8. Examine under low power (250×) for fluorescence.
9. Confirm all positive results by Ziehl-Neelsen stain.

Quality control

A series of slides made from a 7H9 suspension of acid-fast organisms, such as *M. tuberculosis* H37Rv, and gram-positive, non-acid-fast organisms, such as *Staphylococcus aureus*, should be prepared in advance and stored in a closed box. One slide from each control set should be heat-fixed and stained along with the specimen slides each time any slides are stained. The mycobacterial slide should display characteristic fluorescence and cell morphology when examined microscopically; the *E. coli* should not be visible on the slides.

PROCEDURE 41.8

Ziehl-Neelsen Acid-fast Stain

Principle

Heating the slide allows greater penetration of carbolfuchsin into the cell wall. Mycolic acids and waxes complex the basic dye, which then fails to wash out with mild acid decolorization.

Method

1. Heat-fix slides on a hot plate (80-85° C for at least 15 min.
2. Flood smear with carbolfuchsin stain reagent (Appendix B) and steam the slides gently for 1 min. This can be accomplished by flaming from below the rack with a gas burner, or by staining the slides directly on a special hot plate. Do not permit the slides to boil or dry out.
3. Allow the stain to remain on the slides for an additional 4–5 min without heat.
4. Rinse with deionized water and tilt slides to drain.
5. Decolorize with acid alcohol (95% ethanol and 3.0% hydrochloric acid) for 3 min.
6. Rinse slides with deionized water and tilt to drain.
7. Flood slides with methylene blue reagent for 1 min.
8. Rinse with deionized water and allow to air dry.
9. Examine under oil immersion (1000×) for presence of acid-fast bacilli.

Quality control

Prepare control slides in advance, as detailed in Procedure 41.7. Stain one control slide for each slide when slides are stained. Bacilli on the positive smear should display numerous red, small, slightly curved, possibly beaded and tapered ends against a blue background (See Figure 7.5, Chapter 7). The negative smear should display numerous blue (non-acid-fast) bacilli.

PROCEDURE 41.9

Kinyoun Stain

Principle

By increasing the concentration of basic fuchsin and phenol, the need for heating the slide is avoided.

Method

1. Heat-fix slides on an 85° C hot plate for at least 15 min.
2. Flood slides with Kinyoun's carbolfuchsin reagent (Appendix B) and allow to stain for 5 min at room temperature.
3. Rinse with deionized water and tilt slide to drain.
4. Decolorize with acid-alcohol for 3 min and rinse again with deionized water.
5. Redecolorize with acid-alcohol for 1 to 2 min or until no more red color runs from the smear.
6. Rinse with deionized water and drain standing water from slide surface by tipping slide.
7. Flood slide with methylene blue counterstain and allow to stain for 4 min.
8. Rinse with distilled water and allow to air dry.
9. Examine under high dry (400×) magnification, and confirm acid-fast structures under oil immersion (1000×).

Quality control

Follow the same protocol as for Procedure 41.8.

Modified from Kinyoun. 1915.

Table 41.4

Enumeration of Acid-fast Bacilli in Smears

NO. OF ORGANISMS SEEN	REPORT
1-2 per entire smear specimen	Negative; request another
3-9 per entire smear	Rare (1+)
10 or more per entire smear	Few (2+)
1 or more per oil immersion field	Numerous (3+)

When large numbers of typical acid-fast bacilli are seen, it is reasonable to assume that they are *M. tuberculosis*. When atypical rods are seen, they may represent other pathogenic or nonpathogenic mycobacteria or other partially acid-fast organisms. It is desirable to report the number of acid-fast bacilli seen; the criteria recommended by the American Lung Association (Table 41.4) may be used.

When only one or two acid-fast bacilli are seen on the entire smear, it is recommended that they not be reported until confirmation is obtained by examining other smears from the same or another specimen. One study involving sputum and gastric contents found that when more than six acid-fast organisms were seen per high-power field (400×), pathogenic mycobacteria were always recovered from the culture.

41.6.e. Staining material other than sputum and gastric lavages. When repeated specimens of cerebrospinal fluid are examined, a high percentage of specimens from patients with disease will reveal acid-fast bacilli by microscopy or culture. Microscopy is particularly important because of the need to initiate therapy as soon as possible when tuberculous meningitis is suspected. Either the fluorochrome or Ziehl-Neelsen stain can be used for detecting acid-fast bacilli in tissues. The tissue sections should be deparaffinized in three changes of xylene and hydrated before staining with rhodamine-auramine. Fluorochrome stains are ideal for tissue sections in which acid-fast bacilli are usually found in clusters. Fluorochrome positive slides may be restained with Ziehl-Neelsen.

41.6.f. Additional considerations. Species of *Nocardia* and *Rhodococcus* are partially acid-fast; therefore, less stringent destaining (weaker acid or shorter duration or both) is used to detect these organisms. Red-green color-blind people can use Spengler's method to visualize acid-fast bacilli in 10% formalin-fixed smears or tissue sections. With this method,

tive." Typical acid-fast bacilli appear purple to red, slightly curved, short or long rods (2 to 8 μm) they may also appear beaded or banded (*M. kansasii*). For some nontuberculous species, such as *M. avium* complex, they appear pleomorphic, usually coccoid.

Results of microscopic examination should be reported "positive for acid-fast bacilli" or "no acid-fast bacilli found." Positive findings should be based only on typical forms, but atypical cells should be noted.

acid-fast bacilli stain black and non-acid-fast organisms appear yellowish.

The examination of stained smears is considered the least sensitive of the diagnostic methods for tuberculosis; *cultures should be performed on all specimens*. Because of its simplicity and speed, however, the stained smear is an important and useful test, particularly for the detection of smear-positive patients ("infectious reservoirs"), who are the greatest risk to others in their environment.

41.7. Macroscopic Examination

The preliminary identification of mycobacterial isolates depends on their rate of growth, colony morphology, colony texture, and pigmentation. The identification procedures are modified from material published by George Kubica and the Bacteriology Training Section of the Centers for Disease Control (CDC).[17] Quality control organisms should be tested along with unknowns, as listed in Table 41.5. The commonly used quality control organisms can be maintained in broth at room temperature and transferred monthly. In this way they will always be available for inoculation to test media along with suspensions of the unknown mycobacteria being tested.

The first test that must always be performed on colonies growing on mycobacterial media is an acid fast stain to confirm that the colonies are indeed mycobacteria. At this point, inoculate several colonies of the organism to 5 ml of Middlebrook 7H9 broth (available from several commercial suppliers) and incubate the broth at 35° C for 5 to 7 days with daily agitation (with the cap tightened shut) to enhance growth. If there is sufficient growth on the original Löwenstein-Jensen (L-J) medium, the L-J slant can be used for performance of the niacin test, as outlined in Section 41.8.a. The broth subculture can be used for inoculation of all test media, including biochemical tests as well as pigmentation and growth rate determinations (Procedure 41.10). It is up to the microbiologist to determine whether all tests are inoculated initially at the same time or whether the results of growth rate and pigment production are determined before additional tests are set up. Some observations about colony morphology and permissive incubation temperatures of mycobacteria that may be found in clinical specimens are listed in Table 41.6

The rate of growth is an important criterion for determining the initial category of an isolate. Rapid growers will usually produce colonies within 3 to 4 days after subculture. Even a rapid grower, however, may take longer than 7 days to initially produce colonies because of inhibition by the harsh decontaminating procedure. The dilution of the organism used to assess growth rate is critical. Even slow-growing mycobacteria will appear to produce colonies in less than 7 days if the inoculum is too heavy. One organism particularly likely to exhibit false-positive rapid growth is *M. flavescens*. This species therefore serves as an excellent quality control organism for this procedure.

Species of mycobacteria synthesize carotenoids in varying amounts; they are categorized into three groups based on productions of these pigments (Procedure 41.10). Photochromogens produce the yellow pigment when exposed to light (Figure 41.3). To achieve optimum photochromogenicity, the colonies should be young, actively metabolizing, isolated, and well aerated. While some species, such as *M. kansasii*, turn yellow after a few hours of light exposure, others, such as *M. simiae*, may take a prolonged exposure to light. Scotochromogens produce pigmented colonies even in the absence of light and colonies often become darker with prolonged exposure to light. One member of this group, *M. szulgai*, is peculiar in that it is a scotochromogen at 37° C and nonpigmented when grown at 25° C. For this reason, all pigmented colonies should be subcultured to test for photoactivated pigment at both 37° C and 25° C. Nonchromogens are not affected by light. Although commonly nonpigmented, some strains of *M. avium* complex isolated from AIDS patients may exhibit differential colony pigmentation.

41.8. Biochemical Testing

Once an organism has been identified on the basis of acid-fast morphology, growth rate, and pigment production, definitive identification is based on a battery of biochemical tests.[13,34] Many of the biochemical tests are qualitative and based on color reactions. Good growth of the isolate is an important prerequisite for performing these tests.[30] A list of commonly used biochemical tests and the strains suggested for quality control testing are summarized in Table 41.5; biochemical profiles of individual species and species groups are summarized in Tables 41.6 to 41.10.

41.8.a. Niacin test. Niacin or nicotinic acid plays an important role in the oxidation-reduction reac-

Table 41.5
Controls and Media Used and Duration of Tests

NO.	BIOCHEMICAL TEST	CONTROL ORGANISMS		RESULT		MEDIUM USED AND AMOUNT	DURATION OF TEST	REMARKS
		POSITIVE	NEGATIVE	POSITIVE	NEGATIVE			
1	Niacin	*M. tuberculosis*	*M. avium*	Yellow	No change of color	0.5 ml DH_2O	30 min	Room temperature
2	Nitrate	*M. tuberculosis* *M. kansasii*	*M. avium*	Pink or red	No change of color	0.3 ml 7H9	2 h	37° C bath
3	Urease	*M. tuberculosis*	*M. avium*	Pink or red	No change of color	0.5 ml DH_2O	2 h	37° C bath
4	68° C Catalase	*M. avium*	*M. tuberculosis*	Bubbles	No bubbles	0.5 ml phosphate buffer [pH 7]	30 min	68° C bath
5	S.Q. Catalase	*M. kansasii*	*M. avium*	>45 mm	≤40 mm	Commercial medium	14 d	37° C incubator [with CO_2]
6	Tween 80	*M. kansasii*	*M. tuberculosis*	Pink or red	No change of color	1 ml DH_2O	5 d or 10 d	37° C incubator [without CO_2]
7	Tellurite	*M. avium*	*M. tubeculosis*	Smooth fine black precipitate (smokelike action)	Gray clumps (no smokelike action)	Middlebrook 7H9 broth	7 + 3 d	37° C incuabor [with CO_2]
8	Arylsulfatase	*M. fortuitum*	Medium	Pink or red	No change of color	Wayne's arylsulfatase medium	3 d	37° C incubator [without CO_2]
9	5% NaCl	*M. fortuitum*	*M. gordonae*	Substantial growth	Little or no growth	Commercial slant	28 d	37° C incubator [with CO_2]
10	(TCH)	*M. bovis*	*M. tuberculosis*	No growth	Growth	(TCH) flat and L–J	8 wk	37° C incubator [with CO_2]

From Berlin, O.G.W., and Martin, W.J. 1980. Importance of nitrate test in the identification of mycobacteria. Clin. Microbiol. Newsletter. 2:4.

PROCEDURE 41.10

Determination of Pigment Production and Growth Rate

Principle

Certain mycobacteria produce pigmented chemicals (carotenoids), either dependently or independently of exposure to light. This characteristic, in addition to their doubling time under standard conditions, is useful for initial identification.

Method

1. After the broth culture has incubated for 5 to 7 days, adjust the turbidity to that of a McFarland 0.5 standard.
2. Dilute the broth (McFarland 0.5 turbidity) 10^{-4}.
3. Inoculate 0.1 ml of the diluted broth to each of three tubes of Löwenstein-Jensen agar. Completely wrap two of the tubes in aluminum foil so as to block all light. If the isolate was obtained from a skin lesion, or the initial colony was yellow-pigmented (possible *M. szulgai*), six tubes should be inoculated. The second set of tubes, two of them also wrapped with aluminum foil, is incubated at 30° C, or at room temperature if a 30° C incubator is not available.
4. Examine the cultures after 5 and 7 days for the appearance of grossly visible colonies. Examine again at intervals of 3 days. Interpretation:

Rapid growers produce visible colonies in less than 7 days; slow growers require more than 7 days.

5. When colonies are mature, expose the growth from a foil-wrapped tube to a bright light, such as a desk lamp, for 2 h. The cap must be loose during exposure, since pigment production is an oxygen-dependent reaction.[38] The tube is rewrapped and returned to the incubator, and the cap is left loose.
6. The three tubes are examined 24 and 48 h after light exposure. For tubes incubating at 30° C, pigment may require 72 h for development.
7. Results are interpreted as shown in Figure 41.3.

Quality control

Inoculate suspensions of known organisms to 7H9 broths weekly and test these cultures along with unknowns each time the pigment and growth rate tests are performed. A typical photochromogen control is *M. kansasii*, a typical scotochromogen control is *M. flavescens*, and a typical nonphotochromogen control is *M. avium* complex. The *M. flavescens* can also serve as a quality control organism for rapid growth rate.

---

tions that occur during mycobacterial metabolism. While all species produce nicotinic acid, *M. tuberculosis* accumulates the largest amount. *M. simiae* and some strains of *M. chelonae* also produce niacin. Niacin therefore accumulates in the medium in which these organisms are growing. A positive niacin test is preliminary evidence that an organism that exhibits a buff-colored, slow-growing, rough colony may be *M. tuberculosis*. This test is not sufficient, however, for confirmation of the identification. If sufficient growth is present on the initial L-J slant (the egg-base medium enhances accumulation of free

niacin), a niacin test can be performed immediately.[16] If growth on the initial culture was scanty, the subculture used for growth rate determination can be used. If this culture yields only rare colonies, the colonies should be spread around with a sterile cotton swab (after the growth rate has been determined) to distribute the inoculum over the entire slant, which is then reincubated until light growth over the surface of the medium is visible. For reliable results, the niacin test should be performed only from cultures on L-J that are at least 3 weeks old and show at least 50 colonies.

Text continued on p. 623.

Table 41.6
Distinctive Properties of Cultivable Mycobacteria Encountered in Clinical Specimens[a]

GROUP/ COMPLEX[b]	SPECIES	CLINICAL SIGNIFICANCE[c]	GROWTH RATE[d] AT				USUAL COLONY MORPHOLOGY[e]	PIGMENTATION[f]	NIACIN	SUSCEPTIBILITY TO TCH[g] (5 µg/ml)	NITRATE REDUCTION
			45° C	37° C	31° C	24° C					
TB	M. tuberculosis	1	−	S	S	−	R	N	+	−	+
	M. bovis	1	−	S		−	Rt	N	−	+	−
	M. africanum	1	−	S		−	R	N	−	V	−
	M. ulcerans	1	−	−	S	−	R	N	−	−	−
Photochromogens	M. marinum	2		∓	M	M	S/SR	P	∓	−	
	M. kansasii	2		S	S	S	SR/S	P	−	−	+
	M. simiae	3−2	−	S			S	P	+	−	−
	M. asiaticum	3—2	−	S		S		P	−	−	−
Scotochromogens	M. scrofulaceum	3−2		S	S	S	S	S	−	−	−
	M. szulgai	1		S	S	S	S or R	S/P	−	−	+
	M. gordonae	4		S		S	S	S	−	−	−
	M. flavescens	4		M		M	S	S[j]	−	−	+
	M. xenopi	3	S	S			Sf	S	−	−	−
M. avium (complex)	M. avium	2	V	S		±	St/R	N	−	−	−
	M. intracellulare	2	V	S		±	St/R	N	−	−	−
	M. gastri	4		S		S	S/SR/R	N	−	−	−
	M. malmoense	1		S	S	S	S	N	−	−	−
	M. haemophilum	1	−	−	S[k]	S	R	N	−	−	−
	M. shimoidei	2	−	S	−		R	N	−	−	−
M. terrae (complex)	M. terrae	4		S		S	SR	N	−	−	+
	M. triviale	4		M		S	R	N	−	−	+
	M. nonchromogenicum	4		S		S	SR	N	−	−	+
M. fortuitum	M. fortuitum	4-3	−	R		R	Sf/Rf	N	−	−	+
	M. chelonae	4-3	−	R		R	S/R	N	V	−	−
	M. phlei	4	R	R		R	R	S			+
	M. smegmatis	4	R	R		R	R/S	N			+
	M. vaccae	4		R		R	S	S			+

[a] Plus and minus signs indicate the presence or absence, respectively, of the feature; blank spaces indicate either that the information is not currently available or that the property is unimportant. V, Variable; ±, usually present; ∓, usually absent.

[b] For most clinical laboratories, designation to the complex is usually sufficient.

[c] Potential clinical significance: 1, present only as pathogens; 2, present usually as pathogens; 3, present commonly as nonpathogens; 4, present usually as nonpathogens.

[d] S, Slow; M, moderate; R, rapid.

[e] R, Rough, S, smooth; SR, intermediate in roughness; t, thin or transparent; f, filamentous extensions.

SEMIQUANTITATIVE CATALASE (>45 mm)	68° C CATALASE	TWEEN HYDROLYSIS, 5 DAYS	TELLURITE REDUCTION	TOLERANCE TO 5% NaCl	IRON UPTAKE	ARYLSULFATASE, 3 DAYS	GROWTH ON MacCONKEY AGAR	UREASE	PYRAZINAMIDASE, 4 DAYS
−	−	−[h]	∓	−	−	−	−	+	+
−	−	−	∓	−	−	−	−	+	−
−	−	−	−	−	−	−	−	+	−
−	+	−		−		−		−	−
−	−	+	∓	−	−	∓[i]	−	+	+
+	+	+	∓	−	−	−	−	+	−
+	+	−	+	−	−	−	−	+	+
+	+	+	−	−	−	−	−	−	+
+	+	−	∓	−	−	V	−	+	±
+	+	∓[h]	±	−	−	V	−	+	+
+	+	+	−	−	−	V	−	−	∓
+	+	+	∓	+	−	−	−	+	+
−	+	−	∓	−	−	+	−	−	V
−	±	−	+	−	−	−	∓	−	+
−	±	−	+	−	−	−	∓	−	+
−	−	+	∓	−	−	−	−	+	−
−	±	+	+	−	−	−		V	+
−	−	−	−	−	−	−	−	−	+
−	+			−				−	+
+	+	+	−	−	−	−	V	−	V
+	+	+	−	+	−	∓	−	−	V
+	+	+	−	−	−	−	V	−	V
+	+	V	+	+	+	+	+	+	+
+	V	V	+	V[l]	−	+	+	+	+
+	+	+	+	+	+	−	−		
+	+	+	+	+	+	−	−		
+	+	+	+	V	+	−	−		

[f]P, Photochromogenic; S, scotochromogenic; N, nonphotochromogenic. NOTE: *M. szulgai* is scotochromogenic at 37° C and photochromogenic at 25° C.

[g]TCH, Thiophene-2-carboxylic acid hydrazide.

[h]Tween hydrolysis may be + at 10 days.

[i]Arylsulfatase, 14 days, is +.

[j]Young cultures may be nonchromogenic or possess only pale pigment which may intensify with age.

[k]Requires hemin as a growth factor.

[l]*M. chelonae* subsp. *chelonae* is −, *M. chelonae* subsp. *abscessus* is +.

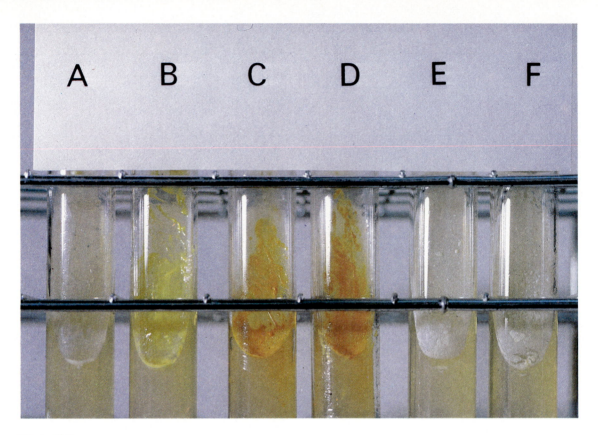

Figure 41.3

Initial grouping of mycobacteria based on pigment production before and after exposure to light. In one test system, subcultures of each isolate are grown on two agar slants. One tube is wrapped in aluminumm foil to prevent exposure of the organism to light, and the other tube is allowed light exposure. After sufficient growth is present, the wrapped tube is unwrapped, and the tubes are examined together. **Photochromogens** are unpigmented when grown in the dark (tube A) and develop pigment after light exposure (tube B). **Scotochromogens** are pigmented in the dark (tube C); the color does not intensify after exposure to light (tube D). **Nonphotochromogens** are nonpigmented when grown in the dark (tube E) and remain so even after light exposure (tube F).

Table 41.7

Differential Characteristics of Photochromogens

PROPERTY	*M. KANSASII*	*M. MARINUM*	*M. SIMIAE*	*M. ASIATICUM*
Rate of growth	S	S(30° C)	S	S
Colonial morphology	SM/R	SM/R	SM	SM
Pigmentation—dark	NC	NC	NC	NC
—light	Y	Y	Y	Y
Niacin	−	−	+	−
Nitrate reduction	+	−	−	−
Catalase S.Q. > 45 mm	+	−	+	+
Tween hydrolysis, 5-day	+	+	−	+
Urease	+	+	+	

S = slow; SM = smooth; R = rough; NC = nonchromogenic; Y = yellow.

Table 41.8
Differential Characteristics of Scotochromogens

PROPERTY	M. SCROFULACEUM	M. SZULGAI	M. GORDONAE	M. FLAVESCENS	M. XENOPI
Rate of growth	S	S	S	S	S
Colonial morphology	SM	SM/R	SM	SM/R	SM
Pigmentation—dark	OR	37° C, OR; 24° C, NC	OR	OR	OR
—light	OR	37° C, OR; 24° C, OR	OR	OR	OR
Nitrate reduction	−	+	−	+	−
Catalase, S.Q. > 45 mm	+	+	+	+	V
Tween hydrolysis, 5-day	−	Wk	+	+	−
Sodium chloride, 5%	−	−	−	+	−
Urease	+	+	V	+	−

S = slow; SM = smooth; R = rough; NC = nonchromogenic; OR = orange, Wk = weak; V = variable.

Table 41.9
Differential Characteristics of Nonpigmented Slow Growers

PROPERTY	M. AVIUM* COMPLEX	M. GASTRI	M. TERRAE COMPLEX	M. MALMOENSE	M. HAEMOPHILUM†
Rate of growth	S	S	S	S	S
Colonial morphology	SM	SM	SM/R	SM	SM
Pigmentation—dark	NC	NC	NC	NC	NC
—light	NC	NC	NC	NC	NC
Niacin	−	−	−	−	−
Nitrate reduction	−	−	+	−	−
Catalase S.Q. > 45 mm	−	−	+	−	−
Catalase 68° C	+	−	+	−	−
Tween hydrolysis 5-day	−	+	+	+	−
Arylsulfatase	−	−	−	−	−
Sodium chloride, 5%	−	−	V	−	
Urease	−	+	−	−	−

S = slow; SM = smooth; R = rough; NC = nonchromogenic.
*M. avium complex includes M. intracellulare.
†Growth between 25° and 30° C; requires hemin for growth.

Table 41.10
Differential Characteristics of Rapid Growers

PROPERTY	M. FORTUITUM*	M. CHELONAE; M. CHELONAE SUBSP. ABSCESSUS	M. SMEGMATIS‡
Rate of growth	Ra	Ra	Ra
Colonial morphology	SM/R	SM/R	SM/R
Pigmentation—dark	NC	NC	NC
—light	NC	NC	NC
Nitrate reduction	+	−	+
Tween hydrolysis, 5-day	V	−	+
Arylsulfatase	+	+	−
Sodium chloride, 5%	+	− / + †	+

Ra = rapid; SM = smooth; R = rough; NC = nonchromogenic; V = variable.
*M. fortuitum complex includes M. chelonae and M. chelonae subsp. abscessus.
†M. chelonae is −; M. chelonae subsp. abscessus is +.
‡Not clinically significant.

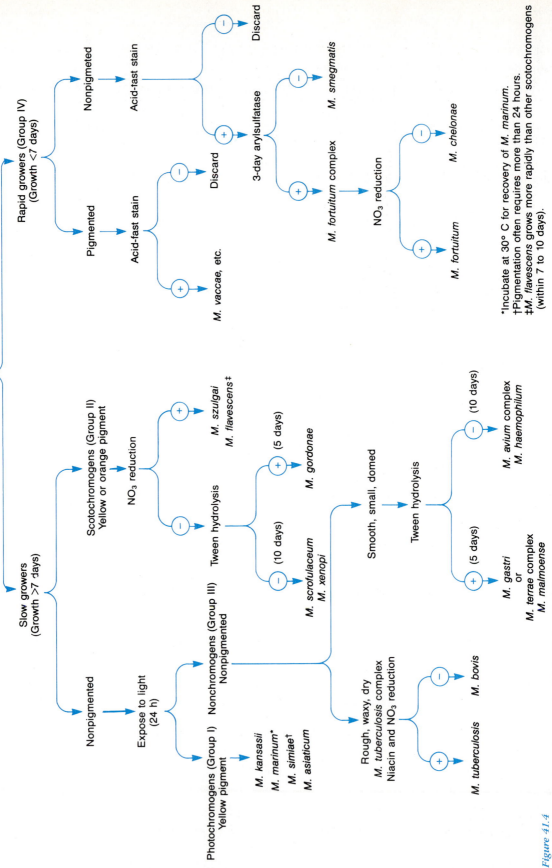

Figure 41.4

The identification of mycobacteria. See Tables 41-6 to 41-12 for additional confirmatory tests.

Classic tests for niacin involve cyanogen bromide, which is hazardous to use and presents disposal problems. For this reason, a method that utilizes reagent-impregnated paper strips should be used (Figure 41.5). The results are comparable and the procedure is simple (Procedure 41.11). Control organisms are inoculated at the same time as the test organisms, as listed in Table 41.5.

41.8.b. Nitrate reduction test.[36] Many species of mycobacteria are able to reduce nitrate to nitrite (Table 41.11).[1] The ability of acid-fast bacilli to reduce nitrate is influenced by age of the colonies, temperature, pH, and enzyme inhibitors. While rapid growers can be tested within 2 weeks, slow growers should be tested after 3 to 4 weeks of luxuriant growth. Commercially available nitrate strips yield acceptable results only with strongly nitrate

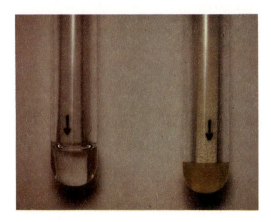

Figure 41.5

Niacin test performed with filter paper strips. The positive test *(right)* displays a yellow color and the negative result remains milky white or clear.

PROCEDURE 41.11

Niacin Test with Commercially Available Paper Strips (Available from Difco Laboratories)

Principle

The accumulation of niacin in the medium due to lack of an enzyme that converts niacin to another metabolite in the coenzyme pathway is characteristic for *M. tuberculosis* and a few other species. Niacin is measured by a colored end product.

Method

1. Add 1 ml sterile distilled water to the surface of the egg-based medium on which the colonies to be tested are growing.
2. Lay the tube horizontal, so that the fluid is in contact with the entire surface. With the pipette used to add the water, scratch or lightly poke through the surface of the agar; this allows niacin in the medium to dissolve in the water.
3. Allow the tube to sit for 15 to 30 min at room temperature. It can incubate longer to achieve a stronger reaction.
4. Remove 0.6 ml of the distilled water (which appears cloudy at this point) to a clean,

12 × 75 mm screw-cap or snap-top test tube. Insert a niacin test strip with the arrow down, following manufacturer's instructions.
5. Cap the tube tightly and incubate at room temperature, occasionally shaking the tube to mix the fluid with the reagent on the bottom of the strip.
6. After 20 min, observe the color of the liquid against a white background (Figure 41.5). Yellow liquid indicates a positive test. The color of the strip should not be considered when evaluating results. If the liquid is clear, the test is negative.
7. Discard the strip into alkaline disinfectant (10% NaOH) to neutralize the cyanogen bromide.
8. Negative tests may be repeated on a fresh 3- to 4-week-old subculture of the isolate.

Quality control

Test positive and negative control organisms (Table 41.5) with each performance of the test.

Table 41.11
Nitrate Reduction Test

GROUP	POSITIVE	NEGATIVE
Slow-growing nonchromogens	*M. tuberculosis*	*M. bovis* *M. simiae*
Slow-growing scotochromogens	*M. szulgai* (weak) *M. flavescens*	*M. scrofulaceum* *M. gordonae*
Rapid-growing nonchromogens	*M. fortuitum*	*M. chelonae*
Photochromogens	*M. kansasii*	*M. marinum* *M. asiaticum* *M. simiae*

positive organisms, such as *M. tuberculosis*. This test (Procedure 41.12) may be tried first because of its ease of performance. The *M. tuberculosis* positive control must be strongly positive in the strip test or the test results will be unreliable. If the paper strip test is negative or if the control test result is not strongly positive, the chemical procedure (Procedure 41.13) must be carried out, using strong and weakly positive controls. Steps and reagents used for performing the classic chemical nitrate procedure are outlined in detail in the CDC manual by Vestal.[34]

41.8.c. Catalase test. Most species of mycobacteria, with the exception of certain strains of *M. tuberculosis* complex, produce the intracellular enzyme **catalase**, which splits hydrogen peroxide into water and oxygen. Catalase is measured in two ways:

1. By the relative activity of the enzyme, as determined by the height of a column of bubbles of oxygen (Figure 41.6) formed by the action of untreated enzyme produced by the organism (semi-

---

PROCEDURE 41.12

Nitrate Reduction Test with Commercially Available Paper Strips
 (Available from Difco Laboratories)

Principle

The presence of the enzyme nitroreductase can be detected by the ability of a suspension of organisms to produce a colored end product from substrates that combine with nitrite, the product of nitroreductase. *M. tuberculosis* and several other species of mycobacteria possess this enzyme.

Method

1. Add 1 ml sterile saline to a sterile 13 × 100 ml screw-cap test tube.
2. Emulsify two very large clumps of growth from a 4-week-old culture in the saline. The solution should be very turbid (milky).
3. Using sterile forceps, carefully insert a nitrite test strip according to the package insert instructions. The strip should touch only the fluid at the bottom of the tube, not the sides.
4. Cap the tube tightly and incubate upright for

2 h at 37° C. Incubation in a water bath will ensure maintenance of adequate temperature.
5. After the first hour, shake the tube gently without tilting.
6. After the 2-h incubation, tilt the tube six times, wetting the entire strip.
7. Place the tube in a slanted position for 10 min with the liquid covering the strip.
8. Observe the top portion of the strip for any blue color change, indicating a positive reaction. A negative reaction (lack of nitroreductase) yields no color change.

Quality control

Test positive and negative control strains (Table 41.5) each time the nitrate test is performed. These strips should be stored refrigerated in the dark. Discolored strips have deteriorated and should not be used.

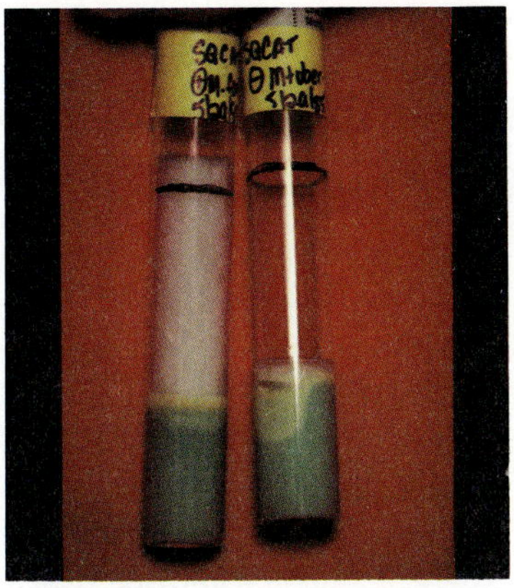

Figure 41.6
Semiquantitative catalase test. The tube on the left contains a
column of bubbles that has risen past the line indicating
45 mm height (a positive test). The tube on the right is the
negative control.

PROCEDURE 41.13

Nitrate Reduction Test Using Chemical Reagents

Principle

As in the conventional nitrate test, the presence of nitrite (product of the nitroreductase enzyme) is detected by production of a red-colored product on the addition of several reagents. If the enzyme has reduced nitrate past nitrite to gas, then addition of zinc dust (which converts nitrate to nitrite) will detect the lack of nitrate in the reaction medium.

Method

1. Prepare the dry crystalline reagent as follows:

Sulfanilic acid (Sigma Chemical Co.)	1 part
N-(1-Naphthyl)ethylenediamine dihydrochloride (Eastman Chemical Co.)	1 part
1-Tartaric acid (Sigma Chemical Co.)	10 parts

   These crystals can be measured out with any small scoop or tiny spoon, since the proportions are by volume, not weight. The mixture should be ground in a mortar and pestle to ensure adequate mixing, because the crystals are of different textures. The reagent can be stored in a dark glass bottle at room temperature for at least 6 months.

2. Add 0.2 ml sterile distilled water to a 16 × 125 mm screw-cap tube. Emulsify two very large clumps of growth from a 4-week culture on Löwenstein-Jensen agar in the water. The suspension should be milky.

3. Add 2 ml nitrate substrate broth (Difco Laboratories or Remel Laboratories) to the suspension and cap tightly.

4. Shake gently and incubate upright for 2 h in a 37° C water bath.

5. Remove from water bath and add a small amount of the crystalline reagent. A wooden stick or a small spatula can be used to add crystals; the amount is not critical.

6. Examine immediately for a pink to red color, indicating the presence of nitrite, demonstrating the ability of the organism to reduce nitrate to nitrite.

7. If no color results, the organisms may have reduced nitrate beyond nitrite (as in the conventional nitrate test, Chapter 9). Add a small amount of powdered zinc to the negative tube. If a red color develops, that indicates that unreduced nitrate was present in the tube and the organism was nitroreductase-negative.

Quality control

Test the quality control organisms, including the weakly positive control (*M. kansasii*, Table 41.5), each time the test is performed.

PROCEDURE 41.14

Semiquantitative (S.Q.) Catalase Test

Principle

The amount of catalase present within cells of species of mycobacteria can be estimated by the height of the column of bubbles of oxygen produced during reduction of hydrogen peroxide.

Method

1. Prepare 10% Tween 80 solution as follows:

Tween 80 (Difco Laboratories)	10 ml
Distilled water	90 ml

   Mix together and autoclave for 10 min at 121° C. Swirl solution after autoclaving to disperse Tween 80. Store in refrigerator. This reagent is also available from Remel Laboratories and can be stored for at least 6 months.

2. Inoculate the surface of a 5-ml L-J agar butt tube (available commercially) with 0.1 ml of the broth subculture originally made for preparing the inoculum for the growth rate and pigment tests (described in Section 41.7). Inoculate tubes with the quality control organisms at the same time.

3. Incubate tubes with caps loose for 2 weeks at 37° C.

4. Prepare hydrogen peroxide reagent fresh for each use:

30% hydrogen peroxide (Superoxol, Merck Chemical Co.)	1 part
10% Tween 80	1 part

   Make 1 ml of the hydrogen peroxide reagent for each test to be performed.

5. Place the tubes upright in a rack that is standing in a tray lined with paper towels soaked with disinfectant. The tray must be autoclavable and waterproof. The column of bubbles produced by this test often tends to overflow; the tray will catch the overflow. If the microbiologist is quick enough, he or she can tighten the cap on a vigorously bubbling tube before it flows out the top.

6. Add 1 ml hydrogen peroxide reagent to each tube and to an uninoculated control tube.

7. Allow tubes to stand and column of bubbles to develop for 5 min before measuring the height of the column of bubbles above the surface of the medium. Alternatively, a line can be drawn on the side of each tube at a height of 45 mm above the agar surface before the reagent is added. Cultures whose bubbles rise above the line are considered positive; those with bubble column heights less than 20 mm are considered negative (Figure 41.6).

8. If the height of the column of bubbles is between 20 and 45 mm, the test should be considered equivocal and repeated.

Quality control

Test positive and negative control strains (Table 41.5) and an uninoculated control tube (above) each time the test is performed.

---

quantitative [S.Q.] catalase test,[20] Procedure 41.14).

2. By the ability of the catalase enzyme to remain active after heating, a measure of the heat stability of the enzyme (heat-stable catalase test,[21] Procedure 41.15).

41.8.d. Hydrolysis of Tween 80.[39] The commonly nonpathogenic slow-growing scotochromogens and nonchromogens produce a lipase that is able to hydrolyze Tween 80 (the detergent polyoxyethylene sorbitan monooleate) into oleic acid and polyoxyethylated sorbitol, whereas pathogenic species do not. Tween 80 hydrolysis (Procedure 41.16) is useful for separating species of photochromogens, nonchromogens, and scotochromogens, as shown in Table 41.12. Because laboratory-prepared media have a very short shelf life, the CDC recommends the use of a commercial Tween 80 hydrolysis substrate (Difco Laboratories or Remel Laboratories) that is stable for up to 1 year.

Heat Stable (68° C, pH 7.0) Catalase Test

Principle

Species of mycobacteria produce catalases that are either resistant to the effect of heat (heat-stable) or that become denatured when heated (heat-labile). This trait can be used for differentiation.

Method

1. Prepare 1/15 M phosphate buffer, pH 7.0 as follows:

   Solution A

Na_2HPO_4 (anhydrous)	9.47 g
Distilled water	1000 ml

   Solution B

KH_2PO_4	9.07 g
Distilled water	1000 ml

   Mix 61.1 ml of solution A with 38.9 ml of solution B and check that the pH is 7.0. Adjust if necessary. Since the suspension will be tested for only a short time, the buffer need not be sterile. Store the two solutions in the refrigerator.

2. Suspend several large clumps of growth from an actively growing agar slant in 0.5 ml of the phosphate buffer in a 16 × 125 mm screw-cap test tube. Prepare control organisms in the same way.

3. Incubate tubes for exactly 20 min in a 68° C heating block or water bath. The temperature must be strictly monitored during the entire incubation.

4. Cool the suspensions to room temperature.

5. Add 0.5 ml of the Tween–hydrogen peroxide solution (same as Procedure 41.14) and observe for formation of bubbles. Negative tubes should be held for 20 min before reporting as negative. Observe carefully, since even a few tiny bubbles are indicative of a positive result. The tubes must not be agitated in any way, since Tween will bubble if shaken.

Quality control

Test positive and negative control strains (Table 41.5) each time the test is performed.

Tween 80 Hydrolysis Test

Principle

Intact Tween 80 binds the phenol red indicator, causing it to assume the structure it would normally assume only at a more acid pH. When Tween 80 is hydrolyzed, it no longer binds the indicator, allowing it to assume its normal configuration at pH 7.0, which is visible to us as pink or red. This pink color, which is the sign of a positive reaction, does not result from a pH shift but results from a breakdown of the Tween 80.

Method

1. Prepare Tween 80 hydrolysis substrate from concentrate according to manufacturer's instructions.

2. Inoculate the substrate with one large clump of actively growing mycobacteria from an agar slant. Inoculate control substrate tubes at the same time.

3. Incubate at 35° C.

4. Examine after 1, 5, and 10 days for a change in the substrate from orange to pink. Compare the color to an uninoculated substrate control. Tubes should not be shaken during reading.

Quality control

Test positive and negative control strains (Table 41.5) and an uninoculated control tube each time the test is performed.

Table 41.12
Tween 80 Hydrolysis Test

GROUP	POSITIVE	NEGATIVE
Photochromogens	M. kansasii	M. simiae
	M. marinum	
	M. asiaticum	
Nonphoto-chromogens	M. gastri	M. bovis
	M. terrae complex	M. avium complex
	M. malmoense	M. xenopi
		M. simiae
		M. haemophilum
Scotochromogens	M. szulgai (slow)	M. scrofulaceum
	M. gordonae	M. xenopi
	M. flavescens	

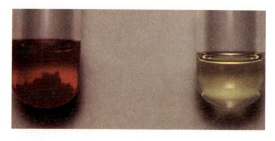

Figure 41.7
A positive arylsulfatase test is shown on the left; the tube containing the negative control is on the right.

PROCEDURE 41.17

Tellurite Reduction Test

Principle

The enzyme tellurite reductase reduces potassium tellurite to metallic tellurite, which is visualized as a black precipitate. Only *M. avium* complex strains and rapid-growing mycobacteria possess a fast-acting enzyme, which is detected in this test.

Method

1. Prepare tellurite stock solution as follows:

Potassium tellurite	0.1 g
Distilled water	50 ml

   Dissolve the tellurite and dispense in 2 ml amounts into 12 × 75 mm screw-cap tubes, sterilize by autoclaving, and store refrigerated. The solution should remain stable for 6 months. Commercially prepared 1% potassium tellurite is available.
2. Inoculate commercial 7H9 broth with a heavy inoculum of organisms and incubate for 7 days at 37° C.
3. Add 2 to 3 drops of the tellurite stock solution to each tube, vortex, and reincubate for 3 more days at 37° C.
4. Examine the sedimented cells in each tube. Formation of a black precipitate indicates a positive reaction. There is no color change with a negative reaction.

Quality control

Test a positive and negative control strain (Table 41.5) each time the test is performed.

41.8.e. Tellurite reduction.[14] Some species of mycobacteria reduce potassium tellurite at variable rates. The ability to reduce tellurite in 3 days distinguishes members of *M. avium* complex from most other nonchromogenic species (Procedure 41.17). All rapid growers reduce tellurite in 3 days.

41.8.f. Arylsulfatase test.[37] The enzyme arylsulfatase, which splits free phenolphthalein from the tripotassium salt of phenolphthalein disulfate, is present in most mycobacteria. Varying the test conditions helps to differentiate different forms of the enzyme (Procedure 41.18). The 3-day test is particularly useful for identifying the potentially pathogenic rapid growers, *M. fortuitum*, *M. triviale*, and *M. chelonae*. Slow-growing *M. marinum* and *M. szulgai* are positive in the 14-day test (Figure 41.7).

41.8.g. Growth inhibition by thiophene-2-carboxylic acid hydrazide (TCH).[35] This test is used to distinguish *M. bovis* from *M. tuberculosis*, since only *M. bovis* is unable to grow in the presence of 2 μg/ml TCH (Procedure 41.19).

41.8.h. Other tests. Tests other than those mentioned here are often performed to make more subtle distinctions between species. They include the ability to grow using only sodium citrate or mannitol as a sole source of carbon, used to distinguish between certain rapid growers. *M. fortuitum* and most other rapid growers are able to convert ferric ammonium citrate to iron oxide. The "iron uptake test" is useful for separating *M. chelonae*, which is unable to convert iron in this way (Figure 41.8). Ability to grow on MacConkey agar without crystal violet can help to identify *M. fortuitum*, which is not inhibited by the medium. Pyrazinamide can be deaminated by *M. tuberculosis* and the *M. avium* complex, as well

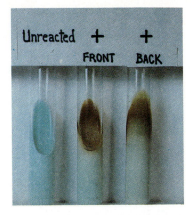

Figure 41.8
Iron uptake test for mycobacteria.

PROCEDURE 41.18

Arylsulfatase Test

Principle

The rate of activity of the ability of arylsulfatase to break down phenolphthalein disulfate into phenolphthalein (which forms a red color in the presence of sodium bicarbonate) and other salts can help differentiate among certain strains of mycobacteria, particularly rapid growers (Table 41.10).

Method

1. Prepare enzyme substrate stock solution as follows:

   Phenolphthalein disulfate tripotassium,   2.6 g
       salt (Sigma Chemical Co.)
   Distilled water   50 ml

   a. Mix thoroughly to make a 0.08 M solution. Sterilize through a 0.2-μm pore size membrane filter. Store refrigerated.
   b. Prepare two flasks of 180 ml each of basal Middlebrook 7H9 or Dubos-Tween-albumin broth (from commercial dry powder). Autoclave for 15 min at 121° C and cool to room temperature. Aseptically add one 20-ml vial of Middlebrook albumin-dextrose-catalase (ADC) enrichment to each flask.
   c. For the 3-day test, aseptically add 2.5 ml of the enzyme substrate stock to one flask, for a final concentration of 0.001 M phenolphthalein substrate.
   d. For the 14-day test, add 7.5 ml of the substrate stock to the other flask, for a concentration of 0.003 M substrate.

e. These two reagents should be dispensed in 2 ml amounts into 16- × 125-mm screw-cap test tubes. Store at room temperature. The substrates are also available commercially (ready-made) from Remel Laboratories.

2. Prepare the alkaline indicator solution (6 N sodium carbonate) as follows:

   Na_2CO_3, anhydrous   10.6 g
   Distilled water   100 ml

   Mix together.

3. Inoculate tubes of the 3-day substrate and the 14-day substrate with 0.1 ml of the broth culture originally set up for determination of growth rates and pigment production. Alternatively, a heavy inoculum of material from an agar slant is acceptable.
4. After 3 days of incubation at 35° C, 6 drops of the sodium carbonate is added to the 3-day 0.001 M substrate.
5. After 14 days of incubation, 6 drops of the sodium carbonate solution is added to the 14-day 0.003 M substrate.
6. Observe for an immediate color change to pink or red after addition of carbonate, indicating a positive result for arylsulfatase (Figure 41.7).

Quality control

Test a positive control strain (Table 41.5) and uninoculated medium as a negative control each time the test is performed.

PROCEDURE 41.19

TCH Susceptibility

Principle

The antimycobacterial compound TCH is inhibitory to *M. bovis*, which can be used to distinguish niacin-positive *M. bovis* from *M. tuberculosis*.

Method

1. Prepare the TCH agar as follows: Prepare Middlebrook 7H10 agar according to manufacturer's instructions, adding the enrichment when the agar has cooled to 55° C. At this time, also add sufficient filter-sterilized TCH (Aldrich Chemical Co.) to make a final concentration of 5 μg/ml. Chapter 13 discusses methods for making such solutions. Mix the agar thoroughly. Also prepare drug-free control agar. Pour the molten agar into quadrants of Felsen Petri dishes, 5 ml per quadrant. Allow the plates to set.

2. Make dilutions of the 7-day-old broth culture that was originally inoculated for preparation of the growth control, 1:1000 and 1:10,000, in sterile water or saline.

3. Inoculate 0.1 ml of each dilution to one drug-containing and one control agar medium. Incubate for 3 weeks in 10% CO_2 at 35° C and examine amount of growth.

4. Organisms are resistant to TCH if growth in the TCH-containing medium is equal to or exceeds 1% of the growth on the control agar. Results are interpreted much as are those of susceptibility tests, described in Chapter 13.

Quality control

Test positive and negative control strains (Table 41.5) each time the test is performed.

as by *M. marinum*, whereas *M. bovis* and *M. kansasii* do not possess the enzyme pyrazinamidase. The inability of *M. chelonae* to grow in 5% NaCl is yet another test for differentiating this organism from *M. fortuitum*. Most rapid growers and some *M. flavescens* strains will grow on medium containing such high salt concentrations. The urease test[31] for hydrolysis of urea by mycobacteria can provide valuable information. As it is currently performed, however, results vary among laboratories, and no reliable method can be recommended.

It is not cost-effective for routine clinical microbiology laboratories to be able to perform all of the procedures necessary for definitive identification of mycobacteria, since excellent reference laboratories are available in every state. With a minimal number of basic procedures, however, the great bulk of all strains isolated can be presumptively identified and those that require further testing can be presumptively identified and forwarded to regional laboratories.

41.9. Antimicrobial Susceptibility Testing

Antituberculosis antimicrobial susceptibility testing, if performed properly, provides important information to the physician for determining the patient's course of treatment.[24] It is a time-consuming procedure that requires meticulous care in the preparation of the medium, selection of adequate samples of colonies, standardization of the inoculum, use of appropriate controls, and interpretation of results.

The susceptibility test may be performed by either the direct or the indirect method. The direct method utilizes a smear-positive concentrate containing more than 50 acid-fast bacilli per 100 oil immersion fields; the indirect method uses a culture as the inoculum source. Isolates of mycobacteria should be tested for susceptibility to primary drugs. In areas where resistant strains of *M. tuberculosis* are commonly seen, susceptibility testing of all isolates is recommended. Laboratories that see very few positive cultures should consider sending isolates to a reference laboratory for testing. Those iso-

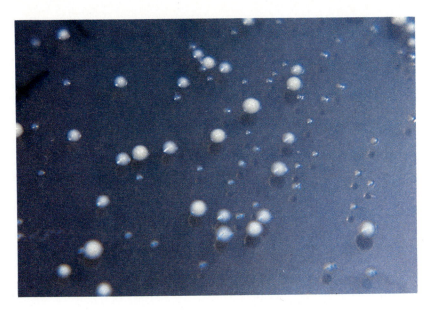

Figure 41.9
Different colony morphologies seen on culture of one strain of *M. avium* complex; the transparent, glossy colonies should be chosen for susceptibility studies because they are known to be more drug resistant.

lates that must be saved for the future possibility of additional studies (such as susceptibilities if the patient does not respond well to treatment) can be frozen in sterile 10% skim milk in distilled water at −70° C.

With the advent of AIDS, several nontuberculous species have been detected with increasing frequency from patients with immune dysfunctions. Many of these species, including *M. avium* complex, *M. fortuitum*, and *M. chelonae*, are very resistant to all conventional antituberculosis drugs. Therefore, new and previously little-used antimycobacterial drugs have been tested in vitro and in vivo. The conventional primary drugs are tested against *M. tuberculosis* complex and some photochromogens and scotochromogens, as outlined in Chapter 13. *M. avium* complex and *M. scrofulaceum* are resistant to these agents. It has been shown that some novel drugs, such as ansamycin (rifabutin), and antileprosy drugs, such as clofazimine (lamprene), are effective against these organisms in vitro. One important consideration to take into account when testing isolates of *M. avium–intracellulare* is that colony morphology relates to virulence in this species. Transparent, glossy colonies are more virulent than

the opaque, dull, white or yellow colonies often seen on isolation media (Figure 41.9). Therefore, isolated colonies of the transparent type should be chosen for in vitro susceptibility testing of these organisms. The rapidly growing species such as *M. fortuitum* and *M. chelonae* are susceptible to amikacin and ciprofloxacin, even though they are resistant to most of the conventional agents. They may exhibit varying susceptibility to erythromycin, cefoxitin, minocycline, and imipenem.

Indirect susceptibility testing can be done by agar dilution, disk elution, a modified agar dilution, a radiometric method that uses the Bactec instrument, and microdilution procedures. With agar dilution, antimycobacterial agents are serially diluted into Middlebrook agar (often in quadrant plates), and dilutions of the organism are inoculated to the surface. Disk elution is a modified agar preparation in which antibiotics elute from disks (obtained from commercial suppliers) that are embedded in the molten agar. The radiometric system involves inoculating either sediments of acid-fast smear-positive specimens or suspensions of organisms grown in culture into Bactec bottles containing Middlebrook 7H12 B broth with antibiotics. Growth in the liquid medium is

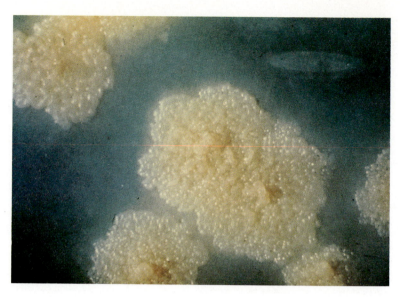

Figure 41.10
M. tuberculosis colonies on L-J agar after 8 weeks of incubation.

monitored radiometrically and the results are interpreted in 4 to 5 days. An increase in the growth index greater than or equal to the growth index measured in concurrently inoculated control bottles without antibiotics indicates resistance. Greater growth in the control suggests susceptibility. Results of trials of this method compare well with conventional testing and yield results much more quickly. A microdilution procedure can be used for rapidly growing mycobacteria. Wells of microbroth dilution plates containing dilutions of the antibiotics to be tested are inoculated in the same manner as for routine susceptibility testing (Chapter 13). Results can usually be read within 2 to 3 days.

41.10. Brief Discussion of Individual Organisms

41.10.a. *M. tuberculosis* complex and related species. This group contains M. tuberculosis, M. bovis, M. africanum, M. microti, and the BCG strain. Except for M. microti, an animal pathogen, all species infect humans. DNA hybridization studies show close homology among all species in the complex.

M. tuberculosis. Colonies of human tubercle bacilli generally appear on egg media after 2 to 3 weeks at 35° C; no growth occurs at 25° or 45° C. Growth first appears as small (1 to 3 mm), dry, friable colonies that are rough, warty, granular, and buff-colored.

After several weeks these increase in size (up to 5 to 8 mm); typical colonies have a flat irregular margin and a "cauliflower" center (Figure 41.10). Because of their luxuriant growth, these mycobacteria are termed **eugonic.** Colonies are easily detached from the medium's surface but are difficult to emulsify. After some experience with mycobacteria has been gained, one can recognize typical colonies of human-type tubercle bacilli without great difficulty. However, final confirmation by biochemical tests must be carried out in all cases.

Virulent strains tend to orient themselves in tight, "serpentine cords," best observed in smears from the condensation water or by direct observation of colonies on a cord medium. Catalase is produced in moderate amounts but not after heating at 68° C for 20 minutes in pH 7 phosphate buffer; human strains resistant to isoniazid (INH) are frequently catalase-negative and yield smooth colonies on egg media. Nitrate reduction is positive. The niacin test is useful in that most *niacin-positive* strains encountered in the diagnostic laboratory prove to be *M. tuberculosis.* Susceptibility to antituberculous drugs is characteristically high.

M. bovis. Bovine tubercle bacilli are rarely isolated in the United States but remain significant pathogens in other parts of the world. They require a longer incubation period—generally 3 to 6 weeks—and ap-

r as tiny (less than 1 mm), translucent, smooth,
-amidal colonies when grown at 35° C. They ad-
-e to the surface of the medium but are emulsified
ily. On the basis of these characteristics, their
-wth is termed **dysgonic.** On 7H10 the colonies
rough and resemble those of *M. tuberculosis.*
bovis grows only at 35° C. It forms serpentine
-ds in smears from colonies on egg media; the
-cin reaction and nitrate reduction tests are neg-
-ve. *M. bovis* is also susceptible to thiophene-2-
-boxylic acid hydrazide (TCH) (unless it is isoni-
-d-resistant), a useful test to differentiate it from
-er mycobacteria. The susceptibility of *M. bovis*
the primary antituberculous drugs is similar to
-t of *M. tuberculosis.*

M. africanum. Rarely isolated in the United
-tes, *M. africanum* resembles *M. tuberculosis.* It
inactive biochemically, showing only positive
-ase and variably positive ability to grow in the
-esence of TCH. This species has been isolated
-m pulmonary cultures of humans as well as from
-nkeys.

M. ulcerans. *M. ulcerans,* probably one of the
-cient species, exhibits discontinuous distribu-
-n. It has been reported from parts of Australia,
-laysia, Africa, and Central America. It is associ-
-d with skin lesions and is considered the caus-
-ve agent of Buruli ulceration, a necrotizing ulcer
-nd in African natives. The organism requires sev-
-l weeks' incubation at 32° C. Unlike *M. marinum,*
-s organism is a **nonchromogen.** It is resistant
isoniazid, ethambutol, para-aminosalicylic acid
-S), and ethionamide, but it is susceptible to ri-
-pin, streptomycin, viomycin, kanamycin, and cy-
serine.

41.10.b. Photochromogens. Four well-defined
-otochromogenic mycobacteria display pigment af-
- exposure to light: *M. kansasii, M. marinum, M.
-iae,* and *M. asiaticum.* All species in this category
facultative pathogens. *M. kansasii* organisms are
-ponsible for pulmonary disease in humans, often
-pearing in white emphysematous men older than
years. The disease with its complications is in-
-tinguishable from that caused by *M. tuberculosis,*
-t it follows a more chronic and indolent course.
-her types of disease, including disseminated in-
-tion, may occur. The disease is not communica-
-, in distinct contrast with that caused by the tu-
-rcle bacillus.

Optimal growth of *M. kansasii* occurs after 2 to

3 weeks at 35° C (slower at 25° C); growth does not
occur at 45° C. Colonies are generally smooth, although there is a tendency to develop roughness.
They are cream-colored when grown in the dark and
become a bright lemon yellow if exposed to light
(Figure 41.11).

If cultures are grown continuously under light (2
to 3 weeks), bright orange crystals of β-carotene form
on the surface of colonies, especially where growth
is heavy. Nonchromogenic and scotochromogenic
variants of *M. kansasii* occur very rarely.

Clinically significant strains of *M. kansasii* are
strongly catalase-positive, even after heating at 68°
C at pH 7 (especially when using the semiquantitative test of Wayne, Procedure 41.14). Low-catalase
strains of *M. kansasii* have been described; these
were not associated with human pathogenicity. Most
strains do not produce niacin, although aberrant
strains have been noted; nitrates are reduced; mature colonies show loose cords.

Stained preparations of *M. kansasii* show characteristically *long, banded, and beaded cells* that are
strongly acid-fast. There is variable susceptibility to
INH and streptomycin, moderate susceptibility to
rifampin, and resistance to PAS, but *M. kansasii* infections typically respond to conventional antituberculous therapy; however, triple therapy, including
rifampin, is desirable.

Primarily associated with granulomatous lesions
of the skin, particularly of the extremities, *M. marinum* infection usually follows exposure of the
abraded skin to contaminated water. Known best for
causing "swimming pool granuloma," this organism
also has been implicated in infections related to
home aquariums, bay water, and industrial exposures involving water. It grows best at *25° to 32° C,*
with sparse to no growth at 35° C (corresponding to
the reduced skin temperature of the extremities),
and it is never isolated from sputum. It may be distinguished from *M. kansasii* by its source, its more
rapid growth at 25° C, negative nitrate reduction,
and weaker catalase production. The drugs most active against *M. marinum* are amikacin and kanamycin. Tetracyclines are inhibitory, chiefly at concentrations slightly below the expected blood levels.

First isolated from monkeys, *M. simiae* has subsequently been recovered from humans with pulmonary disease. Pigmentation may be erratic. It has
a positive niacin reaction, a high thermostable catalase activity, and a negative nitrate test; hydrolyzes

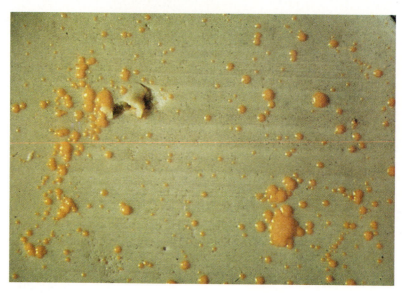

Figure 41.11
M. kansasii colonies exposed to light.

Tween 80 slowly (more than 10 days); and is resistant to all first-line antituberculous drugs. It is sensitive to cycloserine and ethionamide.

M. asiaticum grows at 37° C and yields smooth colonies; photochromogenicity may vary with different growth conditions. This species is rarely encountered in the United States. It has been isolated from cases of pulmonary disease in humans and from monkeys. More isolates are needed in order to better define the characteristics of *M. asiaticum*.

41.10.c. Scotochromogens. The **scotochromogens** are pigmented in the dark (Greek *scotos*, dark), usually a deep yellow to orange, which darkens to an orange or dark red when the cultures are exposed to continuous light for 2 weeks (Figure 41.12). This pigmentation in the dark occurs on nearly all types of media at all stages of growth—characteristics that clearly aid in their identification.

The scotochromogens include the potential pathogens *M. scrofulaceum*, *M. szulgai*, and *M. xenopi*; the so-called tap water scotochromogen, isolated from laboratory water stills, faucets, soil, and natural waters (now classified as *M. gordonae*); and *M. flavescens*. Since the tap water scotochromogen is rarely associated with human disease, it is important to differentiate it from the potentially pathogenic mycobacteria. The former may contaminate equipment used in specimen collection, as in gastric lavage.

M. scrofulaceum is a slow-growing organism, producing smooth, domed to spreading, yellow colonies in both light and darkness. When exposed to continuous light, the colonies may increase in pigment to an orange or brick red; the aluminum foil shield should remain in place (Procedure 41.10) until visible growth occurs in the unshielded tube; then colonies in the shielded tube should be exposed to continuous light. Initial growth may be inhibited by too much light. The hydrolysis of Tween 80 (and urease activity) separates *M. scrofulaceum* from the tap water organisms in that the latter hydrolyze it within 5 days, whereas *M. scrofulaceum* remains negative up to 3 weeks. *M. scrofulaceum* is a cause of cervical adenitis and bone and other infections, particularly in children. It is often resistant to INH and PAS.

M. szulgai has been associated with pulmonary disease, cervical adenitis, cutaneous infection, tenosynovitis, and olecranon bursitis. It gives a positive nitrate reduction test. It is relatively susceptible to ethionamide, rifampin, ethambutol, and higher levels of INH.

M. xenopi has been isolated from the sputum of patients with pulmonary disease. The optimal temperature for its growth is 42° C, and it fails to grow at 22° to 25° C. Four to five weeks' incubation is required to produce tiny dome-shaped colonies of a characteristic yellow color; branching filamentous extensions are seen around colonies on 7H10 agar,

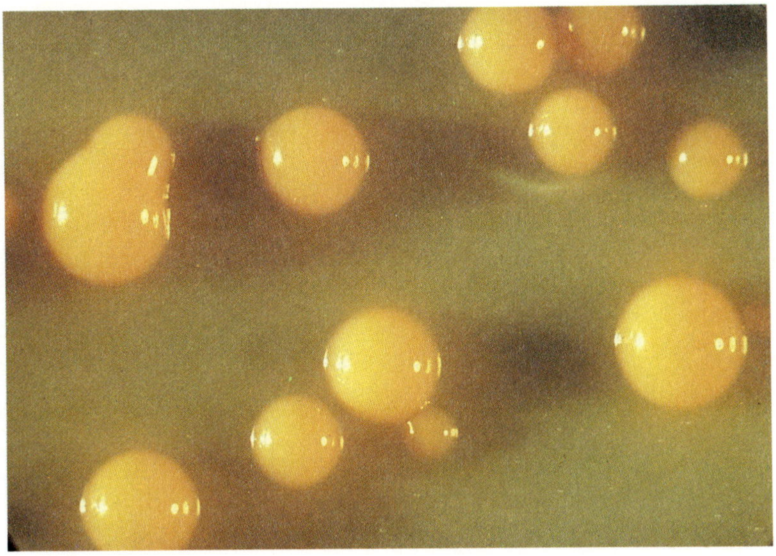

Figure 41.12
Scotochromogen *Mycobacterium gordonae* with yellow colonies.

resembling a miniature bird's nest. Tween 80 hydrolysis and tellurite reduction tests are negative. Therapy with standard antituberculous drugs is generally successful.

Growth of *M. gordonae* appears late on L-J and 7H10 media, usually after 2 weeks and frequently after 3 to 6 weeks, as scattered small yellow-orange colonies in both light and darkness. Hydrolysis of Tween 80 characteristically occurs. *M. flavescens*, another nonpathogenic organism, also produces a yellow-pigmented colony in both light and darkness but is considerably more rapid in growth (usually within 1 week) and reduces nitrate as well as hydrolyzing Tween 80.

41.10.d. Nonchromogens. This group of mycobacteria is made up of a heterogeneous variety of both pathogenic and nonpathogenic organisms that do not usually develop pigment on exposure to light. The *M. avium* complex grow slowly at 35° C (10 to 21 days) and 25° C and usually produce thin, translucent, radially lobed to smooth, cream-colored colonies (Figure 41.13). Isolates often undergo rapid-phase variation to a domed, opaque, yellow colony. This colony is commonly the predominant morphotype initially isolated from patients with AIDS. It has been shown that the rough or opaque colony type is less virulent and that its cell wall is more permeable to antibacterial agents. *M. avium* complex contains two phenotypically similar but genet-

ically distinct species, *M. avium* and *M. intracellulare*. These organisms are encountered most commonly as opportunistic pathogens in patients with AIDS and other immune dysfunctions.[43] DNA probe tests performed against both species have shown that more than 90% of isolates from AIDS patients react with only the *M. avium* probe, whereas two thirds of isolates from non-AIDS patients react with only the *M. intracellulare* probe.[8,9]

Another variant of *M. avium* complex bacilli resembles *M. scrofulaceum* in certain biochemical characteristics; the colonies also become darker yellow with age (unlike other *M. avium* strains). Although biochemical results vary, the majority of isolates of the *M. avium* complex are niacin-negative (with rare exceptions), do not reduce nitrate, and produce only a small amount of catalase. Tween 80 is not hydrolyzed in 10 days, but most of these organisms reduce tellurite within 3 days, a useful test to differentiate these potential pathogens from clinically insignificant nonchromogens.

The *M. avium* complex, while producing serious tuberculosis-like endobronchial lesions in non-AIDS patients, causes disseminated disease in the majority of AIDS patients. However, these organisms may also occur in clinical specimens as nonpathogens. The organisms are resistant to most antituberculosis drugs. Newer agents such as ansamycin and clofazimine may be partially active against these organ-

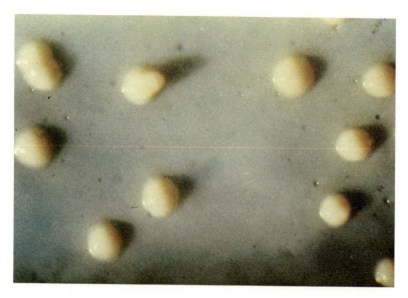

isms. Combinations of drugs, including ethambutol, rifampin, and amikacin, have also had limited success, at least for treatment (but not cure) of the disseminated infection commonly seen in patients with AIDS (Chapter 23). Standard practice has been to use five drugs in combination therapy (if five drugs with in vitro activity can be found).

Mycobacterium gastri ("J" bacillus) has been described as occurring primarily as single-colony isolates from gastric washings. However, it has not been associated with disease in humans. It is closely related to the low catalase-producing strains of *M. kansasii*, from which it may be readily differentiated by the photochromogenic ability of the latter. *M. gastri* may be differentiated from other nonphotochromogens by its ability to hydrolyze Tween 80 rapidly, loss of catalase activity at 68° C, and nonreduction of nitrate.

M. malmoense was first described in 1977 in Sweden, where it was found associated with pulmonary disease. Subsequently, it has been found in human pulmonary disease in Australia and Wales. The organism is nonphotochromogenic and grows slowly (2 to 3 weeks at 37° C and up to 6 weeks at 22° C). Colonies are colorless, smooth, glistening, grayish white, opaque, domed, and circular, 0.5 to 1.5 mm in diameter. The organism does not produce niacin, is nitrate-negative, hydrolyzes Tween 80 and pyra-

zinamide, and produces heat-labile catalase. It is resistant to isoniazid, streptomycin, PAS, and rifampin and is susceptible to ethambutol, cycloserine, kanamycin, and ethionamide.

M. haemophilum is a recently described organism isolated from skin lesions.[28] It requires hemin for growth and may be isolated on chocolate agar, 7H10 agar containing hemolyzed but not whole sheep red blood cells, or L-J medium containing 1% ferric ammonium citrate. Incubation should be at 32° C for a minimum of 2 to 4 weeks. The organism does not grow at 37° C. It should not be expected in specimens of sputum or gastric lavage. It is highly resistant to INH, streptomycin, and ethambutol but is susceptible to PAS.

M. terrae has been called "radish" bacillus. A number of these mycobacteria have been isolated from soil and vegetables as well as from humans, where their pathogenicity remains questionable. The slow-growing (35° C) colonies may be circular or irregular in shape and smooth or granular in texture. They actively hydrolyze Tween 80, reduce nitrate, and are strong catalase producers, but they do not reduce tellurite in 3 days. *M. terrae* is resistant to INH.

M. triviale ("V" bacillus) occurs on egg media as rough colonies that may be confused with *M. tuberculosis* or rough variants of *M. kansasii*. These

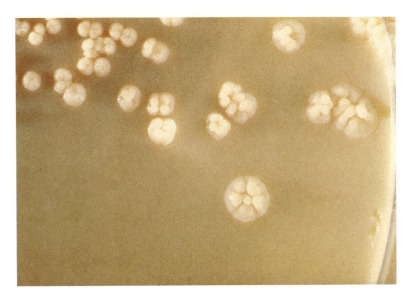

Figure 41.14
Smooth, multilobate colonies of *M. fortuitum* on L-J medium.

bacilli have been recovered from patients with previous tuberculous infections but are considered to be unrelated to human infections. There is one report of human infection with this organism. They are nonphotochromogenic, moderate to strong nitrate reducers, and maintain a high catalase activity at 68° C. They hydrolyze Tween 80 rapidly and do not reduce tellurite.

M. shimoidei was first isolated from a patient in Japan in 1975. It has since been isolated from other patients with pulmonary disease. The organism hydrolyzes Tween 80 and produces heat-stable catalase. Colonies are rough, and growth occurs from 37° to 45° C.

41.10.e. Rapid growers. These mycobacteria are characterized by their ability to grow in 3 to 5 days on a variety of culture media, incubated either at 25° or 35° C. Two members, *M. fortuitum* and *M. chelonae*, are associated with human pulmonary infection, although *M. fortuitum* is also a common soil organism and may frequently be recovered from sputum without necessarily being implicated in a pathological process.

M. fortuitum has been incriminated in progressive pulmonary disease, usually with a severe underlying complication, and has resulted in death. This potential pathogen also grows rapidly (2 to 4 days), is generally nonchromogenic, and may be readily separated from the rapidly growing saprophytes by its positive 3-day arylsulfatase reaction and by growing on MacConkey agar within 5 days, producing a change in the indicator. Both rough and smooth colonies are produced, with increased dye absorption (greening) on L-J medium (Figure 41.14). The niacin test is negative. *M. fortuitum* is usually resistant to PAS, streptomycin, and INH but is susceptible to amikacin and cefoxitin and often the tetracyclines.

M. chelonae (formerly *M. borstelense*) comprises two distinct subspecies: *M. chelonae* subsp. *chelonae*, which fails to grow on 5% NaCl medium, and *M. chelonae* subsp. *abscessus*, which grows on the NaCl medium. *M. fortuitum* and *M. chelonae* are distinguished from each other by the combined use of five tests. *M. fortuitum* is typically nitrate reductase–positive, β-glucosidase–positive, penicillinase-negative, and trehalose-negative and produces acid from fructose. *M. chelonae* has the opposite reactions. *M. chelonae* subsp. *abscessus* has been isolated from pulmonary, postsurgical wound, and other infections. There have been several cases of disseminated disease attributed to this species since 1978. *M. chelonae* subsp. *chelonae* is less common, and it has not been isolated from sputum. Infection occurs at the site of an injury that penetrates the skin.[27]

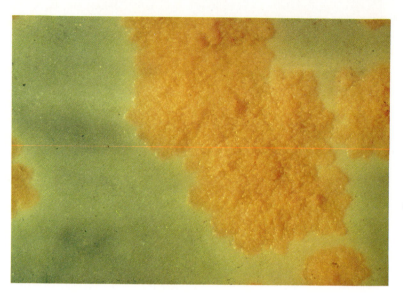

Figure 41.15
M. phlei (rapid grower). Rough colonies.

M. smegmatis, M. phlei (Figure 41.15), and *M. vaccae* are considered saprophytes and are non-pathogenic. *M. smegmatis* and *M. phlei* produce pigmented colonies and show filamentous extensions from colonies growing on cornmeal-glycerol agar. The ability of *M. phlei* ("hay bacillus") to produce large amounts of CO_2 has been utilized to stimulate primary growth of *M. tuberculosis* on 7H10 agar plates incubated in CO_2-impermeable (Mylar) bags. *M. phlei* also produces the growth factor "mycobactin," required by some species of *M. avium* complex and the putative Crohn's disease–associated *Mycobacterium*.

M. fallax resembles *M. tuberculosis,* with cord formation on solid media. The organisms grow rapidly only at 30° C and slowly at 37° C.[22] Several strains have been isolated from humans with pulmonary disease; other strains are found in soil and water. The species is nitrate reductase–positive and –negative for thermostable catalase, arylsulfatase, and urease.

41.10.f. Unclassified *Mycobacterium* associated with Crohn's disease. After long incubation (18 months), colonies are brilliant white and mucoid. With the exception of a weak niacin result, positive 14-day arylsulfatase, and positive thermostable catalase, the isolates are biochemically inactive. Some isolates seem to resemble the animal pathogen, *M.*

paratuberculosis. They have been called *Mycobacterium* sp. "linda." Further studies are ongoing to definitively characterize these organisms and to define their role (if there is one) in Crohn's disease.

41.11. New Approaches to Mycobacterial Identification

New approaches are being explored for identification of the mycobacteria because, as can be appreciated from the number and difficulty of tests necessary and the time required for organisms to grow, the state of the art is somewhat archaic. Thin-layer chromatography and gas-liquid chromatography have seemed logical choices for test systems, because cell wall lipids lend themselves to such procedures. Workers such as Tisdall, de Young, Roberts, and Anhalt[33] and Brennan, Heifers, and Ullom[7] have used chromatographic methods for identification of clinical isolates of mycobacteria.

Patterns produced by mycobacterial nucleic acids after restriction endonuclease treatment and gel electrophoresis have also proved useful for separating the bacilli into species. Those tests are not yet within the realm of routine microbiology laboratories, although a number of large reference laboratories are beginning to use such methods on a routine basis.

Many of the MOTT mycobacterial groups have

been characterized by serotyping schemes and phage typing. In particular, the *M. avium* complex has been studied and defined serologically and by phage typing. Once serovars are established, more sensitive techniques, such as enzyme-linked immunosorbent assay (ELISA), may prove useful for rapid identification of clinically relevant strains.[40]

DNA hybridization methods have been used recently for detection of mycobacteria in clinical specimens. DNA-RNA probes (Gen-Probe) have been used for identifying *M. tuberculosis* complex and *M. avium* complex isolates within several hours of obtaining good growth. Results have been very encouraging and numerous laboratories now incorporate such tests as part of their routine procedures.[8,9]

REFERENCES

1. Berlin, O.G.W., and Martin, W.J. 1980. Importance of nitrate test in the identification of mycobacteria. Clin. Microbiol. Newsletter 2:4.
2. Berlin, O.G.W., and Martin, W.J. 1981. Leprosy or Hansen's disease. Clin. Microbiol. Newsletter 3:135.
3. Berlin, O.G.W., Zakowski, P., Bruckner, D.A., et al. 1984. *Mycobacterium avium*: a pathogen of patients with acquired immunodeficiency syndrome. Diagn. Microbiol. Infect. Dis. 2:213.
4. Berlin, O.G.W., Zakowski, P., Bruckner, D.A., and Johnson, B.L. 1984. New biphasic culture system for isolation of mycobacteria from blood of patients with acquired immune deficiency syndrome. J. Clin. Microbiol. 20:572.
5. Bennedson, J., and Larson, S.O. 1966. Examination for tubercle bacilli by fluorescence microscopy. Scand. J. Respir. Dis. 47:114.
6. Bishop, P.J., and Newman, G. 1970. The history of the Ziehl-Neelsen stain. Tubercle 51:196.
7. Brennan, P.J., Heifers, M., and Ullom, B.P. 1982. Thin-layer chromatography of lipid antigens as a means of identifying nontuberculous mycobacteria. J. Clin. Microbiol. 15:447.
8. Drake, T.A., Herron, R.M., Hindler, J.A., et al. 1988. DNA probe activity of *Mycobacterium avium* complex isolates from patients without AIDS. Diagn. Microbiol. Infect. Dis. 11:125.
9. Drake, T.A., Hindler, J.A., Berlin, O.G.W., and Bruckner, D.A. 1987. Rapid identification of *Mycobacterium avium* complex. J. Clin. Microbiol. 25:1442.
10. Good, R.C. 1985. Opportunistic pathogens in the genus *Mycobacterium*. Annu. Rev. Microbiol. 39:347.
11. Good, R.C., and Snider, D.E., Jr. 1982. Isolation of nontuberculous mycobacteria in the United States, 1980. J. Infect. Dis. 146:829.
12. Inderlied, C.B., Baron, E.J., and Gagné, C. 1984. Disseminated mycobacterial disease in a patient with acquired immune deficiency syndrome. ASCP Check Sample No. MB 84-9 (MB-140). American Society of Clinical Pathologists, Chicago.
13. Kent, P.T., and Kubica, G.P. 1985. Public Health mycobacteriology. A guide for the level III laboratory. Centers for Disease Control, Atlanta, Ga.
14. Kilburn, J.O., Silcox, V.A., and Kubica, G.P. 1969. Differential identification of mycobacteria. V. The tellurite reduction test. Am. Rev. Respir. Dis. 99:94.
15. Kinyoun, J.J. 1915. A note on Uhlenhuth's method for sputum examination for tubercle bacilli. Am. J. Public Health 5:867.
16. Konno, K. 1956. New chemical method to differentiate human-type tubercle bacilli from other mycobacteria. Science 124:985.
17. Kubica, G.P. 1984. Culture examination and identification. Centers for Disease Control, Atlanta, Ga.
18. Kubica, G.P., Dye, W.E., Cohen, M.L., and Middlebrook, G. 1963. Sputum digestion and concentration with N-acetyl-L-cysteine-sodium hydroxide for culture of mycobacteria. Am. Rev. Respir. Dis. 87:775.
19. Kubica, G.P., Gross, W.M., Hawkins, J.E., et al. 1975. Laboratory services for mycobacterial diseases. Am. Rev. Respir. Dis. 112:773.
20. Kubica, G.P., Jones, W.D., Abbott, V.D., et al. 1966. Differential identification of mycobacteria. I. Tests on catalase activity. Am. Rev. Respir. Dis. 94:400.
21. Kubica, G.P., and Pool, G.L. 1960. Studies on the catalase activity of acid fast bacilli. I. An attempt to subgroup these organisms on the basis of their catalase activity at different temperatures and pH. Am. Rev. Respir. Dis. 81:387.
22. Levy-Frebault, V., Rafidinarivo, E., Prome, J.C., et al. 1983. *Mycobacterium fallax* sp. nov. Int. J. Syst. Bacteriol. 33:336.
23. Middlebrook, G., Reggiordo, Z., and Tigertt, W.D. 1977. Automatable radiometric detection of growth of *Mycobacterium tuberculosis* in selective media. Am. Rev. Respir. Dis. 115:1066.
24. Mitchison, D.A. 1979. Basic mechanisms of chemotherapy. Chest 76:771.
25. Morbidity and Mortality Weekly Report. 1987. Tuberculosis and acquired immunodeficiency syndrome—New York City. United States Public Health Service, Centers for Disease Control, Atlanta, Ga. 36:785.
26. Rickman, T.W., and Meyer, N.P. 1980. Increased sensitivity of acid fast smears. J. Clin. Microbiol. 11:618.
27. Righter, J., Hart, G.D., and Howes, M. 1983. *Mycobacterium chelonei*: report of a case of septicemia and review of the literature. Diagn. Microbiol. Infect. Dis. 1:323.
28. Ryan, C.G., and Dwyer, B.W. 1983. New characteristics of *Mycobacterium haemophilum*. J. Clin. Microbiol. 18:976.
29. Siddiqi, S.H. 1988. Bactec T.B. System Product and Procedure Manual. Becton, Dickinson & Co., Towson, Md.
30. Sommers, H.M. 1978. The identification of mycobacteria. Lab. Med. 9:34.
31. Steadham, J.E. 1979. Reliable urease test for identification of mycobacteria. J. Clin. Microbiol. 10:134.
32. Thangaraj, R.H., and Yawalker, S.J. 1987. Leprosy for medical practitioners and paramedical workers. Ciba-Geigy Limited, Basel, Switzerland.
33. Tisdall, P.A., DeYoung, D.R., Roberts, G.D., and Anhalt, J.P. 1982. Identification of clinical isolates of mycobacteria with gas-liquid chromatography: a 10-month follow up study. J. Clin. Microbiol. 16:400.
34. Vestal, A.L. 1975. Procedures for the isolation and identification of mycobacteria. DHEW (CDC 75-8230). Centers for Disease Control, Atlanta, Ga.

35. Vestal, A.L., and Kubica, G.P. 1967. Differential identification of mycobacteria. III. Use of thiacetazone, thiophen-2-carboxylic acid hydrazide and triphenyltetrazolium chloride. Scand. J. Respir. Dis. 48:142.

36. Virtanen, A. 1960. A study of nitrate reduction by mycobacteria. Acta. Tuberc. Scand. Suppl. 48:1.

37. Wayne, L.G. 1961. Recognition of *Mycobacterium fortuitum* by means of the 3 day phenolphthalein sulfatase test. Am. J. Clin. Pathol. 36:185.

38. Wayne, L.G. 1964. The role of air in the photochromogenic behavior of *Mycobacterium kansasii*. Am. J. Clin. Pathol. 42:431.

39. Wayne, L.G., Doubaek, J.R., and Russel, R.L. 1964. Classification and identification of mycobacteria. 1. Tests employing Tween-80 as substrate. Am. Rev. Respir. Dis. 90:588.

40. Yanagihara, D.L., Barr, V.L., Knisely, C.V., et al. 1985. Enzyme-linked immunosorbent assay of glycolipid antigens for identification of mycobacteria. J. Clin. Microbiol. 21:569.

41. Youmans, G.P. 1979. Tuberculosis. W. B. Saunders Co., Philadelphia, Pa.

42. Young, L.J., Inderlied, C.B., Berlin, O.G.W., and Gottlieb, M.S. 1986. Mycobacterial infections in AIDS patients, with an emphasis on the *Mycobacterium avium* complex. Rev. Infect. Dis. 8:1024.

43. Zakowski, P., Fligiel, S., Berlin, O.G.W., and Johnson, B.L. 1982. Disseminated *Mycobacterium avium–intracellulare* infection in homosexual men dying of acquired immunodeficiency. J.A.M.A. 248:2980.

BIBLIOGRAPHY

Chiodini, R.J. 1989. Crohn's disease and the mycobacterioses: a review and comparison of two disease entities. Clin. Microbiol. Rev. 2:90.

Chiodini, R.J., Van Kruiningen, H.J., Merkal, R.S., et al. 1984. Characteristics of an unclassified *Mycobacterium* species isolated from patients with Crohn's disease. J. Clin. Microbiol. 20:966.

Hastings, R.C., Gillis, T.P., Krahenbuhl, J.L., and Franzblau, S.G. 1988. Leprosy. Clin. Microbiol. Rev. 1:330.

Hernandez, R., Munoz, O., and Guiscafre, H. 1984. Sensitive enzyme immunoassay for early diagnosis of tuberculous meningitis. J. Clin. Microbiol. 20:533.

Krasnow, I. 1978. Primary isolation of mycobacteria. Lab. Med. 9:26.

Lowry, P.W., Jarvis, W.R., Oberle, A.D., et al. 1988. *Mycobacterium chelonae* causing otitis media in an ear-nose-throat practice. N. Engl. J. Med. 319:978.

Sommers, H.M., and Good, R.C. 1985. *Mycobacterium*. In Lennette, E.H., Balows, A., Hausler, W.J., Jr., and Shadomy, H.J., editors. Manual of clinical microbiology, ed. 4. American Society for Microbiology, Washington, D.C.

Swenson, J.M., Thornsberry, C., and Silcox, V. 1982. Rapidly growing mycobacteria: testing of susceptibility to 34 antimicrobial agents by broth microdilution. Antimicrob. Agents Chemother. 22:186.

Wallace, R.J., Jr. 1987. Nontuberculous mycobacteria and water: a love affair with increasing clinical importance. Infect. Dis. Clin. North Am. 1:677.

Wallace, R.J., Jr., Nash, D.R., Tsukamura, M., et al. 1988. Human disease due to *Mycobacterium smegmatis*. J. Infect. Dis. 158:52.

Wallace, R.J., Jr., Swenson, J.M., Silcox, V.A., et al. 1983. Spectrum of disease due to rapidly growing mycobacteria. Rev. Infect. Dis. 5:657.

Wayne, L.G., David, H., Hawkins, J.E., et al. 1976. Referral without guilt or how far should a good lab go? ATS News 2:8.

Wayne, L.G., Good, R.C., Krichevsky, M.I., et al. 1981. First report of the cooperative, open-ended study of slowly growing mycobacteria by the International Working Group on Mycobacterial Taxonomy. Int. J. Syst. Bacteriol. 31:1.

Wolinsky, E. 1984. Nontuberculous mycobacteria and associated diseases. pp. 1141-1207. In Kubica, G.P., and Wayne, L.G., editors. The mycobacteria: a sourcebook. Marcel Dekker, New York.

42 Laboratory Methods in Basic Virology

W. Lawrence Drew

42.1. General Principles

42.1.a. Viral structure. With the electron microscope, viruses can be seen to consist of capsid, or protein coat, and a core of nucleic acid. Some viruses, such as members of the herpes family, may also have a lipid-containing envelope. Figure 42.1 shows numerous herpes simplex viruses (HSVs) in various stages of development. Each viral particle has a dark central core and an outer coat of one or more layers, creating a halo effect.

42.1.b. Virus classification. All true viruses have a nucleic acid that is either DNA or RNA. Nucleic acid composition is the basis for a simple system of classifying viruses of clinical importance. The DNA viruses comprise six groups that cause human disease (Table 42.1); the RNA viruses may be divided into 11 such groups (Table 42.2).

42.1.c. Viral replication. Unlike bacteria, viruses can reproduce only within cells, where they utilize cellular "machinery" for synthesis of daughter viruses (Figure 42.2). A typical cycle of viral replication involves the following steps:

1. Attachment of the virus to the cell.
2. Penetration of the cell by the virus.
3. Uncoating of the viral coat, exposing nucleic acid. In this eclipse phase, intact virus is not detectable within the cell by electron microscopy.
4. Viral nucleic acid functions as a template for the production of "messenger" RNA, which codes for the synthesis of viral proteins (structural and enzymatic) using cellular polysomes. In the case of retroviruses, RNA is the template for the pro-

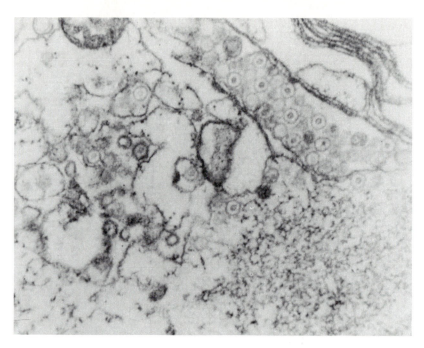

Figure 42.1
Electron micrograph of herpes simplex virus.

Table 42.1
Viruses of Human Importance: DNA

FAMILY	VIRAL MEMBERS
Pox	Variola, vaccinia, molluscum contagiosum
Herpesvirus	Herpes simplex, varicella-zoster, cyto-megalovirus, Epstein-Barr virus
Adenovirus	Types 1 to 8 most implicated in causing human disease
Papovavirus	Human papilloma (wart), progressive multifocal leukoencephalopathy agents (JC, SV40), BK
Hepatitis B	Hepatitis B
Parvovirus	B-19

Table 42.2
Viruses of Human Importance: RNA

FAMILY	VIRAL MEMBERS
Orthomyxovirus	Influenza A, B, C
Paramyxovirus	Parainfluenza, mumps, measles, respiratory syncytial virus
Togavirus	Western and eastern equine encephalitis
Flavivirus	St. Louis encephalitis, yellow fever, dengue
Rubivirus	Rubella
Bunyavirus	California and La Crosse encephalitis, Rift Valley fever
Calcivirus	Calcivirus (? Norwalk agent)
Coronavirus	Coronavirus
Reovirus	Types 1 to 3, rotavirus, Colorado tick fever
Picornavirus	Enterovirus Polio, Coxsackie A, Coxsackie B, Echovirus, enterovirus 68-71, 72 (hepatitis A) Rhinovirus Calicivirus, Norwalk virus
Arenavirus	Lymphocytic choriomeningitis, Lassa, Tacaribe (hemorrhagic fever agents)
Rhabdovirus	Rabies
Filovirus	Marburg, Ebola
Retrovirus	Human T-lymphotropic virus (HTLV-I and -II), human immunodeficiency virus (HIV 1 and 2)

duction of complementary DNA, via the enzyme reverse transcriptase. This intermediary DNA is then the template for production of messenger RNA, and virus synthesis proceeds as described.

5. Synthesis of "daughter" viral nucleic acid using the "parent" viral nucleic acid as template.
6. Assembly of intact viral particles within the cell.
7. Release of viral particles from the cell. In this process of extrusion, cell lipid or membrane may envelop the virus and form its outer coat.

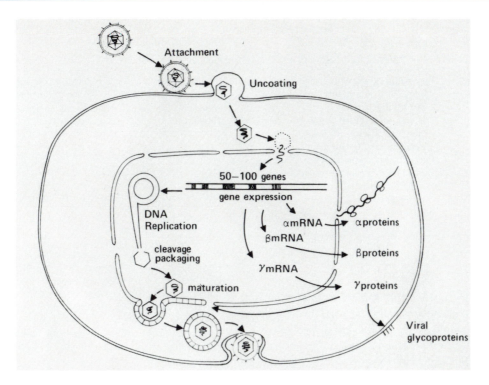

Figure 42.2
Schematic of viral replication.

42.1.d. Viral infection. Within the intact animal, viral infection may be pictured as follows:

1. Invasion of susceptible superficial cells by a specific virus. For example, enteroviruses may initially attack cells lining the gastrointestinal tract.
2. Viral replication within these cells may lead to local spread and may yield sufficient virus progeny to cause viremia.
3. This primary viremia may lead to parasitism of reticuloendothelial cells.
4. Following replication within reticuloendothelial cells, a secondary viremia may occur with parasitism of distal visceral cells, for example, neural cells by poliomyelitis virus.

Symptoms may develop at the time of initial invasion of superficial living cells, as with rhinoviruses and the common cold, or may not appear until after secondary viremia and invasion of visceral target organs, as with poliomyelitis. In the case of "slow" virus infections such as progressive multifocal leukoencephalopathy (PML), symptoms may not develop for many years.

42.2. Etiology of Viral Syndromes

Certain specific syndromes may be caused by several different viruses. This is especially true of respiratory diseases, such as bronchiolitis, which may be caused by either respiratory syncytial or parainfluenza virus (Tables 42.3 and 42.4). Similarly, the spectrum of disease potential for any one virus type is quite broad. For example, influenza virus may cause illness ranging from upper respiratory tract infection (URI) to pneumonia. Table 42.5 illustrates similar considerations in several nonrespiratory diseases.

Despite the broad range of viruses responsible for human illness, Table 42.6 indicates that relatively few are recovered with any frequency in a clinical virology laboratory. This simplifies the problem of recognition for the technologist, since in most instances these commonly isolated viruses develop distinctive cytopathic effect (CPE; described in Section 42.8.f) in tissue culture. If the CPE does not permit ready identification, a few simple immunologic tests suffice for recognition of the commonly isolated viruses. It is apparent from Table 42.6 that if one can

Table 42.3

Most Common Etiologic Agents of Viral
Respiratory Diseases in Infants and Children

Upper respiratory tract infection	Rhinovirus, coronavirus, parainfluenza, adenovirus, respiratory syncytial virus, influenza
Pharyngitis	Adenovirus, coxsackie A, herpes simplex, EB virus, rhinovirus, parainfluenza, influenza
Croup	Parainfluenza, respiratory syncytial virus
Bronchitis	Parainfluenza, respiratory syncytial virus
Bronchiolitis	Respiratory syncytial virus, parainfluenza
Pneumonia	Respiratory syncytial virus, adenovirus, influenza, parainfluenza

Table 42.4

Most Common Etiologic Agents of Viral
Respiratory Disease in Adults

Upper respiratory tract infection	Rhinovirus, coronavirus, adenovirus, influenza, parainfluenza
Pneumonia	Influenza, adenovirus
Pleurodynia	Coxsackie B

Table 42.5

Etiologic Agents of Common Viral Syndromes

SYNDROME	AGENTS
Myocarditis	Coxsackie B
Pleurodynia	Coxsackie B
Herpangina	Coxsackie A
Febrile illness ± rash	Echo, coxsackie
Infectious mononucleosis	EB virus, cytomegalovirus
Aseptic meningitis	Echo, coxsackie A and B
Encephalitis	Herpes simplex, togavirus, rabies, enteroviruses
Hepatitis	Hepatitis A, B, C, non-A non-B (NANB), delta agent

learn to isolate and identify the eight virus groups listed, 96% of all isolates can be reported correctly. Despite the impressive results cited previously, however, more rapid methods of viral diagnosis are highly desirable, especially for slow-growing viruses.

42.3. Cytology

The most readily available rapid technique is cytologic examination for the presence of characteristic viral inclusions. These intracellular structures may represent aggregates of virus within an infected cell or may be abnormal accumulations of cellular materials consequent to the viral-induced metabolic disruption. Papanicolaou (Pap) smears may show these inclusions in single cells or in large syncytial (large aggregates of cells containing more than one nucleus) groups, as in a patient with herpes simplex infection of the cervix (Figure 42.3). Cytology is most commonly used to detect infections with herpes simplex virus or cytomegalorivus, but it is definitely less sensitive than culture. Rabies infection may also be detected by use of the Seller stain for the detection of Negri bodies (rabies inclusions in brain tissue).

42.4. Detection of Viral Antigen

42.4.a. Fluorescent antibody assays for detection of viral antigen. Direct examination of virus-infected tissues or exudates may be performed with specific fluorescein-labeled viral antibody as described in Procedure 42.1. Indirect immunofluorescence (IF) staining of selected clinical specimens can be a rapid (for example, 1 hour) and highly reliable method for

the detection of antigens from a number of viruses, including influenza, parainfluenza, respiratory syncytial virus (RSV), adenoviruses, mumps, measles, rubella, rabies, herpes simplex virus (HSV), varicella-zoster virus (VZ), and cytomegalovirus (CMV)[6,10,16,21] (Table 42.7). In addition, IF has been used successfully in the detection of more unusual agents such as Colorado tick fever, vaccinia, lymphocytic choriomeningitis, orf, and Lassa fever viruses.[8] At the present time, IF methods have not been as widely successful for routine application to the rapid diagnosis of enterovirus infections, and further work in this area is necessary. The recent development of a method for the in vitro production of monoclonal antibodies should lead to greatly enhanced specificity and sensitivity of IF as well as other immunodiagnostic methods in the future.

Strict criteria for the interpretation of fluorescence patterns must be applied. For example, nuclear and cytoplasmic staining are typical patterns for influenza virus, adenoviruses, and the herpesviruses; only cytoplasmic staining is seen with respiratory syncytial, parainfluenza, and mumps vi-

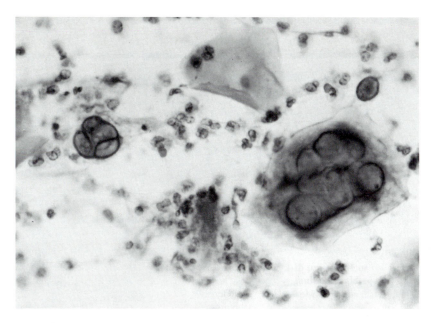

Figure 42.3
Herpes simplex virus cytology.

Table 42.6
Frequency of Occurrence and Average Detection Time for Commonly Isolated Viruses at Mount Zion Hospital and Medical Center

| | ISOLATES | | AVERAGE DETECTION TIME |
VIRUS	NO.	%	(DAYS)
Herpes simplex virus	416	42	2.7
Influenza A	66	7	3.8
Enteroviruses (echo, coxsackie A, B)	79	8	4.2
Cytomegalovirus (CMV)	213	21	5.8*
Respiratory syncytial virus (RSV)	35	3	6.1
Varicella-zoster	41	4	6.1
Adenovirus	80	8	6.4
Parainfluenza 1, 3	29	3	6.4
Other	41	4	4.1
TOTALS	1000	100	

*Can be detected in an average of 2 to 3 days using a shell vial centrifugation and pre-CPE IFA staining procedure.

ruses; staining within multinucleated giant cells is typical of measles viruses. If the pattern of fluorescence is appropriate and proper controls have been employed, the specificity of the test is high.

False-positive results can be obtained if the preceding criteria are not strictly applied. Specimens that contain yeasts, certain bacteria, mucus, or leukocytes can be especially misleading. Also, results of fluorescent antibody (FA) staining of cerebrospinal fluid (CSF) sediment should be viewed with great caution; leukocytes from any source may possess Fc receptors, which can be responsible for nonspecific binding of antibody conjugates. Especially when first utilizing FA staining, it is extremely important for the investigator to attempt isolation of viruses from specimens submitted for FA staining in order to ver-

PROCEDURE 42.1

Rapid Diagnosis of Viral Infection by Direct Fluorescent Antibody Staining

Specimens

Four types of specimens can be used for IF diagnosis: frozen sections, impression smears, lesion scrapings, and resuspended cells in centrifuged sediment.

Frozen sections should be cut to 3 to 4 μm in thickness, and lesion scrapings are best obtained with a scalpel blade and then smeared in spots on the slide. Swabs of lesions may be **rolled** onto the slide; rubbing should be avoided since this can distort cell morphology.

Cell suspensions can usually be readily recovered from urine or other body fluids (e.g., amniotic fluid by centrifugation). In addition, if appropriate vigor has been applied in the collection of swabs from the respiratory tract, conjunctiva, vagina, or skin lesions, the specimens in viral transport media can be utilized. These samples are blended thoroughly on a vortex mixer, and the swabs are removed. The samples are then centrifuged at 1200 to 1500 × g for 30 min, and the supernatant is used for cell culture inoculation. The remaining sediment is suspended in just enough PBS (without phenol red) to yield a slightly turbid suspension, which is spotted on the wells of slides with a Pasteur pipette. The amount of PBS required for resuspension usually varies from 0.1 to 1 ml. All slides are labeled appropriately, allowed to air dry completely, and then fixed in acetone at −20° C for 10 min. If slides must be transported from one laboratory to another, they may be sent air dried at ambient temperature, or acetone-fixed at 4° C. Formalin-fixed tissues are **not** suitable for IF studies.

Slides

Clean, plain, 1-mm thick glass slides can be used for frozen sections or impression smears. For examination of resuspended cells, preprinted slides are preferred to slides prepared by spraying with Fluoroglide.

Conjugates

Fluorescein isothiocyanate−conjugated antisera are reconstituted with PBS, pH 7.4 to 8.0, aliquoted, and stored at −60° C until the time of use. These samples are then titrated at 1:5, 1:10, 1:20, and 1:40 dilutions in PBS to determine optimal working dilutions in infected cell cultures. (Optimal dilution is defined as that which gives 3+ to 4+ specific fluorescence in cells infected with homologous virus and no fluorescence in cells infected with heterologous virus or in uninfected cells.) This optimal dilution is then tested for cross-reactivity with heterologous viruses, as well as for nonspecific fluorescence in impression smears or frozen sections of normal, noninfected human tissues, such as brain and lung. In clinical use, appropriate controls include preimmune conjugates derived from the homologous animal source, conjugated antisera to heterologous viruses, and, when tissue sections or impression smears are used, normal, noninfected tissue controls. The conjugates are used on clinical specimens at a twofold lower dilution than for typing of tissue culture isolates. Slides submitted for VZV or HSV fluorescent antibody examination should be stained with both conjugates. The HSV conjugate used in our laboratory is bivalent, i.e., contains antibody to both types 1 and 2 HSV, and is obtained commercially. The working dilution is determined as described in Procedure 42.4.

Positive and negative controls for each conjugate are necessary. For example, HSV- and VZV-positive controls should be stained with the heterologous conjugate to ascertain the extent (if any) of cross-reactions.

PROCEDURE 42.1—cont'd

Staining

The procedure used is the same as that outlined for identification of cell culture isolates (Procedure 42.4). Appropriately diluted conjugate is overlaid on each specimen, and the slides are incubated at 35° C for 30 to 60 min in a humidified chamber. The slides are then washed with gentle agitation for two 5-min periods in PBS. Coverslips (No. 1) are mounted with buffered glycerol (pH 8.0), and specimens are examined for fluorescence. A halogen-source microscope equipped with epifluorescence is ideal for this purpose, with observation at 600× magnification. If oil immersion is used, low-fluorescence oil is necessary.

Interpretation

Strict criteria for interpreting fluorescence patterns must be applied. For example, nuclear and cytoplasmic staining are typical for influenza virus, adenoviruses, and the herpesviruses (Figure 42.4); cytoplasmic staining only is seen with respiratory syncytial (Figure 42.5), parainfluenza, and mumps viruses; staining within multinucleated giant cells is typical of measles viruses. If the pattern of fluorescence is appropriate, and proper controls have been employed, the specificity of the test is high. In fact, for some agents such as VZV, direct IF is often considerably more

sensitive than culture. Smears that have insufficient (<6) epithelial cells, or that have primarily pus or tissue fragments, are considered unsatisfactory and should be reported as such.

Note: *The technologist should be aware of nonspecific staining reactions. Leukocytes are notorious for nonspecific binding of fluorescein-conjugated antisera; only epithelial cells should be used to interpret direct smears. Tissues also may trap the conjugate and prevent it from being washed away.*

False-positive results can be obtained if the preceding criteria are not strictly applied. Specimens that contain yeasts, mucus, or leukocytes can be especially misleading.

It is extremely important to attempt virus isolation on specimens submitted for fluorescent-antibody staining to verify results, to enhance the overall sensitivity of diagnosis, and to standardize the conjugates properly. When both cultures and IF examination are performed, false-negative IF tests will be observed. In some instances, these false-negative tests result from specimens with very low virus titer, requiring many days for detection in culture. False-negative fluorescent assay results have occurred with critical specimens such as brain biopsy specimens for HSV encephalitis; culture "backup" is therefore mandatory.

ify results, enhance the overall sensitivity of diagnosis, and properly standardize the conjugates.

Schmidt et al.[21] recently revised their experience with detection of HSV antigens in vesicular lesions. Nearly 200 specimens were examined; the immunofluorescence test was positive in more than 80% of the specimens from which HSV was grown; conversely, 90% of the specimens in which herpesvirus was demonstrated by FA yielded a positive culture. On the basis of these results, they concluded that direct immunofluorescence staining can be a reliable and rapid method for diagnosis of HSV infection when performed by experienced personnel using

good reagents and equipment. The few immunofluorescence test results that were positive for HSV but failed to yield infectious virus were not false-positives, since the specimens gave positive staining only with HSV conjugate and not with VZV conjugate, and since clinical symptoms in the patient were compatible with HSV infection. Furthermore, the specimens examined in this study had to be transported statewide, and there was considerable opportunity for the virus to lose viability.

When both cultures and IF examinations are performed, false-negative IF tests will be observed. Table 42.8 indicates that irrespective of the type of

Table 42.7
Detection of Viral Antigens by Fluorescent Antibody

SYNDROME	POSSIBLE VIRAL AGENTS DETECTABLE BY IF	USUAL TISSUE OR CELL SOURCE
Colorado tick fever	Colorado tick fever virus	Erythrocytes
Congenital infections	Rubella virus, cytomegalovirus, herpes simplex virus	Nasopharyngeal, throat, lesion scrapings, tissue, urine sediment
Conjunctivitis, keratitis	Herpes simplex, adenovirus	Conjunctival cells, corneal scrapings
Disseminated disease	Herpes simplex virus, cytomegalovirus, varicella zoster virus	Tissue, lesion scrapings
Encephalitis	Herpes simplex virus	Brain biopsy
	Mumps virus	Throat, urine sediment
	Rabies virus	Brain biopsy, corneal scrapings, neck skin biopsy
Infectious mononucleosis	Epstein-Barr virus	Lymphocytes, lymphoid tissue
Macular or maculopapular exanthems	Measles, rubella, adenoviruses	Nasopharyngeal, throat, urine sediment
Mucocutaneous vesicles and ulcers	Herpes simplex, varicella-zoster viruses	Lesion or vesicle scrapings, mucosal cells
Respiratory tract infection	Influenza A, B; parainfluenza 1, 2, 3; adenovirus; respiratory syncytial virus	Nasopharyngeal, throat, lung biopsy

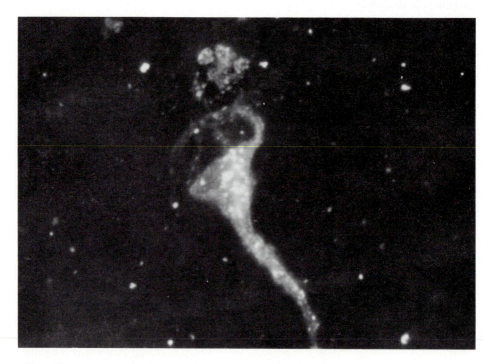

Figure 42.4
Herpes simplex virus, FA stain.

HSV skin lesion, false-negative FA results occur.[17] In some instances, these false-negative test results are from specimens with very low titers of virus, which require many days for detection in culture.

From these results, it is clear that neither immunofluorescence nor culture tests are 100% accurate. In our laboratory, we often perform both tests, especially in critical situations. False-negative results of fluorescence assays have occurred with specimens such as brain biopsy specimens taken for diagnosis of HSV encephalitis; culture backup is therefore mandatory on such critical specimens. Another critical situation may arise when a genital lesion is observed in a pregnant woman near term. Determination that the lesion is herpetic may influence the decision to perform a cesarean section. If the patient has a history of herpes infections and there are clinical features that support this diagnosis, many experts believe that the lesion should be considered as herpetic, irrespective of the results of culture or immunofluorescence tests. FA examination may well be able to confirm immediately the clinical impres-

Table 42.8

Comparison of Viral Culture, Fluorescent Antibody (FA), and Indirect Immunoperoxidase (IP) Techniques for Detection of Herpes Simplex Viral Genital Skin Lesions

	PERCENTAGE POSITIVE BY INDICATED TECHNIQUE		
TYPE OF LESION	**CULTURE**	**FA**	**IP**
Vesicle	93	77	77
Pustule	83	58	75
Ulcer	72	38	55

From Moseley, R.C., Corey, L., Benjamin, D., et al. 1981.

sion and, if time permits, confirmation may be obtained by viral culture methods in as few as 1 or 2 days. Direct immunofluorescence examination should not be performed blindly on specimens of cervix or vagina, since cellular material in these secretions may interfere with the reading of the test.

FA is actually superior to culturing for the detection of RSV antigen.[10,16] This may result in part from the fact that antibody may bind to the virus in the tissue and prevent growth of the virus in culture; yet detection of viral antigens is still possible. The quality of antisera available for this test is now excellent, so we feel that we can confidently rely on the FA result without an accompanying culture.

Schmidt et al.[21] reviewed their experience with both immunofluorescence and culturing for the diagnosis of (VZV) infections. Unlike HSV, which grows rapidly in cell culture, VZV takes an average of 6 days for detection. Also, unlike the generally good correlation observed between detection of HSV by fluorescent antibody test and by positive viral culture results, a poor correlation was found between fluorescent antibody and culture results for VZV. Indeed, 45 specimens were positive for VZV by immunofluorescence detection because the specimen showed staining only with conjugates specific for VZV virus and not with those for HSV or vaccinia virus, and none of these specimens yielded HSV in cell culture. Only 11 specimens were culture positive. Of the 34 patients whose culture results were negative, 28 had clinical diagnoses of herpes zoster or varicella infections, two had diagnoses of possible smallpox, one of possible vaccinia, and three simply had vesicular rashes.

The conclusion was that the culture results were

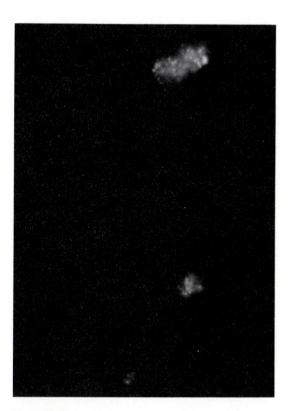

Figure 42.5
RSV, FA stain.

Table 42.9
CMV Culture Procedure—Standard Versus Rapid

	STANDARD	RAPID
Cells	Any diploid fibroblast	MRC-5
Cell growth	Tube	Coverslip in dram vial
Inoculation	Add 2 cells	Centrifuge onto cells
Method of detection	Routine CPE	FA at 2-3 days before CPE
Time for detection	6-21 days	2-3 days

false-negative rather than that the fluorescence examination results were false-positive. The reason that the cultures were false-negative related to the time after onset of disease at which the specimens were collected. All of the cultures positive for virus were from specimens collected within the first 5 days of illness. No positive viral culture results were obtained on specimens taken later than 5 days. We previously published a similar article. Skin lesions from 47 patients were simultaneously examined by viral culture and direct immunofluorescence techniques. The latter procedure established the diagnosis in 24 (86%) of 28 patients, but viral culture results were positive for only 10 of 28 specimens.[6]

As mentioned earlier, the limitations of the fluorescent antibody procedure are the quality of the antisera used in the test and the technical capability of the person reading the result. In trained hands the fluorescent antibody (FA) test is more useful than the viral culture, since the former can be performed on the day the specimen is submitted and since culture results are often falsely negative. However, this is in contrast to our experience with HSV; we have found that the culture method is both rapid and reliable for this virus, and we reserve the FA test for critical situations.

Many of these antigens also may be detected by indirect fluorescent antibody (IFA) techniques. Indeed, the IFA procedure to detect RSV directly is considered by many to be superior to culture if performed by experienced individuals.[16,19] Immunofluorescent antibody may also be used for rapid detection of the presence of a virus such as CMV in tissue culture. By centrifuging urine onto tissue culture monolayers and staining at 24 to 36 hours after inoculation, this virus may be detected without waiting many days for cytopathogenic effect (CPE) to develop (Table 42.9; Figure 42.6).[11] Many laboratories have had difficulty obtaining positive results with the

rapid method. In part, this resulted from the unavailability commercially of monoclonal antibodies to immediate early and delayed early antigens induced by CMV infection. Fortunately there now are several good commercial sources. The other problems have resulted from a failure to adhere strictly to the recommended procedure, especially the use of MRC-5 cells.[11] When the rapid assay is correctly performed it is approximately 90% sensitive when compared with standard tissue culture. On the other hand, standard tissue culture may be negative in 10% of cases where the rapid procedure is positive. Because of these findings, it is prudent to do both procedures on critical samples, for example, biopsies, lavages, and blood, and to perform the rapid procedure alone on urines where multiple samples are often submitted on the same patient. It remains to be proven whether the rapid technique for CMV can be applied to other viruses, for example, influenza. It has been utilized for HSV cultures, but since this virus grows so rapidly anyway (often 1 to 2 days), it seems unnecessary to resort to the more time-consuming "rapid" method. Immunoperoxidase tests have also been used for detection of HSV in tissue culture.[18,20]

42.4.b. Solid-phase immunoassays for detection of viral antigen. Solid-phase immunoassays (SPIAs) for the detection of antigens or antibodies use, as an indicator, a radioactive label (for radioimmunoassay [RIA]) or the action of an enzyme label on a substrate (for enzyme-linked immunosorbent assay [ELISA]). Several excellent reviews on these procedures and their application to viral diagnosis have been published. Chapters 10 and 12 describe the principles of such methods.

SPIA techniques have been successfully applied to the detection of hepatitis B, rotavirus, hepatitis A antibody, adenovirus, HSV, RSV, influenza A virus, CMV, and group A coxsackievirus. Commercial

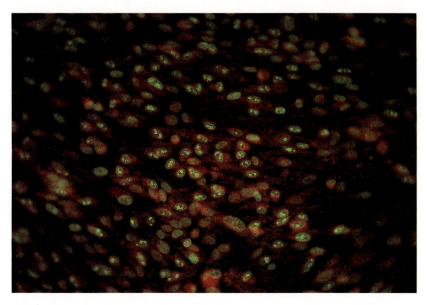

Figure 42.6
Monoclonal antibody to early and immediate early antigen of CMV stained in tissue culture at 36 hours.

kits are available for the detection of rotaviruses as well as hepatitis B surface antigen (HBsAg), hepatitis B surface antibody (HBsAb), hepatitis B core antibody (HBcAb), Hepatitis A virus (HAV), HAV-IgM, and HAV-IgG. ELISA techniques are more sensitive for the detection of rotavirus than is electron microscopy (EM), especially if weakly positive reactions are ignored.[25] In contrast, detection of influenza virus type A antigen by ELISA was only 53% as sensitive as by culturing.[12] Similarly, detection of adenovirus was only 62%, and there were 8% false-positive results.[12] Fluid specimens are most appropriate for detection of viral antigens by ELISA. Serum may be used directly in the test; urine and feces may need homogenization with saline and preliminary clarification by centrifugation to be suitable for the test. Nasopharyngeal or sputum specimens should be collected in appropriate transport media and diluted 1:5 to a final concentration of 20% in N-acetyl-L-cysteine before use in the test.

Enzyme immunoassays provide the advantage of relatively stable and nonradioactive reagents, and the results can be either qualitative or quantitative (Figure 42.7). ELISAs are usually more sensitive than all other assays except RIA. The equipment necessary for ELISAs can be quite simple and objective. Also, ELISA assays lend themselves to au-

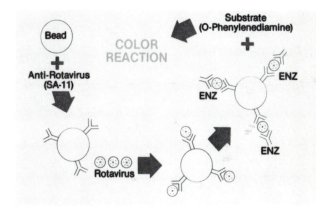

Figure 42.7
Enzyme immunoassay (Rotazyme, Abbott Laboratories) for rotavirus.

tomation. The major drawback of all SPIAs is that the quality, that is, the presence of adequate cellular material, of specimens, such as respiratory, genital, or skin swabs, cannot be assessed. This is in marked contrast to IF. Specific disadvantages of ELISAs include the variability of solid-phase carriers and the carcinogenicity of certain chromogenic substrates. RIAs require expensive equipment and also involve exposure to carcinogens. In addition, disposing of these hazardous materials poses considerable diffi-

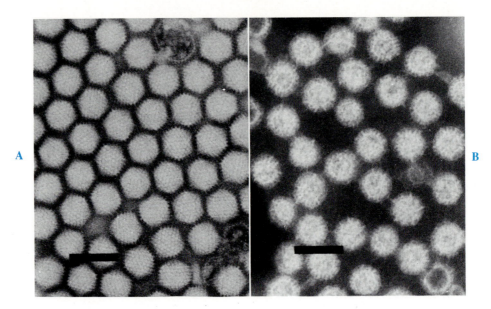

Figure 42.8
Electron micrographs of viruses visualized in feces from patients with diarrhea. **A**, Adenovirus.
B, Rotavirus.

culty. Most SPIAs also require a day or overnight incubation with several washing procedures. For the optimal use of SPIAs in rapid viral diagnosis, several specimens should be examined for antigen in a given run. Thus these techniques are best suited for diseases such as viral gastroenteritis, viral hepatitis, or respiratory infections, in which many specimens are being submitted to the laboratory at a given time. Although a single specimen could be analyzed, quite often an alternative assay (IF, EM, for example) might be more appropriate.

42.5. Nucleic Acid Hybridization

Nucleic acid hybridization techniques for the detection of viral nucleic acids in clinical specimens have been described recently. CMV has been successfully identified in urine by dot blot hybridization (Chapter 10), but this method is less sensitive (although more rapid) than tissue culture.[4] The converse has been reported in blood samples where dot blot hybridization was positive in samples negative by culture, although the specificity of this procedure needs to be confirmed.[22] RNA viruses, specifically rotaviruses, have also been detected by a dot hybridization assay of fecal samples,[9] but the sensitivity and specificity of this procedure must also be established. The relative insensitivity of DNA probes derives

from several obstacles that may be difficult to overcome, including (1) low specific activity, (2) cross-hybridization of the probe with human cellular DNA, (3) nonspecific binding of carrier, that is, vector DNA, to the target viral host DNA, and, possibly, (4) viral strain variation with sufficient genomic mutation for the prevention of probe hybridization. RNA probes have been used to detect complementary DNA of papillomaviruses in cervix samples. This may become the procedure of choice for those viruses since they do not grow in tissue culture.

42.6. Electron Microscopy (EM)

Several reviews of the procedures and utility of EM in diagnostic virology have been published. Relatively few viral diagnostic laboratories have or utilize EM because it can be relatively labor-intensive and insensitive, and alternative simpler procedures can frequently be employed. For example, EM was initially necessary to detect rotavirus in stool but rotavirus antigen assays are suitable alternatives.[1,3,5,14] EM techniques are most applicable for the investigation of viral infections in which the titer of virus in specimens is at least 10^6 to 10^7 particles per milliliter. EM is most commonly utilized for feces examination since rotaviruses as well as adenoviruses, coronaviruses, and caliciviruses may be seen and identified as the cause of the illness (Figure 42.8). The Norwalk agent virus, an important cause of gastroenteritis, is not easily visible by standard EM in feces, and it usually requires enhancement by immune EM to permit detection. Immune EM allows visualization of virus particles that may be present in numbers too small for easy direct detection. The addition of specific antiserum to the test suspension causes the virus particles to form antibody-bound aggregates, which are more easily detected by EM than are single virus particles. Other specimens, such as vesicle fluid, biopsy tissue, solid wart tissue, urine, or serum, can be negatively stained with minimum preparation to yield positive results. If concentrations of viruses are lower in these specimens or others, techniques to enhance visualization are necessary. Enhancement techniques may include pseudoreplication, agar gel diffusion, ultracentrifugation, or immune EM.

42.7. Viral Serology

Up to about a decade ago, serology was utilized as a primary procedure in diagnosing viral infections. More recently, this approach has been replaced in many cases by methods designed to detect the viral agents or their antigens as quickly as possible. However, several situations still exist in which serologic diagnosis can be extremely helpful. These are outlined in Table 42.10.

Certain viruses, for example, hepatitis A and B, rubella, measles, and coronaviruses, are difficult to isolate in tissue culture, and infections caused by them are best diagnosed serologically as discussed here and in Chapter 12. Arboviruses, which cause some types of encephalitis, require suckling mice for isolation; serologic techniques are also the most practical means for diagnosing infections with these viruses (in this chapter, the term "arbovirus" is used in preference to the more correct toga- or bunyavirus because of its familiarity). Serologic studies, especially complement fixation, are much less useful in infants, who may not mount an antibody response detectable by this method.

In practice, we encourage the submission of an acute-phase serum specimen in all patients suspected of having a viral illness. A convalescent serum specimen is requested only if a virus etiology has not been established by culture or other methods.

The specifics of the wide variety of serologic testing procedures cannot be detailed in this chapter but can be found in reference texts such as that edited by Lennette and Schmidt (Bibliography) and in Chapter 12.

Serologic tests in present use include complement fixation (CF), neutralization (Neut), hemagglutination inhibition (HI), passive hemagglutination (PHA), indirect fluorescent antibody (IFA), immune adherence hemagglutination (IAHA), immunoelectron microscopy (IEM), counterimmunoelectrophoresis (CIE), radioimmunoassay (RIA), enzyme-linked immunosorbent assay (ELISA), fluorescent-focus inhibition (FFI), anticomplement immunofluorescence (ACIF), and single radial hemolysis (SRH). Each of these tests can be adapted to demonstrate antibody response or to identify a particular agent.

42.7.a. Tests available. Complement fixation (CF) is a highly satisfactory serologic test. Antibodies measured by this system generally develop slightly later in the course of an illness than those measured by other techniques; this lag provides a greater opportunity to demonstrate titer differences between acute and convalescent sera. Members of some virus groups, such as the adenoviruses, influenza A viruses, and influenza B viruses, possess common antigens demonstrable by complement fixation. Thus, antibody response to infection by any member of the particular group can be observed without resorting to a multiplicity of tests with individual antigens. Unfortunately other members of large virus groups such as enteroviruses do not possess a common antigen and must be tested individually.

The neutralization test (Neut) is essentially a protection test. When a virus is incubated with homologous type-specific antibody, the virus is rendered incapable of producing infection in an indicator host system. The test is technically more exacting than other serologic tests and is the principal method used for identifying virus isolates. A neutralizing antibody response is virus-type-specific and develops with the onset of symptoms. Titers peak rapidly to a plateau and persist for long intervals, and measurable titers may be maintained indefinitely.

The hemagglutination inhibition test (HI) can be performed with a variety of viruses that have the capacity to agglutinate selectively red blood cells of various animal species (chicken, guinea pig, human O group, and others). The hemagglutination capacity of a virus is inhibited by specific immune or con-

Table 42.10

Situations Where Serologic Testing Can Be Helpful

SITUATION	VIRUSES UNDER CONSIDERATION	COMMON METHODS OF CHOICE*
AIDS	Human immunodeficiency virus (HIV)	ELISA, Western blot, IFA
CNS infections	Western equine encephalitis	HI, CF
	Eastern equine encephalitis	HI, CF
	California encephalitis virus	HI, CF, CIE
	St. Louis encephalitis virus	HI, CF
	Lymphocytic choriomeningitis virus	CF, IFA
	Measles	HI, CF
	Epstein-Barr virus	IFA
	Rabies	IFA, FFI, CF
Exanthems	Measles	HI, CF, Neut
	Rubella	HI, SRH, ELISA, RIA
	Parvovirus	CIE, ELISA
Vesicular	Herpes simplex virus	CF, IFA
	Varicella-zoster virus	IFA, IAHA, RIA, ELISA
Hepatitis A	Hepatitis A virus	ELISA, RIA, RIA(IgM)
Hepatitis B	Hepatitis B virus	ELISA
Heterophile-negative infectious mononucleosis syndromes	Cytomegalovirus	IFA, ACIF, PHA, ELISA, CF
	Epstein-Barr virus	IFA, ELISA
Myocarditis-pericarditis	Group B coxsackievirus, types 1-5	Neut
	Influenza A, B	HI, CF
	Cytomegalovirus	IFA, ACIF, PHA, ELISA, CF
Respiratory	Influenza A, B	CF
	Respiratory syncytial virus	
	Parainfluenza 1-3	
	Adenovirus	
	(Also, *M. pneumoniae, Chlamydia*)	
Serology needed to determine immune status (single serum)		
Rubella		HI, SRH, ELISA, RIA
Hepatitis B		RIA, PHA, ELISA
Varicella-zoster		IFA, IAHA, RIA, ELISA

*Neut = neutralizing antibody; RIA = radioimmunoassay; HI = hemagglutination inhibition; CF = complement fixation; CIE = counterimmunoelectrophoresis; IFA = indirect immunofluorescence; FFI = fluorescent-focus inhibition; SRH = single radial hemolysis; PHA = passive hemagglutination; IAHA = immune adherence hemagglutination; ELISA = enzyme-linked immunosorbent assay; ACIF = anticomplement immunofluorescence.

valescent serum. Hemagglutination-inhibiting antibody develops rapidly after the onset of symptoms, plateaus rapidly, declines slowly, and may last indefinitely at low levels.

In the passive hemagglutination (PHA) procedure, certain viruses can be chemically coupled to the surface of erythrocytes, which then serve as indicators of the presence of homologous antibody in serum by the hemagglutination reaction.

For the indirect fluorescent antibody test (**IFA**), virus-infected cells are placed in prepared wells on microscope slides, and then fixed in cold acetone and dried. Serum antibody is applied and, following incubation for antigen-antibody coupling, anti-human globulin-fluorescein conjugate is added to delineate, by fluorescence, the sites of antigen-antibody reaction. It is possible to identify specifically a virus in any adequately prepared specimen

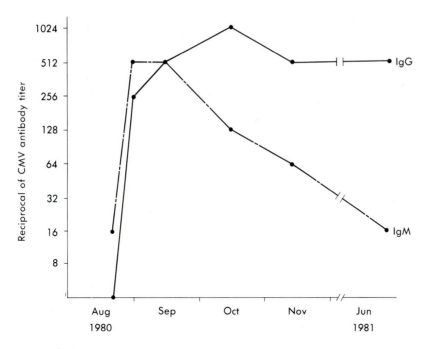

Figure 42.9
Time course of CMV IgM antibody.

containing virus-infected cells, but the current lack of high-titer, specific antisera limits the usefulness of this method.

42.7.b. Interpretation of viral serologic tests

Acute-phase serum. When a virological workup is planned for an individual patient, it is generally useful to obtain at least 2 to 3 ml of acute-phase serum and store it in the freezer. This may become valuable, particularly if virus detection subsequently fails or the interpretation of an isolate is equivocal. In these instances a convalescent-phase serum may be requested 2 to 3 weeks after the first, and appropriate selection of antigens to be tested can be made.

Single sera. In some cases, a single serum may be studied and appropriately interpreted. Virus-specific immunoglobulin M (IgM) antibody usually rises during the first 2 to 3 weeks of infection and persists for several weeks to months, eventually becoming replaced by IgG antibody (Figure 42.9). Thus, an elevated titer of specific IgM antibody suggests a recent primary infection by the virus in question, and this may be further supported by demonstrating a fall in IgM antibody in follow-up sera. Detection of specific IgM has been used with success in the di-

agnosis of infections due to VZV, Epstein-Barr virus (EBV), CMV, rubella, and coxsackieviruses and is currently the procedure of choice for establishment of a recent or acute infection due to hepatitis A or B (hepatitis A IgM and IgM antibody to hepatitis B core antigen, respectively). The methods to be employed in IgM-specific antibody determination vary considerably, including sucrose density gradient centrifugation, column chromatography, staphylococcal protein A absorption, and solid-phase immunoassays such as IF, ELISA, and RIA. These methods vary in sensitivity, convenience, and applicability. Several limitations of interpretation must be kept in mind. It is now recognized that IgM-specific antibody responses are not always restricted to primary infections; reactivation or reinfection may result in IgM responses, particularly in CMV, HSV, EBV, and VZV infections. In addition, patients may continue to produce IgM-specific antibody to rubella or CMV for many months after a primary infection. Heterotypic IgM responses can also occur; for example, antibody responses to CMV in EBV infections and vice versa. Other pitfalls include falsely low or negative IgM titers due to competition by IgG antibody for antigen-binding sites and false-positive reactions due to rheumatoid factor. Both these errors appear to be most common in solid-phase assays employing IF.

Both false-negative and false-positive IgM fluorescent antibody results have been frequently encountered in screening sera from newborns for specific antibody to CMV and rubella virus. In some, but not all, cases, false-positive results can be attributed to rheumatoid factor of maternal origin. False-negative results might occur as a result of competition between high levels of maternal IgG and low levels of fetal IgM in cord sera.

Other uses of single sera include screening infant blood for certain antibodies of the IgG class, known popularly as the TORCH screen. Antibody to *Toxoplasma gondii (To)*, rubella *(r)*, CMV *(c)*, and HSV *(h)* is measured in an effort to determine possible congenital infection with these agents; however, the utility of these tests has been misunderstood (also discussed in Chapter 12). They are more useful in excluding a possible infection than in proving an etiology. If, for example, rubella antibody is absent, then the infant almost certainly does not have congenital rubella infection. To diagnose active rubella infection in such a baby, viral cultures and additional serologic studies are required. Other uses of single sera include CMV antibody screening to eliminate the transmission of CMV antibody–positive blood to seronegative babies or other immunocompromised patients and rubella antibody screening to identify women requiring vaccination.

If there is adequate knowledge of the specific levels of antibody titers achieved in individuals during acute infection and afterward, the height of a titer in a single serum sample may aid in a presumptive diagnosis of recent infection. For example, hemagglutination-inhibition antibody titer of 1:160 or greater to western equine encephalitis or St. Louis encephalitis virus or a complement fixation titer of 1:128 or greater to influenza B virus would be supportive of a recent experience with the agent. However, it is important to remember that such interpretive criteria cannot be applied to all infections, since titers to many viruses can persist at varying levels. Thus, titers in single sera must be interpreted cautiously in most cases.

False-positive serologic results. The majority of serologic interpretations are based upon conversion from seronegativity to positivity or a fourfold or greater rise in antibody titer between paired sera.

However, such apparently significant antibody titer rises may not always be significant. An example of this is the occasional rise of antibody to CMV in patients with influenza A or *Mycoplasma pneumoniae* infections, suggesting stress reactivation of CMV by the latter agents. False-positive serologic responses may also result from cross-reactions to related antigens; for example, an antibody rise to parainfluenza virus may actually result from infection with mumps virus. Also, anamnestic antibody responses may falsely suggest seroconversion or cause an apparent fourfold or greater rise in antibody titer.

42.7.c. Combinations of several serologic tests for diagnosis of clinical syndromes. Selection of antigens for testing with paired sera in cases where a virus is suspected but not detected can sometimes be made on the basis of clinical syndrome, the known local epidemiology of particular viruses, and the age of the patient. This has led to the concept of serologic "batteries" or "panels." Some examples of possible batteries are included in Table 42.10.

CNS syndromes. HSV, mumps, western equine encephalitis, eastern equine encephalitis, St. Louis encephalitis, and California encephalitis viruses and perhaps lymphocytic choriomeningitis virus and EBV may be included in a battery of tests for a central nervous system (CNS) syndrome. Although herpes simplex antigen is included in the panel, a rise in antibody titer is not sufficient to diagnose HSV encephalitis. A large share of viral CNS illness, especially aseptic meningitis, is caused by the enterovirus group, but the multiplicity of serotypes and the cumbersome serologic methods necessary for their diagnosis usually make it impractical to include them in a battery. When one or two enteroviruses have been shown to be epidemic in an area in one summer, it is possible to pick up some additional cases by carrying out neutralization tests on paired sera employing only the enterovirus or enteroviruses in question.

Respiratory syndromes. Depending upon the age of the patient, the antigen panel for testing respiratory syndromes might include influenza A and B, respiratory syncytial virus, parainfluenza 1, 2, and 3, and adenoviruses (and *M. pneumoniae* and *Chlamydia*). For example, respiratory syncytial virus and parainfluenza might be routinely tested for in infants and young children but not in adults.

Exanthems. To test for exanthems, an antigen battery would include measles and rubella. If the dis-

Table 42.11

Interpretation of Epstein-Barr Virus Serology

SITUATION	IgG-VCA	IgM-VCA	EA	EBNA
No past infection	−	−	−	−
Acute infection	+	+	+	−
Convalescent phase	+	+ or −	+ or −	+
Past infection	+	−	−	+
?Chronic or reactivation	+	−	+	+

ease is vesicular, HSV and VZV should be included.

Myocarditis-pericarditis. Antigens from group B coxsackievirus types 1 through 5 and perhaps influenza A and B viruses (depending upon epidemiologic circumstances) would make up the battery tested for myocarditis and pericarditis. Although there are numerous viruses that have been implicated in inflammatory diseases of the heart and its covering membranes, the group B coxsackieviruses types 1 through 5 have been considered to account for nearly 50% of the cases. Unfortunately, much of the clinical illness is expressed at a time when standard methods of virus detection are likely to fail, and serologic diagnosis must be attempted.

42.7.d. Special considerations: EBV, Hepatitis, AIDS. The full interpretation of serologic results may require testing for the presence of antibody to several different antigenic components of a single virus: two notable examples are EBV and hepatitis B. In those instances of EBV infections that cannot be diagnosed by the usual clinical criteria and heterophile antibody tests, the following specific IF antibody tests can be performed (Table 42.11):

1. IgG antibody to viral capsid antigen (VCA), which appears early in infection and usually persists for life
2. Antibody to early antigen (EA), which appears in most patients and persists only during the active phase of infection (weeks to months)
3. Antibody to EBV nuclear antigen (EBNA), detected by anticomplement IF, which appears 2 to 4 weeks after onset and usually persists for life

In the early phase of acute infection, IgM-specific VCA titers are usually elevated; however, reactivation of infection may also provoke a similar response. Presence of **both** VCA and EBNA antibody in an acute- or convalescent-phase serum suggests a past infection. Recent EBV infection is suggested by any of the following:

1. IgM antibody to VCA
2. Presence of VCA antibody and absence of EBNA
3. Rising titer of EBNA
4. Presence of elevated VCA and early antigen antibodies

Hepatitis. A specific diagnosis of hepatitis A, B, C, or non-A, non-B (NANB), and hepatitis D (delta) has considerable importance in determining prognosis and the use of immune globulin or vaccine or both. For example, if a patient with hepatitis A survives (as he usually does) he will not develop chronic viral liver disease and need not take immune serum globulin (ISG) for future travel or contact prophylaxis. His immediate contacts, however, should receive ISG if they have not previously been infected. In contrast, if a patient has acute hepatitis B, he has a risk of chronic liver disease and his sexual contacts should probably receive hepatitis B immune globulin (HBIG) and vaccine if they do not already have evidence of hepatitis B infection. Furthermore, he should be cautioned against blood donation and receiving ISG since delta hepatitis virus may be present in ISG lots. In patients with evidence of past hepatitis B infection, serologic tests for the delta agent may provide additional prognostic information.

Lastly, if tests for hepatitis A, B, C, and D are negative, a diagnosis of hepatitis NANB may be made. This, too, provides prognostic information since, if it is secondary to blood transfusion, significant chronic liver disease occurs in ≥50% of patients. Furthermore, ISG will not prevent disease in contacts, although it may induce a more benign course.

With these points in mind, the following is a summary of the tests that will assist in the diagnosis of the specific type of hepatitis.

The best test to document acute hepatitis A is the presence of hepatitis A–specific IgM antibody

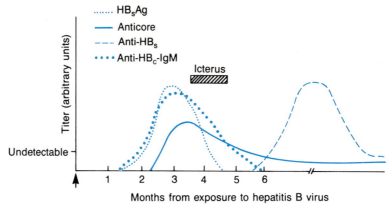

Figure 42.10

Representative antibody response in patient who recovers from acute hepatitis B infection.

in the patient's serum. To determine whether a patient has had hepatitis A in the past, a hepatitis A–specific IgG test should be obtained.

The most reliable distinguishing feature of acute hepatitis B is the presence of IgM anti-HBc in the blood of patients with this disease. This antibody is detected by a variety of immunological techniques, including ELISA and RIA. Chronic carriers of this virus are likely to have HBsAg in their blood (Figure 42.10). Approximately 0.1% of random blood donors are positive for HBsAg. Individuals who have been infected previously by hepatitis B virus and who have cleared the HBsAg have IgG antibody to hepatitis B surface antigen (anti-HBs) and hepatitis B core antibody (anti-HBc) in their serum, indicating that they are immune to repeat infection by this virus. Patients who have been vaccinated against hepatitis B will exhibit anti-HBs but not anti-HBc. Chronic hepatitis is suggested by the persistent presence of HBsAg and by the failure to develop IgG anti-HBs. These patients may also exhibit persistence of hepatitis "e" antigen and failure to develop antibody to this antigen.

The marker of acute hepatitis D is the presence of anti-delta IgM. Later in the course of developing chronic infection/disease, antidelta IgG antibody develops. Delta infection occurs only in patients who are HBsAg-positive, so this test should be ordered only in such patients.

Hepatitis NANB is diagnosed by exclusion, that is, when there are no markers of active infection by the hepatitis A, B, C, and D agents. The newly recognized agent of hepatitis C[18a] can be diagnosed

with molecular techniques. Only preliminary studies have been published.[3a]

AIDS. Human immunodeficiency virus (HIV) infection is most commonly documented by detection of antibody using ELISA or agglutination procedures for screening and more specific procedures (Western blot, IFA) for confirmation. The ELISA test measures antibody to one or more envelope proteins (glycoprotein [gp]120), Western blot assays determine the presence of antibody to each of several viral antigens including the core protein (p24). The IFA detects antibody directed at antigens expressed on the surface of infected cells. The presence of serum antibody does not label a patient as having acquired immunodeficiency syndrome (AIDS). The latter is a clinical diagnosis that depends upon symptomatology, signs, and other laboratory tests. The antibody test does confirm that an individual with clinical findings has been infected by HIV and supports the impression that his illness is due to the virus. The antibody test is also used to identify individuals who may transmit infection to others, for example, by blood or organ donors, pregnant women, and sex partners. HIV antibody may develop slowly, requiring 4 to 8 weeks in most patients but 6 months or more in up to 5% of those infected. Newer serologic tests using HIV antigens derived by genetic engineering techniques may provide more sensitive tests that are consistently positive shortly after infection. Measurement of specific antibodies to differing HIV antigens may have prognostic utility and may assist in "staging" a patient. For example, in early infection, p24 antibody appears as HIV enters into latency. Later this antibody dimishes as p24 antigen reappears and the process of viral replication resumes.

Early detection of viral nucleic acid in infected peripheral blood lymphocytes has been accomplished with **polymerase chain reaction (PCR)** methods, which may gain more widespread use in the future. PCR has proved to be particularly sensitive for detecting HIV infections in neonates.

P24 antigen can be detected in the serum of up to 60% of patients with HIV infection and indicates that active viral replication is probably occurring. This antigen is detectable during acute HIV infection and then disappears as the virus enters the latent proviral state. Its reappearance signifies the resumption of viral replication and is a bad prognostic sign.

Culture of HIV is more difficult than for many other viruses of human importance. The virus is cell-associated, so that peripheral blood mononuclear cells (PBMCs) are better specimens for culture than is serum or plasma. The usual tissue culture cells used for viral isolation culture in a clinical virology laboratory do not support the growth of HIV. The optimum culture system is to use PBMC from HIV-uninfected donors in coculture with the patient's PBMCs. Further, these donor cells should be blast-transformed by exposure to mitogens. While CPE may occur, detection of the virus in tissue culture is classically accomplished by measuring the appearance of reverse transcriptase in the medium. This assay is being replaced by the detection of viral antigens (p24) in the medium, which appear after 5 or more days in culture. Culture appears to detect even latent virus since the procedure will activate provirus. When carefully performed, culture is positive in the great majority of antibody-positive individuals.

42.8. Viral Culture

Tissue culture recovery of viruses can be rapid especially if viral antigens are detected prior to the development of CPE.

42.8.a. Laboratory equipment. Necessary equipment includes the following items:

1. A 35° C aerobic incubator equipped to hold at least two roller drum racks and with sufficient shelf space to store a week's supply of cell cultures.
2. Two or three roller drums with motor-driven bases to rotate the drums.
3. An inverted microscope with $4\times$ and $10\times$ objectives to examine the cell culture flasks and tubes.
4. An ultracold freezing unit $(-70°\ C)$ to store reagents, antigens, and other materials.
5. A laminar flow hood (Chapter 2) in which to carry out cell culture procedures.
6. A conventional horizontal head centrifuge.
7. Refrigerator $(4°\ C)$ with $-20°\ C$ freezer for reagent and media storage.
8. Fluorescent microscope.

Other equipment includes vortex mixers, a 56° C water bath, a vibrating platform, electric pipetters, and a sonic oscillator (helpful but not essential). Many of these items can be shared with other sections of the laboratory.

The remaining equipment is minor and includes such items as disposable pipettes, assorted glassware, hemacytometer, plastic cell culture flasks, and membrane filtration units, along with the usual furnishings for storage of laboratory requisitions and other records.

42.8.b. Selection of specimens for viral culture. Selection of appropriate specimens is complicated since several different viruses may cause the same clinical disease (Table 42.12). For example, several different types of specimens may be submitted from patients with CNS disease: CSF (enterovirus, mumps virus, and perhaps herpes simplex virus [HSV type 2]); throat (enterovirus); stool or rectal swab (enterovirus). In addition, blood should be collected as an acute-phase specimen in case subsequent serologic tests are necessary (mumps virus, HSV, arbovirus). Many considerations, however, allow the clinician to select the most appropriate specimens. For example, during the summer, when enteroviral meningitis is prevalent, throat and stool specimens should certainly be submitted, in addition to CSF. On the other hand, the development of encephalitis in children after the acquisition of several mosquito bites in wooded areas endemic for California encephalitis virus would suggest that a blood specimen for antibody testing would be optimal. Further examples include CNS disease following parotitis (urine and CSF specimens for mumps virus) or a focal encephalitis with a temporal lobe localization preceded by headaches and disorientation (brain biopsy for HSV). In respiratory syndromes it is generally necessary to submit only a throat or nasopharyngeal specimen; stool and urine

Table 42.12
Appropriate Specimens for Viral Isolation*

SYNDROMES AND PROBABLE VIRAL AGENTS	THROAT/ NASOPHARYNX	STOOL	CSF	URINE	OTHER
Respiratory syndrome	+ + + +				
Adenoviruses					
Enteroviruses					
Influenza virus					
Parainfluenza virus					
Respiratory syncytial virus (RSV)					
Rhinoviruses					+ + + nasal
Dermatologic and mucous membrane disease	+				+ + + +
Vesicular					
Enterovirus (hand-foot-and-mouth syndrome)	+ +	+ + +			+ + + (Vesicle fluid or scraping)
Herpes simplex†					
Varicella-zoster†	+ +				
Exanthematous	+ +				
Enterovirus		+ + +			
Measles‡					
Rubella‡					
Parvovirus					Serum for antigen detection
Meningoencephalitis	+ +		+ + +		
Arboviruses					
Enteroviruses		+ + + +			
Herpes simplex					(Brain biopsy)
Lymphocytic choriomeningitis§					
Mumps virus					
Gastrointestinal		+ +			
Adenoviruses‡					
Parvovirus‡					
Rotavirus‖					
Congenital and perinatal	+ +	+	+ +		+ +
Cytomegalovirus				+ + +	(Blood)
Enteroviruses					
Herpes simplex virus					(Vesicle fluid)
Eye syndrome					+ + + +
Adenoviruses	+ +				(Conjunctival swab or scraping)
Herpes simplex virus					
Vaccinia virus					
Varicella-zoster virus					
(Chlamydiae¶)					
CMV infection	+ +			+ + + +	+
Cytomegalovirus (CMV)					(Blood)
Myocarditis, pericarditis, and pleurodynia	+ +	+ + + +			+
Coxsackie B					(Pericardial fluid)

*Specimens indicated beside the disease categories should be obtained in all instances; others should be obtained if the specific virus is suspected.

†Direct fluorescent antibody studies are available for herpes simplex virus and varicella-zoster.

‡Best diagnosed by EM since the adenoviruses responsible for gastroenteritis are not culturable by standard techniques.

§Best diagnosed serologically.

‖Best diagnosed by antigen detection or EM.

¶Chlamydiae were once considered viruses because they are obligate intracellular parasites. They are included here because they can be isolated in cell culture. (See Chapter 38.)

Summary of Procedures for Obtaining and Transporting Specimens for Viral Studies

General

Do not freeze specimens. Obtain specimens as early in the patient's illness as possible. Inoculate tissue cultures at patient's bedside if possible.

Throat

Swab inflamed area. Use Culturette swab (Becton-Dickinson) as for bacteriologic culture.

Nasopharynx

Obtain a nasopharyngeal swab or a nasal wash specimen using a bulb syringe or a suction apparatus and 3-7 ml buffered saline.

Stool

Obtain as for bacteriologic culture. If a specimen cannot be passed, a rectal swab of feces may be obtained with a Culturette.

Cerebrospinal fluid (CSF)

Obtain 1 ml as for bacteriologic culture.

Urine

Obtain a clean-voided specimen (10-20 ml) as for bacteriologic culture and transport in sterile screw-capped tube.

Skin or mucosal lesion

Use Culturette swab to obtain vesicle fluid and scrape cells from base of lesion.

Biopsy material

Use aseptic technique and submit in a sterile container (e.g., urine container).

Blood for culture

Submit at least 3 ml of heparinized blood (green-top Vacutainer tube, Becton-Dickinson). Some laboratories prefer citrated blood because of evidence suggesting that heparin has antiviral properties.

Blood for serologic studies

Submit at least 5 ml of clotted whole blood (red-top Vacutainer tube). In certain viral syndromes (e.g., lower respiratory) an acute-phase specimen should be submitted. If a virus is not isolated, a convalescent specimen should be obtained at least 7 days after the acute specimen. Certain viral illnesses (e.g., rubella, rubeola, hepatitis, and arbovirus encephalitis) are diagnosed most readily by serologic studies.

Transportation

Transport specimens as rapidly as possible, using a messenger service. Specimens should be stored and transported at refrigerator temperature (4° C). Do not freeze. If transportation of swabs will be delayed, place them in a tube of buffered bacteriologic broth medium rather than in the Culturette.

---

isolates would be irrelevant. The procedures for obtaining and transporting specimens for viral studies are summarized in the box. Other considerations follow.

Throat, nasopharyngeal swab, aspirate. For recovering viruses, nasopharyngeal aspirates are superior to swabs, but the latter are considerably more convenient. Throat swabs are probably adequate for recovering entero- and adenoviruses and HSV, whereas nasopharyngeal specimens are definitely superior for recovering respiratory syncytial virus and probably better for parainfluenza viruses. Nasal specimens are optimal for recovering rhinoviruses.

Rectal swabs and stool specimens. Most cases of viral gastroenteritis are now known to be due to viruses that cannot be cultivated in cell cultures. Fecal specimens from such cases may be examined for nonculturable agents, for example, rotavirus, by EM or by antigen detection (see Section 42.4.b). Stool cultures are useful in patients suspected of having enterovirus disease, for example, aseptic meningitis, myopericarditis, and hand-foot-and-mouth disease. Enteroviruses in the feces of such patients support the possibility but do not definitely prove that these agents are causing the illness. Available evidence indicates that stool specimens are more productive than rectal swabs. Generally, infectivity of viruses that are surrounded by a lipid membrane (for example, HSV and CMV) is destroyed by gastric acidity, and therefore they will not be excreted in active form in the feces.

Urine. CMV, mumps, and adenovirus are the viruses most frequently recovered from urine by the laboratory. In cases of CNS disease due to mumps, the virus can be isolated from urine when specimens from other sites are negative. The recovery of CMV from urine is increased twofold to threefold by processing several specimens. Urine specimens submitted for culture of CMV can be inoculated directly into cell cultures. Alternatively, they may be centrifuged, and either the supernatant urine or the sediment, resuspended in a small volume, can be used as inoculum. Recent studies indicate that centrifuging the urine onto the tissue culture monolayer is the best of all these procedures.[11]

Generally, examination of the urine sediment for cytomegalic inclusion-bearing cells is not a sensitive method for diagnosing CMV infections. Viral isolation is at least four times more sensitive in both infants and adults than is examination of urine sediment.

Dermal lesions. Fluid and cells from vesicles are superior to specimens from ulcers or crusts for both culture and direct stains.

"Sterile" fluids. CSF and other "sterile" fluids, for example, pleural, peritoneal, pericardial, and joint fluids, should be inoculated as quickly as possible into tissue culture.

Eye. A nasopharyngeal swab may be used to obtain secretions from the palpebral conjunctiva. Eye scrapings should be obtained by an ophthalmologist or other trained person.

Blood. Viremia may be present in symptomatic severe viral infections, for example, AIDS, severe CMV infection. Leukocytes, in which these and other viruses reside, may be collected more efficiently by a Ficoll-Hypaque-Macrodex sedimentation technique than by the conventional buffy coat method (Procedure 42.2). Anticoagulated blood or a clot can be used for isolation of arboviruses, and serum is suitable for recovering enteroviruses.

Tissue. Tissue explants and cells grown in cell cultures after dispersal of the cells from tissue fragments have provided higher rates of viral isolation than homogenized specimens. Presumably, viral inhibitors may be released into the homogenate, resulting in lower recovery rates in the disrupted cells. Lung (CMV, influenza virus, adenovirus) and brain (HSV) are the most productive tissue sources for viral isolates. As with urine sediment, the cytological detection of CMV inclusions in tissue is at least three to six times less sensitive than viral isolation.

• • •

Proper timing of specimen collection is essential for adequate recovery of viruses. Specimens should be collected early in the acute phase of infection. Studies with respiratory viruses indicate that the mean duration of viral shedding may be 3 to 7 days. Also, HSV and VZV may not be recovered from lesions beyond 5 days after onset. Isolation of an enterovirus from the CSF may be possible only within 2 to 3 days after onset of the CNS manifestations.

42.8.c. Transport of specimens to the laboratory. The shorter the interval between collection of a specimen and its delivery to the laboratory, the greater the potential for isolating an agent. When feasible, inoculate all specimens other than blood, feces, and tissue into culture tubes at the patient's bedside. These are then transported to the laboratory promptly. Any material may be used for swabs; however, calcium alginate may inactivate HSV. In general, the following statements hold, but there may be a few exceptions:

1. Never leave a specimen at room or incubator temperature.
2. When it is impossible to deliver a specimen immediately, it should be refrigerated and packed in shaved ice for delivery to the laboratory within 12 hours of collection.

Several types of media have been used for the transport of viral specimens. Most of these have been selected for this purpose based either on tradition or on data obtained by testing the survival of laboratory strains of virus. A recent double-blind prospective study to compare the recovery of viruses from the upper respiratory tracts or dermal lesions of children, using three types of transport media, showed no statistically significant differences between modified Stuart's (Appendix A), modified Hanks', or Leibovitz-Emory media.[15] It is generally believed that protein (serum, albumin, gelatin) incorporated into a transport medium enhances

PROCEDURE 42.2

Blood Specimens

Principle

Presence of HSV or CMV in blood is often diagnostic of active systemic infection. To optimize the recovery of virus, both mononuclear and polymorphonuclear (PMN) leukocytes, which make up the "buffy coat," should be harvested. Two methods are presented here. One is a modification of the Ficoll-Hypaque (F-H) and Macrodex procedures described by Howell et al.,[13] in which the mononuclear and PMN leukocyte fractions are harvested separately. The other method, described by Zaia et al.,[26] uses dextran (Macrodex) to separate red blood cells (RBCs) from all other cells in the peripheral blood and then uses the resultant cell pellet derived from the plasma as the inoculum. The dextran method was described for, and has been used primarily in, bone marrow transplant populations. Preliminary evidence (in my laboratory) suggests that in patient populations with normal white blood cell and platelet counts, this method may lead to increased toxicity to the cell monolayer.

Method

1. Pipette 5 ml anticoagulated blood and 5 ml sterile phosphate-buffered saline (PBS) into a sterile 15-ml conical centrifuge tube. Mix by gentle inversion.
2. Aspirate approximately 2.5 ml F-H and place into a second sterile conical 15-ml tube.
3. Using a Pasteur pipette, gently layer the diluted blood over the F-H.
4. Centrifuge at $400 \times g$ for 30 min at room temperature with brake off.
5. Handle the layers in the tube as follows:
   a. Plasma layer (top layer): Carefully aspirate and discard the plasma layer, leaving a small amount of the plasma layer above the mononuclear cell layer (this contains lymphocytes, monocytes, and some platelets).
   b. Mononuclear cell layer (second layer from top; only visible band): Harvest this layer. Gently and carefully aspirate the layer and transfer to a sterile 15-ml centrifuge tube. Let stand.
   c. F-H layer (third layer from top): Discard.
   d. RBC and PMN layer (bottom layer): Note the volume. Using a 5-ml pipette, slowly aspirate the layer and place into a sterile 15-ml tube containing 2.5 ml sterile Macrodex solution. A cell pellet will remain, containing some RBCs and PMNs. Add an equal volume of Eagle's minimal essential medium (EMEM) + 5% fetal calf serum (FCS) (PBS may be substituted for EMEM) to the cell pellet. Gently resuspend the pellet and transfer this suspension into the tube containing the Macrodex and RBC-PMN suspension. Allow tube to stand for 2 h. Draw off supernatant and place in separate sterile 15-ml tube. Discard the sediment.
6. Centrifuge both the tube containing the PMN cell fraction and the tube containing the mononuclear cell fraction at 800 to 900 × g for 15 min at room temperature. Aspirate and discard the supernatant. Resuspend each pellet in 10 ml EMEM + 5% FCS by flicking the tube several times.
7. If there is no obvious RBC contamination in either tube, proceed to step 8. If obvious RBC contamination is present in either tube, add 10 ml cold lysing buffer and incubate at 4° C for 30 min. Turn the tube upside down 2 to 3 times during incubation to resuspend any RBCs that may have sedimented to the bottom of the tube. Centrifuge at 800 to 900 × g for 15 min. Aspirate and discard the supernatant and proceed to step 8.
8. Resuspend the cell pellets by flicking the tubes several times. Add 10 ml EMEM or PBS. Centrifuge and repeat the wash 2 to 3 times with EMEM or PBS and resuspend in 2 ml EMEM + 1% FCS. (Shell vials may be inoculated separately with the two cell fractions, or the fractions may be combined during one of the previous wash steps.) Use 0.3 ml to inoculate each of three shell vials and two routine culture tubes.

the survival of viruses in transit; however, two studies have indicated that HSV survives as well in Stuart's or Hanks' protein-free medium.[24] The Culturette (Modified Stuart's Bacterial Transport Medium, Becton-Dickinson) appears to be satisfactory for short-term (that is, up to 4 hours) transport.

Improper storage can significantly reduce viral culture yields. After a freeze-thaw cycle, significant losses in infectivity titer occur with lipid-envelope viruses (HSV, CMV), but not with agents such as adenoviruses and enteroviruses, which have a coat of protein only. For example, a laboratory strain of HSV held for 1 to 3 days at $-20°$ C and then thawed had reductions in infectious titer of 10^2 or more. In contrast, when stored for 1 to 3 days at 4° C in Hanks' or broth medium, there was no loss of infectivity in two thirds of the specimens.[24] In another study only 3 of 45 (7%) strains of CMV failed to produce cytopathic effects after storage for 7 days at 4° C.[23] Storage at room temperature was unsatisfactory. Alternatively, once a specimen is received in the laboratory, cryoprotectants such as sorbitol may be added, but even then viral suspensions must be frozen and thawed under rigid conditions ($-70°$ C when freezing, 25° C/min when thawing) to achieve maximum recovery of the virus. Thus, for short-term (<5 days) transit or storage of specimens for viral culture, specimens should be held at 4° C rather than frozen.

Specific requirements for shipping specimens have been published by the United States Public Health Service (Fed. Reg., vol. 45, no. 141, 21 July 1980) and by the Department of Transportation and Interstate Quarantine regulations (49 CFR, Section 173.386.388, and 42 CFR, Section 72.25, Etiologic Agents). (See Chapter 2, Section 2.5.)

42.8.d. Media and cells used for viral isolation. Several kinds of cell culture systems are routinely used for isolation of viruses (also see Chapter 8). Cell cultures may be primary, low passage, or established cell lines. Primary cells, for example, monkey or human embryonic kidney, are most receptive to viruses after only one or two passages, whereas diploid fibroblast cells may remain virus-sensitive through 20 to 50 passages. Continuous cell lines such as Hep-2 are virus-sensitive even after hundreds of passages.

1. Primary Monkey Kidney. Primary monkey kidney (PMK) is an excellent system for recovery of myxoviruses and many enteroviruses and also may support growth of adenoviruses, respiratory syncytial viruses, and measles viruses. These cells are occasionally contaminated by simian viruses (most commonly SV5 and SV40), a problem minimized by the addition of antisera to these agents in the cell culture media.

2. Human fetal diploid (HFD), for example, foreskin fibroblasts (Figure 42.11). These fibroblastic cells have the dual advantages of being relatively inexpensive and susceptible to a broad spectrum of viruses. They are useful in the isolation of VZV, HSV, adenovirus, picornavirus, and RSV and are the only cells in which CMV is recovered.

3. Hep-2 continuous cell line. These epithelial cells, derived from a human cancer, are an excellent cell system for recovering adenovirus, HSV, and especially RSV.

The availability of commercial cell cultures and media greatly facilitates the work involved in virus isolation. If purchased commercially, upon arrival in the laboratory, tubes are examined microscopically. If an adequate monolayer of cells is present, the growth medium is replaced by 2 to 3 ml of fresh maintenance medium prior to storage at 35° C. If the monolayer is incomplete, the growth medium is replaced by 2 to 3 ml of fresh growth medium. HFD and Hep-2 cultures can be prepared in a clinical laboratory rather than purchased commercially.

The majority of clinically significant viruses can be recovered in the three cell systems described above. Specimens submitted for the isolation of viruses requiring other types of cell cultures (for example, coxsackie A, togaviruses) are forwarded to reference laboratories. Some laboratories prefer additional cell cultures such as RD (rhabdomyosarcoma) or BGM (continuous monkey kidney) for recovering coxsackie A and B viruses, respectively.

Two kinds of media, growth and maintenance, are used for cell culture. These media are prepared with Eagle's minimum essential medium (EMEM) in Earle's balanced salt solution (EBSS). Suppliers are listed in Appendix C, and formulas are given in Appendix A. Growth medium is a serum-rich nutrient medium designed to support rapid cell growth. We use this medium for initiating growth of Hep-2 cells in tubes or for feeding tubes or purchased tissue culture cells that have incomplete cell monolayers. Maintenance medium, on the other hand, is used to keep cells in a steady state of metabolism and is, therefore, less rich in growth factors such as serum.

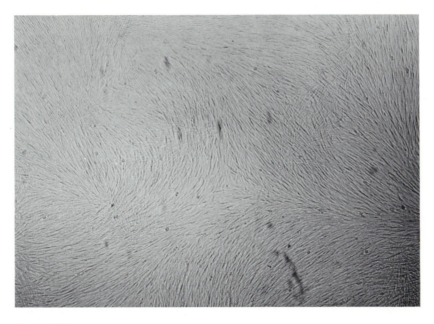

Figure 42.11
Foreskin fibroblast monolayer.

42.8.e. Specimen processing. Because specimens submitted for virus isolation are similar to those submitted for routine bacterial isolation, they can be inoculated in a bacteriology laboratory by the same technologist who handles all the other microbiology cultures. This system assures that viral cultures are set up promptly and that they are processed during evening shifts and on weekends.

Virus specimens are inoculated according to the guidelines presented in Table 42.13. In all cases the volume of fluid inoculated into a single tissue culture tube is 0.25 ml. If not inoculated directly at the patient's bedside, body fluids or swabs taken from sterile or minimally contaminated areas, such as the nasopharynx or throat, may be inserted directly into a tissue culture tube in the laboratory. The type of tissue culture used for this inoculation is selected according to the type of specimen, as outlined in Table 42.13.

After 30 minutes the swab is removed from the culture tube, and 0.25-ml aliquots of the tissue culture fluid from the tube are used as the inocula for additional necessary cultures. Swabs of specimens such as feces that are heavily contaminated with bacteria must first be treated with antibiotic-antifungal mixtures to reduce the chances of tissue culture contamination.

Inoculated cell cultures are transferred daily from the processing area to the virus laboratory where they are incubated at 35° C and examined daily for cytopathogenic effect (CPE) for a period of 10 to 14 days. CPE may be quantitated as follows:

± = < 25% of monolayer exhibits CPE
1+ = 25% of monolayer exhibits CPE
2+ = 50% of monolayer exhibits CPE
3+ = 75% of monolayer exhibits CPE
4+ = 100% of monolayer exhibits CPE

HFD cultures are kept at least 21 days to allow for the isolation of CMV. The longer incubation of these culture cells necessitates weekly media changes (see box on p. 667). Because toxic specimens such as stool, urine, and tissues can cause degeneration of monolayers, media must be changed the day following their inoculation.

Our laboratory does not make a practice of "blind passing" negative specimens. However, cell cultures that show nonspecific or ambiguous CPE are passed into appropriate cell systems by scraping the monolayer off the sides of the culture tube with a 1-ml pipette and inoculating 0.25 ml of the resulting suspension into new cell cultures. If CMV or VZV is suspected in a specimen, such passages should be made by trypsinizing the monolayer. Absence of CPE in the subpassages indicates that the initial changes were not caused by a virus.

Table 42.13
Laboratory Processing of Viral Specimens

SOURCE	SPECIMEN	PROCESSING*	TISSUE CULTURE
Blood	Heparinized blood	Obtain buffy coat by centrifuging at 2500 rpm for 10-15 min. Inoculate directly.	PMK, HFD, Hep-2
Cerebrospinal fluid (CSF)	1 ml CSF	Inoculate directly.	PMK, HFD, Hep-2
Feces (preferred to rectal swab)	Pea-sized aliquot of feces	Place in 2 ml of viral antibiotic mixture (Appendix A). Shake with mixer and hold at RT for 60 min. Centrifuge at 2500 rpm for 15 min and use supernatant fluid for inoculum.	PMK, HFD, Hep-2
Genital, skin	Culturette or swab in HFD tube	Insert swab in HFD tube for 30 min at RT. Use fluid from that tube to inoculate additional tubes.	PMK, Hep-2
Miscellaneous	Culturette, fluids	Swab: insert into PMK tube for 30 min at RT; use fluid from that tube to inoculate additional tubes. Fluid: inoculate directly.	PMK, HFD, Hep-2
Respiratory tract	Culturette, nasopharyngeal or throat swab or washings	Insert swab directly into PMK tube for 30 min at RT. Use fluid from that tube to inoculate additional tubes. If infant specimen, inoculate Hep-2 first.	PMK, HFD, Hep-2
Tissue	Tissue in sterile container	Mince with sterile scalpel and scissors. Prepare 20% suspension in viral antibiotic mixture (Appendix A) and grind with sterile sand. Centrifuge at 2500 rpm for 15 min and use supernatant fluid for inoculum.	PMK, HFD
Urine	Fresh refrigerated urine or frozen with equal volume of sterile 70% sorbitol in distilled water	Inoculate directly† into HFD. Also, treat 5-10 ml urine with 0.3 ml viral antibiotic mixture (Appendix A) for 60 min at RT. Centrifuge at 2500 rpm for 15 min. Discard all but 1 ml of the supernate, resuspend the sediment in the remaining fluid, and use for inoculum.	HFD, PMK (if mumps or adenovirus suspected)

RT = room temperature; PMK = primary monkey kidney; HFD = human fetal diploid.
*All inocula into tissue culture tubes are 0.25 ml volumes.
†Treatment of urine with antibiotics is not necessary for direct inoculation of HFD tube.

42.8.f. Isolation and identification of viruses. In addition to the rapid IFA assay for detecting viruses in tissue culture,[11] there are two standard procedures for detecting the presence of viruses in cell culture: (1) the observation of CPE and (2) hemadsorption/hemagglutination of guinea pig erythrocytes. Often determining the type, rapidity, and selectivity of CPE in cell cultures is enough to enable preliminary or final identification of an isolate.

Tubes of PMK inoculated with respiratory specimens are hemadsorbed routinely at 5 and 10 days after inoculation (or earlier if myxovirus-like CPE is detected) with a 0.4% suspension of guinea pig erythrocytes to aid detection of myxoviruses as de-

---

Changing Media

When changing inoculated tissue culture media, it is important to avoid cross-contamination between specimens. Different pipettes should be used to remove and to add media. Pipettes should also be changed between specimens. It might be helpful to set up a vacuum flask assembly to which the pipettes may be attached when removing media.

When changing uninoculated tissue culture media, one pipette may be used to remove the media and another to add it. Contamination of media with cells of different types should be avoided by using separate containers of media for changing one particular cell type.

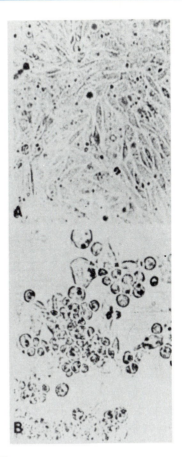

Figure 42.12
Herpes simplex virus cytopathic effect. *A*, normal cell monolayer. *B*, Infected cells.

---

scribed in Procedure 42.3. Hemadsorption may be performed at 3 days' postinoculation during periods of influenza virus prevalence to accelerate detection of this virus.

Examples of viruses that are frequently identifiable on initial isolation include HSV when it produces typical rapid CPE in HFD and Hep-2 cells, and CMV, a slow-growing virus that produces clusters of refractile cells only in human fibroblasts. Table 42.14 lists the viruses most commonly isolated in the clinical laboratory and the cell cultures in which they can be cultivated.

In this section the recognition and identification of these viruses are described. The reader is referred to standard textbooks[1,2] for additional information about these viruses and other less commonly isolated viruses.

Herpes simplex virus (HSV). HSV is the most frequently isolated virus in the clinical laboratory. It grows well in a variety of cell cultures, including HFD and epithelial cell lines such as Hep-2. CPE appears an average of 1 to 3 days after culture inoculation. Typically, the CPE begins in focal areas and may progress to involve the entire monolayer within 24 hours. Infected cells become enlarged "giant cells" and may clump together to form cellular clusters called syncytia (Figure 42.12). Type 2 HSV is especially prone to develop syncytia and in ad-

dition may produce CPE in PMK, a property not shared by type 1 HSV.

The necessity for confirming an isolate as HSV is controversial but may be achieved with specific fluorescent antisera as described in Procedure 42.4 or by an immunoperoxidase method. Fluorescein-conjugated antisera may also be used to identify HSV isolates as type 1 or 2, but the distinction is not always clear-cut.

Varicella-zoster virus (VZV). VZV is a member of the herpesvirus group. Occasionally VZV is confused with HSV because both are likely to be recovered from skin lesions and both can produce CPE in human fibroblasts. Usually the CPE produced by VZV is focal, spreads slowly, and appears several days later than that of HSV. The CPE is characterized by foci of enlarged refractile cells appearing 5 to 7 days after in-

Table 42.14

Cultivation and Identification of Commonly Isolated Viruses

VIRUS	PMK	HEP-2	HFD	CPE DESCRIPTION	RATE OF GROWTH (DAYS)	IDENTIFICATION AND COMMENTS
Adenovirus	+ +*	+ +	+ +	Rounding and aggregation of infected cells in grapelike clusters	2-10	Confirm by FA. Serotype by cell culture neutralization.
Cytomegalo-virus (CMV)	−	−	+ +	Discrete small foci of rounded cells.	5-21	Distinct CPE sufficient to identify. Cell-associated virus; requires trypsin for passage. Confirm by FA.
Enterovirus	+ + + +	±	+ +	Characteristic refractile angular or tear-shaped CPE; progresses to involve entire monolayer.	2-8	Identify by cell culture neutralization test with intersecting pools of hyperimmune sera. Stable at pH 3.
Herpes simplex (HSV)	± (type 2)	+ + + +	+ + + +	Rounded, swollen refractile cells. Occasional syncytia, especially with type 2. Rapidly involves entire monolayer.	1-3 (may take up to 7)	Ether, chloroform labile. Distinct CPE. Confirmation may be performed by FA.
Influenza	+ + + +	−	±	Destructive degeneration with swollen, vacuolated cells.	2-10	Detect by hemadsorption or hemagglutination with guinea pig RBCs. Identify by FA, HAD, or HI.†
Mumps	+ + +	±	±	CPE, usually absent. Occasionally syncytia are seen.	5-10	Detect by hemadsorption with guinea pig RBCs. Confirm by FA or HAD.
Parainfluenza (PIV)	+ + +	−	−	CPE is often minimal or absent. PIV 3 produces fibroblast-like appearance at edges of cell sheet.	4-10	Detect by hemadsorption with guinea pig RBCs. Identify by FA or HAD.
Respiratory syncytial virus (RSV)	+	+ + +	+	Syncytia in Hep-2, PMK. In HFD degeneration of cell sheet in definite foci.	3-10	Distinct CPE in Hep-2 is sufficient for presumptive identification. Confirm by FA.
Rhinovirus	±	−	+ + +	Characteristic refractile rounding of cells. In PMK, CPE is identical to that produced by enteroviruses.	4-10	Labile at pH 3.
Varicella-zoster	−	−	+ +	Discrete foci of rounded, swollen, refractile cells. Slowly involves entire monolayer.		Confirm by FA.

FA = fluorescent antibody; HAD = hemadsorption; HI = hemagglutination inhibition.
*Relative sensitivity of cell cultures for recovering the virus: − = none recovered; ± = rare strains recovered; + = few strains recovered; + + + + = ≥80% of strains recovered.

PROCEDURE 42.3

Hemadsorption of Primary Monkey Kidney (PMK) Monolayers to Detect Myxoviruses

Perform on cultures of respiratory specimens (or urine in the case of suspected mumps) at 3 days' postinoculation during influenza season and at 5 and 10 days' postinoculation, or when CPE first appears during the rest of the year.
Note: *RSV is not detected by this method.*

Preparation of 0.4% Suspension of Guinea Pig Erythrocytes

1. Wash fresh guinea pig erythrocytes three times in dextrose-gelatin-veronal (DGV) buffer (purchased commercially). Centrifuge cells at $500 \times g$ for 5 min after the first two washes, and at $900 \times g$ for 10 min after the last wash.
2. Prepare a 10% suspension of the washed erythrocytes in DGV (3.6 ml DGV and 0.4 ml packed RBCs). Store at 4° C; cells will last approximately 1 week.
3. On the day of testing, prepare a 0.4% suspension of the RBCs by diluting the 10% suspension with PMK maintenance medium (Appendix A) (0.4 ml of 10% suspension plus 9.6 ml medium).

Hemadsorption Procedure

1. To each inoculated PMK culture to be tested, to two uninoculated negative controls, and to two positive controls (influenza A, parainfluenza 2), add 0.2 ml of the 0.4% RBC suspension. Be careful not to cross-contaminate tubes; positive controls should be tested last.
2. Place tubes horizontally in the rack so that the erythrocyte suspension covers the monolayer. Refrigerate at 4° C for 30 min.
3. Invert tubes quickly to dislodge RBCs lying on the cell sheet. Examine each tube microscopically for RBCs that adhere to the monolayer (Figure 42.11). Culture fluids should be inspected for hemagglutination.

Viruses that both hemadsorb and hemagglutinate guinea pig erythrocytes are usually either influenza A or B. Mumps virus and the parainfluenza viruses (PIV) generally produce only hemadsorption. Certain simian viruses, most notably SV5, contaminate monkey kidney tissue cultures and also hemadsorb at 4° C. Examine all tubes as soon as possible after removal from the refrigerator, because the neuraminidase of myxoviruses is active at room temperature, and hemadsorbing viruses will begin to elute if left for extended periods at this temperature.

---

oculation. To confirm the presence of VZV in culture, we employ fluorescent antisera (Procedure 42.4).

Cytomegalovirus (CMV). CMV, another member of the herpesvirus family, is a frequent clinical isolate. As mentioned earlier, CMV is characterized by the slow development of discrete foci of rounded cells in cell culture (Figure 42.13) and its inability to produce CPE in any cells other than human diploid fibroblasts (HFD). CMV is by far the most common virus recovered from urine; rarely an adenovirus, enterovirus, mumps, or herpes simplex virus also may be recovered from urine.

HFD cultures inoculated with specimens of suspected CMV should be held for at least 21 days to enable the CPE of the virus to develop, although 92% of our isolates from infants have been detectable in 10 days and 98% in 14 days of incubation. Direct inoculation of urine into cell culture often enables CPE to develop in less than 10 days. As mentioned earlier, centrifugation of the urine onto the monolayer and staining with monoclonal antibody may enable CMV to be detected after just 24 hours in tissue culture (see Figure 42-6).[11] Because CMV may be confused with certain strains of adenovirus, immunofluorescent confirmation of isolates (FA, Procedure 42.4) should be performed using available antibodies.

Adenoviruses. Adenoviruses, of which there are

PROCEDURE 42.4

Identification of Isolates by Fluorescent Antibody (FA) Method

This method of virus identification is currently used in our laboratory in preference to the hemadsorption inhibition (HadI) and hemagglutination inhibition (HI) methods. FA is also used for identification of measles, VZV, CMV, and adenovirus, as well as for typing of HSV isolates.

Each virus isolate to be identified should have developed 2+ to 3+ CPE (or demonstrate pronounced hemadsorption) without appreciable loss of cells from the glass. Pool three tubes of uninoculated homologous cell cultures with one tube of infected cells to (1) assure adequate cell numbers for making the required numbers of smears and (2) provide contrast between fluorescent infected cells and nonfluorescent uninfected cells.

Method

1. **Determination of working dilution of fluorescent conjugates**
   a. Prepare serial doubling dilutions of the conjugate in phosphate buffered saline (PBS).
   b. Test each conjugate dilution for its ability to stain homologous and heterologous virus-infected cell culture smears as well as normal uninfected cell culture smears.
   c. The working dilution of the antiserum should be the highest dilution, producing 3+ to 4+ fluorescence on the homologous virus smears, no fluorescence on negative smears, and ≤1+ fluorescence on heterologous virus smears.
2. **Preparation of slides**
   a. Discard media from all tubes. Wash monolayers with 2 ml PBS, pH 7.5 (Appendix A).
   b. To washed monolayers, add 1 ml prewarmed 0.25% trypsin (Appendix A). Bathe cell sheets by rotating tubes 10 to 15 s.
   c. Pour off trypsin, and incubate tubes at 35° C for 10 min in a slanted position so that the residual trypsin covers the mono-

layers. After incubation, examine microscopically to assure that the cells are detached from the glass (occasionally PMK cells require an additional 4 to 5 min).
   d. Pool the resulting cell suspensions in 3 ml PBS containing 2% fetal bovine serum (FBS). Disperse cells by vigorous pipetting or shaking on vortex mixer.
   e. Centrifuge pooled cells at 900 × g for 10 min and carefully remove supernatant.
   f. Resuspend the cell pellet in 0.05 ml PBS with 2% FBS. Examine microscopically to assure that cells are not overdiluted or underdiluted and that they are adequately dispersed.
   g. Using a Pasteur pipette, place 2 small (5 mm) drops of the cell suspension on cleaned and labeled slides. Prepare enough smears to test with antisera to all viruses under consideration. Remaining cells can be suspended in a few milliliters of growth medium and stored at −70° C.
   h. Allow slides to air dry and fix for 10 min in acetone. Store at −70° C.
3. **Fluorescent antibody staining procedure**
   Fluorescent antisera should be titrated in advance (see step 1). This staining procedure is used for both direct smears (see Section 42.4.a.) and slides prepared as in step 2.
   a. Circle areas to be stained with permanent ink marker.
   b. Before each run, dilute conjugate to predetermined working dilution with PBS. Allow 0.05 ml diluted conjugate per smear.
   c. Apply diluted conjugates to appropriate areas without touching pipette to slide. Cover circles completely.
   d. Place slides in a moist chamber and cover the chamber to minimize evaporation. Incubate slides at 35° C for 20 min. Be careful not to tilt slides, since conjugates will run together.

PROCEDURE 42.4—cont'd

Method—cont'd

e. After staining, tip slides to drain conjugate from smear, place slides in a slide carrier, and rinse with running PBS, pH 7.2 to 7.5 (Appendix A). Soak in two changes of PBS for a total of 20 min.

f. Rinse slides in distilled water to remove PBS salt crystals.

g. Allow slides to air dry, taking care to protect them from bright light. Mount with 25% buffered glycerol in PBS and cover with No. 1 coverslips.

h. Examine with fluorescent microscope using Schott UG2 exciter filter or equivalent.

Quality control

Each test must include known positive controls for each fluorescent antiserum to be used, controls to detect heterologous staining, and negative controls of uninfected homologous cells. Positive control slides and controls for heterologous staining are prepared by pooling the cells from four tubes of infected cells. Negative control slides are prepared by pooling the cells from four tubes of uninfected cell cultures. Control smears may be prepared in advance, fixed, and stored at −70° C until needed.

Expected results and interpretation of smears

1. Uninfected cell culture smears (negative controls) should exhibit no fluorescence.

2. Positive controls should exhibit 3+ to 4+ fluorescence with homologous antisera. Cross-reactions with heterologous antigens must be minimal, that is, no greater than 1+. This should not present a problem if initial titration of the conjugate was performed properly.

3. Specific staining of an isolate with acceptable control reactions constitutes positive identification.

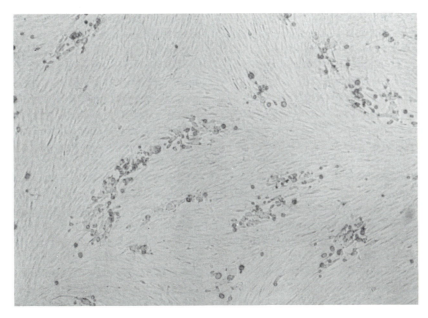

Figure 42.13
CMV cytopathic effect.

more than 30 serotypes, cause a variety of clinical syndromes ranging from pneumonia to acute pharyngitis to conjunctivitis. The virus may be recovered from conjunctiva, stool, body fluids, and urine.

Growth in cell culture tends to be slow, with CPE appearing in an average of 6 days after inoculation. Adenoviruses may be recovered in a variety of cell systems, including PMK and HFD, although human embryonic kidney (HEK) is probably the best culture system. The CPE is characterized by marked rounding and clumping, producing the appearance of grapelike clusters. Continuous cell lines, such as HeLa and Hep-2, are also sensitive to adenovirus growth and are possible substitutes. CPE in Hep-2 has the appearance of rounded, tightly clumped, very granular cell aggregates.

Since adenoviruses possess a common group antigen, isolates are confirmed easily by FA methods. Precise typing, however, requires a cell culture neutralization method (Procedure 42.5).

Because adenoviruses types 1 to 7 are more frequently associated with illness than are other serotypes, a neutralization test with antisera to these specific types can be performed on isolates from respiratory and fecal specimens. If typing of an isolate is not possible with these antisera, the virus is forwarded to a reference laboratory for further identification. Adenoviruses recovered from specimens such as urine and conjunctiva are not usually typed since these sites are not normally colonized with any adenoviruses. If an adenovirus is responsible for respiratory illness, it should be recoverable from respiratory secretions and not from feces alone.

Picornaviruses. The picornaviruses include two major groups of viruses: (1) rhinoviruses, agents of the common cold, and (2) enteroviruses, which include polioviruses, coxsackieviruses types A and B, echoviruses, and miscellaneous other enteroviruses and hepatitis A virus. Both rhinoviruses and enteroviruses tend to be seasonal isolates with peak isolations occurring from late summer to early winter. Epidemics caused by a single type of enterovirus are not uncommon.

Enteroviruses. Presently a large number of enteroviruses are known: poliovirus 1-3, coxsackie A 1-24, coxsackie B 1-6, echovirus 134, enterovirus 68-71, and enterovirus 72 (hepatitis A). Despite this large number, only relatively few tend to be recovered in the clinical laboratory. Of the nonpolio enteroviruses typed in our laboratory, 75% were one

of the following: coxsackie A9, A16, B2-5, and echo 9, 11, and 30. Polioviruses are recovered frequently from recently immunized infants and children.

Most enteroviruses can be isolated in cell culture, although some types of coxsackie A require inoculation of suckling mice. PMK is an excellent cell culture system for recovering these viruses, but they grow in other systems (such as rhabdomyoma [RD], African green monkey kidney [AGMK], and HFD) with varying degrees of success. Tear-shaped or angular refractile CPE is characteristic for the group and is usually detectable 3 to 5 days after inoculation.

Unfortunately, enteroviruses have no group antigen, and except for hepatitis A, identification is based on neutralization tests with intersecting pools of specific antisera. During enterovirus epidemics, it is often useful to attempt identification of an isolate by first testing with antisera to the prevailing virus(es) in an effort to avoid the use of all antisera pools. In addition, enteroviral isolates from small children who have a history of recent oral poliomyelitis immunization can be tested with trivalent poliomyelitis antisera to rule out these agents prior to neutralization attempts with serum pools. A clue to the presence of vaccine strains of polioviruses is the very rapid development of CPE, often in 1 or 2 days. The Lim-Benyesh-Melnick intersecting pools (A-H) of hyperimmune serum are available through the Research Resources Branch of the National Institute of Allergy and Infectious Diseases (NIAID), Department of Health and Human Services, Bethesda, MD 20014. These eight pools identify poliovirus 1-3, coxsackie A7, 9, 16; coxsackie B1, 2, 4-6; and echovirus 1-7, 9, 13-21, 24-27, 29-33. Laboratories may use additional specific antisera to identify coxsackie A24, coxsackie B3, and echo 8 viruses, if desired. These antisera are available but are not included in any of the pools. Instructions for rehydration of the serum pools and performance of the neutralization test are provided by NIAID on receipt of the antisera, and therefore are not included here. A presumptive identification of the isolate usually is possible and can be confirmed using specific antisera.

If an enterovirus cannot be identified by the serum pools and the individual antisera mentioned, the isolate may represent a new virus type or antigenic variant, a mixture of viruses, or a very high titer of virus that is able to overcome the antibody used in the test. Occasionally enteroviruses form

PROCEDURE 42.5

Adenovirus Neutralization Test

This test is used in the typing of adenovirus isolates.

Principle

Serotyping of a virus isolate is based on the ability of specific immune sera to neutralize 100 $TCID_{50}$ (median tissue culture infective dose) of virus and to inhibit its growth (that is, CPE production) in cell culture.

Type-Specific Antisera

We keep antisera to adenovirus types 1 to 7 on hand. If typing of an isolate cannot be accomplished with these, the virus can be forwarded to a reference laboratory for further identification.

Method

1. Inactivate sera at 56° C for 30 min and dilute to a working dilution (determined by the supplier) with maintenance medium.
2. The working dilution should contain a minimum of 20 standard antibody units. If this titration has not been done by the commercial suppliers, it can be performed in the laboratory using 100 $TCID_{50}$ per 0.1 ml of the reference adenovirus type and an equal volume of serial doubling dilutions of the antisera. The highest serum dilution that neutralizes 100 $TCID_{50}$ of the reference virus is 1 standard antibody unit; 20 U are used in the test.

Neutralization Test Procedure

Harvest culture fluids when culture shows 3+ to 4+ CPE. Viral titers in the fluid can be boosted by sonication or alternate cycles of freezing and thawing. The infectivity titer of the fluid may be determined by the Reed-Muench method (con-

sult any standard virology text such as those listed in the Bibliography). A convenient alternative to titrating the virus by the Reed-Muench method is to select arbitrarily the dilution that is most likely to approximate 100 $TCID_{50}$. For adenovirus, a 1:10 dilution of a culture showing 3+ to 4+ CPE is usually adequate; for enteroviruses, a 10^{-2} or 10^{-3} dilution should be used. This alternative is used in our laboratory. To check on this estimate of virus titer, make serial log dilutions of the virus in maintenance medium; 0.1 ml of each dilution (10^0 to 10^{-4}) is inoculated into single tissue culture tubes of Hep-2 or HFD cells, and the virus titer can be calculated approximately from the dilutions that exhibit CPE.

Method

1. Mix 0.2 ml of diluted virus (in this case 10^{-1}) with an equal volume of each antiserum at its working dilution, that is, the dilution containing 20 antibody units.
2. Allow the serum-virus mixture to incubate for 1 h at room temperature.
3. Use 0.2 ml of each serum-virus mixture to inoculate duplicate tubes of appropriate cell cultures.
4. Incubate all inoculated tubes (titration and neutralization assays) at 35° C and examine daily for 7 days.

Interpretation

Inhibition of CPE by specific antisera, when control tubes (in this case, the 10^{-1} dilution) show 2+ to 3+ CPE, constitutes identification of the serotype. Complete inhibition is not always possible, but there should be at least a 2+ difference in CPE between the positive control and the inhibited serotype.

PROCEDURE 42.6

Acid Lability Test to Differentiate Rhinovirus from Enterovirus

Principle

Rhinoviruses are labile at pH 3, while enteroviruses are not.

Preparation of media

1. Eagle's minimum essential medium (EMEM) prepared without sodium bicarbonate (Appendix A) is approximately pH 3; test with pH meter and adjust with 2 N HCl if necessary.
2. The same medium prepared with sodium bicarbonate should be pH 7; check with pH meter and adjust if necessary.

Performance of test

1. Make a 1:10 dilution of the virus to be tested in each of the above media (0.2 ml virus and 1.8 ml medium) and incubate for 3 h at room temperature.
2. Use stock rhinovirus and enterovirus as controls.
3. Make serial $\log_{10}$ dilutions in Hanks' balanced saline solution (Appendix A) of each mixture (10^{-1} to 10^{-5}).
4. Inoculate 0.1 ml of each dilution in each medium, in duplicate, into tubes of human fetal diploid (HFD), incubate at 35° C, and observe for a period of 7 to 10 days for CPE.

Interpretation of results

A 2 log decrease of infectivity due to pH 3 treatment and no decrease at pH 7 indicates that the isolate is a rhinovirus. The isolate is an enterovirus if no reduction of infectivity by pH 3 treatment occurs.

---

aggregates that are incompletely neutralized by antisera. In these cases, there will be an apparent neutralization for several days; then the virus will "break through" the antisera and produce CPE.

Hepatitis A is not recovered in tissue culture and is diagnosed by serologic methods (see Section 42.7.e.).

Rhinoviruses. These viruses are a major cause of the common cold or upper respiratory infection (URI). They differ from enteroviruses in that they are labile at pH 3 and grow better in HFD cells than in cells of monkey origin.

Rhinoviruses are rarely recovered in the clinical laboratory, in part because patients with mild illness usually are not cultured. In addition, they grow best at 33° C rather than at the 35° C of most laboratory incubators. To detect the occasional rhinovirus, all viruses producing picornavirus-like CPE in respiratory specimens are tested for acid lability (Procedure 42.6) unless a picornavirus is isolated from a stool or CSF specimen.

Myxoviruses. Myxoviruses are generally separated into two groups: (1) orthomyxoviruses, including in-

fluenza A, B, and C, and (2) paramyxoviruses, including parainfluenza types 1 to 4, respiratory syncytial virus, and mumps virus. They are identified by hemadsorption inhibition (Procedure 42.7).

Influenza viruses. These viruses are notable for their epidemic potential, particularly influenza A, which affects all age groups and tends to cause pandemics every 10 years and lesser outbreaks almost yearly. Influenza B virus may be recovered sporadically or in association with true outbreaks, while influenza C is rarely if ever isolated. The ability of influenza virus to cause epidemics is related to its antigenic variations, a feature especially notable with type A. The first isolates of an outbreak are likely to be of great interest to the medical community and should be sent to a reference laboratory for strain identification.

Influenza viruses are readily recovered in PMK cell cultures, although occasional strains of type A virus may grow only in embryonated hen's eggs. CPE production varies among different types of influenza A viruses, but it may be observed in 2 to 4 days with certain strains. Influenza virus CPE con-

PROCEDURE 42.7

Hemadsorption Inhibition Test (HadI) to Identify Myxovirus Isolates

Viruses to be considered are influenza A and B, PIV 1, 2, and 3, mumps, and SV5. Treat immune sera to these seven virus agents with receptor-destroying enzyme (RDE) of *Vibrio cholerae* to remove nonspecific inhibitors of hemadsorption (see below).

Principle

Inhibition of hemadsorption by specific antisera.

RDE treatment of immune sera

1. Mix 0.3 ml of each antiserum to be used with an equal volume of RDE and incubate in a 37° C water bath overnight. The RDE should have a titer of 128 units. (For RDE titration procedure, see standard texts.)
2. Inactivate treated sera in a 56° C water bath for 30 min.
3. Dilute serum 1:10 by adding 2.4 ml phosphate-buffered saline (PBS).
4. To remove nonspecific agglutinins, add 0.1 ml 50% guinea pig RBCs for each milliliter of the 1:10 dilution. Refrigerate with occasional agitation at 4° C for 1 h.
5. Centrifuge at 900 × *g* for 10 min. Remove supernatant and use in HadI test. Freeze excess treated sera at −20° C.

Method

1. Scrape cells and fluid together with a 1 ml pipette and pass 0.1 ml into each of 10 tubes

of PMK. After 72-h incubation, hemadsorb one PMK tube to determine whether the virus titer is adequate to perform the inhibition test. Hemadsorption by 50% or greater of the cell sheet generally is adequate.
2. Wash remaining infected monolayers twice with Hanks' balanced salt solution (BSS) plus antibiotics (Appendix A).
3. Add 0.6 ml Hanks' BSS plus 0.2 ml of each RDE-treated antiserum to labeled tubes. The two remaining tubes include one positive control and one to be saved for further studies if necessary.
4. After incubation for 30 min at room temperature, add 0.2 ml of a 0.4% guinea pig erythrocyte suspension to each tube and reincubate cultures at 4° C for 30 min. Place tubes in rack, cell sheet down.

Interpretation of results

Examine tubes as in hemadsorption procedure (Procedure 42.3). Inhibition of hemadsorption by a specific antiserum is sufficient evidence to identify the isolate. This inhibition may not be complete, but it must show at least a 2+ difference from the control.

Note: *Occasional influenza A isolates cannot be identified by this method. In such cases, perform a hemagglutination inhibition (HI) test. Strain identification of influenza A isolates is beyond the scope of the hospital laboratory and should be performed by a reference facility.*

---

sists of destructive degeneration of the cell sheet; infected cells become granular and swollen and eventually detach from the glass.

Parainfluenza viruses (PIVs). PIVs are important agents of acute respiratory illness among infants and small children. Infection with parainfluenza type 1 is seasonal in nature, with peak isolations occurring in fall and early winter, often during epidemics of croup. Type 3 infections occur sporadically throughout the year as well as in seasonal outbreaks.

PIVs, like influenza virus, grow well in PMK but often do not produce CPE. As a result, PMK cells inoculated with respiratory specimens are routinely hemadsorbed at 5 and 10 days' postinoculation (or earlier if CPE is present) with a suspension of guinea pig erythrocytes (Procedure 42.3). If virus is present, these erythrocytes will hemadsorb to the infected monolayer because of the presence of a viral hemagglutinin elaborated at the cell surface (Figure 42.14). This adherence can be minimal in cases

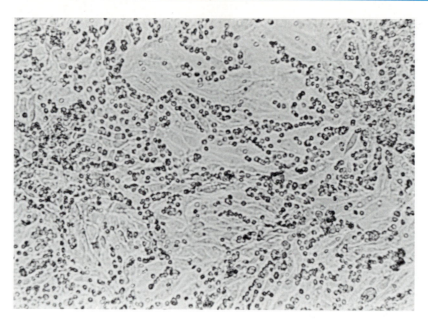

Figure 42.14
Parainfluenza virus hemadsorption.

where large amounts of virus have been liberated into the culture fluid, and the erythrocytes are agglutinated before they can adsorb to the monolayer. Consequently, it is important that both fluids and the monolayer surface be examined in the performance of this test.

Monolayers exhibiting hemadsorption during an influenza outbreak are tested with FA to confirm the presence of influenza A. If this test is negative, the isolate should be passed and tested further with fluorescent antisera to other hemadsorbing viruses, or identified by the hemadsorption inhibition or hemagglutination inhibition tests.

Respiratory syncytial virus. RSV is a major cause of pneumonia and bronchiolitis in infants and small children. RSV is very labile, and best isolation results are obtained when respiratory specimens are inoculated directly into tubes of Hep-2 cells. CPE may take up to 14 days to first appear, but direct inoculation can reduce isolation time to an average of 4 to 5 days. This virus does not hemadsorb and tends to show little or no CPE in PMK and HFD. The slow production of refractile giant cell syncytia in Hep-2 is highly suggestive of RSV in a patient with respiratory disease, and confirmation is optional. Troublesome isolates can be confirmed by FA methods.

Mumps virus. This virus is recovered infrequently in the clinical laboratory, probably because the disease is recognized easily by physicians and preventive vaccination is widespread. It is, however, an important agent of aseptic meningitis in children, and it is occasionally associated with orchitis in adult males. Specimens submitted for isolation of this virus include respiratory swabs, urine, and CSF. PMK tubes inoculated with such specimens should be hemadsorbed with guinea pig erythrocytes (by the same procedure [Procedure 42.3] described for influenza and parainfluenza viruses) since CPE in culture is not regularly caused by mumps virus. When present, CPE consists of a destructive degeneration of the monolayer with occasional syncytia. Isolates are confirmed with fluorescent antisera.

Parvovirus. Parvoviruses recently have been implicated as the cause of erythema infectiosum (fifth disease)[7] and some forms of arthritis, some instances of hemolytic crisis (especially in patients with hemoglobinophathies),[2] and some infections of fetuses or stillborns. They are best diagnosed serologically, although the antigen of the virus causing hemolytic crisis (the serum parvolike virus) has been detected in serum by counterimmunoelectropheresis (CIE) during acute infection.

•   •   •

PROCEDURE 42.8

Cultivation and Subpassage of Hep-2 Cells

1. Remove maintenance medium from stock flask and rinse cell sheet once with 10 to 20 ml PBS, pH 7.5 (Appendix A).
2. Add 1 to 2 ml 0.24% trypsin (Appendix A) to flask and incubate at 35° C for 5 to 10 min.
3. When cells detach from the plastic, add 10 ml of growth medium (Appendix A) and disperse cells by pipetting vigorously. Examine the suspension microscopically to ensure adequate cell dispersal.
4. Seed new 250 ml plastic culture flasks with 2 to 3 ml of this suspension, and then add an additional 20 ml of growth medium per flask.
5. Inoculate cell culture tubes with 0.05 ml of the suspension from step 4, and then add 1 ml of the growth medium to each tube.
6. Close tubes and flasks tightly and incubate horizontally in a stationary position at 35° C for 72 h. Once cells are sufficiently sheeted, replace growth medium in culture tubes with 3 ml maintenance medium (Appendix A). Replace growth medium in flasks with 20 ml of maintenance medium.

PROCEDURE 42.9

Preservation and Storage of Hep-2 Cells by Freezing

1. Repeat steps 1 to 3 in Procedure 42.8.
2. Transfer the cell suspension to a test tube and centrifuge at 1500 rpm for 5 min. Decant supernatant.
3. Resuspend pellet thoroughly in 2 ml of growth medium (Appendix A) containing 10% DMSO (dimethyl sulfoxide) or 50% glycerol. Dispense 1-ml aliquots of this suspension into sterile glass ampules. Seal ampules by flaming and freeze to −70° C slowly.
4. For reconstitution of the frozen cells, the ampule should be thawed rapidly in a 35° C water bath and the contents used to seed a new flask. Add 10 ml of growth medium and incubate the flask at 35° C until a confluent monolayer has formed. Replace growth medium with 20 ml of maintenance medium (Appendix A) and reincubate.

Additional tissue culture techniques are given in Procedures 42.8 to 42.11.

42.8.g. Interpretation of viral culture results. The interpretation of virological data must be based on knowledge of the normal viral flora in the site sampled, the clinical findings, and the epidemiologic behavior of viruses. In some situations, serologic studies may be necessary to support or refute the possible association of a virus isolate with a disease.

Viruses in tissue and body fluids. In general, the detection of any virus in host tissues, CSF, blood, or vesicular fluid can be considered highly significant. Recovery of viruses other than CMV in urine may be diagnostic of significant infection, for example, adenovirus type 2, associated with acute hemorrhagic cystitis, and mumps. However, recovery of CMV from urine can be difficult to interpret. The CMV isolate may merely reflect active, asymptomatic virus replication or may indicate a significant infection in the patient. Viruria in the first 3 weeks of life establishes a diagnosis of congenital CMV infection, whereas the onset of viral excretion after 4 weeks of life reflects intrapartum or postpartum infection. Diagnosis of acquired CMV infections in older patients usually results from a combination of findings, including positive cultures from any site, illness known to be compatible with CMV, reasonable exclusion of other potential etiologic agents, and support by specific serologic or histological data or both.

Virus isolation from other sites. Upper respiratory tract (or specimens obtained by traversing the upper airways), vaginal, and fecal cultures vary greatly in terms of their significance. At one extreme, isolates such as measles, mumps, influenza, parainfluenza, and RSV are very significant since asymptomatic carriage and prolonged shedding of these viruses is un-

PROCEDURE 42.10

Passage of CMV and VZV Isolates

Principle

Most viruses can be passed by subculturing the culture medium. CMV and VZV are cell-associated viruses and must be passed by trypsinizing infected monolayers.

Method

1. Discard media from infected cell sheet and wash the monolayer two times with PBS, pH 7.5 (Appendix A).
2. To washed monolayer, add 2 ml 0.25% trypsin (Appendix A). Bathe cell sheet by rotating tube for 10 to 15 s. Pour off trypsin.
3. Allow monolayer to incubate in residual trypsin for 5 to 10 min at 35° C. (Occasionally a subpassage will rapidly deteriorate because of the presence of excess trypsin in the inoculum. Care must be exercised to assure that most of the trypsin is removed before the incubation step.)
4. After cells detach from the glass, add 1 ml growth medium (Appendix A) to the cell-trypsin suspension and pipette vigorously to disperse cell aggregates.
5. Inoculate fresh monolayers with 0.2 ml of the suspension from step 4.

PROCEDURE 42.11

Preservation and Storage of Viruses by Freezing

CMV and VZV

CMV- and VZV-infected monolayers having 2+ to 3+ CPE are trypsinized as described in Procedure 42.10. Instead of adding growth medium to the trypsin-cell suspension, resuspend cells in 1 to 2ml of growth medium containing 10% DMSO for VZV and 35% sorbitol for CMV. Disperse monolayer by vigorous pipetting and store at −70° C in flame-sealed glass ampules.

Other Viruses

There are two acceptable methods of preparing infected monolayers for storage. DMSO or sorbitol is not necessary for the preservation of viruses other than VZV and CMV.

Methods

1. Scrape monolayers exhibiting 3+ to 4+ CPE (or hemadsorption) into their own culture media, pipette vigorously to disperse cell aggregates, and aliquot 1-ml amounts into glass ampules, which are then flame-sealed and stored at −70° C. For short-term storage, tightly sealed screw-cap vials or test tubes may be used.
2. Trypsinize infected monolayers (Procedure 42.10). Resuspend cells in 2 to 3 ml of fresh growth medium (Appendix A), aliquot 1-ml amounts into glass ampules or test tubes, seal, and freeze at −70° C.

usual. Conversely, other viruses can be shed without symptoms and for periods ranging from several weeks (enteroviruses) to many months (adenoviruses, HSV, CMV). Examples include HSV and CMV in the oropharynx and vagina, adenoviruses in the oropharynx and intestinal tract, and enteroviruses in the intestinal tract. VZV, HSV, CMV, adenoviruses, and EBV may remain latent for long periods and then become reactivated in response to a variety of stressful stimuli, including other infectious agents. In this setting, their detection may have no significance (VZV is an exception) or may merely represent a secondary problem complicating the primary infection (for example, HSV "cold sores" in patients with bacterial sepsis).

Adenovirus isolates are common in infants and young children. Based on the epidemiology and observed serologic responses, it has been found that, in febrile and respiratory syndromes, simultaneous isolation of these agents from both the throat and feces has greater probability of association with that illness; isolation from the throat, but not the feces, has a lesser probability of association, and isolation from the feces alone has the least diagnostic significance. In these latter situations, interpretation of the significance of the culture results can be aided by adenovirus serologic studies.

Enteroviruses are also most commonly found in infants and children, particularly during the late summer and early autumn seasons. A knowledge of the relative frequency of virus shedding among various age groups in a particular locale is extremely helpful in assessing significance of results of throat or stool cultures; for example, the peak prevalence of enteroviruses in the stools of toddlers during the late summer may range from greater than 20% in subtropical climates to 5% in temperate zones. Even in the latter areas, carriage rates may approach 30% in infants during periods of enterovirus activity. Shedding of enteroviruses in the throat is relatively transient (usually 1 to 2 weeks), whereas fecal shedding may last 4 to 16 weeks. Thus, with a clinically compatible illness, isolation of an enterovirus from the throat supports a stronger temporal relationship to the disease than an isolate from the feces alone. When echovirus or coxsackievirus is recovered from the stool only, it may be helpful to study the patient's serum for an antibody rise against that particular viral isolate.

HSV is unusual in a fecal culture; in such cases, it usually represents either severe disseminated infection or infection of the anus or perianal areas. If this virus is obtained from an anal or rectal culture of a sexually active patient with signs of nervous system disease, for example, aseptic meningitis or lumbosacral myeloradiculitis, it may indicate the etiology. Detection of HSV in the upper respiratory tract may have no meaning other than nonspecific stress reactivation unless typical vesicles or ulcers are also seen. Because of the stress-related phenomenon, isolation of HSV in the throat or mucocutaneous lesions of patients with encephalitis cannot be interpreted as causative of the CNS disease. Currently, the definitive way to establish a diagnosis of herpes simplex encephalitis is by direct demonstration of the virus in a brain biopsy specimen. In newborn infants, however, isolation of the virus from any site should raise the possibility that a potentially severe infection exists.

Isolation of adenoviruses, HSV, VZV, and some enteroviruses from the cornea and conjunctiva in cases of inflammatory disease at these sites usually establishes the etiology of the infection.

Significance of negative virological results. There are numerous occasions when the laboratory is asked to perform studies with the intent of ruling out specific viral agents. The ability to exclude the presence of a virus depends greatly on the sensitivity of the detection systems being used. The most important prerequisites include the following:

1. Proper communication with the laboratory *before* initiating studies
2. Procurement of the appropriate specimens in the *early* phase of acute illness
3. Careful attention to the procedures of collection, transportation, and processing of specimens
4. Avoidance of fungal or bacterial contamination of processed cultures.

When all these criteria are fulfilled, it is usually possible to interpret negative data with a high degee of confidence.

REFERENCES

1. Almeida, J.D. 1980. Practical aspects of diagnostic electron microscopy. Yale J. Biol. Med. 53:5.
2. Anderson M.J., and Pattison, J.R. 1984. The human parvovirus. Arch. Virol. 82:137.
3. Chernesky, M.A. 1979. The role of electron microscopy in diagnostic virology. In Lennette, D., Specter, S., and Thompson, K., editors. Diagnosis of viral infections: the role of the clinical laboratory. University Park Press, Baltimore.
3a. Choo, Q.-L., Kuo, G., Weiner, A.J., et al. 1989. Isolation of a cDNA clone derived from a blood-borne non-A, non-B hepatitis genome. Science 244:359.
4. Chou, S., and Merigan, T.C. 1983. Rapid detection and quantitation of human cytomegalovirus in urine through DNA hybridization. N. Engl. J. Med. 308:921.
5. Doane, F.W., and Anderson, N. 1977. Electron and immune electron microscopic procedures for diagnosis of viral infections. In Kurstak, E., and Kurstak, C., editors. Comparative diagnosis of viral diseases, vol. 2. Academic Press, New York.
6. Drew, W.L., and Mintz, L. 1980. Rapid diagnosis of varicella-zoster virus infection by direct immunofluorescence. Am. J. Clin. Pathol. 73:699.
7. Duncan, J.R., Capellini, M.D., Anderson, M.J., et al. 1983. Aplastic crisis due to parvovirus infection in pyruvate kinase deficiency. Lancet 2:14.
8. Emmons, R.W., and Riggs, J.L. 1977. Application of immunofluorescence to diagnosis of viral infections. Methods in Virology 6:1.
9. Flores, J., Boeggeman, E., Purcell, R.H., et al. 1983. A dot hybridization assay for detection of rotaviruses. Lancet 1:555.
10. Fulton, R.E., and Middleton, P.J. 1974. Comparison of immunofluorescence and isolation techniques in the diagnosis of respiratory viral infections of children. Infect. Immun. 10:92.
11. Gleaves, C.A., Smith, T.F., Shuster, E.A., and Pearson, G.R. 1984. Rapid detection of cytomegalovirus in MRC-5 cells inoculated with urine specimens by using low-speed centrifugation and monoclonal antibody to an early antigen. J. Clin. Microbiol. 19:917.

12. Harmon, M.W., and Pawlik, K.M. 1982. Enzyme immuno-assay for direct detection of influenza type A and adenovirus antigens in clinical specimens. J. Clin. Microbiol. 15:5.

13. Howell, C.L., Miller, M.J., and Martin, W.J. 1979. Comparison of rates of virus isolation from leukocyte populations from blood by conventional and Ficoll-Hypaque/Macrodex methods. J. Clin. Microbiol. 10:533.

14. Hsiung, G.D., Fong, C.K.Y., and August, M.J. 1979. The use of electron microscopy for diagnosis of virus infections: an overview. Prog. Med. Virol. 25:133.

15. Huntoon, C.J., House, R.F., Jr., and Smith, T.F. 1981. Recovery of viruses from three transport media incorporated into culturettes. Arch. Pathol. Lab. Med. 105:436.

16. Minnich, L., and Ray, C.G. 1980. Comparison of direct immunofluorescent staining of clinical specimens for respiratory virus antigens with conventional isolation techniques. J. Clin. Microbiol. 12:391.

17. Moseley, R.C., Corey, L., Benjamin, D., et al. 1981. Comparison of viral isolation, direct immunofluorescence, and indirect immunoperoxidase techniques for detection of genital herpes simplex virus infection. J. Clin. Microbiol. 13:913.

18. Nilheden, E., Jeansson, S., and Vahlne, A. 1983. Typing of herpes simplex virus by an enzyme-linked immunosorbent assay with monoclonal antibodies. J. Clin. Microbiol. 17:677.

18a. Polesky, H.F., and Hanson, M.R. 1989. Transfusion-associated hepatitis C virus (non-A, non-B) infection. Arch. Pathol. Lab. Med. 113:232.

19. Popow-Kraupp, T., Kern, G., Binder, G., et al. 1986. Detection of respiratory syncytial virus in nasopharyngeal secretions by enzyme-linked immunosorbent assay, indirect immunofluorescence, and virus isolation: a comparative study. J. Med. Virol. 19:123.

20. Rubin, S.J., and Rogers, S. 1984. Comparison of Cultureset and primary rabbit kidney cell culture for the detection of herpes simplex virus. J. Clin. Microbiol. 19:920.

21. Schmidt, N.J., Gallo, D., Devlin, V., et al. 1980. Direct immunofluorescence staining for detection of herpes simplex and varicella-zoster virus antigens in vesicular lesions and certain tissue specimens. J. Clin. Microbiol. 12:651.

22. Spector, S.A., Rua, J.A., Spector, D.H., et al. 1984. Detection of human cytomegalovirus in clinical specimens by DNA-RNA hybridization. J. Infect. Dis. 150:121.

23. Stagno, S., Pass, R.F., Reynolds, D.W., et al. 1980. Comparative study of diagnostic procedures for congenital cytomegalovirus infection. Pediatrics 65:251.

24. Yeager, A.S., Morris, J.E., and Prober, C.G. 1979. Storage and transport of cultures for herpes simplex virus, type 2. Am. J. Clin. Pathol. 72:977.

25. Yolken, R.H., and Leister, F. 1982. Rapid multiple-determinant enzyme immunoassay for the detection of human rotavirus. J. Infect. Dis. 146:43.

26. Zaia, J.A., Forman, S.J., and Gallagher, M.T., et al. 1984. Prolonged human cytomegalovirus viremia following bone marrow transplantation. Transplantation 37:315.

BIBLIOGRAPHY

Drew, W.L., editor. 1976. Viral infections: a clinical approach. F.A. Davis Co., Philadelphia.

Gardner, P.S., and McQuillin, J. 1974. Rapid virus diagnosis: application of immunofluorescence. Butterworth & Co., London.

Hsiung, G.D., in collaboration with Fong, C.K.Y. 1982. Diagnostic virology (illustrated with light and electron micrographs). Yale University Press, New Haven, Conn.

Lennette, D.A., Specter, S., and Thompson, K.D., editors. 1979. Diagnosis of viral infections: the role of the clinical laboratory. University Park Press, Baltimore.

Lennette, E.H., and Schmidt, N.J., editors. 1979. Diagnostic procedures for viral, rickettsial, and chlamydial infections, ed. 5. American Public Health Association, Washington, D.C.

43 Laboratory Methods in Basic Mycology

Glenn D. Roberts

Historically, the fungi have been regarded as relatively insignificant causes of infection and until recently clinical laboratories offered little more than interest in providing mycological services. During the past few years, however, the literature has shown a sharp increase in the number of case reports of fungal infections. The fungi are now well recognized causes of infection, and physician awareness of their importance is much more common. Some clinical microbiology laboratories have kept pace with the changing times, but unfortunately many still offer only minimal mycological services. The reasons for this are not easily defined, but the lack of emphasis in the area of mycology by medical technology educational programs has played a major role in the scant training in this area of microbiology. In addition, the myth that mycology is too hard to learn has probably been partly responsible for the lack of interest in mycology.

The emergence of continuing education programs presenting the practical aspects of clinical mycology and a number of recent textbooks in the same area, along with the increased number of journal publications, now makes mycology available to all clinical microbiology laboratories where it should be included as an important component.

43.1. Importance of Fungi

There are more than 50,000 valid species of fungi, but only some 50 to 75 are generally recognized as being pathogenic for humans. These organisms normally live a saprophytic existence in nature, enriched by decaying nitrogenous matter, where they are capable of maintaining a separate existence, with a parasitic cycle in humans or animals. The mycoses are not communicable in the usual sense of person-to-person or animal-to-person transfer; humans become an accidental host by the inhalation of spores or by their introduction into tissue through trauma. With the exception of the dimorphic fungi, humans are relatively resistant to infections caused by these organisms. However, an alteration in the immune system of the host (Chapter 23) may lead to infection by fungi that are normally considered to be nonpathogenic. Such infections may occur in patients with debilitating diseases, diabetes, or impaired immunological function resulting from corticosteroid or antimetabolite therapy. Other predisposing factors include long-term intravenous cannulation, gastrointestinal surgical procedures, and long-term antimicrobial chemotherapy. During recent years, there has been an increase in the number of infections caused by saprobic fungi in immunocompromised patients. This has resulted in an obligation for the laboratory to identify and report all organisms recovered from clinical specimens submitted for fungal culture.

43.2. Levels of Laboratory Service

To ensure adequate patient care, mycological services should be offered by all clinical microbiology laboratories. The extent to which these services are offered is dependent on the individual laboratory setting. The following are proposed levels of service:

I. Performance of direct examination of clinical specimens for the presence of fungi and collection, culturing, and transport of appropriate clinical specimens to a reference laboratory.

II. Performance of all functions of level I laboratories as well as the identification of yeasts using commercially available systems, performance of the latex test for cryptococcal antigen, and performance of commercially available fungal immunodiffusion tests.

III. Performance of all functions of level II laboratories as well as the identification of commonly encountered filamentous fungi.

IV. Performance of all functions of laboratories at lower levels, the identification of all fungi, performance of all fungal serologic tests, and antifungal susceptibility tests.

Laboratories should choose the extent to which they are proficient and forward all additional procedures to a qualified reference laboratory. With the current emphasis on cost containment (Chapter 4),

Table 43.1

Fungi Most Commonly Recovered from Clinical Specimens at the Mayo Clinic

BLOOD	CEREBROSPINAL FLUID	GENITOURINARY TRACT	RESPIRATORY TRACT	SKIN
Candida albicans	*Cryptococcus neo-formans*	*Candida albicans*	Yeast, not *Cryptococcus*	*Trichophyton rubrum*
Candida tropicalis	*Candida albicans*	*Candida glabrata*	*Penicillium* species	*Trichophyton menta-grophytes*
Candida parapsilosis	*Candida parapsi-losis*	*Candida tropicalis*	*Aspergillus* species	*Alternaria* species
Cryptococcus neofor-mans	*Candida tropicalis*	*Candida parapsi-losis*	*Aspergillus fumigatus*	*Candida albicans*
Histoplasma capsulatum	*Coccidioides im-mitis*	*Penicillium* species	*Cladosporium* species	*Penicillium* species
Candida lusitaniae	*Histoplasma capsu-latum*	*Candida krusei*	*Alternaria* species	*Scopulariopsis* species
Candida krusei		*Cryptococcus neo-formans*	*Aspergillus niger*	*Epidermophyton floc-cosum*
Saccharomyces species		*Saccharomyces* spe-cies	*Geotrichum candidum*	*Candida parapsilosis*
Candida pseudotropi-calis		*Histoplasma capsu-latum*	*Fusarium* species	*Aspergillus* species
Candida zeylanoides		*Cladosporium* spe-cies	*Aspergillus versicolor*	*Acremonium* species
Trichosporon beigelii		*Aspergillus* species	*Aspergillus flavus*	*Aspergillus versicolor*
Coccidioides immitis		*Trichosporon cuta-neum*	*Acremonium* species	*Cladosporium* species
Candida guilliermondii		*Alternaria* species	*Scopulariopsis* species	*Fusarium* species
			Beauveria species	*Trichosporon cuta-neum*
				Phialophora species

smaller clinical laboratories should carefully consider the extent to which they should provide mycological services.

43.3. Fungi Commonly Encountered in a Clinical Laboratory

Of the more than 50,000 valid species of fungi, less than 100 are likely to be encountered in clinical specimens. Laboratorians just beginning to work in clinical mycology might feel intimidated by this large number; however, it is commonplace for a laboratory to recover many of the same fungi on a day-to-day basis. During a 9-year period, 267,861 clinical specimens were submitted for fungal culture at the Mayo Clinic. Of these, 75,258 (28.1%) were positive for one or more fungi. Table 43.1 presents the fungi most commonly recovered from clinical specimens at the Mayo Clinic. This listing is derived from the 94,358 fungi recovered from various clinical sources, and organisms are listed in order of their frequency of occurrence. It is well known that there are differences in the geographical distribution of certain fungi; however, Table 43.1 should be of value to most laboratories in the interpretation of fungal culture results.

43.4. Collection, Transport, and Culturing of Clinical Specimens

The diagnosis of fungal infections is dependent entirely on the selection and collection of an appropriate clinical specimen for culture. Many fungal infections are similar clinically to mycobacterial infections, and often the same specimen is cultured for both fungi and mycobacteria. Most infections have a primary focus in the lungs; respiratory secretions are almost always included among the specimens selected for culture. It should be emphasized that dissemination to distant body sites often occurs, and fungi may be commonly recovered from nonrespiratory sites. The proper collection of specimens and their transport to the clinical laboratory are of major importance for the recovery of fungi. In many instances, specimens not only contain the etiologic agent but also contain contaminating bacteria or fungi that will rapidly overgrow some of the slower growing pathogenic fungi. Since overgrowth with contaminating organisms is common, it is important to transport the specimens to the clinical laboratory as soon as possible. Although collection methods are discussed in Chapter 6, a few specific comments concerning specimen collection and culturing are included in this chapter.

43.4.a. Respiratory secretions. Respiratory secretions (sputum, induced sputum, bronchial washings, and tracheal aspirations) are perhaps the most commonly submitted specimens for fungal culture. To ensure the optimal recovery of fungi and prevent overgrowth by contaminants, antibacterial antibiotics should be included in the battery of media to be used. Cycloheximide, an antifungal agent that prevents rapid overgrowth by contaminating organisms, should be included in at least one of the culture media used. As much specimen as possible (0.5 ml) should be used to inoculate each medium.

43.4.b. Cerebrospinal fluid. Cerebrospinal fluid (CSF) collected for culture should be filtered through a 0.45-μm pore size membrane filter attached to a sterile syringe. After filtration, the filter is removed and is placed onto the surface of an appropriate culture medium with the "organism" side down. Cultures should be examined daily and the filter moved to another location on an every-other-day basis. If less than 2 ml of specimen is submitted for culture, it should be centrifuged and 1-drop aliquots of the sediment should be placed onto several areas on the agar surface. Media used for the recovery of fungi from CSF should contain no antibacterial or antifungal agents. Once submitted to the laboratory, CSF specimens should be processed promptly. If prompt processing is not possible, samples should be kept at room temperature or placed in a 30° C incubator, since most organisms will continue to replicate in this environment.

43.4.c. Blood. Disseminated fungal infections are more prevalent than previously recognized, and blood cultures provide an accurate method for determining their cause. Only a few fungal blood culture systems have been available over past years, and most are not used by clinical microbiology laboratories. In smaller laboratories, it may be adequate to use a biphasic brain-heart infusion agar-broth blood culture system.[73] However, larger laboratories are encouraged to use a lysis-centrifugation system, the DuPont Isolator tube, since it has been shown to be the optimal fungal blood culture system (Chapter 14). Using this system, red blood cells and white blood cells that may contain the microorganisms are lysed, and centrifugation serves to concentrate fungi and bacteria prior to culturing. The concentrate is inoculated onto the surface of appropriate culture media, and most fungi are detected within the first 4 days of incubation. However, an occasional isolate

of *Histoplasma capsulatum* may require approximately 10 to 14 days for recovery. The optimal temperature for fungal blood cultures is 30° C, and the suggested incubation time is 30 days.

43.4.d. Hair, skin, and nail scrapings. These specimens are usually submitted for dermatophyte culture and are contaminated with bacteria or rapidly growing fungi or both. Samples collected from lesions may be obtained by scraping the skin or nails with a scalpel blade or microscope slide, and infected hairs are removed by plucking them with forceps. These specimens should be placed in a sterile Petri dish or paper envelope prior to culturing; they should not be refrigerated. Either Mycobiotic or Mycosel agar (Chapter 8), which contain chloramphenicol and cycloheximide, is satisfactory for the recovery of dermatophytes from hair, skin, or nails. Cultures should be incubated for a minimum of 30 days at 30° C before being reported as negative.

43.4.e. Urine. Urine samples collected for fungal culture should be processed as soon as possible after collection. Twenty-four-hour urine samples are unacceptable for culture. After considering the arguments concerning the value of quantitating the growth of fungi recovered from urine cultures, I have concluded that quantitation should not be performed except as part of the routine urine culture procedure. All urine samples should be centrifuged and the sediment cultured using a loop to provide adequate isolation of colonies. Since urine is often contaminated with gram-negative bacteria, it is necessary to use media containing antibacterial agents to ensure the recovery of fungi.

43.4.f. Tissue, bone marrow, and sterile body fluids. All tissues should be processed prior to culturing by mincing or grinding or placement in a Stomacher (Tekmar; Chapter 21). Currently the optimal system is the use of the Stomacher, which expresses the cytoplasmic contents of cells by pressure exerted from the action of rapidly moving metal paddles against the tissue in a broth suspension. After processing, at least 1 ml of specimen should be spread onto the surface of appropriate culture media, and incubation should be at 30° C for 30 days.

Bone marrow may be placed directly onto the surface of appropriate culture media and incubated in the manner previously mentioned. Sterile body fluids should be concentrated by centrifugation before culturing, and at least 1 ml of specimen should be placed onto the surface of appropriate culture

Table 43.2
Fungal Culture Media: Indications for Use

MEDIA	INDICATIONS FOR USE
Primary recovery media	
Brain-heart infusion agar	Primary recovery of saprobic and pathogenic fungi
Brain-heart infusion agar with antibiotics	Primary recovery of pathogenic fungi exclusive of dermatophytes
Brain-heart infusion biphasic blood culture bottles	Recovery of fungi from blood
Dermatophyte test medium	Primary recovery of dermatophytes, recommended as screening medium only
Inhibitory mold agar	Primary recovery of pathogenic fungi exclusive of dermatophytes
Mycosel or mycobiotic agar	Primary recovery of dermatophytes
SABHI agar	Primary recovery of saprobic and pathogenic fungi
Yeast-extract phosphate agar	Primary recovery of pathogenic fungi exclusive of dermatophytes
Differential test media	
Ascospore agar	Detection of ascospores in ascosporogenous yeasts such as *Saccharomyces* sp.
Cornmeal agar with Tween 80 and trypan blue	Identification of *C. albicans* by chlamydospore production; identification of *Candida* by microscopic morphology
Cottonseed conversion agar	Conversion of dimorphic fungus *B. dermatitidis* from mold to yeast form
Czapek's agar	Recovery and differential identification of *Aspergillus* sp.
Niger seed agar	Identification of *C. neoformans*
Nitrate reduction medium	Detection of nitrate reduction in confirmation of *Cryptococcus* sp.
Potato dextrose agar	Demonstration of pigment production by *T. rubrum;* preparation of micro-slide cultures
Rice medium	Identification of *M. audouinii*
Trichophyton agars 1-7	Identification of members of *Trichophyton* genus
Urea agar	Detection of *Cryptococcus* sp.; differentiate *T. mentagrophytes* from *T. rubrum;* detection of *Trichosporon* sp.
Yeast fermentation broth	Identification of yeasts by determining fermentation
Yeast nitrogen base agar	Identification of yeasts by determining carbohydrate assimilation

From Koneman, E.W., and Roberts, G.D. 1985. Practical laboratory mycology, ed. 3. Williams & Wilkins, Baltimore.

media. All specimens should be cultured as soon as they are received by the laboratory to ensure the recovery of fungi from these important sources. Chapter 21 discusses laboratory handling of these specimens.

43.5. Culture Media and Incubation Requirements

Any of a number of fungal culture media are satisfactory for use in the clinical microbiology laboratory. Most are adequate for the recovery of fungi, and selection is usually left up to each individual laboratory director. Table 43.2 lists various fungal culture media and the indications for their use. Ideally, a battery of media should be used, and the following recommendations should be met:
1. Media with and without blood enrichment should be used.
2. Media with and without cycloheximide should be used.

3. All media should contain antibacterial agents; if *Nocardia* is suspected, mycobacterial culture media should be used for this purpose.

Culture dishes or screw-capped culture tubes are satisfactory for the recovery of fungi. Culture dishes are optimal, since they provide better aeration of cultures, a large surface area for better isolation of colonies, and greater ease of handling by technologists making microscopic preparations for examination. Agar in culture dishes has a marked tendency to dehydrate during the extended incubation period required for fungi; however, this problem can be minimized by using culture dishes containing at least 40 ml of agar and placing them in an incubator that contains a pan of water to humidify the environment. Dishes should be opened and examined only within a certified biological safety cabinet (Chapter 2). Many laboratories discourage the use of culture dishes; however, the advantages of using them outweigh the disadvantages.

Culture tubes are more easily stored, require less space for incubation, and are easily handled. In addition, they have a lower dehydration rate, and laboratory workers feel that cultures are less hazardous to handle when in tubes. The disadvantages, which include relatively poor isolation of colonies, a reduced surface area for culturing, and a tendency to promote anaerobiosis, discourage their routine use in a clinical microbiology laboratory.

Cultures should be incubated at room temperature or preferably at 30° C for 30 days before reporting as negative. A relative humidity of 40% to 50% can be achieved by placing an open pan of water in the incubator. Cultures should be examined at least three times weekly during incubation.

As previously mentioned, most clinical specimens are contaminated with bacteria and rapidly growing fungi. The need for antibacterial and antifungal agents is obvious. The addition of 0.5 µg/ml of cycloheximide and 0.016 mg/ml of chloramphenicol to media has been traditionally advocated to inhibit the growth of contaminating saprobic molds and bacteria. Better results have been achieved using a combination of 5 µg/ml of gentamicin and 16 µg/ml of chloramphenicol as antibacterial agents.

Certain of the fungi seem to have a requirement for blood, and a concentration of 5% to 10% sheep blood is recommended for inclusion into at least one of the culture media used. Cycloheximide may be added to any of the media that contain or lack antibacterial antibiotics. However, if cycloheximide is included as a part of the battery of culture media used, a medium lacking this ingredient should also be included. Certain of the pathogenic fungi are partially or completely inhibited by this compound; included are *Cryptococcus neoformans*, *Candida krusei* and other species of *Candida*, *Trichosporon beigelii*, *Pseudallescheria boydii*, and species of *Aspergillus*.

The use of antibiotics in fungal culture media is necessary for the optimal recovery of organisms; however, the use of decontamination and concentration methods advocated for the recovery of mycobacteria is not appropriate for fungal cultures.[71]

43.6. Direct Microscopic Examination of Clinical Specimens

Direct microscopic examination of clinical specimens has been used for many years; however, its usefulness should be reemphasized.[69] Since the charge of the clinical microbiology laboratory is to provide a rapid and accurate diagnosis, the mycology laboratory can provide this service in many instances by direct examination of the clinical specimen submitted for culture. Microbiologists are encouraged to become familiar with the diagnostic features of fungi commonly encountered in clinical specimens. This very important procedure can often provide the first microbiological proof of etiology in patients with fungal infection.

Tables 43.3 and 43.4 present the methods available for the direct microscopic detection of fungi in clinical specimens and a summary of the characteristic microscopic features of each method. More information regarding specific procedures is given in Chapter 7. Figures 43.1 to 43.22 present photomicrographs of some of the fungi commonly seen in clinical specimens.

Traditionally, the potassium hydroxide preparation has been the recommended method for the direct microscopic examination of specimens.[66] However, it is currently felt that the calcofluor white stain[30] (Chapter 7) is preferred. Slides prepared by this method may be observed using fluorescent microscopy or brightfield microscopy as used for the potassium hydroxide preparation; the former is optimal since fungal cells will fluoresce.

43.7. Characteristics of Fungi (Informal Glossary)

The fungi, a term that includes both yeasts and molds, differ significantly from the bacteria. The fungi are eukaryotic and contain a definite nucleus with a surrounding nuclear membrane; their cell wall is primarily composed of glucose and mannose polymers (chitin); their cell membrane contains sterols, and the organisms are resistant to antibacterial antibiotics. They show marked susceptibility to polyene antifungal agents, and all reproduce asexually; however, some reproduce sexually as well.

The fungi seen in the clinical laboratory can easily be separated into two groups based on the macroscopic appearance of the colonies formed. The yeasts produce moist, creamy, opaque or pasty colonies on culture media, while the molds (filamentous fungi) produce fluffy, cottony, woolly, or powdery colonies. Certain of the slow-growing pathogenic fungi are dimorphic and produce a mold form at 25° to 30° C and a yeast or spherule form at 35° to 37° C under certain circumstances.

Text continued on p. 699.

Table 43.3

Characteristics of Methods Available for the Direct Microscopic Detection of Fungi in Clinical Specimens

METHOD	USE	TIME REQUIRED	ADVANTAGES	DISADVANTAGES
Acid-fast stain	Detection of myco-bacteria and *No-cardia*	12 min	Detects *Nocardia** and *B. dermatitidis*	Tissue homogenates are difficult to observe because of background staining
Calcofluor white	Detection of fungi	1 min	Can be mixed with KOH; detects fungi rapidly because of bright fluorescence	Requires use of a fluorescence microscope; background fluorescence prominent, but fungi exhibit more intense fluorescence; vaginal secretions are difficult to interpret
Gram stain	Detection of bacteria	3 min	Is commonly performed on most clinical specimens submitted for bacteriology and will detect most fungi, if present	Some fungi stain well; however, others, e.g., *Cryptococcus* sp., stain weakly in some instances; some isolates of *Nocardia* fail to stain or stain weakly
India ink	Detection of *C. neoformans* in CSF	1 min	When positive in CSF, is diagnostic of meningitis	Positive in less than 50% of cases of meningitis; not reliable
Potassium hydroxide (KOH)	Clearing of specimen to make fungi more readily visible	5 min; if clearing is not complete, an additional 5-10 min is necessary	Rapid detection of fungal elements	Experience required since background artifacts are often confusing; clearing of some specimens may require an extended time
Methenamine silver stain	Detection of fungi in histologic section	1h	Best stain to detect fungal elements	Requires a specialized staining method that is not usually readily available to microbiology laboratories
Papanicolaou stain	Examination of secretions for presence of malignant cells	30 min	Cytotechnologist can detect fungal elements	
Periodic acid-Schiff (PAS) stain	Detection of fungi	20 min; 5 min additional if counterstain is employed	Stains fungal elements well; hyphae of molds and yeasts can be readily distinguished	*Norcardia* sp. do not stain well; *B. dermatitidis* appears pleomorphic
Wright stain	Examination of bone marrow or peripheral blood smears	7 min	Detects *H. capsulatum*	Detection is limited to *H. capsulatum*

*Acid-fast bacterium.

From Roberts, G.D., Goodman, N.L., Land, G.A., et al. 1985. Detection and recovery of fungi in clinical specimens. In Lennette, E.H., Balows, A., Hausler, W.J., Jr., and Shadomy, H.J., editors. Manual of clinical microbiology, ed. 4. American Society for Microbiology, Washington, D.C.

Table 43.4

Summary of Characteristic Features of Fungi Seen in Direct Examination of Clinical Specimens

MORPHOLOGICAL FORM FOUND IN SPECIMENS	ORGANISM(S)	SIZE RANGE (DIAMETER, μm)	CHARACTERISTIC FEATURES
Yeastlike	*H. capsulatum*	2-5	Small; oval to round budding cells; often found clustered within histiocytes; difficult to detect when present in small numbers
	S. schenckii	2-6	Small; oval to round to cigar-shaped; single or multiple buds present; uncommonly seen in clinical specimens
	C. neoformans	2-15	Cells exhibit great variation in size; usually spherical but may be football-shaped; buds single or multiple and "pinched off"; capsule may or may not be evident; occasionally pseudohyphal forms with or without a capsule may be seen in exudates or CSF
	M. furfur (in fungemia)	1.5-4.5	Small; bottle-shaped cells, buds separated from parent cell by a septum; emerge from a small collar
	B. dermatitidis	8-15	Cells are usually large, double refractile when present; buds usually single; however, several may remain attached to parent cells; buds connected by a broad base
	P. brasiliensis	5-60	Cells are usually large and are surrounded by smaller buds around the periphery ("mariner's wheel appearance"); smaller cells may be present (2-5 μm) and resemble *H. capsulatum*; buds have "pinched-off" appearance
Spherules	*C. immitis*	10-200	Spherules vary in size; some may contain endospores, others may be empty; adjacent spherules may resemble *B. dermatitidis*; endospores may resemble *H. capsulatum* but show no evidence of budding; spherules may produce multiple germ tubes if a direct preparation is kept in a moist chamber for ≥24 h
	Rhinosporidium seeberi	6-300	Large, thick-walled sporangia containing sporangiospores are present; mature sporangia are larger than spherules of *C. immitis*; hyphae may be found in cavitary lesions

From Roberts, G.D., Goodman, N.L., Land, G.A., et al. 1985. Detection and recovery of fungi in clinical specimens. In Lennette, E.H., Balows, A., Hausler, W.J., Jr., and Shadomy, H.J., editors. Manual of clinical microbiology, ed. 4. American Society for Microbiology, Washington, D.C.

Table 43.4
Summary of Characteristic Features of Fungi Seen in Direct Examination of Clinical Specimens—cont'd

MORPHOLOGICAL FORM FOUND IN SPECIMENS	ORGANISM(S)	SIZE RANGE (DIAMETER, μm)	CHARACTERISTIC FEATURES
	P. boydii (cases other than mycetoma)		Hyphae are septate and are impossible to distinguish from those of other hyaline molds
Yeast and pseudohyphae or hyphae	*Candida* sp.	3-4 (yeast) 5-10 (pseudohyphae)	Cells usually exhibit single budding; pseudohyphae, when present, are constricted at the ends and remain attached like links of sausage; hyphae, when present, are septate
	M. furfur (in tinea versicolor)	3-8 (yeast) 2.5-4 (hyphae)	Short, curved hyphal elements are usually present along with round yeast cells that retain their spherical shape in compacted clusters
Nonseptate hyphae	Zygomycetes; *Mucor, Rhizopus,* and other genera	10-30	Hyphae are large, ribbonlike, often fractured or twisted; occasional septa may be present; smaller hyphae are confused with those of *Aspergillus* sp., particularly *A. flavus*
Hyaline septate hyphae	Dermatophytes Skin and nails	3-15	Hyaline, septate hyphae are commonly seen; chains of arthroconidia may be present
	Hair	3-15	Arthroconidia on periphery of hair shaft producing a sheath are indicative of ectothrix infection; arthroconidia formed by fragmentation of hyphae within the hair shaft are indicative of endothrix infection
		3-15	Long hyphal filaments or channels within the hair shaft are indicative of favus hair infection
	Aspergillus sp.	3-12	Hyphae are septate and exhibit dichotomous, 45-degree angle branching; larger hyphae, often disturbed, may resemble those of Zygomycetes
	Geotrichum sp.	4-12	Hyphae and rectangular arthroconidia are present and are sometimes rounded; irregular forms may be present
	Trichosporon sp.	2-4 by 8	Hyphae and rectangular arthroconidia are present and sometimes rounded; occasionally blastoconidia may be present
Dematiaceous septate hyphae	*Bipolaris* sp. *Cladosporium* sp. *Curvularia* sp. *Drechslera* sp. *Exophiala* sp. *Exserohilum* sp. *Phialophora* sp. *Wangiella dermatitidis*	2-6	Dematiaceous polymorphous hyphae are seen; budding cells with single septa and chains of swollen rounded cells are often present; occasionally aggregates may be present in infection caused by *Phialophora* and *Exophiala* sp.
	Phaeoannellomyces (*Exophiala*) *werneckii*	1.5-5	Usually large numbers of frequently branched hyphae are present along with budding cells

Continued.

Table 43.4
Summary of Characteristic Features of Fungi Seen in Direct Examination of Clinical Specimens—cont'd

MORPHOLOGICAL FORM FOUND IN SPECIMENS	ORGANISM(S)	SIZE RANGE (DIAMETER, μm)	CHARACTERISTIC FEATURES
Sclerotic bodies	*Cladosporium carrionii* *Fonsecaea compacta* *Fonsecaea pedrosoi* *Phialophora verrucosa* *Rhinocladiella aqua-spersa*	5-20	Brown, round to pleomorphic, thick-walled cells with transverse septations; commonly, cells contain two fission planes that form a tetrad of cells; occasionally, branched septate hyphae may be found along with sclerotic bodies
Granules	*Acremonium* *A. falciforme* *A. kiliense* *A. recifei*	200-300	White, soft granules without a cementlike matrix
	Curvularia *C. geniculata* *C. lunata*	500-1,000	Black, hard grains with a cementlike matrix at periphery
	Aspergillus *A. nidulans*	65-160	White, soft granule without a cementlike matrix
	Exophiala *E. jeanselmei*	200-300	Black, soft granules, vacuolated, without a cementlike matrix, made of dark hyphae and swollen cells
	Fusarium *F. moniliforme* *F. solani*	200-500 300-600	White, soft granules without a cementlike matrix
	Leptosphaeria *L. senegalensis*	400-600	Black, hard granules with cementlike matrix present
	L. tompkinsii	500-1,000	Periphery composed of polygonal swollen cells and center of a hyphal network
	Madurella *M. grisea*	350-500	Black, soft granules without a cementlike matrix, periphery composed of polygonal swollen cells and center of a hyphal network
	M. mycetomatis	200-900	Black to brown, hard granules of two types: (1) Rust brown, compact, and filled with cementlike matrix (2) Deep brown, filled with numerous vesicles, 6-14 μm in diameter, cementlike matrix in periphery, and central area of light-colored hyphae.
	Neotestudina *N. rosatti*	300-600	White, soft granules with cementlike matrix present at periphery
	Pseudallescheria *P. boydii*	200-300	White, soft granules composed of hyphae and swollen cells at periphery in cementlike matrix
	Pyrenochaeta *P. romeri*	300-600	Black, soft granules composed of polygonal swollen cells at periphery, center is network of hyphae, no cementlike matrix present

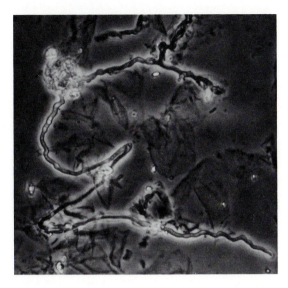

Figure 43.1
Potassium hydroxide preparation of skin, phase-contrast, dermatophyte, showing septate hyphae intertwined among epithelial cells (500 ×).

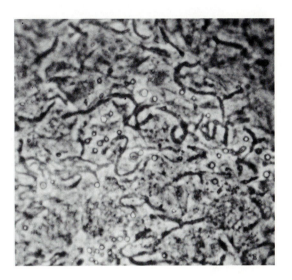

Figure 43.2
Potassium hydroxide preparation of skin, phase-contrast, *M. furfur*, showing spherical yeast cells and short hyphal fragments (500 ×).

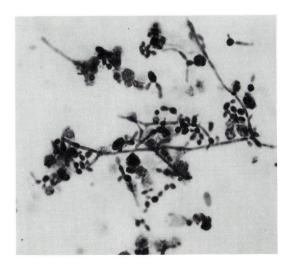

Figure 43.3
Gram stain of urine, *C. albicans*, showing blastoconidia and pseudohyphae.

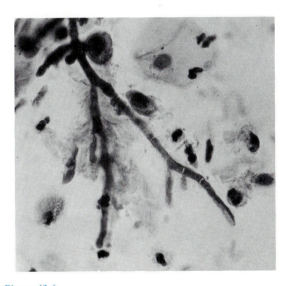

Figure 43.4
Papanicolaou stain of sputum, *A. fumigatus*, showing dichotomously branching septate hyphae.

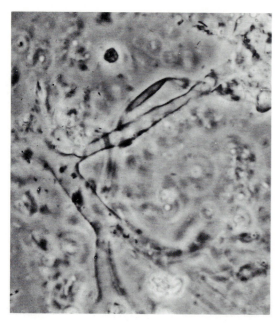

Figure 43.5
Potassium hydroxide preparation of sputum, phase contrast, *Rhizopus* species, showing fragmented portions of nonseptate hyphae of varying size.

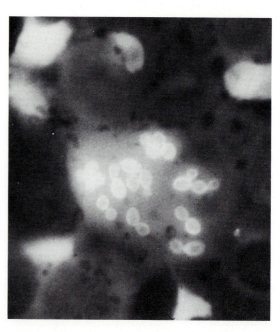

Figure 43.6
Calcofluor white stain of sputum, *H. capsulatum*, showing intracellular yeast cells 2 to 5 μm in diameter.

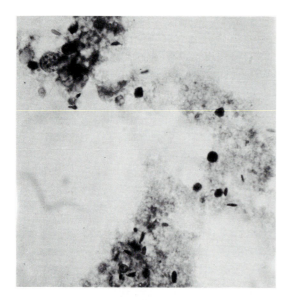

Figure 43.7
Periodic acid–Schiff stain of exudate. *S. schenckii*, showing cigar- to oval-shaped yeast cells.

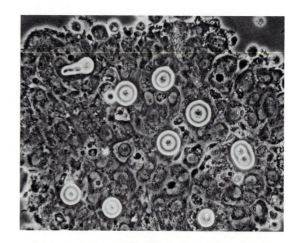

Figure 43.8
Potassium hydroxide preparation of pleural fluid, phase contrast, *C. neoformans*, showing encapsulated, spherical yeast cells of varying sizes.

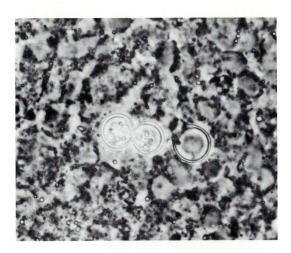

Figure 43.9
Potassium hydroxide preparation of exudate, phase contrast, *B. dermatitidis*, showing large budding yeast cells with a distinct broad base between the cells.

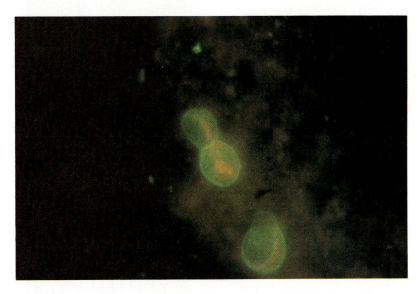

Figure 43.10
Auramine-rhodamine preparation of bone lesion. *Blastomyces dermatitis* showing characteristic broad-based budding yeast cell.

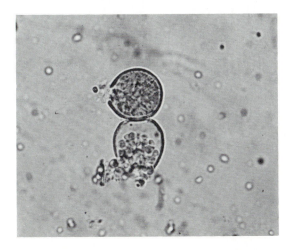

Figure 43.11
Potassium hydroxide preparation of sputum, bright field, *C. immitis*, showing two spherules, filled with endospores, lying adjacent to each other that resemble *B. dermatitidis*.

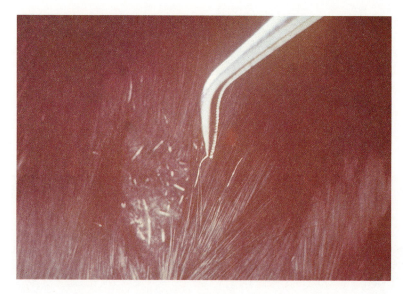

Figure 43.12
Fluorescent hairs. Wood's lamp (mycotic infection).

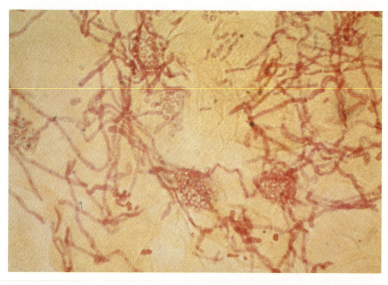

Figure 43.13
M. furfur, microscopic (400 ×). (Courtesy Upjohn Co.)

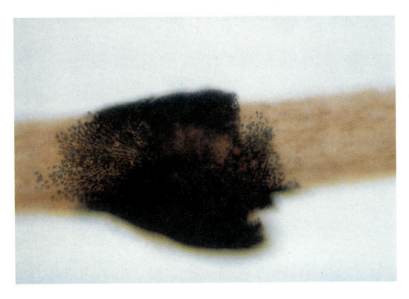

Figure 43.14
P. hortae. Hair (400 ×). (Courtesy Upjohn Co.)

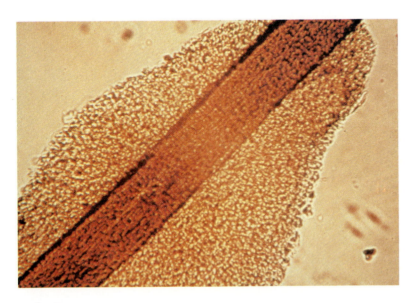

Figure 43.15
Trichosporon beigelii. Hair (40×). (Courtesy Upjohn Co.)

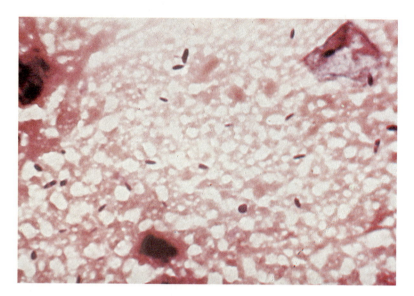

Figure 43.16
Sporothrix schenkii in mouse testis.

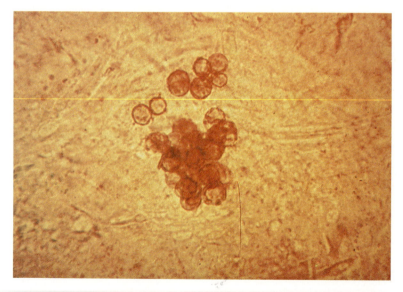

Figure 43.17
Sclerotic bodies of chromoblastomycosis in tissue (400×). (Courtesy Upjohn Co.)

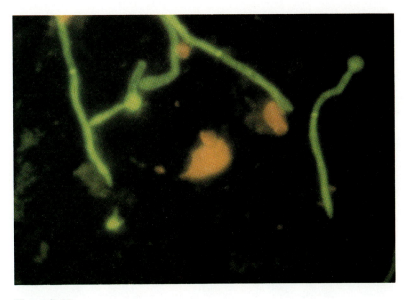

Figure 43.18
Candida albicans in urine; calcofluor white stain.

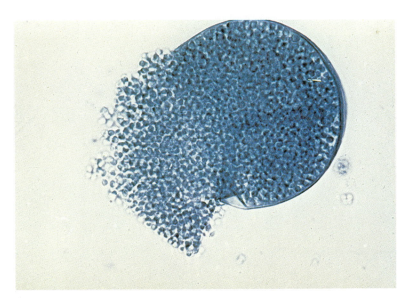

Figure 43.19
Coccidioides immitis. Ruptured spherule with endospores.

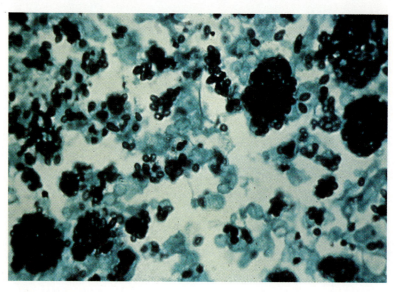

Figure 43.20
Histoplasma capsulatum in lung. Methenamine silver stain (430 ×).

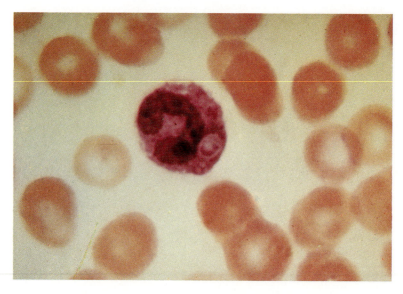

Figure 43.21
Histoplasma capsulatum in neutrophil on peripheral blood smear (1000 ×).

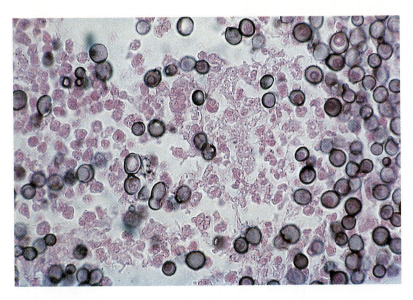

Figure 43.22
Blastomyces dermatitides in tissue. Methenamine silver stain (430 ×).

The identification of the yeasts requires not only recognition of certain microscopic features, but also the use of biochemical tests to provide a definitive species identification. The definitive identification of the molds requires recognition of the characteristic microscopic features of the organism. The following paragraphs describe the basic microscopic morphological features of fungi, and representative photomicrographs are used to illustrate them.

The yeasts are unicellular organisms that reproduce by budding; their microscopic morphological features usually appear similar for different genera and are not particularly helpful in their separation. The basic structural units of the molds are tubelike projections known as hyphae (Figures 43.23 to 43.26). As the **hyphae** grow, they become intertwined to form a loose network called the **mycelium,** which penetrates the substrate from which it obtains the necessary nutrients for growth. The nutrient-absorbing and water-exchanging portion of the fungi is called the vegetative mycelium. The portion projecting above the substrate surface is known as the aerial mycelium; aerial mycelia often give rise to fruiting bodies from which the asexual spores are borne. Recognition of certain types of vegetative hyphae is helpful in placing the organism into a certain group. For example, dermatophytes often produce several types of hyphae, including antler hyphae

(Figure 43.27) that are curved, freely branching, and antlerlike in appearance. Racquet hyphae are often found that are enlarged, club-shaped hyphae with the smaller end attached to the large end of an adjacent club-shaped hyphal strand (Figure 43.28). In addition, certain of the dermatophytes produce spiral hyphae that are coiled or corkscrewlike turns seen within the hyphal strand (Figure 43.29). These structures are not characteristic for any certain group of organisms; however, they are frequently found in the dermatophytes.

The features by which most fungi are identified are related to the mode of sporulation and the morphology and arrangement of the spores produced. Fungi may reproduce sexually, asexually, or by both means. Sexual reproduction is associated with the production of specialized structures that result in nuclear fusion and the production of specialized spores. Some species of fungi produce sexual spores in a large saclike structure called an ascocarp (Figure 43.30). This, in turn, contains smaller sacs called asci, each of which contains four or eight ascospores. This type of sexual reproduction is sometimes seen in the fungi recovered in the clinical microbiology laboratory. Most of the fungi of clinical importance reproduce asexually. There is a consensus that perhaps all fungi possess a sexual form; however, this form has not been observed on artificial culture me-

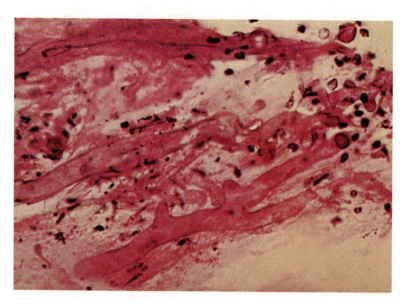

Figure 43.23
Zygomycosis. Note large, nonseptate branched hyphae.

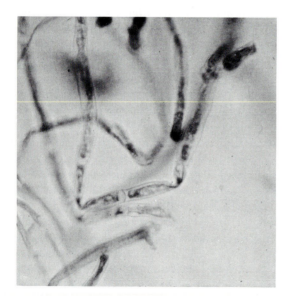

Figure 43.24
Hyaline hyphae showing septations (430 ×).

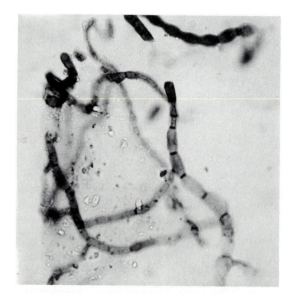

Figure 43.25
Dematiaceous hyphae showing pigmentation and septations
(430 ×).

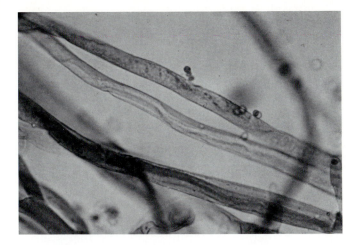

Figure 43.26
Hyaline hyphae lacking septations (aseptate).

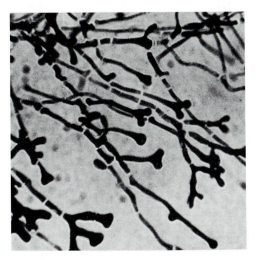

Figure 43.27
Antler hyphae showing swollen hyphal tips resembling antlers, with lateral and terminal branching (favic chandeliers) (500 ×).

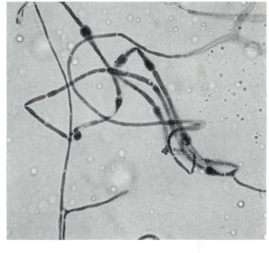

Figure 43.28
Racquet hyphae showing a swollen area resembling a tennis racquet.

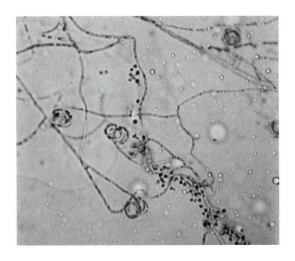

Figure 43.29
Spiral hyphae exhibiting corkscrewlike turns (430 ×).

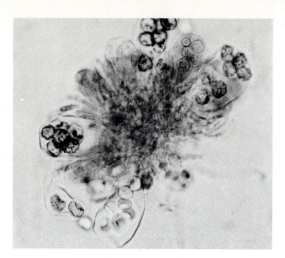

Figure 43.30
Ascocarp showing dark-appearing ascospores (430 ×).

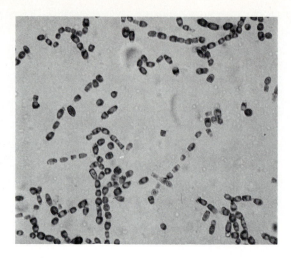

Figure 43.31
Arthroconidia formation produced by the breaking down of a hyphal strand into individual rectangular units (430 ×).

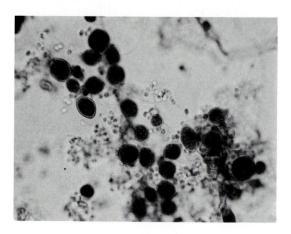

Figure 43.32
Chlamydospores composed of thick-walled spherical cells (430 ×).

dia for most of the clinically important species. Asexual sporulation is the type of sporulation seen in most fungi encountered in a clinical laboratory. The type of spores, their morphology and arrangement are important criteria for establishing the definitive identification of an organism.

The simplest type of sporulation is the development of the spore directly from the vegetative hyphae. Three types of spores are recognized. **Arthroconidia** are formed directly from the hyphae by fragmentation through the points of septation. When mature, they appear as square, rectangular, or barrel-shaped, thick-walled cells (Figure 43.31). These result from the simple fragmentation of the hyphae into spores, which are easily dislodged and disseminated into the environment. **Chlamydospores** are round, thick-walled resistant spores formed directly from the differentiation of the hyphae in which there is a concentration of protoplasm and nutrient material (Figure 43.32). These spores appear to be resistant resting spores produced by the rounding up and enlargement of the terminal cells of the hyphae. **Blastoconidia**, most often found in the yeasts, are cells produced by budding with the daughter cells being pinched off from portions of the mother cell through a constricted area (Figure 43.33). In some species of yeasts, most commonly *Candida*, blastoconidia may elongate and remain attached and form structures called pseudohyphae (Figure 43.34).

A variety of other types of spores occur with many species of fungi. Conidia are asexual spores produced singly or in groups by specialized vegetative hyphal strands called conidiophores. In some instances, the conidia are freed from their point of attachment by pinching off, or abstriction. Some conidiophores terminate in a swollen structure called a vesicle. From the surface of the vesicle are formed secondary small flask-shaped phialides, which in turn give rise to long chains of conidia. This type of fruiting structure is characteristic of the aspergilli (Figure 43.35). A single slender, tubular conidiophore (phialide) that supports a cluster of conidia, held together as a gelatinous mass, is characteristic of certain fungi, includ-

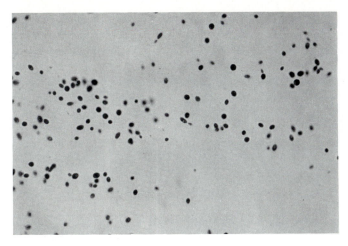

Figure 43.33
Blastoconidia (budding cells) characteristic of the yeasts (430 ×).

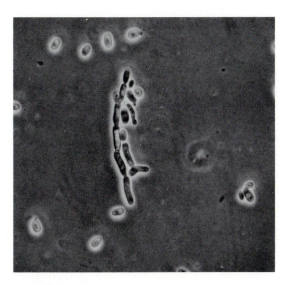

Figure 43.34
Pseudohyphae consisting of elongated cells with constrictions where attached (430 ×).

ing the genus *Acremonium* (Figure 43.36). In other instances, conidiophores branch into a structure known as a penicillus where each branch terminates in secondary branches (metulae) and phialides from which chains of conidia are borne (Figure 43.37). Species of *Penicillium* and *Paecilomyces* are representative of this type of sporulation. In other instances, fungi may produce conidia of two sizes: **microconidia** are small, unicellular, round, elliptical, or pyriform in shape (Figure 43.38); **macroconidia** are large, usually multiseptate, and club- or spindle-

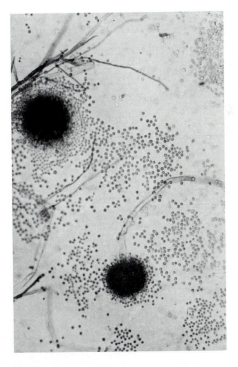

Figure 43.35
Conidia (asexual spores) produced on specialized structures (conidiophores) of *Aspergillus* (430 ×).

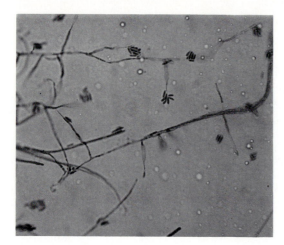

Figure 43.36
Simple tubular phialide with a cluster of conidia at its tip, characteristic of *Acremonium* (430 ×).

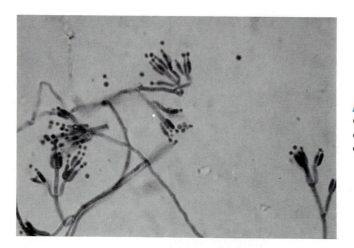

Figure 43.37
Complex method of sporulation where conidia are borne on phialides produced on secondary branches (metulae), characteristic of *Penicillium* (430 ×).

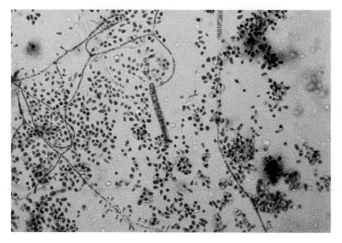

Figure 43.38
Numerous small, spherical microconidia contrasted with a large, elongated macroconidium (430 ×).

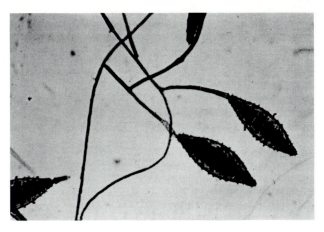

Figure 43.39
Large, rough-walled macronidia of *M. canis* (430 ×).

shaped (Figure 43.39). Microconidia may be borne directly on the side of the hyphal strand or at the end of a long or short conidiophore. Macroconidia are usually borne on a short to long conidiophore and may be smooth-walled or rough-walled. Microconidia and macroconidia are seen in many fungal species and are not specific, except as they are used to differentiate the different genera of dermatophytes.

One group of fungi, the **Zygomycetes,** produce structures different from the ones previously described. The hyphae are sparsely septate, and asexual spores are produced in a large saclike structure called a *sporangium*, which is borne on the tip of a supporting structure (sporangiophore) (Figure 43.40). Sporulation takes place by progressive cleavage during maturation within the sporangium; the spores are produced and released by the rupture of the sporangial wall. This type of sporulation is characteristic of the Zygomycetes.

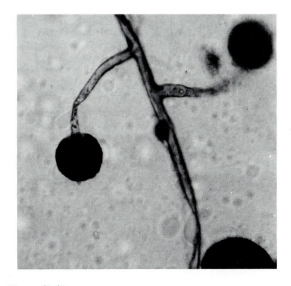

Figure 43.40
Large, saclike sporangium that contains sporangiospores, characteristic of the zygomycetes (250 ×).

43.8. Classification of Fungi

The botanical taxonomical scheme for grouping the fungi has very little value in a clinical microbiology laboratory. Table 43.5 is a simplified taxonomical scheme illustrating the major groups to which the clinically important fungi belong. Using this classification scheme, the fungi can be included within four major divisions: Zygomycota, Ascomycota, Basidiomycota, and Deuteromycota.[13] The division Zygomycota includes organisms that have aseptate hy-

phae and reproduce asexually by spores produced inside of sporangia and reproduce sexually by the production of zygospores. *Mucor, Rhizopus*, and *Absidia* are the most common members of this group. The Ascomycota includes organisms that have septate hyphae, produce conidia, or reproduce sexually by means of ascospores produced within an ascus. Common members of this group include *Pseudallescheria boydii* and species of *Aspergillus*. The Basidiomycota includes a group of organisms that have

Table 43.5
Phylogenetic Position of Medically Significant Fungi

CLASS	ORDER	FAMILY	GENUS/SPECIES
Phylum Zygomycota			
Zygomycetes	Entomophthorales	Entomophthoraceae	*Basidiobolus*
	Mucorales	Mucoraceae	*Absidia*
			Cunninghamella
			Mucor
			Rhizopus
			Syncephalastrum
Phylum Ascomycota			
Hemiascomycetes	Endomycetales	Endomycetaceae	*Endomyces (Geotrichum* sp.)*
		Saccharomycetaceae	*Kluyveromyces (Candida pseudotropicalis)*
Loculoascomycetes	Myriangiales	Saccardinulaceae	*Piedraia hortae*
	Microascales	Microascaceae	*Pseudallescheria boydii*
Plectomycetes	Eurotiales	Eurotiaceae	*Emericella (Aspergillus nidulans)*
			Sortorya (Aspergillus fumigatus)
		Gymnoascaceae	*Ajellomyces (Histoplasma capsulatum, Blastomyces dermatitidis)*
			Arthroderma (Trichophyton sp. and *Microsporum* sp.)*
Phylum Basidiomycota			
Teliomycetes	Ustilaginales	Filobasidiaceae	*Filobasidiella (Cryptococcus neoformans)*

*Genus/species designations for the sexual, imperfect forms are shown in parentheses.
Modified from Chandler, F.W., Kaplan, W., and Ajello, L., 1980. Histopathology of mycotic disease. Year Book Medical Publishers, Chicago.

septate hyphae and reproduce asexually by conidia or sexually by means of basidiospores. *Filobasidiella (Cryptococcus)* is the major genus within this division that is encountered in a clinical laboratory. The major group to which most of the clinically important fungi belong is the Deuteromycota. This group of organisms has septate hyphae and reproduces asexually with the production of conidia. Whether they reproduce sexually is not known. As previously mentioned, the botanical taxonomical scheme has little role in the clinical laboratory. Clinicians find more value in categorizing the fungi into three or four categories of mycoses: (1) the superficial or cutaneous mycoses; (2) subcutaneous mycoses; (3) the systemic mycoses; and (4) the opportunistic mycoses.

The superficial or cutaneous mycoses are fungal infections that involve the hair, skin, or nails without invasion of the tissue. The group of fungi in this category that are most commonly recovered are the dermatophytes; also included are agents of infections such as tinea versicolor, tinea nigra, and piedra, which involve the outermost keratin layer of the skin.

Subcutaneous mycoses are infections confined to the subcutaneous tissue without dissemination to distant sites. Examples include sporotrichosis, chromoblastomycosis, and mycetoma.

The systemic mycoses are caused primarily by fungi belonging to the genera *Blastomyces, Coccidioides, Histoplasma,* and *Paracoccidioides*. Infec-

Table 43.5
Phylogenetic Position of Medically Significant Fungi—cont'd

CLASS	ORDER	FAMILY	GENUS/SPECIES
Form Phylum Deuteromycota			
Blastomycetes		Cryptococcaceae	*Candida*
Hyphomycetes	Moniliales	Moniliaceae	*Acremonium*
			Aspergillus
			Blastomyces
			Chrysosporium
			Coccidioides
			Epidermophyton
			Geotrichum
			Gliocladium
			Histoplasma
			Microsporum
			Paecilomyces
			Paracoccidioides
			Penicillium
			Sepedonium
			Scopulariopsis
			Sporothrix
			Trichoderma
			Trichophyton
		Dematiaceae	*Alternaria*
			Aureobasidium
			Bipolaris
			Cladosporium
			Curvularia
			Drechslera
			Exserohilum
			Fonsecaea
			Helminthosporium
			Madurella
			Nigrospora
			Phaeoannellomyces
			Phialophora
			Rhinocladiella
			Stemphylium
			Ulocladium
			Wangiella
		Tuberculariaceae	*Epicoccum*
			Fusarium
Coelomycetes	Sphaeropsidales		*Phoma*

tions caused by these organisms involve the lungs primarily, but also may become widely disseminated and involve any organ of the body.

The group of fungi included in the opportunistic mycoses includes an ever-expanding list of organisms. These infections are commonly found in patients who are immunocompromised, usually by an underlying disease process or by immunosuppressive agents. Fungi previously thought to be nonpathogenic can cause infection in the compromised host; commonly encountered infections include aspergillosis, zygomycosis, candidosis, and cryptococcosis.

This type of classification allows the clinician to categorize organisms logically into groups having clinical relevance. Table 43.6 presents an example of the clinical classification of fungi that will be useful to the clinician. This type of classification also plays little role in the identification of fungi in the clinical microbiology laboratory.

Table 43.6
Clinical Classification of Pathogenic Fungi

CUTANEOUS	SUBCUTANEOUS	OPPORTUNISTIC	SYSTEMIC
Superficial mycoses	Chromoblastomycosis	Aspergillosis	Aspergillosis
Tinea	Sporotrichosis	Candidosis	Blastomycosis
Piedra	Mycetoma (eumycotic)	Cryptococcosis	Candidosis
Candidosis	Phaeohyphomycosis	Geotrichosis	Coccidioidomycosis
Dermatophytosis		Zygomycosis	Histoplasmosis
			Cryptococcosis
			Geotrichosis
			Paracoccidioidomycosis
			Zygomycosis

43.9. Clinical Laboratory Working Schema

To assist persons working in clinical microbiology laboratories with the identification of clinically important fungi, Koneman and Roberts[46] have suggested the use of a practical working schema designed to (1) assist in the recognition of fungi most commonly encountered in clinical specimens, (2) assist with the recognition of fungi recovered on culture media that belong to the strictly pathogenic fungi, and (3) provide a pathway that is easy to follow and that allows a positive identification of an organism to be made on the basis of a few colonial and microscopic features of the organism. Table 43.7 presents these features; however, it must be recognized that the table includes only those organisms commonly seen in the clinical laboratory. With practice, most laboratorians should be able to recognize the fungi commonly encountered on a day-to-day basis. The identification of others will require the use of various texts containing photomicrographs useful for their identification.

The use of this schema requires that one first examine the culture for the presence or absence of septae. If the hyphae appear to be predominantly nonseptate, zygomycetes should be considered. If the hyphae are septate, they must be examined further for the presence or absence of pigment. If a dark pigment is present in the conidia or the hyphae, the organism is considered to be dematiaceous and the conidia are then examined for their morphological features and their arrangement on the hyphae. If the hyphae are nonpigmented, they are considered to be hyaline. They are then examined for the type and the arrangement of the conidia produced. The molds are identified by recognition of their characteristic microscopic features.

The yeasts may be presumptively identified by the presence or absence of hyphae, pseudohyphae, blastoconidia, and arthroconidia on cornmeal agar. The identification of yeasts is discussed later within the chapter.

43.10. Extent of Identification of Fungi Recovered from Clinical Specimens

The question of when and how far to go with identification of fungi recovered from clinical specimens presents an interesting situation. The current emphasis on cost containment (Chapter 4) and the ever-increasing number of opportunistic fungi causing infection in compromised patients cause one to consider whether all fungi recovered from clinical specimens should be thoroughly identified and reported. Murray et al.[59] in 1977 were concerned with the time and expense associated with the identification of yeasts from respiratory tract specimens. Since these are the specimens most commonly submitted for fungal culture, they questioned whether it was important to provide an identification for every organism recovered. After evaluating the clinical usefulness of information provided by the identification of yeast recovered from respiratory tract specimens, they suggested that (1) the routine identification of yeasts recovered in culture from respiratory secretions is not warranted, but that all yeasts should be screened for the presence of *Cryptococcus neoformans*; (2) all respiratory secretions submitted for fungal culture, regardless of the presence or absence of oropharyngeal contamination, should be cultured since pathogens such as *H. capsulatum*, *Blastomyces dermatitidis*, *Coccidioides immitis*, and *Sporothrix schenckii* may be recovered; and (3) the routine identification of yeast in respiratory secretions is of little or no

Table 43.7
Commonly Encountered Fungi of Clinical Laboratory Importance: A Practical Working Schema

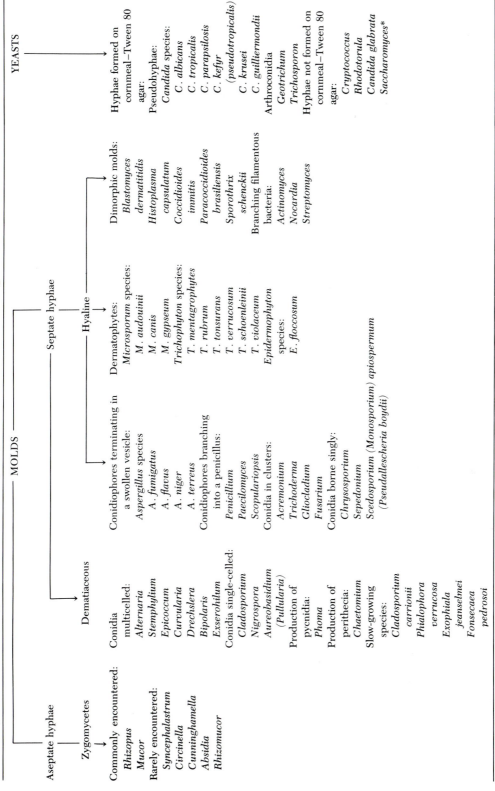

Aseptate hyphae

Zygomycetes

Commonly encountered:
Rhizopus
Mucor

Rarely encountered:
Syncephalastrum
Circinella
Cunninghamella
Absidia
Rhizomucor

MOLDS — Septate hyphae

Dematiaceous

Conidia multicelled:
Alternaria
Stemphylium
Epicoccum
Curvularia
Drechslera
Bipolaris
Exserohilum

Conidia single-celled:
Cladosporium
Nigrospora
Aureobasidium
(*Pullularia*)

Production of pycnidia:
Phoma

Production of perithecia:
Chaetomium

Slow-growing species:
Cladosporium carrionii
Phialophora verrucosa
Exophiala jeanselmei
Fonsecaea pedrosoi

Hyaline

Dermatophytes:
Microsporum species:
M. audouinii
M. canis
M. gypseum
Trichophyton species:
T. mentagrophytes
T. rubrum
T. tonsurans
T. verrucosum
T. schoenleinii
T. violaceum
Epidermophyton species:
E. floccosum

Conidiophores terminating in a swollen vesicle:
Aspergillus species
A. fumigatus
A. flavus
A. niger
A. terreus

Conidiophores branching into a penicillus:
Penicillium
Paecilomyces
Scopulariopsis

Conidia in clusters:
Acremonium
Trichoderma
Gliocladium
Fusarium

Conidia borne singly:
Chrysosporium
Sepedonium
Scedosporium (Monosporium) apiospermum
(*Pseudallescheria boydii*)

Dimorphic molds:
Blastomyces dermatitidis
Histoplasma capsulatum
Coccidioides immitis
Paracoccidioides brasiliensis
Sporothrix schenckii

Branching filamentous bacteria:
Actinomyces
Nocardia
Streptomyces

YEASTS

Hyphae formed on cornmeal–Tween 80 agar:

Pseudohyphae:
Candida species:
C. albicans
C. tropicalis
C. parapsilosis
C. kefyr
(*pseudotropicalis*)
C. krusei
C. guilliermondii

Arthroconidia
Geotrichum
Trichosporon

Hyphae not formed on cornmeal–Tween 80 agar:
Cryptococcus
Rhodotorula
Candida glabrata
*Saccharomyces**

From Koneman, E. W., and Roberts, G. D. 1985. Practical laboratory mycology, ed. 3. Williams & Wilkins, Baltimore.
*Rudimentary hyphae may be present.

value to the clinician and probably represents "normal flora" with the exception of *C. neoformans*.

When and how far to proceed with an identification of the molds is a much more difficult question to answer. A consensus of a number of clinical mycologists is that all commonly encountered molds should be identified and reported regardless of the clinical source. Those organisms that fail to sporulate after a reasonable time should be reported as being present but the identification need not be attempted if the dimorphic fungi have been ruled out or if the clinician feels that the organism is not clinically significant. Ideally, all laboratories should identify all fungi recovered from clinical specimens; however, the limits of practicality and economic considerations play a definite role in making a decision as to how far to go with their identification. Each individual laboratory director, in consultation with the clinicians being served, will have to make this decision after considering the patient population, laboratory practice, and economic impact.

43.11. Laboratory Safety Considerations

Although there are risks associated with the handling of fungi recovered from clinical specimens, a commonsense approach concerning their handling will protect the laboratory from contamination and workers from infection.

It is necessary that all mold cultures and clinical specimens be handled in a Class II biological safety cabinet (Chapter 2), *with no exceptions*. Some laboratory directors feel that it is necessary to handle mold cultures within an enclosed biological safety cabinet equipped with gloves; however, this is not necessary if a laminar flow biological safety cabinet is used. It is permissible, however, to handle yeast cultures on the bench top; they must be treated as infectious agents. The use of an incinerator-burner or a gas flame is suitable for the decontamination of a loop used for transfer of yeast cultures. Cultures of organisms suspected of being pathogens should be sealed with tape to prevent laboratory contamination and should be autoclaved as soon as a definitive identification of the organism is made.

Few problems concerning laboratory contamination or infection of laboratory personnel will be associated with the handling of fungi if common safety precautions and careful handling of cultures are observed.

43.12. General Considerations for the Identification of Molds

The identification of molds is made using a combination of (1) the growth rate, (2) colonial morphological features, and (3) microscopic morphological features. In most instances the latter provides the most definitive means for identification. The determination of the growth rate of a culture is one of the most helpful observations made when examining a mold culture. However, this information may be of limited value since the growth rate of certain fungi is variable, depending upon the amount of inoculum present in a clinical specimen. In general, the growth rate for the dimorphic fungi, including *B. dermatitidis*, *C. immitis*, *H. capsulatum*, and *Paracoccidioides brasiliensis*, is slow; 1 to 4 weeks are usually required before colonies become visible. In some instances, however, cultures of *B. dermatitidis* and *C. immitis* may be detected within 3 to 5 days. This is a somewhat unusual circumstance and is encountered only when large numbers of the organism are present on the culture medium. In contrast, colonies of the Zygomycetes may appear within 24 hours, while the other hyaline and dematiaceous fungi often exhibit growth within 1 to 5 days. The growth rate of an organism is an important observation, but it must be used in combination with other features before the definitive identification of an organism can be made.

The colonial morphological features are also of limited value in identifying the molds, because of natural variation among isolates and variation of colonies on different culture media. Although it may be possible to recognize certain species recovered repeatedly in the laboratory based on their colonial morphological features, this is an unreliable criterion and should be used only to supplement the information obtained by microscopic examination of the culture. When examining the colonial morphological features, the type of culture media used and the incubation conditions must be considered. For example, *H. capsulatum*, which appears as a white to tan mold on brain heart infusion agar, may appear yeastlike in appearance when grown on the same medium containing blood enrichment. It is recommended that the colonial morphological features be used to supplement the information obtained from the growth rate and microscopic morphological features.

PROCEDURE 43.1

Wet Mount

1. With a wire bent at a 90-degree angle, cut out a small portion of an isolated colony. The portion should be removed from a point intermediate between the center and the periphery. The portion removed should contain a small amount of the supporting agar.
2. Place the portion of the culture onto a slide to which has been added a drop of lactophenol cotton (Appendix B) or aniline blue (Figure 43.41).
3. Place a coverslip into position and apply gentle pressure with a pencil eraser or other suitable object to disperse the growth and agar. Examine microscopically.

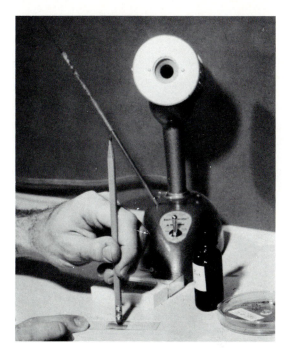

Figure 43.41
Performance of a wet mount, showing dispersion of growth under coverslip using pressure.

In general, the microscopic morphological features of the molds are stable and exhibit minimal variation. The definitive identification is based on the characteristic shape, method of production, and arrangement of spores; however, the size of the hyphae also provides helpful information. The large ribbonlike hyphae of the zygomycetes are easily recognized, while small hyphae, 1 to 2 μm in size, may suggest the presence of one of the dimorphic fungi.

The fungi may be prepared for microscopic observation using several techniques. The procedure traditionally used by most laboratories is the wet mount examination (Procedure 43.1). The wet mount can be prepared easily and quickly and often is sufficient to make the identification for many of the fungi commonly encountered in the clinical laboratory.

The major disadvantage of the wet mount is that the characteristic arrangement of spores is disrupted when pressure is applied to the coverslip. This method is suitable in many instances since characteristic spores are often seen but, when their arrangement cannot be determined, it is not adequate to make a definitive identification.

The easiest, most economical and most suitable

PROCEDURE 43.2

Scotch or Cellophane Tape Preparation

1. Touch the adhesive side of a small length of transparent tape to the surface of the colony.
2. Adhere the length of tape to the surface of a microscope slide to which has been added a drop of lactophenol cotton or aniline blue (Figure 43.42).
3. Observe microscopically for the characteristic shape and arrangement of the spores.

method for the microscopic identification of fungi is the Scotch (cellophane) tape preparation (Procedure 43.2). This method is recommended for routine use in clinical microbiology laboratories of all sizes.

The transparent tape preparation allows one to

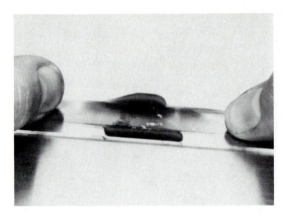

Figure 43.42
Scotch tape preparation, showing placement of tape onto slide containing lactophenol cotton blue.

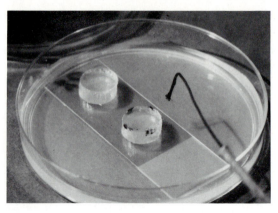

Figure 43.43
Microslide culture, showing inoculation of agar plug.

PROCEDURE 43.3

Microslide Culture

1. Cut a small block of a suitable agar medium that has been previously poured into a Petri dish to a depth of approximately 2 mm. The block may be cut using a sterile scalpel blade or with a sterile test tube that has no lip (which produces a round block).
2. Place a sterile microscope slide onto the surface of a Petri dish containing sterile 2% agar. Alternatively, place a round piece of filter paper or paper towel into a sterile Petri dish, add two applicator sticks, and position the microscope slide on top.
3. Add the agar block to the surface of the sterile microscope slide.
4. With a right-angle wire, inoculate the four quadrants of the agar plug with the organisms (Figure 43.43).
5. Apply a sterile coverslip onto the surface of the agar plug.
6. If the filter paper applicator stick method is used, add a small amount of sterile water to the bottom of the Petri dish. Replace the lid of the culture and allow it to incubate at 30° C.
7. After a suitable incubation period, remove the coverslip (working inside of a biological safety cabinet) and place it on a microscope slide containing a drop of lactophenol cotton or aniline blue. It is often helpful to place the coverslip near the opening of an incinerator-burner to allow rapid drying of the organism on the coverslip to occur before adding it to the stain.
8. Observe microscopically for the characteristic shape and arrangement of spores.
9. The remaining agar block may be used later (if the microslide culture is unsatisfactory for the microscopic identification) if it is allowed to incubate further. The agar plug is then removed and discarded, and a drop of lactophenol cotton or aniline blue is placed on the area of growth and a coverslip is positioned into place. Many laboratorians like to make two cultures on the same slide so that if characteristic microscopic features are not observed on examination of the first culture, the second will be available after an additional incubation period.

observe the organism microscopically approximately the way it grows in culture. The spores are usually intact, and the microscopic identification of an organism can be made with ease. If the tape is not pressed firmly enough to the colonies' surface, the sample may not be adequate for an identification. In instances where spores are not observed, a wet mount should be made as a backup step. There have been situations where the macroconidia of *H. capsulatum* were seen in wet mount preparations when the Scotch tape preparation revealed only hyphal fragments. On the contrary, there have been instances where cultures have sporulated heavily and revealed only the presence of conidia when the Scotch tape preparation is observed. In this type of situation, a second Scotch tape preparation should be made from the periphery of the colony where sporulation is not as heavy.

Some laboratories prefer to use the microslide culture (Procedure 43.3) for making the microscopic identification of an organism. This method might appear to be the most suitable since it allows one to observe microscopically the fungus growing directly underneath the coverslip. Microscopic features should be easily discerned, structures should be intact, and a large number of representative areas of growth are available for observation.

Although this method is ideal for making a definitive identification of an organism, it is the least practical of all the methods described. It should be reserved for those instances where an identification cannot be made on the basis of a Scotch tape preparation or wet mount. CAUTION: do not make slide cultures of slowly growing organisms suspected of being dimorphic pathogens such as *H. capsulatum*, *B. dermatitidis*, *C. immitis*, *P. brasiliensis*, or *S. schenckii*. Microslide cultures should be observed only after a coverslip has been removed from the agar plug and not while it is in position on top of the agar plug. The latter method of observation is highly dangerous in the case of the species mentioned and should not be used in the clinical laboratory.

43.13 Superficial and Cutaneous Mycoses

The superficial fungal infections are produced by fungi of very low virulence. They exhibit little tissue invasion and evoke minimal host response, the infections they produce are asymptomatic, and aesthetically displeasing lesions are usually produced. Lesions usually exhibit hyperpigmentation, hypo-

pigmentation, or nodular mass production on the hair shaft distal to the skin. Most are uncommonly seen except for tinea versicolor.

43.13.a. Tinea versicolor (pityriasis versicolor). Tinea versicolor is a skin infection characterized by superficial brownish scaly areas on light-skinned persons and lighter areas on dark-skinned persons. The lesions occur on the smooth surfaces of the body, namely, the trunk, arms, shoulders, and face. It has a worldwide distribution. It is caused by *Malassezia furfur*, an organism not usually cultured in the clinical laboratory. Recovery of the organism is not required to establish a diagnosis, and it is seldom attempted; if one wishes to culture the organism, an agar medium overlaid with a fatty acid (olive oil) is used. Most often, the diagnosis of *M. furfur* is made by the direct microscopic examination of skin scales. Here the organism will easily be recognized as oval- or bottle-shaped cells that exhibit monopolar budding in the presence of a cell wall with a septum at the site of the bud scar (Figures 43.2 and 43.13). In addition, small hyphal fragments are observed. *Malassezia pachydermatis*, another species, may be recovered from skin lesions of patients; it requires no lipid additives.

It should be mentioned that *M. furfur* is currently being seen as the cause of disseminated infection in infants and young children and even adults given lipid replacement therapy.[55] The organism is readily cultured from blood or skin lesions without the use of a fatty acid additive. The morphological form seen in the direct microscopic examination of specimens from these patients is the yeast form without the presence of pseudohyphae.

43.13.b. Tinea nigra. Tinea nigra is an infection manifested by blackish-brown macular patches on the palm of the hand or sole of the foot. Lesions have been compared with silver nitrate staining of the skin. The etiologic agent is *Phaeoannellomyces werneckii*, a dematiaceous fungus. Initial colonies of *P. werneckii* may be black, shiny, and yeastlike in appearance. With age, colonies become filamentous with velvety-gray aerial hyphae. Microscopically, the yeastlike growth consists of olive-colored budding cells that are one- or two-celled. Older colonies exhibit one- or two-celled conidia that are produced by annelides, that bear successive rings (annelations).

43.13.c. Piedra. Black piedra is a fungal infection of the hair of the scalp and rarely of axillary and pubic hair. The etiologic agent is a dematiaceous fungus called *Piedraia hortae*. The disease occurs primarily in tropical areas of the world; cases have been reported in Africa, Asia, and in Latin America. Portions of hair are examined (in wet mounts using potassium hydroxide that is gently heated) for the presence of nodules composed of cemented mycelium. When mature nodules are crushed, oval asci, containing two to eight aseptate ascospores, 19 to 55 μm long by 4 to 8 μm in diameter, are seen (Figures 43.14 and 43.44). The asci are spindle-shaped and have a filament at each pole. The organism is easily cultured on any fungal culture medium lacking cycloheximide.

White piedra is an uncommon fungal infection found in both tropical and temperate regions of the world. It is characterized by the development of soft, yellow or pale brown aggregations around hair shafts in the axillary, facial, genital, and scalp regions of the body. The etiologic agent is *T. beigelii*. It frequently invades the cortex of the hair and causes damage. White nodules are removed and observed using the potassium hydroxide preparation after applying light pressure to the coverslip so that crushing of the nodule occurs. Hyaline hyphae, 2 to 4 μm in width, and arthroconidia are found in the preparation of the cementlike material binding the hyphae together. The organism may be identified in culture by blastoconidia and arthroconidia formation. *T. beigelii* may be distinguished from the other species in the genus by its inability to ferment carbohydrates and ability to aerobically utilize certain substrates. *T. beigelii* may produce systemic infection in immunocompromised hosts, particularly patients with leukemia.

43.14. Cutaneous Infections (Dermatomycoses)

Dermatomycoses are fungal infections that involve the superficial areas of the body, including the hair, skin, and nails. The genera *Trichophyton, Microsporum,* and *Epidermophyton* are the only fungi associated with the dermatomycoses. Such cutaneous mycoses are perhaps the most common fungal infections of humans and are usually referred to as **tinea** (Latin for "worm" or "ringworm"). The gross appearance of the lesion is that of an outer ring of an active, progressing infection with central healing within the ring. These infections may be characterized by another Latin noun to designate the area of the body involved. For example, tinea corporis

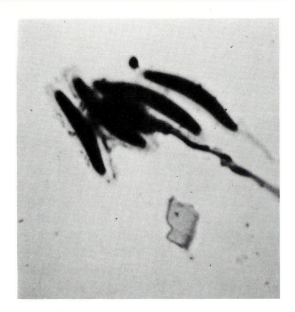

Figure 43.44
Piedra, showing curved, fusiform ascospores of *P. hortae* (430 ×).

(body), tinea cruris (groin), tinea capitis (scalp and hair), tinea barbae (beard), and tinea unguium (nail) are used to designate the type of infection observed. The group of fungi commonly called dermatophytes break down and utilize keratin as a source of nitrogen but are usually incapable of penetrating the subcutaneous tissue. The genus *Trichophyton* is capable of invading the hair, skin, and nails, whereas the genus *Microsporum* involves only the hair and skin; the genus *Epidermophyton* involves the skin and nails.

43.14.a. Common species. Common species of dermatophytes recovered from clinical specimens, in order of frequency, include *Trichophyton rubrum, Trichophyton mentagrophytes, Epidermophyton floccosum, Trichophyton tonsurans, Microsporum canis, Trichophyton verrucosum, Trichophyton violaceum,* and *Trichophyton schoenleinii*.[4]

Since the dermatophytes generally present a similar microscopic appearance within infected hair, skin, or nails, the final identification can be made only by culture. A summary of the colonial and microscopic morphological features of these fungi is presented in Table 43.8. Figure 43.45 presents an identification schema that will be of use to the clinical microbiologist for the identification of commonly encountered dermatophytes.

Descriptions of the common species of fungi caus-

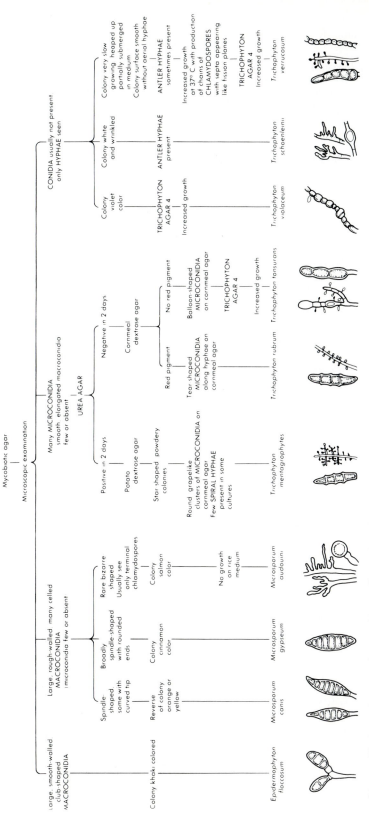

Figure 43.45

Dermatophyte identification schema. (From Koneman, E.W., and Roberts, G.D. 1985. Practical laboratory mycology, ed. 3. Williams & Wilkins, Baltimore.)

Table 43.8
Characteristics of More Commonly Isolated Dermatophytes

DERMATOPHYTE	COLONIAL MORPHOLOGY	GROWTH RATE	MICROSCOPIC IDENTIFICATION
Microsporum audouinii	Downy white to salmon pink colony; reverse tan to salmon pink	2 weeks	Sterile hyphae: terminal chlamydospores, favic chandeliers, and pectinate bodies; macroconidia rarely seen—bizarre-shaped if seen; microconidia rare or absent
Microsporum canis	Colony usually membranous with feathery periphery; center of colony white to buff over orange-yellow; lemon yellow or yellow-orange apron and reverse	1 week	Thick-walled, spindle-shaped, multiseptate, rough-walled macroconidia some with a curved tip; microconidia rarely seen
Microsporum gypseum	Cinnamon-colored, powdery colony; reverse light tan	1 week	Thick-walled rough, elliptical multiseptate macroconidia; microconidia few or absent
Epidermophyton floccosum	Center of colony tends to be folded and is khaki green; periphery is yellow; reverse yellowish brown with observable folds	1 week	Macroconidia large, smooth-walled, multiseptate, clavate, and borne singly or in clusters of two or three; microconidia not formed by this species
Trichophyton mentagrophytes	Different colonial types; white to pinkish, granular and fluffy varieties; occasional light yellow periphery in younger cultures; reverse buff to reddish brown	7-10 days	Many round to globose microconidia most commonly borne in grapelike clusters or laterally along the hyphae; spiral hyphae in 30% of isolates; macroconidia are thin-walled, smooth, club-shaped, and multiseptate; numerous or rare depending upon strain
Trichophyton rubrum	Colonial types vary from white downy to pink granular; rugal folds are common; reverse yellow when colony is young; however, wine red color commonly develops with age	2 weeks	Microconidia usually teardrop, most commonly borne along sides of the hyphae; macroconidia usually absent, but when present are smooth, thin-walled, and pencil-shaped
Trichophyton tonsurans	White, tan to yellow or rust, suedelike to powdery; wrinkled with heaped or sunken center; reverse yellow to tan to rust red	7-14 days	Microconidia are teardrop or club-shaped with flat bottoms; vary in size but usually larger than other dermatophytes; macroconidia rare and balloon forms found when present
Trichophyton schoenleinii	Irregularly heaped, smooth white to cream colony with radiating grooves; reverse white	2-3 weeks	Hyphae usually sterile; many antler-type hyphae seen (favic chandeliers)
Trichophyton violaceum	Port wine to deep violet colony, may be heaped or flat with waxy-glabrous surface; pigment may be lost on subculture	2-3 weeks	Branched, tortuous hyphae that are sterile; chlamydospores commonly aligned in chains
Trichophyton verrucosum	Glabrous to velvety white colonies; rare stains produce yellow-brown color; rugal folds with tendency to sink into agar surface	2-3 weeks	Microconidia rare; large and tear-drop when seen; macroconidia extremely rare, but form characteristic "rat-tail" types when seen; many chlamydospores seen in chains, particularly when colony is incubated at 37°C

From Koneman, E.W., and Roberts, G.D. 1985. Practical laboratory mycology, ed. 3. Williams & Wilkins, Baltimore.

ing dermatomycoses in the United States follow; other geographically limited species that are uncommonly encountered are described in the references cited.

Figure 43.45 begins with the microscopic features of the dermatophytes as they might be observed in an initial examination of the culture. In many instances the primary recovery medium fails to function well as a sporulation medium. It is commonly necessary to subculture the initial growth onto cornmeal agar or potato dextrose agar so that sporulation will occur.

The genus *Trichophyton* is recognized by the presence of microconidia borne either laterally along the side of the hyphae or in clusters. Microconidia are usually numerous, except for some of the slower growing species such as *T. violaceum*, *T. schoenleinii*, and *T. verrucosum*, which rarely exhibit sporulation. Macroconidia are uncommonly produced by most species of *Trichophyton*. When present, they are smooth-walled, elongated, pencil- to cigar-shaped, and are borne from short, delicate conidiophores.

The genus *Epidermophyton* is characterized by the presence of large, club-shaped, multisegmented, smooth-walled macroconidia that are commonly produced either singly or in clusters of two to three from the tips of short conidiophores; microconidia are not produced. This organism is easily identified.

The genus *Microsporum* is characterized by the production of large, rough-walled, multisegmented macroconidia that are produced singly from short conidiophores or are produced directly from the hyphae. Macroconidia may be numerous and are usually spindle-shaped to elongated. Microconidia are uncommonly produced except for the occasional isolate where their production may predominate.

43.14.b. Genus *Trichophyton.* Species of this genus are widely distributed and are the most important and common causes of infections of the feet and nails; they may be responsible for tinea corporis (Figure 43.46), tinea capitis, and tinea barbae. They are most commonly seen in adult infections, which vary considerably in their clinical manifestations. Most cosmopolitan species are anthropophilic, or "man-loving"; few are zoophilic, primarily infecting animals.

Generally, hairs infected with members of the genus *Trichophyton* do not fluoresce under a Wood's lamp (Figure 43.12); the demonstration of fungal elements inside, surrounding, and penetrating the

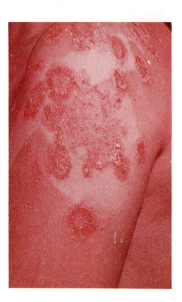

Figure 43.46
T. verrucosum, ringworm of skin. (Courtesy Upjohn Co.)

hair shaft, or within a skin scraping is necessary to make a diagnosis of the dermatophyte infection. The recovery and identification of the causative organism are necessary for confirmation.

Microscopically, the genus *Trichophyton* is characterized by smooth, club-shaped, thin-walled macroconidia with eight to ten septa ranging in size from 4×8 μm to 8×15 μm. The macroconidia are borne singly at the terminal ends of hyphae or on short conidiophores; the microconidia predominate and are usually spherical, pyriform (teardrop-shaped), or clavate (club-shaped), and 2 to 4 μm in size. Only the common species of *Trichophyton* are described in this chapter.

T. rubrum and *T. mentagrophytes* are the most common species recovered in the clinical laboratory. *T. rubrum* is a slow-growing organism that produces a flat or heaped-up colony that is generally white to reddish with a cottony or velvety surface. The characteristic cherry-red color is best observed on the reverse side of the colony; however, this is produced only after 3 or 4 weeks of incubation. Occasional strains may lack the deep red pigmentation on first isolation. Colonies may be of two types, fluffy and granular. Microconidia are uncommon in most of the fluffy strains but are more common in the granular strains and occur as small, teardrop-shaped conidia often borne laterally along the sides of the hyphae (Figure 43.47). Macroconidia are seen uncommonly,

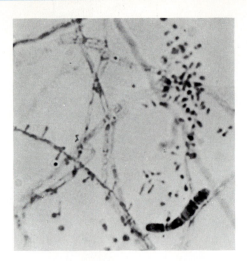

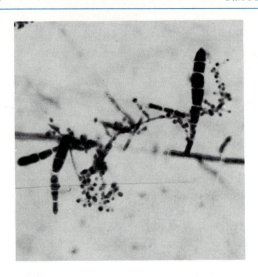

Figure 43.47
T. rubrum, showing an elongated macrocondium and numerous pyriform microconidia borne singly on hyphae (750 ×).

Figure 43.48
T. mentagrophytes, showing numerous microconidia in grapelike clusters. Also shown are several thin-walled macroconidia (500 ×).

although they are sometimes found in the granular strains, where they appear as thin-walled, smooth-walled, multicelled, pencil-shaped conidia with three to eight septa. *T. rubrum* has no specific nutritional requirements. It does not perforate hair in vitro (Procedure 43.4) or produce urease.

T. mentagrophytes produces two distinct colonial forms: the downy variety recovered from cases of tinea pedis and the granular variety recovered from lesions acquired by contact with animals.

T. mentagrophytes produces rapidly growing colonies that appear as white, cottony or downy colonies to cream-colored or yellow colonies that are coarsely granular to powdery. Granular colonies may show evidence of red pigmentation. The reverse side of the colony is usually rose-brown, occasionally orange to deep red, and may be confused with *T. rubrum*. The white, downy colonies produce only a few spherical microconidia; the granular colonies sporulate freely, with numerous small, spherical microconidia produced in grapelike clusters and thin-walled, smooth-walled, cigar-shaped macroconidia measuring 6 × 20 μm to 8 × 50 μm in size, with two to five septa (Figure 43.48). Macroconidia characteristically exhibit a definite narrow attachment to their base. Spiral hyphae may be found in one third of the isolates recovered.

T. mentagrophytes produces urease within 2 to 3 days after inoculation onto Christensen's urea agar

PROCEDURE 43.4

Hair Perforation Test[5]

1. Place a filter paper disk into the bottom of a sterile Petri dish.
2. Cover surface of paper disk with sterile distilled water.
3. Add a small portion of sterilized prepubertal hair into the water.
4. Inoculate a portion of the colony to be studied directly onto the hair.
5. Incubate at 25° C for 10 to 14 days.
6. Observe hairs at regular intervals by placing them into a drop of water on a microscope slide. Position a coverslip and examine microscopically for the presence of conical perforations of the hair shaft (Figure 43.49).

(Chapter 9). In addition, *T. mentagrophytes* perforates hair, in contrast to *T. rubrum*, which does not. This latter criterion may be used when there is difficulty in distinguishing between the two species.

T. tonsurans, along with *Microsporum audouinii*, is responsible for an epidemic form of tinea capitis occurring most commonly in children, but occurring

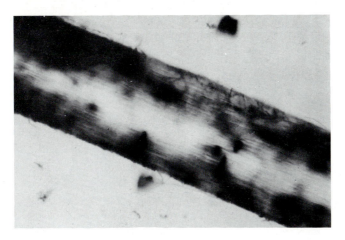

Figure 43.49
Hair perforation by *T. mentagrophytes;* wedge-shaped areas illustrate hair perforation (100 ×).

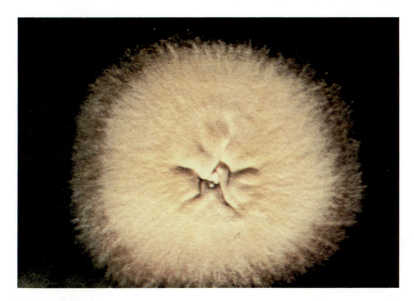

Figure 43.50
T. tonsurans colony.

occasionally in adults. It has displaced *M. audouinii* as a primary cause of tinea capitis in most of the United States. The fungus causes a low-grade superficial lesion of varying severity and produces circular, scaly patches of alopecia (loss of hair). The stubs of hair remain in the epidermis of the scalp after the brittle hairs have broken off and may give the typical "black dot" ringworm appearance. Since the infected hairs do not fluoresce under a Wood's lamp, a careful search for the embedded stub should be carried out by the physician with the use of a bright light.

The direct microscopic examination of infected hairs in a potassium hydroxide preparation (Chapter 7) reveals the hair shaft to be filled with masses of large (4 to 7 μm) arthroconidia in chains, characteristic of an **endothrix** type of invasion. Cultures of *T. tonsurans* develop slowly and are typically buff to brown, wrinkled and suedelike in appearance (Figure 43.50). The colony surface shows radial folds,

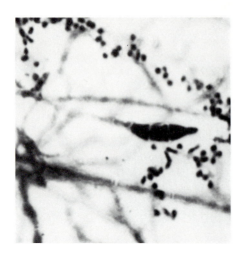

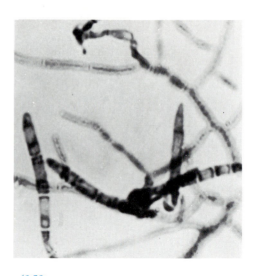

Figure 43.51
T. tonsurans, showing numerous microconidia borne singly or in clusters. A single macroconidium (rare) is also present (600 ×).

Figure 43.52
T. verrucosum, showing multicelled, smooth thin-walled macroconidia, which are rarely seen (500 ×).

often developing a craterlike depression in the center with deep fissures. The reverse side of the colony is yellowish to reddish brown. Microscopically, numerous microconidia with flat bases borne on the sides of hyphae are observed. With age, the microconidia tend to become pleomorphic, are swollen to elongated, and are referred to as "balloon forms" (Figure 43.51). Chlamydospores are abundant in old cultures; swollen and fragmented hyphal cells resembling arthroconidia may be seen. *T. tonsurans* grows poorly on media lacking vitamins; however, growth is greatly enhanced by the presence of thiamine.

T. verrucosum causes a variety of lesions in cattle and in humans; it is most often seen in farmers who acquire their infection from cattle. The lesions are found chiefly on the beard, neck, wrist and back of the hands; they are deep, pustular, and inflammatory. With pressure, short stubs of hair may be recovered from the purulent lesion. Direct examination of the outside of the hair shaft reveals sheaths of isolated chains of large (5 to 10 μm) spores (**ectothrix**) and hyphae within the hair (**endothrix**). Masses of these conidia may also be seen in exudate from the lesions.

T. verrucosum grows very slowly (14 to 30 days), and growth is enhanced at 35° to 37° C. Growth is also enhanced on media enriched with thiamine and inositol. *T. verrucosum* may be suspected when col-

onies appear to embed themselves into the agar surface. Kane and Smitka[38] described a new medium for the early detection and identification of *T. verrucosum*. The ingredients for this medium are 4% casein and 0.5% yeast extract. The organism is recognized by its early hydrolysis of casein and very slow growth rate. Chains of chlamydospores are formed regularly at 37° C. The early detection of hydrolysis, formation of characteristic chains of chlamydospores (Figure 43.52), and the restrictive slow growth rate of *T. verrucosum* differentiate it from *T. schoenleinii*, another slowly growing organism. Colonies are small, heaped, and folded, occasionally flat and disk-shaped. At first they are glabrous and waxy, with a short aerial mycelium. Colonies range from gray and waxlike to a bright ochre. The reverse of the colony is most often nonpigmented but may be yellow.

Chlamydospores in chains and antler hyphae may be the only forms observed microscopically. Chlamydospores are produced abundantly at 35° to 37° C. Microconidia may be produced by some cultures if the medium is enriched with yeast extract or a vitamin. Conidia, when present, are borne laterally from the hyphae and are large and clavate. Macroconidia are rarely formed, vary considerably in size and shape, and are referred to as "rat tail."

T. schoenleinii causes a severe type of infection called "favus" (Figure 43.53). It is characterized by

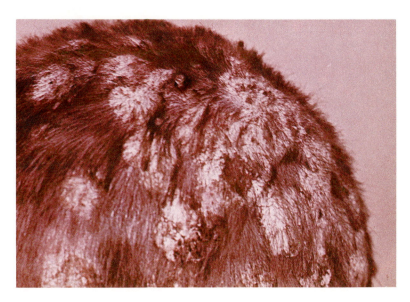

Figure 43.53
Scalp infection. *T. schoenleinii*. (Courtesy Upjohn Co.)

the formation of yellowish cup-shaped crusts or scutulae, resulting in considerable scarring of the scalp and sometimes permanent alopecia. A distinctive invasion of the infected hair, the favic type, is demonstrated by the presence of large inverted cones of hyphae and arthroconidia at the base of the hair follicle and branching hyphae throughout the length of the hair shaft. Longitudinal tunnels or empty spaces appear in the hair shaft where the hyphae have disintegrated. In potassium hydroxide preparations, these tunnels are readily filled with fluid; air bubbles may also be seen in these tunnels. *T. schoenleinii* is a slowly growing organism (30 days or longer) and produces a white to light gray colony that has a waxy surface. Colonies have an irregular border that consists mostly of submerged hyphae and that tends to crack the agar. The surface of the colony is usually nonpigmented or tan, furrowed, and irregularly folded. The reverse side of the colony is usually tan or nonpigmented. Microscopically, conidia are not formed commonly. The hyphae tend to become knobby and club-shaped at the terminal ends, with the production of many short lateral and terminal branches (antler hyphae; Figure 43.54). Chlamydospores are generally numerous. All strains of *T. schoenleinii* may be grown in a vitamin-free medium and grow equally well at room temperature or at 35° to 37° C.

T. violaceum produces an infection of the scalp and body and is seen primarily in persons living in the Mediterranean region, the Middle and Far East, and Africa. Hair invasion is of the endothrix type; the typical "black dot" type of tinea capitis is observed clinically. Direct microscopic examination of the potassium hydroxide preparation of the nonfluorescing hairs shows dark, thick hairs filled with masses of arthroconidia arranged in chains, similar to those seen in *T. tonsurans* infections.

Colonies of *T. violaceum* are very slow-growing, beginning as cream-colored, glabrous, cone-shaped, and later becoming heaped up, verrucous (warty), and violet to purple in color and waxy in consistency. Colonies may often be described as being "port wine" in color. The reverse side of the colony is purple or nonpigmented. Older cultures may develop a velvety area of mycelium and sometimes lose their pigmentation. Microscopically, microconidia and macroconidia are generally not present; only sterile, distorted hyphae and chlamydospores are found. In some instances, however, swollen hyphae containing cytoplasmic granules may be seen (Figure 43.55). The growth of *T. violaceum* is enhanced on media containing thiamine.

43.14.c. Genus *Microsporum.* The genus *Microsporum* is immediately recognized by the presence of large (8×8 to 15 μm $\times 35$ to 150 μm)

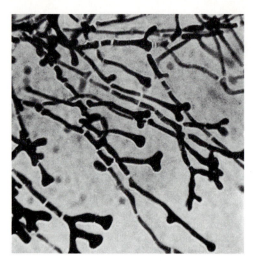

Figure 43.54
T. schoenleinii, showing swollen hyphal tips with lateral and terminal branching (favic chandeliers). Microconidia and macroconidia are absent (500 ×).

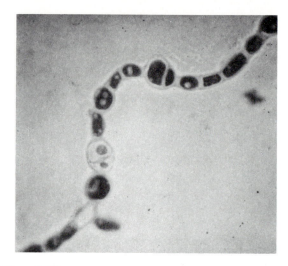

Figure 43.55
T. violaceum, showing chains of swollen cells containing cytoplasmic granules. Microconidia and macroconidia are usually absent (500 ×).

spindle-shaped, rough-walled macroconidia with thick (up to 4 μm) walls that contain 4 to 15 septa. The microconidia, when present, are small (3 to 7 μm) and club-shaped and are borne on the hyphae, either laterally or on short conidiophores. Species of *Microsporum* develop either slowly or rapidly and produce aerial hyphae that may be velvety, powdery, glabrous, or cottony, varying in color from whitish, buff, to a cinnamon brown, with varying shades on the reverse side of the colony.

M. *audouinii* was, in past years, the most important cause of epidemic tinea capitis among schoolchildren in the United States. This organism is anthropophilic and is spread directly by means of infected hairs on hats, caps, upholstery, combs, or barber clippers. The majority of infections are chronic; some heal spontaneously, whereas others may persist for several years. Infected hair shafts fluoresce yellow-green using a Wood's lamp (Figure 43.12). Colonies of M. *audouinii* generally grow more slowly than other members of the genus *Microsporum* (10 to 21 days), and they produce a velvety aerial mycelium that is colorless to light gray to tan. The reverse side often appears salmon-pink to reddish-brown. Colonies of M. *audouinii* do not usually sporulate in culture. The addition of yeast extract may stimulate growth and the production of macroconidia in some instances. Most commonly,

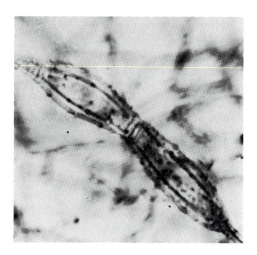

Figure 43.56
M. *audouinii*, showing a distorted macroconidium. Macroconidia and microconidia are usually absent (1800 ×).

atypical vegetative forms such as terminal chlamydospores and antler and racquet hyphae are the only clues to the identification of this organism. It is common to identify M. *audouinii* by exclusion of all the other dermatophytes as a cause of infection (Figure 43.56).

M. *canis* is primarily a pathogen of animals; it is the most common cause of ringworm infection in

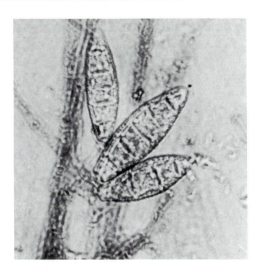

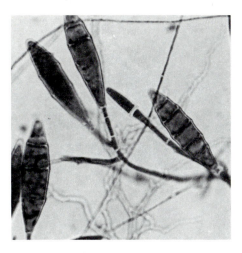

Figure 43.57
M. canis, showing several spindle-shaped, thick-walled,
multicelled macroconidia (500 ×).

Figure 43.58
M. gypseum, showing ellipsoidal, multicelled macroconidia
(750 ×).

dogs and cats in the United States. Children and adults acquire the disease through contact with infected animals, particularly puppies and kittens, although human-to-human transfer has been reported. Hairs infected with *M. canis* fluoresce a bright yellow-green using a Wood's lamp, which is a useful tool for screening pets as possible sources of human infection. Direct examination of a potassium hydroxide preparation of infected hairs reveals small spores (2 to 3 μm) outside the hair, although culture procedures must be performed to provide specific identification.

Colonies of *M. canis* grow rapidly, are granular or fluffy with a feathery border, are white to buff, and characteristically have a lemon-yellow or yellow-orange fringe at the periphery. On aging, the colony becomes dense and cottony and a deeper brownish-yellow or orange and frequently shows an area of heavy growth in the center. The reverse side of the colony is bright yellow, becoming orange or reddish-brown with age. Rarely strains are recovered that show no reverse side pigment. Microscopically, *M. canis* shows an abundance of large (15 μm × 60 to 125 μm), spindle-shaped, multisegmented (four to eight) macroconidia with curved ends (Figure 43.57). These are thick-walled with warty (echinulate) projections on their surfaces. Microconidia are usually few in number; however, large numbers may occasionally be seen.

Microsporum gypseum, a free-living saprophyte of the soil (geophilic) that only rarely causes human or animal infection, may be seen occasionally in the clinical laboratory. Infected hairs generally do not fluoresce using a Wood's lamp. However, microscopic examination of the infected hairs shows them to be irregularly covered with clusters of spores (5 to 8 μm), some in chains. These arthroconidia of the ectothrix type are considerably larger than those of other *Microsporum* species.

M. gypseum grows rapidly as a flat, irregularly fringed colony with a coarse powdery surface that appears to be buff or cinnamon color. The underside of the colony is conspicuously orange to brownish. Microscopically, macroconidia are seen in large numbers and are characteristically large, ellipsoidal, have rounded ends, and are multisegmented (three to nine) with echinulated surfaces (Figure 43.58). Although they are spindle-shaped, these macroconidia are not as pointed at the distal ends as those of *M. canis*. The appearance of the colonial and microscopic morphological features is sufficient to make the distinction between *M. gypseum* and *M. canis*.

43.14.d. Genus *Epidermophyton*. *E. floccosum*, the only member of the genus *Epidermophyton*, is a common cause of tinea cruris and tinea pedis. In direct examination of skin scrapings using the potassium hydroxide preparation, the fungus is seen as fine branching hyphae. *E. floccosum* grows slowly,

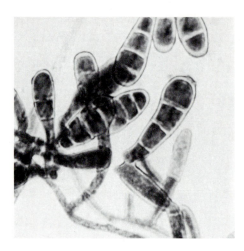

Figure 43.59
E. floccosum, showing numerous smooth, multiseptate, thin-walled macroconidia that appear club-shaped (1000 ×).

and growth appears as an olive-green to khaki color, with the periphery surrounded by a dull orange-brown color. After several weeks, colonies develop a cottony white aerial mycelium that completely overgrows the colony and is sterile.

Microscopically, numerous smooth, thin-walled, club-shaped, multiseptate (2 to 4 μm) macroconidia are seen (Figure 43.59). They are rounded at the tip and are borne singly or in groups of two or three on a conidiophore. Microconidia are absent, spiral hyphae are rare, and chlamydospores are usually numerous.

This organism is very susceptible to cold temperatures and for this reason it is recommended that specimens submitted for dermatophyte culture not be refrigerated prior to culture.

43.15. Subcutaneous Mycoses

Subcutaneous mycoses are infections that involve the skin and subcutaneous tissue, generally without dissemination to other organs of the body. This classification is artificial; for example, sporotrichosis occasionally involves lungs, other viscera, meninges, or joints and may disseminate. The other agents causing subcutaneous infections may also produce disseminated infection occasionally. The etiologic agents are found in several unrelated fungal genera, all of which may exist as saprophytes in nature. Humans and animals serve as accidental hosts after trau-

matic inoculation of the fungal spores into cutaneous and subcutaneous tissues. Three subcutaneous mycoses are considered here: sporotrichosis, chromoblastomycosis, and mycetoma.

43.15.a. Sporotrichosis. Sporotrichosis is a chronic infection of worldwide distribution caused by the dimorphic fungus, *S. schenckii*, whose natural habitat is living or dead vegetation. Humans acquire the infection through trauma (thorns, splinters), usually to the hand, arm, or leg. The primary lesion begins as a small, nonhealing ulcer, commonly of the index finger or the back of the hand. With time, the infection is characterized by the development of nodular lesions of the skin or subcutaneous tissues at the point of contact and later involves the lymphatic channels and lymph nodes draining the region. The subcutaneous nodules break down and ulcerate to form an infection that becomes chronic. Only rarely is the disease disseminated; pulmonary infection may be seen. The infection is an occupational hazard for farmers, nursery workers, gardeners, florists, and miners. It is commonly known as "rose gardener's" disease.

Exudate from unopened subcutaneous nodules or from open draining lesions is often submitted for culture and direct microscopic examination. Direct examination of this material is usually of little diagnostic value because it is difficult to demonstrate the characteristic yeast forms, even with special stains; reasons for this are unclear.

Colonies of *S. schenckii* grow rapidly (3 to 5 days) and are usually small, moist, and white to cream-colored in appearance. On further incubation, these become membranous, wrinkled, and coarsely matted, with the color becoming irregularly dark brown or black and the colony becoming leathery in consistency (Figure 43.60). It is common for the clinical microbiology laboratory to mistake a young culture of *S. schenckii* for that of a yeast until the microscopic features are observed.

Microscopically, hyphae are delicate (1 to 2 μm thick), septate, exhibit branching, and bear one-celled conidia, 2 to 5 μm in diameter. These are borne bouquetlike, in clusters from the tips of single conidiophores. Each conidium is attached to the conidiophore by an individual, delicate, threadlike structure (denticle) that may require examination under oil immersion to be visible. As the culture ages, single-celled, thick-walled, black pigmented conidia may also be borne along the sides of the

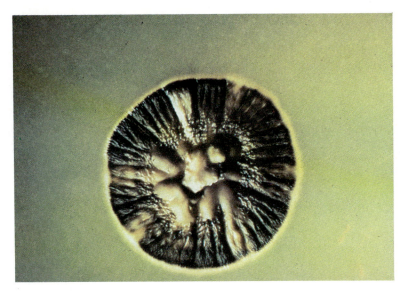

Figure 43.60
S. schenkii colony. (Courtesy Upjohn Co.)

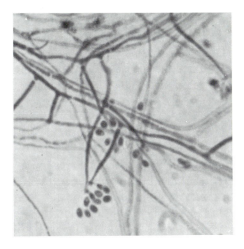

Figure 43.61
S. schenckii, mycelial form, showing pyriform to ovoid microconidia borne in a flowerette at the tip of the conidiophore (750 ×).

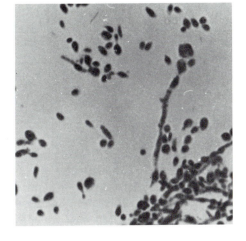

Figure 43.62
S. schenckii, yeast form, showing cigar-shaped and oval budding cells (500 ×).

hyphae, simulating the arrangement of microconidia produced by *T. rubrum*. The common designations for these types of sporulation are the "flowerette" and "sleeve" arrangements, respectively (Figure 43.61).

Because of similar morphological features, saprophytic species of the genus *Sporothrix* may be confused with *S. schenckii*, and it is necessary to distinguish between them. During incubation of a culture at 37° C, the colony of *S. schenckii* transforms to a soft, cream-colored to white, yeastlike colony. Microscopically, singly or multiply budding, spherical, oval, or cigar-shaped yeast cells are observed without difficulty (Figure 43.62). Conversion from

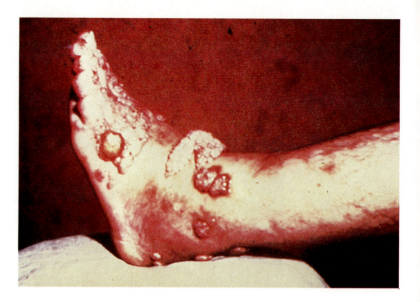

Figure 43.63
Phialaphora infection of foot. (Courtesy Upjohn Co.)

the mold form to the yeast form is easily accomplished and usually occurs within 1 to 5 days after transfer of the culture to a medium containing blood enrichment; most isolates of *S. schenckii* are converted to the yeast form within 12 to 48 hours at 37° C.

42.15.b. Chromoblastomycosis. Chromoblastomycosis is a chronic fungal infection acquired via traumatic inoculation of spores, primarily in the extremities. The infection is characterized by the development of a papule at the site of the traumatic insult that spreads to form warty or tumorlike lesions characterized as "cauliflower-like" (Figure 43.63). There may be secondary infection and ulceration. The lesions are usually confined to the feet and legs but may involve the head, face, neck, and other body surfaces. Histologic examination of lesion tissue reveals characteristic **sclerotic** bodies, copper-colored, septate cells that appear to be dividing (Figure 43.17). Brain abscess caused by the etiologic agents of chromoblastomycosis has been reported with some frequency.[9]

The disease is widely distributed, but most cases occur in tropical and subtropical areas of the world. Occasional cases are reported from temperate zones, including the United States. The infection is seen most often in areas where agricultural workers fail to wear protective clothing and suffer thorn or splinter puncture wounds through which the spores enter from the soil.

The group of fungi known to cause chromoblastomycosis are dematiaceous. All are slow-growing and produce heaped-up and slightly folded, darkly pigmented colonies with a grayish-velvety appearance. The reverse side of the colonies is jet black.

The taxonomy of the organisms that cause chromoblastomycosis is complex.[56] Their identification is based on distinct microscopic morphological features. Three genera, *Cladosporium*, *Phialophora*, and *Fonsecaea*, are known to cause chromoblastomycosis.

The genus *Cladosporium* includes those species that produce long chains of conidia (blastoconidia) that have a dark septal scar present.

The genus *Phialophora* includes those species that produce short, flask-shaped to tubular phialides, usually with a well-developed collarette. Clusters of conidia are produced by the phialides through an apical pore.

The genus *Fonsecaea* includes those organisms that exhibit a mixed type of sporulation, which uniquely includes one-celled primary conidia that are produced on either side of conidiophores resembling a series of bent knees. Conidia are produced sympodially. The primary conidia give rise to secondary conidia that appear to occur in loose heads. This is known as the rhinocladiella type of sporulation and predominates, depending upon the strain isolated. A mixture of the rhinocladiella and cladosporium types may occur; moreover, phialides with

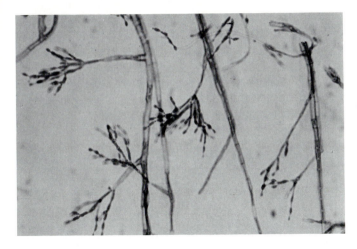

Figure 43.64
Cladosporium species, showing *Cladosporium* type of sporulation with chains of elliptical conidia (430 ×).

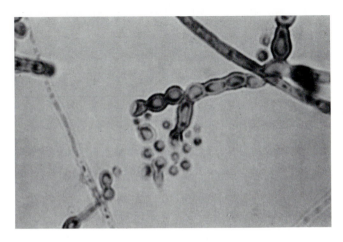

Figure 43.65
P. verrucosa, showing flask-shaped phialide with a distinct collarette and conidia near its tip (750 ×).

collarettes may also be present. Two species, *Fonsecaea pedrosoi* and *Fonsecaea compacta*, are etiologic agents of chromoblastomycosis. Both are morphologically distinct: *F. pedrosoi* is differentiated from *F. compacta* by the production of loose heads, in contrast to the more compact heads produced by *F. compacta*.

The diagnostic features of the three genera are summarized as follows:

1. *Cladosporium (Cladosporium carrionii):* *Cladosporium* type of sporulation with long chains of elliptical conidia (2 to 3 μm × 4 to 5 μm) borne from erect, tall, branching conidiophores (Figure 43.64).
2. *Phialophora (Phialophora verrucosa):* Tubelike or flask-shaped phialides, each with a distinct collarette. Conidia are produced endogenously and

occur in clusters at the tip of the phialide (Figure 43.65).

3. *Fonsecaea (F. pedrosoi and F. compacta):* Conidial heads with sympodial arrangement of conidia, with primary conidia giving rise to secondary conidia (Figure 43.66). Cladosporium type of sporulation may occur and phialides with collarettes may also be present.

The laboratory diagnosis of chromoblastomycosis is made easily. Scrapings from crusted areas added to 10% potassium hydroxide show the presence of the sclerotic bodies, which appear rounded, brown, and 4 to 10 μm in diameter and resemble "copper pennies" (Figure 43.17).

43.15.c. Mycetoma. Mycetoma is a chronic granulomatous infection that usually involves the lower extremities but may occur in any part of the body.

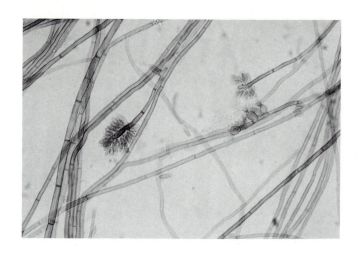

Figure 43.66
F. pedrosoi, showing conidial heads with sympodial arrangement of conidia (430 ×).

The infection is characterized by swelling, purplish discoloration, tumorlike deformities of the subcutaneous tissue, and multiple sinus tracts that drain pus containing yellow, white, red, or black granules. The infection gradually progresses to involve the bone, muscle, or other contiguous tissue and ultimately requires amputation in most cases. Occasionally there may be dissemination to other organs, including the brain; however, this type of infection is relatively uncommon.

Mycetoma is common among persons who live in tropical and subtropical regions of the world, whose outdoor occupations and failure to wear protective clothing predispose them to trauma.

Two types of mycetoma are described, actinomycotic mycetoma, which is caused by species of the aerobic actinomycetes, including *Nocardia, Actinomadura*, and *Streptomyces* (Chapter 33); and eumycotic mycetoma, caused by a heterogeneous group of species having true septate hyphae.[54] The most common etiologic agent of mycetoma in the United States is *P. boydii*, a member of the Ascomycota (because it produces ascospores). The organism is a common saprobe and is found in soil and sewage; humans acquire the infection by traumatic implantation of the organism into the skin and subcutaneous tissues.

Macroscopic examination of granules from lesions of mycetoma caused by *P. boydii* reveal them to be white to yellow, and 0.2 to 2 mm in diameter. Microscopically, the granules of *P. boydii* consist of loosely arranged, intertwined hyphae.

P. boydii is a hyaline organism that grows rapidly (5 to 10 days) on common laboratory media. Initial growth begins as a white, fluffy colony that changes in several weeks to a brownish-gray (mousey) mycelium. The reverse of the colony is black. *P. boydii* has undergone several name changes in the past and is an example of an organism that reproduces both asexually and sexually. The asexual form is called *Scedosporium apiospermum* and microscopically produces elliptical (sperm-shaped), single-celled conidia borne singly from the tips of long or short conidiophores (annellophores) (Figure 43.67). Clusters of conidiophores with conidia produced at the ends sometimes occur and are referred to as "coremia."

P. boydii is the sexual form of the organism. The sexual form exhibits cleistothecia, which are saclike structures that contain asci and ascospores. When the latter are fully developed, the large (50 to 200 μm), thick-walled cleistothecia rupture and liberate the asci and ascospores (Figure 43.68). The ascospores are oval and delicately pointed at each end and resemble the conidia of the asexual form. Isolates of *P. boydii* may be induced to form cleistothecia by culturing on plain water agar.

P. boydii is also involved in causing a variety of infections elsewhere in the body. Included are infections of the nasal sinuses and septum, meningitis, arthritis, endocarditis, mycotic keratitis, external otomycosis, and brain abscess. Most of these more serious infections occur primarily in immunocompromised patients.

It should be mentioned that it is impossible to predict the specific etiologic agent of mycetoma.

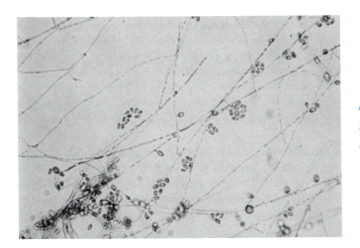

Figure 43.67
S. apiospermum, showing asexually produced conidia borne singly on long or short conidiophores (annellophores) (430 ×).

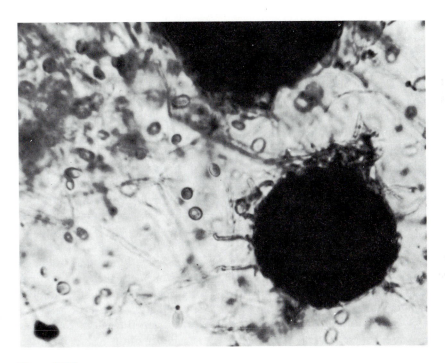

Figure 43.68
P. boydii, showing cleistothecia and numerous ascospores (750 ×).

Culture media containing antibiotics should not be used alone for culturing clinical specimens, since species of the aerobic actinomycetes are susceptible to antibacterial antibiotics and may be inhibited by these agents incorporated into routine culture media. For further information on other fungi involved in mycetoma, one may refer to references listed at the end of this chapter.

43.16. Systemic Mycoses

Systemic fungal infections may involve any of the internal organs of the body as well as lymph nodes, bone, subcutaneous tissue, and skin. Asymptomatic infection is common, may go unrecognized clinically, and may be detected only by serologic testing; in some cases roentgenographic examination may reveal healed lesions. Symptomatic infections may present signs of only a mild or more severe but self-limited disease, with positive supportive evidence from cultural or immunological findings. Disseminated or progressive infection may reveal severe symptoms, with spread of the initial disease to several organs as well as to the bone, skin, and subcutaneous tissues. Some cases of disseminated infection may exhibit little in the way of signs or symptoms of disease for long periods, only to exacerbate later.

Traditionally, the systemic mycoses have included blastomycosis, coccidioidomycosis, histoplasmosis, and paracoccidioidomycosis. The fungi responsible for these infections, although unrelated generically and dissimilar morphologically, have one characteristic in common—that of dimorphism. The dimorphic fungi involved exist in nature as the saprobic form, sometimes called the mold form, which is quite distinct from the parasitic, or invasive form, sometimes called the tissue form. Distinct morphological differences may be observed with the dimorphic fungi both in vivo and in vitro. Temperature (35° to 37° C), certain nutritional factors, and stimulation of growth in tissue independent of temperature are among the factors necessary to initiate the transformation of the mold form to the parasitic form.

43.16.a. General features of dimorphic fungi. As a general rule, the dimorphic fungi are regarded as slow-growing organisms that require 7 to 21 days for visible growth to appear. However, exceptions to this rule occur with some frequency. Cultures of *B. dermatitidis* and *H. capsulatum* are recovered in as short a time as 4 to 5 days when large numbers of organisms are present in the clinical specimen. In contrast, single colonies of *B. dermatitidis* and *H. capsulatum* sometimes require 21 to 30 days of incubation before they are detected. *C. immitis* is consistently recovered within 3 to 5 days of incubation, but when large numbers of colonies are present, colonies may be detected within 48 hours. Single colonies may require 14 to 21 days before visible growth can be detected. Cultures of *P. brasiliensis* are commonly recovered within 5 to 25 days, with a usual incubation period of 10 to 15 days. As one can see, the growth rate, if slow, might lead one to suspect the presence of a dimorphic fungus; however, a great deal of variation in the time for recovery exists.

Textbooks present descriptions for the dimorphic fungi that the reader assumes are typical for each particular organism. As is true in other areas of microbiology, a great deal of variation in the colonial morphological features also occurs, commonly because of the type of medium used. One must be aware of this variation and must not rely heavily on colonial morphological features for the identification of members of this group of fungi.

The color of the colony is sometimes helpful but varies widely; colonies of *B. dermatitidis* and *H. capsulatum* are described as being fluffy white with a change in color to tan or buff with age. Some isolates initially appear darkly pigmented with colors ranging from gray or dark brown to red. On media containing blood enrichment, these organisms appear heaped, wrinkled, glabrous and neutral in color, and yeastlike in appearance; often tufts of aerial hyphae project from the top of the colony. Some colonies may appear pink to red because of the adsorption of hemoglobin from the blood in the medium. *C. immitis* is described as being fluffy white with scattered areas of hyphae that are adherent to the agar surface so as to give an overall "cobweb" appearance to the colony. However, numerous morphological forms, including textures ranging from woolly to powdery and pigmentation ranging from pink-lavender or yellow to brown or buff, have been reported. While the growth rate and colonial morphological features may help one to recognize the presence of a dimorphic fungus, they should be used in combination with the microscopic morphological features to make a tentative identification. The definitive identification of a dimorphic fungus has traditionally been made by observing both the mold and parasitic forms of the organism. Cultures of the mold form are easily recovered at 25° to 30° C; however, the tissue form is usually not recovered from the clinical specimen. Previously the definitive identification was made by the in vitro conversion of a mold form to the corresponding yeast or spherule form by animal inoculation or by in vitro conversion on a blood-enriched medium incubated at 35° to 37° C. The conversion of dimorphic molds to the yeast form (except for *C. immitis*) can be accomplished with some difficulty, as outlined in Procedure 43.5.

Since the conversion of the dimorphic molds to the corresponding yeast or spherule forms is technically cumbersome to perform and long delays are often experienced, the effort to convert the dimorphic fungi is not recommended and should be replaced by a relatively new procedure, *exoantigen testing* (Procedure 43.6). This technique is used in many laboratories to make a definitive identification of *B. dermatitidis*, *C. immitis*, *H. capsulatum*, and *P. brasiliensis*. The exoantigen test relies on the principle that soluble antigens are produced and can be extracted from fungi; they are concentrated and subsequently reacted with serum known to contain antibodies directed against the specific antigenic components of the organism being tested. Reagents and materials for the exoantigen test are currently available commercially and provide all laboratories with the capability of identifying the dimorphic fungi with ease and rapidity.

The exoantigen test is now considered by most laboratories to be the most conclusive method for making a definitive identification of the dimorphic fungi.

The inclusion of only the dimorphic fungi in the group of systemic mycoses is a bit artificial, since other fungi, including *C. neoformans* and species of *Candida* and *Aspergillus*, also cause disseminated infection. They are not discussed in this portion of the chapter, since they are not dimorphic as previously defined and since they usually cause infection only in immunocompromised patients. They are discussed in a subsequent section on the opportunistic mycoses.

43.16.b. Blastomycosis. Blastomycosis is a chronic suppurative and granulomatous infection caused by the dimorphic fungus *B. dermatitidis*. The disease is most commonly found on the continent of North America and extends southward from Canada to the Mississippi, Ohio, and Missouri River valleys, Mexico and Central America. Some isolated cases have also been reported from Africa. The largest number of cases occur in the Mississippi, Ohio, and Missouri River valley regions.

Blastomycosis begins as a respiratory infection and is probably acquired by inhalation of the conidia or hyphal fragments of the organism. The exact ecological niche for this organism in nature has not been determined; however, patients with a history of exposure to soil or wood have the highest incidence of infection. The infection may spread and involve the lungs, long bones, soft tissue, and skin. It is not transmitted from person to person and generally occurs as sporadic cases. Several outbreaks have been reported, however, and have been related to a common exposure. Blastomycosis is more common in men and seems to be associated with outdoor occupations.

PROCEDURE 43.5

In Vitro Conversion of Dimorphic Molds

Principle

Dimorphic molds exist in the yeast form in infected tissue. Proof that a mold is actually one of the systemic dimorphic fungi can be achieved by simulating the environment of the host and converting the mold to the yeast or spherule form.

Method

1. Transfer a large inoculum of the mold form of the culture onto the surface of a fresh, moist slant of brain-heart infusion agar containing 5% to 10% sheep blood. If *B. dermatitidis* is suspected, a tube of cottonseed conversion medium[90] should be inoculated.
2. Add a few drops of sterile distilled water to provide moisture if the surface of the culture medium appears to be dry.
3. Leave the cap of the screw-capped tube slightly loose to allow the culture to have adequate oxygen exchange.
4. Incubate cultures at 35° to 37° C for several days; observe for the appearance of yeast-like portions of the colony. It may be necessary to make several subcultures of any growth that appears, since several transfers are often required to accomplish the conversion of many isolates. Cultures of *B. dermatitidis*, however, are usually easily converted and require 24 to 48 h on cottonseed agar medium. *C. immitis* may be converted in vitro to the spherule form using a chemically defined medium[84]; however, this method is of little use to the clinical laboratory and it should not be attempted.

Quality control

Because of their hazardous nature, it is not recommended that stock cultures be tested routinely. The exoantigen test (Procedure 43.6) can serve as a confirmatory identification of the dimorphic fungi.

PROCEDURE 43.6

Exoantigen Test[41,43,79,80]

Principle

Antibodies developed against particular mycelial antigens will react specifically in a gel immunodiffusion precipitin test. The mold forms of the dimorphic fungi can be identified definitively by an antigen-antibody reaction, negating the need for conversion to the yeast phase.

Method

1. A mature fungus culture on a Sabouraud's dextrose agar slant is covered with an aqueous solution of merthiolate (1:5000 final concentration), which is allowed to remain in contact with the culture for 24 h at 25° C. It is necessary that the entire surface of the colony be covered so that effective killing of the organism is ensured.

2. Filter the aqueous solution through a 0.45 μm size membrane filter. This should be performed inside a biological safety cabinet.

3. Five milliliters of this solution is concentrated using a Minicon Macrosolute B-15 Concentrator (Amicon Corporation). The solution is concentrated 50× when testing with *H. capsulatum* and *B. dermatitidis* antiserum and 5× and 25× for reaction with *C. immitis* antiserum.

4. The concentrated supernatant is used in the microdiffusion test. The supernatant is placed into wells punched into a plate of buffered, phenolized agar adjacent to the control antigen well and is tested against positive control antiserum obtained from commercial sources (Immunomycologics, Meridian Diagnostics, and Scott-Nolan Laboratories).

5. The immunodiffusion test is allowed to react for 24 h at 25° C, and the plate is observed for the presence of precipitin bands of identity with the reference reagents. The sensitivity of the exoantigen test for the identification of *B. dermatitidis* may be increased by incubating the immunodiffusion plates at 37° C for 48 h; however, bands appear sharper at 25° C after 24 h. It is recommended that any culture suspected of being *B. dermatitidis* be incubated at both temperatures.

6. *C. immitis* may be identified for the presence of the CF, TP, or HL antigens, while *H. capsulatum* and *B. dermatitidis* may be identified by the presence of H or M bands, or both, and the A band, respectively. Detailed instructions for the performance and interpretation of the tests are included with the manufacturers' package insert.

Quality control

Extracts from known fungi are tested each time the test is performed. Lines of identity with the unknown strain are necessary for identification.

The diagnosis of blastomycosis may easily be made when a clinical specimen is observed by direct microscopy. *B. dermatitidis* appears as large, spherical, thick-walled cells 8 to 20 μm in diameter, usually with a single bud that is connected to the parent cell by a broad base.

B. dermatitidis usually requires 5 days to 4 weeks or longer for growth to be detected. On enriched culture media, the mold form develops initially as a glabrous- or waxy-appearing colony that may become off-white to white in color. With age, the aerial hyphae often turn gray to brown; however, on media enriched with blood, colonies appear to have a more waxy, yeastlike appearance. Tufts of hyphae often project upward from the colonies and are referred to as the "prickly state" of the organism.

Microscopically, hyphae of the mold form are septate and delicate and measure 1 to 2 μm in diameter. Commonly, ropelike strands of hyphae are seen; however, these are found with most of the dimorphic fungi. The characteristic microscopic morphological features are single, pyriform conidia produced on long to short conidiophores that resemble lollipops (Figure 43.69). The production of conidia in some

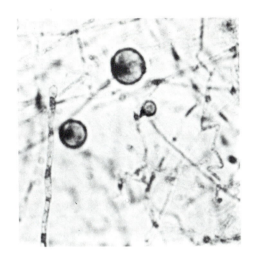

Figure 43.69
B. dermatitidis, mycelial form, showing oval conidia borne laterally on branching hyphae (1000 ×).

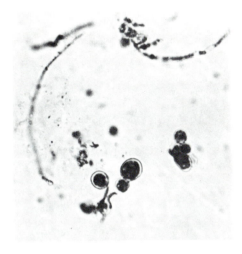

Figure 43.70
B. dermatitidis, yeast form, showing thick-walled, oval to round, single-budding yeastlike cells (500 ×).

isolates is minimal or absent, particularly on a medium containing blood enrichment.

Colonies of the yeast form develop within 7 days and appear waxy and wrinkled, and cream to tan in color.[90] Microscopically, large, thick-walled yeast cells with buds attached by a broad base are seen (Figure 43.70). During the conversion process, swollen hyphal forms and immature cells with rudimentary buds may be present.

As previously mentioned, the definitive identification of *B. dermatitidis* is based on the characteristic microscopic features of the mold form and the presence of a specific A band in the exoantigen test. In some instances, *H. capsulatum*, *P. boydii*, and *T. rubrum* might be confused microscopically with *B. dermatitidis*. The relatively slow growth rate of *B. dermatitidis* and careful examination of the microscopic morphological features will usually differentiate these fungi from *B. dermatitidis*.

43.16.c. Coccidioidomycosis. Coccidioidomycosis is a fungal infection that is primarily limited to the desert southwestern portion of the United States as well as semiarid regions of Mexico and Central and South America. Although the geographical distribution of the organism is well-defined, cases of coccidioidomycosis may be seen in any part of the world because of the ease of travel. The infection is acquired by inhalation of the infective arthroconidia of *C. immitis*. Approximately 60% of the cases are

asymptomatic and self-limited respiratory tract infections. The infection, however, may become disseminated, with extension to other organs, meninges, bone, skin, lymph nodes, and subcutaneous tissue. Fewer than 1% of persons who acquire coccidioidomycosis ever become seriously ill; dissemination does, however, occur most frequently in persons of dark-skinned races.

In direct microscopic examinations of sputum or other body fluids, *C. immitis* appears as a nonbudding, thick-walled spherule, 20 to 200 μm in diameter, containing either granular material or numerous small (2 to 5 μm in diameter) endospores (Figure 43.71). The endospores are freed by rupture of the cell wall of spherules; therefore, empty and collapsed "ghost" spherules may be present. Small, immature spherules measuring 10 to 20 μm may be confused with *B. dermatitidis* when two are lying adjacent. In instances where the identification of *C. immitis* is questionable, a wet preparation of the clinical specimen may be made using sterile saline, and the edges of the coverglass may be sealed with petrolatum and incubated overnight. When spherules are present, multiple hyphal strands will be produced from the endospores.

Cultures of *C. immitis* represent a biohazard to laboratory workers, and strict safety precautions must be followed when examining cultures. Mature colonies may appear within 3 to 5 days of incubation

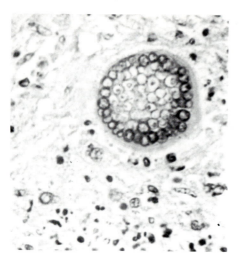

Figure 43.71
C. immitis, tissue form, showing spherule containing numerous spherical endospores (1000 ×).

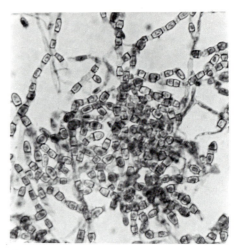

Figure 43.72
C. immitis, mycelial form, showing numerous thick-walled, rectangular or barrel-shaped alternate arthroconidia (500 ×).

and may be present on most media, including those used for bacteriology. *Laboratory workers should be cautioned not to open cultures of fluffy white molds unless they are placed in a biological safety cabinet*. Colonies of *C. immitis* often appear as delicate, cobweblike growth after 3 to 21 days of incubation. Some portions of the colony will exhibit aerial hyphae whereas others will have the hyphae adherent to the agar surface. Most isolates appear fluffy white; however, colonies of varying colors have been observed. On blood agar, some colonies exhibit a greenish discoloration, whereas others appear yeastlike, smooth, wrinkled, and tan in color. Isolates of *C. immitis* have been reported to range in color from pink to yellow to purple and black.[36]

Microscopically, some cultures show small septate hyphae that often exhibit right-angle branches and racquet forms. With age, the hyphae form arthroconidia that are characteristically rectangular or barrel-shaped in appearance. The arthroconidia are larger than the hyphae from which they are produced and stain darkly with lactophenol cotton or aniline blue. The arthroconidia are separated from one another by clear or lighter staining nonviable cells and are referred to as *alternate arthroconidia* (Figure 43.72). Arthroconidia have been reported to range in size from 1.5 to 7.5 μm in width and 1.5 to 30 μm in length, whereas most are 3 to 4.5 μm in width and 3.1 μm in length. Variation has been

reported in the shape of arthroconidia and ranges from rounded to square to curved; however, most are barrel-shaped. Even if alternate arthroconidia are observed microscopically, the definitive identification should be made using only the exoantigen test.

If a culture is suspected of being C. immitis, *it should be sealed with tape to prevent chances of laboratory-acquired infection*. Since *C. immitis* is the most infectious of all the fungi, extreme caution should be used when handling cultures of this organism. Safety precautions should be observed (see box on p. 735).

Some members of the Gymnoascasceae are found in the environment and may resemble *C. immitis* microscopically. Some species produce alternate arthroconidia that tend to be more rectangular, and it is necessary to consider them when making an identification. *Geotrichum candidum* and species of *Trichosporon* produce hyphae that disassociate into arthroconidia (Figures 43.73 and 43.74). The colonial morphological features of older cultures may resemble *C. immitis*. Microscopically, the arthroconidia do not appear to be alternate and are even-staining. Confusion rarely occurs between members of the Gymnoascasceae and *C. immitis*. It is also important to remember that there are occasional strains of *C. immitis* that fail to sporulate and may be identified only by the exoantigen test.

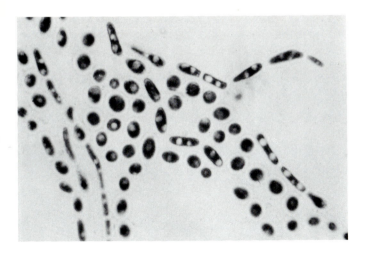

Figure 43.73
Trichosporon species, showing arthroconidia and an occasional blastoconidium.

43.16.d. Histoplasmosis. Histoplasmosis is a chronic, granulomatous infection that is primary in the lung and eventually invades the reticuloendothelial system. Approximately 95% of cases are asymptomatic and self-limited. Chronic pulmonary infections occur, and dissemination to the lymphatic tissue, liver, spleen, kidneys, meninges, and heart has been reported. Ulcerative lesions of the upper respiratory tract may occur. Histoplasmosis is another infection that is prevalent in the Ohio, Mississippi River, and Missouri River valleys, where conditions are optimal for growth of the organism in soil enriched with bird manure or bat guano.

Outbreaks of histoplasmosis have been associated with activities that disperse the microconidia or hyphal fragments into the air. Infection is acquired via inhalation of these infective units from the environment. The severity of the disease is generally related directly to the inoculum size. Numerous cases of histoplasmosis have been reported in persons cleaning a chicken house or barn that has been undisturbed for long periods or from working in or cleaning those areas that have served as roosting places for starlings and similar birds.

It is estimated that 500,000 persons are infected annually by *H. capsulatum*, the etiologic agent of histoplasmosis. It is perhaps one of the most common fungal infections seen in the midwestern and southern parts of the United States.

The direct microscopic examination of respiratory tract specimens and other similar specimens is usually unsatisfactory for the detection of *H. capsulatum*. The organism, however, may be detected by an astute laboratorian when examining Wright- or Giemsa-stained specimens of bone marrow or peripheral blood. *H. capsulatum* is found intracellularly within mononuclear cells as small, round to oval yeast cells 2 to 5 μm in diameter.

H. capsulatum is easily cultured from clinical

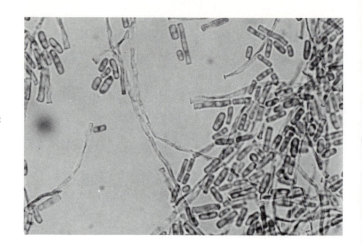

Figure 43.74
G. candidum, showing numerous arthroconidia. Note that arthroconidia do not alternate with a clear cell as in the case of *C. immitis* (430 ×).

specimens; however, it may be overgrown by bacteria or rapidly growing molds. A procedure useful for the recovery of *H. capsulatum*, *B. dermátitidis*, and *C. immitis* from contaminated specimens utilizes a yeast extract phosphate medium[7] and a drop of concentrated ammonium hydroxide (NH_4OH) placed on one side of the inoculated plate of medium. In the past, it has been recommended that specimens not be kept at room temperature before culture, since *H. capsulatum* would not survive. It has been shown that *H. capsulatum* will survive transit in the mail for as long as 16 days.[31] It is, however, recommended that specimens be cultured as soon as possible to ensure the optimal recovery of *H. capsulatum* and other dimorphic fungi.

　H. capsulatum is considered to be a slow-growing mold at 25° to 30° C and usually requires 2 to 4 weeks or more for colonies to appear. It is not uncommon to recover the organism in 7 days or less if large numbers of cells are present in the clinical specimen. Isolates of *H. capsulatum* have been reported to be recovered from blood cultures in a mean time of 8 days.[8] Textbooks describe the colonial morphology of *H. capsulatum* as being a white, fluffy mold that turns brown to buff with age. Some isolates ranging from gray to red have also been reported. The organism commonly produces wrinkled, moist, heaped, yeastlike colonies that are soft and cream, tan, or pink in color. Tufts of hyphae often project upwards from the colonies as described with *B. dermatitidis*.

　Microscopically, the hyphae of *H. capsulatum* are small (1 to 2 μm in diameter) and are often inter-

twined to form ropelike strands. Commonly, large (8 to 14 μm in diameter) spherical or pyriform, smooth-walled macroconidia are seen in young cultures. With age, the macroconidia become roughened or tuberculate and provide enough evidence to make a tentative identification (Figure 43.75). The macroconidia are produced either on short or long lateral branches of the hyphae. Some isolates produce round to pyriform, smooth microconidia (2 to 4 μm in diameter) in addition to the characteristic tuberculate macroconidia. Some isolates of *H. capsulatum* fail to sporulate despite numerous attempts to induce sporulation.

　Conversion of the mold form to the yeast form is usually difficult and requires several successive transfers at 3- to 5-day intervals. Yeast colonies appear bacteria-like, mucoid, and membranous and are white to tan. Microscopically, a mixture of swollen hyphae and small budding yeast cells 2 to 5 μm in size are observed (Figure 43.76). These are similar to the intracellular yeast cells seen in mononuclear cells in infected tissue. The yeast form of *H. capsulatum* cannot be recognized unless the corresponding mold form is present on another culture or unless the yeast form is converted directly to the mold form by incubation at 25° to 30° C after yeast cells have been observed. The observation of both the mold and yeast form of *H. capsulatum* is satisfactory for the definitive identification. However, the exoantigen test is recommended as the most definitive means of providing an identification of this organism.

　Sepedonium, a saprobic organism found growing

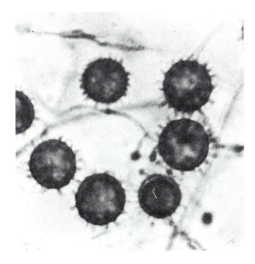

Figure 43.75
H. capsulatum, mycelial form, showing characteristic tuberculate macroconidia (1000 ×).

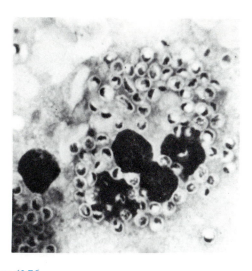

Figure 43.76
H. capsulatum, yeast form, showing intracellular, oval yeast cells, deeply stained (2000 ×).

on mushrooms, is always mentioned as being confused with *H. capsulatum*, since it produces similar tuberculate macroconidia. This organism is almost never recovered from clinical specimens, does not have a yeast form, and fails to produce the characteristic H or M bands seen in the exoantigen test with *H. capsulatum*.

43.16.e. **Paracoccidioidomycosis.** Paracoccidioidomycosis is a chronic granulomatous infection that begins as a primary pulmonary infection. It is often asymptomatic and then disseminates to produce ulcerative lesions of the mucous membranes. Ulcerative lesions are commonly present in the nasal and oral mucosa, gingivae, and less commonly in the conjunctivae. Lesions occur most commonly on the face in association with oral mucous membrane infection (Figure 43.77). The lesions are characteristically ulcerative, with a serpiginous active border and a crusted surface. Lymph node involvement in the cervical area is common. Pulmonary infection is seen most often, and progressive chronic pulmonary infection is found in approximately 50% of cases. Dissemination to other anatomic sites, including the lymphatic system, spleen, intestines, liver, brain, meninges, and adrenal glands, occurs in some patients.

The infection is most commonly found in South America, with the highest prevalence in Brazil, Venezuela, and Colombia. It also has been seen in many other areas, including Mexico, Central America, and Africa. Occasional imported cases have been seen in the United States and Europe.

The exact mechanism by which paracoccidioidomycosis is acquired is unclear; however, it is speculated that its origin is pulmonary and that it is acquired by inhalation of the organism from the environment. Since mucosal lesions are an integral part of the disease process, it is also speculated that the infection may be acquired through trauma to the oropharynx caused by vegetation that is commonly chewed by residents of the endemic areas. The exact ecological niche of the organism in nature is undetermined.

Specimens submitted for direct microscopic examinations are important for the diagnosis of paracoccidioidomycosis. Large, round or oval, multiply budding yeast cells (8 to 40 μm in diameter) are usually recognized in sputum, mucosal biopsy, and other exudates. Characteristic multiply budding yeast forms resemble a "mariner's wheel." The yeast cells surrounding the periphery of the parent cell range from 8 to 15 μm in diameter.

Colonies of *P. brasiliensis* grow very slowly (21 to 28 days) and are heaped, wrinkled, moist, and yeastlike. With age, colonies may become covered with a short aerial mycelium and turn tan to brown in color. The surface of colonies is often heaped with crater formations.

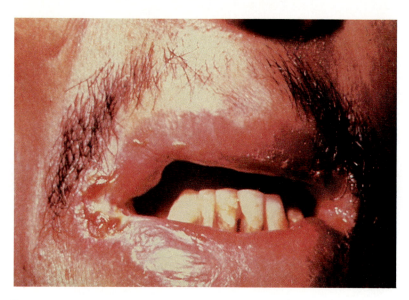

Figure 43.77
Lesions of paracoccidioidomycosis about lips. Note purulent exudate at right edge of mouth. (Courtesy Upjohn Co.)

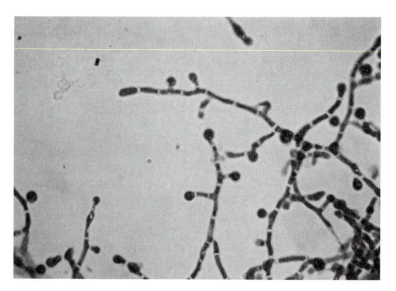

Figure 43.78
Paracoccidioides brasiliensis, mycelial form, showing septate hyphae and pyriform conidia singly borne (430 ×).

Microscopically, the mold form is similar to that seen with *B. dermatitidis.* Small hyphae (1 to 2 μm in diameter) are seen, along with numerous chlamydospores. Small, delicate (3 to 4 μm globose or pyriform conidia may be seen arising from the sides of the hyphae or on very short conidiophores (Figure 43.78). Most often, cultures reveal only fine septate hyphae and numerous chlamydospores.

After conversion on a blood-enriched medium, the colonial morphology of the yeast form is characterized by smooth, soft-wrinkled, yeastlike colonies that are cream to tan in color. Microscopically,

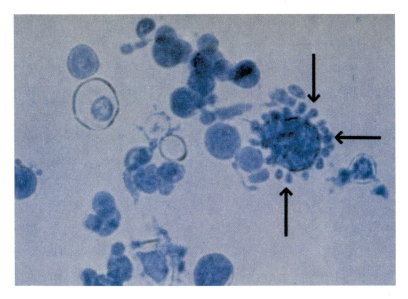

Figure 43.79
P. brasiliensis. Numerous small buds.

the colonies are composed of yeast cells 10 to 40 μm in diameter that are surrounded by narrow-necked yeast cells around the periphery, as previously described (Figure 43.79).

If in vitro conversion to the yeast form is unsuccessful, the exoantigen test[79] (Procedure 43.6) should be used to make the definitive identification of *P. brasiliensis*.

Table 43.9 presents a summary of the colonial and microscopic morphological features of the dimorphic fungi.

43.17. Opportunistic Mycoses

The opportunistic mycoses are a group of fungal infections that occur almost exclusively in immunocompromised patients. The type of patient who acquires an opportunistic fungal infection is one who is compromised by some underlying disease process such as lymphoma, leukemia, diabetes mellitus, or an underlying defect of the immune system. Patients are often on treatment with corticosteroids, cytotoxic drugs, or other immunosuppressive agents. A host of fungi previously thought to be nonpathogenic are known to be the etiologic agents of the opportunistic fungal infections. Since most of the organisms known to cause infection in this group of patients are commonly encountered in the clinical laboratory as saprobes, it is impossible for the laboratory to determine the clinical significance of an isolate recovered from

the specimens of immunocompromised patients. It is necessary for the laboratory to identify and report completely the presence of all fungi recovered from immunocompromised patients, since every organism is a potential pathogen.

While there is an ongoing list of opportunistic mycoses, a certain few are seen with the greatest frequency and include aspergillosis, zygomycosis, candidosis (candidiasis), and cryptococcosis. The etiologic agents of each will be discussed; however, the fungi associated with the less common opportunistic mycoses are presented in Section 43.22, Saprobic Fungi Commonly Encountered in the Clinical Laboratory.

43.17.a. Aspergillosis. Several species of aspergilli are among the most frequently encountered organisms in the clinical laboratory; some are pathogenic whereas others are infrequently associated with infection or do not cause infection at all. The aspergilli are widespread in the environment, where they colonize grain, leaves, soil, and living plants. Conidia of the aspergilli are easily dispersed into the environment, and humans become infected by inhaling them. These organisms are capable not only of causing disseminated infection, as is seen in immunocompromised patients, but also of causing a whole host of other types of infections, including invasive lung infection, pulmonary mycetoma, allergic bronchopulmonary aspergillosis, external otomycosis,

Table 43.9

Summary of the Characteristic Features of Fungi Known to be the Most Common Causes
of Fungal Infection of Man

INFECTION	ETIOLOGIC AGENT	GROWTH RATE (DAYS)	CULTURAL CHARACTERISTICS AT 30°C	
			BLOOD-ENRICHED MEDIUM	MEDIUM LACKING BLOOD ENRICHMENT
Blastomycosis	*Blastomyces dermatitidis*	5-30	Colonies are cream to tan, soft, moist, wrinkled, waxy, flat to heaped, and yeastlike; "tufts" of hyphae often project upward from colonies	Colonies are white to cream to tan, some with drops of exudate present, fluffy to glabrous, and adherent to the agar surface
Cryptococcosis	*Cryptococcus neoformans*	3-10	Colonies are usually dome-shaped, dry, cream to tan, and smaller than those on media lacking blood enrichment	Colonies are dry to mucoid and shiny, dome-shaped, smooth and cream to tan in color; however, some isolates appear golden to orange on certain media, i.e., inhibitory mold agar
Histoplasmosis	*Histoplasma capsulatum*	5-45	Colonies are heaped, moist, wrinkled, yeastlike, soft, and cream, tan or pink in color; "tufts" of hyphae often project upward from colonies	Colonies are white, cream, tan or gray, fluffy to glabrous; some colonies appear yeastlike and adherent to the agar surface; many variations in colonial morphology occur
Paracoccidioidomycosis	*Paracoccidioides brasiliensis*	21-28	Colonies are heaped, wrinkled, moist, and yeastlike; with age, colonies may become covered with short aerial mycelium and may turn brown	
Candidosis	*Candida albicans* and other *Candida* species	2-4	Colonies vary in their morphology but are usually white to tan, shiny to dull, flat to heaped, smooth to wrinkled, and moist to dry; some colonies produce pseudohyphal fringes at the periphery; colonies growing on blood-enriched media are somewhat smaller and drier than on non-blood-containing media	

From Thomson, R.B., and Roberts, G.D. 1982. A practical approach to the diagnosis of fungal infections of the respiratory tract. Clin. Lab. Med. 2:321.

MICROSCOPIC MORPHOLOGICAL FEATURES		SCREENING TESTS	MICROSCOPIC MORPHOLOGICAL FEATURES OF TISSUE FORM	CONFIRMATORY TESTS FOR IDENTIFICATION
BLOOD-CONTAINING MEDIUM	**NON-BLOOD-CONTAINING MEDIUM**			
Hyphae 1-2 μm in diameter are present; some are aggregated in ropelike clusters; sporulation is rare	Hyphae 1-2 μm in diameter are present; single pyriform conidia are produced on short to long conidiophores; some cultures produce few conidia	Not available	8-15 μm, broad-based budding cells with double-contoured walls are seen; cytoplasmic granulation is often obvious	1. Broad-based budding cells may be seen after in vitro conversion on cottonseed agar 2. Exoantigen test positive with A band 70% exhibit A bands
Cells are usually spherical, vary in size, and may be encapsulated; cells may have more than one "pinched-off" bud present on parent cell		1. Urease production 2. Phenol oxidase production 3. Nitrate reductase production	2-15 μm, single or multiply budding spherical cells that vary in size are seen; evidence of encapsulation may be present	1. Carbohydrate utilization 2. Pigment on niger seed agar
Hyphae 1-2 μm in diameter are present; some are aggregated in ropelike clusters; sporulation is rare	Young cultures usually have a predominance of smooth-walled macroconidia that become tuberculate with age; macroconidia may be pyriform or spherical; some isolates produce small pyriform microconidia in the presence or absence of macroconidia	Not available	2-5 μm, small, oval to spherical budding cells often seen inside of mononuclear cells	Exoantigen test positive with H, M, or H and M band
Hyphae 1-2 μm in diameter are present; some isolates produce conidia similar to those of *B. dermatitidis*; chlamydospores may be numerous, and multiple budding yeast cells 10-25 μm in diameter may be present		Not available	10-25 μm, multiply budding cells (buds 1-2 μm) resembling a "mariner's wheel" may be present; buds are attached to the parent cell by a narrow neck	Exoantigen test positive for bands 1, 2, 3
Most species produce either blastoconidia, pseudohyphae, or true hyphae; chlamydospores are produced by *C. albicans* and certain isolates of *C. tropicalis*		Germ tube production by *C. albicans*	Blastoconidia 2-5 μm in diameter and pseudohyphae are present	1. Germ tube production for *C. albicans* 2. Carbohydrate utilization

Continued.

Table 43.9

Summary of the Characteristic Features of Fungi Known to be the Most Common Causes of Fungal Infection of Man—cont'd

INFECTION	ETIOLOGIC AGENT	GROWTH RATE (DAYS)	CULTURAL CHARACTERISTICS AT 30°C	
			BLOOD-ENRICHED MEDIUM	MEDIUM LACKING BLOOD ENRICHMENT
Zygomycosis	*Rhizopus* species, *Mucor* species, and other Zygomycetes	1-3	Colonies are extremely fast growing, woolly, and gray to brown to gray-black in color	
Aspergillosis	*Aspergillus fumigatus* *Aspergillus flavus* *Aspergillus niger* *Aspergillus terreus* *Aspergillus* species	3-5	Colonies of *A. fumigatus* are usually blue-green to gray-green while those of *A. flavus* and *A. niger* are yellow-green and black, respectively; colonies of *A. terreus* resemble powdered cinnamon; other species of *Aspergillus* exhibit a wide range of colors; blood-enriched media usually have little effect on the colonial morphological features	
Coccidioidomycosis	*Coccidioides immitis*	2-21	Colonies may be white and fluffy to greenish on blood-enriched media; some isolates are yeastlike, heaped, wrinkled, and membranous	Colonies usually are fluffy white but may be pigmented gray, orange, brown, or yellow; mycelium is adherent to the agar surface in some portions of the colony

mycotic keratitis, onychomycosis, sinusitis, endocarditis, and central nervous system infection. Most often, immunocompromised patients acquire a primary pulmonary infection that rapidly disseminates and causes infection in virtually every organ.

It is difficult to assess the significance of members of the genus *Aspergillus* in a clinical specimen. They are found frequently in cultures of respiratory secretions, skin scrapings, and other specimens. Table 43.10 presents the Mayo Clinic experience with the recovery of species of *Aspergillus* from clinical specimens. It has been reported that *Aspergillus* is significant in only 10% of cases[82]; however, this depends upon the hospital setting and type of patient population seen.

Since aspergilli are recovered frequently, it is imperative that the organism be demonstrated by the direct microscopic examination of fresh clinical specimens and that the organism be recovered repeatedly from patients with an appropriate clinical picture to ensure that the organism is clinically significant. Most species of *Aspergillus* are susceptible to cycloheximide; therefore, specimens for recovery of *Aspergillus* or subcultures should not be cultured onto media containing this ingredient.

Aspergillus fumigatus is most commonly recovered from immunocompromised patients; moreover, it is the species most often seen in the clinical laboratory. In addition, *Aspergillus flavus* is commonly recovered from immunocompromised patients and represents a frequent isolate in the clinical microbiology laboratory. The recovery of *A. fumigatus* or *A. flavus* from surveillance nasal cultures is strongly correlated with subsequent invasive aspergillosis.[88]

MICROSCOPIC MORPHOLOGICAL FEATURES		SCREENING TESTS	MICROSCOPIC MORPHOLOGICAL FEATURES OF TISSUE FORM	CONFIRMATORY TESTS FOR IDENTIFICATION
BLOOD-CONTAINING MEDIUM	NON-BLOOD-CONTAINING MEDIUM			
1. *Rhizopus* species—rhizoids are produced at the base of a sporangiophore 2. *Mucor* species—no rhizoids are produced		Not available	Large ribbonlike (10-30 μm), twisted; often distorted pieces of aseptate hyphae may be present; septa may occasionally be seen	Identification is based on characteristic morphological features
1. *A. fumigatus*—uniserate heads with phialides covering the upper one half to two thirds of the vesicle 2. *A. flavus*—uniserate or biserate or both with phialides covering the entire surface of a spherical vesicle 3. *A. niger*—biserate with phialides covering the entire surface of a spherical vesicle; conidia are black 4. *A. terreus*—biserate with phialides covering the entire surface of a hemispherical vesicle; aleuriospores are formed on submerged hyphae		Not available	Septate hyphae 5-10 μm in diameter that exhibit dichotomous branching	Identification is based on microscopic morphological features and colonial morphology; *A. fumigatus* can tolerate elevated temperatures at ≥15°C
Chains of alternate, barrel-shaped arthroconidia are characteristic; some arthroconidia may be elongated; hyphae are small and often arranged in ropelike strands and racquet forms are seen in young cultures		Not available	Round spherules 30-60 μm in diameter containing 2-5 μm endospores are characteristic	Exoantigen test positive for III, F, or TP bands

Table 43.10
Recovery of *Aspergillus* from Clinical Specimens During a 10-Year Period at Mayo Clinic

ORGANISM	TYPE OF CLINICAL SPECIMEN				
	RESPIRATORY SECRETIONS	GASTRO-INTESTINAL	GENITO-URINARY	SKIN, SUBCUTANEOUS TISSUE	BLOOD, BONE, CNS, ETC.
Aspergillus clavatus	97/93*	1/1	—	1/1	—
A. flavus	1298/740	10/10	11/11	177/131	2/2
A. fumigatus	3247/2656	11/9	14/14	175/137	8/8
A. glaucus	307/503	1/1	—	8/8	1/1
A. nidulans	52/48	—	—	5/3	—
A. niger	1484/1376	18/18	17/17	151/124	11/11
A. terreus	164/146	—	—	23/21	3/3
A. versicolor	1237/1202	6/6	24/22	226/224	16/16
Other species of *Aspergillus*	3463/3418	14/18	32/32	319/314	16/16

Numerator = number of cultures; *denominator* = number of patients.

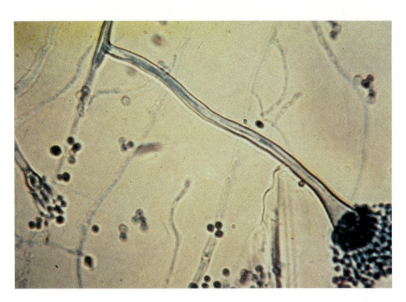

Figure 43.80
A. fumigatus conidiophore and conidia (400 ×).

The absence of a positive nasal culture does not preclude infection, however. *Aspergillus niger* is seen commonly in the clinical laboratory, but its association with clinical disease is somewhat limited. *Aspergillus terreus*, a previously uncommon isolate, is recognized currently as a significant cause of infection in immunocompromised patients, but its frequency of recovery is much lower than the previously mentioned species.

Specimens submitted for direct microscopic examination may contain septate hyphae that show evidence of dichotomous branching. In addition, some hyphae may show the presence of rounded, thick-walled cells.

A. fumigatus is a rapidly growing mold (2 to 6 days) that produces a fluffy to granular, white to blue-green colony. Mature sporulating colonies most often exhibit the blue-green powdery appearance. Microscopically, *A. fumigatus* is characterized by the presence of septate hyphae and short or long conidiophores having a characteristic cell at their base. The tip of the conidiophore expands into a large, dome-shaped vesicle that has bottle-shaped phialides occurring in a single row and around the upper half or two thirds of its surface. Long chains of small (2 to 3 μm in diameter), spherical, rough-walled, green conidia form a columnar mass on the vesicle (Figure 43.80). Cultures of *A. fumigatus* are ther-

motolerant and are able to withstand temperatures up to 45° C.

A. flavus, somewhat more rapidly growing (1 to 5 days), produces a yellow-green colony. Microscopically, vesicles are globose and phialides are produced directly from the vesicle surface (uniserate) or from a primary row of branches (metulae; biserate). The phialides give rise to short chains of yellow-orange elliptical or spherical conidia that become roughened on the surface with age (Figure 43.81).

A. niger, sometimes referred to as being dematiaceous, produces mature colonies within 2 to 6 days. Growth begins initially as a yellow colony that soon develops a black, dotted surface as conidia are produced. With age, the colony becomes jet black and powdery while the reverse remains buff or cream color.

Microscopically, *A. niger* exhibits septate hyphae, long conidiophores that support spherical vesicles that give rise to large metulae and smaller phialides from which long chains of brown, rough-walled conidia are produced (Figure 43.82). The entire surface of the vesicle is involved in sporulation.

A. terreus, less commonly seen in the clinical laboratory, produces colonies that are tan and resemble cinnamon. Vesicles are hemispherical, as seen microscopically, and phialides cover the entire surface and are produced from a primary row of

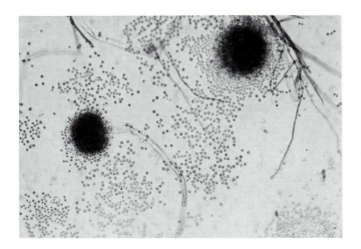

Figure 43.81
A. flavus, showing spherical vesicles that give rise to metulae and phialides that produce chains of conidia (430 ×).

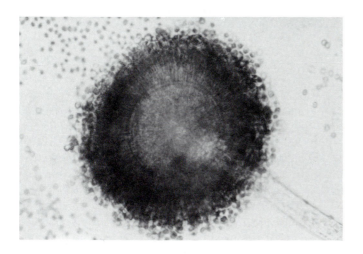

Figure 43.82
A. niger, showing larger spherical vesicle that gives rise to metulae, phialides, and chains of dark brown conidia (750 ×).

branches (metulae; biserate). Phialides produce globose to elliptical conidia arranged in chains. This species produces the unique structures of larger aleuriospores, which are found on submerged hyphae. The reader is referred to the chapter by Swatek et al.[85] for further information regarding other species.

43.17.b. Zygomycosis. Zygomycosis is a somewhat less common infection when compared with aspergillosis; however, it is a significant cause of morbidity and mortality in immunocompromised patients. The organisms involved have a worldwide distribution and are commonly found on decaying vegetable matter or in soil. The infection is generally acquired by inhalation of spores followed by subsequent development of infection. Immunocompromised patients, particularly those having uncon-

trolled diabetes and patients receiving prolonged corticosteroid, antibiotic, or cytotoxic therapy, are at greatest risk. The organisms involved in causing zygomycosis have a marked propensity for vascular invasion and rapidly produce thrombosis and necrosis of tissue. One of the most common forms observed is the rhinocerebral form where the nasal mucosa, palate, sinuses, orbit, face, and brain are involved; each shows massive necrosis with vascular invasion and infarction. Other types of infection involve the lungs and gastrointestinal tract; some patients develop disseminated infection. Organs including the liver, spleen, pancreas, and kidney may be involved. The Zygomycetes have also been reported to be the etiologic agent of infection in the skin of burn patients and in subcutaneous tissue of patients undergoing surgery.

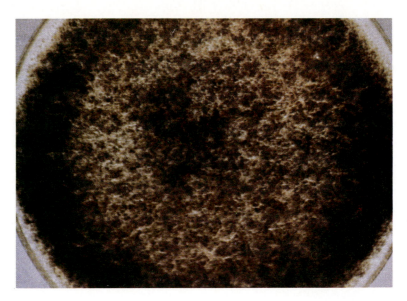

Figure 43.83
Rhizopus colony.

The rapid diagnosis of zygomycosis may be made by examination of tissue specimens or exudate from infected lesions using the potassium hydroxide preparation. Branching, predominantly nonseptate hyphae will be observed. It is highly important that the laboratory notify the clinician of these findings since Zygomycetes grow very rapidly and vascular invasion occurs at about the same rate.

The colonial morphological features of the Zygomycetes allow one to immediately suspect organisms belonging to this group. Colonies characteristically produce a fluffy, white to gray or brown hyphal growth that diffusely covers the surface of the agar within 24 to 96 hours (Figure 43.83). The hyphae appear to be coarse and fill the entire culture dish or tube rapidly with loose grayish hyphae dotted with brown or black sporangia. It is impossible to distinguish between the different genera and species of Zygomycetes based on their colonial morphological features since most are identical in appearance.

Microscopically, the Zygomycetes characteristically produce large ribbonlike hyphae that are irregular in diameter and nonseptate; however, occasional septa may exist in older cultures. The specific identification of these organisms is confirmed by observing the characteristic saclike fruiting structures *(sporangia)*, which produce internally spherical, yellow or brown spores *(sporangiospores)* (Figure 43.84). Each sporangium is formed at the tip of

a supporting structure *(sporangiophore)*. During maturation, the sporangium becomes fractured and sporangiospores are released into the environment. Sporangiophores are usually connected to each other by occasionally septate hyphae called *stolons*, which attach at contact points where rootlike structures (**rhizoids**) anchor the organism to the agar surface. The identification of the three most common Zygomycetes, *Mucor*, *Rhizopus*, and *Absidia*, is based on the presence or absence of rhizoids and the position of the rhizoids in relation to the sporangiophores. *Mucor* is characterized by sporangiophores that are singularly produced or branched and have at their tip a round sporangium filled with sporangiospores. *Mucor* does not have rhizoids or stolons and this distinguishes it from the other genera of Zygomycetes (Figure 43.84).

Rhizopus has unbranched sporangiophores with rhizoids that appear at the point where the stolon arises (Figure 43.85).

Absidia, an uncommon isolate in the clinical laboratory, is characterized by the presence of rhizoids that originate between sporangiophores (Figure 43.86). The sporangia are pyriform and have a swollen portion of the sporangiophore at the junction of the sporangium. Usually a septum is formed in the sporangiophore just below the sporangium.

The other genera of Zygomycetes that may be encountered in the clinical laboratory include *Sak-*

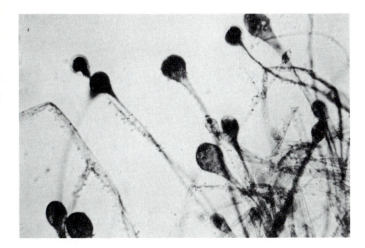

Figure 43.84
Mucor species, showing numerous sporangia in the absence of rhizoids (430 ×).

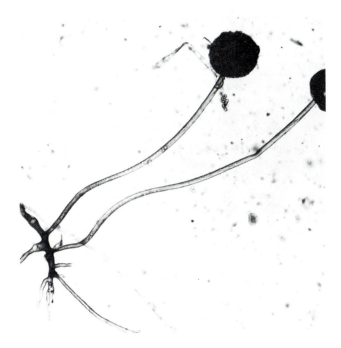

Figure 43.85
Rhizopus species, showing sporangium on long sporangiophore arising from nonseptate hyphae. Note presence of characteristic rhizoids at the base of the sporangiophore (250 ×).

senaea, Cunninghamella, Conidiobolus, and *Basidiobolus.* For additional information on these and other species, the reader is referred to the chapter by Greer and Rogers.[27]

43.17.c. Candidosis (candidiasis). Candidosis is the most frequently encountered opportunistic fungal infection. It is caused by a number of species of *Candida* with *Candida albicans* being the most fre-

quent etiologic agent, followed by *Candida tropicalis* and *Candida (Torulopsis) glabrata.* A number of other species have been involved in infection in immunocompromised patients; however, their incidence is not nearly as high, as previously mentioned. *C. albicans* and others are a part of the normal endogenous microbial flora, and infections are believed to be endogenous in origin. The organisms

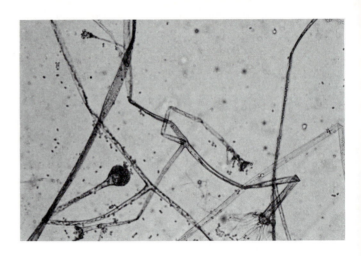

Figure 43.86
Absidia species, showing sporangia on long sporangiophores arising from nonseptate hyphae. Note that rhizoids are produced between sporangiophores and not at their bases (250 ×).

may be recovered from the oropharynx, gastrointestinal tract, genitourinary tract, and skin. *Candida* species are responsible for a number of different types of infections in normal and immunocompromised patients. Included are intertriginous candidosis where skin folds are involved, paronychia, onychomycosis, perlèche, vulvovaginitis, thrush, pulmonary infection, eye infection, endocarditis, meningitis, fungemia, and disseminated infection. The latter two types of infection are most commonly seen in immunocompromised patients, while the others mentioned may occur in normal hosts. Onychomycosis and esophagitis produced by *C. albicans* are very common in patients having acquired immunodeficiency syndrome (AIDS).

The clinical significance of *Candida* recovered from specimens is difficult to evaluate, since it is considered to be part of the normal flora of humans.[77] A study at Mayo Clinic evaluated the clinical significance of yeasts recovered from respiratory secretions, except for *Cryptococcus neoformans*, and concluded that they are part of the normal flora and that their routine identification is unnecessary.[59] The repeated recovery of different species of yeasts from multiple specimens from the same patient usually indicates colonization. The simultaneous recovery of the same species of yeast from several body sites, including urine, is a good indicator of disseminated infection and the subsequent development of fungemia.

The direct microscopic examination of clinical specimens containing *Candida* will reveal budding yeast cells (blastoconidia) 2 to 4 μm in diameter or pseudohyphae showing regular points of constriction, resembling lengths of sausages; or true septate hyphae. The blastoconidia, hyphae, and pseudohyphae are strongly gram-positive. It is advisable to report the approximate number of such forms since the presence of large numbers in a fresh clinical specimen may be of diagnostic significance.

The colonial and microscopic morphological features of the species of *Candida* are of little value in making a definitive identification. *C. albicans*, however, may be identified by the production of germ tubes (Figure 43.87) or the presence of chlamydospores (Figure 43.88). Other species of *Candida* must be identified by the utilization of, and sometimes fermentation of, specific carbohydrate substrates. Specific detailed procedures for the identification of yeast, including *Candida* species, will be presented later in this section.

43.17.d. Cryptococcosis. Cryptococcosis, specifically caused by *C. neoformans*, is a subacute or chronic fungal infection that has several manifestations. In the immunocompromised patient, it is not uncommon to see disseminated disease with or without meningitis; meningitis occurs in approximately two thirds of patients with disseminated infection. Disseminated cryptococcosis is becoming a very common clinical entity in patients with AIDS. Occasionally, patients with disseminated infection will exhibit painless skin lesions that may ulcerate. Other uncommon manifestations of cryptococcosis include endocarditis, hepatitis, renal infection, and pleural effusion. It is of interest to note that a review of patient records at the Mayo Clinic revealed over 100

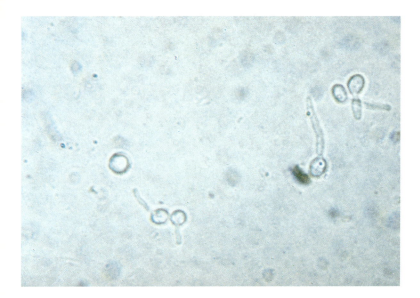

Figure 43.87
C. albicans. Germ tubes.

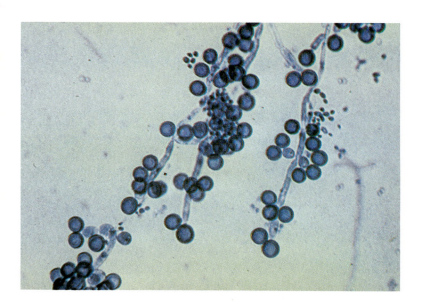

Figure 43.88
C. albicans. Blastoconidia and chlamydo-spores.

cases of colonization of the respiratory tract with *C. neoformans* without subsequent development of infection. Follow-up on these patients was as long as 6 years; none in this group was considered to be immunocompromised. This makes the clinical significance of *C. neoformans* somewhat difficult to assess; however, its presence in clinical specimens from immunocompromised patients should be considered to be significant. In many instances the clinical symptoms are suppressed by corticosteroid ther-

apy, and culture or serologic evidence provides the earliest proof of infection. There is a strong association of cryptococcal infection with such debilitating diseases as leukemia and lymphoma and the immunosuppressive therapy that may be required for these and other underlying diseases. The presence of *C. neoformans* in clinical specimens in some instances precedes the symptoms of an underlying disease. The infection is probably more frequent than is commonly recognized; it is estimated that there may be 300 new cases each year in the United States.[33]

Four serotypes of *C. neoformans* have been described (A, B, C, and D) with somewhat different geographic distribution.[49] The organism has been proved to be a basidiomycete by the discovery of its sexual form. The name of the sexual form is *Filobasidiella*, with two species. *F. neoformans* and *F. bacillisporus;* the latter includes serotypes B and C.[48] The term *Cryptococcus* will continue to be used since it is well established by tradition. Despite the discovery of two species of *Cryptococcus*, there is no difference in disease produced or in the response to chemotherapy between the two species.

C. neoformans exists as a saprobe in nature. It is most often found associated with the excreta of pigeons. The hypothesis that pigeon habitats serve as reservoirs for human infection is substantiated by numerous reports; the pigeon manure apparently serves as an enrichment for *C. neoformans* because of its chemical makeup. It is believed that *C. neoformans* is widely distributed in nature, becomes aerosolized, and is inhaled prior to infection.

Traditionally, the India ink preparation has been the most widely used method for the rapid detection of *C. neoformans* in clinical specimens. An evaluation of 39 consecutive patients with cryptococcal meningitis seen at Mayo Clinic showed that only 40% gave positive India ink preparations of the cerebrospinal fluid. The purpose of the India ink preparation is to delineate the large capsule of *C. neoformans*, since the ink particles cannot penetrate the capsular polysaccharide material. *Because of the low positivity rate of the India ink preparation, it is not recommended as a routine tool in the clinical microbiology laboratory. It should be replaced with the cryptococcal latex test for antigen that will be described in a subsequent section.* The India ink preparation is commonly positive in specimens from patients having AIDS. Laboratories examining large numbers of specimens from these patients may wish to retain the use of this procedure in combination with the cryptococcal latex test for antigen.

The microscopic examination of other clinical specimens, including respiratory secretions, can be of value in making a diagnosis of cryptococcosis. *C. neoformans* appears as a spherical, single or multiple budding, thick-walled, yeastlike organism 2 to 15 μm in diameter, usually surrounded by a wide, refractile polysaccharide capsule. Perhaps the most important characteristic of *C. neoformans* is the extreme vari-

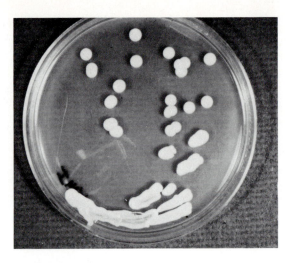

Figure 43.89
C. neoformans, showing colonies that appear shiny and mucoid because of the presence of a polysaccharide capsule.

ation in the size of the yeast cells; this is unrelated to the amount of polysaccharide capsule present. It is important to remember that not all isolates of *C. neoformans* exhibit a capsule.

C. neoformans is easily cultured on routine fungal culture media without cycloheximide. The organism is inhibited by the presence of cycloheximide at 25° to 30° C. For the optimal recovery of *C. neoformans* from cerebrospinal fluid, it is recommended that a 0.45-μm pore size membrane filter be used with a sterile syringe. The filter is placed on the surface of the culture medium and is removed at daily intervals so that growth under the filter can be visualized. An alternative to the membrane filter technique is the use of centrifugation. Contrary to a prior report[89] the centrifugation of cerebrospinal fluid has no effect on the viability of the organism.

Colonies of *C. neoformans* usually appear on culture media within 1 to 5 days and begin as a smooth white to tan colony that may become mucoid and cream to brown in color. It is important to recognize the colonial morphology on different culture media since variation does occur; for example, on inhibitory mold agar, *C. neoformans* appears as a golden yellow, nonmucoid colony. Textbooks typically characterize the colonial morphology as being *Klebsiella*-like because of the large amount of polysaccharide capsule material present (Figure 43.89). In reality, most isolates of *C. neoformans* do not have large capsules and may not have the typical mucoid appearance.

The microscopic examination of colonies of *C. neoformans* may be of help in providing a tentative identification of *C. neoformans* since the cells will be spherical and exhibit a wide variation in their size. A presumptive identification of *C. neoformans* may be based on urease production, rapid phenol oxidase production, and failure to utilize an inorganic nitrate substrate. The final identification of *C. neoformans* is based on typical carbohydrate utilization patterns and pigment production on niger seed agar. Specific tests useful for the identification of *C. neoformans* and other species of cryptococci will be presented in a subsequent section.

43.18. General Considerations for the Identification of Yeasts

During the past few years, a significant increase in the number of fungal infections caused by yeasts has been reported in the literature. Numerous species of *Candida* and other yeasts have been implicated. These infections are primarily seen in immunocompromised patients (including those with AIDS), and some of the yeasts have proved to be resistant to antifungal therapy.[6,20,26,53] It is now recognized that these infections are associated with patients having surgery and patients on long-term intravenous therapy without adequate catheter care. Microbiologists should be aware that any of the genera and species of yeast can be potential pathogens in this group of patients.

Just how far the laboratory should go with a complete identification of all yeast species is of question. It is recommended that:
1. All yeasts recovered from sterile body fluids, including cerebrospinal fluid, blood, urine, paracentesis, and other fluids, should be identified to the species level.
2. Yeasts from all seriously ill or immunocompromised patients or in whom a mycotic infection is suspected should be identified to the species level.
3. Yeasts from respiratory secretions should not be identified on a routine basis; however, they should be screened for the presence of *C. neoformans*.
4. Yeasts recovered in large amounts from any clinical source should be identified to the species level.
5. Yeasts recovered from several successive specimens, except respiratory secretions, should be identified to the species level. Each laboratory

director will have to decide how much time, effort, and expense is to be spent on the identification of yeasts in the laboratory.

The development of commercially available yeast identification systems provides laboratories of all sizes with the capability of accurate and standardized methods.[24,50] These systems have extensive computer-based data bases that include information based on thousands of isolates of yeasts. Variations in the reactions of carbohydrates and other substrates utilized are considered in the identification of yeasts provided by these systems. Commercially available systems are recommended for all laboratories; however, they should be used in conjunction with some rapid screening tests that will provide the presumptive identification of *C. neoformans* and a definitive identification of *C. albicans*. In addition, some laboratories might prefer the use of conventional systems[21]; therefore, the information presented within this section discusses rapid screening methods for the presumptive identification of yeasts, commercially available systems, and a conventional schema that will provide for the identification of commonly encountered species of yeast seen in the clinical laboratory.

43.19. Rapid Screening Tests for the Identification of Yeast

43.19.a. Rapid urease test. The rapid urease test (Procedure 43.7) is a most useful tool for screening for urease-producing yeasts recovered from respiratory secretions and other clinical specimens. Alternatives to this method include the heavy inoculum of the tip of a slant of Christensen's urea agar and subsequent incubation at 35° to 37° C. In many instances, a positive reaction will occur within several hours; however, 1 to 2 days of incubation may be required. It is of interest to note that strains of *Rhodotorula*, *Candida*, and *Trichosporon* occasionally hydrolyze urea. Therefore the microscopic morphological features will be of help in interpreting the usefulness of the urease test for the detection of *Cryptococcus*. Another alternative method is the rapid selective urease test (Procedure 43.8) developed by Zimmer and Roberts.[93] An evaluation of this method showed that the urease activity of 99.6% of 286 isolates of *C. neoformans* was detected within 15 minutes. This test appears to be useful in detecting *C. neoformans* from specimens cultured onto Sabouraud's dextrose agar. It has not been evaluated using isolates tested from other media.

PROCEDURE 43.7

Rapid Urease Test [70]

Principle

The hydrolysis of urea by the enzyme urease produces ammonia and carbon dioxide. The ammonia produces alkaline conditions in the medium and changes the indicator (phenol red) from yellow to pink.

Method

1. Reconstitute a vial of dehydrated Difco urea broth with 3 ml of sterile distilled water on the day of use.
2. Dispense three to four drops into each well of a microdilution plate. Determine the exact number of wells to be used for the day and use only the number necessary.
3. Transfer a heavy inoculum of a yeast colony (not including pink yeasts) to a well containing the urea broth. Colonies tested should be no older than 7 days and should be free of contamination with bacteria. In some instances it might be necessary to make a subculture to obtain enough growth to provide the inoculum for the test.
4. Include positive and negative controls using *C. neoformans* and *C. albicans*, respectively.
5. Seal the microdilution wells with plastic tape and incubate 4 h at 37° C.
6. Observe for the production of a pink to purple color, which is indicative of urease production.

Quality control

C. neoformans and *C. albicans* are used as the positive and negative controls, respectively.

Expected results

C. neoformans should produce urease while *C. albicans* will not.

Performance schedule

Controls should be performed with each test run.

PROCEDURE 43.8

Rapid Selective Urease Test [93]

Principle

Benzalkonium chloride (1%) is added to the test medium to disassociate the cell wall of yeasts to allow the endogenous urease to be released into the test medium. The hydrolysis of urea is detected by the presence of ammonia, which changes the indicator to pink because of the alkaline conditions produced.

Method

1. Sweep a cotton-tipped applicator impregnated with the dehydrated urea substrate over the surface of two or three colonies so that the tip is well covered with the organism.
2. Place the applicator containing the yeast into a tube containing three drops of 1% benzalkonium chloride (pH 4.86 ± 0.01) and whirl firmly against the bottom of the tube to place the organisms into contact with the cotton fibers.
3. Add a cotton plug to the tube and incubate at 45° C for up to 30 min.
4. Examine after 10, 15, 20, and 30 min for the presence of a color change from yellow to purple. A red or purple color indicates urease production by *C. neoformans*.

Quality control

Same as for Procedure 43.7.

PROCEDURE 43.9

Nitrate Reduction Test[34]

Principle

Benzalkonium chloride (1%) is added to the test medium to disassociate the cell wall of yeasts to allow the endogenous nitrate reductase to be released into the test medium. The test reagents turn pink in the presence of nitrite. Addition of zinc dust to detect unreacted nitrate prevents a false-negative reaction resulting from complete reduction of nitrate to ammonia (and thus a lack of nitrite).

Method

1. Sweep the tip of an applicator impregnated with the nitrate reduction test reagents across two or three colonies of yeast.
2. Swirl the applicator containing the yeast against the bottom of an empty test tube to get the yeast cells in contact with the cotton fibers.
3. Incubate the tube and swab at 45° C for 10 min.

4. Remove the swab and add two drops each of N-naphthylethylenediamine and sulfanilic acid reagents to the tube and replace the applicator. A change in color to red indicates a positive test. If no color appears after 10 min, add a pinch of zinc dust. A change in color to red indicates the presence of previously unreacted nitrate and a negative test.

Quality control

Cryptococcus albidus and *C. neoformans* are used as positive and negative controls, respectively.

Expected results

C. albidus will reduce inorganic nitrate while *C. neoformans* will not.

Performance schedule

Controls should be performed with each test run.

All of the tests mentioned are useful for helping to provide a tentative identification of *C. neoformans;* however, they must be supplemented with new additional tests before a preliminary identification can be reported. These include the rapid nitrate reduction test and the levodopa test for the detection of phenol oxidase production.

43.19.b. Rapid nitrate reductase test. A characteristic feature of *C. neoformans* is that it does not utilize an inorganic nitrate substrate. A rapid method described by Hopkins and Land (Procedure 43.9) is recommended for the detection of nitrate reductase by species of cryptococci; however, it is not useful for the pink yeasts, including *Rhodotorula*.

43.19.c. Levodopa–ferric citrate test. *C. neoformans* is the only member of the genus *Cryptococcus* known to produce the enzyme phenol oxidase. Phenol oxidase will react with dihydroxyphenylalanine in the presence of ferric citrate to form the dark pigmented compound, melanin.[40] If an organism suspected of being *C. neoformans* produces urease, fails

to reduce nitrate, and produces phenol oxidase, a presumptive identification of *C. neoformans* may be reported; all this can be accomplished within 3 to 4 hours (Procedure 43.10).

A commercially available product, C/N-Screen (Flow Laboratories) is useful for the presumptive identification of *C. neoformans*. Levodopa is used as a substrate for the detection of phenol oxidase production. The major disadvantage of this product is that it requires 48 to 72 hours before positive reactions are visible.[14]

Although it is ideal to use all three screening tests to make a presumptive identification of *C. neoformans*, it is not always possible to perform all three since the inoculum size available may be limited. In instances where inoculum is limited, the laboratorian must use the tests that he or she feels can be performed and then make a subculture so that additional tests can be performed at a subsequent time. The Mycology Laboratory at Mayo Clinic has found that it is often just as fast to inoculate the organism

PROCEDURE 43.10

Levodopa–Ferric Citrate Test

Principle

C. neoformans is the only species of cryptococci that produces 3,4-dihydroxyphenylalanine-phenol oxidase. When reacted with L-β-3,4-dihydroxyphenylalanine and an iron compound (ferric citrate), *C. neoformans* oxidizes *O*-diphenol to melanin, which produces a brown to black color.

Method

1. Remove the number of frozen levodopa–ferric citrate disks necessary for testing. Place in a Petri dish and moisten disks with two or three drops of distilled water before testing. Disks may be obtained commercially from Remel Laboratories.
2. Smear a liberal amount of the test organism onto the surface of each moistened disk.
3. Incubate disks at 37° C and examine at 30-min intervals for up to 6 h. Other reactions produced by *C. neoformans* should occur in less than 3 h.

Quality control

C. neoformans and *C. albidus* are used as positive and negative controls, respectively.

Expected results

C. neoformans should exhibit a positive test (brown color development on the disk surface) while *C. albidus* will not.

Performance schedule

Controls should be performed with each test run.

PROCEDURE 43.11

Germ-Tube Test

Principle

Strains of *C. albicans* produce germ tubes from their yeast cells when placed in a liquid nutrient environment and incubated at 35° C for 3 hours (similar to the in vivo state).

Method

1. Suspend a very small inoculum of yeast cells obtained from an isolated colony in 0.5 ml of sheep serum (or normal human serum).
2. Incubate the tubes at 35° to 37° C for no longer than 3 h.
3. After incubation, remove a drop of the suspension and place on a microscope slide. Examine under low-power magnification for the presence of germ tubes. A germ tube is defined as an appendage that is one-half the width and three to four times the length of the yeast cell from which it arises (Figure 43.90). In most instances, there is no point of constriction at the origin of the germ tube from the cell.

Quality control

C. albicans and *C. tropicalis* are used as positive and negative controls, respectively.

Expected results

C. albicans will produce germ tubes, usually within 2 h, while *C. tropicalis* will not.

Performance schedule

Controls should be performed with each test run.

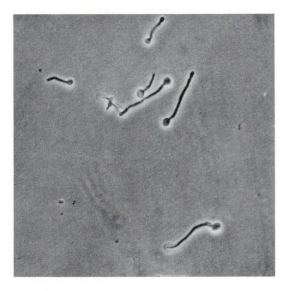

Figure 43.90
C. albicans, germ-tube test, showing yeast cells with germ tubes present (430 ×).

onto the surface of a plate of niger seed agar; results may be obtained during the same day of incubation. This will be discussed further within this section.

43.19.d. Germ-tube test (species of *Candida*). The germ-tube test (Procedure 43.11) is the most economical method used in the clinical laboratory for the identification of yeasts.[3] Approximately 75% of the yeasts recovered from clinical specimens are *C. albicans*, and the germ-tube test usually provides a definitive identification of this organism within 3 hours.

Germ tubes appear as hyphal-like extensions of yeast cells, produced usually without a constriction at the point of origin from the cell. In the past, it has been emphasized that *Candida stellatoidea* also produces germ tubes, and the distinction between *C. albicans* should be made. The latest edition of the text entitled *The Yeasts: A Taxonomic Study*, by Kreger-Van Rij,[47] indicates that *C. stellatoidea* is no longer a valid species and has been combined with *C. albicans*. The germ-tube test is specific for the identification of *C. albicans* with the exception of an occasional isolate of *C. tropicalis* that may rarely produce germ tubes.

Another method of identification of *C. albicans* is based on the presence of chlamydospores (see Figure 43.88) on cornmeal agar containing 1% Tween

80 and trypan blue incubated at room temperature for 24 to 48 hours. In addition, the appearance of spiderlike colonies on eosin methylene blue agar is characteristic of *C. albicans* and may be used to make a final identification by persons having experience with this method.

43.20. Commercially Available Yeast Identification Systems

As previously mentioned, commercially available yeast identification systems have provided laboratories of all sizes with standardized identification methods. The methods for the most part are rapid, and results are available within 72 hours. The major advantage is that the systems provide an identification based on a data base of thousands of yeast biotypes that considers a number of variations and substrate utilization patterns. Another advantage is that manufacturers of these products provide computer consultation services to help the laboratorian with the identification of isolates that give an atypical result.

43.20.a. API-20C yeast system. The API-20C yeast identification system has perhaps the most extensive computer-based data set of all commercial systems available. The system consists of a strip that contains 20 microcupules, 19 of which contain dehydrated carbohydrate substrates for determining carbohydrate utilization profiles of yeasts (Figure 43.91). Reactions are compared to growth in the first cupule, which lacks a carbohydrate substrate. Reactions are read and results are converted to a seven-digit biotype profile number, and the yeast identification is made from a profile register (Analytab Products). Chapter 9 discusses the principle of such systems. Most of the yeasts are identified within 48 hours using this system; however, species of *Cryptococcus* and *Trichosporon* may require up to 72 hours. It should be mentioned that the API-20C yeast identification system, as well as all the other commercially available products, requires that the microscopic morphological features of yeast grown on cornmeal agar containing 1% Tween 80 and trypan blue be used in conjunction with the carbohydrate utilization patterns. This is particularly helpful when more than one possibility for an identification is provided and the microscopic morphological features can be used to distinguish between the possibilities given by the profile register. Several evaluations of the API-20C yeast identification system

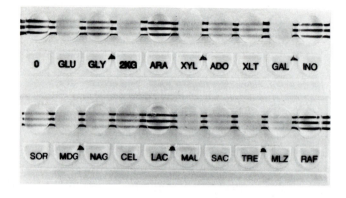

Figure 43.91
API-20C yeast identification system.

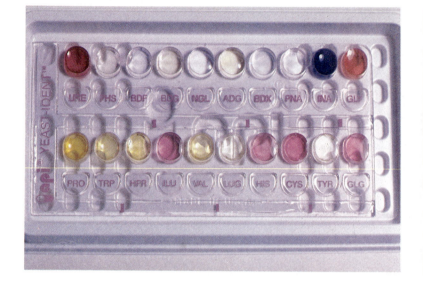

Figure 43.92
API Yeast-Ident system.

have been made and results have all been favorable.[12,51,72]

43.20.b. API Yeast-Ident system. The API Yeast-Ident system is a recently introduced product that utilizes both miniaturized conventional and chromogenic tests for the identification of yeasts and yeast-like organisms.[65] It consists of a series of 20 cupules containing dehydrated substrates or nutrient medium (Figure 43.92). Inoculated strips are incubated for 4 hours at 30° C, and reactions are monitored by various indicator systems after the addition of a specific reagent, cinnamaldehyde, to certain substrates. Reactions are based on the degradation of carbohydrate substrates or the enzymatic hydrolysis of other substrates. The system is designed to provide an identification within 4 hours. Since this is a recent product, the data base is not as extensive as that of the API-20C system; however, in time the system should have an adequate data base for comparison of reactions. This system was not designed to replace the API-20C system, but rather to supplement it and to provide laboratories the option of using either system.

Salkin et al,[74] studied 489 isolates of yeasts and found that 55% were accurately identified; however, only the first choice on the profile index was used. Additional tests suggested by the manufacturer were not used. Sixty-three percent (312 isolates) of the yeasts studied were commonly encountered species, while the remainder (177 isolates) were uncommon. Yeast-Ident correctly identified 62% and 43%, respectively, of the isolates in these two groups. Pfaller et al.[64] evaluated the Yeast-Ident system using 221 isolates of yeasts and determined that it correctly

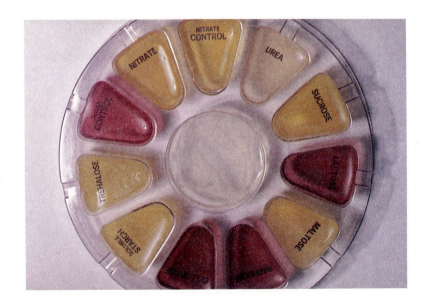

Figure 43.93
Uni-Yeast Tek (Flow Laboratories) system.

identified 132 (60%). Only 69% and 49%, respectively, of the common and uncommon yeast species were identified. Both studies concluded that Yeast-Ident is not an acceptable method for the identification of yeasts.

43.20.c. Uni-Yeast Tek system. The Uni-Yeast Tek yeast identification system (Flow Laboratories) consists of a sealed, multicompartment plate containing media to determine carbohydrate utilization, nitrate utilization, urease production, and cornmeal agar morphology (Figure 43.93). In addition, media for performing the germ-tube test and the phenoloxidase test may be obtained from the manufacturer and used in conjunction with this system. Past evaluations of this product showed that it was satisfactory for the identification of commonly encountered yeasts.[10,14] However, in a more recent study of 489 yeasts, the Uni-Yeast Tek system correctly identified only 40% of isolates. The authors did not recommend the system as useful.[74] A major disadvantage of this system is that it requires up to 7 days for the complete identification of some yeasts. It, too, has a profile index provided by the manufacturer that is generated with computer-based data.

The use of commercially available yeast identification systems is recommended for all laboratories. In general, the systems are easy to use, easy to interpret, and relatively inexpensive when compared with testing using conventional methods. In most instances, they are faster than conventional systems

and certainly require less media preparation prior to testing.

43.20.d. AutoMicrobic system. The Auto-Microbic system was evaluated favorably for the identification of yeasts in the early 1980s.[32,61] A more recent evaluation, however, showed that the system identified 83% (184 isolates) of 221 yeasts studied; the authors concluded that it was unacceptable as a method for the identification of clinically important yeasts.[64]

43.20.e. Abbott Quantum II system. The Abbott Quantum II system was evaluated in 1974[17] and was shown to be satisfactory for the identification of yeasts. However, recent studies[44,75] have shown the system to be between 80% and 86% accurate. Neither of the latter studies concludes that the system is satisfactory.

Laboratories that utilize these automated systems for yeast identification because they are in the laboratory for other reasons should reconsider their use for this purpose.

43.21. Conventional Yeast Identification Methods

A few laboratories still prefer to use conventional methods for the identification of yeasts. Regardless of the type of identification system used, the germ-tube test is a beginning step in screening a large number of isolates. As previously mentioned, approximately 75% of yeasts recovered in the clinical

PROCEDURE 43.12

Cornmeal Agar Morphology

Principle

Polysorbate (Tween) 80 is added to cornmeal agar to reduce the surface tension to allow for development of pseudohyphal, hyphal, and blastoconidial growth of yeasts. Certain species of yeasts develop characteristic morphological features on this medium.

Method

1. Obtain an isolated colony from the primary culture medium.
2. Inoculate a plate of cornmeal agar containing 1% Tween 80 and trypan blue by making three parallel cuts about 1/2 inch apart at a 45-degree angle to the culture medium. A sterile coverslip may be added to one area.
3. Incubate the cornmeal agar plate at 30° C for 48 h.
4. After 48 h, remove and examine the areas where the cuts into the agar were made for the presence of blastoconidia, arthroconidia,

pseudohyphae, hyphae, or chlamydospores.[21] Table 43.11 presents the microscopic morphological features of the commonly encountered yeasts on cornmeal Tween 80 agar. This method is required for use with commercial systems for yeast identification.

Quality control

C. albicans is tested for production of characteristic features.

Expected results

C. albicans will produce chlamydospores and clusters of blastoconidia arranged at regular intervals along the pseudohyphae.

Performance Schedule

Test a strain of *C. albicans* each time new media are received in the laboratory or produced, and monthly thereafter.

---

laboratory can be identified using the germ-tube test.

43.21.a. **Cornmeal agar morphology.** The second major step using this practical identification schema is to use cornmeal agar morphology as a means to determine if the yeast produces blastoconidia, arthroconidia, pseudohyphae, true hyphae, or chlamydospores (Procedure 43.12). In the past, cornmeal agar morphology was used successfully for the detection of characteristic chlamydospores produced by *C. albicans*. This method is currently satisfactory for the definitive identification of *C. albicans* when the germ-tube test is negative. In other instances, microscopic morphological features on cornmeal agar differentiate the genera *Cryptococcus, Saccharomyces, Candida, Geotrichum,* and *Trichosporon*. Previously, it was believed that the morphological features of the common species of *Candida* were distinct enough to provide a presumptive identification. This can be accomplished for *C. albicans, C. (Torulopsis) glabrata, C. krusei, C. parapsilosis, C.*

tropicalis, and *C. pseudotropicalis* if one keeps in mind that there are numerous other species, uncommonly recovered in the clinical laboratory, that might resemble microscopically any of the previously mentioned species. In general, this method performs well since the previously mentioned genera and species are more commonly seen in clinical laboratories. For the uncommonly encountered isolates, cornmeal agar morphology will have less value. It is, however, recommended for use with most commercially available yeast identification systems and plays a major role in the differentiation between genera that yield similar biochemical profiles.

43.21.b. **Carbohydrate assimilation (utilization).** Carbohydrate utilization profiles are the most commonly used conventional methods for the definitive identification of yeast recovered in a clinical laboratory. A number of different methods have been advocated for use in determining carbohydrate utilization patterns by clinically important yeast, and all work equally as well.[2,51,53,67] Procedure 43.13 out-

Carbohydrate Assimilation Tests

Principle

Yeasts and yeastlike fungi utilize specific carbohydrate substrates. Organisms are inoculated onto a carbohydrate-free medium. Carbohydrate-containing filter paper disks are added and utilization is determined by the presence of growth around the disk. Characteristic carbohydrate utilization profiles are used to identify species of yeasts.

Method

1. Prepare a suspension of the yeast in saline or distilled water to a density equivalent to a McFarland No. 4 standard.
2. Cover the surface of a yeast nitrogen base agar plate containing bromcresol purple with the suspension of the yeast cells.
3. Remove the excess inoculum and allow the surface of the agar medium to dry.
4. With sterile forceps, place selected carbohydrate disks (Difco Laboratories and BBL Laboratories) onto the surface of the agar. These should be spaced approximately 30 mm apart from each other.
5. Incubate the carbohydrate utilization plate at 30° C for 24 to 48 h.
6. Remove the plate and observe for the presence of a color change around the carbohydrate-containing disks or the presence of growth surrounding them.

Quality control

Choose a combination of control yeasts that utilize each of the carbohydrates being tested. Often two or three organisms may be necessary to control each carbohydrate (use published tables[46]). Test control yeasts with each new lot number of carbohydrate disks and monthly thereafter.

Table 43.11

Characteristic Microscopic Features of Commonly Encountered Yeasts on Cornmeal Tween 80 Agar

ORGANISM	ARTHROCONIDIA	BLASTOCONIDIA	PSEUDOHYPHAE OR HYPHAE
Candida albicans	—	Spherical clusters at regular intervals on pseudohyphae	Chlamydospores present on pseudohyphae
C. glabrata	—	Small, spherical and tightly compacted	—
C. krusei	—	Elongated; clusters occur at septa of pseudohyphae	Branched pseudohyphae
C. parapsilosis	—	Present but not characteristic	Sagebrush appearance; large (giant) hyphae present
C. kefyr (pseudotropicalis)	—	Elongated, lie parallel to pseudohyphae	Pseudohyphae present but not characteristic
C. tropicalis	—	Produced randomly along hyphae or pseudohyphae	Pseudohyphae present but not characteristic
Cryptococcus	—	Round to oval, vary in size, separated by a capsule	Rare
Saccharomyces	—	Large and spherical	Rudimentary hyphae sometimes present
Trichosporon	Numerous; resemble *Geotrichum*	May be present bud difficult to find	Septate hyphae present

PROCEDURE 43.14

Phenol Oxidase Detection using Niger Seed Agar

Principle

C. neoformans is the only species of cryptococci that produces 3,4-dihydroxyphenylalanine-phenol oxidase. When reacted with L-β-3,4-dihydroxyphenylalanine and an iron compound (ferric citrate), C. neoformans oxidizes O-diphenol to melanin, which produces a brown to black color.

Method

1. Place a heavy inoculum onto the surface of a plate of niger seed agar medium.
2. Incubate at 25° C for up to 7 days.
3. Observe daily for the presence of a dark brown or black pigment, which is indicative of phenol oxidase specifically produced by C. neofor-

mans (Figure 43.94). Many isolates of C. neoformans will produce phenol oxidase on this medium within 2 to 24 hours.

Quality control

C. neoformans and C. albidus are used as positive and negative controls, respectively.

Expected results

C. neoformans should exhibit a positive test (brown color development on the disk surface) while C. albidus will not.

Performance schedule

Controls should be performed with each test run.

---

lines the method previously found to be most useful by the Mayo Clinic Mycology Laboratory.

Once the carbohydrate utilization profile is obtained, reactions may be compared to those listed in tables in most mycology laboratory manuals.[46] In most instances, carbohydrate utilization tests provide the definitive identification of an organism, and additional tests are unnecessary. Carbohydrate fermentation tests are preferred by some laboratories and are simply performed using purple broth containing different carbohydrate substrates. In general, carbohydrate fermentation tests are unnecessary and are not recommended for routine use.

43.21.c. Phenol oxidase detection using niger seed agar (Procedure 43.14). As has been mentioned previously, the levodopa–ferric citrate test is a useful screening test for the presumptive identification of C. neoformans. It is felt that a simplified Guizotia abyssinica medium (niger seed medium) is the definitive method for detection of phenol oxidase production.[62] Most isolates of C. neoformans readily produce phenol oxidase; however, some isolates have been described that are deficient in their ability to produce this enzyme. In addition, there have been instances where cultures of C. neoformans have been shown to contain both phenol oxidase–

producing and phenol oxidase–deficient colonies within the same culture. It is necessary to use all the criteria, including the nitrate reductase test, urease production, carbohydrate utilization, and the phenol oxidase test, before making a final identification of C. neoformans.

43.22. Saprobic fungi commonly encountered in the clinical laboratory. As shown in Table 43.1, there are a number of fungi seen in the clinical microbiology laboratory that have not been discussed thus far. They are considered by many to be laboratory contaminants, but in reality they must be regarded as potential pathogens since infections with a number of these organisms have been reported, including Fusarium,[6] P. boydii,[18,23] Bipolaris,[1,26,57] Exserohilum,[1,26,57] Trichosporon,[35] Aureobasidium pullulans,[37] Geotrichum,[39] and others.[60] It is necessary for the laboratory to identify and report all organisms that are present in clinical specimens so that the clinician can determine their significance to the patient. In many instances, the presence of saprobic fungi is unimportant; however, that is not always the case. The following section will present the molds most commonly recovered from clinical specimens and a brief description of their colonial and morphological features. In addition, Tables 43.12 and

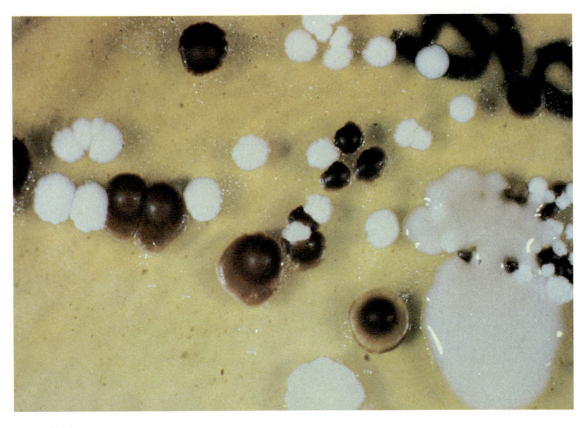

Figure 43.94
Niger seed agar. *C. neoformans* (dark colonies) and *C. albicans*.

Table 43.12
Common Filamentous Fungi Implicated in Human Mycotic Infections

ETIOLOGIC AGENT	TIME REQUIRED FOR IDENTIFICATION	PROBABLE RECOVERY SITES	CLINICAL IMPLICATION
Acremonium	2-6 days	Skin, nails, respiratory secretions, cornea, vagina, gastric washings	Skin and nail infections, mycotic keratitis, mycetoma
Alternaria species	2-6 days	Skin, nails, conjunctiva, and respiratory secretions	Skin and nail infections, sinusitis, conjunctivitis, hypersensitivity pneumonitis, skin abscess
Aspergillus flavus	1-4 days	Skin, respiratory secretions, gastric washings, nasal sinuses	Skin infections, allergic bronchopulmonary infection, sinusitis, myocarditis, disseminated infection, renal infection, subcutaneous mycetoma

From Koneman, E.W. and Roberts, G.D. 1984. Mycotic disease. In Henry, J.B., editor. Clinical diagnosis and management by laboratory methods. W.B. Saunders Co., Philadelphia.

Continued.

Table 43.12
Common Filamentous Fungi Implicated in Human Mycotic Infections—cont'd

ETIOLOGIC AGENT	TIME REQUIRED FOR IDENTIFICATION	PROBABLE RECOVERY SITES	CLINICAL IMPLICATION
Aspergillus fumigatus	2-6 days	Respiratory secretions, skin, ear, cornea, gastric washings, nasal sinuses	Allergic bronchopulmonary infection, fungus ball, invasive pulmonary infection, skin and nail infections, external otomycosis, mycotic keratitis, sinusitis, myocarditis, renal infection
Aspergillus niger	1-4 days	Respiratory secretions, gastric washings, ear, skin	Fungus ball, pulmonary infection, external otomycosis, mycotic keratitis
Aspergillus terreus	2-6 days	Repiratory secretions, skin, gastric washings, nails	Pulmonary infection, disseminated infection, endocarditis, onychomycosis, allergic bronchopulmonary infection
Bipolaris species	2-6 days	Respiratory secretions, skin, nose, bone	Sinusitis, brain abscess, peritonitis, subcutaneous abscess, pulmonary infection, osteomyelitis, encephalitis
Blastomyces dermatitidis	6-21 days (recovery time) (additional 3-14 days required for confirmatory identification)	Respiratory secretions, skin, oropharyngeal ulcer, bone, prostate	Pulmonary infection, skin infection, oropharyngeal ulceration, osteomyelitis, prostatitis, arthritis, CNS infection, disseminated infection
Cladosporium species	6-10 days	Respiratory secretions, skin, nails, nose, cornea	Skin and nail infections, mycotic keratitis; chromoblastomycosis, brain abscess, and tinea nigra palmaris caused by *Cladosporium carrioni*, *C. bantianum*, and *C. werneckii*, respectively
Coccidioides immitis	3-21 days	Respiratory secretions, skin, bone, cerebrospinal fluid, synovial fluid, urine, gastric washings	Pulmonary infection, skin infection, osteomyelitis, meningitis, arthritis, disseminated infection
Drechslera species	2-6 days	Respiratory secretions, skin, peritonitis (following dialysis)	Pulmonary infection (rare)
Epidermophyton floccosum	7-10 days	Skin, nails	Tinea cruris, tinea pedis, tinea corporis, onychomycosis
Exserohilum species	2-6 days	Eye, skin, nose, bone	Keratitis, subcutaneous abscess, sinusitis, endocarditis, osteomyelitis
Fusarium species	2-6 days	Skin, respiratory secretions, cornea	Mycotic keratitis, skin infection (in burn patients)
Geotrichum species	2-6 days	Respiratory secretions, urine, skin, stool, vagina, conjunctiva, gastric washings, throat	Bronchitis, skin infection, colitis, conjunctivitis, thrush, wound infection
Histoplasma capsulatum	10-45 days (recovery time) (additional 7-21 days required for confirmatory identification)	Respiratory secretions, bone marrow, blood, urine, adrenals, skin, cerebrospinal fluid, eye, pleural fluid, liver, spleen, oropharyngeal lesions, vagina, gastric washings, larynx	Pulmonary infection, oropharyngeal lesions, CNS infection, skin infection (rare), uveitis, peritonitis, endocarditis, brain abscess, disseminated infection

Table 43.12

Common Filamentous Fungi Implicated in Human Mycotic Infections—cont'd

ETIOLOGIC AGENT	TIME REQUIRED FOR IDENTIFICATION	PROBABLE RECOVERY SITES	CLINICAL IMPLICATION
Microsporum audouinii	10-14 days (recovery time) (additional 14-21 days required for confirmatory identification)	Hair	Tinea capitis
Microsporum canis	5-7 days	Hair, skin	Tinea corporis, tinea capitis, tinea barbae, tinea manuum
Microsporum gypseum	3-6 days	Hair, skin	Tinea capitis, tinea corporis
Mucor species	1-5 days	Respiratory secretions, skin, nose, brain, stool, orbit, cornea, vitreous humor, gastric washings, wounds, ear	Rhinocerebral infection, pulmonary infection, gastrointestinal infection, mycotic keratitis, intraocular infection, external otomycosis, orbital cellulitis, disseminated infection
Penicillium species	2-6 days	Respiratory secretions, gastric washings, skin, urine, ear, cornea	Pulmonary infection, skin infection, external otomycosis, mycotic keratitis, endocarditis
Pseudallescheria (Petriellidium) boydii	2-6 days	Respiratory secretions, gastric washings, skin, cornea	Pulmonary fungus ball, mycetoma, mycotic keratitis, endocarditis, disseminated infection
Phialophora species	6-21 days	Respiratory secretions, gastric washings, skin, cornea, conjunctiva	Some species produce chromoblastomycosis or mycetoma; mycotic keratitis, conjunctivitis, intraocular infection
Rhizopus species	1-5 days	Respiratory secretions, skin, nose, brain, stool, orbit, cornea, vitreous humor, gastric washings, wounds, ear	Rhinocerebral infection, pulmonary infection, mycotic keratitis, intraocular infection, orbital cellulitis, external otomycosis, disseminated infection
Scopulariopsis species	2-6 days	Respiratory secretions, gastric washings, nails, skin, vitreous humor, ear	Pulmonary infection, nail infection, skin infection, intraocular infection, external otomycosis
Sporothrix schenckii	3-12 days (recovery time) (additional 2-10 days required for confirmatory identification)	Respiratory secretions, skin, subcutaneous tissue, maxillary sinuses, synovial fluid, bone marrow, bone, cerebrospinal fluid, ear, conjunctiva	Pulmonary infection, lymphocutaneous infection, sinusitis, arthritis, osteomyelitis, meningitis, external otomycosis, conjunctivitis, disseminated infection
Trichophyton mentagrophytes	7-10 days	Hair, skin, nails	Tinea barbae, tinea capitis, tinea corporis, tinea cruris, tinea pedis, onychomycosis
Trichohyton rubrum	10-14 days	Hair, skin, nails	Tinea pedis, onychomycosis, tinea corporis, tinea cruris
Trichophyton tonsurans	10-14 days	Hair, skin, nails	Tinea capitis, tinea corporis, onychomycosis, tinea pedis
Trichophyton verrucosum	10-18 days	Hair, skin, nails	Tinea capitis, tinea corporis, tinea barbae
Trichophyton violaceum	14-18 days	Hair, skin, nails	Tinea capitis, tinea corporis, onychomycosis

Table 43.13

Common Yeastlike Organisms Implicated in Human Infection*

ETIOLOGIC AGENT	PROBABLE RECOVERY SITES	CLINICAL IMPLICATION
Candida albicans	Respiratory secretions, vagina, urine, skin, oropharynx, gastric washings, blood, stool, transtracheal aspiration, cornea, nails, cerebrospinal fluid, bone, peritoneal fluid	Pulmonary infection, vaginitis, urinary tract infection, dermatitis, fungemia, mycotic keratitis, onychomycosis, meningitis, osteomyelitis, peritonitis, myocarditis, endocarditis, endophthalmitis, disseminated infection, thrush, arthritis
Candida glabrata	Respiratory secretions, urine, vagina, gastric washings, blood, skin, oropharynx, transtracheal aspiration, stool, bone marrow, skin (rare)	Pulmonary infection, urinary tract infection, vaginitis, fungemia, disseminated infection, endocarditis
Candida tropicalis	Respiratory secretions, urine, gastric washings, vagina, blood, skin, oropharynx, transtracheal aspiration, stool, pleural fluid, peritoneal fluid, cornea	Pulmonary infection, vaginitis, thrush, endophthalmitis, endocarditis, arthritis, peritonitis, mycotic keratitis, fungemia
Candida parapsilosis	Respiratory secretions, urine, gastric washings, blood, vagina, oropharynx, skin, transtracheal aspiration, stool, pleural fluid, ear, nails	Endophthalmitis, endocarditis, vaginitis, mycotic keratitis, external otomycosis, paronychia, fungemia
Saccharomyces species	Respiratory secretions, urine, gastric washings, vagina, skin, oropharynx, transtracheal aspiration, stool	Pulmonary infection (rare), endocarditis
Candida krusei	Respiratory secretions, urine, gastric washings, vagina, skin, oropharynx, blood, transtracheal aspiration, stool, cornea	Endocarditis, vaginitis, urinary tract infection, mycotic keratitis
Candida guilliermondii	Respiratory secretions, gastric washings, vagina, skin, nails, oropharynx, blood, cornea, bone, urine	Endocarditis, fungemia, dermatitis, onychomycosis, mycotic keratitis, osteomyelitis, urinary tract infection
Rhodotorula species	Respiratory secretions, urine, gastric washings, blood, vagina, skin, oropharynx, stool, cerebrospinal fluid, cornea	Fungemia, endocarditis, mycotic keratitis
Trichosporon species	Respiratory secretions, skin, oropharynx, stool	Pulmonary infection, brain abscess, disseminated infection, piedra
Cryptococcus neoformans	Respiratory secretions, cerebrospinal fluid, bone, blood, bone marrow, urine, skin, pleural fluid, gastric washings, transtracheal aspiration, cornea, orbit, vitreous humor	Pulmonary infection, meningitis, osteomyelitis, fungemia, disseminated infection, endocarditis, skin infection, mycotic keratitis, orbital cellulitis, endophthalmic infection
Cryptococcus albidus subsp. *albidus*	Respiratory secretions, skin, gastric washings, urine, cornea	Meningitis, pulmonary infection
Candida kefyr (pseudotropicalis)	Respiratory secretions, vagina, urine, gastric washings, oropharynx	Vaginitis, urinary tract infection
Cryptococcus luteolus	Respiratory secretions, skin, nose	Not commonly implicated in human infection
Cryptococcus laurentii	Respiratory secretions, cerebrospinal fluid, skin, oropharynx, stool	Not commonly implicated in human infection
Cryptococcus albidus subsp. *diffluens*	Respiratory secretions, urine, cerebrospinal fluid, gastric washings, skin	Not commonly implicated in human infection
Cryptococcus terreus	Respiratory secretions, skin, nose	Not commonly implicated in human infection

*Arranged in order of occurrence in the clinical laboratory.

From Koneman, E.W., and Roberts, G.D. 1984. Mycotic disease. In Henry, J.B., editor. Clinical diagnosis and management by laboratory methods. W.B. Saunders Co., Philadelphia.

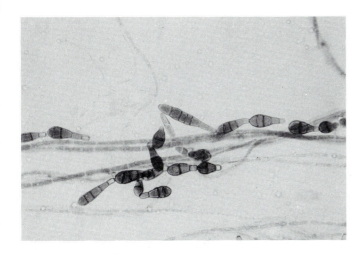

Figure 43.95
Alternaria species, showing muriform, dematiaceous conidia with horizontal and longitudinal septa.

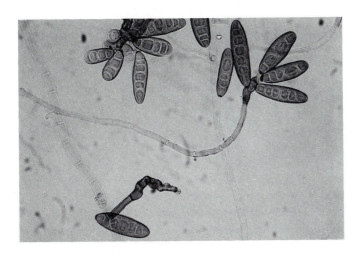

Figure 43.96
Bipolaris species, showing dematiaceous multicelled conidia produced sympodially (430 ×).

43.13 present the common molds and yeasts implicated in causing human infection, the time required for their identification, most likely site for their recovery, and the clinical implications of each.

43.23. Dematiaceous (Darkly Pigmented) Molds

43.23.a. *Alternaria* **species.** Colonies of *Alternaria* are rapidly growing and appear to be fluffy and gray to gray-brown or dark to gray-green in color. Microscopically, hyphae are septate and golden-brown-pigmented, and conidiophores are simple but sometimes branched. Conidiophores bear a chain of large brown conidia resembling a drumstick and contain both horizontal and longitudinal septa (Figure 43.95). It is difficult to observe chains of conidia since they are easily dislodged as the culture mount is prepared.

43.23.b. *Bipolaris* **species.** Colonies of *Bipolaris* are gray-green to dark brown and slightly powdery. Hyphae are dematiaceous and septate, as observed microscopically. Conidiophores are twisted at the ends where conidia are attached; conidia are arranged sympodially, are oblong to fusoid, and the hilum protrudes only slightly (Figure 43.96). Germ tubes are formed at one or both ends of the conidium when the fungus is incubated in water at 25° C for up to 24 hours.

43.23.c. *Cladosporium.* Colonies of *Cladosporium* most commonly appear as velvety or suedelike, heaped, and folded. Microscopically, hyphae are septate and brown in color. Conidiophores are long and branched and give rise to chains of darkly pigmented conidia. Conidia are usually single-celled and exhibit prominent attachment scars (disjunctors)

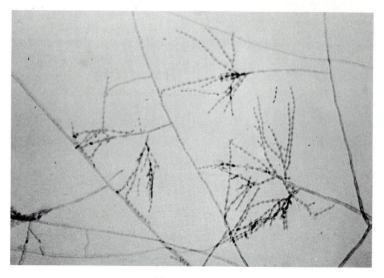

Figure 43.97
Cladosporium species, showing branching chains of dematiaceous blastoconidia that are easily dislodged during the preparation of a microscopic mount (430 ×).

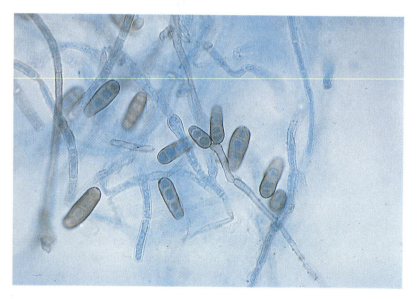

Figure 43.98
Drechslera species, showing dematiaceous multicelled conidia. Most isolates produce only a few conidia.

that may resemble "shield" cells (Figure 43.97). This organism also fails to reveal chains of conidia on wet mounts because of the ease of dislodging of conidia.

43.23.d. *Drechslera* *Drechslera* is a dematiaceous organism that has been described erroneously as *Helminthosporium* or *Bipolaris* in many text-

books. Colonies of *Drechslera* are fluffy to velvety and gray to brown or black in color. Microscopically, the hyphae are septate and darkly pigmented, and conidiophores are twisted where the large multiseptate elongate conidia are attached. A zigzag appearance is produced by the production of conidia on

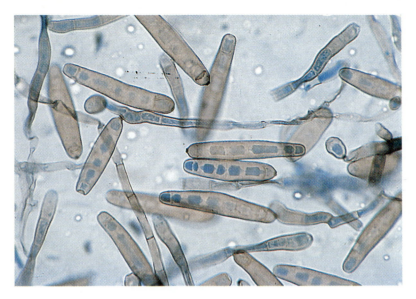

Figure 43.99
Exserohilum species, showing elongated multicelled conidia with prominent hila.

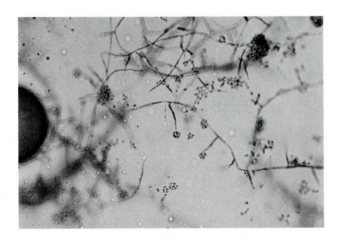

Figure 43.100
Acremonium species, showing single unbranched phialides that give rise to clusters of elliptical conidia at their tips (500 ×).

alternate sides of the conidiophore where growth continued until a conidium was formed on the alternate side (Figure 43.98). However, sporulation is generally sparse with this organism, and it is not commonly seen.

43.23.e. ***Exserohilum***. Colonies of *Exserohilum* resemble those of *Bipolaris*. Hyphae are dematiaceous and septate when viewed under the microscope. Conidiophores are twisted at the ends where conidia are attached sympodially. Conidia are ellipsoid to fusoid and exhibit a prominent hilum that is truncated and protruding (Figure 43.99).

43.24. Hyaline Molds

43.24.a. ***Acremonium***. Colonies of *Acremonium* are rapidly growing and often appear yeastlike when initial growth is observed. Mature colonies become white to gray to rose or reddish orange in color. Microscopically, small septate hyphae that produce single unbranched tubelike phialides are observed. Phialides give rise to clusters of elliptical, single-celled conidia contained in a cluster at the tip of the phialide (Figure 43.100).

43.24.b. ***Fusarium***. Colonies of *Fusarium* are fluffy to cottony and may appear in colors of pink,

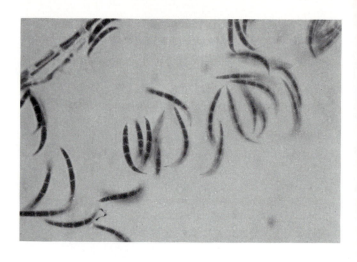

Figure 43.101
Fusarium species, showing characteristic multicelled, sickle-shaped macroconidia (500 ×).

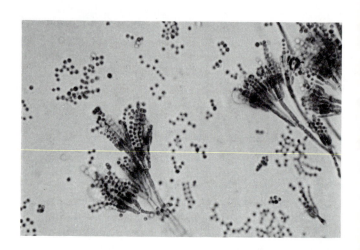

Figure 43.102
Penicillium species, showing typical brushlike conidiophores (penicillus) (430 ×).

purple, yellow, green, and other shades. Microscopically, the hyphae are small and septate and give rise to phialides that produce either single-celled microconidia, usually borne in gelatinous heads similar to those seen in *Acremonium*, or large macroconidia that are sickle- or boat-shaped and contain numerous septa (Figure 43.101). It is common to find numerous chlamydospores produced by some cultures of *Fusarium*.

43.24.c. *Penicillium*. Colonies of *Penicillium* may be shades of green, blue-green, pink, white, or other colors. The surface of the colonies may be velvety to powdery due to the presence of conidia. Microscopically, hyphae are hyaline and septate and produce brushlike conidiophores. Conidiophores exhibit branching metulae from which phialides pro-

ducing chains of conidia arise (Figure 43.102).

43.24.d. *Scopulariopsis*. Colonies of *Scopulariopsis* initially appear white but later become light brown and powdery in appearance. Colonies often resemble those of *M. gypseum*. Microscopically, *Scopulariopsis* resembles a large *Penicillium* at first glance. The hyaline and septate conidiophores are branched and produce a penicillium-like structure. Conidia are produced from annellides. Annellides may be produced singly directly from the hyphae. Conidia are large, have a flat base, and are rough-walled (Figure 43.103).

A number of other saprobic fungi may be encountered in the clinical laboratory but are seen less commonly than those previously mentioned. The chapters by McGinnis[56] and Swatek et al.[85] provide

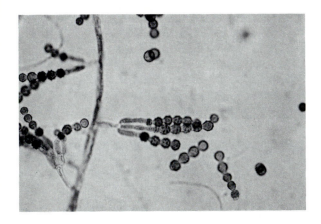

Figure 43.103
Scopulariopsis species, showing a large penicillus with echinulate conidia having a flat base (430 ×).

more detailed information on their identification. In many instances, it will be necessary to use reference texts to make an identification.

43.25. Fungal Serologic Tests

A confirmed diagnosis of mycotic infection is based on the recovery and identification of a specific etiologic agent from a clinical specimen. However, the presence and identification of characteristic etiologic agents in clinical specimens observed microscopically also allow for the definitive diagnosis. There are instances, however, when either cultural proof or pathologic proof of infection cannot be obtained, and other laboratory information must be utilized. Fungal serologic tests often provide this supplemental information for the diagnosis of mycotic infections, and in some instances provide the only means of diagnosis.[68]

Most clinical microbiology laboratories do not offer fungal serologic testing since the methods require precise technical expertise, difficult reagent preparation, and costly reagents. In the past few years, commercial sources for reagents have become available, and now fungal serologic tests can be offered by laboratories if they wish. Most often, these tests are performed by reference laboratories.

The usefulness of fungal serologic tests is hampered by false-negative results when blood is drawn at an inappropriate time or if blood is drawn from immunocompromised patients before antibodies are produced to the infection. Antigens used in fungal serologic testing are not purified and contain many cross-reacting components in common with other fungi. Antigens of *H. capsulatum*, *B. dermatitidis*,

and *C. immitis* often cross-react and provide for difficulty in interpretation of results. It is recommended that a battery of antigens be used for testing to simplify the interpretation of these cross-reactions. As with other tests, false-negative and false-positive results can occur, but in most instances fungal serologic tests provide helpful and reliable results, particularly when used in combination with cultural and histopathologic proof of the etiologic agent.

The most simple and useful fungal serologic test available to the clinical laboratory is the cryptococcal latex test for antigen. Determination of the presence of cryptococcal polysaccharide by this method has proved to be extremely reliable and sensitive.[91] All laboratories are encouraged to provide this test on a routine basis because of its simplicity, sensitivity, and reliability. As previously mentioned, when compared with the India ink preparation, positive results are obtained in approximately 90% of the cases of cryptococcal meningitis when cerebrospinal fluid from the first lumbar puncture is tested. All false-positive reactions due to interference factors have been eliminated using an enzymatic method[25,81] that makes the test highly specific. However, the latex test is positive in serum from patients having disseminated *Trichosporon* infection.[58] The decision of whether to offer additional tests other than the cryptococcal latex test for antigen depends on the individual situation for each laboratory. Table 43.14 presents a summary of the common fungal serologic tests available and information regarding their interpretation. More detailed methods can be found in the text by Palmer et al.[63] and the chapter written

Table 43.14

Commonly Available Fungal Serologic Tests

INFECTION	ANTIGEN(S)	TEST(S)	INTERPRETATION
Aspergillosis	*Aspergillus fumigatus* *Aspergillus niger* *Aspergillus flavus*	Immunodiffusion	One or more precipitin bands suggestive of active infection; precipitin bands shown to correlate with complement-fixation titers—the greater the number of bands, the higher the titer; when cultural proof is present in the presence of a positive test, it is diagnostic of active infection Precipitins can be found in 95% of the fungus ball cases and 50% of the allergic bronchopulmonary cases; sometimes positive in invasive infection, depending on the immunologic status of the patient
Blastomycosis	*Blastomyces dermatitidis*		
	Yeast form	Complement-fixation	Titers of 1:8 to 1:16 are highly suggestive of active infection; titers of 1:32 or greater are indicative; cross-reactions occur in patients having coccidioidomycosis or histoplasmosis; however, titers are usually lower; a decreasing titer is indicative of regression; most patients (75%) having blastomycosis have negative tests
	Yeast culture filtrate	Immunodiffusion	Preliminary results show that it is more sensitive than complement-fixation—80% detection rate
Candidosis	*Candida albicans*	Immunodiffusion, counterimmunoelectrophoresis, latex agglutination	Test difficult to interpret because precipitins are found in 20%-30% of the normal population, and reports in the literature are conflicting; clinical correlation must exist for the test to be useful
Coccidioidomycosis	Coccidioidin	Complement-fixation	Titers of 1:2 to 1:4 have been seen in active infection; low titers should be followed by repeat testing at 2 to 3-week intervals; titers of greater than 1:16 are usually indicative of active infection; cross-reactions occur in patients having histoplasmosis, and false-negative results occur in patients with solitary pulmonary lesions; titer parallels severity of infection
	Coccidioidin	Immunodiffusion	Results correlate with complement-fixation test and can be used as a screening test—should be confirmed by performing complement-fixation test
	Coccidioidin	Latex agglutination	Precipitins occur during first 3 weeks of infection and are diagnostic, but not prognostic; useful as a screening test for precipitins in early infection; false-positive tests frequent when diluted serum or cerebrospinal fluid specimens are used

From Koneman, E.W., and Roberts, G.D. 1984. Mycotic disease. In Henry, J.B., editor. Clinical diagnosis and management by laboratory methods. W.B. Saunders Co., Philadelphia.

Table 43.14
Commonly Available Fungal Serologic Tests—cont'd

INFECTION	ANTIGEN(S)	TEST(S)	INTERPRETATION
Cryptococcosis	No antigen—latex particles coated with hyperimmune anticryptococcal globulin	Latex agglutination for cryptococcal antigen	Presence of cryptococcal polysaccharide in body fluids is indicative of cryptococcosis; rheumatoid factor presents false-positive reactions and RA test must be performed as a control; decrease in antigen titer indicates regression; positive tests (in CSF) have been seen in 95% of cryptococcal meningitis cases and 30% of non-meningitis cases; serum is less frequently positive than CSF; disseminated infections usually present positive results in serum; test may be performed using serum, CSF, and urine; test more sensitive than India ink preparation
Histoplasmosis	Histoplasmin and yeast form of *Histoplasma capsulatum*	Complement-fixation	Titers of 1:8 to 1:16 are highly suspicious of infection; however titers of 1:32 or greater are usually indicative of active infection; cross-reactions occur in patients having aspergillosis, blastomycosis, and coccidioidomycosis, but titers are usually lower; several follow-up serum samples should be tested—drawn at 2- to 3-week intervals
Rising titers indicate progressive infection and decreasing titers indicate regression; some disseminated infections are nonreactive to the complement-fixation test
Recent skin tests in persons who have had prior exposure to *H. capsulatum* will cause an elevation in the complement-fixation titer; this occurs in 17%-20% of persons tested
The yeast antigen gives positive reactions in 75%-80% of cases, and the histoplasmin gives positive reactions in 10%-15% of cases; in 10% of cases both are positive simultaneously
	Histoplasmin	Immunodiffusion	H and M bands appearing simultaneously are indicative of active infection
M band may appear alone and can indicate early infection or chronic infection; also the M band may appear after a recent skin test
The H band appears later than the M band and disappears earlier, and its disappearance may indicate regression of the infection
	Histoplasmin	Latex agglutination	Test is unreliable; many false-positive and false-negative tests may be observed; any positive test should be confirmed by the complement-fixation test
Sporotrichosis	Yeast of *Sporothrix schenckii*	Agglutination	Titers of 1:80 or greater usually indicative of active infection; some cutaneous infections present negative tests; however, extracutaneous infections present positive tests

Table 43.15
In Vitro Antifungal Activities of Four Antifungal Agents Against Pathogenic Fungi*

ORGANISM	AMPHOTERICIN B		FLUCYTOSINE (5-FC)		MICONAZOLE		KETOCONAZOLE
	MIC (µg/ml)	MFC (µg/ml)	MIC (µg/ml)	MFC (µg/ml)	MIC (µg/ml)	MFC (µg/ml)	MIC (µg/ml)
Pathogenic yeasts							
Cryptococcus neoformans	0.05-0.78†	0.1-12.5	0.10-100‡	0.39->100	0.05-3.13	0.05-25	0.1-32
Candida albicans	0.2-0.78§	0.39-0.78	0.05-12.5‡	0.10->100	0.1-2.0§	0.1-10	<0.1-80
Candida spp. not *C. albicans*	0.2-1.56§	0.39-6.25	0.10-50‡	0.20->100	<0.1-2.0	0.1->10	<0.1-64
Candida glabrata	0.1-0.4	0.2-0.78	0.05-1.56	0.4->100	0.5-10	2-10	1-64
Trichosporon sp.	0.78-3.13	1.56-3.13	25-100	>100	0.2-25	0.2->100	
Geotrichum sp.	0.4-1.56	0.78-3.13	1.56-12.5	25->100	0.1-2	0.5->10	
Filamentous fungi							
Pseudallescheria boydii	1.56->100‡	>100	Resistant		0.05‖	0.05	0.1-4‡
Aspergillus sp. including *A. fumigatus*	0.05-8	6.25->100	0.2-1.56‡	>100	0.4->100	0.8->100	0.1-100¶
Blastomyces dermatitidis	0.05-0.2	0.1-0.4	Resistant		≤0.25	ND	0.1-2
Cladosporium trichoides	3.13->100	3.13->100	3.13-12.5‡	12.5->100	0.5->64	ND	0.1-64
Coccidioides immitis	0.1-0.78	0.78-1.56	Resistant		0.25-1.0	ND	0.1-0.8
Histoplasma capsulatum	0.05-1.0	0.05-0.2	Resistant		≤0.25	ND	0.1-0.5
Phialophora sp. and other dematiaceous fungi	0.05->128	6.25->128	Variable susceptibility	Resistant	0.05-32	ND	0.1-64
Sporothrix schenckii	1.56-12.5	3.13->100	Resistant		1-2	ND	0.1-16
Zygomycetes	0.78-1.56	1.56->100	Variable susceptibility	Resistant			
Dermatophytic fungi							
Epidermophyton floccosum					0.5-10	2-10	0.1-8
Microsporum sp.					0.5-10	0.5->10	0.1-64
Trichophyton sp.					0.5-10	0.5-10	<0.05-128
Control organisms							
S. cerevisiae ATCC 36375	0.1	0.2	0.05	0.10	0.20	0.39	0.20
C. pseudotropicalis ATCC 28838			0.05	0.10	0.10	0.20	0.05

*Based upon both data obtained at the Medical College of Virginia, Virginia Commonwealth University, Richmond, and a review of the literature. In vitro data for nystatin is not included because of the narrow clinical spectrum of this agent; however, most isolates of *Candida* species should be clinically susceptible (MIC [minimum inhibitory concentration] of ≤10 µg/ml) to nystatin. MFC, Minimal fungicidal concentration; ND, not determined.
†Expected ranges of MICs and MFCs.
‡Resistance not uncommon.
§Resistance reported but rare.
‖Only limited data available.
¶In vitro susceptibility of *Aspergillus* sp. to ketoconazole is highly species dependent.
From Shadomy, S., Espinel-Ingroff, A., and Cartwright, R.Y. 1985. Susceptibility testing with antifungal drugs. In Lennette, E.H., Balows, A., Hausler, W.J., Jr., and Shadomy, H.J., editors. Manual of clinical microbiology, ed. 4. American Society for Microbiology, Washington, D.C.

by Kaufman and Reiss.[42] Perhaps these new methods and others[6,19,41] will be available in a few years.

43.26. Antifungal Susceptibility Testing

Antifungal susceptibility tests are performed to provide information that will allow the physician to select the appropriate antifungal agent useful for treating a specific infection. Unfortunately, antifungal susceptibility testing has not progressed as far as tests used for determining susceptibility of bacteria to antimicrobial agents. There is no standard method used by all laboratories and there is disagreement concerning specific conditions of incubation and other variables necessary for performing the test. The National Committee for Clinical Laboratory Standards is examining the issue and standards for testing are expected to be proposed.

Despite the problems associated with antifungal susceptibility testing, many physicians believe that these tests are important for the selection of an appropriate antifungal agent and as a method to detect the development of resistance of certain organisms during chemotherapy. The method described by Shadomy et al.[76] is perhaps the most commonly used procedure in the United States. A laboratory not equipped for such studies should be prepared to send an important isolate to a reference laboratory for testing. Table 43.15 provides information on the susceptibility of the various fungi to amphotericin B, 5-fluorocytosine, miconazole, and ketoconazole, the common antifungal agents available at the present time. Susceptibility testing of itraconazole and fluconazole is slowly coming into use.

REFERENCES

1. Adam, R.D., Paquin, M.L., Petersen, E.A. et al. 1986. Phaeohyphomycosis caused by the fungal genera *Bipolaris* and *Exserohilum*. A report of 9 cases and review of the literature. Medicine 65:203.
2. Adams, E.D., Jr., and Cooper, B.H. 1984. Evaluation of modified Wickenham medium for identification of medically important yeasts. Am. J. Med. Technol. 40:377.
3. Ahearn, D.G. 1973. Identification and ecology of yeasts of medical importance. In Prior, J.E., and Friedman, H., editors. Opportunistic pathogens. University Park Press, Baltimore.
4. Ajello, L. 1968. A taxonomic review of the dermatophytes and related species. Sabouraudia 6:147.
5. Ajello, L., and Georg, L.K. 1957. In vitro hair cultures for differentiating between atypical isolates of *Trichophyton mentagrophytes* and *Trichophyton rubrum*. Mycopathologia 8:3.
6. Anaissie, E. Kantarjian, H., and Jones, P. 1987. Fungal infections caused by *Fusarium* in cancer patients. Am. J. Clin. Oncol. 10:86.
7. Bille, J., Edson, R.S., and Roberts, G.D. 1984. Clinical evaluation of the lysis-centrifugation blood culture system for detection of fungemia and comparison with a conventional biphasic broth blood culture system. J. Clin. Microbiol. 19:126.
8. Bille, J., Stockman, L., Roberts, G.D., et al. 1983. Evaluation of a lysis-centrifugation system for recovery of yeasts and filamentous fungi from blood. J. Clin. Microbiol. 18:469.
9. Binford, C.H., Thompson, R.K., Gorham, M.E., and Emmons, C.W. 1952. Mycotic brain abscess due to *Cladosporium trichoides*, a new species. Am. J. Clin. Pathol. 22:535.
10. Bowman, P.I., and Ahearn, D.G. 1975. Evaluation of the Uni-Yeast-Tek kit for the identification of medically important yeasts, J. Clin. Microbiol. 2:354.
11. Brock, E.G., Reiss, E., Pine, L., and Kaufman, L. 1984. Effect of periodate-oxidation on the detection of antibodies against the M-antigen of histoplasmosis by enzyme immunoassay (EIA) inhibition. Curr. Microbiol. 10:177.
12. Buesching, W.J., Kurek, K., and Roberts, G.D. 1979. Evaluation of the modified API 20C system for identification of clinically important yeasts. J. Clin. Microbiol. 9:565.
13. Chandler, F.W., Kaplan, W., and Ajello, L. 1980. Color atlas and text of the histopathology of mycotic diseases. Year Book Medical Publishers, Chicago.
14. Cooper, B.H. 1980. Clinical laboratory evaluation of a screening medium (CN screen) for *Cryptococcus neoformans*. J. Clin. Microbiol. 11:672.
15. Cooper, B.H. 1980. Taxonomy classification and nomenclature of fungi. In Leannette, E.H., Balows, A., Hausler, W.J., Jr., and Truant, J.P., editors. Manual of clinical microbiology, ed. 3. American Society for Microbiology, Washington, D.C.
16. Cooper, B.H., Johnson, J.B., and Thaxton, E.S. 1978. Clinical evaluation of the Uni-Yeast-Tek system for rapid presumptive identification of medically important yeasts. J. Clin. Microbiol. 7:349.
17. Cooper, B.H., Prowant, S., Brunson, D., and Alexander, B.A. 1984. Collaborative evaluation of the Abbott automated yeast identification system. J. Clin. Microbiol. 11:853.
18. Davis, W.A., Isner, J.M., Bracey, A.W., et al. 1980. Disseminated *Petriellidium boydii* and pacemaker endocarditis. Am. J. Med. 69:929.
19. deRepentigny, L., Marr, L.D., Keller, et al. 1985. Comparison of enzyme immunoassay and gas-liquid chromatography for the rapid diagnosis of invasive candidiasis in cancer patients. J. Clin. Microbiol. 21:972.
20. Dick, J.D., Merz, W.G., and Saral, R. 1980. Incidence of polyene-resistant yeasts recovered from clinical specimens. Antimicrob. Agents Chemother. 18:158.
21. Dolan, C.T. 1971. A practical approach to identification of yeast-like organisms. Am. J. Clin. Pathol. 55:580.
22. Douer, D., Goldschmied-Reouven, Segea, S., and Benbassat, I. 1987. Human *Exserohilum* and *Bipolaris* infections: report of *Exserohilum* nasal infection in a neutropenic patient with acute leukemia and review of the literature. J. Med. Vet. Mycol. 25:235.
23. Enggano, I.L., Hughes, W.T., Kalasinsky, D.K., et al. 1984. *Pseudallescheria boydii* in a patient with acute lymphoblastic leukemia. Arch. Pathol. Lab. Med. 108:619.

24. Gray, L.D., and Roberts, G.D. 1988. Identification of medically important yeasts. Clin. Microbiol. Newsletter 10:73.

25. Gray, L.D., and Roberts, G.D. 1988. Experience with the use of pronase to eliminate interference factors in the latex agglutination test for cryptococcal antigen. J. Clin. Microbiol. 26:2450.

26. Gray, L.D., and Roberts, G.D. 1988. Laboratory diagnosis of systemic fungal diseases. Inf. Dis. Clin. N. Amer. 2:779.

27. Greer, D.L., and Rogers, A.L. 1985. Agents of zygomycosis (phycomycosis). In Lennette, E.H., Balows, A., Hausler, W.J., Jr., and Shadomy, H.J., editors. Manual of clinical microbiology, ed. 4. American Society for Microbiology, Washington, D.C.

28. Guerra-Romero, L., Edson, R.S., Cockerill, F.R. III, et al. 1987. Comparison of duPont Isolator and Roche Septi-Chek for detection of fungemia. J. Clin. Microbiol. 25:1623.

29. Guinet, R.J., Chanas, J., Goullier, A., et al. 1983. Fatal septicemia due to amphotericin B–resistant *Candida lusitaniae*. J. Clin. Microbiol. 18:443.

30. Hageage, G.J., and Harrington, B.J. 1984. Use of calcofluor white in clinical mycology. Lab. Med. 15:109.

31. Harari, A.R., Hempel, H.O., Kimberlin, C.L., and Goodman, N.L. 1982. Effects of time lapse between sputum collection and culturing on isolation of clinically significant fungi. J. Clin. Microbiol. 15:425.

32. Hasyn, J.J., and Buckley, H.R. 1982. Evaluation of the Automicrobic System for the identification of yeasts. J. Clin. Microbiol. 16:901.

33. Hoeprich, P.D. 1977. Cryptococcosis. In Hoeprich, P.D., editor. Infectious diseases. Harper & Row, Hagerstown, Md.

34. Hopkins, J.M., and Land, G.A. 1977. Rapid method for determining nitrate utilization by yeasts. J. Clin. Microbiol. 5:497.

35. Hoy, J., Hsu, K.C., Rolston, K., et al. 1986. *Trichosporon beigelii* infection: a review. Rev. Infect. Dis. 8:959.

36. Huppert, M., Sun, S.H., and Bailey, J.W. 1967. Natural variability in *Coccidioides immitis*. In Ajello, L., editor. Coccidioidomycosis. University of Arizona Press, Tucson.

37. Kaczmarski, E.B., Liu Yin, J.A., Tooth, J.A., et al. 1986. Systemic infection with *Aureobasidium pullulans* in a leukemic patient. J. Infect. 13:209.

38. Kane, J., and Smitka, C. 1978. Early detection and identification of *Trichophyton verrucosum*. J. Clin. Microbiol. 8:740.

39. Kassamali, H., Anaissie, E., Ro, J., et al. 1987. Disseminated *Geotrichum candidum* infection. J. Clin. Microbiol. 25:1782.

40. Kaufman, L. 1984. Antigen detection: its role in the diagnosis of mycotic disease and the identification of fungi. In Sanna, A., and Morace, G., editors. New horizons in microbiology. Elsevier Science Publishing Co., Amsterdam.

41. Kaufman, C.S., and Merz, W.G. 1982. Two rapid pigmentation tests for identification of *Cryptococcus neoformans*. J. Clin. Microbiol. 15:339.

42. Kaufman, L., and Reiss, E. 1985. Serodiagnosis of fungal diseases. In Lennette, E.H., Balows, A., Hausler, W.J., Jr., and Shadomy, H.J., editors. Manual of clinical microbiology, ed. 4. American Society for Microbiology, Washington, D.C.

43. Kaufman, L., and Standard, P. 1978. Improved version of the exoantigen test for identification of *Coccidioides immitis* and *Histoplasma capsulatum* cultures. J. Clin. Microbiol. 8:42.

44. Kiehn, T.E., Edwards, F.F., Tom, D., et al. 1985. Evaluation of the Quantum II Yeast Identification system. J. Clin. Microbiol. 22:216.

45. Koneman, E.W., and Roberts, G.D. 1984. Mycotic disease. In Henry, J.B., editor. Clinical diagnosis and management by laboratory methods. W.B. Saunders Co., Philadelphia.

46. Koneman, E.W., and Roberts, G.D. 1985. Practical laboratory mycology, ed. 3. Williams & Wilkins, Baltimore.

47. Kreger-Van Rij, N.J.N. 1984. The yeasts: a taxonomic study. Elsevier Science Publishing Co., New York.

48. Kwon-Chung, K.J., Bennett, J.E., and Theodore, T.S. 1978. *Cryptococcus neoformans* sp. nov.: serotype B-C of *Cryptococcus neoformans*. Int. J. Sys. Bacteriol. 28:616.

49. Kwon-Chung, K.S. 1976. A new species of *Filobasidiella*, the sexual state of *Cryptococcus neoformans* B and C serotypes. Mycologia 68:942.

50. Land, G.A., Fleming, W.H. III, Beadles, T.A., and Foxworth, J.H. 1979. Rapid identification of medically important yeasts. Lab. Med. 10:533.

51. Land, G.A., Harrison, B.A., Hulme, K.L., et al. 1979. Evaluation of the new API 20C strip for yeast identification against a conventional method. J. Clin. Microbiol. 10:357.

52. Land, G.A., Stotler, R., Land, K.J., and Staneck, J.L. 1984. Updating and evaluation of the Vitek AMS yeast identification system. J. Clin. Microbiol. 4:649.

53. Libertin, C.R., Wilson, W.R., and Roberts, G.D. 1985. *Candida lusitaniae*—an opportunistic pathogen. Diag. Microbiol. Infect. Dis. 3:69.

54. Mahgoub, E.S., and Murray, I.G. 1973. Mycetoma. William Heineman Medical Books, London.

55. Marcon, M.J., and Powell, D.A. 1987. Epidemiology, diagnosis and management of *Malassezia furfur* systemic infection. Diagn. Microbiol. Infect. Dis. 7:161.

56. McGinnis, M.R. 1985. Dematiaceous fungi. In Lennette, E.H., Balows, A., Hausler, W.J., Jr., and Shadomy, H.J., editors. Manual of clinical microbiology, ed. 4. American Society for Microbiology, Washington, D.C.

57. McGinnis, M.R., Rinaldi, M.G., and Winn, R.E. 1986. Emerging agents of phaeohyphomycosis: pathogenic species of *Bipolaris* and *Exserohilum*. J. Clin. Microbiol. 24:250.

58. McManus, E.J., and Jones, J.M. 1985. Detection of *Trichosporon beigelii* antigen cross-reactive with *Cryptococcus neoformans* capsular polysaccharide in serum from a patient with disseminated *Trichosporon* infection. J. Clin. Microbiol. 21:681.

59. Murray, P.R., Van Scoy, R.E., and Roberts, G.D. 1977. Should yeasts in respiratory secretions be identified? Mayo Clin. Proc. 52:42.

60. Musial, C.E., Cockerill, F.R. III, and Roberts, G.D. 1988. Fungal infections of the immunocompromised host: clinical and laboratory aspects. Rev. Infect. Dis. 1:349.

61. Oblack, D.L., Rhodes, J.C., and Martin, W.J. 1981. Clinical evaluation of the AutoMicrobic system yeast biochemical card for rapid identification of medically important yeasts. J. Clin. Microbiol. 13:351.

62. Paliwal, D.K., and Randhawa, H.S. 1978. Evaluation of a simplified *Guizotia abyssinica* seed medium for differentiation of *Cryptococcus neoformans*. J. Clin. Microbiol. 7:346.

63. Palmer, D.F., Kaufman, L., Kaplan, W., and Cavallano, J.J. 1977. Serodiagnosis of mycotic diseases. Charles C Thomas, Publisher, Springfield, Ill.

64. Pfaller, M.A., Preston, T., Bale, M., et al. 1988. Comparison of the Quantum II, API Yeast Ident and Automicrobic Systems for identification of clinical yeast isolates. J. Clin. Microbiol. 26:2054.

65. Pincus, D.H., Leun, I.L., Baecher, C., et al. 1985. Development of a same day yeast identification system. Abstracts of the Annual Meeting of the American Society for Microbiology, No. 344.

66. Roberts, G.D. 1975. Detection of fungi in clinical specimens by phase-contrast microscopy. J. Clin. Microbiol. 2:261.

67. Roberts, G.D. 1976. Laboratory diagnosis of fungal infections. Hum. Pathol. 7:161.

68. Roberts, G.D. 1979. Serodiagnosis of mycotic infections. Ill. Med. J. 156:406.

69. Roberts, G.D., Goodman, N.L., Land, G.A., et al. 1985. Detection and recovery of fungi in clinical specimens. In Lennette, E.H., Balows, A., Hausler, W.J., Jr., and Shadomy, H.J., editors. Manual of clinical microbiology, ed. 4. American Society for Microbiology, Washington, D.C.

70. Roberts, G.D., Horstmeier, C.D., Land, G.A., and Foxworth, J.H. 1978. Rapid urea broth test for yeasts. J. Clin. Microbiol. 7:584.

71. Roberts, G.D., Karlson, A.G., and DeYoung, D.R. 1976. Recovery of pathogenic fungi from clinical specimens submitted for mycobacterial culture. J. Clin. Microbiol. 3:47.

72. Roberts, G.D., Wang, H.S., and Hollick, G.E. 1976. Evaluation of the API 20C microtube system for the identification of clinically important yeasts. J. Clin. Microbiol. 3:302.

73. Roberts, G.D., and Washington, J.A. II. 1975. Detection of fungi in blood cultures. J. Clin. Microbiol. 1:309.

74. Salkin, I.F., Schadow, K.H., Bankaitis, L.A., et al. 1985. Evaluation of Abbott Quantum II Yeast Identification System. J. Clin. Microbiol. 22:442.

75. Salkin, I.F., Land, G.A., Hurd, N.J., et al. 1987. Evaluation of Yeast Ident and Uni-Yeast-Tek Yeast Identification Systems. J. Clin. Microbiol. 25:624.

76. Shadomy, S., Espinel-Ingroff, A., and Cartwright, R.Y. 1985. Susceptibility testing with antifungal drugs. In Lennette, E.H., Balows, A., Hausler, W.J., Jr., and Shadomy, H.J., editors. Manual of clinical microbiology, ed. 4. American Society for Microbiology, Washington, D.C.

77. Silva-Hutner, M., and Cooper, B.H. 1985. Yeasts of medical importance. In Lennette, E.H., Balows, A., Hausler, W.J., Jr., and Shadomy, H.J., editors. Manual of clinical microbiology, ed. 4. American Society for Microbiology, Washington, D.C.

78. Smith, C.D., and Goodman, N.L. 1975. Improved culture method for the isolation of *Histoplasma capsulatum* and *Blastomyces dermatitidis* from contaminated specimens. Am. J. Clin. Pathol. 68:276.

79. Standard, P.G., and Kaufman, L. 1980. A rapid and specific method for the immunological identification of mycelial form cultures of *Paracoccidioides brasiliensis*. Curr. Microbiol. 4:297.

80. Standard, P.G., and Kaufman, L. 1982. Safety considerations in handling exoantigen extracts from pathogenic fungi. J. Clin. Microbiol. 15:663.

81. Stockman, L., and Roberts, G.D. 1983. Corrected version. Specificity of the latex test for cryptococcal antigen: a rapid, simple method for eliminating interference factors. J. Clin. Microbiol. 17:945.

82. Strimlan, C.V., Dines, D.E., Rodgers-Sullivan, R.F., et al. 1980. Respiratory tract *Aspergillus*—clinical significance. Minn. Med. 63:25.

83. Summerbell, R.C., Rosenthal, S.A., and Kane, J. 1988. Rapid method for differentiation of *Trichophyton rubrum*, *Trichophyton mentagrophytes*, and related dermatophyte species. J. Clin. Microbiol. 26.2279.

84. Sun, S.H., Huppert, M., and Vukovich, K.R. 1976. Rapid in vitro conversion and identification of *Coccidioides immitis*. J. Clin. Microbiol. 3:186.

85. Swatek, F., Halde, C., Rinaldi, M.J., and Shadomy, H.J. 1985. *Aspergillus* and other opportunistic saprophytic hyaline hyphomycetes. In Lennette, E.H., Balows, A., Hausler, W.J., Jr., and Shadomy, H.J., editors. Manual of clinical microbiology, ed. 4. American Society for Microbiology, Washington, D.C.

86. Terreni, A.A., Strohecker, J.S., and Dowa, H. Jr. 1987. *Candida lusitaniae* septicemia in a patient on extended home intravenous hyperalimentation. J. Med. Vet. Mycol. 25:63.

87. Thomson, R.B., and Roberts, G.D. 1982. A practical approach to the diagnosis of fungal infections of the respiratory tract. Clin. Lab. Med. 2:321.

88. Treger, T.R., Visscher, D.W., Bartlett, M.S., and Smith, J.W. 1985. Diagnosis of pulmonary infection caused by *Aspergillus*: usefulness of respiratory cultures. J. Infect. Dis. 152:572.

89. Utz, J.P. 1967. Recognition and current management of the systemic mycoses. Med. Clin. North Am. 51:519.

90. Weeks, R.J. 1964. A rapid simplified medium for converting the mycelial phase of *Blastomyces dermatitidis* to the yeast phase. Mycopathologia 22:153.

91. Wu, T.C., and Koo, S.Y. 1983. Comparison of three commercial cryptococcal latex kits for detection of cryptococcal antigen. J. Clin. Microbiol. 18:1127.

92. Zackheim, H.S., Halde, C., Goodman, R.S., et al. 1985. Phaeohyphomycotic cyst of the skin caused by *Exophiala jeanselmei*. J. Am. Acad. Dermatol. 12:207.

93. Zimmer, B.L., and Roberts, G.D. 1979. Rapid selective urease test for presumptive identification of *Cryptococcus neoformans*. J. Clin. Microbiol. 10:380.

BIBLIOGRAPHY

Beneke, E.S., and Roger, A.L. 1980. Medicine mycology manual, ed. 4. Burgess Publishing Co., Minneapolis.

Emmons, C.W., Binford, C.H., Utz, J.P., and Kwon-Chung, K.J. 1977. Medical mycology, ed. 3. Lea & Febiger, Philadelphia.

Koneman, E.W., and Roberts, G.D. 1985. Practical laboratory mycology, ed. 3. Williams & Wilkins, Baltimore.

Larone, D.H. 1987. Medically important fungi: a guide to identification, ed. 2. Elsevier Science Publishing Co., Inc., New York.

Lennette, E.H., Balows, A., Hausler, W.J., Jr., and Shadomy, H.J. 1985. Manual of clinical microbiology, ed. 4. American Society for Microbiology, Washington, D.C.

McGinnis, M.R. 1980. Laboratory handbook of medical mycology. Academic Press, New York.

Rippon, J.W. 1988. Medical mycology—the pathogenic fungi and pathogenic actinomycetes, ed. 3. W.B. Saunders Co., Philadelphia.

44 Laboratory Methods for Diagnosis of Parasitic Infections

Lynne Shore Garcia

DIAGNOSTIC TECHNIQUES

The field of parasitology is often associated with tropical areas; however, many parasitic organisms that infect humans are worldwide in distribution and occur with some frequency in the temperate zones. Many organisms endemic elsewhere are seen in the United States in persons who have lived or traveled in those areas. The influx of a number of refugee populations into the United States has also served as both a source of infected patients and possible transmission of certain parasites. Another factor to be considered is the increase in numbers of compromised patients, particularly those who are immunodeficient or immunosuppressed. Those persons are very much at risk for certain parasitic problems. Consequently, clinicians and laboratory personnel should be aware of the possibility that these organisms may be present and should be trained in the ordering and the performance of appropriate procedures for their recovery and identification. The clinician must be able to recognize and interpret the relevance of the laboratory data, and

Table 44.1

Body Sites and Possible Parasites Recovered*

SITE	PARASITES	SITE	PARASITES
Blood			*Blastocystis hominis*
Red cells	*Plasmodium* sp.		*Isospora belli*
	Babesia sp.		*Ascaris lumbricoides*
White cells	*Leishmania donovani*		*Enterobius vermicularis*
	Toxoplasma gondii		Hookworm
Whole blood/plasma	*Trypanosoma* sp.		*Strongyloides stercoralis*
	Microfilariae		*Trichuris trichiura*
Bone marrow	*Leishmania donovani*		*Hymenolepis nana*
Central nervous sys-	*Taenia solium* (cysticercosis)		*Taenia saginata*
tem	*Echinococcus* sp.		*Taenia solium*
	Naegleria fowleri		*Diphyllobothrium latum*
	Acanthamoeba/Hartmanella sp.		*Opisthorchis sinensis (Clonorchis)*
	Toxoplasma gondii		*Paragonimus westermani*
	Trypanosoma sp.		*Schistosoma* sp.
Cutaneous ulcers	*Leishmania* sp.	Liver, spleen	*Echinococcus* sp.
Eye	*Acanthamoeba* spp.		*Entamoeba histolytica*
Intestinal tract	*Entamoeba histolytica*		*Leishmania donovani*
	Entamoeba coli	Lung	*Pneumocystis carinii*
	Entamoeba hartmanni		*Paragonimus westermani*
	Endolimax nana	Muscle	*Taenia solium* (cysticerci)
	Iodamoeba bütschlii		*Trichinella spiralis*
	Giardia lamblia		*Onchocerca volvulus*
	Chilomastix mesnili	Skin	*Leishmania* sp.
	Dientamoeba fragilis		Microfilariae
	Trichomonas hominis	Urogenital system	*Trichomonas vaginalis*
	Cryptosporidium sp.		*Schistosoma* sp.

*This table does not include every possible parasite that could be found in a particular body site. However, the most likely organisms have been listed.

the laboratorian must be able to review the pros and cons of each procedure, selecting those that will provide the most accurate diagnostic test results.

Although common names are frequently used to describe parasitic organisms, these names may represent different parasites in different parts of the world. To eliminate these problems, a binomial system of nomenclature is used in which the scientific name consists of the genus and species. On the basis of life histories and morphology, systems of classification have been developed to indicate the relationship among the various parasite species.

Parasites of humans are classified into five major subdivisions. These include the Protozoa (amebas, flagellates, ciliates, sporozoans, coccidia, microsporidians), the Platyhelminthes or flatworms (cestodes, trematodes), the Acanthocephala or thorny-headed worms, the Nematoda or roundworms, and the Arthropoda (insects, spiders, mites, ticks). The main

groups presented here include Protozoa, Nematoda, Platyhelminthes, and Arthropoda. This information is presented in the box on pp. 779-780. This classification scheme is designed to provide some order and meaning to a widely divergent group of organisms. No attempt has been made to include every possible organism, but only those that are considered to be clinically relevant in the context of human parasitology. It is hoped this table will provide some insight into the parasite groupings, thus leading to a better understanding of organism morphology, parasitic infections, and the appropriate clinical diagnostic approach.

The identification of parasitic organisms is dependent on morphological criteria; these criteria are in turn dependent on correct specimen collection and adequate fixation. Improperly submitted specimens may result in failure to find the organisms or in their misidentification. Tables 44.1 and 44.2 con-

Table 44.2

Body Sites and Specimen Collection

SITE	SPECIMEN OPTIONS	COLLECTION METHOD
Blood	Smears of whole blood	Thick and thin films (first choice)
	Anticoagulated blood	Anticoagulated blood (second choice)
		EDTA (first choice)
		Heparin (second choice)
Bone marrow	Aspirate	Sterile
Central nervous system	Spinal fluid	Sterile
Cutaneous ulcers	Aspirates from below surface	Sterile plus air-dried smears
	Biopsy	Sterile; nonsterile to histology
Eye	Corneal scraping	Sterile saline, air-dried smear
	Corneal biopsy	Sterile saline
Intestinal tract	Fresh stool	½ pint waxed container
	Preserved stool	5% or 10% formalin, MIF, SAF, Schaudinn's PVA
	Sigmoidoscopy material	Fresh, PVA, or Schaudinn's smears
	Duodenal contents	Entero-Test or aspirates
	Anal impression smear	Cellophane tape (pinworm examination)
	Adult worm/worm segments	Saline, 70% alcohol
Liver, spleen	Aspirates	Sterile, collected in 4 separate aliquots (liver)
	Biopsy	Sterile, nonsterile to histology
Lung	Sputum	True sputum (not saliva); no preservative (10% formalin if time delay)
	Lavage (centrifuged sediment)	No preservative
	Transbronchial aspirate	Air-dried smears
	Tracheobronchial aspirate	Same as above
	Brush biopsy	Same as above
	Open lung biopsy	Same as above
Muscle	Biopsy	Fresh-squash preparation, nonsterile to histology
Skin	Scrapings	Aseptic, smear or vial
	Skin snip	No preservative
	Biopsy	Nonsterile to histology
Urogenital system	Vaginal discharge	Saline swab, Culturette (no charcoal), culture medium
	Urethral discharge	Same as above
	Prostatic secretions	Same as above
	Urine	Single unpreserved specimen (24-h unpreserved specimen)

tain information on the body sites and possible parasites recovered and the most commonly used specimen collection approaches.

The information presented in this chapter should provide the reader with appropriate laboratory techniques and examples of morphological criteria to permit the correct identification of the more common human parasites. Several excellent resource texts are also available.*

44.1. Fecal Specimens

44.1.a. Collection. The ability to detect and identify intestinal parasites (particularly protozoa) is di-

*References 4, 7, 12, 19, 21, 35, 38, 44.

rectly related to the quality of the specimen submitted to the laboratory. Certain guidelines (below) are recommended to ensure proper collection and accurate examination of specimens.

Collection of fecal specimens for intestinal parasites should always be performed *prior to* radiologic studies involving barium sulfate. Because of the excess crystalline material in the stool specimen, the intestinal protozoa may be impossible to detect for at least 1 week after the use of barium. Certain medications may also prevent the detection of intestinal protozoa; these include mineral oil, bismuth, nonabsorbable antidiarrheal preparations, antimalarials, and some antibiotics (for example, tetracyclines). The organisms may be difficult to detect for several

Classification of Human Parasites

Protozoa

1. Amebas—intestinal
   Entamoeba histolytica
   Entamoeba hartmanni
   Entamoeba coli
   Entamoeba polecki
   Entamoeba gingivalis
   Endolimax nana
   Iodamoeba bütschlii
2. Flagellates—intestinal
   Giardia lamblia
   Chilomastix mesnili
   Dientamoeba fragilis
   Trichomonas hominis
   Trichomonas tenax
   Enteromonas hominis
   Retortamonas intestinalis
3. Ciliates—intestinal
   Balantidium coli
4. Coccidia, Microsporidia, *Blastocystis hominis*—intestinal
   Coccidia
     Cryptosporidium sp.
     Isospora belli
     Sarcocystis hominis
     Sarcocystis suihominis
     Sarcocystis "lindemanni"
   Microsporidia
     Encephalitozoon
     Nosema
     Pleistophora
     Enterocytozoon
   Blastocystis hominis
5. Amebas, flagellates—from other body sites
   Amebas
     Naegleria fowleri
     Acanthamoeba culbertsoni
   Flagellates
     Trichomonas vaginalis
6. Coccidia, sporozoa—from other body sites
   Coccidia
     Toxoplasma gondii
   Sporozoa
     *Pneumocystis carinii**

*May be reclassified with the fungi (Edman, J.C., Kovacs J.A., Masur, H., et al. 1988. Ribosomal RNA sequence shows *Pneumocystis carinii* to be a member of the fungi. Nature 334:519.

7. Sporozoa, flagellates—from blood and tissues
   Sporozoa (malaria and *Babesia*)
     Plasmodium vivax
     Plasmodium ovale
     Plasmodium malariae
     Plasmodium falciparum
     Babesia sp.
   Flagellates (leishmaniae, trypanosomes)
     Leishmania tropica complex
     Leishmania mexicana complex
     Leishmania braziliensis complex
     Leishmania donovani
     Trypanosoma gambiense
     Trypanosoma rhodesiense
     Trypanosoma cruzi
     Trypanosoma rangeli

Nematodes

1. Intestinal
   Ascaris lumbricoides
   Enterobius vermicularis
   Ancylostoma duodenale
   Necator americanus
   Strongyloides stercoralis
   Trichuris trichiura
2. Tissue
   Trichinella spiralis
   Visceral larva migrans (*Toxocara canis* or *T. cati*)
   Cutaneous larva migrans (*Ancylostoma braziliense* or *A. caninum*)
   Angiostrongylus cantonensis
   Angiostrongylus costaricensis
   Gnathostoma spinigerum
   Anisakis sp. (larvae from saltwater fish)
   Phocanema sp. (larvae from saltwater fish)
3. Filarial worms—blood
   Wuchereria bancrofti
   Brugia malayi
   Loa loa
   Onchocerca volvulus
   Mansonella ozzardi
   Mansonella streptocerca

Continued.

Classification of Human Parasites—cont'd

Mansonella perstans
Dirofilaria immitis (usually lung lesion/
  dog heartworm)
Dirofilaria sp.

Cestodes

1. Intestinal
   Diphyllobothrium latum
   Dipylidium caninum
   Hymenolepis nana
   Hymenolepis diminuta
   Taenia solium
   Taenia saginata
2. Larval forms—tissue
   Taenia solium
   Echinococcus granulosus
   Echinococcus multilocularis
   Multiceps multiceps
   Diphyllobothrium sp.

Trematodes

1. Intestinal
   Fasciolopsis buski
   Echinostoma ilocanum
   Heterophyes heterophyes
   Metagonimus yokogawai
2. Liver/lung
   Opisthorchis sinensis
   Opisthorchis viverrini
   Fasciola hepatica
   Paragonimus westermani
3. Blood
   Schistosoma mansoni
   Schistosoma haematobium
   Schistosoma japonicum
   Schistosoma intercalatum
   Schistosoma mekongi

Arthropods

1. Arachnida
   Scorpions
   Spiders (black widow, brown recluse)
   Ticks *(Dermacentor, Ixodes, Argas, Ornitho-doros)*
   Mites *(Sarcoptes)*
2. Crustacea
   Copepods *(Cyclops)*
   Crayfish, lobsters, crabs
3. Pentastomida
   Tongue worms
4. Diplopoda
   Millipedes
5. Chilopoda
   Centipedes

Insecta

Anoplura: sucking lice *(Pediculus, Phthirus)*
Dictyoptera: cockroaches
Hemiptera: true bugs *(Triatoma)*
Coleoptera: beetles
Hymenoptera: bees, wasps, etc.
Lepidoptera: butterflies, moths, etc.
Diptera: flies, mosquitos, gnats, midges *(Phle-botomus, Aedes, Anopheles, Glossina, Simulium)*
Siphonaptera: fleas *(Pulex, Xenopsylla)*

---

weeks after the medication is discontinued. Fecal specimens should be collected in clean, wide-mouthed containers; most laboratories use a waxed, cardboard half-pint container with a tight-fitting lid. The specimen should not be contaminated with water that may contain free-living organisms. Contamination with urine should also be avoided to prevent destruction of motile organisms in the specimen. All specimens should be identified with the patient's name, physician's name, hospital number if applicable, and the time and date collected. Every fecal specimen represents a potential source of infectious material (for example, bacteria, viruses, and parasites) and should be handled accordingly.

The number of specimens required to demonstrate intestinal parasites will vary depending on the quality of the specimen submitted, the accuracy of the examination performed, and the severity of the infection. For a routine examination for parasites *prior to treatment, a minimum of three fecal specimens* is recommended—two specimens collected from normal movements and one specimen collected after a cathartic, such as magnesium sulfate or Fleet Phospho-Soda. A cathartic with an oil base should not be used, and all laxatives are contraindicated if the patient has diarrhea or significant abdominal pain. Stool softeners are inadequate for producing a purged specimen. The examination of at least six specimens ensures detection of 90% of infections; six are usually recommended when amebiasis is suspected.

Many organisms do not appear in fecal specimens in consistent numbers on a daily basis; thus collection of specimens on *alternate days* tends to yield a higher percentage of positive findings. The series of three specimens should be collected within no more than 10 days and a series of six within no more than 14 days.

The number of specimens to be examined after therapy will vary depending on the diagnosis; however, a series of three specimens collected as previously outlined is usually recommended. A patient who has received treatment for a protozoan infection should be checked 3 to 4 weeks after therapy. Patients treated for helminth infections may be checked 1 to 2 weeks after therapy, and those treated for *Taenia* infections 5 to 6 weeks after therapy. Since the age of the specimen directly influences the recovery of protozoan organisms, the *time the specimen was collected* should be recorded on the laboratory request form. Freshly passed specimens are mandatory for the detection of trophic amebas or flagellates. *Liquid specimens should be examined within 30 minutes of passage* (not 30 minutes from the time they reach the laboratory), or the specimen should be placed in polyvinyl alcohol fixative (PVA) or another suitable preservative (see following section on preservation of specimens). *Semiformed or soft specimens should be examined within 1 hour of passage;* if this is not possible, the stool material should be preserved. Although the time limits are not as critical for the examination of a formed specimen, it is recommended that the material be examined on the day of passage. If these time limits cannot be met,

portions of the sample should be preserved. Stool specimens should not be held at room temperature but should be refrigerated at 3° to 5° C and stored in closed containers to prevent desiccation. At this temperature eggs, larvae, and protozoan cysts remain viable for several days. Fecal specimens should never be incubated or frozen prior to examination. When the proper criteria for collection of fecal specimens are not met, the laboratory should request additional samples.

Collection kit for outpatient use. A number of commercial collection systems are presently available, and one can select which vials are appropriate for a particular institution. Most manufacturers will package the kit according to individual specifications. (See PVA Fixative below for representative suppliers.)

CAUTION: PVA solution contains a large amount of mercury; for safety reasons and protection of the patient, each vial containing PVA or any type of preservative should have a child-proof cap and should be marked *Poison*. In some areas of the country it may be helpful to label the vials in more than one language, depending on the population using the medical facility.

A PVA-preserved portion of the specimen may be used for the complete examination, although many laboratories prefer to use the sample in 10% formalin for the concentration procedure. Other laboratories may prefer to use Schaudinn's fixative for collection. The unpreserved portion of the specimen (many laboratories do not request this sample unless an occult blood procedure is requested) may be examined to determine the specimen type (for example, liquid, soft, or formed).

44.1.b. Preservation. Depending on specimen-to-laboratory transportation time, the laboratory workload, and the availability of trained personnel, it may often be impossible to examine the specimen within specified time limits. To maintain protozoan morphology and prevent further development of certain helminth eggs and larvae, the fecal specimen should be placed in an appropriate preservative for examination at a later time. A number of preservatives are available; four of these methods—PVA (Appendix A), formalin (Appendix A), Merthiolate (thimerosal)-iodine-formalin (MIF), and sodium acetate–formalin (SAF)—will be discussed. When selecting an appropriate fixative, it is important to realize the limitations of each. PVA and

SAF are the only fixatives included here from which a permanent stained smear can be easily prepared. The stained smear is extremely important in providing a complete and accurate examination for intestinal protozoa. The other fixatives mentioned permit the examination of the specimen as a wet mount only, a technique much less accurate than the stained smear for the identification of protozoa.

Although there has been a great deal of interest in developing a preservative without the use of mercury compounds, studies indicate that substitute compounds may not provide the quality of preservation necessary for good protozoan morphology on the permanent stained smear. Copper sulfate is the compound that has been tried most frequently, but it does not provide results equal to those seen with mercuric chloride. Work will probably continue in this area in order to provide a solution to the problem of mercury disposal, a problem many laboratories are trying to solve.

PVA fixative. PVA fixative solution is highly recommended as a means of preserving protozoan cysts and trophozoites for examination at a later time.[6] The use of PVA also permits specimens to be shipped by regular mail service to a laboratory for subsequent examination. PVA, which is a combination of modified Schaudinn's fixative and a water-soluble resin, should be used in the ratio of three parts PVA to one part fecal material. Perhaps the greatest advantage in the use of PVA is that permanent stained slides can be prepared from PVA-preserved material.[6] This is not the case with many other preservatives; some permit the specimen to be examined as a wet preparation only, a technique that may not be adequate for the correct identification of protozoan organisms. PVA can be prepared in the laboratory (Appendix A) or purchased commercially.* This fixative remains stable for long periods (months to years) when kept in *sealed containers* at room temperature. Commercial packaging and distribution of these vials have essentially eliminated the problem of moisture loss and shelf life.

Protozoan cysts, helminth eggs, and larvae are well preserved for long periods in *10% formalin* (Appendix A). It is recommended that hot formalin (60° C) be used for helminth eggs to prevent further development of the eggs to the infective stage; this is important when bulk specimens are being saved for teaching purposes. Formalin should be used in the ratio of at least 3 parts formalin to 1 part fecal material; thorough mixing of the fresh specimen and fixative is necessary to ensure good preservation.

MIF solution. The Merthiolate (thimerosal)iodine-formalin solution of Sapèro and Lawless[45] can be used as a stain preservative for most kinds and stages of intestinal parasites and may be helpful in field surveys. Helminth eggs, larvae, and certain protozoa can be identified without further staining in wet mounts, which can be prepared immediately after fixation or several weeks later. This type of wet preparation may not be adequate for the diagnosis of all intestinal protozoa. Although some workers prepare a permanent stained smear from MIF-preserved material, another fixative preparation may be preferred for the precise morphology necessary for protozoan identification on the permanent stained smear. There are certain disadvantages with the MIF method, which may include the instability of the iodine component of the fixative.

SAF fixative. SAF fixative contains formalin combined with sodium acetate, which acts as a buffer. It is a liquid fixative much like 10% aqueous formalin. When the sediment is used to prepare permanent stained smears, there may be some difficulty in getting material to adhere to the slide. Mayer's albumin has been recommended as an adhesive.[46,47] This fixative tends to give better results when used with hematoxylin rather than trichrome stain.

44.1.c. **Macroscopic examination.** The consistency of the stool (formed, semiformed, soft, or liquid) may give an indication of the protozoan stages present. When the moisture content of the fecal material is decreased during *normal passage* through the intestinal tract, the trophozoite stages of the protozoa encyst to survive. **Trophozoites** (motile forms) of the intestinal protozoa are usually found in soft or liquid specimens and occasionally in a semiformed specimen; the cyst stages are normally found in formed or semiformed specimens, rarely in liquid stools.

---

*Elvanol, grades 71-24, 71-30, and 90-25, can be obtained from E.I. duPont de Nemours & Co., Inc. (or their local representatives) in a minimum of 50-pound bags. One could check with a local chemical supply house to see if small quantities might be available. When ordering PVA powder, be sure to specify the pretested powder for use in PVA fixative. The PVA powder should be water-soluble and of medium viscosity. Prepared liquid PVA (ready for use) can be obtained from Hardy Media, Medical Chemical Corporation, Meridian Diagnostics, Remel, Trend Scientific, Medical Media Lab, and Bio Spec.

Helminth eggs or larvae may be found in any type of specimen, although the chances of finding any parasitic organism in a liquid specimen will be reduced because of the dilution factor.

Occasionally adult helminths, such as *Ascaris lumbricoides* or *Enterobius vermicularis* (pinworm), may be seen in or on the surface of the stool. Tapeworm proglottids may also be seen on the surface, or they may actually crawl under the specimen and be found on the bottom of the container. Other adult helminths, such as *Trichuris trichiura* (whipworm), hookworms, or perhaps *Hymenolepis nana* (dwarf tapeworm), may be found in the stool, but usually this occurs only after medication. The presence of blood in the specimen may indicate a number of things and should always be reported. Dark stools may indicate bleeding high in the gastrointestinal tract, whereas fresh (bright red) blood most often is the result of bleeding at a lower level. In certain parasitic infections blood and mucus may be present; a soft or liquid stool may be highly suggestive of an amebic infection. These areas of blood and mucus should be carefully examined for the presence of trophic amebas. Occult blood in the stool may or may not be related to a parasitic infection and can result from a number of different conditions. Ingestion of various compounds may give a distinctive color to the stool (iron, black; barium, light tan to white).

44.1.d. Microscopic examination. The identification of intestinal protozoa and helminth eggs is based on recognition of specific morphological characteristics; these studies require a good binocular microscope, good light source, and the use of a calibrated ocular micrometer.

The microscope should have $5\times$ and $10\times$ oculars (wide-field oculars are often recommended) and three objectives: low power ($10\times$), high-dry ($40\times$ to $44\times$), and oil immersion ($97\times$ to $99\times$). The microscope should be kept covered when not in use, and all lenses should be carefully cleaned with lens paper. The light source should provide light of variable intensity in the blue-white range.

Calibration of microscope. Parasite identification depends on several parameters, one of which is size; any laboratory doing diagnostic work in parasitology should have a calibrated microscope available for precise measurements.

Measurements are made by means of a micrometer disk placed in the ocular of the microscope; the disk is usually calibrated as a line divided into 50 units. Since the divisions in the disk represent different measurements, depending on the objective magnification used, the ocular disk divisions must be compared with a known calibrated scale, usually a stage micrometer with a scale of 0.1- and 0.01-mm divisions. Specific directions may be found in the work of Garcia and Bruckner.[21]

NOTE: After each objective power has been calibrated on the microscope, *the oculars containing the disk or these objectives cannot be interchanged with corresponding objectives or oculars on another microscope*. Each microscope that will be used to measure organisms must be calibrated as a unit; *the original oculars and objectives that were used to calibrate the microscope must also be used when an organism is measured*.

In order to comply with quality control requirements, each calibrated microscope should be recalibrated once a year. The calibrations do change, and a slight error can be magnified, particularly using the oil-immersion objective, where measurements can be critical to accurate speciation.

44.1.e. Diagnostic procedures. A combination of techniques yields a greater number of positive specimens than does any one technique alone. Procedures recommended for a complete ova and parasite examination are discussed in the following section.

Direct smears. Normal mixing in the intestinal tract usually ensures even distribution of helminth eggs or larvae and protozoa. However, examination of the fecal material as a direct smear may or may not reveal organisms, depending on the parasite density. The direct smear is prepared by mixing a small amount of fecal material (approximately 2 mg) with a drop of physiologic saline; this mixture provides a uniform suspension under a 22- $\times$ 22-mm coverslip. Some workers prefer a 1½- $\times$ 3-inch (4×7 cm) glass slide for the wet preparations, rather than the standard 1- $\times$ 3-inch (2.5×7 cm) slide most often used for the permanent stained smear. A 2-mg sample of fecal material forms a low cone on the end of a wooden applicator stick. If more material is used for the direct mount, the suspension is usually too thick for an accurate examination; less than 2 mg results in the examination of too thin a suspension, thus decreasing the chances of finding any organisms. If present, blood and mucus should always be examined as a direct mount. The entire 22 $\times$ 22 mm coverslip should be systematically examined using the low-power objective (10×) and low light intensity; any suspect objects may then be examined under high-dry power (43×). The use of the oil immersion objective on mounts of this kind is not recommended unless the coverslip (no. 1 thickness coverslip is recommended when the oil immersion objective is used) is sealed to the slide with a cotton-tipped applicator stick dipped in equal parts of heated paraffin and petroleum jelly. Many workers believe the use of oil immersion on this type of preparation is impractical, especially since morphological detail is most easily seen and the diagnosis confirmed with oil immersion examination of the permanent stained smear.

The direct wet mount is used primarily to detect motile trophozoite stages of the protozoa. These organisms are very pale and transparent, two characteristics that require the use of low light intensity. Protozoan organisms in a saline preparation usually appear as refractile objects. If suspect objects are seen on high-dry power, one should allow at least 15 seconds to detect motility of slow-moving protozoa. Heat applied by placing a hot penny on the edge of a slide may enhance the motility of trophic protozoa.

NOTE: *With few exceptions, protozoan organisms should not be identified on the basis of a wet mount alone. Permanent stained smears should be examined to confirm the specific identification of suspected organisms.*

Helminth eggs or larvae and protozoan cysts may also be seen on the wet film, although these forms are more often detected after fecal concentration procedures.

After the wet preparation has been thoroughly checked for trophic amebas, a drop of iodine may be placed at the edge of the coverslip, or a new wet mount can be prepared with iodine alone. A weak iodine solution is recommended; too strong a solution may obscure the organisms. Several types of iodine solutions are available: Dobell and O'Connor's, Lugol's (Appendix B), and D'Antoni's (Appendix B). *Gram's iodine used in bacteriologic work is not recommended for staining parasitic organisms.*

NOTE: Many laboratories believe that the benefits gained in organism recovery and identification from receipt of preserved stool specimens far outweigh the disadvantages of not receiving a fresh specimen that can be examined for motile organisms. This is particularly true with the intestinal protozoa.

Protozoan cysts correctly stained with iodine contain yellow-gold cytoplasm, brown glycogen material, and paler refractile nuclei. The chromatoidal bodies may not be as clearly visible as they were in the saline mount.

Several staining solutions are available that may be used to reveal nuclear detail in the trophozoite stages. Nair's[41] buffered methylene blue stain is effective in showing nuclear detail when used at a low pH; a pH range of 3.6 to 4.8 allows more active penetration of the organism with the biological dye. After 5 to 10 minutes, Nair's buffered methylene blue stain stains the cytoplasm a pale blue and the nuclei a darker blue. Methylene blue (0.06%) in an acetate buffer (Appendix A) at pH 3.6 usually gives satisfactory results; the mount should be examined within 30 minutes.

Concentration procedures. Often a direct mount of fecal material fails to reveal the presence of parasitic organisms in the gastrointestinal tract. Fecal concentration procedures should be included for a complete examination for parasites; these procedures allow the detection of small numbers of organisms that may be missed using only the direct mount. Helminth eggs can usually be identified when recovered from a concentration procedure. Generally the identification of intestinal protozoa should be considered tentative and confirmed with the permanent stained smear. Those protozoa that might be routinely identified from a concentration procedure include cysts of *Giardia lamblia, Entamoeba histolytica, Entamoeba coli,* and *Iodamoeba bütschlii* (trophozoites are rarely identified from a concentrate). There are commercially available concentrating devices that may assist a laboratory in standardizing the methodology.*

A number of concentration procedures are available; they are either *flotation* or *sedimentation techniques* designed to separate the parasitic components from excess fecal debris through differences in specific gravity. A flotation procedure (Procedure 44.1) permits the separation of protozoan cysts and certain helminth eggs through the use of a liquid with a high specific gravity. The parasitic elements are recovered in the surface film, whereas the debris will be found in the bottom of the tube. This tech-

---

*Evergreen Scientific (FPC, fecal parasite concentrator), Hardy Media, Meridian Diagnostics, Inc., Trend Scientific (FeKal, CON-Trate System).

PROCEDURE 44.1

Zinc Sulfate Flotation Procedure (Modified)

Principle

Parasitic cysts and some helminth eggs will rise to the surface of a liquid with a high specific gravity, such as zinc sulfate, due to their buoyant properties in that solution.

Method

1. Prepare a fecal suspension of ¼ to ½ teaspoon of feces (more if the specimen is diarrheal) in 10 to 15 ml of tap water.
2. Filter this material through two layers of gauze into a small tube (Wassermann tube). Fill the tube with tap water to within 2 to 3 mm of the top, and centrifuge for 1 min at 500 × g.
3. Decant the supernatant fluid, fill the tube with water, and resuspend the sediment by stirring with an applicator stick. Centrifuge for 1 min at 500 × g.
4. Decant the water, add 2 to 3 ml zinc sulfate solution, resuspend the sediment, and fill the tube with zinc sulfate solution to within 0.5 cm of the top.
5. Centrifuge for 1 to 2 min at 500 × g. Do not "brake" the centrifuge; allow the tubes to come to a stop without interference or vibration.
6. Without removing the tubes from the centrifuge, touch the surface film of the suspension with a wire loop (diameter 5 to 7 mm; loop should be parallel with the surface of the fluid). *Do not go below the surface of the film with the loop.* Add the material in the loop to a slide containing a drop of dilute iodine or saline.

Note: *Material recovered from the zinc sulfate flotation procedure must be examined within several minutes; prolonged contact with the high specific gravity solution leads to organism distortion. Protozoan cysts may be more distorted using this method, and the technique is unsuitable for stool specimens containing large amounts of fatty material. The specific gravity of the zinc sulfate should be 1.18 and should be checked frequently with a hydrometer. If this technique is used to concentrate formalin-preserved material, the specific gravity should be increased to 1.20. Zinc sulfate solution (ZnSO$_4$, specific gravity 1.18); consists of approximately 330 g of dry crystals in 670 ml of distilled water. A 33% solution usually approximates the correct specific gravity but may be adjusted to 1.18 by the addition of zinc sulfate or distilled water.*

Quality control

The specific gravity of the solution should be checked. Formalin-fixed stools containing known parasites can be purchased and should be concentrated along with patient specimens to check for the detection of the parasites.

Expected results

Known parasites should be detected readily.

Performance schedule

The specific gravity of the zinc sulfate should be checked when prepared and at least monthly thereafter. Quality control samples should be concentrated at least four times yearly. Participation in a proficiency survey program that includes formalin-preserved stools would fulfill this need.

---

nique yields a cleaner preparation than does the sedimentation procedure; however, some helminth eggs (operculated eggs or very dense eggs, such as unfertilized *Ascaris* eggs) and some protozoa do not concentrate well with the flotation method. The specific gravity may be increased, although this may produce more distortion in the eggs and protozoa.

Any laboratory that uses only a flotation procedure may fail to recover all the parasites present; to ensure detection of all organisms in the sample, both the surface film and the sediment should be carefully examined.

NOTE: Directions for any flotation technique must be followed exactly to produce reliable results.

PROCEDURE 44.2

Formalin-Ether Sedimentation Techniques

Principle

Formalin fixes the eggs, larvae, and cysts, so that they are no longer infectious, as well as preserving their morphology. Fecal debris is extracted into the ether phase of the solution, freeing the sedimented parasitic elements from at least some of the artifactual material in stool.

Method

1. Transfer ¼ to ½ teaspoon of fresh stool into 10 ml of 10% formalin in a 15-ml shell vial, unwaxed paper cup, or 16 × 125 mm tube (container may vary depending on individual preferences) and comminute thoroughly. Let stand 30 min for adequate fixation.
2. Filter this material (funnel or pointed paper cup with end cut off) through two layers of gauze into a 15-ml centrifuge tube.
3. Add physiologic saline to within ½ inch (1.5 cm) of the top and centrifuge for 1 min at 500 × g.
4. Decant, resuspend the sediment (should have 0.5 to 1 ml sediment) in saline to within ½ inch (1.5 cm) of the top, and centrifuge again for 1 min at 500 × g. This second wash may be eliminated if the supernatant fluid after the first wash is light tan or clear.

5. Decant and resuspend the sediment in 10% formalin (fill the tube only half full). If the amount of sediment left in the bottom of the tube is very small, do not add ether in step 6; merely add the formalin, then spin, decant, and examine the remaining sediment.
6. Add approximately 3 ml of ether (*do not use near open flames*), stopper, and shake vigorously for 30 seconds. Hold the tube so that the stopper is directed away from your face; remove stopper carefully to prevent spraying of material caused by pressure within the tube.
7. Centrifuge for 2 to 3 min at 500 × g. Four layers should result: a small amount of sediment in the bottom of the tube, containing the parasites; a layer of formalin; a plug of fecal debris on top of the formalin layer; and a layer of ether at the top.
8. Free the plug of debris by ringing with an applicator stick, and decant all the fluid. After proper decanting, a drop or two of fluid remaining on the side of the tube will drain down to the sediment. Mix the fluid with the sediment and prepare a wet mount for examination.

The formalin-ether sedimentation procedure may be used on PVA-preserved material. Steps 1 and 2 differ as follows:

Sedimentation procedures (using gravity or centrifugation) allow the recovery of all protozoa, eggs, and larvae present; however, the sediment preparation contains more fecal debris. If a single technique is selected for routine use, the *sedimentation procedure (Procedure 44.2) is recommended* as the easiest to perform and least subject to technical error.

Permanent stained smears. The detection and correct identification of intestinal protozoa are frequently dependent on the examination of the permanent stained smear. These slides not only provide the microscopist with a permanent record of the protozoan organisms identified but also may be used for consultations with specialists when unusual morphological characteristics are found. In view of the number of morphological variations possible, organisms may be found that are very difficult to identify and do not fit the pattern for any one species.

The smaller protozoan organisms are often seen on the stained smear and missed with only the direct smear and concentration methods. Although an experienced microscopist can occasionally identify certain organisms on a wet preparation, most identifications should be considered tentative until confirmed by the permanent stained slide. For these

1. Fixation time with PVA should be at least 30 min. Mix contents of PVA bottle (stool-PVA mixture: 1 part stool to 2 or 3 parts PVA) with applicator sticks. Immediately after mixing, pour approximately 2 to 5 ml (amount will vary depending on the viscosity and density of the mixture) of the stool-PVA mixture into a 15-ml shell vial, 16- × 125-mm tube, or such, and add approximately 10 ml physiologic saline.
2. Filter this material (funnel or paper cup with pointed end cut off) through two layers of gauze into a 15-ml centrifuge tube.

Steps 3 through 8 will be the same for both fresh and PVA-preserved material.

Note: *Tap water may be substituted for physiologic saline throughout this procedure; however, saline is recommended. Some workers prefer to use 10% formalin for all the rinses (steps 3 and 4).*

Note: *The introduction of ethyl acetate as a substitute for diethyl ether (ether) in the formalin-ether sedimentation concentration procedure provides a much safer chemical for the clinical laboratory. Tests comparing the use of these two compounds on formalin-preserved and PVA-preserved material indicate that the differences in organism recovery and identification are minimal and probably do not reflect clinically relevant differences.*

When examining the sediment in the bottom of the tube:

1. Prepare a saline mount (1 drop of sediment and 1 drop of saline solution mixed together), and scan the whole 22 × 22 mm coverslip under low power for helminth eggs or larvae.
2. Iodine may then be added to aid in the detection of protozoan cysts and should be examined under high-dry power. If iodine is added prior to low-power scanning, be certain that the iodine is not too strong; otherwise, some of the helminth eggs will stain so darkly that they will be mistaken for debris.
3. Occasionally a precipitate is formed when iodine is added to the sediment obtained from a concentration procedure with PVA-preserved material. The precipitate is formed from the reaction between the iodine and excess mercuric chloride that has not been thoroughly rinsed from the PVA-preserved material. The sediment can be rinsed again to remove any remaining mercuric chloride, or the sediment can be examined as a saline mount without the addition of iodine.[21]

Quality control

The same recommendations for testing prepared known samples as were mentioned for the zinc flotation procedure are applicable.

reasons, *the permanent stain is recommended for every stool sample submitted for a routine examination for parasites.*

A number of staining techniques are available; individual selection of a particular method may depend on the degree of difficulty and amount of time necessary for staining. The older classical method is the long Heidenhain's iron-hematoxylin method; however, for routine diagnostic work most laboratories select one of the shorter procedures, such as the trichrome method or one of several methods using iron-hematoxylin. Other procedures are available; however, those included here generally tend to give the best and most reliable results with both fresh and PVA-preserved specimens.

PREPARATION OF FRESH MATERIAL. When the specimen arrives, use an applicator stick or brush to smear a small amount of stool on two clean slides and immediately immerse them in Schaudinn's fixative. If the slides are prepared correctly, one should be able to read newsprint through the fecal smear. The smears should fix for a minimum of 30 minutes; fixation time may be decreased to 5 minutes if the Schaudinn's solution is heated to 60° C.

If a liquid specimen is received, mix 3 or 4 drops of PVA with 1 or 2 drops of fecal material on a slide, spread the mixture, and allow the slides to dry for several hours at 35° C or overnight at room temperature. The formulas for saturated mercuric chloride and Schaudinn's fixative are presented in Appendix A.

PREPARATION OF PVA-PRESERVED MATERIAL. Stool specimens preserved in PVA should be allowed to fix at least 30 minutes. After fixation, the sample should be thoroughly mixed and a small amount of the material poured onto a paper towel to absorb excess PVA. This is an important step in the procedure; allow the PVA to soak into the paper towel for 2 to 3 minutes before preparing the slides. With an applicator stick apply some of the stool material from the paper towel to two slides and let them dry for several hours at 37° C or overnight at room temperature. The PVA-stool mixture should be spread to the edges of the glass slide; this causes the film to adhere to the slide during staining. It is also important to dry the slides thoroughly to prevent the material from washing off during staining.

TRICHROME STAIN. This stain was originally developed by Gomori[24] for tissue differentiation and was adapted by Wheatley[57] for intestinal protozoa (Procedure 44.3). It is an uncomplicated procedure that produces well-stained smears from both fresh and PVA-preserved material.

The trichrome stain can be used repeatedly, and stock solution may be added to the jar when the volume is decreased. Periodically, the staining strength can be restored by removing the lid and allowing the 70% alcohol carried over from the preceding jar to evaporate. Each lot number or batch of stain (either purchased commercially or prepared in the laboratory) should be checked to determine the optimum staining time, which is usually a few minutes longer for PVA-preserved material.

The 90% acidified alcohol is used as a destaining agent that will provide good differentiation; however, prolonged destaining (more than 3 seconds) may result in a poor stain. To prevent continued destaining, the slides should be quickly rinsed in 100% alcohol and then dehydrated through two additional changes of 100% alcohol.

INTERPRETATION OF STAINED SMEARS. Many problems in interpretation may arise when poorly stained smears are examined; these smears are usually the result of inadequate fixation or incorrect specimen collection and submission. An old specimen or inadequate fixation may result in organisms

that fail to stain or that appear as pale pink or red objects with very little internal definition. This type of staining reaction may occur with *E. coli* cysts, which require a longer fixation time; mature cysts in general need additional fixation time and therefore may not be as well stained as immature cysts. Degenerate forms or those that have been understained or destained too much may stain pale green.

When the smear is well fixed and correctly stained, the background debris will be green, and the protozoa will have a blue-green to purple cytoplasm with red or purple-red nuclei and inclusions. The differences in colors between the background and organisms provide more contrast than in hematoxylin-stained smears.

Helminth eggs and larvae usually stain dark red or purple; they are usually distorted and difficult to identify. White blood cells, macrophages, tissue cells, yeast cells, and other artifacts still present diagnostic problems, since their color range on the stained smear approximates that of the parasitic organisms (Figures 44.1 to 44.3).

IRON-HEMATOXYLIN STAIN. Although the original method produces excellent results, most laboratories that use an iron-hematoxylin stain select one of the shorter methods. A number of procedures are available; both of those presented here can be used with either fresh or PVA-preserved material. Both background debris and the organisms stain gray-blue to black, with the cellular inclusions and nuclei appearing darker than the cytoplasm.

The method described by Spencer and Monroe[49] (Appendix B) is a bit longer than the trichrome procedure. Although the slides do not require destaining, decolorizing in 0.5% hydrochloric acid after a longer initial staining time may provide better differentiation.

Another iron-hematoxylin method, described by Tompkins and Miller[56] (Appendix B) includes the use of phosphotungstic acid as a destaining agent. This procedure also gives good, reproducible results.

General information. The most important step in preparing a well-stained fecal smear is adequate fixation of a specimen that has been submitted within specified time limits. To ensure best results, the acetic acid component of Schaudinn's fixative should be added just prior to use; fixation time (room temperature) may be extended overnight with no adverse effects on the smears.

After fixation it is very important to completely

PROCEDURE 44.3

Trichrome Stain

Principle

The internal elements that distinguish among cysts and trophozoites can be best visualized with a stain that enhances the morphological features. In addition, such a stained smear provides a permanent record of the results.

Method

1. Formula

Chromotrope 2R	0.6 g
Light green SF	0.3 g
Phosphotungstic acid	0.7 g
Acetic acid (glacial)	1 ml
Distilled water	100 ml

2. Preparation. The stain is prepared by adding 1 ml of glacial acetic acid to the dry components. Allow the mixture to stand for 15 to 30 min to "ripen"; then add 100 ml of distilled water. This preparation gives a highly uniform and reproducible stain; the stain should be purple. Store in Coplin jars.

3. Procedure
   a. Prepare fresh fecal smears or PVA smears as described.
   b. Place in 70% ethanol for 5 min.* (This step may be eliminated for PVA smears.)
   c. Place in 70% ethanol plus D'Antoni's iodine (dark reddish brown) for 2 to 5 min.
   d. Place in two changes of 70% ethanol—one for 5 min* and one for 2 to 5 min.

   e. Place in trichrome stain solution for 10 min.
   f. Place in 90% ethanol, acidified (1% acetic acid) for up to 3 s (do not leave the slides in this solution any longer).
   g. Dip once in 100% ethanol.
   h. Place in two changes of 100% ethanol for 2 to 5 min each.*
   i. Place in two changes of xylene or toluene for 2 to 5 min each.*
   j. Mount in Permount or some other mounting medium; use a no. 1 thickness coverglass.

Quality control

Using the same timing and reagents as for patient samples, stain slides prepared from fixed stool samples with known parasites, available commercially or as part of a proficiency testing survey program. Negative preserved stool (PVA) seeded with buffy coat cells from sedimented whole blood can also be used.[21]

Expected results

Background debris will be green and protozoa will show blue-green to purple cytoplasm. The nuclei and inclusions will be red or purple-red and sharply delineated from background.

Performance schedule

Stain quality control samples when new stain solution is prepared and at least four times yearly.

*At this stage, slides can be held several hours or overnight.

remove the mercuric chloride residue from the smears. The 70% alcohol-iodine mixture removes the mercury complex; the iodine solution should be changed often enough (at least once a week) to maintain a dark reddish-brown color. If the mercuric chloride is not completely removed, the stained smear may contain varying amounts of highly refractive granules, which may prevent finding or identifying any organisms present.

Good results in the final stages of dehydration (100% alcohol) and clearing (xylene) depend on the use of fresh reagents. It is recommended that solutions be changed at least weekly and more often if large numbers of slides (10 to 50 per day) are being stained. Stock containers and staining dishes should have well-fitting lids to prevent evaporation and absorption of moisture from the air. If the clearing agent turns cloudy on addition of the slides from

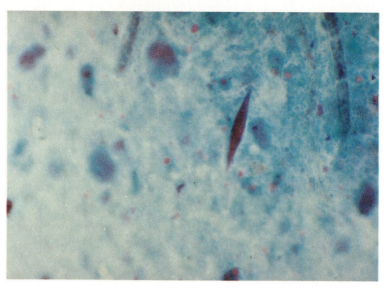

Figure 44.1
Charcot-Leyden crystals.

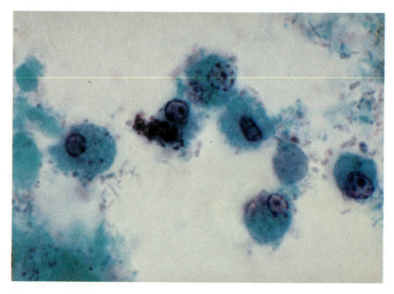

Figure 44.2
Polymorphonuclear leukocytes.

100% alcohol, there is water in the solution. When clouding occurs, immediately return the slides to 100% alcohol, replace all dehydrating and clearing agents with fresh stock, and continue with the dehydration process.

   Modified acid-fast stain for Cryptosporidium *sp.* Although a number of different procedures have been tried for the recovery and identification of *Crypto-*
sporidium sp. in humans, the best approach seems to be hot or cold modified acid-fast stains (Appendix B). The hot modified acid-fast method presented here consistently provides excellent results (see Chapter 7, Figure 7.6).[22] In patients with few oocysts in the stool, the highly specific and sensitive fluorescent method using a monoclonal antibody reagent is more likely to reveal the organisms.[20,50]

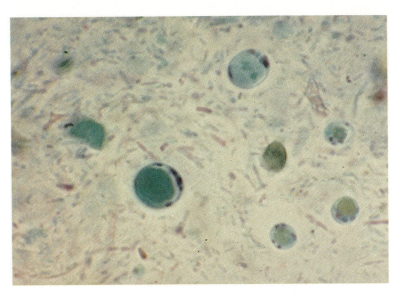

Figure 44.3
Blastocystis hominis (larger objects) and yeast cells (smaller, more homogenous objects).

44.2. Additional Techniques for Gastrointestinal Tract Specimens

44.2.a. Sigmoidoscopy material. When repeated fecal examinations fail to reveal the presence of *Entamoeba histolytica*, material obtained during sigmoidoscopy may be valuable in the diagnosis of amebiasis. However, this procedure does not take the place of routine fecal examinations; a series of at least three (six is preferable) fecal specimens should be submitted for each patient having a sigmoidoscopy examination. Material from the mucosal surface should be obtained by aspiration or scraping, not with a cotton-tipped swab. If swabs must be used, most of the cotton should be removed (leave just enough to safely cover the end) and should be tightly wound to prevent absorption of the material to be examined.

The specimen should be processed and examined immediately; the number of techniques used will depend on the amount of material obtained. If the specimen is sufficient for both wet preparations and permanent stained smears, proceed as follows. The direct mount should be examined immediately for the presence of moving trophozoites; it may take time for the organisms to become acclimated to this type of preparation; thus motility may not be obvious for several minutes. Care should be taken not to confuse protozoan organisms with macrophages or other tissue cells; any suspect cells should be con-

firmed with the use of the permanent stained slide. The smears for permanent staining should be prepared at the same time the direct mount is made by gently smearing some of the material onto several slides and immediately placing them into Schaudinn's fixative. The slides can then be stained by any of the techniques mentioned for routine fecal smears. If the material is bloody, contains a lot of mucus, or is a "wet" specimen, 1 or 2 drops of the sample can be mixed with 3 or 4 drops of PVA right on the slide. Allow the smears to dry (overnight if possible) prior to staining.

44.2.b. Duodenal contents. In some instances repeated fecal examinations may fail to confirm a diagnosis of *G. lamblia* and *Strongyloides stercoralis* infections. Since these two parasites are normally found in the duodenum, the physician may submit duodenal drainage fluid to the laboratory for examination. The specimen should be submitted without preservatives and should be received and examined within 1 hour after being taken. The amount of fluid may vary. It should be centrifuged and the sediment examined as wet mounts for the detection of motile organisms. Several mounts should be prepared and examined; because of the dilution factor, the organisms may be difficult to recover with this technique.

Another convenient method of sampling duodenal contents, which eliminates the necessity for intubation, is the use of the Entero-Test. This device consists of a gelatin capsule containing a weighted, coiled length of nylon yarn. The end of the line protrudes through the top of the capsule and is taped to the side of the patient's face. The capsule is then swallowed, the gelatin dissolves, and the weighted string is carried by peristalsis into the duodenum. After approximately 4 hours the string is recovered and the bile-stained mucus attached to the string is examined as a wet mount for the presence of organisms. This type of specimen should also be examined immediately after the string is recovered. When the mucus is examined from either duodenal drainage or the Entero-Test capsule, typical "falling leaf" motility of *G. lamblia* trophozoites is usually not visible. The flagella usually are visible as a rapid "flutter," with the organism remaining trapped in the mucus.

44.2.c. Estimation of worm burdens.

Although these procedures are not routinely performed, circumstances may arise when it is helpful to know the degree of infection in a patient or perhaps to follow the effectiveness of therapy. In certain helminth infections that have little clinical significance, the patient may not be given treatment if the numbers of parasites are small. The parasite burden may be estimated by counting the number of eggs passed in the stool.

The dilution egg-count technique developed by Stoll and Hausheer[51] has been widely used to estimate the number of adult worms present in several helminth infections, specifically hookworm, *Ascaris*, and *Trichuris*. The value of this type of procedure is based on repeated egg counts to detect changes in the numbers present. The direct smear method of Beaver[2,3] has also proved to be helpful in estimating the parasite burden.

Generally *T. trichiura* and hookworm are the only helminth infections in which the egg count will determine whether the patient will receive therapy; low egg counts usually correlate with a lack of clinical symptoms. Approximately 30,000 eggs of *T. trichiura* per gram indicate the presence of several hundred worms, a worm burden that usually causes definite symptoms. From 2000 to 5000 hookworm eggs per gram indicate a clinically significant infection.

NOTE: The presence of even one *Ascaris* is potentially dangerous; when irritated, the parasite tends to migrate while in the gastrointestinal tract, and this migratory habit may cause severe clinical symptoms in the patient.

44.2.d. Recovery of larval-stage nematodes.

Nematode infections that give rise to larval stages, which hatch either in the soil or in tissues, may be diagnosed by using culture techniques designed to concentrate the larvae. These procedures are used in hookworm, *Strongyloides*, and *Trichostrongylus* infections. Some of these techniques, which permit the recovery of infective-stage larvae, may be helpful since the eggs of many species are identical, and specific identifications are based on larval morphology.

Harada-Mori paper strip culture. As a means of detecting light infections and providing specific identifications, the Harada-Mori filter paper strip culture technique is very useful. The method was originally introduced by Harada and Mori[25] in 1955 and has been modified by several workers. Fecal specimens should not be refrigerated prior to culture; some of the nematodes are susceptible to cold and do not undergo further development. Since infective-stage larvae may be recovered from the culture system, gloves should be worn to handle the filter paper strip and other equipment.

Baermann technique. When the stools from a patient suspected of having strongyloidiasis are repeatedly negative, the Baermann technique may be helpful in recovering larvae. The apparatus is designed to allow the larvae to migrate from the fecal material through several layers of damp gauze into water, which is centrifuged, thus concentrating the larvae in the bottom of the tube.[21] Specimens for this technique should be collected after a mild saline cathartic, not a stool softener.

44.2.e. Hatching procedure for schistosome eggs.

When schistosome eggs are recovered from either urine or stool, they should be carefully examined to determine viability. The presence of living miracidia within the eggs indicates an active infection, which may require therapy. The viability of the miracidium larvae can be determined in two ways:

1. The cilia on the flame cells (primitive excretory cells) may be seen on high-dry power and are usually actively moving.
2. The larvae may be released from the eggs with the use of a hatching procedure.[21]

The eggs usually hatch within several hours when placed in 10 volumes of dechlorinated or spring water. The eggs, which are recovered in the urine, are easily obtained from the sediment and can be examined under the microscope to determine viability.

PROCEDURE 44.4

Examination of Cellophane Tape Preparations*

Principle

The female adult pinworm deposits her eggs during the night on the surface of the skin surrounding the anus. The eggs will adhere to the sticky surface of clear cellophane tape, on which they can be visualized microscopically.

Method

1. Place a strip of cellophane tape on a microscope slide, starting ½ inch (1.5 cm) from one end and, running toward the same end, continuing around this end across the slide; tear off the strip even with the other end. Place a strip of paper, ½ × 1 inch (1.5 × 2.5 cm), between the slide and the tape at the end where the tape is torn flush.
2. To obtain the sample from the perianal area, peel back the tape by gripping the label, and, with the tape looped adhesive side outward over a wooden tongue depressor held against the slide and extended about 1 inch (2.5 cm)

beyond it, press the tape firmly against the right and left perianal folds.
3. Spread the tape back on the slide, adhesive side down.
4. Place name and date on the label.
Note: *Do not use Magic transparent tape, but use regular clear cellophane tape.*
5. Lift one side of the tape and apply 1 *small drop* of toluene or xylene; press the tape down onto the glass slide.
6. The tape is now cleared; examine under low power and low illumination. The eggs should be visible if present; they are described as football-shaped with one slightly flattened side.

Quality control

The laboratory should retain control slides with known pinworm eggs for comparison, as well as take part in proficiency testing programs that include parasite unknowns.

*Refers to cellulose (Scotch) tape.

44.2.f. Cellophane tape preparations. *Enterobius vermicularis* is a roundworm that is worldwide in distribution. It is very common in children and is known as the "pinworm" or the "seatworm." The adult female migrates from the anus during the night and deposits her eggs on the perianal area. Since the eggs are deposited outside the gastrointestinal tract, examination of a stool specimen may produce negative results. Although some laboratories use the anal swab technique, pinworm infections are most frequently diagnosed by using the cellophane tape method (Procedure 44.4) for egg recovery. Another collection procedure is illustrated in Figure 44.4. Occasionally the adult female may be found on the surface of a formed stool or on the cellophane tape. Specimens should be taken in the morning *before bathing* or going to the bathroom. For small children, it is best to collect the specimen early in the morning, just before the child awakens.

A series of at least *four to six consecutive negative tapes* should be obtained before ruling out infection with pinworms. However, most laboratories rarely receive more than one or two tapes, and the clinician may decide to treat the patient on the basis of symptoms or recurrent symptoms after the initial diagnosis.

44.2.g. Identification of adult worms. Most adult worms or portions of worms that are submitted to the laboratory for identification are *A. lumbricoides, E. vermicularis,* or segments of tapeworms. The adult worms present no particular problems in identification (Section 44.14); however, identification of the *Taenia* species tapeworms is dependent on the gravid proglottids, which contain the fully developed uterine branches. Identification as to species is based on the number of lateral uterine branches that arise from the main uterine stem in the gravid proglottids. Often the uterine branches are not clearly visible;

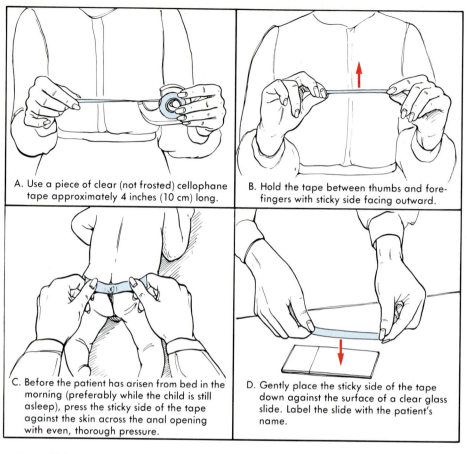

A. Use a piece of clear (not frosted) cellophane tape approximately 4 inches (10 cm) long.

B. Hold the tape between thumbs and forefingers with sticky side facing outward.

C. Before the patient has arisen from bed in the morning (preferably while the child is still asleep), press the sticky side of the tape against the skin across the anal opening with even, thorough pressure.

D. Gently place the sticky side of the tape down against the surface of a clear glass slide. Label the slide with the patient's name.

Figure 44.4

A method for collection of a cellulose (Scotch) tape preparation for pinworm diagnosis. This method dispenses with the tongue depressor (Procedure 44.4), requiring only tape and a glass microscope slide.

one technique that can be used is the injection of the branches with India ink (Procedure 44.5), allowing them to be easily seen and counted.

44.3. Urogenital Specimens (Trichomoniasis)

The identification of *Trichomonas vaginalis* is usually based on the examination of wet preparations of vaginal and urethral discharges and prostatic secretions. These specimens are diluted with a drop of saline and examined under low power with reduced illumination for the presence of actively motile organisms; urine sediment can be examined in the same way. As the jerky motility of the organisms begins to diminish, it may be possible to observe the undulating membrane, particularly under high-dry power (Figure 44.5). Stained smears are usually not

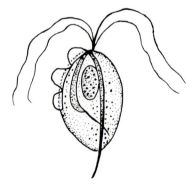

Figure 44.5

Trichomonas vaginalis trophozoite. (Illustration by Nobuko Kitamura.)

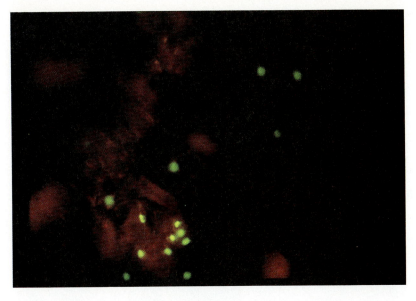

Figure 44.6
Fluorescein-conjugated monoclonal antibody–stained *T. vaginalis* in vaginal discharge (Courtesy Meridian Diagnostics, Inc., Cincinnati, Ohio.)

PROCEDURE 44.5

Identification of Adult Tapeworms

Principle

The uterus of gravid tapeworm proglottids (*Taenia* spp.) can be injected with India ink for visualization of the branches; the number of branches determines the species of tapeworm.

Method

1. Using a 1-ml syringe and 25- to 26-gauge needle, inject India ink into the central stem or into the uterine pore, filling the uterine branches with ink.
2. Press the proglottid between two slides, hold it up to the light, and count the branches (see Figure 44.66). (Besides Permount, Euparol is another mounting medium that can be used for tapeworm proglottids.)

Note: *Caution should be used in handling proglottids of* Taenia *species, since the eggs of* T. solium *are infective for humans.*

necessary for the identification of this organism; often the number of false-positive and false-negative results reported on the basis of stained smears would strongly suggest the value of confirmation (that is, observation of the motile organisms).

Some studies indicate that the most sensitive method of detecting *T. vaginalis* is culture. This technique may not be the most practical, and expense may limit its availability. Although commercial media are available, positive control strains should be used each time patient material is cultured. More sensitive and specific methods using monoclonal antibodies are also available. The specimen is smeared onto a glass slide, allowed to air dry, and then transported to the laboratory prior to testing by fluorescent methodology (Figure 44.6).[8]

44.4. Sputum (Paragonimiasis)

When sputum is submitted for examination, it should be "deep sputum" from the lower respiratory passages, not a specimen that is mainly saliva. The specimen should be collected early in the morning (before eating or brushing teeth) and immediately delivered to the laboratory. Sputum is usually examined as a saline or iodine wet mount under low and high-dry microscope power. If the quantity is

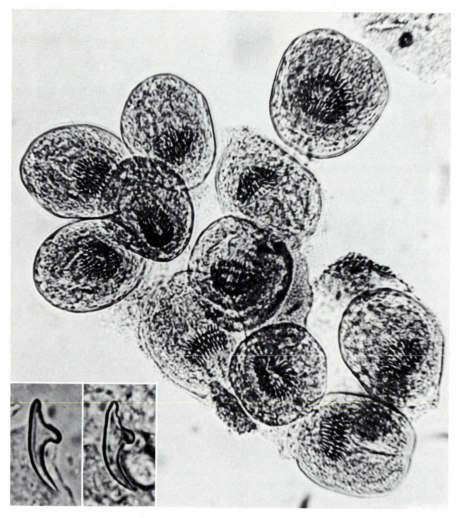

Figure 44.7
Echinococcus granulosus, hydatid sand. *Inset*, two individual hooklets (300 × ; inset 1000 ×).

sufficient, the formalin-ether sedimentation technique can be used. A very mucoid or thick sputum can be centrifuged after the addition of an equal volume of 3% sodium hydroxide. With any technique, the sediment should be carefully examined for the presence of brownish spots or "iron filings," which may be *Paragonimus* eggs.

NOTE: Care should be taken not to confuse *Entamoeba gingivalis*, which may be found in the mouth and might be seen in the sputum, with *E. histolytica* from a pulmonary abscess. *E. gingivalis* will contain ingested polymorphonuclear neutrophils (PMN); *E. histolytica* will not.

44.5. Aspirates

The diagnosis of certain parasitic infections may be based on procedures using aspirated material. These techniques include microscopic examination, animal inoculation, and culture.

Examination of aspirated material from lung or liver abscesses may reveal the presence of *E. histolytica*; however, the demonstration of these parasites is often extremely difficult for several reasons. Hepatic abscess material taken from the peripheral area, rather than the necrotic center, may reveal organisms, although they may be trapped in the thick pus and not exhibit any motility. The Amoebiasis Research Unit, Durban, South Africa, has rec-

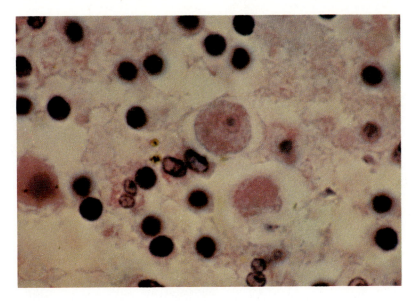

Figure 44.8
Naegleria in brain tissue. Hematoxylin and eosin stain.

ommended using proteolytic enzymes, such as 10 units of streptodornase per milliliter of thick pus, to free the organisms from the aspirate material.[21] The enzyme is incubated with the specimen for 30 minutes at 37° C with repeated shaking, the suspension is centrifuged, and the sediment is examined as for other direct examination methods.

Aspiration of cyst material (usually liver or lung) for the diagnosis of hydatid disease is usually performed when open surgical techniques are used for cyst removal. The aspirated fluid is submitted to the laboratory and examined for the presence of hydatid sand (scolices) or hooklets; the absence of this material does not rule out the possibility of hydatid disease, since some cysts are sterile (Figure 44.7).

Material from lymph nodes, spleen, liver, bone marrow, or spinal fluid may be examined for the presence of trypanosomes or leishmanial forms. Part of the specimen should be examined as a wet preparation to demonstrate motile organisms. Impression smears can also be prepared and stained with Giemsa stain (see Section 44.11). This type of material can also be cultured (see Section 44.8 for specific details).

Specimens obtained from cutaneous ulcers should be aspirated from below the ulcer bed rather than the surface; this type of sample will be more likely to contain the intracellular leishmanial organisms and will be free of bacterial contamination. A few drops of sterile saline may be introduced under the ulcer bed (through uninvolved tissue) by needle (25-gauge) and syringe (1 or 2 ml). The aspirated fluid should be examined as stained smears and should be inoculated into appropriate media (see Section 44.8).

44.6. Spinal Fluid

Cases of primary meningoencephalitis are infrequently seen, but the examination of spinal fluid may reveal the causative agent, *Naegleria fowleri* (Figure 44.8), if present. The spinal fluid may range from cloudy to purulent (with or without red blood cells). The cell count ranges from a few hundred to more than 20,000 white blood cells per milliliter, primarily neutrophils; the failure to find bacteria in this type of spinal fluid should alert one to the possibility of primary meningoencephalitis. Motile amebas may be found in unstained spinal fluid; however, one should be very careful not to confuse organisms with various blood and tissue cells that may also be motile, particularly if the spinal fluid is in a counting chamber.

The classification, transmission, virulence, and disease pathogenesis of the free-living amebic genera *Naegleria*, *Hartmannella*, and *Acanthamoeba* are receiving considerable attention at this time. The question of increasing infections has not been answered, although studies of thermally polluted or enriched waters indicate the presence of such amebas in these

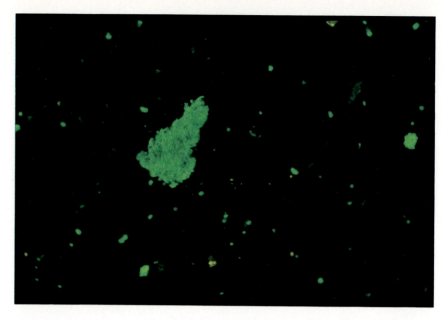

Figure 44.9
P. carinii cysts and trophozoites stained with a monoclonal antibody–fluorescent stain. (Courtesy Meridian Diagnostics, Inc., Cincinnati, Ohio.)

situations. Studies have also shown that these organisms have been recovered from asymptomatic human carriers (nasal passages, nasopharyngeal secretions) and have been implicated in chronic or subacute meningoencephalitis as well as acute primary amebic meningoencephalitis.

44.7. Biopsy Material

In some cases biopsy material may be used to confirm the diagnosis of certain parasitic infections. Most of these specimens are sent for routine tissue processing (fixation, embedding, sectioning, and staining). However, fresh material may be sent directly to the laboratory for examination; it is imperative that these specimens be received immediately to prevent deterioration of any organisms present. *Pneumocystis carinii* is recognized as an important cause of pulmonary infection in patients who are immunosuppressed as a result of therapy or patients with congenital or acquired immunological disorders, including acquired immunodeficiency syndrome (AIDS).[37] The organisms can be demonstrated in stained impression smears of lung material obtained by open, transbronchial, or brush biopsy. *Pneumocystis* can be seen in stained smears of tracheobronchial aspirates, although preparations of lung tissue are more likely to reveal the organisms. Bronchoalveolar lavage has a lower yield than trans-

bronchial biopsy, but it is helpful when biopsy is contraindicated. The usefulness of induced sputum has been evaluated, and it is becoming more widely used, particularly when obtained from patients with AIDS and when coupled with the monoclonal antibody diagnostic procedure (Figure 44.9).[5,23,30,52] Sputum specimens are generally considered unacceptable for the detection of *Pneumocystis*.

Regardless of the technique used, multiple specimens may have to be examined to confirm the presence of *P. carinii* organisms. Although a number of different stains are available, the stain most often recommended is Gomori's methenamine silver (GMS), which clearly stains *Pneumocystis* organisms in dark brown or black (Figure 44.10, *A*). Preparation of the silver stain is relatively complex (Procedure 44.6), and positive control slides should be included with each specimen to ensure accurate identification of the smears. Although the silver stain yields the most definitive results, toluidine blue O stains are much easier and faster to perform and yield reliable results in the hands of skilled technologists (Figure 44.10, *B*). One modified toluidine blue O method developed at the National Institutes of Health is described in Procedure 44.7.

Cryptosporidium sp. are coccidial protozoa usually found in the intestinal tract. Respiratory cryptosporidiosis has also been reported as well as in-

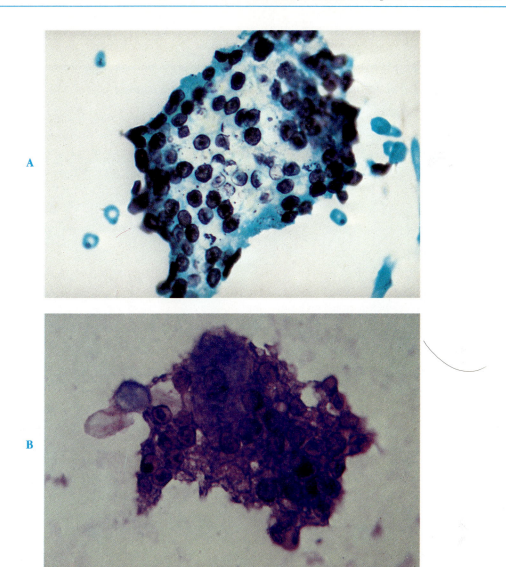

Figure 44.10
A, Cysts of *P. carinii* in bronchial lavage, stained with modified Gomori methenamine silver stain
(1000 ×). **B,** Toluidine blue O stained cysts of *P. carinii* in smear made from centrifuged sediment
from bronchial lavage specimen (1000 ×).

fection of the gallbladder and biliary tree. Human
cryptosporidiosis has been confirmed from gastrointestinal biopsies (and more recently from stool)
from patients whose immune responses were diminished (including AIDS patients) and those with normal immune systems. Cryptosporidia differ from
other coccidia in that they are limited to the mi-
crovillus layer of gastrointestinal cells. Tissue diagnosis has been based on electron microscopy studies

and Giemsa-stained smears from jejunal biopsy material and routine tissue processing (paraffin embedding and sectioning). This organism has definitely
become more widely recognized as a potential pathogen in both immunosuppressed and immunocompetent hosts, and other diagnostic procedures have
been developed to facilitate organism recovery and
identification, that is, modified acid-fast staining
methods of stool (modified Kinyoun's stain, Appen-

PROCEDURE 44.6

Gomori Methenamine Silver Stain (GMS) (80° C Methenamine–Silver Nitrate Stain)

Principle

Hot, acidified metal ions will precipitate on the cell walls of parasites and fungi, rendering them visible in specimen material.

Method

1. Prepare reagents as follows:
    a. Chromic acid (5% solution)

Chromic acid (Fisher Scientific)	50 g
Distilled deionized water	1000 ml

   Weigh out 50 g chromic acid and dissolve in 1 L distilled water. Solution usable for up to 1 year.

    b. Methenamine (3% solution)

Hexamethylenetetramine (Fisher Scientific)	12 g
Distilled deionized water	400 ml

   Weigh out 12 g hexamethylenetetramine and dissolve in 400 ml distilled water. Solution usable for up to 6 months.

    c. Silver nitrate (5% solution)

Silver nitrate (Fisher Scientific)	5 g
Distilled deionized water	100 ml

   Weigh out 5 g silver nitrate and dissolve in 100 ml distilled water. Solution is usable for up to 6 months.

    d. Stock methenamine-silver nitrate

Methenamine (3% solution)	400 ml
Silver nitrate (5% solution)	20 ml

   A white precipitate forms when reagents are added together but immediately clears with mixing. Store at 4° C. The solution is usable for up to 1 month.

    e. Borax (5% solution)

Borax (sodium borate) (Fisher Scientific)	5 g
Distilled deionized water	100 ml

   Dissolve sodium borate in distilled water. Solution usable for up to 1 year.

    f. Sodium bisulfite (1% solution)

Sodium bisulfite (Fisher Scientific)	10 g
Distilled deionized water	1000 ml

   Weigh out sodium bisulfite and add to distilled water. Solution usable for up to 1 year.

    g. Gold chloride (0.2% solution)

Gold chloride (chloroauric acid; Fisher Scientific)	0.5 g
Distilled deionized water	250 ml

   Weigh out gold chloride and add to distilled water. Solution usable for up to 1 year.

    h. Sodium thiosulfate (2% solution)

Sodium thiosulfate (Fisher Scientific)	20 g
Distilled deionized water	1000 ml

   Solution usable for up to 1 year.

    i. Stock light green solution

Light green SF-Yellowish (Harleco)	0.2 g
Distilled deionized water	100 ml
Glacial acetic acid	0.2 ml

   Solution usable for up to 1 year.

    j. Working light green solution

Stock light green solution	10 ml
Distilled deionized water	40 ml

   Solution usable for up to 1 month.

    k. Fill two Coplin jars each with absolute ethanol and 95% ethanol. These jars may be sealed with screw caps and the reagents can be reused until they become cloudy.
    l. Fill two Coplin jars with xylene. These jars may be sealed and the xylene can be reused.

Modified by the UCLA parasitology laboratory from Pintozzi, R. 1978. J. Clin. Pathol. 31:803.

2. Immediately before each staining procedure, prepare working methenamine–silver nitrate as follows:

Stock methenamine–silver nitrate	25 ml
Distilled deionized water	25 ml
Borax (5% solution)	2 ml

This solution must be prepared fresh in a Coplin jar for each set of slides stained. It is not reusable, even for a second staining procedure performed immediately afterward.

3. Staining procedure
   a. Turn on water bath allowing 45 to 60 min to reach 80° C.
   b. Prepare smears and air dry. Heat-fix all smears at 70° C for 10 min on a heating block.
   c. Fix smears in absolute *methanol* for a minimum of 3 min.
   d. Place two Coplin jars, one containing 5% chromic acid (approximately 50 ml) and the other containing working methenamine solution into 80° C water bath for 5 min.
   e. Place smears into heated 5% chromic acid. Incubate in water bath at 80° C for 2 min.
   f. Remove slides from chromic acid and place in Coplin jar with distilled water. Rinse slides in three changes of distilled water.
   g. Place slides in 1% sodium bisulfite for 30 s.
   h. Rinse in three changes of distilled water.
   i. Place slides in heated methenamine working solution. Incubate in water bath at 80° C for 4½ min.
   j. Place slides in Coplin jar with distilled water. Rinse in three changes of distilled water.
   k. Wipe the back of slides with a paper towel to remove excess methenamine.
   l. Tone in 0.2% gold chloride for 30 s; background lightens in this step.
   m. Rinse in three changes distilled water.
   n. Place slides in 2% sodium thiosulfate for 30 s to remove unreduced silver.
   o. Rinse in three changes of distilled water.
   p. Counterstain in light green working solution for 30 s.
   q. Rinse in three changes of distilled water.
   r. Dehydrate and clear for 30-s intervals in two changes each of 95% ethanol, 100% ethanol, and xylene, respectively.
   s. Place coverslips on slides with Permount while the slides are still wet with xylene. Slides are ready to be read.

4. Interpretation: Background will be green and *Pneumocystis* cysts will appear gray to black. They are spherical, may be punched in and cup shaped, and may show black parentheses-like structures in the center (Figure 44.10, *A*). The cysts tend to occur in groups.

Quality control

Specimens from positive patients should be smeared onto numerous slides, which are fixed and stored. One positive control slide should be stained along with each batch of patient slides. The proper appearance of cysts on the control slide is a requirement for interpretation and reporting of the patient slides.

PROCEDURE 44.7

Modified Toluidine Blue O Stain for Pneumocystis carinii

Principle

The thick cyst wall of parasites and the cell wall of some fungi, after sulfation treatment, will absorb and retain toluidine blue O stain.

Method

1. Prepare the specimen as follows:
   a. For tissue, make touch preparations on clean slides by touching the cut surface of tissue to the slide and squeezing the tissue down to express infectious agents. Allow the smears to air dry.
   b. For sputum, if thin and watery, simply make thin smears. If thick and mucuslike, combine with equal amount of sputolysin (diluted 1:10 in water), vortex, and allow to stand 30 min before revortexing and preparing thin smears.
   c. For bronchoalveolar lavage or washing, centrifuge for at least 10 min at 3000 rpm. Pour off supernatant. Prepare slides from sediment; if thick, treat as sputum. If possible, choose mucoid-appearing flecks.
2. Prepare solution A, sulfation reagent
   a. Add 15 ml 1 N NaOH to 35 ml ether (USP) in a separating funnel and shake vigorously for 1 min. Release the stopcock oc-

casionally to relieve pressure. Drain the NaOH phase out the bottom of the funnel. Repeat this procedure once again to remove impurities and preservatives from the ether.
   b. Add 10 ml distilled water to the 35 ml ether (USP) in the separating funnel and shake vigorously for 1 min. Release the stopcock occasionally to relieve pressure. Repeat this procedure once again. The ether should be fully saturated with water at this point. Allow the two solutions to separate and discard the water layer (the lower phase) by allowing it to run out the bottom of the funnel. Allow a few milliliters of the ether phase to run out also, to ensure that no water is left.
   c. Transfer the remaining 25 ml of water-saturated ether to a 100-ml Erlenmeyer flask immersed in an ice water bath. Allow to cool for 5 min. Place the ice bath under a chemical fume hood. Slowly add 25 ml concentrated sulfuric acid while continuously shaking the flask. Mix contents well and pour the reagent into a Coplin jar.

Modified by Beverly Tenenbaum, North Shore University, Manhasset, N.Y., from Witebsky, F.G., et al. 1988. Modified toluidine blue O stain for *Pneumocystis carinii*: further evaluation of some technical factors. J. Clin. Microbiol. 26:774.

dix B; see Section 44.12.d). The organisms may also be visible as refractile bodies in smears made directly or from concentrated feces.

Biopsy specimens from the intestinal tract, particularly in AIDS patients, may reveal microsporidian organisms, although electron microscopy may be necessary for confirmation. Microsporidiosis is still considered to be rare; effective diagnostic methods using stool specimens have not yet been developed.[13,31,53]

Corneal scrapings or biopsy specimens can be examined by routine histology, calcofluor white

stain, or culture for the presence of *Acanthamoeba*.[21,59] Although these infections are relatively rare, the medical community has become much more aware of *Acanthamoeba* keratitis, especially among contact lens wearers, during the last few years.*

Skin biopsy specimens for the diagnosis of cutaneous amebiasis or cutaneous leishmaniasis should be submitted for tissue processing. A portion of the

---

*References 1, 9, 10, 16, 18, 32, 40.

The solution is stored at room temperature and prepared fresh weekly. The jar is sealed with stopcock grease to prevent evaporation. After 10 slides have been stained, discard the reagent and use fresh reagent.

3. Prepare solution B, Toluidine blue O.

   a. In a Coplin jar under a fume hood, place: 0.06 g toluidine blue O (Fisher Scientific Co., Aldrich, and others) and add 15 ml distilled water. Swirl vigorously to dissolve the dye in the water. Add, in order:

Hydrochloric acid (concentrated)	0.5 ml
Absolute ethanol	35 ml

   Screw the cap of the Coplin jar tightly closed. The stain solution can be kept at room temperature and reused for 1 month. Add fresh stain when the level drops.

4. Fix slides for 1 min in absolute *ethanol*. Allow to dry.

5. Place slides in solution A for 10 min, dipping them twice when they are initially immersed. Stir with a glass stirring rod after each 5-min period.

6. Place them into a Coplin jar filled with tap water. Allow the jar to sit under running cold tap water for 5 min.

7. Place slides into solution B for 3 min.

8. Dehydrate slides by dipping them for approximately 10 seconds into a jar of 95% alcohol or until they are clean.

9. Dip slides into a jar of absolute ethanol for another 10 sec for further decolorizing.

10. Clear slides by dipping them into a jar of xylene (10 s).

11. Mount coverslips with Permount or similar mounting medium. Slides can be examined immediately.

12. Observe for cysts of *Pneumocystis*, which appear reddish blue or purple against a blue background (Figure 44.10, *B*). The organisms are often seen in clumps, particularly in areas of frothy looking material. If there is no difference in color between cysts and background, try using toluidine blue from another source. Cysts are occasionally punched in, appearing crescent-shaped.

Quality control

Stain a known positive control slide with each patient specimen run.

tissue for the diagnosis of leishmaniasis can be teased apart with sterile needles and inoculated into appropriate culture media (see Section 44.8).

The diagnosis of onchocerciasis *(Onchocerca volvulus)* may be confirmed by the examination of "skin snips," very thin slices of skin, which are teased apart in saline to release the microfilariae.

Biopsy specimens taken from lymph nodes are submitted for routine tissue processing; impression smears can also be prepared and stained with Giemsa stain (see Section 44.11). The diagnosis of trichinosis is usually based on clinical findings; however, con-firmation may be obtained by the examination of a muscle biopsy (Figure 44.11). The encapsulated larvae can be seen in small pieces of fresh tissue, which are pressed between two slides and examined under low power of the microscope. At necropsy the larvae are most abundant in the diaphragm, masseter muscle, or tongue. Larvae can also be recovered from tissue that has undergone digestion in artificial digestive fluid at 37° C. Figure 44.12 shows the life cycle of this organism.

Tapeworm larvae may occasionally be recovered from a muscle specimen and should be carefully dis-

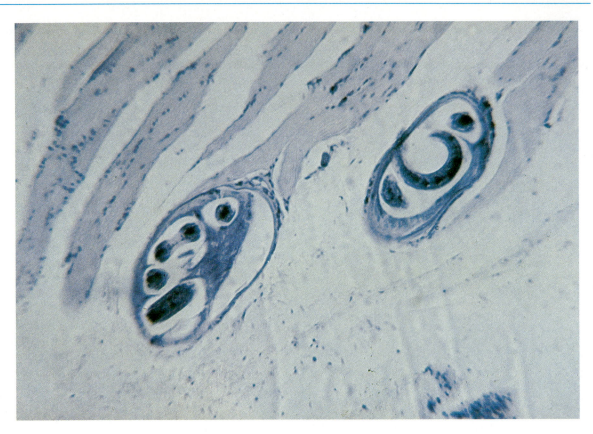

Figure 44.11
Trichinella spiralis larvae (encysted in muscle).

Figure 44.12
Life cycle of *Trichinella spiralis*.

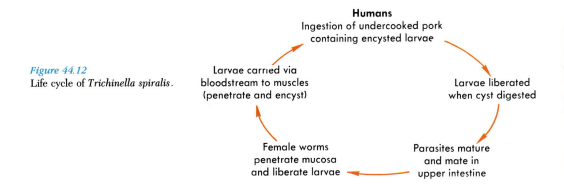

Humans
Ingestion of undercooked pork
containing encysted larvae

Larvae carried via
bloodstream to muscles
(penetrate and encyst)

Larvae liberated
when cyst digested

Female worms
penetrate mucosa
and liberate larvae

Parasites mature
and mate in
upper intestine

sected from the capsules. They should then be pressed between two slides and examined under low power for the presence of a scolex with four suckers and a circle of hooks. If no hooks are present, it may be a species other than *Taenia solium*.

In some cases of schistosomiasis, the eggs may not be recovered in the stool or urine; however, examination of the rectal or bladder mucosa may reveal eggs of the appropriate species. The mucosal tissue should be compressed between two slides and examined under low power and decreased illumination. The eggs should be carefully examined to determine viability (Section 44.2.e). Small pieces of tissue may be digested with 4% sodium hydroxide for 2 to 3 hours at 60° to 80° C. The eggs, which are recovered by sedimentation or centrifugation, can be examined under the microscope.

44.8. Culture Techniques

Most clinical laboratories do not provide culture techniques for the diagnosis of parasitic organisms; however, the lack of culture procedures should not prevent the correct identification of the majority of parasites. Isolation of intestinal amebas yields a higher number of positive results, provided fresh specimens are received by the laboratory within specified time limits. Most of the intestinal amebas do not culture as well as *E. histolytica;* however, once the organisms are established in culture, they must be speciated on the basis of morphology. Accurate identification of the organisms can be determined by the examination of permanent stained smears of culture sediment material, although the morphology may not appear typical from stained culture sediment.

Many different media have been developed for the culture of protozoan organisms (some of which are available commercially), and specific directions for their preparation are available in the literature. Types of media that have been widely used include: amebas—Balamuth's aqueous egg yolk infusion[35] and Boeck and Drbohlav's Locke-egg-serum medium[36]; *T. vaginalis*—Lash's casein hydrolysate serum medium[21] and Feinberg medium[17]; *Acanthamoeba*[21]; leishmaniae and trypanosomes—Novy-MacNeal-Nicolle medium,[21] diphasic blood agar medium (NIH method),[21] and Schneider's *Drosophila* medium.[27] Techniques for the culture and isolation of other organisms (*G. lamblia*, *Plasmodium* species, and some of the helminths) are more difficult and are often reserved for research purposes. One method for culture of free-living amebas is given in Procedure 44.8.

44.9. Animal Inoculation

Most laboratories have neither the time nor facilities for animal care to provide animal inoculation procedures for the diagnosis of parasitic infections. Host specificity for many parasites also limits the kinds of laboratory animals available for these procedures. Occasionally animal studies may be requested; included here are several procedures that can be used.

The hamster is the animal of choice for inocula-tion procedures designed to recover leishmanial organisms. After intraperitoneal or intratesticular inoculation, the infection may develop very slowly over a period of several months; in some cases a generalized infection develops more quickly, and the animal may die in several days. Splenic and testicular aspirates should be examined for the presence of intracellular organisms; stained smears should be prepared and carefully examined with the oil immersion lens.

Mice are generally used for the isolation of *Toxoplasma gondii*, although most cases are diagnosed on clinical and serologic findings. Mice that are inoculated through the peritoneum develop a fulminating infection that leads to death within a few days. Organisms can be easily recovered from the ascitic fluid and should be examined as stained smears. Giemsa stain is recommended for both intraperitoneal and intratesticular inoculation studies (specific staining techniques are found in Section 44.11).

44.10. Serodiagnosis

Although serologic procedures for the diagnosis of parasitic diseases have been available for many years, they are generally not performed by most clinical laboratories. The procedures vary both in sensitivity and specificity and at times may be difficult to interpret. The Centers for Disease Control (CDC) offers several serologic procedures for diagnostic purposes, some of which are still in the experimental stages and not available elsewhere. For a discussion of specific procedures, see Chapter 12. Although commercial antigens and diagnostic kits are available, results from different reagents have been variable.[28] Developmental work using monoclonal reagents is in progress, and some commercially prepared kits and components are now available.[21]

The enzyme-linked immunosorbent assay (ELISA) procedure is presently being evaluated for a number of parasitic infections. A significant contribution of the ELISA method will be detection of antigen in the body fluids of patients with parasitic diseases. With purified antigens the usefulness of techniques such as radioimmunoassay, ELISA, FIAX, and defined antigen substrate spheres (DASS) will be greatly expanded. At the present time immunodiagnostic procedures are most widely used for amebiasis, toxoplasmosis, leishmaniasis, Chagas' dis-

PROCEDURE 44.8

Cultivation of N. fowleri *and* Acanthamoeba *Species*[21]

Principle

Free-living amebae can be cultivated on nonnutrient agar on a lawn of bacteria, which provide the nutrients.

Method

1. Prepare Page's saline:

NaCl	60 mg
$MgSO_4 \cdot 7H_2O$	2 mg
$CaCl_2 \cdot 2H_2O$	2 mg
Na_2HPO_4	71 mg
KH_2PO_4	68 mg
Distilled water	500 ml

    Autoclave at 15 psi for 15 min; store in glass bottle in refrigerator; solution is usable for up to 6 mo.

2. Prepare Nonnutrient agar:

Page's saline	100 ml
Difco agar	1.5 g

    a. Dissolve agar in Page's saline with gentle heating—stir or swirl.

    b. Aliquot 20 ml into screw-capped tubes (20 × 150 mm).

    c. Autoclave at 15 psi for 15 min; label deeps with 12-mo expiration date; store in refrigerator.

Plate Preparation

Melt agar deeps and pour into Petri dishes as needed. Plates may be stored in the refrigerator up to 3 mos.

Culture

1. Warm two agar plates per specimen in a 37° C incubator for 30 mins.

2. Add 0.5-ml Page's saline to a slant culture of *Escherichia coli*

3. Gently scrape surface of slant (do not break agar surface) and uniformly suspend the bacteria. Add 2 to 3 drops of suspension to middle of warm agar plate.

4. Spread the bacteria on the agar surface with a bacteriological loop.

5. Inoculate 2 to 3 drops of specimen sediment (ground tissue in Page's saline or centrifuged CSF) in the center of the agar plate.

6. Seal the edges of each plate with cellophane tape to prevent drying, and incubate in air for 7 days; one plate at 37° C and one plate at 42° C.

7. Examine the surface of the agar with the low-power objective of a microscope (100×) daily for motile amebas. Amebas may become visible within 48 h.

8. If viable amebas are found, they may be fixed and permanently stained by emulsifying a loopful scraped from the surface of the plate in a tiny amount of Page's saline in a small test tube.

9. Add 3 parts polyvinyl-alcohol (see PVA Fixative), and prepare a thin smear as for staining PVA-fixed fecal specimens.

10. Stain the smear with trichrome stain and observe for trophozoites.

Culture Examination

Examine plates every day (7 days) with 10× objective; cysts will be visible within 4 to 5 days, trophozoites earlier. Positive areas of agar can be cut out and placed face down on new plate coated with bacteria (culture transfer).

Quality control

Positive control strains (available from ATCC) should always be cultured in parallel with patient specimens to confirm efficacy of culture system.

*Modified from Page, F.C. 1976. An illustrated key to freshwater and soil amoeba. Freshwater Biological Association Scientific Publication 34, Ferry Moose Ambeside, Cumbria, England.

ease, trichinosis, schistosomiasis, cysticercosis, and hydatid disease.

44.11. Detection of Blood Parasites

44.11.a. Laboratory diagnosis of malaria. Malaria is one of the few acute parasitic infections that can be life-threatening. For this reason any laboratory that offers this type of diagnostic service must be willing to provide technical expertise on a 24-hour basis, 7 days per week.

The definitive diagnosis of malaria is based on the demonstration of the parasites in the blood. Two types of blood films are used. The "thick smear" (Figure 44.13) allows the examination of a larger amount of blood and is used as a screening procedure; the "thin film" allows species identification of the parasite.

Blood films are usually prepared when the patient is admitted; samples should be taken at intervals of 6 to 18 hours for at least three successive days. Two to three hundred microscopic fields should be examined before a film is signed out as negative. If possible, the smears should be prepared from blood obtained from the finger or earlobe; the blood should flow freely. If patient contact is not possible and the quality of the submitted slides may be poor, a tube of fresh blood should be requested (ethylenedi-aminetetraacetic acid [EDTA] anticoagulant is recommended), and smears should be prepared immediately after the blood is received. It is even better to use the blood remaining in the needle from a venipuncture for smear preparation because this blood has not been in contact with any anticoagulant.

To prepare the thick film, place 2 or 3 small drops of fresh blood on an alcohol-cleaned slide. With the corner of another slide, and using a circular motion, mix the drops and spread the blood over an area about 2 cm in diameter. Continue stirring for about 30 seconds to prevent formation of fibrin strands, which may obscure the parasites after staining. If the blood is too thick or any grease remains on the slide, the blood will flake off during staining. Allow the film to air dry (room temperature) in a dust-free area. Never apply heat to a thick film since heat will fix the blood, causing the red blood cells to remain intact during staining; the result is stain retention and subsequent inability to identify any parasites present.

The thin blood film is used primarily for specific parasite identification, although the number of or-

ganisms per field is much reduced compared with the thick film. The thin film is prepared in exactly the same manner one used for the differential blood count. After the film has air dried (do not apply heat), it may be stained. The necessity for fixation before staining depends on the stain selected.

44.11.b. Staining blood films. For accurate identification of blood parasites, it is very important that a laboratory develop proficiency in the use of at least one good staining method. As a general rule, blood films should be stained as soon as possible, since prolonged storage results in stain retention. The stains used are generally of two types. One has the fixative in combination with the staining solution, so that both fixation and staining occur at the same time. Wright stain (Appendix B) is an example of this type of staining solution. Giemsa stain (Appendix B) represents the other type of staining solution, in which the fixative and stain are separate; thus, the thin film must be fixed prior to staining (Procedures 44.9 and 44.10). There are also methods available for the identification of malarial parasites with the use of acridine orange (Appendix B) and other DNA-binding dyes, the smears being examined using fluorescence microscopy.

When slides are removed from either type of staining solution, they should be dried in a vertical position. After being air dried, they may be examined under oil immersion by placing the oil directly on the uncovered blood film.

Specimens may be submitted from patients with *Plasmodium falciparum* infections who do not yet have gametocytes in the blood. Consequently, a low-level parasitemia with delicate ring forms might be missed without extensive oil immersion examination of the blood films (at least 200 to 300 oil immersion fields).

NOTE: Remember that automated differential instruments used in hematology laboratories are not designed to recognize intracellular (red blood cell) parasites. Any suspected parasitic infection or presumptive diagnosis of fever of unknown origin mandates a manual blood smear examination.[21]

There have been many studies using immunodiagnostic procedures for the diagnosis of malaria; However, these procedures are not routinely performed in most laboratories. Sulzer and Wilson[54] have reported the use of thick-smear antigens prepared from washed parasitized blood cells. This type of antigen is used in the indirect fluorescent antibody (IFA) procedure, which has a 95% sensitivity and a

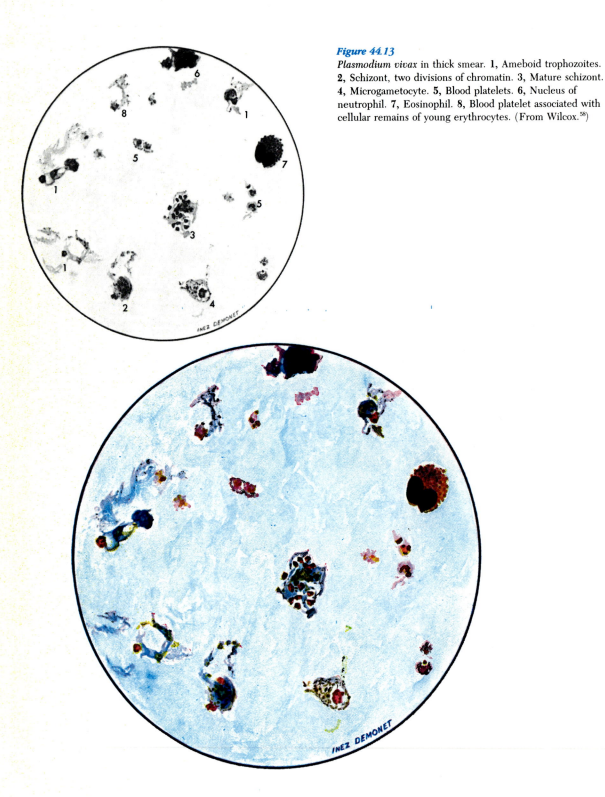

Figure 44.13
Plasmodium vivax in thick smear. **1,** Ameboid trophozoites. **2,** Schizont, two divisions of chromatin. **3,** Mature schizont. **4,** Microgametocyte. **5,** Blood platelets. **6,** Nucleus of neutrophil. **7,** Eosinophil. **8,** Blood platelet associated with cellular remains of young erythrocytes. (From Wilcox.[58])

PROCEDURE 44.9

Staining Thin Films

Principle

By spreading the blood cells in a thin layer, the size of red cells, inclusions, and extracellular forms can be more easily visualized.

Method

1. Fix blood films in absolute methanol (acetone-free) for 30 s.
2. Allow slides to air dry.
3. Immerse slides in a solution of 1 part Giemsa stock (commercial liquid stain or stock prepared from powder) to 10 to 50 parts of Triton-buffered water (pH 7.0 to 7.2). Stain 10 to 60 min (see note below). Fresh working stain should be prepared from stock solution each day.
4. Dip slides briefly in Triton X-100 buffered water.
5. Drain thoroughly in vertical position and allow to air dry.

Note: *A good general rule for stain dilution versus staining time is that if dilution is 1:20, stain for 20 min; if 1:30, stain for 30 min; and so forth.*

However, a series of stain dilutions and staining times should be tried to determine the best dilution/time for each batch of stock stain.

Expected results

Giemsa stain colors the components of blood as follows: erythrocytes, pale gray-blue; nuclei of white blood cells, purple and pale purple cytoplasm; eosinophilic granules, bright purple-red; neutrophilic granules, deep pink-purple. Parasitic forms are blue to purple, with reddish nuclei. Their characteristic morphologies are used for differentiation. Inexperienced workers may confuse platelets with parasites.

Quality control

Known positive blood films should be stained periodically along with patient specimens. The laboratory should maintain control slides for comparison and participate in a proficiency testing program for blood parasites.

PROCEDURE 44.10

Staining Thick Films

Principle

A large amount of blood can be examined for parasitic forms by lysing the red cells and staining for parasites. The lack of methanol fixation allows lysis of red cells by the aqueous stain solution. Although parasites can be found in the larger volume of blood, definitive morphologic criteria necessary for specific organism identification may be more difficult to see.

Method

The procedure to be followed for thick films is the same as for thin films, except that the first two steps are omitted. If the slide has a thick film at one end and a thin film at the other, fix only the thin portion, and then stain both parts of the film simultaneously.

Quality control

Follow the same program as outlined for Procedure 44.9.

false-positive rate of 1% at a titer of 1:16.[55] Indirect hemagglutination assay (IHA) has also been used and evaluated by a number of workers. The newly developed polymerase chain reaction has even been used for amplification and subsequent detection of malarial DNA in blood.

In some areas of the world where *P. falciparum* is endemic, there are also high incidences of hemoglobin S (HbS), thalassemia, and glucose-6-phosphate dehydrogenase (G-6-PD)-deficiency carriers. The young heterozygous carrier of HbS gains some protection against *P. falciparum*. Apparently, G-6-PD deficiency and thalassemia are also associated with increased resistance.

Miller and coworkers[39] reported that Duffy-positive human erythrocytes are easily infected with *Plasmodium knowlesi;* however, Duffy-negative human erythrocytes are resistant to infection. They suggest that the resistance of many west Africans and approximately 70% of American blacks to *Plasmodium vivax* may be related to the high incidence of Duffy-negative erythrocytes in these groups. In east Africa, where there is a higher incidence of Duffy-positive red cells, *P. vivax* is more common.

IDENTIFICATION OF ANIMAL PARASITES
44.12. Intestinal Protozoa

The protozoa are unicellular organisms, most of which are microscopic. They possess a number of specialized organelles, which are responsible for life functions and which allow further division of the group into classes.

The class Sarcodina contains the organisms that move by means of cytoplasmic protrusions called pseudopodia. Included in this group are free-living organisms, as well as nonpathogenic and pathogenic organisms found in the intestinal tract and other areas of the body.

The Mastigophora, or flagellates, contain specialized locomotor organelles called flagella: long, thin cytoplasmic extensions that may vary in number and position depending on the species. Different genera may live in the intestinal tract, the bloodstream, or various tissues. Diagnosis of the blood- and tissue-dwelling flagellates is discussed in Section 44.11.

The class Ciliata contains a number of species that move by means of cilia, short extensions of cytoplasm that cover the surface of the organism. This group contains only one organism that infects humans: *Balantidium coli* infects the intestinal tract and may produce severe symptoms.

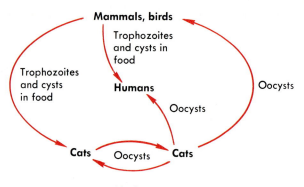

Figure 44.14
Life cycle of *Toxoplasma gondii*.

Members of the class Sporozoa are found in the blood and other tissues and have a complex life cycle that involves both sexual and asexual generations. The four species of *Plasmodium*, the cause of malaria, are found in this group; their diagnosis is discussed in Section 44.11. Members of the genera *Isospora* and *Cryptosporidium* and the microsporidia can be found in the intestinal mucosa. These organisms have been seen with increasing frequency in specimens from immunosuppressed patients, particularly those with AIDS.[11,42,43]

Isospora and *Cryptosporidium* are passed in the stool as oocysts; the other members of the protozoa exist in the intestinal tract in the trophozoite or cyst stages. In the case of *Enterocytozoon* (one of the genera of microsporidia that can infect humans), there are spore stages in the life cycle that are probably passed in the stool.[15] However, at the present time there are no practical diagnostic tests capable of revealing these organisms. Considering the spore size (approximately 1 to 4 µm), the clinical laboratory may have to wait until monoclonal antibodies are produced for detection of spores. The coccidian parasite *T. gondii* is acquired by humans via ingestion, although its life cycle includes stages in several animal hosts, particularly cats (Figure 44.14). The trophozoites may be seen in squash preparations from lymph nodes or brain tissue, usually examined by pathologists.

The important characteristics of the intestinal protozoa are found in Tables 44.3 to 44.8. The clinically important intestinal protozoa are generally considered to be *E. histolytica, Dientamoeba fragilis, G. lamblia, I. belli, Cryptosporidium,* and *B. coli. E. histolytica* is the most important species and may invade other tissues of the body, resulting in

Text continued on p. 816.

Table 44.3
Morphologic Criteria Used to Identify Intestinal Amebic Trophozoites

	ENTAMOEBA HISTOLYTICA	*ENTAMOEBA HARTMANNI*	*ENTAMOEBA COLI*	*ENDOLIMAX NANA*	*IODAMOEBA BÜTSCHLII*
Size (diameter or length)*	12-60 μm; usual range, 15-20 μm; invasive forms may be >20 μm	5-12 μm; usual range, 8-10 μm	15-50 μm; usual range, 20-25 μm	6-12 μm; usual range, 8-10 μm	8-20 μm usual range, 12-15 μm
Motility	Progressive with hyaline, fingerlike pseudopods, motility may be rapid	Usually nonprogressive	Sluggish, nondirectional, with blunt pseudopods	Sluggish, usually nonprogressive	Sluggish, usually nonprogressive
Number of nuclei	One; difficult to see in unstained preparations, usually not seen	One; usually not seen in unstained preparations	One; often visible in unstained preparations	One; occasionally visible in unstained preparations	One; usually not visible in unstained preparations
Nucleus					
Peripheral chromatin (stained)	Fine granules, uniform in size, usually evenly distributed; may have beaded appearance	May appear as solid ring rather than beaded; nucleus may stain more darkly than *E. histolytica*, although morphology is similar	May be clumped and unevenly arranged on membrane; may also appear as solid, dark ring with no beads or clumps	No peripheral chromatin	No peripheral chromatin
Karyosome (stained)	Small, usually compact; centrally located but may also be eccentric	Usually small and compact; may be centrally located or eccentric	Large, not compact; may or may not be eccentric; may be diffuse and darkly stained	Large, irregularly shaped; may appear "blotlike"; many nuclear variations common	Large, may be surrounded by refractile granules that are difficult to see
Cytoplasm					
Appearance (stained)	Finely granular, "ground-glass" appearance; clear differentiation of ectoplasm and endoplasm; if present, vacuoles usually small	Finely granular	Granular with little differentiation into ectoplasm and endoplasm; usually vacuolated	Granular, vacuolated	Coarsely granular; may be highly vacuolated
Inclusions (stained)	Noninvasive organism may contain bacteria; presence of red blood cells diagnostic	May contain bacteria; no red blood cells	Bacteria, yeast, other debris	Bacteria	Bacteria, yeast, other debris

*These sizes refer to wet preparation measurements. Organisms on a permanent stained smear may be 1 to 1.5 μm smaller because of artificial shrinkage.

Table 44.4
Morphologic Criteria Used to Identify Intestinal Flagellate Trophozoites

	DIENTAMOEBA FRAGILIS	TRICHOMONAS HOMINIS	GIARDIA LAMBLIA	CHILOMASTIX MESNILI	ENTEROMONAS HOMINIS	RETORTAMONAS INTESTINALIS
Shape and size*	Shaped like amebas; 5-15 μm; usual range, 9-12 μm	Pear-shaped; 8-20 μm; usual range, 11-12 μm	Pear-shaped; 10-20 μm; usual range, 12-15 μm	Pear-shaped; 6-24 μm; usual range, 10-15 μm	Oval; 4-10 μm; usual range, 8-9 μm	Pear-shaped or oval; 4-9 μm; usual range, 6-7 μm
Motility	Usually nonprogressive; pseudopodia angular, serrated, or broad-lobed and almost transparent	Jerky and rapid	"Falling leaf," organisms may be trapped in mucus; only flagella flutter seen	Stiff, rotary	Jerky	Jerky
Number of nuclei	Percentage may vary, but approximately 40% of organisms have 1 nucleus and 60% 2 nuclei; not visible in unstained preparations; no peripheral chromatin, karyosome composed of cluster of 4-8 granules	One; not visible in unstained mounts	Two; not visible in unstained mounts	One; not visible in unstained mounts	One; not visible in unstained mounts	One; not visible in unstained mounts
Number of flagella (usually difficult to see)	No visible flagella	3-5 anterior, 1 posterior	4 lateral, 2 ventral, 2 caudal	3 anterior, 1 in cytostome	3 anterior, 1 posterior	1 anterior, 1 posterior
Other features	Cytoplasm finely granular and may be vacuolated with ingested bacteria, yeasts, and other debris	Axostyle (slender rod) protrudes beyond posterior end and may be visible; undulating membrane extends length of body	Sucking disk occupying 1/3 to 1/2 of ventral surface; pear-shaped front view, spoon-shaped side view	Prominent cytostome extending 1/3 to 1/2 length of body; spiral groove across ventral surface	One side of body flattened; posterior flagellum extends free posteriorly or laterally	Prominent cytostome extending approximately 1/2 length of body

*These sizes refer to wet preparation measurements. Organism on a permanent stained smear may be 1 to 1.5 μm smaller because of artificial shrinkage.

Table 44.5
Morphological Criteria Used To Identify Intestinal Amebic Cysts

	ENTAMOEBA HISTOLYTICA	ENTAMOEBA HARTMANNI	ENTAMOEBA COLI	ENDOLIMAX NANA	IODAMOEBA BÜTSCHLII
Size*	10-20 μm; usual range, 12-15 μm	5-10 μm; usual range, 6-8 μm	10-35 μm; usual range, 15-25 μm	5-10 μm; usual range 6-8 μm	5-20 μm; usual range, 10-12 μm
Shape	Usually spherical	Usually spherical	Usually spherical, occasionally oval, triangular, or other shapes; may be distorted on stained slide if fixation poor	Spherical, ovoidal, or ellipsoidal	Ovoidal, ellipsoidal, or other shapes
Number of nuclei	Mature cyst, 4; immature, 1 or 2 nuclei may be seen; nuclear characteristics difficult to see on wet preparation	Mature cyst, 4; immature, 1 or 2 nuclei may be seen; 2 nucleated cysts very common	Mature cyst, 8; occasionally 16 or more nuclei may be seen; immature cysts with 2 or more nuclei occasionally seen	Mature cyst, 4; immature cysts, 2 (very rarely seen and may resemble cysts of *Enteromonas hominis*)	Mature cyst, 1
Nucleus					
Peripheral chromatin (stained)	Peripheral chromatin present; fine, uniform granules, evenly distributed; nuclear characteristics may not be as clearly visible as in trophozoite	Fine granules evenly distributed on membrane; nuclear characteristics may be difficult to see	Coarsely granular and may be clumped and unevenly arranged on membrane; nuclear characteristics not as clearly defined as in trophozoite; may resemble *E. histolytica*	No peripheral chromatin	No peripheral chromatin
Karyosome (stained)	Small, compact, usually centrally located	Small, compact, usually centrally located	Large, may or may not be compact or eccentric; occasionally appears to be centrally located	Smaller than karyosome seen in trophozoite, but generally larger than those of genus *Entamoeba*	Large, usually eccentric refractile granules may be on one side of karyosome ("basket nucleus")
Cytoplasm					
Chromatoidal bodies (stained)	May be present; bodies usually elongate with blunt, rounded, smooth edges	Often present; bodies elongate with blunt, rounded, smooth edges	May be present (less frequently than *E. histolytica*); splinter-shaped with rough, pointed ends	No chromatoidal bodies present; occasionally small granules or inclusions seen; also, fine linear structures may be faintly visible on well-stained smears	No chromatoidal bodies present; occasionally small granules may be present
Glycogen (stained)	May be diffuse or absent in mature cyst; clumped chromatin mass may be present in early cysts (stains reddish brown in iodine)	May or may not be present, as in *E. histolytica*	May be diffuse or absent in mature cysts; clumped mass occasionally seen in immature cysts (stains reddish brown in iodine)	Usually diffuse if present (stains reddish-brown in iodine)	Large, compact, well-defined mass (stains reddish brown in iodine)

*These sizes refer to wet preparation measurements. Organisms on a permanent stained smear may be 1 to 1.5 μm smaller because of artificial shrinkage.

Table 44.6
Morphologic Criteria Used To Identify Intestinal Flagellate Cysts

	DIENTAMOEBA FRAGILIS	*TRICHOMONAS HOMINIS*	*GIARDIA LAMBLIA*	*CHILOMASTIX MESNILI*	*ENTEROMONAS HOMINIS*	*RETORTAMONAS INTESTINALIS*
Shape	No cyst	No cyst	Oval, ellipsoidal, or may appear round	Lemon-shaped with anterior hyaline knob	Elongate or oval	Pear-shaped or slightly lemon-shaped
Size*			8-19 μm; usual range, 11-12 μm	6-10 μm; usual range, 8-9 μm	4-10 μm; usual range, 6-8 μm	4-9 μm; usual range 4-7 μm
Number of nuclei			Four; not distinct in unstained preparations; usually located at one end	One, not visible in unstained preparations	One to four; usually 2 lying at opposite ends of cyst; not visible in unstained mounts	One; not visible in unstained mounts
Other features			Longitudinal fibers in cyst may be visible in unstained preparations; deep-staining fibers usually lie across longitudinal fibers; there is often shrinkage, and cytoplasm pulls away from cyst wall; may also be "halo" effect around outside of cyst wall	Cytostome with supporting fibrils, usually visible in stained preparation; curved fibril along side of cytostome usually referred to as "shepherd's crook"	Resembles *E. nana* cyst; fibrils or flagella usually not seen	Resembles *Chilomastix* cyst; shadow outline of cytostome with supporting fibrils extending above nucleus

*These sizes refer to wet preparation measurements. Organisms on a permanent stained smear may be 1 to 1.5 μm smaller because of artificial shrinkage.

Table 44.7

Morphologic Criteria of *Balantidium coli*

	TROPHOZOITE	CYST
Shape and size*	Ovoid with tapering anterior end; 50-100 μm in length, 40-70 μm wide, usual range, 40-50 μm	Spherical or oval; 50-70 μm; usual range, 50-55 μm
Motility	Rotary or boring or both; may be rapid	
Number of nuclei	1 large kidney-shaped macronucleus; 1 small round micronucleus, which is difficult to see even in stained smear; macronucleus may be visible in unstained preparation	1 large macronucleus visible in unstained preparation
Other features	Body covered with cilia, which tend to be longer near cytostome; cytoplasm may be vacuolated	Macronucleus and contractile vacuole visible in young cysts; in older cysts, internal structure appears granular

*These sizes refer to wet preparation measurements. Organisms on a permanent stained smear may be 1 to 1.5 μm smaller because of artificial shrinkage.

Table 44.8

Morphologic Criteria Used To Identify Intestinal Protozoa (Coccidia, Microsporidia, *Blastocystis hominis*)

SPECIES	SHAPE/SIZE	OTHER FEATURES
Cryptosporidium sp.	Oocyst generally round, 4-6 μm, each mature oocyst containing 4 sporozoites	Oocyst, usual diagnostic stage in stool; various other stages in life cycle can be seen in biopsy specimens taken from gastrointestinal tract (brush border of epithelial cells) (intestinal tract)
Isospora belli	Ellipsoidal oocyst; range 20-30 μm in length, 10-19 μm in width; sporocysts rarely seen broken out of oocysts but measure 9-11 μm	Mature oocyst contains 2 sporocysts with 4 sporozoites each; usual diagnostic stage in feces is immature oocyst containing spherical mass of protoplasm (intestinal tract)
Sarcocystis hominis S. *suihominis* S. *bovihominis*	Oocyst thin-walled and contains 2 mature sporocysts, each containing 4 sporozoites; frequently thin oocyst wall ruptures; ovoidal sporocysts each measure 10-16 μm in length and 7.5-12 μm in width	Thin-walled oocyst or ovoid sporocysts occur in stool (intestinal tract)
S. *"lindemanni"*	Shapes and sizes of skeletal and cardiac muscle sarcocysts vary considerably	Sarcocysts contain from several hundred to several thousand trophozoites, each of which measures from 4-9 μm in width and 12-16 μm in length. The sarcocysts may also be divided into compartments by septa, not seen in *Toxoplasma* cysts (tissue/muscle)
Microsporidia	Small, oval spores (1-4 μm) can be found in routine histological sections; however, electron microscopy has been used most successfully	Spores shed in enterocytes have not yet been identified in stool specimens. The development of monoclonal antibodies may provide a more sensitive detection method
Blastocystis hominis	Organisms are generally round, measure approximately 6-40 μm, and are usually characterized by a large, central body (looks like a large vacuole)	The more amebic form can be seen in diarrheal fluid, but will be difficult to identify

severe symptoms and possible death. *D. fragilis* has been associated with diarrhea, nausea, vomiting, and other nonspecific abdominal complaints. *G. lamblia* is probably the most common protozoan organism found in persons in this country and is known to cause symptoms ranging from mild diarrhea, flatulence, and vague abdominal pains to acute, severe diarrhea to steatorrhea and a typical malabsorption syndrome. There have been a number of documented water-borne and food-borne outbreaks during the past several years, and the beaver has been implicated as an animal reservoir host for *G. lamblia*. It is speculated that other animals may be involved as well. With present improved culture techniques and the ability to harvest material for antigen, serologic tests for giardiasis have been developed for both antibody and antigen. An ELISA method has also been marketed.

Another organism, *Blastocystis hominis* (Figures 44.3 and 44.15), is also now considered to be potentially pathogenic for humans. It has been reclassified as a protozoan, and there are reports of *B. hominis* as an agent of human enteric disease.[48,60,61] However, another report indicated that *B. hominis* is an incidental finding where other proven pathogens may be present in low numbers.[34] We recommend that its presence in large numbers be reported.

Sarcocystis sp. appears in Table 44.8 but will not be discussed in detail. According to the literature, extraintestinal human sarcocystosis is rare, with a much lower incidence than that seen with the intestinal infection.

The identification of intestinal protozoan parasites is difficult, at best, and the importance of the permanent stained slide should be reemphasized (Procedure 44.3). It is important to remember that many artifacts (vegetable material, debris, cells of human origin) may mimic protozoan organisms on a wet mount (Figure 44.15). The important diagnostic characteristics will be visible on the stained smear, and the *final identification of protozoan parasites should be confirmed with the permanent stain*.

44.12.a. **Amebas.** Occasionally when fresh stool material is examined as a direct wet mount, motile trophozoites may be observed. *E. histolytica* is described as having directional and progressive motility, whereas the other amebas tend to move more slowly and at random. The cytoplasm usually appears finely granular, less frequently coarsely granular, or vacuolated. Bacteria, yeast cells, or debris may be present in the cytoplasm. The presence of red blood cells in the cytoplasm is usually considered to be diagnostic for *E. histolytica* (Figures 44.16 and 44.17).

Nuclear morphology is one of the most important criteria used for identification; nuclei of the genus *Entamoeba* contain a relatively small karyosome and have chromatin material arranged on the nuclear membrane (Figures 44.16 to 44.25). The nuclei of the other two genera, *Endolimax* and *Iodamoeba*, tend to have very large karyosomes with no peripheral chromatin on the nuclear membrane (Figures 44.26 to 44.30).

The trophozoite stages may often be pleomorphic and asymmetrical, whereas the cysts are usually less variable in shape, with more rigid cyst walls. The number of nuclei in the cysts may vary, but their general morphology is similar to that found in the trophozoite stage. There are various inclusions in the cysts, such as chromatoidal bars or glycogen material, which may be helpful in identification.

44.12.b. **Flagellates.** Four common species of flagellates are found in the intestinal tract: *G. lamblia*, *Chilomastix mesnili*, *T. hominis*, and *D. fragilis* (Figures 44.31 to 44.38). Several other smaller flagellates, such as *Enteromonas hominis* and *Retortamonas intestinalis* (Figure 44.31), are rarely seen, and none of the flagellates in the intestinal tract, with the exception of *G. lamblia* and *D. fragilis*, are considered pathogenic. *T. vaginalis* is pathogenic but occurs in the urogenital tract. *Trichomonas tenax* is occasionally found in the mouth and may be associated with poor oral hygiene.

With the exception of *Dientamoeba*, the flagellates can be recognized by their characteristic rapid motility, which has been described as a "falling leaf" motion for *Giardia* and a jerky motion for the other species. Most of the flagellates have a characteristic pear shape and possess different numbers and arrangements of flagella, depending on the species. The sucking disk and axonemes of *Giardia*, the cytostome and spiral groove of *Chilomastix*, and the undulating membrane of *Trichomonas* are all distinctive criteria for identification (Figures 44.31 to 44.35).

Until recently *Dientamoeba* was grouped with the amebas; however, electron microscopy studies have confirmed its correct classification with the flagellates, specifically the trichomonads. *Dientamoeba* has no known cyst stage and is characterized by hav-

Text continued on p. 834.

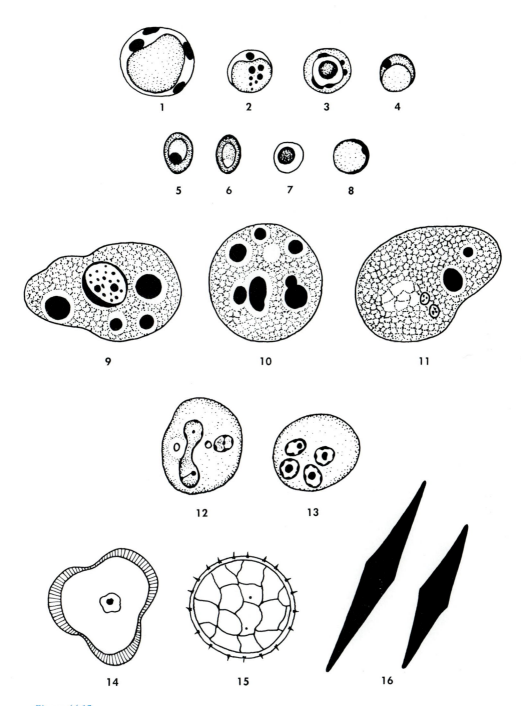

Figure 44.15

Various structures that may be seen in stool preparations. **1, 2, 4,** *Blastocystis hominis*. **3, 5-8,** Various yeast cells. **9,** Macrophage with nucleus. **10, 11,** Deteriorated macrophage without nucleus. **12, 13,** Polymorphonuclear leukocytes. **14, 15,** Pollen grains. **16,** Charcot-Leyden crystals. (Adapted from Markell, E.K., and Voge, M. 1981. Medical parasitology, ed. 5. W.B. Saunders Co., Philadelphia, Illustration by Nobuko Kitamura.)

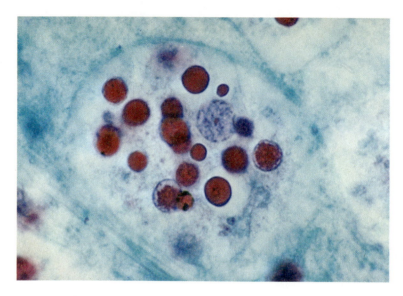

Figure 44.16
Entamoeba histolytica trophozoite (contains ingested red blood cells).

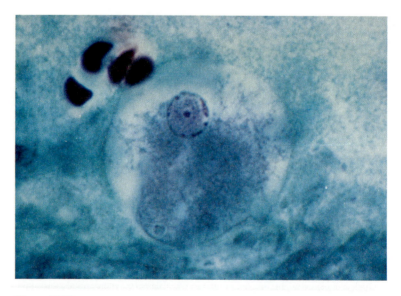

Figure 44.17
Entamoeba histolytica trophozoite.

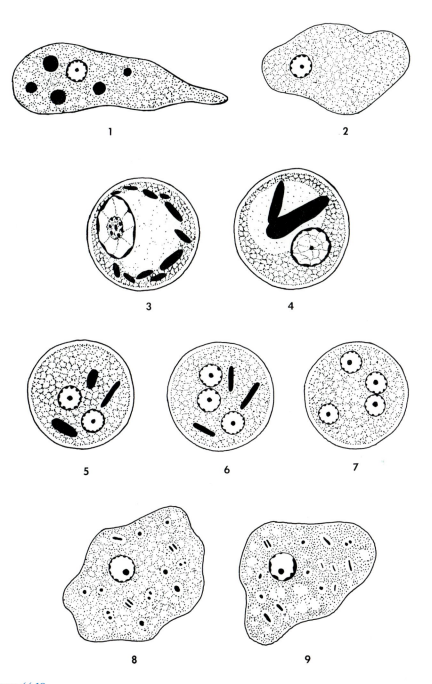

Figure 44.18
1, 2, Trophozoites of *Entamoeba histolytica*. **3, 4,** Early cysts of *E. histolytica*. **5-7,** Cysts of *E. histolytica*. **8, 9,** Trophozoites of *Entamoeba coli*. (**1-18** from Garcia, L.S., and Bruckner, D.A. 1988. Diagnostic medical parasitology. Elsevier, New York. Illustrations **4** and **11** by Nobuko Kitamura.)

Continued.

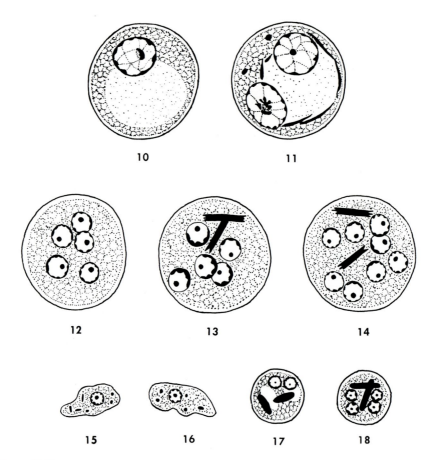

Figure 44.18, cont'd
10, 11, Early cysts of *E. coli.* **12-14,** Cysts of *E. coli.* **15, 16,** Trophozoites of *Entamoeba hartmanni.*
17, 18, Cysts of *E. hartmanni.*

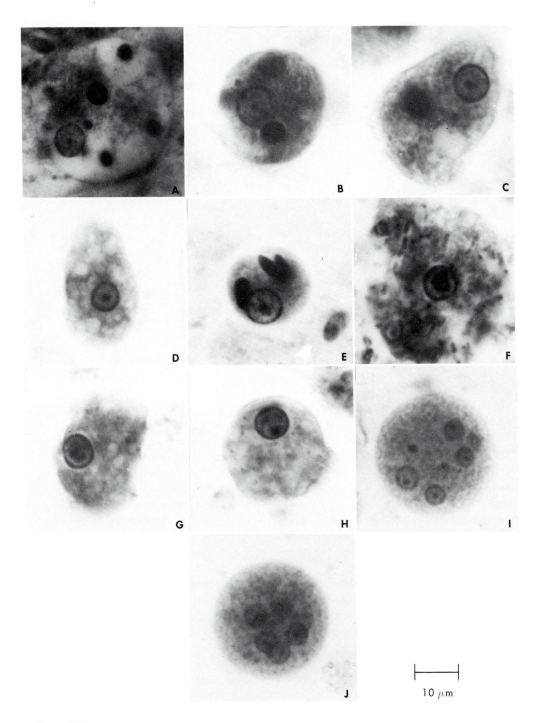

10 μm

Figure 44.19
A-D, Trophozoites of *Entamoeba histolytica*. **E,** Early cysts of *E. histolytica*. **F-H,** Trophozoites of *Entamoeba coli*. **I, J,** Cysts of *E. coli*.

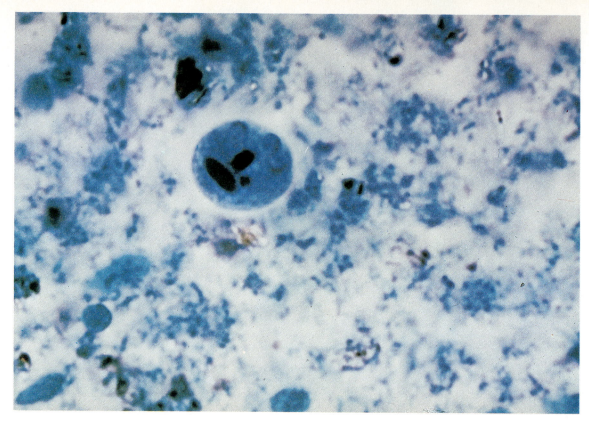

Figure 44.20
E. histolytica cyst.

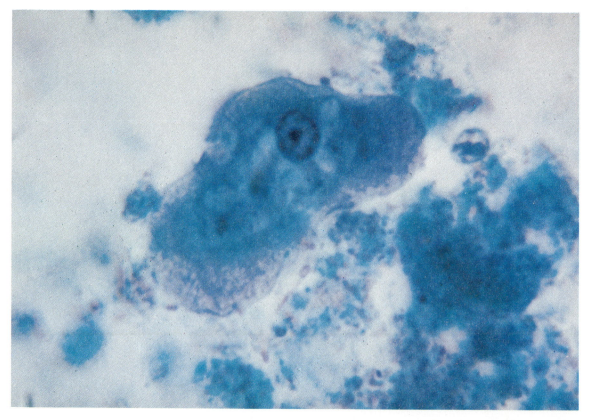

Figure 44.21
Entamoeba coli trophozoite.

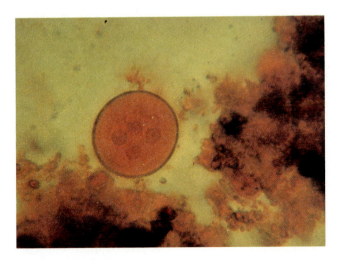

Figure 44.22
E. coli cyst, iodine stain.

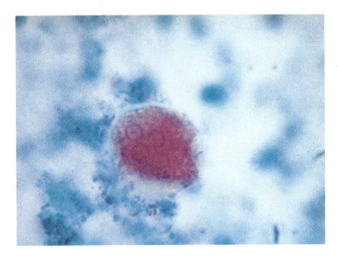

Figure 44.23
E. coli cyst, trichrome stain (poor preservation).

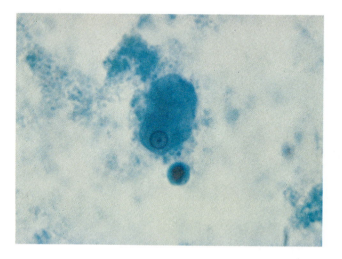

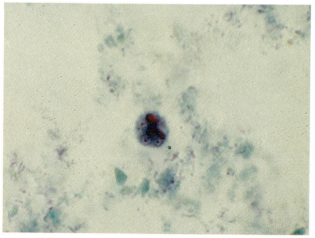

Figure 44.24
Entamoeba hartmanni trophozoite. *Bottom, E. hartmanni* cyst.

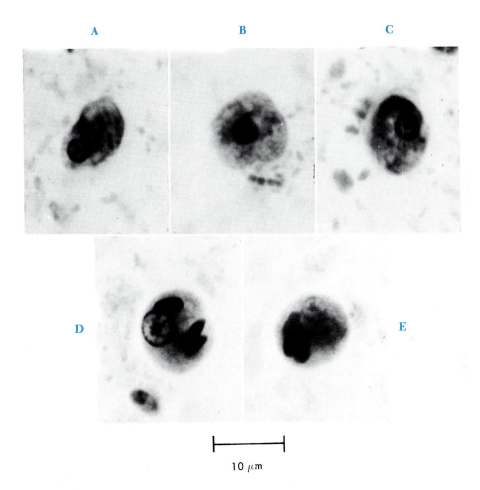

10 μm

Figure 44.25
A-C, Trophozoites of *Entamoeba hartmanni*. **D, E,** Cysts of *E. hartmanni*.

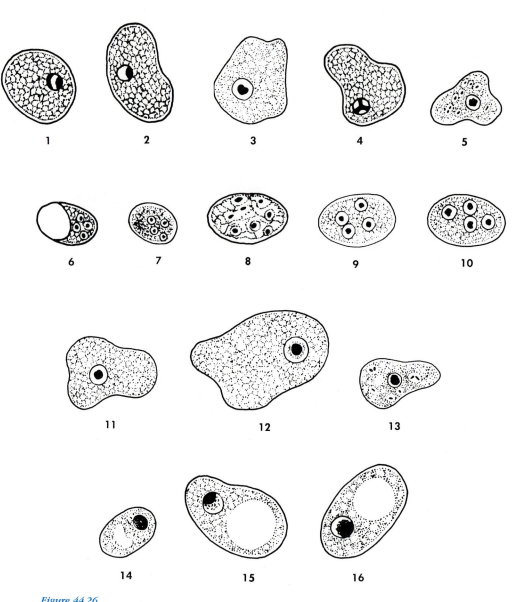

Figure 44.26
1-5, Trophozoites of *Endolimax nana*. **6-10,** Cysts of *E. nana*. **11-13,** Trophozoites of *Iodamoeba bütschlii*. **14-16,** Cysts of *I. bütschlii*. (From Garcia, L.S., and Bruckner, D.A. 1988. Diagnostic medical parasitology. Elsevier, New York.)

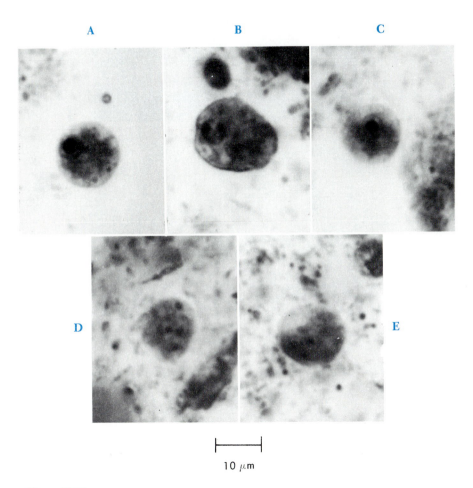

10 μm

Figure 44.27
A-C, Trophozoites of *Endolimax nana*, **D, E**, Cysts of *E. nana*.

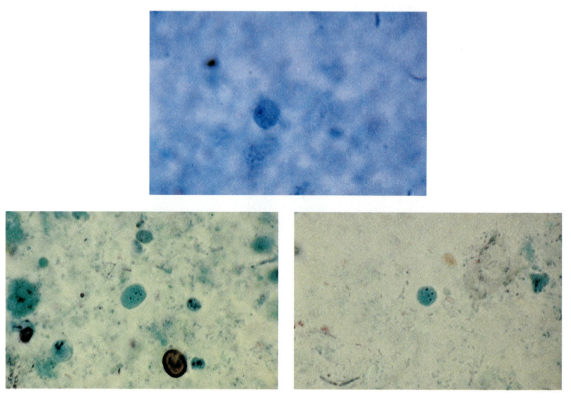

Figure 44.28
Top, Endolimax nana trophozoite. Bottom left, E. nana cyst. Bottom right, E. nana cyst.

A   B   C

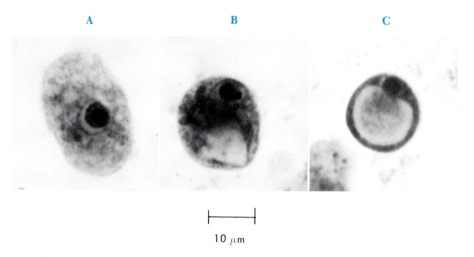

10 μm

Figure 44.29
A, Trophozoites of *Iodamoeba bütschlii*. **B, C,** Cysts of *I. bütschlii*.

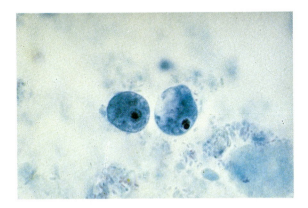

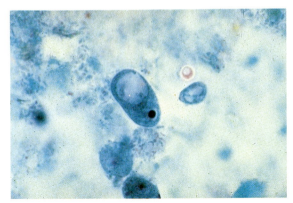
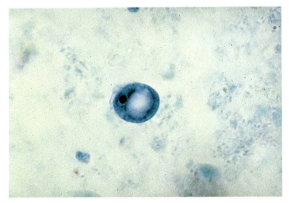

Figure 44.30
Top, Iodamoeba bütschlii trophozoites. Bottom left, I. bütschlii cyst. Bottom right, I. bütschlii cyst.

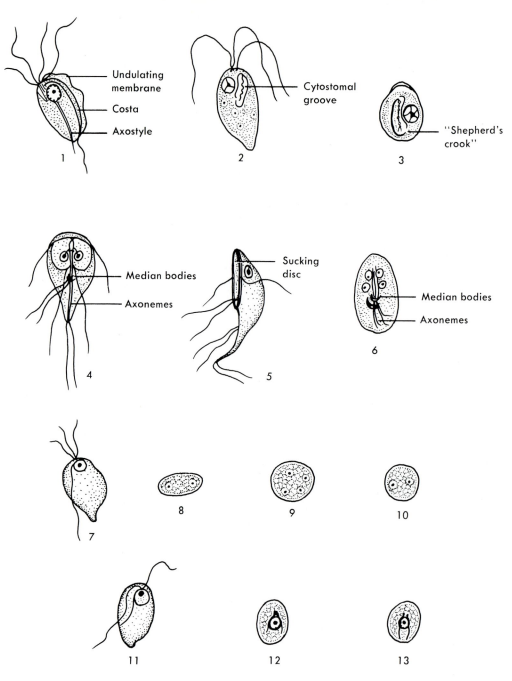

Figure 44.31

1, Trophozoite of *Trichomonas hominis*. **2,** Trophozoite of *Chilomastix mesnili*. **3,** Cyst of *C. mesnili*. **4,** Trophozoite of *Giardia lamblia* (front view). **5,** Trophozoite of *G. lamblia* (side view). **6,** Cyst of *G. lamblia*. **7,** Trophozoite of *Enteromonas hominis*. **8-10,** Cysts of *E. hominis*. **11,** Trophozoite of *Retortamonas intestinalis*. **12, 13,** Cysts of *R. intestinalis*. (From Garcia, L.S., and Bruckner, D.A. 1988. Diagnostic medical parasitology. Elsevier, New York. Illustration **5** by Nobuko Kitamura; illustrations **7** to **13** adapted from Markell, E.K., and Voge, M. 1981. Medical parasitology, ed. 5. W.B. Saunders Co., Philadelphia.)

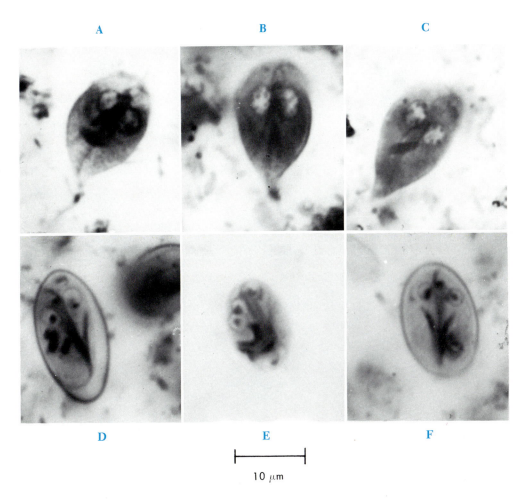

10 μm

Figure 44.32
A-C, Trophozoites of *Giardia lamblia*. **D-F,** Cysts of *G. lamblia*.

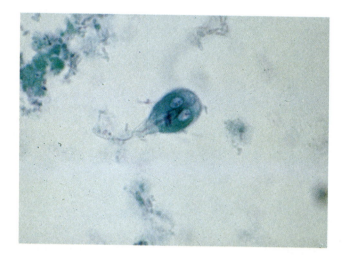

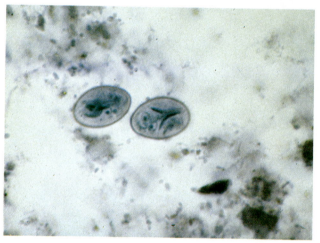

Figure 44.33
Top, *Giardia lamblia* trophozoite. Bottom left, *G. lamblia* cyst.

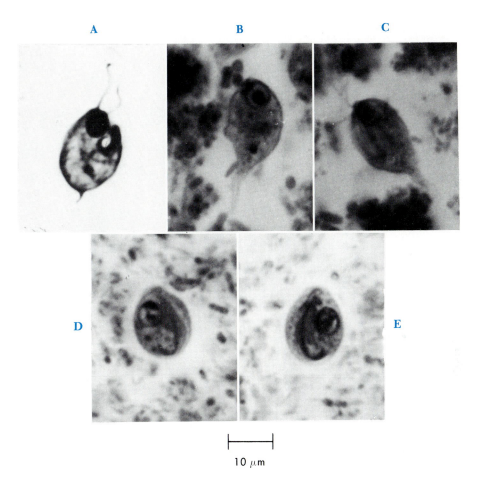

10 μm

Figure 44.34
A-C, Trophozoites of *Chilomastix mesnili* (**A,** silver stain). **D, E,** Cysts of *C. mesnili*.

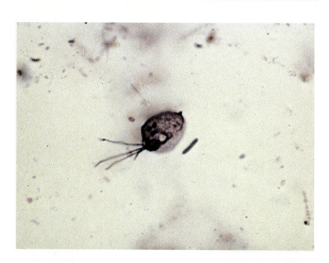

Figure 44.35
Top, Chilomastix mesnili trophozoite, silver stain.
Bottom left, C. mesnili cyst.

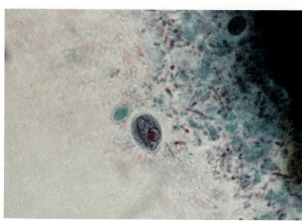

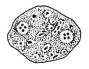 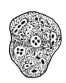

Figure 44.36
Trophozoites of *Dientamoeba fragilis*. (From Garcia, L.S., and
Bruckner, D.A. 1988. Diagnostic medical parasitology.
Elsevier, New York.)

ing one or two nuclei, which have no peripheral
chromatin and which have four to eight chromatin
granules in a central mass. This organism is quite
variable in size and shape and may contain large
numbers of ingested bacteria and other debris. *Dientamoeba* is inconspicuous in the wet mount and is
consistently overlooked without the use of the
stained smear (Figures 44.36 to 44.38).

Organisms can be recovered in fecal specimens
from asymptomatic persons, but reports in the literature describe a wide range of symptoms, which
include intermittent diarrhea, abdominal pain, nausea, anorexia, malaise, fatigue, poor weight gain, and
unexplained eosinophilia.

44.12.c. Ciliates. *Balantidium coli* is the largest
protozoan and the only ciliate that infects humans
(Figure 44.39). The living trophozoites have a ro-
tatory, boring motion, which is usually rapid. The
surface of the organism is covered by cilia, and the
cytoplasm contains both a kidney-shaped macronu-
cleus and a smaller, round micronucleus that is often
difficult to see. The number of nuclei in the cyst
remains the same as that in the trophozoite. *B. coli*
infections are rarely seen in this country; however,
the organisms are quite easily recognized (Figure
44.40).

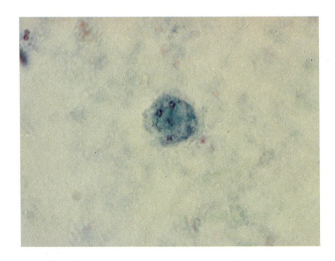

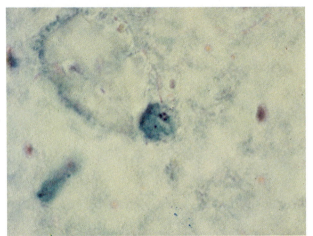

Figure 44.37
Top, *Dientamoeba fragilis*, two nuclei. *Bottom left*,
D. fragilis, one nucleus.

44.12.d. Coccidia. *Isospora belli* is now considered to be the only valid species of the genus *Isospora* that infects humans, since *Isospora hominis* has been placed in the genus *Sarcocystis*. *I. belli* is released from the intestinal wall as immature oocysts, so all stages from the immature oocyst containing a mass of undifferentiated protoplasm to those oocysts containing fully developed sporocysts and sporozoites are found in the stool (Figure 44.41). If passed in the immature condition, they mature within 4 or 5 days to form sporozoites. *I. belli* infections are becoming increasingly important as a cause of diarrhea in immunodeficient and immunosuppressed patients.[43] Many of the recently reported infections have occurred in patients with AIDS. The diagnosis of *Isospora* infection is usually accomplished by find-

ing oocysts in stool concentrates or rarely by direct wet mount examination during routine ova and parasite examinations. Multiple stool examinations are recommended since the oocysts are not continually shed in the stool during infections. Oocysts can be stained with rhodamine-auramine (Appendix B), modified acid-fast procedures, or Giemsa. The oocyst wall and sporocyst will fluoresce bright yellow when stained with rhodamine-auramine. With the modified acid-fast stain (Appendix B), the oocyst will appear pink with bright red sporocysts.[43] Giemsa (Appendix B) stains both the oocyst and the sporocyst pale blue; however, trichrome stain is not recommended because it stains the oocyst poorly or not at all. Multiple biopsies of the jejunal-duodenal brush border can also lead to diagnosis, since in many pa-

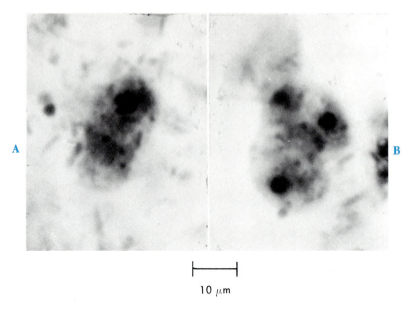

10 μm

Figure 44.38
A, B, Trophozoites of *Dientamoeba fragilis*.

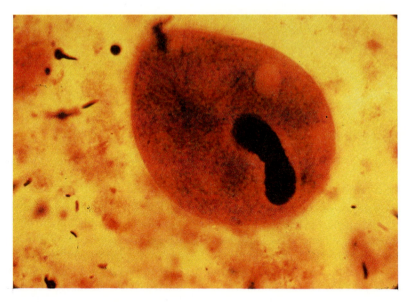

Figure 44.39
Balantidium coli trophozoite, iodine stain.

tients apparently only the asexual stages are seen.

Cryptosporidium sp. is another coccidian parasite that has been implicated in intestinal disease, primarily in immunosuppressed patients and particularly those with AIDS.[22,42] These organisms may not be host-specific, are probably transmitted by the

fecal-oral route, and may also infect persons with a competent immune system. The developmental stages occur within a vacuole of host cell origin, which is located at the microvillous surface of the host epithelial cell (Figure 44.42). Although the infection is generally self-limiting in the immunocom-

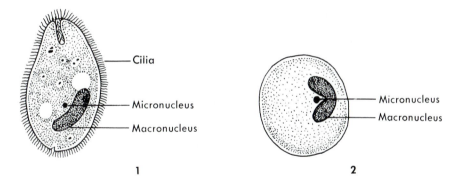

Figure 44.40

1, Trophozoite of *Balantidium coli*. **2,** Cyst of *B. coli*. (From Garcia, L.S., and Bruckner, D.A. 1988. Diagnostic medical parasitology. Elsevier, New York.)

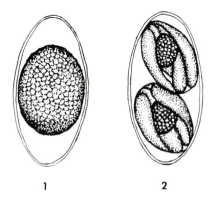

Figure 44.41

1, Immature oocyst of *Isospora belli*. **2,** Mature oocyst of *I. belli*. (Illustration by Nobuko Kitamura.).

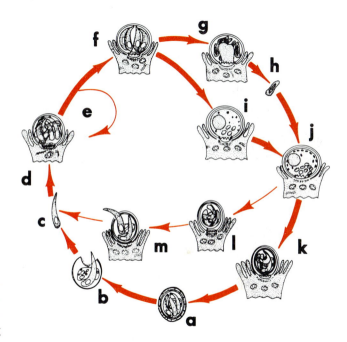

Figure 44.42

Proposed life cycle of *Cryptosporidium*. (*a*) Sporulated oocyst in feces. (*b*) Excystation in intestine. (*c*) Free sporozoite in intestine. (*d*) Type I meront (6 or 8 merozoites). (*e*) Recycling of Type I merozoite. (*f*) Type II meront (4 merozoites). (*g*) Microgametocyte, with approximately 16 microgametes. (*h*) Microgamete fertilizes macrogamete (*i*) to form zygote (*j*). Approximately 80% of the zygotes form thick-walled oocysts (*k*) which sporulate within the host cell. About 20% of the zygotes do not form an oocyst wall; their sporozoites are surrounded only by a unit membrane (*l*). Sporozoites within "autoinfective," thin walled oocysts (*l*) are released into the intestinal lumen (*m*) and reinitiate the endogenous cycle (at *c*). (Life cycle from William L. Current, Lilly Research Laboratories, Greenfield, Indiana.)

petent person, the presence of autoinfective oocysts may explain why a small inoculum can lead to an overwhelming infection in compromised patients and why they may have persistent, life-threatening infections in the absence of documentation of repeated exposure to oocysts. In the immunodeficient individual, *Cryptosporidium* is not always confined to the gastrointestinal tract but has been associated with cholecystitis (biliary tree and gallbladder epithelium) and respiratory tract infections.

Previously, the majority of cases had been diagnosed by light or electron microscopic examination of small or large bowel biopsy material. However, recent cases have been diagnosed from stool specimens and suggest that the use of specific stains and concentration techniques may be more sensitive than intestinal biopsies in diagnosing *Cryptosporidium*. The oocysts range from 4 to 6 μm and can be confused with yeast or overlooked without special

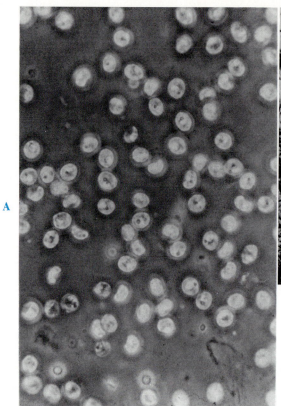

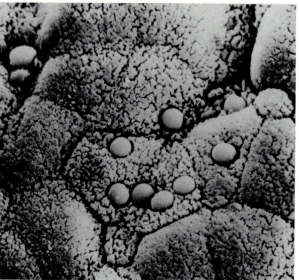

A

B

Figure 44.43

Cryptosporidium. **A,** Oocysts recovered from a Sheather's sugar flotation; organisms measure 4-6 μm. **B,** Scanning electron microscopy view of organisms at brush border of epithelial cells. (From Garcia, L.S., and Bruckner, D.A. 1988. Diagnostic medical parasitology. Elsevier, New York.)

techniques, various modified acid fast stains being one of the best approaches.[22] In wet preparations where iodine is added, yeast cells will stain with the iodine, but *Cryptosporidium* does not take up the stain. However, in light infections with few oocysts and many artifacts in the stool, this difference will be very difficult to visualize. The most widely used concentration method for obtaining the oocysts from stool is Sheather's sugar flotation (Figure 44.43),[21] although they may be visible in routine stool concentrates.

NOTE: The number of oocysts per stool specimen will vary considerably, both from patient to patient and from specimen to specimen during an infection in a single patient. Since therapy for this infection is less than optimal, even with the use of spiramycin, one should check multiple specimens before accepting the patient as being cured of the infection. With the development of very specific monoclonal reagents directed against components of the oocyst wall (Figure 44.44), the ability to screen large numbers of specimens is now available.[20,50]

44.12.e. Microsporidia. The microsporidia are obligate intracellular parasites that can infect both animals and humans, probably through the gastrointestinal tract. The four genera that have been implicated in human infection are *Encephalitozoon*, *Nosema*, *Pleistophora*, and *Enterocytozoon*.[31,53]

The number of documented cases is rare; however, *Enterocytozoon bieneusi* has been reported in a patient with AIDS.[15]

The diagnosis can be made by identifying the spores in biopsy or autopsy specimens; all body organs have been involved, including the eye. The resistant spores measure approximately 1 to 4 μm, and they do not stain well with hematoxylin-eosin. They are occasionally acid-fast and have a periodic acid–Schiff (PAS)–positive polar granule at the anterior end.[53] Definitive diagnosis can also be made using electron microscopy. It is anticipated that additional cases will be diagnosed, particularly if more sensitive diagnostic methods are developed for organism identification in stool.

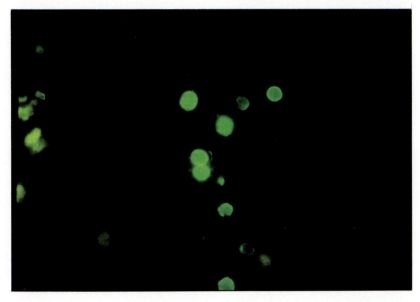

Figure 44.44
Cryptosporidium oocysts stained with monoclonal antibody–conjugated fluorescent reagent. (Merifluor, Meridian Diagnostics, Inc., Cincinnati, Ohio.)

44.13 Blood Protozoa

44.13.a. Malaria. Malaria is caused by four species of the protozoan genus *Plasmodium: P. vivax, P. falciparum* (Figure 44.45), *P. malariae*, and *P. ovale* (Table 44.9). Humans become infected when the sporozoites are introduced into the blood from the salivary secretion of the infected mosquito when the mosquito vector takes a blood meal. These sporozoites then leave the blood and enter the parenchymal cells of the liver, where they undergo asexual multiplication. This development in the liver prior to red cell invasion is called the preerythrocytic cycle; if further liver development takes place after red cell invasion, it is called the exoerythrocytic cycle. The length of time for the preerythrocytic cycle and the number of asexual generations vary depending on the species; however, the schizonts eventually rupture, releasing thousands of merozoites into the bloodstream, where they invade the erythrocytes. The early forms in the red cells are called **ring forms** or young trophozoites (Figure 44.46). As the parasites continue to grow and feed, they become actively ameboid within the red cell. They feed on hemoglobin, which is incompletely metabolized; the residue that is left is called malarial pigment and is a compound of hematin and of protein.

During the next phase of the cycle the chromatin (nuclear material) becomes fragmented throughout the organism, and the cytoplasm begins to divide, each portion being arranged with a fragment of nuclear material. These forms are called mature schizonts and are composed of individual merozoites. The infected red cell then ruptures, releasing the merozoites and also metabolic products into the bloodstream. If large numbers of red cells rupture simultaneously, a malarial paroxysm may result from the amount of toxic materials released into the bloodstream. In the early stages of infection or in a mixed infection with two species, rupture of the red cells is usually not synchronous; consequently, the fever may be continuous or daily rather than intermittent. After several days, a 48- or 72-hour periodicity is usually established.

After several generations of erythrocytic schizogony, the production of gametocytes begins. These forms are derived from merozoites, which do not undergo schizogony but continue to grow and form the male and female gametocytes that circulate in the bloodstream. When the mature gametocytes are ingested by the appropriate mosquito vector, the sexual cycle is initiated within the mosquito with the eventual production of the sporozoites, the infective stage for humans (Figure 44.47).

The asexual and sexual forms just described cir-

Text continued on p. 844.

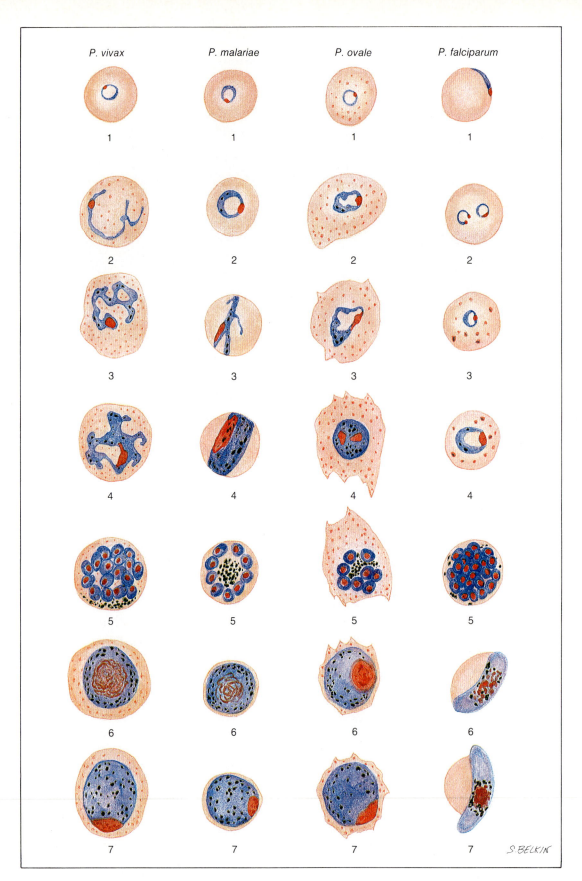

Figure 44.45
For legend see opposite page.

Figure 44.45
The morphology of malaria parasites.

Plasmodium vivax

1 Early trophozoite (Ring form)
2 Late trophozoite with Schuffner's dots (note enlarged RBC)
3 Late trophozoite with ameboid cytoplasm (very typical of *P. vivax*)
4 Late trophozoite with ameboid cytoplasm
5 Mature schizont with merozoites (18) and clumped pigment
6 Microgametocyte with dispersed chromatin
7 Macrogametocyte with compact chromatin

Plasmodium malariae

1 Early trophozoite (Ring form)
2 Early trophozoite with thick cytoplasm
3 Early trophozoite (Band form)
4 Late trophozoite (Band form) with heavy pigment
5 Mature schizont with merozoites (9) arranged in a rosette
6 Microgametocyte with dispersed chromatin
7 Macrogametocyte with compact chromatin

Plasmodium ovale

1 Early trophozoite (Ring form) with Schuffner's dots
2 Early trophozoite (note enlarged RBC)
3 Late trophozoite in RBC with fimbriated edges
4 Developing schizont with irregular shaped RBC
5 Mature schizont with merozoites (8) arranged irregularly
6 Microgametocyte with dispersed chromatin
7 Macrogametocyte with compact chromatin

Plasmodium falciparum

1 Early trophozoite (accolé or appliqué form)
2 Early trophozoite (one ring is in the headphone configuration/double chromatin dots)
3 Early trophozoite with Mauer's dots
4 Late trophozoite with larger ring and Mauer's dots
5 Mature schizont with merozoites (24)
6 Microgametocyte with dispersed chromatin
7 Macrogametocyte with compact chromatin

Note: Without the appliqué form, Schuffner's dots, multiple rings/cell, and other developing stages, differentiation among the species can be very difficult. It is obvious that the early rings of all four species can mimic one another very easily. *Remember: One set of negative blood films cannot rule out a malaria infection*. (Reprinted by permission of the publisher from Garcia, L.S., and Bruckner, D.A. 1988. Diagnostic medical parasitology, p. 98. Copyright 1988 by Elsevier Science Publishing Co., Inc.)

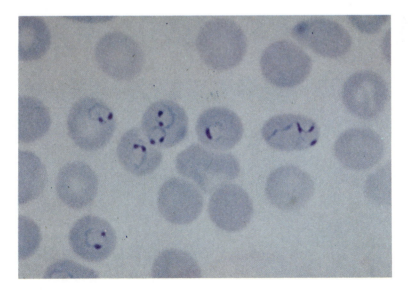

Figure 44.46
Plasmodium falciparum early ring forms.

Table 44.9
Microscopic Identification of Plasmodia of Humans in Giemsa-Stained Thin Blood Smears

	PLASMODIUM VIVAX	PLASMODIUM MALARIAE	PLASMODIUM FALCIPARUM	PLASMODIUM OVALE
Appearance of parasitized red blood cells: size and shape	1½ to 2 times larger than normal; oval to round	Normal shape; size may be normal or slightly smaller	Both normal	60% of cells larger than normal and oval; 20% have irregular, frayed edges (fimbriated)
Schüffner's dots (eosinophilic stippling)	Usually present in all infected cells except early ring forms	None	None; occasionally commalike red dots are present (Maurer's dots)	Present in all stages including early ring forms, dots may be larger and darker than in *P. vivax*
Color of cytoplasm	Decolorized, pale	Normal	Normal, bluish tinge at times	Decolorized, pale
Multiple infections	Occasional	Rare	Common	Occasional
All developmental stages present in peripheral blood	All stages present	Ring forms few, as ring stage brief; mostly growing and mature trophozoites and schizonts	Young ring forms and very rarely older stages in moribund patients; few gametocytes	All stages present
Appearance of parasite: young trophozoite (early ring form)	Ring is ⅓ diameter of cell; cytoplasmic circle around vacuole; heavy chromatin dot	Ring often smaller than in *P. vivax*, occupying ⅙ of cell; heavy chromatin dot; vacuole at times "filled-in"; pigment forms early	Delicate, small ring with small chromatin dot (frequently 2); scanty cytoplasma around small vacuoles; sometimes at edge of red cell (appliqué form) or filamentous slender form; may have multiple rings per cell	Ring is larger and more ameboid than in *P. vivax*, otherwise similar to *P. vivax*
Growing trophozoite	Multishaped irregular ameboid parasite; streamers of cytoplasm close to large chromatin dot; vacuole retained until close to maturity; increasing amounts of brown pigment	Nonameboid rounded or band-shaped solid forms; chromatin may be hidden by coarse dark brown pigment	Heavy ring forms fine pigment grains	Ring shape maintained until late in development

	P. vivax	*P. malariae*	*P. falciparum*	*P. ovale*
Mature trophozoite	Irregular ameboid mass; 1 or more small vacuoles retained until schizont stage; fills almost entire cell; fine brown pigment	Vacuoles disappear early; cytoplasm compact, oval, band-shaped, or nearly round, almost filling cell; chromatin may be hidden by peripheral coarse dark brown pigment	Not seen in peripheral blood (except in severe infections); development of all phases following ring form occurs in capillaries of viscera	Compact; vacuoles disappear; pigment dark brown, less than in *P. malariae*
Schizont (presegmenter)	Progressive chromatin division; cytoplasmic bands containing clumps of brown pigment	Similar to *P. vivax* except smaller, darker, larger pigment granules peripheral or central	Not seen in peripheral blood (see above)	Smaller and more compact than *P. vivax*
Mature schizont	16 (12-24) merozoites, each with chromatin and cytoplasm, filling entire red cell, which can hardly be seen	8 (6-12) merozoites in rosettes or irregular clusters filling normal-sized cells, which can hardly be seen; central arrangement of brown-green pigment	Not seen in peripheral blood (rare exceptions)	¾ of cells occupied by 8 (8-12) merozoites in rosettes or irregular clusters
Macrogametocyte	Rounded or oval homogeneous cytoplasm; diffuse delicate light brown pigment throughout parasite; eccentric compact chromatin	Similar to *P. vivax*, but fewer in number, pigment darker and more coarse	Sex differentiation difficult; "crescent" or "sausage" shapes characteristic; may appear in "showers"; black pigment near chromatin dot, which is often central	Smaller than *P. vivax*
Microgametocyte	Large pink to purple chromatin mass surrounded by pale or colorless halo; evenly distributed pigment	Similar to *P. vivax*, but fewer in number, pigment darker and more coarse	See above	Smaller than *P. vivax*
Main criteria	Large, pale red cell; trophozoite irregular; pigment usually present; Schüffner's dots not always present; several phases of growth seen in one smear; gametocytes appear early	Red cell normal in size and color; trophozoites compact, stain usually intense, band forms not always seen; coarse pigment; no stippling of red cells; gametocytes appear late	Development following ring stage takes place in blood vessels in internal organs; delicate ring forms and crescent-shaped gametocytes are only forms normally seen in peripheral blood	Red cell enlarged, oval, with fimbriated edges; Schüffner's dots seen in all stages

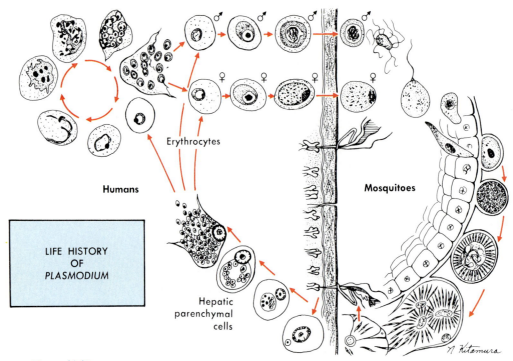

Figure 44.47
Life cycle of *Plasmodium*. (Adapted from Wilcox, A. 1960. Manual for the microscopical diagnosis of malaria in man. U.S. Public Health Service, Washington, D.C. Illustration by Nobuko Kitamura.)

culate in the human bloodstream in three species of *Plasmodium*. However, in *P. falciparum* infections, as the parasite continues to grow the red cell membrane becomes sticky, and the cells tend to adhere to the endothelial lining of the capillaries of the internal organs; thus, only the ring forms and crescent-shaped gametocytes occur in the peripheral blood. Interference with normal blood flow in these vessels gives rise to additional problems, which are responsible for the different clinical manifestations of this type of malaria.

44.13.b. Babesiosis. *Babesia* are tick-borne (also can be transmitted via a blood transfusion) sporozoan parasites that have generally been considered parasites of animals (Texas cattle fever) rather than humans. However, there are now documented human cases, some infections occurring in splenectomized patients and others in patients with intact spleens.[4] *Babesia* organisms infect the red blood cells and appear as pleomorphic ringlike structures when stained with any of the recommended stains used for blood films (Figure 44.48). They may be confused with the ring forms in *Plasmodium* infections; however, in a *Babesia* infection there are often many rings (four or

five) per red cell and the individual rings are quite small compared with those found in malaria infections.[26]

44.13.c Hemoflagellates. Hemoflagellates are blood and tissue flagellates, two genera of which are medically important for humans: *Leishmania* and *Trypanosoma*. Some species may circulate in the bloodstream or at times may be present in lymph nodes or muscle. Other species tend to parasitize the reticuloendothelial cells of the hematopoietic organs. The hemoflagellates of human beings have four morphological types (Figure 44.49): amastigote (leishmanial form, or Leishman-Donovan body), promastigote (leptomonal form), epimastigote (crithidial form), and trypomastigote (trypanosomal form).

The amastigote form is an intracellular parasite in the cells of the reticuloendothelial system and is oval, measuring approximately 1.5 to 5 μm, and contains a nucleus and kinetoplast. Species of the genus *Leishmania* usually exist as the amastigote form in humans and in the promastigote form in the insect host. The life cycle is essentially the same for all three species, and the clinical manifestations vary

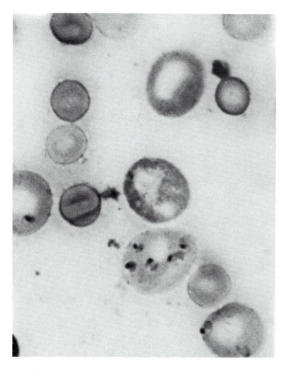

Figure 44.48
Babesia in red blood cells. (Photomicrograph by Zane Price. From Markell, E.K., and Voge, M. 1981. Medical parasitology, ed. 5. W.B. Saunders Co., Philadelphia.)

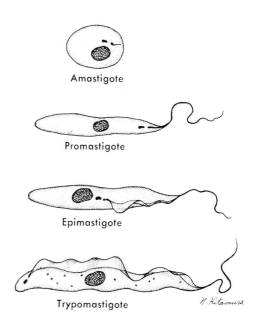

Figure 44.49
Characteristic stages of species of *Leishmania* and *Trypanosoma* in human and insect hosts. (Illustration by Nobuko Kitamura.)

depending on the species involved. As the vector takes a blood meal, the promastigote form is introduced into a human, thus initiating the infection. Depending on the species, the parasites then move from the site of the bite to the organs of the reticuloendothelial system (liver, spleen, bone marrow) or to the macrophages of the skin (Figure 44.50).

Species based on clinical grounds are morphologically the same; however, there are differences in serologies and in growth requirements for culture. There is a great deal of biological variation among the many strains that make up these groups. *Leishmania tropica* causes oriental sore or cutaneous leishmaniasis of the Old World; *Leishmania braziliensis* causes mucocutaneous leishmaniasis of the New World; and *L. donovani* causes visceral leishmaniasis (Dumdum fever, or kala-azar) (Figure 44.51). Additional species have been delineated based on the buoyant density of kinetoplast DNA, the isoenzyme patterns, and serologic testing.

In tissue impression smears or sections *Histoplasma capsulatum* must be differentiated from the Leishman-Donovan (L-D) bodies. *H. capsulatum* does not have a kinetoplast and stains with both periodic acid–Schiff (PAS) stain and Gomori methenamine silver stain, neither of which stains L-D bodies. Diagnosis of leishmanial organisms is based on the demonstration of the L-D bodies or the recovery of the promastigote in culture.

Three species of trypanosomes are pathogenic for humans: *Trypanosoma gambiense* (Figure 44.52) causes West African sleeping sickness; *Trypanosoma rhodesiense* causes East African sleeping sickness; and *Trypanosoma cruzi* causes South American trypanosomiasis, or Chagas' disease (Figure 44.53). The first two species are morphologically similar and produce African sleeping sickness, an illness characterized by both acute and chronic stages. In the acute stage of the disease the organisms can usually be found in the peripheral blood or lymph node aspirates. As the disease progresses to the chronic stage the organisms can be found in the cerebrospinal fluid (CSF) (comatose stage: "sleeping sickness"). *T. rhodesiense* produces a more severe infection, usually resulting in death within 1 year.

In the early stages of infection with *T. cruzi*, the trypomastigote forms appear in the blood but do not multiply (Figure 44.54, *A*). They then invade the endothelial or tissue cells and begin to divide, producing many L-D bodies, which are most often found in cardiac muscle (Figure 44.54, *B*). When these forms are liberated into the blood, they trans-

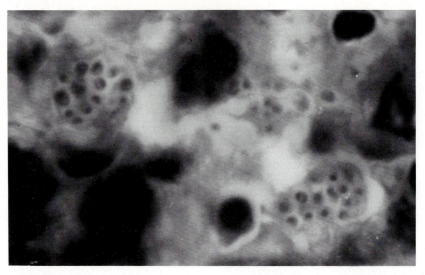

Figure 44.50
Leishmania donovani parasites in Küpffer cells of liver (2000 ×).

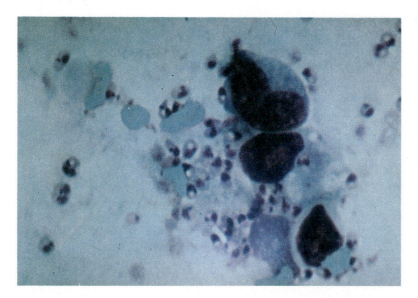

Figure 44.51
Leishmania donovani amastigotes.

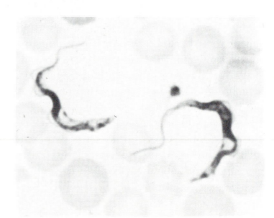

Figure 44.52
Trypanosoma gambiense in blood film (1600 ×).

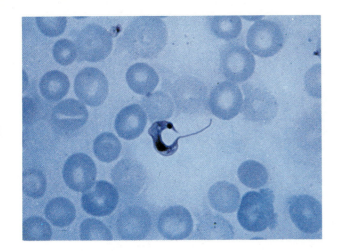

Figure 44.53
Trypanosoma cruzi trypomastigote.

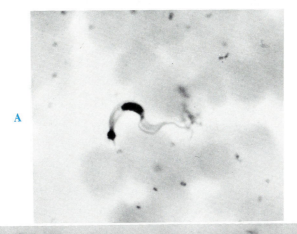

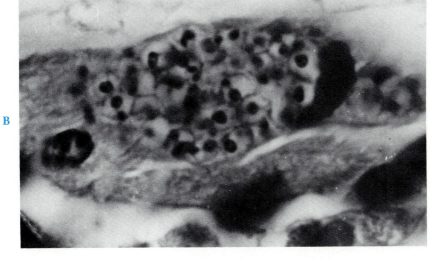

Figure 44.54
A, *Trypanosoma cruzi* in blood film (1600 ×). **B,** *Trypanosoma cruzi* parasites in cardiac muscle
(2500 ×). (From Markell, E.K., and Voge, M.: Medical parasitology, ed. 5, Philadelphia, 1981, W.B.
Saunders Co.)

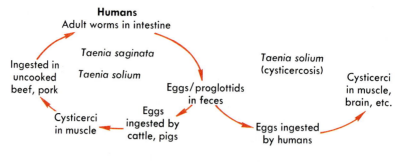

Figure 44.55
Life cycle of *Taenia saginata* and *Taenia solium*.

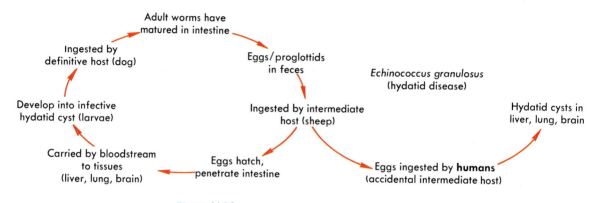

Figure 44.56
Life cycle of *Echinococcus granulosus* (hydatid disease).

form into the trypomastigote forms, which are then carried to other sites, where tissue invasion again occurs.

Diagnosis of the infection is based on demonstration of the parasites, most often on wet unstained or stained blood films. Both thick and thin films should be examined; these can be prepared from peripheral blood or buffy coat. The sediment recovered from CSF can also be examined for the presence of trypomastigotes. Specific techniques for culture, animal inoculation, handling of aspirate and biopsy material, and serologic procedures are presented in earlier sections of this chapter.

Another technique often used in endemic areas for the diagnosis of Chagas' disease is **xenodiagnosis**. Triatomids, the insect vector, are raised in the laboratory and are determined to be free from infection with *T. cruzi*. These insects are allowed to feed on the blood of an individual suspected of having Chagas' disease, and after 2 weeks the intestinal contents are checked for the presence of the epimastigote forms. For additional information, consult Maekelt.[33]

44.14. Intestinal Helminths

The intestinal helminths that infect humans belong to two phyla: the Nematoda, or roundworms, and the platyhelminths, or flatworms. The platyhelminths, most of which are hermaphroditic, have a flat, bilaterally symmetrical body. The two classes, Trematoda and Cestoda, contain organisms that are parasitic for human beings.

The trematodes (flukes) are leaf-shaped or elongate and slender organisms (blood flukes: *Schistosoma* species) that possess hooks or suckers for attachment. Members of this group, which parasitize humans, are found in the intestinal tract, liver, blood vessels, and lungs.

The cestodes (tapeworms) typically have a long, segmented, ribbonlike body, which has a special attachment portion, or scolex, at the anterior end. Adult forms inhabit the small intestine; however, humans may be host to either the adult or the larval forms, depending on the species. The cestodes, as well as the trematodes, require (with few exceptions) one or more intermediate hosts for the completion of the life cycle (Figures 44.55 and 44.56).

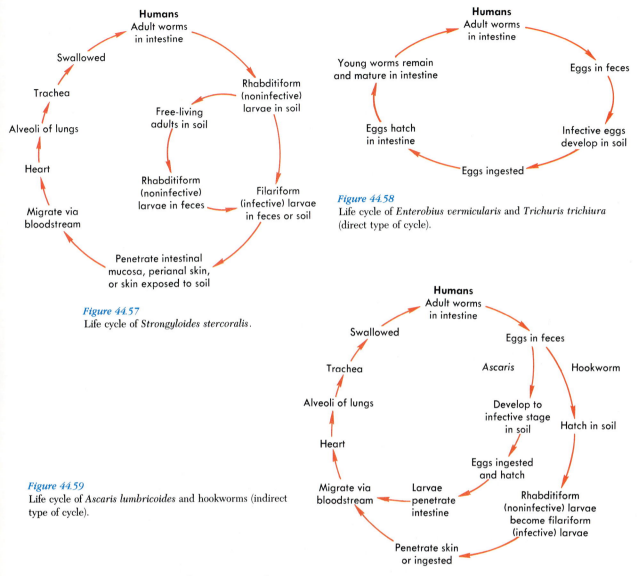

Figure 44.57
Life cycle of *Strongyloides stercoralis*.

Figure 44.58
Life cycle of *Enterobius vermicularis* and *Trichuris trichiura* (direct type of cycle).

Figure 44.59
Life cycle of *Ascaris lumbricoides* and hookworms (indirect type of cycle).

The Nematodes, or roundworms, are elongate, cylindrical worms with a well-developed digestive tract. The sexes are separate, the male usually being smaller than the female. Intermediate hosts are required for larval development in certain species; a large number of species parasitize the intestinal tract and certain tissues of humans (Figures 44.57 to 44.59).

Diagnosis of most intestinal helminth infections is based on the detection of the characteristic eggs and larvae in the stool; occasionally adult worms or portions of worms may also be found. No permanent stains are required, and most diagnostic features can easily be seen on direct wet mounts or in mounts of the concentrated stool material.

44.14.a. Nematodes. The majority of nematodes are diagnosed by finding the characteristic eggs in the stool (Figures 44.60 and 44.61). The eggs of *Ancylostoma duodenale* and *Necator americanus* are essentially identical, so an infection with either species is reported as "hookworm eggs present." *Trichostrongylus* eggs may easily be mistaken for those of hookworms; however, the eggs of *Trichostrongylus* are somewhat larger, and one end tends to be more pointed.

S. stercoralis is passed in the feces as the noninfective rhabditiform larva (Figure 44.62). Although hookworm eggs are normally passed in the

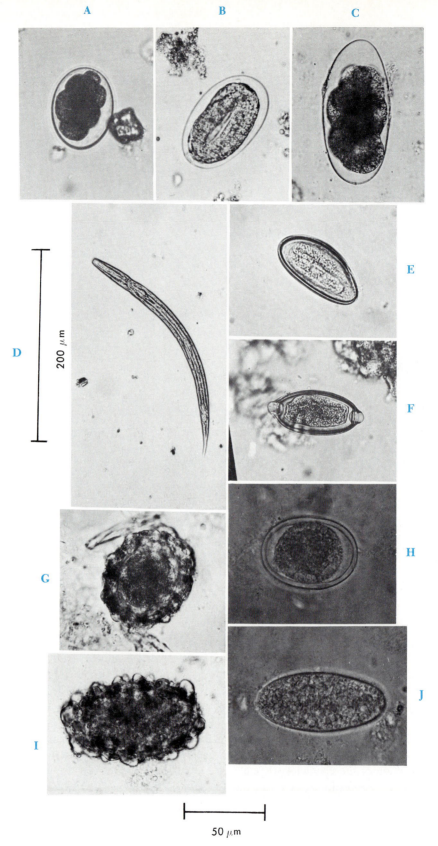

A   B   C

E

D   200 μm

F

G   H

I   J

50 μm

Figure 44.60
For legend see opposite page.

Figure 44.60
A, Immature hookworm egg. **B,** Embryonated hookworm egg. **C,** *Trichostrongylus orientalis,*
immature egg. **D,** *Strongyloides stercoralis,* rhabditiform larva (200 μm). **E,** *Enterobius vermicularis*
egg. **F,** *Trichuris trichiura* egg. **G,** *Ascaris lumbricoides,* fertilized egg. **H,** *A. lumbricoides,* fertilized
egg, decorticate. **I,** *A. lumbricoides,* unfertilized egg. **J,** *A. lumbricoides,* unfertilized egg, decorticate.

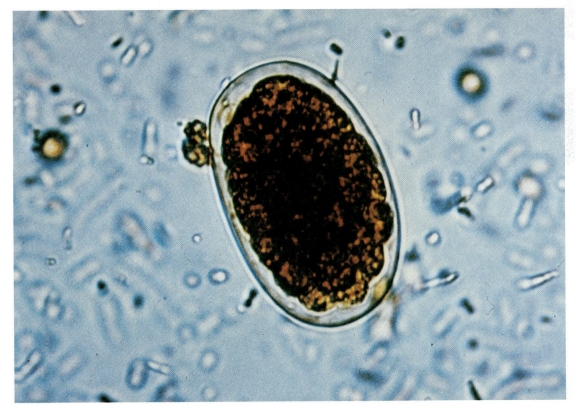

Figure 44.61
Hookworm egg, iodine stain.

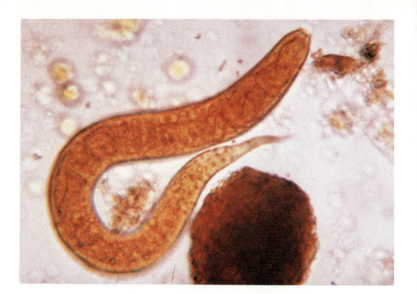

Figure 44.62
Strongyloides stercoralis larva, iodine stain.

Figure 44.63
Rhabditiform larvae. **A,** *Strongyloides.* **B,** Hookworm.
C, *Trichostrongylus. bc,* Buccal cavity; *es,* esophagus; *gp,*
genital primordia; *cb,* beadlike swelling of caudal tip.
(Illustration by Nobuko Kitamura.)

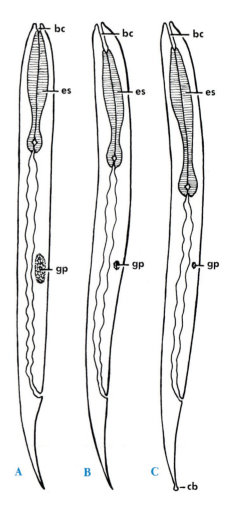

stool, these eggs may continue to develop and hatch
if the stool is left at room temperature for several
days. These larvae may be mistaken for those of
Strongyloides. Figure 44.63 shows the morphological differences between the rhabditiform larvae of
hookworm and *Strongyloides.* Recovery of *Strongyloides* larvae in duodenal contents is mentioned
in Section 44.2.

The appropriate techniques for recovery of *E.
vermicularis* (pinworm) eggs are given in Section
44.2.f. Other worms will not deposit eggs in the same
site; the characteristic morphology of pinworm eggs
is shown in Figure 44.64. Eggs of the other nematodes are fairly easy to find and to differentiate from
one another.

44.14.b. Cestodes. With the exception of *Diphyllobothrium latum,* tapeworm eggs are embryonated and contain a six-hooked oncosphere (Figure
44.65 and Table 44.10). *Taenia saginata* and *T. solium* cannot be speciated on the basis of egg morphology; gravid proglottids (Figure 44.66) or the
scolices must be examined. *T. saginata* (beef tape-

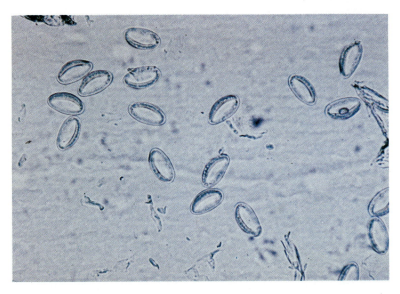

Figure 44.64
Enterobius vermicularis eggs (cellophane [Scotch] tape preparation).

worm) proglottids have approximately 15 to 30 main lateral branches, and the scolex has no hooks; the proglottids of *T. solium* have 7 to 12 main lateral branches, and the scolex has a circle of hooks.

H. nana has an unusual life cycle in that the ingestion of the egg can lead to the adult worm in humans (Figure 44.67). The eggs of *H. nana* (more common) and *Hymenolepis diminuta* are very similar; however, *H. nana* eggs are smaller and have polar filaments, which are present in the space between the oncosphere and the egg shell (Figure 44.65).

Eggs of *Dipylidium caninum* are occasionally found in humans (particularly children) and are passed in the feces in packets of 5 to 15 eggs each (Figures 44.65 and 44.68). The proglottids may also be found; they may resemble cucumber seeds or, when dry, may look like rice grains (white).

The fish tapeworm, *D. latum*, does not have embryonated eggs; these eggs have a somewhat thicker shell and are operculated, much like the trematode eggs (Figure 44.65). Humans acquire the parasite by eating undercooked or raw fish (Figure 44.69).

44.14.c. Trematodes. Humans acquire most fluke infestations by ingesting the encysted metacercariae (Figure 44.70). Most of the trematodes have operculated eggs, which are best recovered by the sedimentation concentration technique rather than the flotation method. Many of these eggs are very similar, both in size and morphology, and often careful measurements must be taken to speciate the eggs (Figure 44.71). The eggs of *Clonorchis (Opisthorchis)*, *Heterophyes*, and *Metagonimus* are very similar and quite small; they are easily missed if the concentration sediment is examined with the $10\times$ objective only. The eggs of *Fasciola hepatica* and *Fasciolopsis buski* are also very similar but much larger than those just mentioned.

Paragonimus westermani eggs are not only found in the stool but also may be found in sputum (Figure 44.71). These eggs are very similar in size and shape to the egg of the fish tapeworm, *D. latum*. Schistosomiasis, a great source of morbidity in much of the developing world, is acquired during activities (such as bathing, swimming, doing laundry, planting rice, and fishing) that involve contact with water infested with the intermediate snail host of the parasite. The free-swimming cercarial form attaches to a vertebrate host and penetrates through intact skin (Figure 44.72). In temperate zones, such as in the areas near the Great Lakes, cercariae of other trematodes that normally infect birds or other animals can penetrate human skin and cause a strong local reaction (swimmer's itch), although they cannot go on to develop into adult worms in the unnatural human host. Probably the easiest trematode eggs to

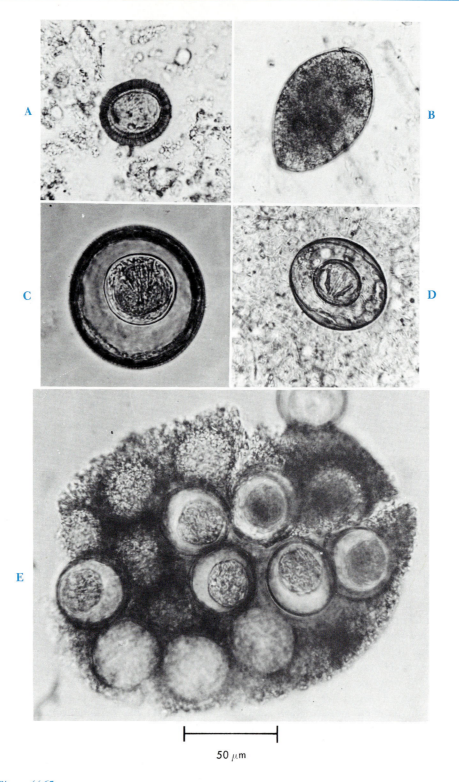

50 μm

Figure 44.65

A, *Taenia* species egg. **B,** *Diphyllobothrium latum* egg. **C,** *Hymenolepis diminuta* egg. **D,** *Hymenolepis nana* egg. **E,** *Dipylidium caninum* egg packet.

Table 44.10

Differential Characteristics of Some Important Tapeworms of Humans

	TAENIA SAGINATA	*TAENIA SOLIUM*	*HYMENOLEPIS NANA*	*DIPHYLLOBOTHRIUM LATUM*
Length	4-8 m	3-5 m	2.5-4 cm	4-10 m
Scolex				
Shape	Quadrilateral	Globular	Usually not seen	Almondlike
Size	1 × 1.5 mm	1 × 1 mm		3 × 1 mm
Rostellum and hook-lets	No	Yes		No
Suckers	4	4		2 (grooves)
Terminal proglottids (gravid)				
Size	19 × 7 mm, longer than wide	11 × 5 mm	Usually not seen	3 × 11 mm, wider than long
Primary lateral uterine branches	15-30 on each side	6-12 on each side		Rosette-shaped
Color	Milky white	Milky white		Ivory
Appearance in feces	Usually appear singly	5 or 6 segments		Varies from a few inches to a few feet in length
Ova				
Shape	Spheroid	Spheroid	Broadly oval	Oval
Size	35 μm	35 μm	30 × 47 μm	45 × 70 μm
Color	Rusty brown	Rusty brown	Pale	Yellow-brown
Embryo with hooklets	Yes	Yes	Yes	No
Operculum	No	No	No	Yes (difficult to see)

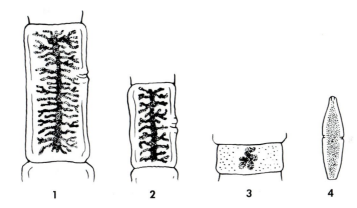

Figure 44.66
Gravid proglottids. **1,** *Taenia saginata*. **2,** *Taenia solium*. **3,** *Diphyllobothrium latum*. **4,** *Dipylidium caninum*. (From Garcia, L.S., and Bruckner, D.A. 1988. Diagnostic medical parasitology. Elsevier, New York.)

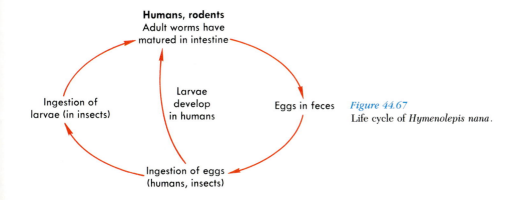

Figure 44.67
Life cycle of *Hymenolepis nana*.

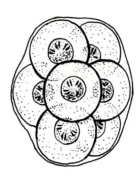

Figure 44.68
Dipylidium caninum egg packet. (Illustration by Nobuko Kitamura.)

Figure 44.69
Life cycle of *Diphyllobothrium latum*.

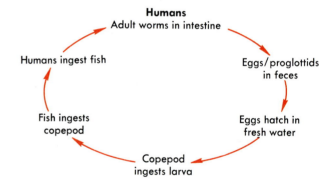

Figure 44.70
Life cycle of trematodes acquired by humans through ingestion of raw fish, crabs, or crayfish and vegetation.

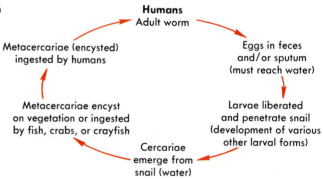

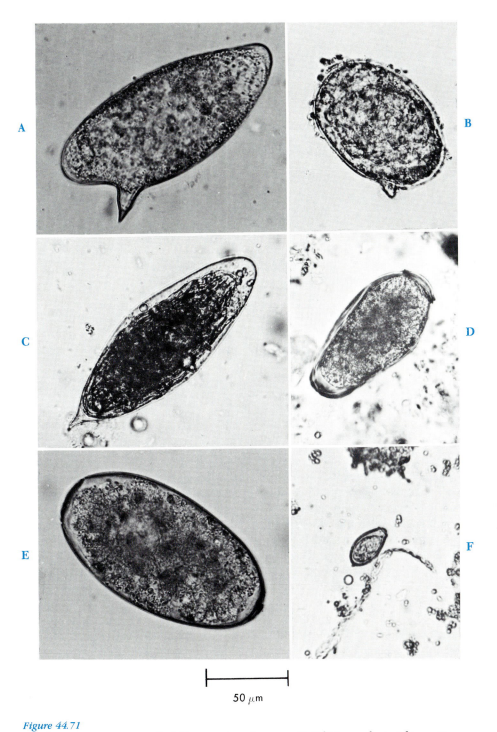

Figure 44.71
A, *Schistosoma mansoni* egg. **B,** *Schistosoma japonicum* egg. **C,** *Schistosoma haematobium* egg.
D, *Paragonimus westermani* egg. **E,** *Fasciola hepatica* egg. **F,** *Clonorchis (Opisthorchis) sinensis* egg.

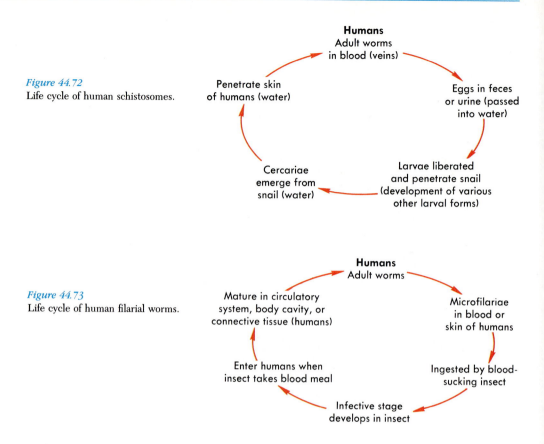

Figure 44.72
Life cycle of human schistosomes.

Figure 44.73
Life cycle of human filarial worms.

identify are those of the schistosomes: *S. mansoni* eggs are characterized by having a very prominent lateral spine, *S. haematobium* a terminal spine, and *S. japonicum* a small lateral spine that may be difficult to see. These eggs are nonoperculated. Schistosome eggs stain acid fast. Specific procedures for their recovery and identification are found in Section 44.2.e.

44.15. Blood Helminths

44.15.a. Filariae. The filarial worms are long, thin nematodes that inhabit parts of the lymphatic system and the subcutaneous and deep connective tissues. A life cycle has been included here to show the various stages present in the human host (Figure 44.73). Most species produce microfilariae, which can be found in the peripheral blood; two species, *O. volvulus* and *Dipetalonema streptocerca*, produce microfilariae found in the subcutaneous tissues and dermis.

Diagnosis of filarial infections is often based on clinical grounds, but demonstration of the parasite is the only accurate means of confirming the diagnosis (Figure 44.74). Fresh blood films may be prepared; actively moving microfilariae can be observed in a preparation of this type. If the patient has a light infection, thick blood films can be prepared and stained. The Knott concentration procedure[29] and the membrane filtration technique[13,14] may also be helpful in recovering the organisms. Microfilariae of some strains tend to exhibit nocturnal periodicity; thus, the time the blood is drawn may be critical in demonstrating the parasite. The microfilariae of *O. volvulus* and *D. streptocerca* are found in "skin snips," very thin slices of skin, which are teased apart in normal saline to release the organisms. Differentiation of the species is dependent on (1) the presence or absence of the sheath and (2) the distribution of nuclei in the tail region of the microfilaria (Figure 44.75).

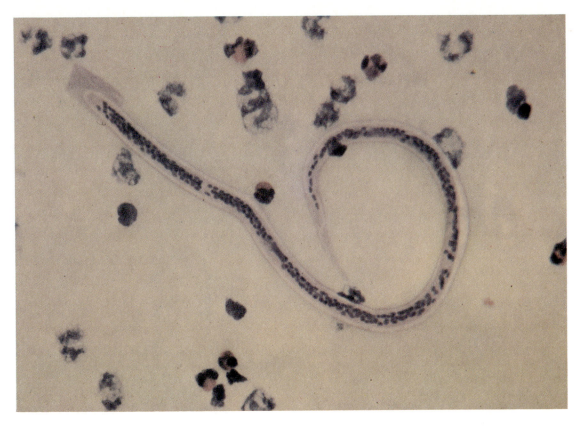

Figure 44.74
Microfilaria of *Wuchereria bancrofti* in thick blood film. (From Markell, E.K., and Voge, M. 1981. Medical parasitology, ed. 5. W.B. Saunders Co., Philadelphia.)

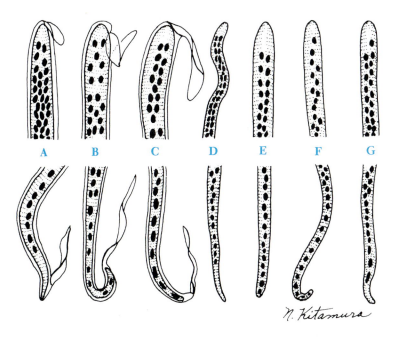

Figure 44.75
Anterior and posterior ends of microfilariae found in humans. **A,** *Wuchereria bancrofti*. **B,** *Brugia malayi*. **C,** *Loa loa*. **D,** *Onchocerca volvulus*. **E,** *Dipetalonema perstans*, **F,** *Dipetalonema streptocerca*. **G,** *Mansonella ozzardi*.

REFERENCES

1. Auran, J.D., Starr, M.B., and Jakobiec, F.A. 1987. *Acanthamoeba* keratitis. Cornea 6:2.

2. Beaver, P.C. 1949. A nephelometric method of calibrating the photoelectric meter for making egg-counts by direct fecal smear. J. Parasitol. 35(Sect. 2):13.

3. Beaver, P.C. 1950. The standardization of fecal smears for estimating egg production and worm burden. J. Parasitol. 36:451.

4. Beaver, P.C., Jung, R.C., and Cupp, E.W. 1984. Clinical parasitology, ed. 9. Lea & Febiger, Philadelphia.

5. Bigby, T.V., Margolskee, D., Curtis, J.L., et al. 1986. The usefulness of induced sputum in the diagnosis of *Pneumocystis carinii* pneumonia in patients with the acquired immunodeficiency syndrome. Am. Rev. Respir. Dis. 133:515.

6. Brooke, M.M., and Goldman, M. 1949. Polyvinyl alcohol-fixative as a preservative and adhesive for protozoa in dysenteric stools and other liquid material. J. Lab. Clin. Med. 34:1554.

7. Brooke, M.M., and Melvin, D. 1969. Morphology of diagnostic stages of intestinal parasites of man. DHEW Publ. No. (HSM)72-8116. U.S. Government Printing Office, Washington, D.C.

8. Chang, T.H., Tsing, S.Y., and Tzeng, S. 1986. Monoclonal antibodies against *Trichomonas vaginalis*. Hybridoma 5:43.

9. Cohen, E.J., Buchanan, H.W., Laughrea, P.A., et al. 1985. Diagnosis and management of *Acanthamoeba* keratitis. Am. J. Ophthalmol. 100:389.

10. Cohen, E.J., Parlato, C.J., Arentsen, J.J., et al. 1987. Medical and surgical treatment of *Acanthamoeba* keratitis. Am. J. Ophthalmol. 103:615.

11. Cohen, J.D., Ruhlig L., Jayich, S.A., et al. 1984. *Cryptosporidium* in acquired immunodeficiency syndrome. Dig. Dis. Sci. 29:773.

12. Committee on Education, American Society of Parasitologists. 1977. Procedures suggested for use in examination of clinical specimens for parasitic infection. J. Parasitol. 63:959.

13. Dennis, D.T., and Kean, B.H. 1971. Isolation of microfilariae: report of a new method. J. Parasitol. 57:1146.

14. Desowitz, R.S., and Hitchcock, J.C. 1974. Hyperendemic bancroftian filariasis in the Kingdom of Tonga: the application of the membrane filter concentration technique to an age-stratified blood survey. Am. J. Trop. Med. Hyg. 23:877.

15. Desportes, I., Le Charpentier, Y., Galian, A., et al. 1985. Occurrence of a new microsporidian: *Enterocytozoon bieneusi* n.g., n.sp., in the enterocytes of a human patient with AIDS. J. Protozool. 32:250.

16. Donzis, P.B., Mondino, B.J., Weissman, B.A., and Bruckner, D.A. 1987. Microbial contamination of contact lens care systems. Am. J. Ophthalmol. 104:325.

17. Feinberg, J.G., and Whittington, M.J. 1957. A culture medium for *Trichomonas vaginalis* Donne and species of *Candida*. J. Clin. Pathol. 10:327.

18. Fritsche, T.R., and Bergeron, D.L. 1987. *Acanthamoeba* keratitis. Clinical Microbiol. Newsletter 9:109.

19. Garcia, L.S., and Ash, L.R. 1979. Diagnostic parasitology: clinical laboratory manual. ed. 2. The C.V. Mosby Co., St. Louis.

20. Garcia, L.S., Brewer, T.C., and Bruckner, D.A. 1987. Fluorescence detection of *Cryptosporidium* oocysts in human fecal specimens by using monoclonal antibodies. J. Clin. Microbiol. 25:119.

21. Garcia, L.S., and Bruckner, D.A. 1988. Diagnostic medical parasitology. Elsevier, New York.

22. Garcia, L.S., Bruckner, D.A., Brewer, T.C., and Shimizu, R.Y. 1983. Techniques for the recovery and identification of *Cryptosporidium* oocysts from stool specimens. J. Clin. Microbiol. 18:185.

23. Gill, V.J., Evans, G., Stock, F., et al. 1987. Detection of *Pneumocystis carinii* by a fluorescent antibody stain using a combination of three monoclonal antibodies. J. Clin. Microbiol. 25:1837.

24. Gomori, G. 1950. A rapid one-step trichrome stain. Am. J. Clin. Pathol. 20:661.

25. Harada, Y., and Mori, O. 1955. A new method for culturing hookworm. Yonago Acta Med. 1:177.

26. Healy, G.R., and Ruebush, T.K. II. 1980. Morphology of *Babesia microti* in human blood smears. Am. J. Clin. Pathol. 73:107.

27. Hendricks, L., and Wright, N. 1979. Diagnosis of cutaneous leishmaniasis by in vitro cultivation of saline aspirates in Schneider's Drosophila medium. Am. J. Trop. Med. Hyg. 28(6):962.

28. Kagan, I.G. 1980. Serodiagnosis of parasitic diseases. In Lennette, E.H., Balows, A., Hausler, W.J., Jr., and Truant, J.P., editors: Manual of clinical microbiology, ed. 3. American Society for Microbiology, Washington, D.C.

29. Knott, J.I. 1939. A method for making microfilarial surveys on day blood. Trans. R. Soc. Trop. Med. Hyg. 33:191.

30. Kovacs, J.A., Ng, V.L., Masur, H., et al. 1988. Diagnosis of *Pneumocystis carinii*. Improved detection in sputum using monoclonal antibodies. N. Engl. J. Med. 318:589.

31. Ledford, D.K., Overman, M.D., Gonzalvo, A., et al. 1985. Microsporidiosis myositis in a patient with acquired immunodeficiency syndrome. Ann. Intern. Med. 102:628.

32. Lindquist, T.D., Sher, N.A., and Doughman, D.J. 1988. Clinical signs and medical therapy of early *Acanthamoeba* keratitis. Arch. Ophthalmol. 106:73.

33. Maekelt, G.A. 1964. A modified procedure of xenodiagnosis for Chagas' disease. Am. J. Trop. Med. Hyg. 13:11.

34. Markell, E.K., and Udkow, M.P. 1986. *Blastocystis hominis*: pathogen or fellow traveler? Am. J. Trop. Med. Hyg. 35:1023.

35. Markell, E.K., and Voge, M. 1981. Medical parasitology, ed. 5. W.B. Saunders Co., Philadelphia.

36. Markell, E.K., Voge, M., and John, D.T. 1986. Medical Parasitology, ed. 6. W.B. Saunders Co., Philadelphia.

37. McCauley, D.I., Naidick, D.P., Leitman, B.S., et al. 1982. Radiographic pattern of opportunistic lung infections and Kaposi sarcoma in homosexual men. Am. J. Radiol. 139:653.

38. Melvin, D.M., and Brooke, M.M. 1974. Laboratory procedures for the diagnosis of intestinal parasites. DHEW Publication No. (CDC) 75-8282, U.S. Government Printing Office, Washington, D.C.

39. Miller, L.H., Mason, S.J., Dvorak, J.A., et al. 1975. Erythrocyte receptors for (*Plasmodium knowlesi*) malaria: Duffy blood group determinants. Science 189:561.

40. Moore, M.B., McCulley, J.P., Luckenbach, M., et al. 1985. *Acanthamoeba* keratitis associated with soft contact lenses. Am. J. Ophthalmol. 100:396.

41. Nair, C.P. 1953. Rapid staining of intestinal amoebae on wet mounts. Nature 172:1051.

42. Navin, T.R., and Juranek, D.D. 1984. Cryptosporidiosis: clinical, epidemiologic and parasitologic review. Rev. Infect. Dis. 6:313.

43. Ng, E., Markell, E.K., Fleming, R.L., and Fried, M. 1984. Demonstration of *Isospora belli* by acid-fast stain in a patient with acquired immune deficiency syndrome. J. Clin. Microbiol. 20:384.

44. Parasitology Subcommittee, Microbiology Section of Scientific Assembly, American Society for Medical Technology. 1978. Recommended procedures for the examination of clinical specimens submitted for the diagnosis of parasitic infections. Am. J. Med. Technol. 44:1101.

45. Sapèro, J.J., and Lawless, D.K. 1953. The MIF stain-preservation technique for the identification of intestinal protozoa. Am. J. Trop. Med. Hyg. 2:613.

46. Scholten, T.H. 1972. An improved technique for the recovery of intestinal protozoa. J. Parasitol. 58:633.

47. Scholten, T.H., and Yang, J. 1974. Evaluation of unpreserved and preserved stools for the detection and identification of intestinal parasites. Am. J. Clin. Pathol. 62:563.

48. Sheehan, D.J., Raucher, B.G., and McKitrick, J.C. 1986. Association of *Blastocystis hominis* with signs and symptoms of human disease. J. Clin. Microbiol. 24:548.

49. Spencer, F.M., and Monroe, L.S. 1976. The color atlas of intestinal parasites, ed. 2. Charles C Thomas, Publisher, Springfield, Ill.

50. Sterling, C.R., and Arrowood, M.J. 1986. Detection of *Cryptosporidium* sp. infections using a direct immunofluorescent assay. Pediatr. Infect. Dis. 5:S139.

51. Stoll, N.R., and Hausheer, W.C. 1926. Concerning two options in dilution egg counting: small drop and displacement. Am. J. Hyg. 6:134.

52. Stover, D.E., Zaman, M.B., Hadju, S.I., et al. 1984. Bronchoalveolar lavage in the diagnosis of diffuse pulmonary infiltrates in the immunosuppressed host. Ann. Intern. Med. 101:1.

53. Strano, A.J., Cali, A., and Neafie, R.C. 1976. Microsporidiosis. pp. 336-339. In Binford, C.H., and Connor, D.H., editors: Pathology of tropical and extraordinary diseases. Armed Forces Institute of Pathology, Washington, D.C.

54. Sulzer, A.J., and Wilson, M. 1967. The use of thick-smear antigen slides in the malaria indirect fluorescent antibody test. J. Parasitol. 53:1110.

55. Sulzer, A.J., Wilson, M., and Hall, E.C. 1969. Indirect fluorescent antibody tests for parasitic diseases. V. An evaluation of a thick-smear antigen in the IFA for malaria antibodies. Am. J. Trop. Med. Hyg. 18:199.

56. Tompkins, V.N., and Miller, J.K. 1947. Staining intestinal protozoa with iron-hematoxylin-phosphotungstic acid. Am. J. Clin. Pathol. 17:755.

57. Wheatley, W.B. 1951. A rapid staining procedure for intestinal amoebae and flagellates. Am. J. Clin. Pathol. 21:990.

58. Wilcox, A. 1960. Manual for the microscopical diagnosis of malaria in man. Public Health Service, Washington, D.C.

59. Wilhelmus, K.R., Osato, M.S., Font, R.L., et al. 1986. Rapid diagnosis of *Acanthamoeba* keratitis using calcofluor white. Arch. Ophthalmol. 104:1309.

60. Zierdt, C.H. 1978. *Blastocystis hominis*, an intestinal protozoan parasite of man. Public Health Lab. 36:146.

61. Zierdt, C.H. 1988. *Blastocystis hominis*, a long-misunderstood intestinal parasite. Parasitology Today 4:15.

Appendix A   Formulas and Preparation of Culture Media and Reagents

The basic principles governing the preparation of laboratory media were discussed in Chapter 8. The importance of testing each batch of media for proper performance was discussed in Chapter 3. Various specialized media formulations and uses have been mentioned throughout the text where appropriate; these media are presented in this chapter. The media formulas included in this chapter are those that can be used for more than one purpose or those that are so complicated that they cannot easily be placed within a chapter. Unless stated otherwise, storage of prepared media at 2° to 8° C best preserves their usefulness. Tubed media should be stored tightly capped; tubed media that must be stored for long periods can be made airtight by dipping the tightly capped end into melted paraffin several times. Alternatively, several layers of Parafilm (American Can Co.) can be wrapped tightly around the cap end.

Liquid media that have been stored for any length of time should be heated in a boiling water bath or in flowing steam (Arnold steam sterilizer) for a few minutes to drive off dissolved gases and then cooled quickly to room temperature (in cold water, for example) before using. Agar tubes should be melted and allowed to resolidify to reconstitute sufficient moisture. Agar plates should be wrapped tightly in sealed plastic bags (polyethylene or other plastic) or wrapped individually (shrink-sealers for plates are available from Scientific Device Laboratory) and stored upside down so that moisture does not collect on the agar surface. If agar plates of a particular medium will be used infrequently, tubes of the medium can be prepared (20 ml per tube) and stored, to be melted down and poured into Petri plates one at a time as needed. In the formulas given in this chapter and throughout the text, specific manufacturers of components have been mentioned if they were specified in the original reference, or if they are commonly available from that source. The substitution of similar ingredients should be confirmed by testing quality control strains of organisms before assuming that such media are equivalent. Instructions for proper preparation of all dry powder media are printed on the container or provided by the manufacturer in a supplemental publication, such as the *Difco Manual*, and *Oxoid Manual*. Almost every medium used for clinical microbiology, however, can be purchased prepared from at least one manufacturer. Specialty media can also be purchased, often at a slightly increased price. The most well-known large media suppliers are listed in Appendix C. Laboratories may often be able to find local suppliers for prepared media that are not cost effective for in-house preparation.

ACETATE AGAR

Acetate agar medium is prepared in the same manner as Simmons citrate agar except that 0.25% sodium acetate is used in place of citrate. It is used to determine whether an organism is able to utilize acetate as its sole carbon source. Growth on the slant and development of a **blue** color indicate a positive test. A negative test is no growth or color change. This test is useful in differentiating *Escherichia coli* from shigellae in that the latter do not utilize acetate.

ACETATE BUFFER SOLUTION FOR STAINING TROPHOZOITES

Stock Solution A

0.2 M acetic acid solution

Acetic acid	11.55 ml
Distilled water	1000.0 ml

Stock Solution B

0.2 M sodium acetate solution

$C_2H_3O_2Na$	16.4 g
or	
$C_2H_3O_2Na \cdot 3H_2O$	27.2 g
Distilled water	1000.0 ml

Proportions of solutions A and B for specific pH are as follows: mix the indicated quantity of stock solutions A and B and dilute with distilled water to a total of 100 ml.

Desired pH	Stock Solution A (ml)	Stock Solution B (ml)
3.6	46.3	3.7
3.8	44.0	6.0
4.0	41.0	9.0
4.2	36.8	13.2
4.4	30.5	19.5
4.6	25.5	24.5

ALKALINE PEPTONE WATER FOR RECOVERY OF *VIBRIO CHOLERAE*

Peptone	10 g
NaCl	5 g
Distilled water	1000 ml

Adjust to pH 9.0 with 1 N NaOH and autoclave for 15 min at 121° C.

AMIES TRANSPORT MEDIUM WITH CHARCOAL FOR MAINTENANCE OF FASTIDIOUS ORGANISMS IN ORIGINAL SPECIMENS

(Amies. 1967. Can. J. Public Health 58:296.)

1. Add 4 g of agar to 1 L of distilled water, heat until dissolved, and while hot add:

Sodium chloride	3 g
Potassium chloride	0.2 g
Sodium thioglycollate	1 g
Disodium phosphate, anhydrous	1.15 g
(or disodium phosphate · 12 H_2O)	2.9 g
Monopotassium phosphate	0.2 g
Calcium chloride, 1% aqueous, freshly prepared	10 ml
Magnesium chloride · 6 H_2O, 1% aqueous	10 ml
(Final pH 7.3)	

2. Stir until dissolved, and then add 10 g of pharmaceutical neutral charcoal. Dispense 5 to 6 ml per 13- × 100-mm screw-capped tube (or vial), with frequent stirring to keep the charcoal in suspension. Avoid cooling or gelling.
3. Sterilize at 121° C for 20 min. *Prior to solidification*, invert tubes to distribute the charcoal evenly. Store in refrigerator.
4. It should be emphasized that prolonged heating in open flasks should be avoided, since the reducing agent (sodium thioglycollate) is volatile.

ANAEROBIC INDICATORS USED TO VISUALLY DEMONSTRATE ANAEROBIC ATMOSPHERE WITHIN A JAR, CHAMBER, OR OTHER SYSTEM

FILDES AND MCINTOSH INDICATOR

Prepare the following solutions:
1. 6% aqueous glucose (add a small crystal of thymol as a preservative).
2. Add 6 ml of 0.1 N sodium hydroxide to 94 ml of distilled water.
3. Add 3 ml of aqueous methylene blue (0.5%) to 100 ml of distilled water.

For use, mix 1 ml of each solution in a test tube, boil the mixture until colorless, then place in a loaded anaerobic jar before sealing. A blue color at the end of incubation indicates that anaerobiosis was not achieved.

SMITH MODIFIED METHYLENE BLUE INDICATOR

(Smith. 1964. ASM Meeting, Washington, D.C.)

Mix thoroughly 1 pound (450 g) of sodium bicarbonate (commercial grade is satisfactory) with 50 g of glucose and 20 mg of methylene blue. For use, add about 1 inch (2.5 cm) to a 16- × 100-mm test tube, half fill with tap water, invert to mix, and place within the anaerobic jar. The solution will slowly become colorless during incubation at 35° C; if more rapid decolorization is required, the solution may be heated to boiling and cooled rapidly immediately before placing in the jar. The indicator should be **colorless** at the end of incubation if anaerobiosis was maintained.

ANDRADE'S INDICATOR

(Modified from MacFaddin. 1980. Biochemical Tests for Identification of Medical Bacteria. Williams & Wilkins, Baltimore.)

Distilled water	100 ml
Acid fuchsin	0.5 g
1 N NaOH	16 ml

Dissolve the fuchsin in distilled water, and add the sodium hydroxide. If the fuchsin is not sufficiently decolorized after several hours, an additional 1 or 2 ml of sodium hydroxide is added. Continue to add NaOH (drop by drop) until the desired straw-yellow color is reached. Add Andrade's indicator to carbohydrate broth base used for phenol red carbohydrates (see Phenol Red Broth Base) without the phenol red to a final concentration of 1% (10 ml indicator per liter broth base). Adjust the pH to 7.1 to 7.2 before adding carbohydrates. See Carbohydrate Media for further information.

ASCOSPORE AGAR

Potassium acetate	10 g
Yeast extract	2.5 g
Dextrose	1 g
Agar	30 g
Distilled water	1000 ml

Dissolve, tube, and autoclave at 121° C for 15 min. Ascospores are obtained in 2 to 6 days at room temperature (23° to 25° C).

BACTEROIDES BILE ESCULIN AGAR (BBE AGAR)

Trypticase soy agar	40 g
Oxgall	20 g
Esculin	1 g
Ferric ammonium citrate	0.5 g
Hemin solution (5 mg/ml)	2 ml
Gentamicin solution (40 mg/ml)*	2.5 ml
Distilled water	1000 ml

Adjust pH to 7.0, heat to dissolve, dispense in 100-ml bottles, autoclave at 121° C for 15 min, and cool to 50° C. Pour plates.

BASIC FUCHSIN AGAR

See Thionine Agar.

BEEF EXTRACT AGAR

Add 2.5% agar to beef extract broth, dissolve by boiling, adjust to pH 7.6, tube and autoclave at 121° C for 15 min, and slant before solidifying.

---

*Garamycin injectable (Schering Corp.) may be used.

The medium is used for pure culture preparation of *Candida* species prior to the carrying out of fermentation tests.

BEEF EXTRACT BROTH

Beef extract	3 g
Peptone	10 g
Sodium chloride	5 g
Distilled water	1000 ml

Dissolve ingredients by boiling, adjust to pH 7.2, tube in 10-ml amounts in 18- × 150-mm tubes, and autoclave at 121° C for 15 min. For use as a fermentation base broth, add 100 ml of a 0.04% aqueous solution of bromthymol blue before tubing and sterilizing.

The medium is used for differentiation of *Candida* species by carbohydrate fermentation tests.

BILE

See Oxgall.

BILE ESCULIN AGAR

Beef extract	3 g
Peptone	5 g
Oxgall	40 g
Esculin	1 g
Ferric citrate	0.5 g
Agar	15 g
Distilled water	1000 ml

1. Suspend 64 g of the dehydrated medium in water, heat to boiling to dissolve, and tube in screw-capped tubes.
2. Sterilize by autoclaving at 121° C for 15 min.
3. Cool to 55° C, add aseptically 50 ml of filter-sterilized horse serum (optional), and mix well.
4. Dispense in sterile tubes, and cool in a slanted position.

This medium is useful in the selective detection of group D streptococci. After inoculation, these organisms form brownish black colonies surrounded by a black zone. *Listeria monocytogenes* also reacts positively, as do some other organisms. Other forms of agar and broth media also are available.

BIRDSEED AGAR

Guizottia abyssinica seeds (niger or thistle seeds)	70 g
Creatinine	0.78 g
Dextrose	10 g
Chloramphenicol (one 50 mg capsule)	0.05 g
Agar	20 g
Distilled water	1000 ml

Diphenyl	100 mg
95% Ethyl alcohol	10 ml

1. Grind seed to powder in blender. Add 300 ml of water and autoclave at 115° C for 10 min.
2. Filter through gauze, and bring volume to 1 L.
3. Add other ingredients except diphenyl, and autoclave at 121° C for 15 min.
4. Cool to 50° C.
5. Add diphenyl to 10 ml of 95% ethanol, and add aseptically to medium.
6. Stir and pour into plates.

BISMUTH SULFITE AGAR

Beef extract	5 g
Peptone	10 g
Dextrose	5 g
Disodium phosphate	4 g
Ferrous sulfate	0.3 g
Bismuth sulfite indicator	8 g
Agar	20 g
Brilliant green	0.025 g
Distilled water	1000 ml

Bismuth sulfite agar medium is highly recommended for the isolation of *Salmonella typhi*, as well as other salmonellae. It may be used for both streak and pour plates.

BLOOD AGAR PLATES FOR STREAKING

Blood agar base medium	500 ml
Sterile blood	20 ml

Sterilize the base medium (trypticase soy agar [BBL] or tryptic soy agar [Difco] is recommended*), cool to 48° to 50° C, and add 5% sterile defibrinated sheep, horse, or rabbit blood, aseptically. Rotate to mix thoroughly, and pour into sterile Petri dishes in approximately 20 ml amounts. When agar is set, invert and incubate one or two plates per 100- to 200-ml batch overnight to test for sterility. Discard test plates. Blood agar plates may be refrigerated for 1 week without deterioration, but they should be packaged to minimize water loss, which could amount to 7% per week if unprotected.

The pouring should be done carefully to avoid air bubbles. If bubbles appear in the poured plate, pass a Bunsen flame over the agar before it sets. This causes the bubbles to break.

An alternative to pouring media from an Erlen-

---

*Brucella agar is an excellent base for blood agar for anaerobic bacteria. Columbia agar and Schaedler agar have also been recommended for this purpose.

meyer flask is the use of a Kelly bottle with a release clamp on a piece of rubber tubing connected to a bell device at the other end. This assembly is mounted on a ring stand. Release of pressure on the clamp permits the heated medium to flow evenly into the plate. An advantage of this system is that bubbles (when present) rise to the top of the liquid medium in the bottle prior to its being poured into the plate.

BLOOD CYSTINE DEXTROSE AGAR

(Francis. 1928. J.A.M.A. 91:1155; Rhamy. 1933. Am. J. Clin. Pathol. 3:121.)

Beef heart infusion	500 g
Proteose peptone	10 g
Glucose	10 g
Sodium chloride	5 g
Cystine	1 g
Agar	15 g
Distilled water	1000 ml

Blood cystine dextrose agar medium may be used satisfactorily for the cultivation of *Francisella tularensis*.

To prepare this medium, dissolve 16.8 g of dehydrated product in 300 ml of distilled water. Adjust the medium to pH 7.3 and autoclave for 20 min at 15 pounds' pressure. Cool to a temperature of 60° to 70° C, add 18 ml of whole rabbit blood or dehydrated hemoglobin, mix well, and distribute into test tubes aseptically. Cool in a slanted position.

BORDET-GENGOU MEDIUM

Potatoes, infusion from	125 g
Sodium chloride	5.5 g
Agar	20 g
Distilled water	1000 ml

Sterilize at 15 pounds for 15 min. Cool to 50° C and add 15% to 20% sterile sheep, rabbit, or human blood aseptically.

The medium is recommended for cultivation of *Bordetella pertussis*.

BRAIN-HEART INFUSION BLOOD AGAR (BHIBA)

Brain-heart infusion agar	26 g
Agar, powdered	2.5 g
Distilled water	500 ml
(Final pH ≈ 7.4)	

Suspend the ingredients in the water, and dissolve by boiling. Autoclave for 15 min at 121° C. Cool to about 45° C, and add aseptically 30 ml of defibrinated animal blood. Mix well, and distribute aseptically in approximately 20-ml amounts in cotton-plugged and sterilized 25- × 150-mm Pyrex test tubes (without lips). Slant, allow to harden, and refrigerate. The medium may also be poured into plates, 40 ml/90 mm diameter Petri dish.

This medium is used for the isolation of fastidious fungi.

BRAIN-HEART INFUSION BROTH

Calf brain infusion	200 g
Beef heart infusion	250 g
Proteose peptone	10 g
Dextrose	2 g
Sodium chloride	5 g
Disodium phosphate	2.5 g
Distilled water	1000 ml

(Final pH ≈ approximately 7.4)

Brain-heart infusion broth is recommended for cultivating the pneumococcus for the liquid bile solubility test.

BRILLIANT GREEN AGAR

Yeast extract	3 g
Proteose peptone No. 3	10 g
Sodium chloride	5 g
Lactose	10 g
Sucrose	10 g
Phenol red	0.08 g
Brilliant green	0.0125 g
Agar	20 g
Distilled water	1000 ml

(Final pH 6.9)

Brilliant green agar is a highly selective medium recommended for the isolation of salmonellae other than *Salmonella typhi*. It is not recommended for the isolation of shigellae.

BROMCRESOL PURPLE BROTH BASE FOR IDENTIFICATION OF STREPTOCOCCI

See Procedure 25.4, Chapter 25.

BRUCELLA AGAR

Pancreatic digest of casein USP	10 g
Peptic digest of animal tissues USP	10 g
Yeast autolysate	2 g
Dextrose	1 g
Sodium chloride	5 g
Sodium bisulfite	0.1 g
Agar	15 g
Distilled water	1000 ml

(Final pH 7.0 ± 0.02)

Heat with agitation until dissolved. Dispense and

autoclave at 121° C for 15 min. Cool to 50° C and pour plates.

CAMPYLOBACTER MEDIA

The basic plate medium (Campy-BAP) consists of *Brucella* agar base and 5% sheep erythrocytes with the following amounts of antimicrobials per liter:

Vancomycin	10 mg
Trimethoprim	5 mg
Polymyxin B	2500 IU
Amphotericin B	2 mg
Cephalothin	15 mg

The liquid medium (Campy-thio) is thioglycollate broth with 0.16% agar and the antimicrobials listed above. See Chapter 30 for more information.

CARBOHYDRATE BROTH

Prepare the following ingredients:

Solution A

Heart infusion broth	22.5 g
Distilled water	900.0 ml

Solution B

Carbohydrate	10 g
Distilled water	100 ml

Solution C

Indicator, 1 ml, comprised of

Bromcresol purple	1.6 g
Ethanol (95%)	100.0 ml

Add solutions A, B, and C together; dispense in 3-ml amounts in 13- × 100-mm screw-capped tubes. Autoclave for 10 min at 121° C. A positive reaction is recorded when the indicator changes from purple to yellow.

CARBOHYDRATE MEDIA FOR FERMENTATION TESTS

When some carbohydrates are sterilized by heating in alkaline broth, they are more or less broken down into simple carbohydrates. It has been found definitely advantageous to sterilize sugar solutions by filtration through Seitz or membrane filters and to add these aseptically to the broth base in the required amounts. Although several carbohydrates can withstand autoclave temperature and pressure, one is advised to sterilize the following by *filtration*: xylose, lactose, sucrose, arabinose, trehalose, rhamnose, and salicin. These may be prepared as 5% or

10% solutions, depending on solubility, then sterilized by filtration and added aseptically to the base containing an indicator, to give 0.5% to 1% final concentration.

Other less heat-susceptible carbohydrates may be added to the broth base containing indicator (e.g., bromcresol purple) before autoclaving at 116° to 118° C (10 to 12 pounds' pressure) for 15 min. Ten Broeck, in 1920, found that unheated serum contains an enzyme that hydrolyzes maltose to glucose. Serum to be added to maltose broth should therefore be heated for 1 h at 60° C to inactivate the enzyme. Incubate the carbohydrate broth to test sterility.

CARY AND BLAIR TRANSPORT MEDIUM FOR FECES

Disodium phosphate	1.1 g
Sodium chloride	5 g
Sodium thioglycollate	1.5 g
Agar	5 g
Distilled water	991 ml

Add the ingredients to a chemically clean flask rinsed with Sörensen's 0.067 M buffer (pH 8.1) (see Sörensen pH Buffer Solutions in this appendix). Heat with frequent agitation until the solution just becomes clear. Cool to 50° C. Add 9 ml of freshly prepared aqueous 1% CaCl₂, and adjust the pH to 8.4.

Distribute 7 ml into previously rinsed and sterilized 9-ml screw-capped vials. Steam for 15 min, cool, and tighten caps.

CASEIN MEDIUM FOR SEPARATION OF *NOCARDIA* AND *STREPTOMYCES*

(Centers for Disease Control)

Prepare separately:

Solution A

Skimmed milk (dehydrated or instant nonfat milk)	10 g
Distilled water	100 ml

Autoclave at 121° C for 20 min

Solution B

Distilled water	100 ml
Agar	2 g

Autoclave at 121° C for 20 min.

Cool both solutions to approximately 45° C, mix, and pour into sterile Petri dishes.

TEST FOR HYDROLYSIS

Streak or make point inoculations of each culture on casein plates, using half of a plate for each organism. Incubate at 25° C (or 35° C if it does not grow at room temperature). Observe for clearing of casein in 7 and 14 days. *Nocardia asteroides* does not hydrolyze casein. *N. brasiliensis* and *Streptomyces* species hydrolyze casein.

CETRIMIDE AGAR

(Lowbury and Collins. 1955. J. Clin. Pathol. 8:47.)

Peptone	20 g
Magnesium chloride	1.4 g
Potassium sulfate	10 g
Agar, dried	13.6 g
Cetrimide	0.3 g
Distilled water	1000 ml
Glycerol	10 ml
(Final pH 7.2)	

Suspend the powder in the water, add 10 ml of glycerol, heat with frequent agitation, and boil for 1 min. Dispense in 5-ml amounts in 15- × 125-mm screw-capped tubes, autoclave at 118° to 121° C for 15 min, and slant to give a generous slant.

This medium is used for the selective isolation or identification of *Pseudomonas aeruginosa*, whose growth is not inhibited by the cetrimide. Other members of the genus (except *P. fluorescens*) and related nonfermentative organisms are inhibited.

Cetrimide is cetyl trimethyl ammonium bromide (hexadecyltrimethylammonium bromide). This agent is called cetrimide per USP. It is available from Sigma and other suppliers. However, lots of cetrimides differ in their properties. For this reason, it is critical that cetrimide agar prepared from a new lot be tested with several quality control strains to ascertain that it is acceptable. Cetrimide agar is also available commercially. See Chapter 23 for additional selective agars for *P. aeruginosa*.

(BUFFERED) CHARCOAL YEAST EXTRACT AGAR (BCYE)*

(Modified from Pasculle et al. 1980. J. Infect. Dis. 441:727.)

Yeast extract	10 g
Activated charcoal (Norit A or SG)	2 g
L-Cysteine HCl · H₂O	0.4 g
Ferric pyrophosphate, soluble	0.25 g
ACES buffer (Calbiochem, Behring, or Sigma)	10 g

---

*Available in prepared plates from Remel and other suppliers.

Agar	17 g
α-Ketoglutarate, monopotassium salt (Sigma)	1 g
Purified water	980 ml

1. Dissolve the cysteine and ferric pyrophosphate separately in 10 ml of purified water. Place in a 37° C water bath for about 15 min to aid dissolution.
2. Add the ACES buffer to 200 ml of purified water, and heat-stir at lowest temperature for 30 min. Membrane filter sterilize, and store in a sterile container.
3. Add yeast extract, agar, and Norit to a flask containing 750 ml purified water.
4. Boil, add a stir bar, and sterilize by autoclaving for 15 min at 121° C.
5. Place the sterilized agar in a 50° to 52° C water bath for 1 h.
6. Place the melted agar on a heated stirrer, and rotate the stir bar slowly to avoid frothing.
7. Add filtered ACES buffer slowly to stirring agar. NOTE: Preheat ACES buffer in a 50° C water bath before adding.
8. Add the cysteine and then the ferric pyrophosphate to the stirred agar, using a syringe with an attached disk filter (e.g., Gelman Acrodisc 0.20 μm) in order to filter-sterilize the small volume added.
9. Check the pH, and adjust it to 6.9 ± 0.05 using 1 N KOH. NOTE: 35 to 40 ml of KOH is required.
10. Pour into plates (15 to 20 ml per plate). NOTE: Swirl the bulk agar after pouring each plate to keep charcoal in suspension.
11. Incubate plates at room temperature for 24 to 48 h, and store packaged at 2° to 8° C for a maximum of 8 weeks.

SELECTIVE BUFFERED CHARCOAL YEAST EXTRACT AGAR (SEMISELECTIVE MEDIUM FOR *LEGIONELLA PNEUMOPHILA* [BMPA-α])

(Edelstein. 1981. J. Clin. Microbiol. 14:298.)

Prepare buffered charcoal yeast extract agar base as described above. After the pH has been adjusted, add antimicrobial agents to the following final concentrations (using methods outlined in Chapter 13):

Anisomycin	80 μg/ml
Polymyxin B	80 U/ml
Cefamandole	4 μg/ml

This medium is also available in prepared plates from Remel and other suppliers.

DIFFERENTIAL BUFFERED CHARCOAL YEAST EXTRACT AGAR (DIFF/BCYE)

(Vickers et al. 1981. J. Clin. Microbiol. 13:380.)

Yeast extract	10 g
Activated charcoal (Norit A or SG)	1.5 g
L-Cysteine HCl	0.4 g
Ferric pyrophosphate (soluble)	0.25 g
ACES buffer	10 g
Agar	17 g
Bromcresol purple	0.01 g
Bromthymol blue	0.01 g
Polymyxin B (optional)	50,000 U
Vancomycin (optional)	0.001 g
Purified water approx.	1000 ml

1. Dissolve the cysteine and ferric pyrophosphate separately in 10 ml of purified water. Place in a 37° C water bath for about 15 min to aid dissolution.
2. Add the ACES buffer to 200 ml of purified water, and heat-stir at lowest temperature for 30 min. Membrane filter-sterilize, and store in a sterile container.
3. Prepare separately 1% solutions (w/v) of bromcresol purple and bromthymol blue in 0.1 N KOH (1 g in 100 ml 0.1 N KOH). Membrane filter-sterilize, and store at 2° to 8° C.
4. Prepare a sterile solution of polymyxin B (50,000 U/ml) and vancomycin (1000 μg/ml), and store in aliquots at −20° C.
5. Add yeast extract, agar, and Norit to a flask containing 750 ml of purified water.
6. Boil, add a stir bar, and sterilize by autoclaving for 15 min at 121° C.
7. Place the sterilized agar in a 50° to 52° C water bath for 1 h.
8. Place the melted agar on a heated stirrer, and rotate the stir bar slowly to avoid frothing.
9. Add filtered ACES buffer slowly to stirring agar. NOTE: Preheat ACES buffer in a 50° C water bath before adding.
10. Add the cysteine and then the ferric pyrophosphate to the stirring agar using a syringe with an attached disk filter (e.g., Gelman Acrodisc 0.20 μm to filter-sterilize the small volume added.
11. Check the pH, and adjust it to 6.9 ± 0.05 using 1 N KOH. NOTE: 35 to 40 ml of KOH is required.
12. Add 1 ml each of the sterile 1% bromcresol pur-

ple and 1% bromthymol blue dye solutions to the adjusted agar.

13. Optional: Add the polymyxin B and vancomycin agents to the adjusted agar at final concentrations of 50,000 U and 1000 μg, respectively, per liter of medium.

14. Pour into plates (15 to 20 ml per plate). NOTE: Swirl the bulk agar after pouring each plate to keep charcoal in suspension.

15. Incubate the plates at room temperature for 24 to 48 h, and store packaged at 2° to 8° C for a maximum of 8 weeks.

CHLAMYDIA MEDIA

GROWTH MEDIUM FOR MCCOY CELL CULTURES USED FOR CULTIVATION OF *CHLAMYDIA TRACHOMATIS*

RPMI 1640 (Flow Laboratories)	500 ml
Inactivated fetal bovine serum (Gibco)	50 ml
Glutamine (Sigma, 200 mmol/ml)	5 ml
Gentamicin (Schering Corp., 1,000 μg/ml)	1.4 ml

Add all ingredients together. Aseptically adjust pH to 7.4.

MAINTENANCE MEDIUM FOR MCCOY CELL CULTURES USED FOR CULTIVATION OF *C. TRACHOMATIS*

RPMI 1640 (Flow Laboratories)	500 ml
Inactivated fetal bovine serum (Gibco)	25 ml
Glucose solution (filter-sterilized, 1.1 g in 100 ml of distilled water)	25 ml
Glutamine (Sigma, 200 mmol/ml)	5 ml
Amphotericin B (E.R. Squibb & Sons, 250 μg/ml)	5.6 ml
Gentamicin (Schering Corp., 1000 μg/ml)	5.6 ml

Add all ingredients together. Aseptically adjust pH to 7.4.

CHLAMYDOSPORE AGAR

Chlamydospore agar (BBL)	18.5 g
Distilled water	500 ml

Suspend the dehydrated product in a 1-L Erlenmeyer flask, dissolve by heating, and tube in approximately 15 ml amounts in screw-capped, 20- × 150-mm test tubes. Autoclave at 121° C for 15 min with caps loosened. When cool, tighten caps and store at room temperature. When needed, melt a tube in a water bath, pour into a sterile Petri plate, and allow to solidify.

CHOCOLATE AGAR

Chocolate agar is agar to which blood or hemoglobin has been added and then heated until the medium becomes brown or chocolate-colored. The recommended method of preparing this is as follows.

Suspend sufficient proteose No. 3 agar (Difco), Eugonagar (BBL), or GC agar base (BBL, Difco, Gibco) in distilled water to make a double-strength base. Mix thoroughly, and heat to boiling for 1 min with frequent agitation. Autoclave at 121° C for 15 min. At the same time, autoclave an equal volume of 2% hemoglobin (BBL, Difco, Gibco), which is made by the gradual addition of distilled water to the dehydrated hemoglobin, to obtain a *smooth suspension*. Cool both solutions to approximately 50° C, add the supplement (Iso-VitaleX enrichment [BBL] or supplement B or C [Difco] is recommended), combine aseptically, and then pour into sterile, disposable Petri plates. Best results are obtained when plates are *freshly prepared*. One or two plates per 100- to 200-ml batch should be incubated at 35° C overnight to determine sterility and later discarded.

Chocolate agar slants may be prepared individually by the method just described, slanting the medium after it has been tubed in 5- to 10-ml amounts in sterile screw-capped tubes. To prepare a large number of slants, use a flask containing 50 to 100 ml of agar, proceeding as before.

CHOCOLATE AGAR WITH ISOVITALEX AND VANCOMYCIN FOR RECOVERY OF *HAEMOPHILUS DUCREYI*

Chocolate agar is prepared as has been described, using 1% IsoVitaleX enrichment. Before plates are poured, vancomycin (Upjohn Co.) is added for a final concentration of 3 μg/ml.

CHOPPED MEAT GLUCOSE (CMG)

Ground beef, fat-free	500 g
Distilled water	1000 ml
Sodium hydroxide, 1 N	25 ml

1. Mix ingredients, bring to boil, and simmer with frequent stirring for 20 min.

2. Cool to room temperature, skim off fat, and filter through three layers of gauze. Squeeze out gauze, retaining both meat particles and filtrate (filtered through coarse and fine paper).

3. Restore filtrate to 1 L with distilled water, and add:

Trypticase	30 g

Yeast extract	5 g
Dipotassium phosphate	5 g
Resazurin solution (25 mg/100 ml water)	4 ml

4. Boil, cool, adjust to pH 7.8, and add 0.5% glucose and 0.5 g of cystine.
5. Dispense 6- to 7-ml amounts into tubes containing meat particles (step 2), 1 part meat to 4 or 5 parts broth, and autoclave at 121° C for 20 min.

This medium is recommended as a "backup" medium for the primary isolation of anaerobes and also for growing pure cultures for gas-liquid chromatographic analysis (available in prereduced tubes from commercial suppliers). It may also be obtained as a dehydrated medium, cooked meat phytone (BBL, Gibco).

CHOPPED-MEAT MEDIUM

To 1 pound of finely ground beef heart and other muscle (fat-free) add 500 ml of boiling sodium hydroxide (N/15 to N/20) and boil for 20 min. Cool, strain off the fat, and filter through muslin. Adjust the fluid to pH 7.5, and add 1% peptone. Add approximately 2 inches (5 cm) of meat and a small ball of steel wool to each tube, and add enough broth to overlay the meat by about 1 inch (2.5 cm). Heat tubes for 30 min in boiling water, and sterilize by autoclaving at 121° C for 15 min. The medium should be boiled for a few minutes to drive off dissolved oxygen if it is not to be used the same day, unless prereduced tubed media are used. Incubation in an anaerobic jar or under a petrolatum seal may be required for cultivation or maintenance of certain *Clostridium* species, except for prereduced tubed media.

CIN AGAR (*YERSINIA ENTEROCOLITICA* SELECTIVE AGAR)

(Schiemann. 1982. Appl. Environ. Microbiol. 43:14.)

1. Agar base (available commercially from Difco, Oxoid, and other suppliers) contains the following ingredients:

Yeast extract	2 g
Peptone	17 g
Proteose peptone (Difco)	3 g
Mannitol	20 g
Sodium deoxycholate	0.5 g
Sodium cholate	0.5 g
Sodium chloride	1 g
Sodium pyruvate	2 g
Magnesium sulfate, heptahydrate	10 mg
Agar (Bacto, Difco)	13.5 g

Neutral red	30 mg
Crystal violet	1 mg
Irgasan	4 mg

2. Add the ingredients to 1000 ml distilled water. Heat to boiling to dissolve the powder.
3. Autoclave for 15 min at 121° C and cool to between 45° and 50° C.
4. Aseptically add:

Cefsulodin	4 mg
Novobiocin	2.5 mg

5. Mix thoroughly and dispense into 90-mm diameter Petri plates, 20 ml per plate. Wrap plates tightly in plastic and store refrigerated for up to 1 month.

The antibiotics are available as premixed supplement solutions (CN, Difco, containing cefsulodin and novobiocin; SR109, Oxoid, containing irgasan, cefsulodin, and novobiocin). Colonies of *Yersinia* appear bright pink or red; most other bacteria are inhibited. One exception is certain strains of *Aeromonas hydrophila;* CIN agar has been found to aid in selective isolation of *Aeromonas* from stool.

CITRATE AGAR

(Simmons. 1926. J. Infect. Dis. 39:209.)

Agar	20 g
Sodium chloride	5 g
Magnesium sulfate	0.2 g
Ammonium dihydrogen phosphate	1 g
Dipotassium phosphate	1 g
Sodium citrate	2 g
Bromthymol blue	0.08 g
Distilled water	1000 ml
(Final pH 6.9)	

Citrate agar is used to determine the utilization of citrate as the sole carbon source. Development of a blue color indicates a positive test.

COLUMBIA AGARS

COLUMBIA AGAR BASE

Polypeptone (BBL) or Pantone (Difco)	10 g
Biosate (BBL) or Bitone (Difco)	10 g
Myosate (BBL) or tryptic digest of beef heart	3 g
Cornstarch	1 g
Sodium chloride	5 g
Agar	13.5 g
Distilled or demineralized water	1000 ml
(Final pH 7.3 ± 0.2)	

Heat with agitation until the medium boils. Dispense and autoclave at 121° C for 15 min.

Columbia CNA Agar

Polypeptone peptone (BBL)	10 g
Biosate peptone (BBL)	10 g
Myosate peptone (BBL)	3 g
Cornstarch	1g
Sodium chloride	5 g
Agar, dried	3.5 g
Colistin	10 mg
Nalidixic acid	15 mg
Distilled water	1000 ml

  (Final pH 7.3 ± 0.2)

1. Suspend 42.5 g of dehydrated medium in water, heat with frequent agitation, and boil for 1 min.
2. Sterilize by autoclaving at 121° C for 15 min.
3. Cool to 50° C, add 5% defibrinated sheep blood, and pour plates.

This medium is excellent for the selective growth of gram-positive cocci, particularly streptococci, when gram-negative bacilli, especially *Proteus* species, tend to overgrow on conventional blood agar plates. This medium may be inhibitory for certain strains of staphylococci.

Cornmeal Agar

Yellow cornmeal	125 g
Agar	50 g
Distilled water	3000 ml

Heat the cornmeal in water at 60° C for 1 h, filter through paper, make up to volume, and add 50 g of agar. Expose to flowing steam for 1 h, filter through absorbent cotton, dispense in tubes, and autoclave at 121° C for 30 min. Cornmeal agar suppresses vegetative growth of many fungi while stimulating sporulation. With the addition of 1% Tween 80, it is useful in stimulating production of chlamydospores of *Candida albicans*. Some workers find that "homemade" media such as this give more consistent results.

Cycloserine-Cefoxitin Fructose Agar (CCFA)

(George et al. 1979. J. Clin. Microbiol. 9:214.)

Prepare 1 L of egg yolk agar base, substituting 6 g of fructose for the glucose and adding 3 ml of 1% neutral red in ethanol. This base is dispensed in 100-ml quantities and sterilized at 121° C for 15 min. After cooling to 50° C, cycloserine basic salt is added to a final concentration of 500 mg/ml, and cefoxitin basic salt is added to a final concentration of 16 mg/

ml. The egg yolk suspension is added as indicated for egg yolk agar. Alternatively, one may leave out the egg yolk suspension (the medium is effective without the egg yolk, but the lecithinase and lipase reactions cannot be determined directly, of course). This is a highly selective and differential medium for *Clostridium difficile*.

Cystine Tellurite Blood Agar

(Frobisher. 1937. J. Infect. Dis. 60:99.)

1. Melt 100 ml of sterile 2% infusion agar in a flask, and cool to 45° to 50° C. Care should be taken to maintain this temperature throughout the following steps in the preparation of the medium.
2. Add aseptically 15 ml of sterile 0.3% solution of potassium tellurite in distilled water. The tellurite solution may be sterilized by autoclaving.
3. Add aseptically 5 ml of sterile blood, and mix well.
4. Add 3 to 5 mg of cystine. The dry powder is used and need not be sterilized. Since different lots of cystine vary, the optimal amount necessary to produce the best growth of *Corynebacterium diphtheriae* may vary from 3 to 5 mg/100 ml.
5. Thoroughly mix the medium, and pour into sterile Petri dishes. Since the cystine does not go entirely into solution, shake the flask frequently while pouring the plates.

This medium is used for the isolation of *C. diphtheriae*.

Cystine Trypticase Agar (CTA)

(Vera. 1948. J. Bacteriol. 55:531.)

Cystine	0.5 g
Trypticase	20 g
Agar	3.5 g
Sodium chloride	5 g
Sodium sulfite	0.5 g
Phenol red	0.017 g
Distilled water	1000 ml

  (Final pH 7.3)

CTA is an excellent all-purpose medium for the growth of pathogenic organisms. It can be used for the maintenance of cultures (including fastidious organisms, held at 25° C), the determination of motility, and (with the addition of carbohydrates) the determination of fermentation reactions of fastidious organisms, including *Neisseria*. Sterilize at 115° to 118° C (no more than 12 pounds pressure) for 15 min.

FERMENTATION MEDIA FOR *NEISSERIA*

1. Suspend 4.3 g of dehydrated CTA medium (available commercially or see Cystine Trypticase Agar) in 150 ml of distilled water, and heat to boiling with frequent agitation.
2. Adjust to pH 7.4 to 7.6 with 1 N NaOH, dispense in 50-ml amounts in 250 ml Erlenmeyer flasks, and sterilize at no more than 118° C (12 pounds) for 15 min.
3. Prepare 20% solutions of glucose, lactose, maltose, and sucrose in distilled water; tube and sterilize by membrane filtration.
4. Add 2.5 ml of each carbohydrate to separate flasks of the 50 ml cooled CTA medium.
5. Mix and dispense in 2 ml amounts in sterile screw-capped tubes (13 × 100 mm) and refrigerate at 4° C.

DECARBOXYLASE TEST MEDIA

(Moeller. 1955. Acta Pathol. Microbiol. Scand. 36:161.)

Basal medium (BBL, Difco, Gibco)	1000 mg
Peptone (Orthana special*)	5 g
Beef extract	5 mg
Bromcresol purple (1.6%)	0.625 ml
Cresol red (0.2%)	2.5 ml
Glucose	0.5 g
Pyridoxal	5 mg
Distilled water	1000 ml
(Adjust to pH 6)	

Divide the basal medium into four 250-ml amounts; one portion is tubed without addition of any of the amino acids (control). To another portion add 1% L-lysine dihydrochloride (Sigma or other chemical supplier), to a third add 1% L-arginine monohydrochloride, and to the fourth add 1% L-ornithine dihydrochloride. Adjust the ornithine portion to pH 6 with 1 N NaOH before sterilization. Tube the media in 3- to 4-ml amounts in small (13 × 100 mm) screw-capped tubes. Autoclave at 121° C for 10 min.

Inoculate all four tubes from an agar slant culture, and overlay each tube with 4 to 5 mm of sterile mineral oil.† If oil is not added, the reactions are not valid after 24 h. Some workers recommend the addition of 0.3% agar to the basal medium in place of an oil overlay.

*Proteose peptone No. 3, 0.3%, has been found to be a suitable alternative.

†Sterilize in test tubes at 121° C for 45 min.

Incubate all four tubes at 35° C, and read daily for not more than 4 days (most positive reactions with the enteric bacilli occur in 1 to 2 days). A *positive* reaction is indicated by alkalinization of the medium with a change in color from yellow (caused by the initial fermentation of glucose) to *violet* (caused by the decarboxylation of the amino acid). Therefore a *yellow* color after several days' incubation indicates a *negative* test, or the absence of the enzymes decarboxylase or dihydrolase. All positive tests should be compared with the control tube, which remains grayish purple.

These media are used primarily for differentiating members of the Enterobacteriaceae.

DIAMOND'S MEDIUM FOR *TRICHOMONAS*

(Diamond. 1957. J. Parasitol. 43:488; Phillips and Nash. 1985. Culture Media. pp. 1051-1107. In Lennette et al., editors. Manual of clinical microbiology, ed. 4. American Society for Microbiology, Washington, D.C.)

1. Prepare base medium as follows:

Trypticase (BBL)	20.0 g
Yeast extract	10.0 g
Maltose	5.0 g
L-Cysteine	2.0 g
L-Ascorbic acid	0.2 g
Ion agar No. 2 (Difco)	1.0 g
Distilled water	900.0 ml

2. Heat the solution to boiling and adjust the pH to 6.5.
3. Autoclave for 15 min at 121° C and cool to 45° C.
4. Aseptically add:

Inactivated sheep or horse serum	100.0 ml
Streptomycin sulfate	1.5 g
Potassium penicillin G	1,000,000 U
Amphotericin B	2.0 mg in 1 ml aqueous solution

5. Dispense into sterile screw-capped tubes. Shelf life should be approximately 6 weeks refrigerated.
6. Warm tubes to 35° C before inoculating.

DNA AGAR FOR TESTING *STAPHYLOCOCCUS AUREUS* FOR THERMOSTABLE NUCLEASE

(Zarzour and Belle. 1978. J. Clin. Microbiol. 7:133.)

Deoxyribonucleic acid (Difco)	0.3 g

Agar (Bacto agar, Difco)	10 g
NaCl	10 g

1. Add the above components to 1 L of 0.05 M TRIS buffer pH 9.0 (hydroxymethylaminomethane, Sigma).
2. Add 1 ml of 0.01 M anhydrous $CaCl_2$ (Mallinckrodt) and boil until dissolved.
3. Cool to 45° C and add 3 ml of 0.1 M toluidine blue O (Allied Chemical and Dye Corp.). Mix thoroughly.
4. Pour 15 to 20 ml into 90-mm diameter Petri dishes.

After the agar has set, it may be stored at 4° C, tightly wrapped in plastic, for approximately 60 days.

Plates should be reincubated at 35° to 37° C for 1 h before inoculating. Control organisms should be run on the same plate as test organisms.

DESOXYCHOLATE AGAR

(Leifson. 1935. J. Pathol. Bacteriol. 40:581.)

Peptone	10 g
Lactose	10 g
Sodium citrate	1 g
Ferric citrate	1 g
Sodium chloride	5 g
Dipotassium phosphate	2 g
Sodium desoxycholate	1 g
Agar	16 g
Neutral red	0.033 g
Distilled water	1000 ml
(Final pH 7.2)	

Desoxycholate agar is used for the isolation of gram-negative enteric bacilli and the differentiation of lactose-fermenting and non-lactose-fermenting species.

EDWARD-HAYFLICK AGAR FOR ISOLATION OF MYCOPLASMA

(Clyde, Kenny, and Schachter. 1984. Cumitech 19; Laboratory diagnosis of chlamydial and mycoplasmal infections. Drew, coordinating editor. American Society for Microbiology, Washington, D.C.)

1. Prepare base medium as follows:

Mycoplasma Broth Base (BBL)	21 g
Distilled water	700 ml
Noble agar (Difco)	8.5 g

Stir the solids into boiling water until they dissolve. Dispense 350 ml into each of two 500 ml bottles and autoclave according to manufacturer's instructions. Store the agar at 4° C.

2. Before use, melt the agar base and cool to 56° C. Add the following supplements to each 500-ml bottle of base:

Aqueous yeast extract (prepared as described under "New York City medium")	50 ml
Horse serum (gamma globulin— free, available commercially)	100 ml
Penicillin G sodium or	500,000 U
Ampicillin	1 mg/ml
Amphotericin B	0.25 g
Polymyxin B	250,000 U

After addition of supplements, agar is poured into 90-mm diameter plastic Petri plates. Plates are poured thick (approximately 25 ml per plate) to prevent dehydration. They may be stored (tightly wrapped in plastic) up to 2 weeks at 4° C. Since lots of ingredients vary, be certain to test each new batch of agar with a quality control strain of *Mycoplasma* of known titer.

EGG YOLK AGAR

Add 10 ml of sterile yolk emulsion (Colab Laboratories or Difco Laboratories) to 90 ml of melted and cooled blood agar base (below), and pour the plates.

BLOOD AGAR BASE

Proteose peptone No. 2	40 g
Sodium orthophosphate (Na_2HPO_4)	5 g
Potassium dihydrophosphate (KH_2PO4)	1 g
Sodium chloride	2 g
Magnesium sulfate	0.1 g
Glucose	2 g
Hemin solution (see below; 5 mg/ml)	1 ml
Agar	25 g
Distilled water	1000 ml
(Adjust to pH 7.6)	

Autoclave at 121° C for 15 min. This medium is used for the isolation and identification of members of the genus *Clostridium* and certain other anaerobes.

ELLINGHAUSEN, McCULLOUGH, JOHNSON, AND HARRIS (EMJH) MEDIUM FOR CULTIVATION OF LEPTOSPIRES

(Johnson and Harris. 1967. J. Bacteriol. 94:27.)

1. Prepare stock solutions as follows:

a.	NH_4Cl	25 g
	Distilled water	100 ml

b. $ZnSO_4 \cdot 7 H_2O$ 0.4 g
    Distilled water   100 ml
c. $CaCl_2 \cdot 2 H_2O$ 1 g
    Distilled water   100 ml
d. $MgCl_2 \cdot 6 H_2O$ 1 g
    Distilled water   100 ml
e. $FeSO_4 \cdot 7 H_2O$ 0.5 g
    Distilled water   100 ml
f. $CuSO_4 \cdot 5 H_2O$ 0.3 g
    Distilled water   100 ml
g. Glycerol   10 ml
    Distilled water   90 ml
h. Tween 80   10 ml
    Distilled water   90 ml
i. Thiamine (Sigma)   0.5 g
    Distilled water   100 ml
j. Vitamin B_{12} (Sigma)   0.02 g
    Distilled water   100 ml

2. Prepare basal medium as follows:

Na_2HPO_4	1 g
KH_2PO_4	0.3 g
NaCl	1 g
Stock NH_4Cl solution (solution a)	1 ml
Stock thiamine (solution i)	1 ml
Stock glycerol (solution g)	1 ml
Distilled water	997 ml

Adjust to pH 7.4 and autoclave for 20 min at 121° C.

3. Prepare albumin supplement as follows:

Bovine albumin, fraction V (Sigma)	20 g
Distilled water	100 ml

Add the albumin to the water in a 500-ml flask and place on a stirring platform. As the solution stirs, slowly add the following stock solutions:

Calcium chloride (solution c)	2 ml
Magnesium chloride (solution d)	2 ml
Zinc sulfate (solution b)	2 ml
Copper sulfate (solution f)	0.2 ml
Iron sulfate (solution e)	20 ml
Vitamin B_{12} (solution j)	2 ml
Tween 80 (solution h)	25 ml

Adjust the pH to 7.4 and add enough distilled water to bring the volume to 200 ml. Sterilize by filtration through a 0.45-μm pore size membrane filter.

4. Add 1 part albumin supplement to 9 parts of basal medium.

EOSIN-METHYLENE BLUE AGAR (EMB)

Peptone	10 g
Lactose	5 g
Sucrose	5 g
Dipotassium phosphate	2 g
Agar	13.5 g
Eosin Y	0.4 g
Methylene blue	0.065 g
Distilled water	1000 ml

The agar concentration may be increased to 5% (use an additional 3.65 g of agar) to inhibit the spreading of *Proteus*. Levine EMB agar, preferred by some workers, does not contain sucrose.

Lactose-fermenting, gram-negative bacteria may be distinguished from non-lactose-fermenting types by their appearance. Colonies of *Escherichia coli* usually have a characteristic metallic sheen. If the sucrose-containing medium is used, *Proteus* colonies also show this characteristic, provided they are inhibited from spreading by the higher agar concentration.

ESCULIN AGAR, MODIFIED

Esculin	1 g
Ferric citrate	0.5 g
Heart infusion agar (blood agar base)	40 g
Distilled water	1000 ml

Heat to dissolve. Cool to 55° C, and adjust pH to 7.0. Dispense in 5-ml amounts in 16- × 125-mm screw-capped tubes. Autoclave at 121° C for 15 min. Cool in a slanted position.

Esculin hydrolysis is indicated when the medium turns black.

FETAL BOVINE SERUM AGAR WITH VANCOMYCIN FOR ISOLATION OF *HAEMOPHILUS DUCREYI*

(Greenwood and Robertson. 1983. Haemophilus ducreyi. ASCP Check Sample MB 83-8 (MB-129). American Society for Clinical Pathology.)

Heart infusion agar base (Difco Laboratories)	80 g
Bacto agar (Difco)	10 g
Fetal bovine serum, not inactivated	200 ml
Vancomycin HCl (1500 μg/ml; Sigma)	4 ml
Distilled water	1800 ml

Measure heart infusion agar into a 4-L flask. Add 200 ml of cold distilled water and stir to a smooth paste. Add remaining water and heat the mixture on a hot plate, stirring until it boils. Autoclave for 15 min at 121° C. Cool to 50° C and add the fetal bovine serum and vancomycin aseptically. Mix solution thoroughly and pour agar plates of approximately 20 ml each.

FLETCHER'S SEMISOLID MEDIUM FOR *LEPTOSPIRA*

1. Sterilize 1.76 L of distilled water by autoclaving at 121° C for 30 min.
2. Cool to room temperature, and add 240 ml of sterile normal rabbit serum.
3. Inactivate by incubation at 56° C for 40 min.
4. Add 120 ml of melted and cooled (no greater than 56° C) 2.5% meat extract agar at pH 7.4.
5. Dispense 5-ml amounts in sterile, 16 × 120 mm, screw-capped test tubes and 15-ml amounts in sterile, 25-ml, diaphragm-type, rubber-stoppered vaccine bottles.
6. Inactivate at 56° C for 60 min on two successive days.

FORMALIN PRESERVATION SOLUTION FOR PARASITES (10% FORMALIN)

Formaldehyde (USP)	100 ml
0.85% saline solution	900 ml

Dilute 100 ml of formaldehyde with 900 ml of 0.85% saline solution (distilled water may be used instead of saline).

FUCHSIN (BASIC) MEDIUM

See Thionine Agar

GELATIN MEDIUM

To veal extract or infusion broth add 12% gelatin. Heat in an Arnold sterilizer or a double boiler until the gelatin is thoroughly dissolved. Adjust to pH 7. Tube and autoclave at 121° C (15 pounds' pressure) for 15 min. Sodium thioglycollate, 0.05%, may be added for cultivation of certain species of clostridia in an external aerobic environment.

GELATIN MEDIUM (DILUTE) FOR DIFFERENTIATION OF *NOCARDIA* AND *STREPTOMYCES*

(Centers for Disease Control.)

Gelatin	4 g
Distilled water	1000 ml
(Adjust to pH 7)	

Dispense in tubes, approximately 5 ml per tube. Autoclave at 121° C for 5 min. Inoculate with a small fragment of growth from a Sabouraud dextrose agar slant. Incubate at room temperature for 21 to 25 days. Examine for quantity and type of growth.

Nocardia asteroides exhibits no growth or very sparse, thin, flaky growth. *N. brasiliensis* shows good growth and round compact colonies. *Streptomyces* species show poor to good growth (stringy or flaky).

GN BROTH

(Hajna. 1955. Pub. Health Lab. 13:83.)

Peptone	20 g
Glucose	1 g
D-Mannitol	2 g
Sodium citrate	5 g
Sodium desoxycholate	0.5 g
Dipotassium phosphate	4 g
Monopotassium phosphate	1.5 g
Sodium chloride	5 g
Distilled water	1000 ml
(Final pH 7)	

Dissolve the dehydrated medium in distilled water and autoclave at 116° C (10 pounds' steam pressure) for 15 min or steam for 30 min at 100° C.

This broth medium is used as an enrichment for isolating salmonellae and shigellae in fecal specimens.

HEKTOEN ENTERIC AGAR

Proteose peptone	12 g
Bile salts	9 g
Yeast extract	3 g
Lactose	12 g
Salicin	2 g
Sucrose	12 g
Sodium chloride	5 g
Sodium thiosulfate	5 g
Ferric ammonium citrate	1.5 g
Agar	14 g
Acid fuchsin	0.1 g
Bromthymol blue	0.065 g
Distilled water	1000 ml

Suspend 76 g of dehydrated medium, if using the commercial product, in 1000 ml of distilled water. Heat to boiling, and continue until the medium dissolves. *Do not autoclave.* Cool to 50° C, and pour into Petri dishes.

This medium is useful for the isolation and differentiation of gram-negative enteric pathogens. The coliforms are usually salmon to orange, whereas the salmonellae and shigellae are bluish-green.

HEMIN SOLUTION

Hemin solution is used as a medium supplement in a final concentration of 5 μg/ml. To prepare, dissolve 0.5 g of hemin (Sigma and others) in 10 ml of commercial ammonia water (or 1 N sodium hydroxide), bring volume to 100 ml with distilled water, and autoclave at 121° C for 15 min. A stock solution is 5 mg/ml.

As a supplement for anaerobic media, 1 ml of hemin solution is added per liter of agar or broth.

HORSE BLOOD–BACITRACIN AGAR (SELECTIVE) FOR RECOVERY OF *HAEMOPHILUS* SPECIES FROM RESPIRATORY CULTURES

(Klein and Blazevic. 1970. Am. J. Med. Technol. 36:97.)

Heart infusion agar (Difco)	40 g
Cornstarch (Argo)	1 g
Distilled water	1000 ml

Add ingredients to water and heat to boiling to dissolve. Autoclave for 15 min at 121° C. Cool to 45° C in a water bath. Add the following ingredients aseptically:

Fildes enrichment (Difco)	20 ml
Defibrinated horse blood (GIBCO)	50 ml
Supplement B (Difco)	10 ml
Bacitracin standard laboratory powder (Upjohn)	375 µg/ml

Pour into Petri plates, approximately 20 ml per plate. Do not flame surfaces of plates to remove bubbles, since the heat may destroy the V factor. Store tightly wrapped in the refrigerator.

HUMAN BLOOD BILAYER MEDIUM (HBT) FOR SELECTIVE AND DIFFERENTIAL ISOLATION OF *GARDNERELLA VAGINALIS*

(Totten et al. 1982. J. Clin. Microbiol. 15:141.)

1. Prepare basal agar layer as follows:

Columbia agar base with colistin and nalidixic acid (CNA) (BBL)	44 g
Proteose peptone No. 3 (Difco)	10 g
Distilled water	1000 ml

Suspend the agar in the water, mix thoroughly, and heat to boiling to dissolve. Autoclave for 15 min at 121° C and cool to 55° C. Add amphotericin B to a final concentration of 2 µg/ml and 0.075 ml Tween 80 (BBL). Mix thoroughly and pour one third of the CNA agar into 90-mm diameter Petri plates, 7 ml per plate.

2. Prepare overlayer as follows: Add freshly outdated human blood of any type (obtained from the hospital blood bank, negative for human immunodeficiency virus [HIV] and hepatitis B antibodies) to the remaining molten CNA agar base with Tween 80 and amphotericin to make a final concentration of 5% blood. Pour directly over the basal agar in the Petri plates, 14 ml per plate.

3. Plates should be stored in the refrigerator, wrapped tightly in plastic bags. They should last approximately 1 month, but should be discarded if they appear hemolyzed.

INDOLE-NITRITE MEDIUM

Trypticase	20 g
Disodium phosphate	2 g
Glucose	1 g
Agar	1 g
Potassium nitrate	1 g
Distilled water	1000 ml
(pH 7.2)	

This medium is used to demonstrate indole production and nitrate reduction by aerobes and anaerobes.

KANAMYCIN-VANCOMYCIN BLOOD AGAR (KVBA)

1. Preparation of base:

Trypticase soy agar	40 g
Agar	2.5 g
Distilled water	1000 ml
Kanamycin base (Bristol Laboratories)	100 mg

Sterilize by autoclaving at 121° C for 15 min, and cool to 50° C.

2. Add aseptically*:

Defibrinated sheep blood	50 ml
Vancomycin (Eli Lilly)	7.5 mg
Vitamin K_1 solution (see Vitamin K_1 Solution)	1 ml

Mix well, pour plates (approximately 20 ml per plate), and store at room temperature.

This medium is extremely useful for primary inoculation of clinical specimens for selective isolation of anaerobes, particularly *Bacteroides*, but a nonselective medium (*Brucella* blood agar plate) should always be used as well.

KANAMYCIN-VANCOMYCIN-LAKED BLOOD AGAR (KVLBA)

KVLBA is the same as KVBA, except that the final concentration of kanamycin is 75 µg/ml and the blood is laked (hemolyzed) by freezing whole blood overnight and then thawing. This medium is particularly useful for isolating the pigmented *Bacteroides*.

---

*Hemin may also be added (1 ml of hemin solution).

KELLY'S MEDIUM (NONSELECTIVE MODIFIED) FOR ISOLATION OF *BORRELIA BURGDORFERI* AND OTHER SPIROCHETES

(Steere et al. 1983. N. Engl. J. Med. 308:733.)

1. Prepare basal medium as follows:

CMRL-1066 with glutamine, 10 × tissue culture medium (GIBCO)	100 ml
Sterile distilled water	900 ml
Proteose peptone No. 2 (Difco)	5 g
Tryptone (Difco)	1 g
Bacto autolyzed yeast (Difco)	1 g
HEPES buffer, acid form (Sigma)	6 g
Glucose α-D(+) (Sigma)	3 g
Sodium citrate (Sigma)	0.7 g
Sodium pyruvate (Sigma)	0.8 g
Sodium bicarbonate (Sigma)	2.2 g
N-Acetyl glucosamine (Sigma)	0.4 g
$MgCl_2 \cdot 6 H_2O$ (Sigma)	0.3 g

Add all ingredients together, adjust pH to 7.6 with 5 N NaOH. Filter-sterilize through a 0.45-μm pore size membrane filter.

2. Prepare gelatin solution as follows:

Gelatin (Fisher Scientific)	14 g
Distilled water	200 ml

Add together and heat gently to cause gelatin to just go into solution. Autoclave for 15 min at 121° C. Allow to cool to 50° to 55° C.

3. Add the gelatin to the basal medium. To this medium add 143 ml of a 35% solution of bovine serum albumin (Sigma) in sterile distilled water and 86 ml of membrane-filtered, heat-inactivated rabbit serum (GIBCO).

4. Dispense aseptically into 8 ml screw-capped test tubes, at least 7 ml per tube. The large volume of medium in the tube prevents excessive oxygenation of the medium.

KELLY'S MEDIUM (SELECTIVE MODIFIED) FOR ISOLATION OF *BORRELIA BURGDORFERI*

Johnson et al. 1984. J. Clin. Microbiol. 19:81.)

1. Prepare basal medium as follows:

1066 Connaught Medical Research Laboratories medium with glutamine, 10 × (GIBCO)	100 ml
Double distilled water	900 ml
Neopeptone (Difco)	5 g
Bovine serum albumin fraction V (Sigma)	50 g
N-2-Hydroxyethylpiperazine-N'-2-ethane sulfonic acid buffer (Sigma)	6 g
Sodium citrate	0.7 g
Glucose	5 g
Sodium pyruvate (Sigma)	0.8 g
N-Acetylglucosamine (Sigma)	0.4 g
Sodium bicarbonate	2.2 g

Add all ingredients separately, dissolving each ingredient completely before the next is added. Adjust pH to 7.6 with 1 N NaOH.

2. Prepare gelatin solution as follows:

Gelatin (Difco)	14 g
Distilled water	200 ml

Warm the solution gently while stirring until gelatin just goes into solution.

3. Add the warm gelatin solution to the basal medium.

4. Sterilize the entire solution by filtration through a 0.45-μm membrane filter.

5. Add 70 ml of partially hemolyzed sterile rabbit serum to produce a final serum concentration of 6%.

6. Add kanamycin laboratory standard powder (Bristol Laboratories) to a final concentration of 8 μg/ml and 5-fluorouracil laboratory standard powder (Roche Laboratories) to a final concentration of 230 μg/ml, using methods described in Chapter 13.

7. Final pH of the medium should be 7.7.

KLIGLER'S IRON AGAR

See Triple Sugar Iron Agar.

LÖWENSTEIN-JENSEN (L-J) MEDIUM

Salt solution	
Monopotassium phosphate	2.4 g
Magnesium sulfate · 7 H_2O	0.24 g
Magnesium citrate	0.6 g
Asparagine	3.6 g
Glycerol, reagent grade	12 ml
Distilled water	600 ml
Potato flour	30 g
Homogenized whole eggs	1000 ml
Malachite green (2% aqueous)	20 ml

Add the potato flour to the flask of salt solution, and autoclave the mixture at 121° C for 30 min. Clean fresh eggs, no more than 1 week old, by vigorous scrubbing in 5% soap solution, and allow them to remain in it for 30 min. Place the eggs in running cold water until the water becomes clear. Immerse the washed eggs in 70% alcohol for 15 min, remove, and break into a sterile flask; homogenize completely by shaking with glass beads. Then filter the homogenate through four layers of sterile gauze.

Add 1 L of the homogenized egg suspension to the flask of cooled potato flour–salt solution. Add the malachite green to this emulsion, and mix thoroughly. Dispense the medium aseptically with a sterile aspirator bottle in 6-ml amounts into sterile, screw-capped 150-mm glass tubes. Inspissate the tubes at 85° C for 50 min, and check for sterility by incubating at 35° C for 48 h. Store in a refrigerator, where the medium will keep for at least 1 month if the tubes are tightly sealed to prevent loss of moisture.

This medium is used for the cultivation of *Mycobacterium tuberculosis*.

Lysine-Iron Agar

(Edwards and Fife. 1961. Appl. Microbiol. 9:478.)

Peptone	5 g
Yeast extract	3 g
Glucose	1 g
L-Lysine	10 g
Ferric ammonium citrate	0.5 g
Sodium thiosulfate	40 mg
Bromcresol purple	20 mg
Agar	15 g
Distilled water	1000 ml
(Adjust to pH 6.7)	

Dispense 4-ml amounts into 13- × 100-mm tubes, and sterilize at 121° C for 12 min. Slant tubes to obtain a deep butt and a short slant. This medium is inoculated by using a straight wire to stab the butt twice and to streak the slant. Incubation is at 35° C for 18 to 24 h. If necessary, incubate for 48 h.

This medium is useful for determining whether members of the family Enterobacteriaceae can decarboxylate or deaminate lysine. However, this medium is not to be considered as a substitute for the Moeller method. A *positive* reaction is indicated by an alkaline or *purple* reaction in the butt of the tube. The absence of lysine decarboxylase is indicated by an acidic or *yellow (negative)* reaction in the butt of the tube caused by fermentation of glucose. Tryptophane deaminase is indicated by the formation of a *red* slant and is characteristic of the tribe Proteeae. It should be noted that H_2S-producing *Proteus* species do not blacken this medium. Furthermore, *Morganella morganii* does not consistently produce a red slant after 24 h incubation.

MacConkey Agar

Peptone	17 g
Proteose peptone	3 g
Lactose	10 g
Bile salts	1.5 g
Sodium chloride	5 g
Agar	13.5 g
Neutral red	0.03 g
Crystal violet	0.001 g
Distilled water	1000 ml

The agar concentration may be increased to 5% (use an additional 3.65 g of agar) to inhibit the spreading of *Proteus*. The medium is inhibitory for gram-positive bacteria and differential rather than selective. Coliforms (lactose-fermenting) produce red colonies on the medium, whereas nonlactose fermenters produce colorless colonies.

Malonate (Sodium) Broth

(Leifson. 1933. J. Bacteriol. 26:329. Ewing et al. 1957. Pub. Health Lab. 15:153.)

Yeast extract	1 g
Ammonium sulfate	2 g
Dipotassium sulfate	0.6 g
Monopotassium phosphate	0.4 g
Sodium chloride	2 g
Sodium malonate	3 g
Glucose	0.25 g
Bromthymol blue	0.025 g
Distilled water	1000 ml
(Final pH 6.7)	

Sterilize in small tubes in 3-ml amounts at 121° C for 15 min. Inoculate from TSI slants or broth cultures; incubate cultures at 35° C for 48 h.

The medium is used to test for utilization of sodium malonate by members of the Enterobacteriaceae. A *positive* test is shown by a change of the indicator from green to a *Prussian blue*.

Mannitol Salt Agar

Beef extract	1 g
Proteose peptone No. 3	10 g
Sodium chloride	75 g
Mannitol	10 g
Agar	15 g
Phenol red	0.025 g
Distilled water	1000 ml

Sterilize the medium at 15 pounds' pressure for 15 min, cool to 48° C, and pour into sterile Petri dishes. Use 15 to 20 ml per plate.

This medium is used for the selective isolation of pathogenic staphylococci, since many other bacteria are inhibited by the high salt concentration. Colonies of potentially pathogenic staphylococci are surrounded by a *yellow* halo, indicating mannitol fermentation.

MARTIN-LEWIS AGAR

This agar is the same as Thayer-Martin agar except that anisomycin is substituted for nystatin and the concentration of vancomycin is increased from 3 to 4 µg/ml. Notice that some strains of *Neisseria gonorrhoeae* may be susceptible to vancomycin at either concentration. See Chapter 26.

MCBRIDE MEDIUM, MODIFIED, FOR THE CULTIVATION OF *LISTERIA*

(J. Lab. Clin. Med. 1960. 55:153.)

Phenylethanol agar*	35.5 g
Glycine, anhydride	10 g
Lithium chloride	0.5 g
Distilled water	1000 ml

Dissolve with the aid of heat and sterilize at 121° C for 20 min.

MERCURIC CHLORIDE (SATURATED) FIXATIVE FOR PROTOZOA

Mercuric chloride (HgCl$_2$)	110 g
Distilled water	1000 ml

Mix in a 2-L flask; place flask in large beaker as a water bath; boil (use a hood if available) until the HgCl$_2$ is dissolved; let stand until crystals form.

METHYL RED–VOGES-PROSKAUER MEDIUM (MR-VP) (CLARK AND LUBS MEDIUM)

Buffered peptone	7 g
Glucose	5 g
Dipotassium phosphate	5 g
Distilled water	1000 ml
(Final pH 6.9)	

This medium is used for the methyl red test and the Voges-Proskauer test (production of acetylmethylcarbinol). See Chapter 27 for a description of performance of the test.

MIDDLEBROOK 7H10 AGAR WITH OADC ENRICHMENT

The preparation of 7H10 oleic acid–albumin agar as originally described is extremely tedious and complicated. Its preparation may be simplified by the use of a combination of six stock solutions prepared

in advance, as described in the handbook *Tuberculosis Laboratory Methods of the Veterans Administration*.* However, for the average diagnostic microbiology laboratory, it is strongly recommended that **commercially prepared** 7H10-OADC complete medium be used whenever possible. For purposes of orientation, the ingredients of each medium are listed, but the directions are intended solely for preparation from dehydrated medium and prepared enrichment.

MIDDLEBROOK 7H10 AGAR

Ammonium sulfate	0.5 g
D-Glutamic acid	0.5 g
Sodium citrate	0.4 g
Disodium phosphate	1.5 g
Monopotassium phosphate	1.5 g
Ferric ammonium phosphate	0.04 g
Magnesium sulfate	0.05 g
Pyridoxine	0.001 g
Biotin	0.0005 g
Malachite green	0.001 g
Agar	15 g

MIDDLEBROOK OADC ENRICHMENT

Oleic acid	0.5 g
Bovine albumin, fraction V	50 g
Glucose	20 g
Beef catalase	0.04 g
Sodium chloride	8.5 g
Distilled water	1000 ml

To rehydrate the 7H10 agar, suspend 20 g in 1 L of cold distilled water containing 0.5% reagent grade glycerol and heat to boiling to dissolve completely. Distribute in 180-ml amounts in flasks; sterilize by autoclaving at 121° C for 10 min; cool to 50° to 55° C; add 20 ml of OADC enrichment aseptically to each flask, and dispense in sterile plastic Petri dishes. Store at 4° C in the dark for no longer than 2 months in a plastic bag to prevent dehydration.

MIDDLEBROOK 7H11 AGAR FOR SUSCEPTIBILITY TESTING OF MYCOBACTERIA

Middlebrook 7H10 agar base (Difco)	19 g
Casein hydrolysate (Sigma)	1 g
Glycerol (Difco)	5 ml
Distilled water	1000 ml

Add ingredients together and heat gently to dissolve. Autoclave for 10 min at 121° C. Allow to cool

---

*Available from several commercial media suppliers. See Phenylethanol Agar.

*Obtainable from the Superintendent of Documents, U.S. Government Printing Office, Washington, D.C.

to 55° C, and add 100 ml of OADC Enrichment (Difco). Mix gently and pour into Felson quadrant Petri plates (Falcon Laboratories) containing anti-microbial agent–impregnated filter paper disks, as described in Chapter 13. Add 5 ml agar to each quadrant.

MILK MEDIA

SKIMMED MILK

Fresh, clean, skimmed cow's milk may be used. This is dispensed in tubes and sterilized either by tyndallization (flowing steam for 30 min on 3 successive days) or in the autoclave at 10 pounds' pressure for 10 min.

Commercial dehydrated skimmed milk is also completely satisfactory. The concentration used is 10% in distilled water. The method of sterilization is as before.

LITMUS MILK

Skimmed milk powder	100 g
Litmus	5 g
Distilled water	1000 ml

Autoclave at 10 pounds' pressure for 10 min.

Reactions in litmus milk. Pink color of litmus indicates an acid reaction caused by fermentation of lactose. A purple or blue color (alkaline) indicates no fermentation of lactose. White color (reduction) results when litmus serves as an electron acceptor and is reduced to its leuco base. Coagulation (clot) is caused by precipitation of casein by the acid produced from lactose. Coagulation may also be caused by the conversion of casein to paracasein by the enzyme rennin. Peptonization (dissolution of the clot) indicates digestion of the curd or milk proteins by proteolytic enzymes.

LITMUS MILK WITH A REDUCING AGENT FOR DETERMINATION OF LITMUS MILK REACTIONS OF *CLOSTRIDIUM* SPECIES

Skimmed milk powder	100 g
Peptone	10 g
Sodium thioglycollate	0.5 g
Litmus	5 g
Distilled water	1000 ml

Autoclave as above.

METHYLENE BLUE MILK FOR IDENTIFICATION OF ENTEROCOCCI

Skimmed milk powder	10 g
Methylene blue (1% aqueous)	10 ml
Distilled water	90 ml

MOTILITY TEST MEDIA

MOTILITY TEST MEDIUM*

Beef extract	3 g
Gelysate peptone	10 g
Sodium chloride	5 g
Agar	4 g
Distilled water	1000 ml
(Final pH 7.3)	

1. Suspend 22 g of dehydrated medium in water, and add 0.05 g triphenyltetrazolium. Heat with frequent agitation; boil 1 min to dissolve ingredients.
2. Dispense in screw-capped tubes, and sterilize by autoclaving at 121° C for 15 min.
3. Tighten caps when cool; store at room temperature.

This medium is stabbed once to a depth of approximately 1 cm below the surface and read after 1 to 2 days' incubation at 35° C. Motile organisms spread out from the line of inoculation; nonmotile organisms grow only along the stab.

If the results are negative, follow with further incubation at 21° to 25° C for 5 days. For special purposes, such as enhancement of the motility and flagellar development in poorly motile cultures, it is often advisable to pass cultures first through a semi-solid medium containing 0.2% agar tubed in Craigie tubes or in U tubes. Subsequent passages may be made in 0.4% agar medium.

Motility media containing concentrations higher than 0.3% agar produce gels through which many motile organisms cannot spread. Spreading in a semisolid medium is judged by macroscopic examination of the medium for a diffuse zone of growth emanating from the line of inoculation. Many aerobic pseudomonads fail to grow deep in semisolid medium in a test tube. Organisms possessing "paralyzed" flagella are nonmotile and cannot spread in the medium. Some filamentous organisms spread in or on semisolid media but are nonmotile and non-flagellated. Although cultures may grow at 37° C or higher temperatures, the flagellar proteins of some organisms are not synthesized optimally at this temperature; hence, motility medium should be incu-

---

*Discussion adapted from Paik. 1980. In Lennette et al., editors. Manual of clinical microbiology, ed. 3. American Society for Microbiology, Washington, D.C.

bated at temperatures near 18° to 20° C. These observations require judicious interpretation of motility and limit, to some extent, the reliability of using spreading in semisolid agar as the sole taxonomic criterion to delineate related species.

MOTILITY TEST SEMISOLID AGAR FOR *LISTERIA*

Bacto-tryptose (Difco)	10 g
Sodium chloride	5 g
Agar	5 g
Glucose	1 g
Distilled water	1000 ml

Dissolve with the aid of heat, distribute in tubes, and sterilize at 121° C for 20 min.

Inoculate by stabbing with a 24-h broth culture. Incubate the tubes at 25° and 35° C, and observe for growth away from the stab line (motile).

MUELLER-HINTON AGAR

(Proc. Soc. Exp. Biol. Med. 1941. 48:330.)

Beef, infusion from	300 g
Peptone	17.5 g
Starch	1.5 g
Agar	17 g
(Final pH 7.4)*	

Suspend the medium in distilled water, mix thoroughly, and heat with frequent agitation. Boil for about 1 min, dispense, sterilize by autoclaving at 116° to 121° C (12 to 15 pounds' steam pressure) for **no longer than 15 min,** and cool by placing immediately in a 50° C water bath before pouring.

The medium is used primarily for the disk-agar diffusion method of testing for antimicrobial susceptibility of microorganisms. Commercial dry powder is recommended for consistent results. It has also been used to detect starch hydrolysis by *Streptococcus bovis* (Lee. 1976. J. Clin. Microbiol. 4:312). Five percent defibrinated animal blood may be added as enrichment.

MUELLER-HINTON BROTH (CATION-SUPPLEMENTED)

(National Committee for Clinical Laboratory Standards. 1983. M7-T, Methods for Dilution Antimicrobial Susceptibility Tests for Bacteria that Grow Aerobically. NCCLS, Villanova, Pa.)

1. Prepare Mueller-Hinton broth as recommended by the manufacturer. After autoclaving, cool to 4° C in the refrigerator or in an ice bath.

*Check by using a surface electrode, if available, after gelling, or with other methods as discussed in Chapter 8.

2. Prepare stock magnesium solution as follows:

$MgCl_2 \cdot 6 H_2O$	8.36 g
Deionized water	100 ml

Sterilize by membrane filtration and store at 4° C. The Mg^{++} concentration is 10 mg/ml.

3. Prepare stock calcium solution as follows:

$CaCl_2 \cdot 2 H_2O$	3.68 g
Deionized water	100 ml

Sterilize by membrane filtration and store at 4° C. The Ca^{++} concentration is 10 mg/ml.

4. Add 1.25 ml of cold magnesium stock solution and 2.5 ml of cold calcium solution per liter of cold Mueller-Hinton broth for a final concentration of:

10-12 mg/L Mg^{++} and 20-25 mg/L Ca^{++}.

MYCOPLASMA MEDIA

Also see Edward-Hayflick agar, SP-4 mycoplasma *medium*, Ureaplasma *agar, and* Ureaplasma broth.

MYCOPLASMA HOMINIS AGAR AND BROTH

(Clyde, Kenny, and Schachter. 1984. Cumitech 19: Laboratory Diagnosis of Chlamydial and Mycoplasmal Infections. Drew, Coordinating Editor. American Society for Microbiology, Washington, D.C.)

1. Prepare 1% phenol red by dissolving 1 g of phenol red (sodium salt) in 100 ml of water. Autoclave for 15 min at 121° C.

2. Prepare stock penicillin solution by dissolving 1,000,000 U of penicillin G (sterile for injection) in 50 ml sterile water. Store in aliquots of 1.2 ml at −20° C.

3. Prepare basal medium as follows:

Soy peptone	20 g
NaCl	5 g
Phenol red (1%)	1 ml
Distilled water	1000 ml

Adjust the pH to 7.3. A second broth base medium without phenol red indicator should also be prepared at the same time. For preparation of agar, add 10 g of agarose per liter after adjusting pH and mix to dissolve. Dispense the media in 100-ml bottles, 70 ml per bottle. Sterilize both broth and agar base solutions at 121° C for 15 min. Store at 4° C.

4. To broth base or to melted and cooled (to 50° C) agar base, add the following supplements:

Horse serum (unheated, sterile)	20 ml
Stock penicillin	1 ml
Fresh yeast extract (prepared as described for New York City medium, below)	10 ml

5. Dispense the broths aseptically into 16- × 125-mm screw-capped test tubes (5 ml per tube) and tighten caps. Store at 4° C for no longer than 1 week.

6. Pour agar into 35-mm diameter Petri dishes, 5 ml per dish. Store tightly wrapped in plastic at 4° C and use plates within 1 week of preparation.

New York City Medium for Isolation of *Mycoplasma hominis* and *Neisseria gonorrhoeae*

(Adapted from Phillips and Nash. 1985. Culture Media. In Lennette et al., editors. Manual of Clinical Microbiology, ed. 4. American Society for Microbiology, Washington, D.C.)

1. Prepare basal medium as follows:
   a. Agar base

Bacto-agar (Difco)	20 g
Distilled water	400 ml

   Place the solution in an Arnold steam sterilizer (Chapter 8) or heat with continuous stirring on a hotplate until the agar has melted.

   b. Cornstarch

Cornstarch (Argo)	1 g
Distilled water	40 ml

   Mix thoroughly on a magnetic stirrer–hot plate before heating. Heat on the hot plate with continuous stirring or in an Arnold steam sterilizer until the mixture is smooth and creamy.

   c. Peptone and salt solution

Proteose peptone No. 3 (Difco)	15 g
Dipotassium phosphate (Sigma)	4 g
Monopotassium phosphate (Sigma)	1 g
Sodium chloride	5 g
Distilled water	200 ml

   Bring peptone and salts to boiling on a magnetic stirrer–hot plate.

   d. Add melted agar, cornstarch, and peptone and salts solutions together in a liter flask. Mix thoroughly on a magnetic stirrer–hot plate.

Autoclave for 15 min at 121° C. The final pH should be 7.1 ± 0.1.

2. Prepare the following supplements:
   a. Yeast dialysate

Baker's yeast (available from grocery stores)	908 g
Distilled water	2500 ml

   Mix the yeast and the water to a smooth paste in a 4-L flask. Autoclave the mixture for 10 min at 121° C and allow to cool to room temperature. Soak 2-inch (5 cm) diameter dialysis tubing in water to soften it, and make at least two knots in one end of the tubing. Pour the yeast mixture into the other end of the dialysis tubing (a total length of about 1 yard of tubing is needed; several different lengths can be prepared), tie the tops of each length of tubing, and rinse the outside of the tubing and the knots to remove any yeast. Dialyze all of the lengths of tubing together against 2 L of cold distilled water in a 4-L flask for 48 h (in a cold room). Discard the dialysis tubing and the yeast mixture inside and dispense the dialysate (the solution remaining in the flask) in 25-ml amounts (in autoclavable 50-ml bottles or large screw-capped glass tubes). Autoclave the dialysate for 15 min at 121° C and store frozen at −20° C. The dialysate is stable at this temperature.

   b. Glucose solution

Glucose (Difco)	50 g
Distilled water	100 ml

   Mix thoroughly; filter-sterilize by passing through a 0.45-μm pore size membrane filter, and dispense aseptically in 10-ml amounts into sterile 16- × 125-mm glass screw-capped tubes. Store refrigerated.

   c. 3% hemoglobin solution
   Add 6 ml of the sedimented red blood cells that remain in a collection bag after the plasma has been removed (packed human erythrocytes, available from the hospital blood bank) to 200 ml sterile distilled water at room temperature. The cells will lyse, creating the 3% hemoglobin solution.

   d. Citrated horse plasma

Sodium citrate (Sigma)	1200 g
NaCl	64 g

Distilled water to   8 L

Place 600 ml of the citrate solution in a blood collection bottle for horses and draw blood up to 6 L, making a final concentration of 10% citrate in the blood.

e. Antibiotic mixture

Vancomycin	2 µg/ml
Colistin (polymyxin)	5.5 µg/ml
Amphotericin B	1.2 µg/ml
Trimethoprim lactate	3 µg/ml

Prepare the antibiotic mixture in 5 ml total volume, using methods outlined in Chapter 13. If a larger quantity is prepared initially, it should be stored frozen at temperatures below −20° C in aliquots of 5 ml each.

3. To the 640 ml basal medium that has been melted from a previously prepared solution or freshly autoclaved and cooled to 55° C, the supplements are added in the following amounts:

Citrated horse plasma	120 ml
3% hemoglobin solution	200 ml
50% glucose solution	10 ml
Yeast dialysate	25 ml
Antibiotic mixture	5 ml

4. Mix all ingredients thoroughly (the final volume is 1 L) and pour into Petri plates, approximately 20 ml per plate. Store plates tightly wrapped in plastic bags in the refrigerator. Medium is stable for approximately 10 weeks.

MODIFIED NEW YORK CITY MEDIUM (HENDERSON FORMULATION) FOR ISOLATION OF *NEISSERIA GONORRHOEAE*

See Chapter 19.

NITRATE BROTH FOR NITRATE REDUCTION TEST

Tryptone	5 g
Neopeptone	5 g
Distilled water	1000 ml
Potassium nitrate (reagent grade)	1 g
Glucose	0.1 g

Before adding the potassium nitrate and glucose, boil the other ingredients in the water and adjust pH to 7.3 to 7.4. Dispense 5 ml per tube and sterilize at 15 pounds' pressure for 15 min. The reagents and tests for nitrate reduction are listed in Chapter 9.

NUTRIENT AGAR

Beef extract	3 g
Peptone or Gelysate pancreatic digest of gelatin	5 g
Agar	15 g
Distilled water	1000 ml
(Final pH 6.8)	

Autoclave at 121° C for 15 min.

ONPG (β-GALACTOSIDASE) TEST

See Chapter 27, Procedure 27.4.

OXGALL (40%)

Dissolve 40 g oxgall in 100 ml of distilled water, autoclave at 121° C for 15 min, and refrigerate. Oxgall is available from media and chemical suppliers. Oxgall is also the concentrated component of bile; 2% oxgall equals 20% bile.

OXIDATIVE-FERMENTATIVE (O-F) BASAL MEDIUM

(Hugh and Leifson. 1953. J. Bacteriol. 66:24.)

See Chapter 28, Procedure 28.1, for preparation and use of this medium.

PHENOL RED BROTH BASE

Trypticase	10 g
Sodium chloride	5 g
Phenol red	0.018 g
(Final pH 7.4)	

Phenol red broth base can be used as a base for determining carbohydrate fermentation reactions. Carbohydrates can be added to the medium in 0.5% to 1% concentrations before dispensing and sterilization. Durham tubes should be inserted into the tubed medium for detection of gas formation.

See Carbohydrate Broth for further information.

PHENYLALANINE AGAR

(Ewing et al. 1957. Pub. Health Lab. 15:153.)

Yeast extract	3 g
DL-Phenylalanine (or L-phenylalanine)	2 g
	1 g
Disodium phosphate	1 g
Sodium chloride	5 g
Agar	12 g
Distilled water	1000 ml

Dispense 3-ml amounts in small tubes, and sterilize at 121° C for 10 min. Allow to solidify in a slanted position.

This medium is used to test for deamination of phenylalanine to phenylpyruvic acid by members of the Enterobacteriaceae.

After incubation of the culture for 18 to 24 h at 35° C, allow 4 to 5 drops of fresh 10% ferric chloride solution to run down over the growth on the slant. If acid has been formed, a *green* color immediately develops on the slant and in the fluid at the base of the slant.

PHENYLETHANOL (PHENYLETHYL ALCOHOL, PEA) AGAR

(Lilley and Brewer. 1953. J. Am. Pharm. Assoc. [Scient. Ed.] 42:6.)

Trypticase	15 g
Phytone	5 g
Sodium chloride	5 g
Beta-phenylethyl alcohol	2.5 g
Agar	15 g
Distilled water	1000 ml
(Final pH 7.3)	

Suspend the powder in the water, mix thoroughly, heat with agitation, and boil 1 min. Dispense in 16- × 150-mm screw-capped tubes. Sterilize at 118° to 121° C (12 to 15 pounds' pressure) for 15 min. If desired, 5% blood may be added to the cooled medium (45° to 50° C) before pouring plates.

Phenylethyl alcohol agar is useful for the isolation of gram-positive cocci and the inhibition of gram-negative bacilli (particularly *Proteus*) when these are found in mixed culture. This medium also supports the growth of most strict anaerobic gram-negative bacilli while inhibiting facultative anaerobic gram-negative bacilli.

PHOSPHATE-BUFFERED SALINE

See under Viral Media: Reagents and Solutions.

POTATO-DEXTROSE AGAR

Potatoes, infusion from	200 g
Glucose	20 g
Agar	20 g
Distilled water	1000 ml

Boil potatoes in water for 15 min, filter through cotton, and make up to volume with water. Add dry ingredients, and dissolve agar with heat. No pH adjustment is required. Dispense as desired, and autoclave at 121° C for 10 min. The agar is used to stimulate spore production of fungi.

PURPLE BROTH BASE FOR TESTING CARBOHYDRATE FERMENTATION BY ENTEROBACTERIACEAE

Peptone: protease or peptic digest of animal tissue USP	10 g
Beef extract	1 g
Sodium chloride	5 g
Bromcresol purple	0.015 g
Distilled water	1000 ml
(Final pH 6.8)	

Autoclave at 121° C for not more than 15 min. Add sugars and alcohols to 1% (w/v). See Carbohydrate Broth for further information.

PVA FIXATIVE FOR PARASITOLOGIC EXAMINATION

(Modified from Brooke and Goldman. 1949. J. Lab. Clin. Med. 34:1554.)

PVA, Elvanol 71-24	10 g
95% ethyl alcohol	62.5 ml
Mercuric chloride, saturated aqueous	125 ml
Glacial acetic acid	10 ml
Glycerin	3 ml

1. Mix liquid ingredients in a 500-ml beaker.
2. Add PVA powder (stirring not recommended).
3. Cover beaker with a large Petri dish, heavy waxed paper, or foil and allow to soak overnight.
4. Heat solution slowly to 75° C. When this temperature is reached, remove beaker and swirl mixture until a homogeneous, slightly milky solution is obtained (30 seconds).

RESAZURIN

Use as an Eh indicator in PRAS media. Dissolve one tablet (Difco) in 44 ml of distilled water. Store the stock solution at room temperature.

RICE GRAIN MEDIUM

White rice	8 g
Distilled water	25 ml

Place in a 125 ml Erlenmeyer flask, and autoclave at 121° C for 15 min.

Rice grain medium is used for differentiation of *Microsporum* species. *M. canis* and *M. gypseum* grow and sporulate well in this medium; *M. audouinii* grows poorly. Conidial formation is stimulated in some of the *Trichophyton* species.

RINGER'S SOLUTION FOR DISSOLVING CALCIUM ALGINATE SWABS

Sodium chloride	8.5 g
Potassium chloride	0.2 g
Calcium chloride · 2 H$_2$O	0.2 g
Sodium carbonate	0.01 g
Distilled water	1000 ml
(pH 7.0)	

Sterilize by autoclaving at 121° C for 15 min. To use in dissolving calcium alginate swabs, prepare in one-quarter strength, and add 1% sodium hexametaphosphate. Approximately 10 min of shaking usually suffices for complete dissolution of the swab.

SABHI AGAR

(Gorman. 1967. Am. J. Med. Technol. 33:151.)

Calf brain, infusion from	100 g
Beef heart, infusion from	125 g
Proteose peptone	5 g
Neopeptone	5 g
Glucose	21 g
Sodium chloride	2.5 g
Disodium phosphate	1.25 g
Agar	15 g
Distilled water	1000 ml
(Final pH 7.0)	

1. Suspend 59 g of commercial powder in 1000 ml of distilled water and heat to boiling to dissolve medium completely.
2. Sterilize by autoclaving at 121° C for 15 min.
3. Cool to 50° to 55° C, and add 1 ml of sterile chloramphenicol solution (100 mg/ml), prepared using methods discussed in Chapter 13.
4. Mix well, and dispense in sterile, cotton-plugged 25- × 150-mm Pyrex test tubes.
5. Slant, allow to harden, and refrigerate.

Sabhi is an equal mixture of Sabouraud dextrose agar and brain-heart infusion agar and has proved useful for isolation of clinically significant fungi, particularly from specimens containing bacteria, such as sputum.

SABOURAUD DEXTROSE AGAR (SAB)

Sabouraud dextrose agar	32.5 g
Agar, powdered	2.5 g
Distilled water	500 ml

Suspend ingredients in water, dissolve by heating to boiling, and dispense in approximately 20-ml amounts in cotton-plugged, 25- × 150-mm Pyrex test tubes (without lips). If antimicrobial agents are to be added, this may be done after heating the medium and before autoclaving. The following amounts are recommended (CDC):

Cycloheximide	250 mg dissolved in 5 ml acetone
Chloramphenicol	25 mg dissolved in 5 ml 95% ethanol

Mix well, and distribute into tubes or bottles as indicated. Autoclave at 118° C for *no longer than 10 min*. Slant, allow to harden, and refrigerate. This selective medium is used primarily for primary isolation of dermatophytes. It is available commercially as Mycobiotic agar (Difco) and Mycosel agar (BBL). Zygomycetes are unable to grow on this medium.

SABOURAUD DEXTROSE BROTH

Dextrose	40 g
Peptone	10 g
Distilled water	1000 ml

Dissolve ingredients, dispense in 10-ml amounts in 18- × 150-mm tubes, and autoclave at 121° C for 10 min. Sabouraud dextrose broth is useful for differentiation of *Candida* species.

SALMONELLA-SHIGELLA (SS) AGAR

Beef extract	5 g
Peptone	5 g
Lactose	10 g
Bile salts mixture	8.5 g
Sodium citrate	8.5 g
Sodium thiosulfate	8.5 g
Ferric citrate	1 g
Agar	13.5 g
Brilliant green	0.33 g
Neutral red	0.025 g
Distilled water	1000 ml

Dissolve by boiling. *Do not autoclave*.

Salmonella-Shigella agar is used primarily as a selective medium for isolation of salmonellae and shigellae, while inhibiting coliform bacilli. It can also differentiate lactose-fermenting from non-lactose-fermenting strains.

Schaudinn's Fixative for Parasites (Stock Solution)

Saturated aqueous solution of $HgCl_2$	600 ml
Ethyl alcohol (95%)	300 ml

Immediately before use add 5 ml of glacial acetic acid per 100 ml of stock solution.

Scott's Modified Castañeda Media and Thioglycollate Broth for Blood Cultures

Agar Bottle—Slant

Trypticase soy agar*	40 g
Agar, granulated	15 g
Distilled water	1000 ml

Heat in autoclave at 121° C for 5 min to melt agar or heat on a hot plate with a magnetic stirring bar.

Agar Bottle—Broth

Trypticase soy broth†	30 g
Sodium polyanethole sulfonate (SPS)	5 ml
Distilled water	1000 ml

Thioglycollate Medium

Thioglycollate broth‡	30 g
Sucrose	100 g
Sodium polyanethole sulfonate (SPS)	5 ml
Distilled water	1000 ml

(pH of all media after autoclaving should be 7.2 ± 0.2)

1. Dispense agar medium (slant) in the melted state in approximately 20-ml amounts into each of 50 clean, nonchipped, 4-ounce, square, clear-glass, screw-capped bottles (10 ml in 2-ounce bottles).§
2. Insert the disposable rubber diaphragms in the special screw caps, which are then applied loosely on the bottle tops.
3. Dispense the thioglycollate medium into 50 clean bottles, approximately 75 ml per bottle (30 ml in 2-ounce bottles), and apply screw caps as noted earlier.
4. Make up trypticase broth in a 2-L flask and plug. Prepare a dispensing buret (a 300-ml Salvarsan tube* or satisfactory substitute) to the end of which are attached a 2-foot (60 m) length of rubber tubing, a needle holder, and a 1½-inch (4 cm), 21-gauge needle, in that order. Insert the attached needle, together with a portion of the rubber tubing, in the top of the buret, and make fast by plugging, thus assuring a closed unit during sterilization.
5. Autoclave all media and equipment at 118° to 121° C for 12 to 15 min.
6. As soon as the pressure reaches zero, open the autoclave, remove all bottles rapidly, and tightly fasten the screw caps. The hands must be protected from the hot bottles by asbestos gloves.
7. Place the bottles containing the agar on their sides on a cool table top to permit hardening of the agar layer. After about 1 h, place bottles upright, and sterilize tops with alcohol sponges.† (The agar does not become detached from the sides of the bottles.)
8. Clamp the sterile dispensing buret to a ring stand. Using aseptic technique, fill the buret with sterile trypticase broth.
9. To each agar slant bottle add 60 ml of broth (25 ml in 2-ounce bottles) by puncturing the rubber diaphragm with the sterile needle. The partial vacuum in each bottle will readily permit addition of this amount.
10. Incubate agar slant bottles at 35° C for 48 h to ensure sterility. The thioglycollate bottles do not need incubation for a sterility check.
11. Inspect bottles, label, and store at room temperature (shelf-life is 6 months).

Selenite-F Enrichment Medium

(Leifson. 1936. Am. J. Hyg. 24:423.)

Sodium hydrogen selenite (anhydrous)	0.4%
Sodium phosphate (anhydrous)	1%
Peptone	0.5%
Lactose	0.4%

(Final pH 7.0)

Dissolve ingredients in distilled water. Sterilize gently; 30 min in flowing steam in an autoclave is sufficient. It is important to note that the medium should not be autoclaved. This medium is used for

---

* Available in dehydrated form from Difco, BBL, and Gibco.
† Available from Roche Diagnostics.
‡ BBL Microbiology Systems.
§ Blood culture bottles (St. Louis Health Department type) with special screw caps and disposable rubber diaphragms, 4-ounce and 2-ounce sizes, can be obtained from several suppliers.

* Arthur H. Thomas Co.
† At the Wilmington Medical Center the use of a loose application of a piece of steam autoclave tape (No. 1222-3M) to the bottle top, which is then fastened down after sterilization, obviates the need for disinfection of the diaphragm when filling with broth (step 8) or when collecting the blood culture.

the selective isolation of *Salmonella* and some strains of *Shigella*.

SODIUM BICARBONATE

Sodium bicarbonate is used as a medium supplement for anaerobes in a final concentration of 1 mg/ml. To prepare, dissolve 2 g in 100 ml of distilled water, and filter-sterilize. The stock solution is 20 mg/ml. For use, add 0.5 ml to 10 ml of medium.

SODIUM CHLORIDE BROTH (6.5%)

Brain-heart infusion broth	100 ml
Sodium chloride	6 g

Brain-heart infusion broth contains 0.5% sodium chloride. Thus, by adding an additional 6%, the desired concentration is obtained. The medium is selective for enterococci and other salt-tolerant organisms and is useful in identification as well.

SÖRENSEN pH BUFFER SOLUTIONS

Buffer solutions may be added to culture media to prevent a significant change in hydrogen-ion concentration. Sörensen buffers, prepared from potassium and sodium phosphates, are readily prepared from the anhydrous salts or purchased from commercial sources.

Solution A
M/15 Na$_2$PO$_4$

Dissolve 9.464 g of the anhydrous salt, previously dried at 130° C, in distilled water, to make 1 L of solution.

Solution B
M/15 KH$_2$PO$_4$

Dissolve 9.073 g of the anhydrous salt, previously dried at 110° C, in distilled water to make 1 L of solution. Mix solutions A and B as indicated.

pH	SOLUTION A (ml)	SOLUTION B (ml)
5.29	0.25	9.75
5.59	0.5	9.5
5.91	1	9
6.24	2	8
6.47	3	7
6.64	4	6
6.81	5	5
6.98	6	4
7.17	7	3
7.38	8	2
7.73	9	1
8.04	9.5	0.5

SP-4 *MYCOPLASMA* MEDIUM FOR PRIMARY ISOLATION OF *MYCOPLASMA*

1. Prepare base as follows:

Mycoplasma broth base (BBL)	3.5 g
Tryptone (Difco)	10 g
Bacto-Peptone (Difco)	5 g
Dextrose (50% aqueous solution, filter-sterilized)	10 ml
Distilled water	615 ml

Stir the solids into boiling water to dissolve them and adjust the pH to 7.5. Autoclave according to the manufacturer's instructions. Cool to 56° C before adding supplements. To prepare the agar necessary for making biphasic media, add 8.5 g Noble agar (Difco) to the basal medium ingredients.

2. Add the following supplements for each 625 ml of base to make a final volume of 1 L:

CMRL 1066 tissue culture medium with glutamine, 10× (GIBCO)	50 ml
Aqueous yeast extract (prepared as described in New York City Medium)	35 ml
Yeastolate (Difco; 2% solution)	100 ml
Fetal bovine serum (heat-inactivated at 56° C for 30 min)	170 ml
Penicillin G sodium	1,000,000 U
or Ampicillin	1 mg/ml
Amphotericin B	0.5 g
Polymyxin B	500,000 U

Dispense 1 ml of SP-4 agar aseptically into the bottom of sterile 4-ml screw-capped vials. Allow the agar to set and dispense 2 ml of SP-4 broth above the agar layer in each vial. Seal caps tightly and store at −20° C indefinitely.

STARCH AGAR MEDIUM

Bacto-agar	20 g
Bacto-peptone	5 g
Beef extract	3 g
Sodium chloride	5 g
Soluble starch	20 g
Distilled water	1000 ml
(Final pH 7.2)	

1. Dissolve the agar in 300 ml of water with heat.
2. Dissolve the beef extract and peptone in 200 ml of water.
3. Mix the solutions in steps 1 and 2, and make up to 1000-ml volume.
4. To this mixture add the starch, dissolve, and autoclave at 121° C for 15 min.

The medium may be dispensed in tubes (15- to 20-ml amounts) or flasks convenient for pouring plates and should be stored in a refrigerator. For pouring of plates, melt the medium in tubes or flasks as required. If poured plates of starch agar are refrigerated, the medium becomes opaque.

Starch agar is useful in developing smooth cultures by streaking borderline rough strains on the surface of the medium. It also may be used for testing cultures for starch hydrolytic activity.

STOCK CULTURE AND MOTILITY MEDIUM

(Hugh. 1974. In ASM Man. Clin. Microbiol., Ed. 2, p. 263.)

Casitone	10 g
Yeast extract	3 g
Sodium chloride	5 g
Agar	3 g
Distilled water	1000 ml

1. Suspend the ingredients in distilled water; heat to boiling to completely dissolve agar.
2. Dispense in 13- × 100-mm screw-capped tubes, 4 ml per tube.
3. Sterilize by autoclaving at 121° C for 15 min; store as butts.

This medium is used for motility testing by stabbing the inoculum once into the agar and incubating overnight at 35° C. Motility is indicated by growth spreading out from the line of stab. By deleting the salt from the formula, the medium is also excellent for preserving stock cultures of nonfermenting and fermenting gram-negative rods (up to 6 months). After inoculation and overnight incubation, the caps are sealed with Parafilm or tape, and the tubes refrigerated.

STUART'S TRANSPORT MEDIUM (MODIFIED FOR USE WITH DACRON OR RAYON SWABS)

Sodium glycerophosphate	10 g
Sodium thioglycollate	1 g
Calcium chloride dihydrate	0.1 g
Distilled water	1000 ml

Mix thoroughly. Dispense into 16- × 125-mm screw-capped test tubes, 0.5 ml per tube. Autoclave for 10 min at 121° C. Tighten caps and store tubes at room temperature.

SUCROSE (5%) BROTH OR AGAR FOR TESTING VIRIDANS STREPTOCOCCI

See Chapter 25.

TELLURITE REDUCTION TEST MEDIUM FOR MYCOBACTERIA

Medium

1. Suspend 4.7 g of Middlebrook 7H9 dehydrated base in 900 ml of distilled water, and add 0.5 ml of Tween 80.
2. Autoclave at 121° C for 15 min, cool to 55° C, and add aseptically 100 ml ADC enrichment (Difco, BBL).
3. Dispense aseptically in 5-ml amounts in 20- × 150-mm screw-capped tubes, check for sterility, and refrigerate.

Tellurite Solution

1. Dissolve 0.2 g of potassium tellurite in 100 ml of distilled water.
2. Dispense in 2- to 5-ml amounts, and sterilize by autoclaving at 121° C for 10 min.

This medium is used to test the ability of certain nonphotochromogens to reduce tellurite rapidly to the *black*, metallic tellurium. To perform the test, incubate the test organism for a minimum of 7 days (until the broth becomes turbid) in the broth medium. Add 2 drops of tellurite solution to each broth culture and incubate (37° C) for 4 more days. A *black precipitate* indicates a positive reaction.

TETRATHIONATE BROTH

Proteose peptone (Difco)	5 g
Bile salts	1 g
Calcium carbonate	10 g
Sodium thiosulfate	30 g
Distilled water	1000 ml

Dispense the medium in 10-ml amounts, and heat to boiling. *Before use* add 0.2 ml of iodine solution (6 g of iodine crystals and 5 g of potassium iodide in 20 ml of water) to each tube.

This is a selective liquid enrichment medium for use in the isolation of *Salmonella*, except *S. typhi*. The sterile base *without iodine* may be stored in a refrigerator indefinitely.

THAYER-MARTIN AGAR

GC agar base (Difco) (double-strength)	72 g
Agar	10 g
Distilled water	1000 ml

1. Suspend the dehydrated medium in water, mix well, and heat with agitation. Boil for 1 min.
2. Sterilize by autoclaving at 121° C for 15 min.
3. At the same time, autoclave a suspension of 20 g of dehydrated hemoglobin in 1000 ml water for 15 min (suspension must be *smooth* before sterilizing).
4. Cool both to 50° C, mix aseptically, and then add 20 ml of IsoVitaleX enrichment (BBL) and 20 ml of V-C-N inhibitor (BBL). Pour plates, using 20 ml per plate. Refrigerate.

This medium is recommended for the isolation of *Neisseria gonorrhoeae* from all sites that might contain a mixed flora, as well as for the recovery of *N. meningitidis* from nasopharyngeal and throat cultures.

MODIFIED THAYER-MARTIN MEDIUM FOR ISOLATION OF *N. GONORRHOEAE* AND *N. MENINGITIDIS*

(Modified from the Difco Manual, Ed. 10. Difco Laboratories, Detroit.)

Trimethoprim lactate and increased agar content inhibit swarming *Proteus* species.

1. Prepare GC medium base as follows:

Bacto GC medium base (Difco)	36 g
Dextrose	1.5 g
Bacto agar (Difco)	10 g
Bacto supplement VX (Difco)	10 ml

Suspend the GC medium base, the agar, and the dextrose in 500 ml of distilled water. Heat to boiling to dissolve the ingredients and autoclave for 15 min at 121° C. Cool the solution to 55° C in a water bath and aseptically add the supplement VX. Allow the medium to remain in the water bath until all components have been added together.

2. Prepare Bacto hemoglobin as follows:

| Bacto hemoglobin (Difco) | 10 g |
| Distilled water | 500 ml |

Place the hemoglobin in a dry liter beaker on a stirring platform with a stir bar. Add the distilled water in 100-ml amounts, stirring vigorously. Break up clumps with a spatula. Transfer to a

liter flask and autoclave for 15 min at 121° C. Cool to 55° C in a water bath.

3. Aseptically add the warm GC medium base to the hemoglobin solution, swirling to mix thoroughly.
4. Rehydrate a vial of Bacto antimicrobic vial CNVT (containing 7500 µg of colistin sulfate, 12,500 U of nystatin, 3000 µg of vancomycin, and 5000 µg of trimethoprim lactate) by aseptically adding 10 ml of sterile distilled or deionized water to the vial. Mix well.
5. Add the CNVT to the warm agar base mixture, mix thoroughly, and pour into Petri plates, approximately 20 ml per plate.

THIOGLYCOLLATE MEDIUM WITHOUT INDICATOR* (THIO)

(Brewer. 1940 and 1943. J. Bacteriol. 39:10 and 46:395.)

Peptone	20 g
L-Cystine	0.25 g
Glucose	6 g
Sodium chloride	2.5 g
Sodium thioglycollate	0.5 g
Sodium sulfite	0.1 g
Agar	0.7 g
Distilled water	1000 ml
(Final pH 7.2)	

Dispense the medium in 15-ml amounts in 16- × 125-mm test tubes, making a column of medium 7 cm high. Autoclave for 15 min at 121° C. Store at room temperature.

ENRICHED THIO

Enriched THIO is prepared by adding to the freshly prepared and autoclaved medium (or to previously prepared medium that has been boiled for 10 min and then cooled) vitamin K_1 solution, 0.1 µg/ml; sodium bicarbonate, 1 mg/ml; and hemin, 5 µg/ml. Rabbit or horse serum (10%) or Fildes enrichment (5%) may also be added. See Vitamin K_1 Solution and Hemin Solution for preparation of these supplements. Enriched thioglycollate medium is often used for susceptibility testing of anaerobes by the broth-disk elution method.

---

*This may be enriched by the addition of 10% normal rabbit or horse serum when cool.

THIONINE OR BASIC FUCHSIN AGAR

(Huddleson et al. 1939. Brucellosis in Man and Animals, The Commonwealth Fund, New York.)

Trypticase soy agar may be used as a base for differential media containing thionine and basic fuchsin.

Prepare the dyes, thionine and basic fuchsin, in 0.1% stock solutions in sterile distilled water. These stock solutions may be stored indefinitely. Before adding to the media, heat the dye solutions in flowing steam in an autoclave for 20 min, shake well, and while still hot, add to melted agar. In trypticase soy agar the final concentration of the dye should be 1:100,000 (10 ml/L of medium). Thoroughly mix the dyes (added individually) and the melted agar, and pour immediately into Petri dishes, one set containing thionine and one containing basic fuchsin. Place the plates in a 35° C incubator until the water of condensation disappears, at which time they are ready for use. Inoculate plates within 24 h of preparation.

Streak the surface of plates with a heavy suspension of *Brucella* prepared from a 48- to 72-h trypticase soy agar slant culture. It is advisable to streak plates in duplicate, incubating one set aerobically and the other in 10% CO_2. Incubate plates for 72 h, and observe for inhibition of growth by thionine or basic fuchsin or both. See Chapter 29 for further information.

TINSDALE AGAR, MOORE AND PARSONS, MODIFIED

Proteose No. 3 (Difco) or Thiotone peptic digest of animal tissue USP (BBL)	20 g
L-Cystine	0.24 g
Sodium chloride	5 g
Sodium thiosulfate	0.43 g
Agar, dried	14 g
or not dried	20 g
Distilled water	1000 ml
(Final pH 7.4)	

1. Heat with agitation, and boil for 1 min.
2. Autoclave at 121° C for 15 min. Cool to 56° C, and to each 100 ml of base add:

Sterile serum (e.g., bovine)	10 ml
Potassium tellurite, 1% aqueous	3 ml

3. Alternatively, the thiosulfate may be dissolved in 1.7 ml of water and added separately. It must be prepared fresh each time the medium is prepared. The cystine may be dissolved in 6 ml of 0.1 N HCl and added separately, in which case it may be necessary to add 6 ml of 0.1 N NaOH to make sure that the final pH is correct.

TODD-HEWITT BROTH, MODIFIED

(J. Pathol. Bacteriol. 1932. 35:973.)

Beef heart infusion	1000 ml
Neopeptone	20 g

Adjust to pH 7 with normal sodium hydroxide and add:

Sodium chloride	2 g
Sodium bicarbonate	2 g
Disodium phosphate	0.4 g
Glucose	2 g
(Final pH 7.8)	

Mix the chemicals in broth, and bring to a slow boil. Boil for 15 min, filter through paper, dispense in tubes, and autoclave at 115° C for 10 min.

Modified Todd-Hewitt broth is used for growing streptococci for serologic identification.

TOLUIDINE BLUE AGAR FOR THERMONUCLEASE TEST

(Lachica, et al. 1971. Appl. Microbiol. 21:585.)

1. Prepare agar base stock as follows:

Deoxyribonucleic acid	0.3 g
Calcium chloride, anhydrous (0.01 M)	1.0 ml
Sodium chloride	10.0 g
Agar (Difco Bacto agar)	10.0 g
TRIS buffer (0.05 M, pH 9.0; Sigma)	1000.0 ml

Heat the solution to boiling and then cool to 45° C in a water bath. Add:

Toluidine blue (0.1 M)	3.0 ml

2. Dispense into sterile glass screw-capped tubes, 18.0 ml per tube. Allow to solidify, and store in the refrigerator. Agar deeps will retain activity for 6 months.
3. Before use, melt the agar in a boiling water bath or by steaming and pour into a 90-mm diameter Petri plate. When the plate has set, proceed as in Procedure 9.8, Chapter 9.

TRANSPORT MEDIA

See Amies Transport Medium, Cary and Blair Transport Medium, and Stuart's Transport Medium.

TRIPLE SUGAR IRON (TSI) AGAR

(Hajna, 1945. J. Bacteriol. 49:516.)

Peptone	20 g
Sodium chloride	5 g

Lactose	10 g
Sucrose	10 g
Glucose	1 g
Ferrous ammonium sulfate	0.2 g
Sodium thiosulfate	0.2 g
Phenol red	0.025 g
Agar	13 g
Distilled water	1000 ml
(Final pH 7.3)	

TSI agar is used for determining carbohydrate fermentation and hydrogen sulfide production as a first step in the identification of gram-negative bacilli.

This medium is considered to be a modification of KIA. The only difference between the two is that sucrose is not included in KIA. It should be stressed that pH changes in the butt and in the slant of the medium must be recorded only after 18 to 24 h of incubation. See Chapter 9 for further information on inoculation of these media and interpretation of the reactions.

TRYPTICASE SOY AGAR

Trypticase	15 g
Phytone	5 g
Sodium chloride	5 g
Agar	15 g
Distilled water	1000 ml
(Final pH 7.3)	

Trypticase soy agar is an excellent blood agar base and can be used for the isolation and maintenance of all organisms, except some with very special nutritional requirements.

TRYPTICASE SOY BROTH

Trypticase	17 g
Phytone	3 g
Sodium chloride	5 g
Dipotassium phosphate	2.5 g
Glucose	2.5 g
Distilled water	1000 ml
(Final pH 7.3)	

Trypticase soy broth is excellent for the rapid (6- to 8-h) growth of most organisms and supports growth of pneumococci and streptococci without the addition of blood or serum. It also supports growth of *Brucella*. However, fermentation of the glucose present will cause a drop in pH, and acid-sensitive organisms, particularly pneumococci, may die in 18 to 24 h.

TRYPTOPHAN BROTH

Tryptophan broth is a popular medium for the detection of indole production. Trypticase (BBL) or tryptone (Difco) is recommended, in 1% aqueous solution. Follow label directions for preparation.

TYROSINE OR XANTHINE AGAR

Nutrient agar	23 g
Tyrosine	5 g
or xanthine	4 g
Demineralized water	1000 ml

1. Dissolve the nutrient agar in the water.
2. Add tryosine or xanthine, and mix to distribute the crystals evenly.
3. Adjust to pH 7.0, and autoclave at 121° C for 15 min.
4. Dispense in plates, 20 ml per plate, with the crystals evenly distributed.

Tyrosine and xanthine agar are recommended for differentiation of species of aerobic actinomycetes. Its use is similar to that of casein agar.

TWEEN 80—ALBUMIN BROTH FOR CULTIVATION OF SPIROCHETES

See Ellinghausen, McCullough, Johnson, and Harris Medium.

UREASE TEST MEDIA

UREA AGAR

(Christensen. 1946. J. Bacteriol. 52:461.)

Peptone	1 g
Glucose	1 g
Sodium chloride	5 g
Monopotassium phosphate	2 g
Phenol red	0.012 g
Agar	20 g
Distilled water	1000 ml
(Final pH 6.8-6.9)	

Prepare the agar base, and sterilize in the autoclave at 121° C for 15 min in flasks containing 100- to 200-ml amounts. Store until needed. Prepare a 29% solution of urea. Sterilize by filtration. Add the sterile urea solution in a final concentration of 10% to a flask of the agar base that has been melted and cooled to a temperature of 50° C. Mix well, and distribute aseptically in sterile small tubes in amounts of 2 to 3 ml. Allow the medium to solidify in a slanting position in such a way as to obtain an agar butt of 1/2 inch and an agar slant of 1 inch.

Urea agar can be used to demonstrate urease production by species of *Proteus*. It also detects the small amounts of urease produced by other enteric bacilli, thus differentiating them from urease-negative *Salmonella* and *Shigella*. Urea agar may be used to detect urease production by *Cryptococcus* species and other aerobic bacteria.

UREASE TEST BROTH

(McKay et al. 1947. Am J. Clin. Pathol. 17:479. Rustigian and Stuart. 1941. Proc. Soc. Exp. Biol. Med. 47:108. Stuart et al. 1945. J. Bacteriol. 49:437.)

Urea	20 g
Monopotassium phosphate	9.1 g
Disodium phosphate	9.5 g
Yeast extract	0.1 g
Phenol red	0.01 g
(Final pH 6.8)	

Use 3.87 g/100 ml of distilled water. *Do not heat.* When the powder has dissolved, sterilize by filtration. Distribute the broth in 0.5- to 2-ml amounts in small sterile tubes. Large amounts may be used if desired, but reactions are slower. If a filter is not available, it is possible to sterilize the medium in an autoclave, if the tubes are not tightly packed and the steam pressure is held at 5 pounds for 20 min or at 8 pounds for 7 min.

In addition, the medium generally gives reliable results without sterilization, if prepared and inoculated immediately. This strongly buffered medium is suitable for determining urease reactions of the strongly positive *Proteus*, *Morganella*, and *Providencia* species. There is a similar medium for detection of urease production in other bacteria that employs the following concentrations of phosphates:

Monopotassium phosphate	0.091 g
Disodium phosphate	0.095 g

Urease test broth may be inoculated from TSI agar (or KIA), trypticase soy agar, or other agar slants having heavy growth. It is recommended that large inocula be employed when it is desirable to obtain results rapidly. Incubate at 35° C. Normally the finished medium is a pale pink or pinkish yellow and has a neutral pH of about 6.8 to 7.0. In cultures that attack urea, ammonia is formed during incubation and makes the reaction of the medium alkaline, with a deep magenta or bluish-red color.

Urease test broth may be used in the same manner for the detection of urease activity of such organisms as members of the genera *Brucella*, *Bacillus*, *Sarcina*, *Mycobacterium*, and anaerobes. In-cubation usually should be longer than for enteric bacilli.

NOTE: Both prepared broth and dehydrated base should be stored in the refrigerator. If the seal on the bottle has been broken, the bottle should preferably be stored with desiccant in a sealed container.

See Chapter 9 for a rapid urease test procedure.

UREAPLASMA AGAR AND BROTH FOR CULTIVATION OF *U. UREALYTICUM*

Several components of both *Ureaplasma* agar and broth must be made in advance, as described below.

1. Prepare MES buffer as follows:

2-(*N*-Morpholino) ethanesulfonic acid (acid form; Behring Diagnostics)	195 g
Distilled water	800 ml

Adjust pH to 6.0 at 37° C with concentrated NaOH (6 M), make volume up to 1 L with water, and sterilize through a membrane filter. Store at room temperature in the dark.

2. Prepare 1% phenol red by dissolving 1 g of phenol red (sodium salt) in 100 ml of water. Autoclave for 15 min at 121° C.

3. Prepare urea by dissolving 60 g of ultrapure urea (Schwartz/Mann) in 1 L of distilled water to make a 1-M solution. Filter-sterilize and store at room temperature.

4. Prepare stock penicillin solution by dissolving 1,000,000 U of penicillin G (sterile for injection) in 50 ml of sterile water. Store in aliquots of 1.2 ml at −20° C.

5. Prepare sodium sulfite solution as follows:

Sodium sulfite (use a fresh bottle of powder with no evidence of caking)	0.063 g
Distilled water	500 ml
Phenol red solution (1%)	0.5 ml

Dispense 10 ml each into 16- × 125-mm screw-capped test tubes. Autoclave for 15 min at 121° C, and as soon as they are removed from the autoclave, tighten the caps. Store at room temperature. The tubes should be purple; if air has leaked into the medium, the indicator will turn orange because of oxidation of sodium sulfite to the neutral sodium sulfate.

6. Prepare agar base as follows:

Soy peptone	20 g
NaCl	5 g
MES buffer	4.25 g

Phenol red (1%)	1 ml
Distilled water	1000 ml
Agarose (Difco)	10 g

Heat the water to dissolve the agarose, and then add the other ingredients. Adjust to pH 6.0 at 37° C with 1 N NaOH. Distribute the agar base into 100-ml bottles, 70 ml per bottle. Autoclave at 121° C for 15 min. Store bottles at room temperature.

UREAPLASMA AGAR MEDIUM

Prepare agar medium by aseptically adding the components as follows:

Agar base (melted and cooled to 50° C)	70 ml
Yeast dialysate (prepared as in New York City Agar, above)	10 ml
Sterile horse serum, unheated	20 ml
Urea (1 M)	0.2 ml
Stock penicillin solution	1 ml
Lincomycin solution (10,000 µg/ml, made fresh)	0.5 ml

Pour into 35-mm diameter plastic Petri plates, 5 ml per plate. Store tightly wrapped in plastic for no longer than 2 weeks at 4° C.

UREAPLASMA BROTH FOR CULTIVATION OF *U. UREALYTICUM*

1. Prepare urea broth base as follows:

Soy peptone	20 g
NaCl	5 g
Phenol red (1%)	1 ml
Distilled water	1000 ml

Add ingredients together and adjust pH to 6.0 with 1 N HCl. Dispense into 100-ml bottles, 87.5 ml per bottle, and autoclave for 15 min at 121° C.

2. To each bottle, add the following supplements:

1 M MES buffer, pH 6.0	1 ml
1 M urea	0.5 ml
Sterile horse serum, unheated	10 ml
Stock penicillin solution	1 ml
Lincomycin (freshly made)	50 µg/ml

Store the bottle in the refrigerator for no longer than 2 weeks. Dispense in 4-ml vials, 3 ml per vial. Just before use, add 1 ml of sodium sulfite (100 mM) per 100 ml of broth (0.03 ml per vial).

VIRAL MEDIA: REAGENTS AND SOLUTIONS

ANTIBIOTIC MIXTURES FOR TREATMENT OF VIRAL CULTURE SPECIMENS

Antibiotic Mixture for Urine Specimens

Gentamicin is used in preference to penicillin and streptomycin because of its broader antibacterial spectrum. Amphotericin B is used to control fungal contamination.

| Gentamicin (50 mg/ml) | 4 ml |
| Amphotericin B (250 µg/ml) | 10 ml |

Dispense 0.3-ml aliquots into test tubes (enough for 40 tubes) and store at −20° C until needed. To each tube of thawed mixture, add 5 to 10 ml of urine.

Antibiotic Mixture for Other Viral Specimens

MEM without bicarbonate in EBSS (1 × concentrate)	100 ml
Gentamicin (10 mg/ml)	1.5 ml
Amphotericin B (250 µg/ml)	3 ml
7.5% NaHCO₃	3 ml

Dispense 5-ml aliquots into sterile tubes containing eight glass beads. This mixture is used to suspend tissues and to treat stool and other specimens that require decontamination before inoculation.

CELL CULTURE MEDIA

The following cell culture media, used to grow and maintain culture cells, are prepared with Eagle's minimum essential medium (MEM) without bicarbonate in Earle's balanced salt solution (EBSS). Both maintenance and growth media are prepared in 1000-ml volumes, aliquoted into sterile, plastic 250-ml flasks, and stored at 4° C until needed. Routine quality control includes pH determination, assay for milliequivalents of Na^+, Cl^-, and culture for bacterial, mycoplasmal, and fungal contamination.

Growth Medium

MEM without bicarbonate in EBSS (10 × concentrate)	100 ml
Gentamicin (50 mg/ml)	0.2 ml
Amphotericin B (250 µg/ml)	10 ml
7.5% NaHCO₃	10 ml
Glutamine (200 mM)	10 ml
Fetal bovine serum (inactivated 30 min at 56° C)	100 ml
Distilled water (sterile) to bring final volume to	1000 ml

We have found it convenient to prepare this medium by adding the concentrate of MEM in EBSS to 1 L of sterile distilled water from which 230 ml has been removed and then adding appropriate amounts of the remaining ingredients.

Maintenance Medium for Primary Monkey Kidney (PMK) Cells

MEM without bicarbonate in EBSS (10 × concentrate)	100 ml
Gentamicin (50 mg/ml)	1 ml
Amphotericin B (250 μg/ml)	10 ml
7.5% NaHCO₃	10 ml
Distilled water (sterile) to bring final volume to	1000 ml

Glutamine is omitted from this medium because it is toxic to monkey cells. Fetal bovine serum is omitted because it may contain substances inhibitory to myxoviruses.

Maintenance Medium for HFD and Hep-2 Cells

MEM without bicarbonate in EBSS (10 × concentrate)	100 ml
Gentamicin (50 mg/ml)	1 ml
Amphotericin B (250 μg/ml)	10 ml
Glutamine (200 mM)	10 ml
7.5% NaHCO₃	30 ml
Fetal bovine serum (inactivated 30 min at 56° C)	30 ml
Distilled water (sterile) to bring final volume to	1000 ml

HANKS' BALANCED SALT SOLUTION (BSS) WITH ANTIBIOTICS FOR WASHING CELL MONOLAYERS AND MAKING DILUTIONS OF VIRUS

Hanks' BSS without bicarbonate (1 × concentrate)	00 ml
Gentamicin (50 mg/ml)	0.1 ml
Amphotericin B (250 μg/ml)	0.5 ml
7.5% NaHCO₃	0.47 ml

PHOSPHATE-BUFFERED SALINE (PBS) SOLUTIONS

PBS (pH 7.5) for Diluting Trypsin and Washing Monolayers

NaCl	8 g
KCl	0.2 g
KH₂PO₄	0.12 g
NaH₂PO₄ (anhydrous)	91 g
Distilled water (sterile) to bring final volume to	1000 ml

PBS (pH 7.2 to 7.5) for Fluorescent Antibody Wash

1. Stock solution (10 ×): Dissolve the following in 2000 ml distilled water. Shake well after each addition of salt.

NaH₂PO₄ · H₂O	6.65 g
Na₂HPO₄	35 g
NaCl	255 g

Distilled water (sterile) to bring final volume to 3000 ml. Add 40% NaOH until pH is 7.2 to 7.5.

2. Working solution (1 ×)

10 × stock solution	1.5 liter
Distilled water (sterile)	13.5 liter

70% SORBITOL (HOLDING MEDIUM FOR CMV SPECIMENS)

Sorbitol	70 g
Distilled water (sterile)	100 ml

Filter-sterilize, and store at 4° C. To use, mix equal volumes of 70% sorbitol solution and urine specimen and freeze at −70° C. Solid specimens, such as tissue, can be immersed in the solution and then frozen to −70° C before shipping on dry ice.

0.25% TRYPSIN

Trypsin (2.5%)	5 ml
PBS (pH 7.5)	45 ml

Dispense in 2-ml aliquots and refrigerate (4° C).

VITAMIN K₁ SOLUTION

Vitamin K₁ solution is used as a medium supplement in a final concentration of 0.1 μg/ml for liquid media and 10 μg/ml for agar media. To prepare, weigh out 0.2 g of vitamin K₁(Sigma Chemical Co. and other suppliers) on a small piece of sterile aluminum foil, and aseptically add it to 20 ml of absolute ethanol in a sterile tube or bottle. The stock solution is 10 mg/ml. The stock solution can be further diluted for use in sterile distilled water. Refrigerate in a tightly closed container protected from light.

Add 1 ml of stock solution per liter of agar and 0.01 ml/L of broth (dilute stock solution in water).

XANTHINE AGAR

See Tyrosine Agar.

XYLOSE LYSINE DEOXYCHOLATE (XLD) AGAR

(Taylor. 1965. Am J. Clin. Pathol. 44:471.)

This medium may be prepared by use of the dehydrated xylose lysine agar base (BBL, Difco, Gibco, Inolex) and adding the sodium thiosulfate, ferric ammonium citrate, and sodium deoxycholate (procedure recommended by some workers) or by utilizing the complete (XLD) agar.

Xylose	3.5 g
L-Lysine	5 g
Lactose	7.5 g
Sucrose	7.5 g
Sodium chloride	5 g
Yeast extract	3 g
Phenol red	0.08 g
Agar, dried	13.5 g
Sodium deoxycholate	2.5 g
Sodium thiosulfate	6.8 g
Ferric ammonium citrate	0.8 g
Distilled water	1000 ml
(Final pH 7.4)	

Suspend the medium in distilled water, and heat with frequent agitation just to the boiling point. *Do not boil*. Transfer immediately to a 50° C water bath, and pour plates as soon as the medium has cooled. The medium should be red-orange and clear, or nearly so. Excessive heating or prolonged holding at 50° C may cause precipitation, which could lead to some differences in colony morphology.

This medium is useful for the isolation of enteric pathogens, especially shigellae.

YERSINIA SELECTIVE AGAR

See CIN Agar.

Appendix B Formulas for Commonly Used Stains

Although a number of the more important staining formulas and procedures are presented in this chapter, space does not permit a comprehensive review of the subject. Many other staining procedures are presented throughout the text where appropriate. Further details are available in the *Manual of Clinical Microbiology** and other references. The solubilities of some of the more widely used stains and dyes, in water and in alcohol, are shown in Table B.1. Most stains are also available commercially (readymade).

Table B.1
Solubility of Stains

| STAIN | PERCENT SOLUBLE AT 26° C | |
	IN WATER	IN 95% ETHANOL
Bismarck brown	1.36	1.08
Congo red	0	0.19
Crystal violet (chloride)	1.68	13.87
Eosin Y	44.2	2.18
Fuchsin, basic (chloride)	0.26	5.93
Malachite green (oxalate)	7.60	7.52
Methylene blue (chloride)	3.55	1.48
Neutral red (chloride)	5.64	2.45
Safranin O	5.45	3.41
Thionin	0.25	0.25

Data from Conn, J.G. 1928. Biological stains, Commission on Standardization of Biological Stains. W.F. Humphrey Press, Geneva, N.Y.

*Lennette, E.H., et al., editors. 1980 and 1985. Manual of clinical microbiology, eds. 3 and 4. American Society for Microbiology, Washington, D.C.

ACID-FAST STAINS

See also Rhodamine-Auramine Fluorochrome Stain for Acid-Fast Cells.

HOT MODIFIED ACID-FAST STAIN FOR *CRYPTOSPORIDIUM*

1. Spin an aliquot of 10% formalinized stool for 2 min at 300 × g.
2. Remove upper layer of sediment with pipette and place a thin layer onto a microscope slide.
   NOTE: If the stool specimen contains a lot of mucus, 10 drops of 10% KOH can be added to the sediment (step 2), vortexed, rinsed with 10% formalin, and respun before smear preparation. Some laboratories use this approach routinely before smear preparation.
3. Heat fix the smear at 70° C for 10 min.
4. Place slide on staining rack and flood with carbolfuchsin (Ziehl-Neelsen formula, p. A-36).
5. Heat to steaming and allow to stain for 5 min. If the slide begins to dry, more stain is added without additional heating.
6. Rinse the smear with tap or distilled water.
7. Decolorize with 5% aqueous sulfuric acid for 30 s (thicker smears may require a longer time).
8. Rinse smear with tap or distilled water, drain, and flood smear with methylene blue counterstain (above) for 1 min.
9. Rinse with tap or distilled water, drain, and air dry.

KINYOUN CARBOLFUCHSIN STAIN

See also Chapters 7 and 41.

(Kinyoun. 1915. Am. J. Pub. Health 5:867.)

Carbolfuchsin

Basic fuchsin	4 g
Phenol	8 ml
Alcohol (95%)	20 ml
Distilled water	100 ml

Dissolve the basic fuchsin in the alcohol, and add the water slowly while shaking. Melt the phenol in a 56° C water bath, and add 8 ml to the stain, using a pipette with a rubber bulb.

Decolorizer

Ethanol (95%)	97 ml
Concentrated HCl	3 ml

Add the hydrochloric acid to the alcohol slowly, working under a chemical fume hood.

Counterstain

Methylene blue	0.3 g
Distilled water	100 ml

1. Stain the fixed smear for 3 to 5 min (no heat necessary).
2. Wash in distilled, filtered water and shake off excess water.
3. Flood with decolorizer for approximately 1 min. Check to see that no more red color runs when the slide is tipped. Add a bit more decolorizer for very thick slides or those that continue to bleed red dye.
4. Wash thoroughly with filtered water as above and shake off excess.
5. Flood with counterstain for approximately 1 min.
6. Wash with distilled water and drain by standing slides upright. Do not blot dry.

By the addition of a detergent or wetting agent the staining of acid-fast organisms may be accelerated. Tergitol No. 7 (Sigma Chemical Co.) may be used. Add 1 drop of Tergitol No. 7 to every 30 to 40 ml of the Kinyoun carbolfuchsin stain.

Acid-fast bacteria stain red with carbolfuchsin stains. The background color is dependent on the counterstain; methylene blue imparts a blue color to non-acid-fast material, whereas brilliant green results in green background, and picric acid results in yellow. More information about the appearance of acid-fast organisms is found in Chapters 33 and 41.

PARTIAL ACID-FAST STAINS

Kinyoun Stain Used for Partial Acid-fast Stain

1. Emulsify a very small amount of the organisms to be stained in a drop of distilled water on the slide. A known positive control and a negative control should be stained along with the unknown strain.
2. Allow to air dry and heat fix.
3. Flood the stain with Kinyoun's carbolfuchsin (above) and allow the stain to remain on the slide 3 min.
4. Rinse with tap water, shake off excess water, and decolorize briefly (no longer than 3 to 5 seconds) with 3% acid alcohol (above).
5. Counterstain with Kinyoun's methylene blue (above) for 30 s.
6. Rinse again with tap water. Allow the slide to air dry, and examine the unknown strain compared to the controls. Partially acid-fast organisms show reddish to purple filaments, compared to non-acid-fast organisms that are blue only.

Other Partial Acid-fast Stains

Other modifications include performing the standard Ziehl-Neelsen procedure (below) with the substitution of 1% aqueous sulfuric acid or 0.5% acid alcohol for the standard 3% acid alcohol decolorizer. Partially acid-fast organisms, such as *Nocardia* species, will stain red to reddish-purple.

ZIEHL-NEELSEN STAIN

Carbolfuchsin

Basic fuchsin	0.3 g
Ethanol (95%)	10 ml
Phenol, melted crystals	5 ml
Distilled water	95 ml

Dissolve fuchsin in alcohol and mix the phenol slowly into the distilled water before adding both solutions together. It is helpful to allow the stain to stir overnight on a warm hotplate or in the 37° C incubator. Stain should be filtered through coarse paper before use.

Decolorizer

Hydrochloric acid, concentrated	3 ml
Ethanol (95%)	97 ml

Counterstain

Methylene blue	0.3 g
Distilled water	100 ml

Some workers may prefer 0.5% aqueous brilliant green or a saturated solution of picric acid as a counterstain; the latter is pale and does not selectively stain cellular material.

The technique for performance of the stain is given in Chaper 7.

ACRIDINE ORANGE STAIN

(McCarthy and Senne. 1980. J. Clin. Microbiol. 11:281.)

1. Prepare stock stain solution as follows:

Acridine orange (Fisher Scientific Co.)	1 g
Distilled water	100 ml

   Store in the dark at 4° C. Solution is stable for 6 months.
2. Prepare working stain solution daily by adding 0.05 ml of stock solution to 5 ml of 0.2 M acetate buffer (pH 4.0).
3. Prepare smears as usual and air dry. Fix with absolute methanol or heat fix.
4. Flood slides with working stain solution and allow to stand for 1 min.
5. Rinse with tap water and air dry.
6. Examine under oil immersion (1000 ×) and ultraviolet light for bacteria.

   Bacteria and yeast stain bright red-orange, and leukocytes stain pale apple green. Slides may be screened under low power for suspicious areas. Smears may be Gram stained directly without prior decolorization as long as all immersion oil is removed with xylene.

AURAMINE-RHODAMINE STAIN

See Chapter 7 and Rhodamine-Auramine Stain.

CALCOFLUOR WHITE

See Chapters 7 and 43.

CAPSULE STAINS

ANTHONY METHOD

1. Make a thin even smear of a culture in skimmed milk or litmus milk by spreading with a glass slide or an inoculating needle bent at a right angle. If it is not a milk culture, a loopful of the material may be mixed with a loopful of skimmed milk and then spread to give a uniform background.
2. Air dry. Do not fix with heat.
3. Stain with 1% aqueous crystal violet for 2 min.
4. Wash with a solution of 20% copper sulfate.
5. Air dry in a vertical position, and examine under the oil immersion lens. The capsule is unstained

against a purple background; the cells are deeply stained.

HISS METHOD

Mix a loopful of physiologic saline suspension of growth with a drop of normal serum on a glass slide. Allow the smear to air dry and heat fix. Flood the smear with crystal violet (1% aqueous solution). Steam the preparation gently for 1 min, and rinse with copper sulfate (20% aqueous solution). Capsules appear as faint blue halos around dark blue to purple cells.

INDIA INK METHOD*

In the India ink method, the capsule displaces the colloidal carbon particles of the ink and appears as a clear halo around the microorganism. The procedure is especially recommended for demonstrating the capsule of *Cryptococcus neoformans*.

1. To a small loopful of saline, water, or broth on a clean slide, add a *minute amount* of growth from a young agar culture, using an inoculating needle. Spinal fluid may be used directly.
2. Mix well; then add a small loopful of India ink and immediately cover with a thin coverglass, allowing the fluid to spread as a thin film beneath the coverglass.
3. Examine immediately under the oil immersion objective, reducing the light considerably by lowering the condenser. Capsules, when present, stand out as *clear halos* against a dark background.

MUIR METHOD

Muir Mordant

Tannic acid, 20% aqueous solution	2 parts
Saturated aqueous solution of mercuric chloride	2 parts
Saturated aqueous solution of potassium alum	5 parts

1. Prepare a thin even film of bacteria; allow to dry in air.
2. Cover the film with a piece of filter paper the size of the smear, and flood the slide with Ziehl-Neelsen carbolfuchsin.
3. Heat to steaming with a low Bunsen flame for 30 s.

---

*Not all India inks are suitable. Pelikan India ink made by Gunther Wagner of Hanover, Germany, is recommended; add about 0.3% thimerasol (Sigma Chemical Co.) as a preservative.

4. Rinse gently with 95% ethanol and then with water.
5. Add the mordant for 15 to 30 s; wash well with water.
6. Decolorize with ethanol to a faint pink; wash with water.
7. Counterstain with 0.3% methylene blue for 30 s.
8. Air dry and examine under the oil immersion lens. The cells are stained red, and the capsules blue.

CARBOLFUCHSIN COUNTERSTAIN FOR *LEGIONELLA PNEUMOPHILA*

See also Gram Stains.

Solution A

Basic fuchsin	0.3 g
Ethyl alcohol	10 ml

Solution B

Phenol (melted crystals)	5 ml
Distilled water	95 ml

Prepare the counterstain by mixing solutions A and B together. Stain the smears according to the standard Gram stain. Counterstain with carbolfuchsin solution for 1 min. Examine the smears microscopically using an oil immersion objective (100 ×).

FLAGELLA STAINS

GRAY METHOD

(Gray. 1926. Bacteriol. 12:273.)

Mordant

Potassium alum, saturated aqueous solution	5 ml
Tannic acid, 20% aqueous solution	2 ml
Mercuric chloride, saturated aqueous solution	2 ml

Mix and add 0.4 ml of a saturated alcoholic solution of basic fuchsin. Make up fresh mordant for use each day.

1. Using a grease-free, well-cleaned slide that has been flamed and cooled, spread a drop of distilled water on the slide to cover an area of approximately 2 cm².
2. Select part of a colony from a younger agar culture or take a small amount of growth from a slant with an inoculating needle and *touch gently* into the drop of water at several places on the slide; then gently rotate the slide.
3. Allow to air dry. *Do not heat or blot*.

4. Add the mordant, and allow it to act for 10 min.
5. Wash gently with distilled water or clean tap water.
6. Add Ziehl-Neelsen carbolfuchsin, and leave it on for 5 to 10 min.
7. Wash with tap water, air dry, and examine under oil.

SILVER STAIN FOR FLAGELLA

Solution A (Mordant or Prestain)

Saturated aqueous solution of aluminum potassium sulfate (approximately 14 g/100 ml of water; maintain as stock)	25 ml
Tannic acid, 10%	50 ml
Ferric chloride solution, 5% (maintain as stock)	5 ml

Combine and store in dark bottle at room temperature. The solution will remain stable for several months.

Solution B (Silver Stain)

1. Prepare 100 ml of 5% silver nitrate solution.
2. Add concentrated ammonium hydroxide (2 to 5 ml) dropwise to 90 ml of the 5% silver nitrate solution until the brown precipitate formed just redissolves.
3. Add some of the remaining 5% silver nitrate dropwise to the solution until a faint cloudiness persists.
4. Store the solution in a dark bottle at room temperature. The solution will remain stable for several months.

Staining Procedure

1. Label and flame commercially cleaned slides to burn off any residue. While the slides are hot, a heavy line may be drawn with wax pencil to reduce the amount of stain needed (optional).
2. Using growth from 18 to 24-h cultures on heart infusion or trypticase soy agar slants incubated at 35° C, prepare a light suspension of organisms in 3 ml of sterile distilled water. (NOTE: Do not use any fluid for suspension other than distilled water or nutrient broth.) Suspension should be only slightly cloudy and less than 0.5 McFarland standard.
3. Place one large loopful of culture suspension on the flamed slide, and allow it to run to the end. Allow to air dry. Do not fix.
4. Place the slide on staining rack, and flood with

solution A. Leave it for 4 min, and then rinse with distilled water.

5. Flood the slide with solution B, and heat just until steam is emitted by running a burner under the slide on a rack. Remove the burner, allow the slide to stain 4 min, rinse with distilled water, and slant to dry.

DIRECT FLUORESCENT ANTIBODY STAINS FOR *BORDETELLA PERTUSSIS* AND *LEGIONELLA*

See Chapters 29 and 39.

GIEMSA STAINS

GIEMSA STAIN FOR CHLAMYDIAE

(Schachter. 1980. In Lennette et al., editors: Manual of clinical microbiology, ed. 3. American Society for Microbiology, Washington, D.C.)

Giemsa stain is prepared by dissolving 0.5 g of powder in 33 ml of glycerol at 55° to 60° C for 1½ to 2 h. To this is added 33 ml of absolute methanol, acetone free. The solution is mixed thoroughly and allowed to sediment and then is stored at room temperature as stock. Dilutions of the stock stain are made with neutral distilled water or buffered water in a ratio of 1 part of stock Giemsa solution to 40 or 50 parts of diluent.

The smear is air dried, fixed with absolute methanol for at least 5 min, and again dried. It is then covered with the diluted Giemsa stain (freshly prepared each day) for 1 h. The slide is then rinsed rapidly in 95% ethanol to remove excess dye, dried, and examined for the presence of the typical basophilic intracytoplasmic inclusion body.

GIEMSA STAIN FOR MALARIA

Giemsa stain is available commercially as a concentrated stock solution or as a powder for those who wish to make their own stain; there seems to be very little difference between the two preparations.

NOTE: Remember that automatic differential instruments used in hematology are not designed to recognize intracellular (red blood cell) parasites. Any suspected parasitic infection or presumptive diagnosis of fever of unknown origin (FUO) mandates a manual blood smear examination.

Stock Giemsa Stain

Giemsa stain powder, certified	600 mg
Methanol, absolute and certified neutral, acetone free	50 ml
Glycerine, neutral, certified	50 ml

Grind well small portions of stain and glycerine in mortar and collect mixtures in a 500- or 1,000-ml flask until all measured material is mixed. Stopper flask with cotton plug, cover with heavy paper, place in 55° to 60° C water bath for 2 h, making sure that the water reaches the level of the stain. Shake gently at 30-min intervals. Allow to cool; add alcohol.

Use a portion of the measured alcohol to wash out the mortar and add to the flask. Store in brown bottle. Allow to stand for 2 to 3 weeks. Filter before use.

10% Stock Solution of Triton X-100

Triton X-100	10 ml
Distilled water	100 ml

Stock Buffers

1. Disodium phosphate buffer:

Na$_2$HPO$_4$ anhydrous	9.5 g
Distilled water	1,000 ml

2. Sodium acid phosphate buffer:

NaH$_2$PO$_4$ · H$_2$O	9.2 g
Distilled water	1,000 ml

Buffered Water: pH Range 7.0 to 7.2

Check with pH meter before use.

Disodium phosphate buffer	61 ml
Sodium acid phosphate buffer	39 ml
Distilled water	900 ml

Triton–Buffered Water Solutions

1. 0.01% Triton buffered water

Stock 10% aqueous Triton X-100	1 ml
Buffered water	1,000 ml

   Use for thin blood films or combination of thin and thick blood films.

2. 0.1% Triton buffered water

Stock 10% Triton X-100	10 ml
Buffered water	1,000 ml

   Use for thick blood films.

GIMÉNEZ STAIN FOR CHLAMYDIAE AND RICKETTSIAE

(Hendrickson. 1985. Reagents and stains. In Lennette et al., editors: Manual of clinical microbiology, ed. 4. American Society for Microbiology, Washington, D.C.; and Giménez. 1984. ASM News 50:292.)

1. Prepare stock carbolfuchsin as follows:

Basic fuchsin (total dye content >94%)	10 g
95% ethanol	100 ml
4% aqueous phenol	250 ml
Distilled water	650 ml

Hold this solution at 37° C for at least 48 h before using.

2. Prepare 0.2 M phosphate buffers as follows:
   a. NaH$_2$PO$_4$ 2.84 g
      Distilled water   100 ml
   b. Na$_2$HPO$_4$ 2.76 g
      Distilled water   100 ml
3. Prepare 0.1 M working phosphate buffer solution (pH 7.45) as follows:
   0.2 M NaH$_2$PO$_4$ 3.5 ml
   0.2 M Na$_2$HPO$_4$ 15.5 ml
   Distilled water   19 ml
4. Prepare working buffered stain solution as follows:
   Stock carbolfuchsin stain   3 ml
   Working phosphate buffer   10.5 ml
   This working stain solution must be filtered immediately (Whatman No. 2 paper filters) and again before each use (see below). It is usable for approximately 3 days.
5. Prepare malachite green counterstain as follows:
   Malachite green oxalate   0.8 g
   Distilled water   100 ml
6. Air dry the smear and heat fix.
7. Drop working stain solution through a filter (Whatman no. 2) directly onto the slide. Allow to stand for 1 to 2 min.
8. Wash thoroughly with tap water.
9. Cover the smear with malachite green and allow to stand for 6 to 9 s; then wash with tap water.
10. Cover the smear a second time with malachite green for 6 to 9 s. Again wash thoroughly with tap water.
11. Examine slides under oil immersion (1000 ×) for characteristic red-staining organisms and a green background.

GRAM STAINS

Although the reagents given below have yielded the most reproducible results, the dilution of the safranin counterstain and the makeup of the decolorizer vary among users. The classic (and longest) method is given in Chapter 7. A rapid modification is presented below. Another counterstain is found under Carbolfuchsin Counterstain for *Legionella pneumophila*.

GRAM STAIN (HUCKER MODIFICATION)

Stock Crystal Violet

   Crystal violet (85% dye)   20 g
   Ethanol (95%)   100 ml

Stock Oxalate Solution

   Ammonium oxalate   1 g
   Distilled water   100 ml

Working Crystal Violet Solution

Dilute the stock crystal violet solution 1:10 with distilled water, and mix with 4 vol of stock oxalate solution. Store in a glass-stoppered bottle.

Gram Iodine Solution

   Iodine crystals   1 g
   Potassium iodide   2 g

Dissolve these completely in 5 ml of distilled water; then add:
   Distilled water   240 ml
   Sodium bicarbonate, 5% aqueous solution   60 ml

Mix well; store in an amber-glass bottle.

Decolorizer

   Ethanol (95%)   250 ml
   Acetone   250 ml

Mix; store in a glass-stoppered bottle.

Counterstain (Stock Safranin)

   Safranin O   2.5 g
   Ethanol (95%)   100 ml

Working Safranin Counterstain Solution

Dilute stock safranin 1:5 or 1:10 with distilled water; store in a glass-stoppered bottle.

The principles of the Gram stain are discussed in Chapter 7. The following procedure is for the *rapid method*:

1. Prepare a thin film of the material to be examined; dry and fix with methanol or heat.
2. Flood the slide with crystal violet stain, and allow it to remain on the slide for 10 s.
3. Pour off the stain, and wash off the remainder with the iodine solution.
4. Flood with iodine solution, and allow to mordant for 10 s.
5. Rinse off with running water. Shake off excess.
6. Decolorize with alcohol-acetone solution or 95% alcohol (an alcohol-acetone solution may prove to be too rapid) until no further color flows from the slide. This usually takes from 10 to 20 s, depending on the thickness of the smear. Care should be taken not to overdecolorize the film, since this may result in an incorrect reading of the stain.

7. Counterstain with safranin for 10 s; then wash off with water.
8. Blot between clean sheets of bibulous paper and examine under oil immersion.

BASIC FUCHSIN GRAM STAIN COUNTERSTAIN FOR PALE-STAINING BACTERIA

Basic fuchsin	0.5 g
Distilled water	500 ml

Mix thoroughly and filter through coarse paper before use. Use instead of safranin in the Gram stain. Organisms known to stain poorly (*Legionella, Bordetella*, etc.) may require as long as 3 min of the counterstain, whereas most gram-negative bacteria stain readily in 10 s. This counterstain works particularly well for staining anaerobic bacteria.

GROCOTT'S GOMORI METHENAMINE–SILVER NITRATE STAIN FOR ACTINOMYCETES AND FUNGI IN TISSUE SECTIONS

See also Chapter 44.

Solution A

Borax, 5%	8 ml
Distilled water	100 ml

Solution B

Silver nitrate, 10%	7 ml
Methenamine, 3%	100 ml

Add equal parts of solutions A and B to make a working methenamine–silver nitrate solution. These solutions should be made up fresh.

Stock Light Green Solution

Light green SF (yellow)	0.2 g
Distilled water	100 ml
Glacial acetic acid	0.2 ml

Deparaffinize and bring to distilled water. Oxidize in 5% chromic acid for 1 h. Wash in running tap water for a few seconds. Rinse in 1% sodium bisulfite for 1 min to remove residual chromic acid. Wash in tap water for 5 to 10 min. Wash in three or four changes of distilled water. Place in working methenamine–silver nitrate solution in oven (58° to 60° C) for 30 to 60 min. When the section turns yellowish brown, use paraffin-coated forceps to remove the slide from the silver nitrate solution. Dip the slide in distilled water, and check with a microscope for adequate silver impregnation. Fungi should be dark brown at this stage. Rinse in six changes of distilled water. Tone in 0.1% gold chloride for 2 to 5 min. Rinse in distilled water. Remove the unreduced silver with 2% sodium thiosulfate for 2 to 5 min. Wash in tap water. Counterstain for 1 min with fresh 1:5 dilution in distilled water of stock light green solution. Dehydrate, clear, and mount.

IODINE SOLUTIONS FOR WET MOUNT PREPARATIONS

Iodine solutions are used to stain protozoan cysts in wet mounts. A weak rather than a strong iodine solution is best. The strong iodine tends to coagulate the fecal particles and to destroy the refractile nature of the organism.

Several iodine solutions can be used satisfactorily. These have been widely used and are simply prepared. The one recommended by Dobell and O'Connor is a weak iodine that should be prepared fresh about every 10 days for best results. Lugol iodine must be diluted about five times with distilled water, since the full-strength solution is too strong. Lugol iodine should be prepared fresh about every 3 weeks. Gram iodine used for bacteriologic work is not satisfactory for staining protozoan cysts. See Chapter 44 for further information.

DOBELL AND O'CONNOR IODINE SOLUTION

(Dobell and O'Connor. 1921. Intestinal protozoa of man. William Wood, New York.)

Iodine (powdered crystals)	1 g
Potassium iodide	2 g
Distilled water	100 ml

The KI is dissolved in the distilled water, and the iodine crystals are added slowly and shaken thoroughly. Filter or decant.

Lugol Iodine Solution

Iodine (powdered crystals)	5 g
Potassium iodide	10 g
Distilled water	100 ml

I is dissolved in the distilled water, and the iodine crystals are added slowly and shaken until dissolved. Filter, and place in tightly stoppered bottle. Dilute to 1:5 with distilled water for use in staining protozoan cysts.

Method. A small portion of feces is comminuted in a drop of the iodine solution, mounted with a coverslip, and sealed with a heated paraffin-petrolatum mixture.

In a correctly stained cyst the glycogen appears reddish-brown, the cytoplasm appears yellow, and the nuclei stand out as lighter refractile bodies. The location of karyosomes may be more easily determined, but the chromatid bodies are less visible than in saline solution. Since glycogen is a reserve food, it does not usually appear in older cysts.

MODIFIED D'ANTONI'S IODINE

(Markell, E.K., and Voge, M. 1981. Medical parasitology, ed. 5. W.B. Saunders Co., Philadelphia.)

Distilled water	100 ml
Potassium iodide (KI)	1 g
Powdered iodine crystals	1.5 g

The potassium iodide solution should be saturated with iodine, with some excess remaining in the bottle. Store in brown glass–stoppered bottles in the dark. The solution is ready for use immediately and should be decanted into a brown-glass dropping bottle; when the solution lightens, it should be discarded and replaced with fresh stock. The stock solution remains good as long as an excess of iodine remains on the bottom of the bottle. The iodine solutions eventually lighten in color and lose their staining strength; fresh solutions should be prepared every 2 to 3 weeks.

IRON-HEMATOXYLIN STAINS

STANDARD IRON-HEMATOXYLIN STAIN

Hematoxylin Solution

Hematoxylin	10 g
Absolute ethanol	1,000 ml

Keep the stain in a stoppered flask and allow to ripen in sunlight for at least a week.

Iron Solution

Ferrous ammonium sulfate	10 g
Ferric ammonium sulfate	10 g
HCl, concentrated	10 ml
Distilled water	1,000 ml

Working Solution

Mix equal parts of hematoxylin and iron solutions; this working solution will last for about 7 days.

1. Prepare fresh fecal smears or PVA-preserved smears as described in Chapter 44.
2. Place in 70% ethanol for 5 min.*
3. Place in 70% ethanol plus D'Antoni's iodine (solution should be dark reddish brown; formula above) for 2 to 5 min.

4. Place in 70% ethanol for 5 min.*
5. Wash in running tap water for 10 min.
6. Place in working solution of iron-hematoxylin staining solution for 4 to 5 min.
7. Wash in running tap water for 10 min.
8. Place in 70% ethanol for 5 min.*
9. Place in 95% ethanol for 5 min.
10. Place in two changes of 100% ethanol for 5 min each.*
11. Place in two changes of xylene or toluene for 5 min each.*
12. Mount in Permount or some other mounting medium; use a No. 1 thickness coverglass.

TOMPKINS AND MILLER IRON-HEMATOXYLIN STAIN

1. Prepare fresh fecal smears or PVA-preserved smears as described in Chapter 44.
2. Place in 70% ethanol plus D'Antoni's iodine (solution should be dark reddish brown; formula above) for 2 to 5 min.
3. Place in 50% ethanol for 3 min.
4. Wash in running tap water for 3 min.
5. Place in 4% ferric ammonium sulfate mordant for 5 min.
6. Wash in tap water for 1 min.
7. Place in 0.5% aqueous hematoxylin for 2 min.
8. Wash in tap water for 1 min.
9. Place in 2% aqueous phosphotungstic acid for 2 to 5 min.
10. Wash in running tap water for 10 min.
11. Place in 70% ethanol (plus a few drops of saturated aqueous lithium carbonate) for 3 min.
12. Place in 95% ethanol for 5 min.
13. Place in two changes of 100% ethanol for 5 min each.*
14. Place in xylene or toluene for 5 min.*
15. Mount in Permount or some other mounting medium; use a No. 1 thickness coverglass.

KOH STAIN

See Potassium Hydroxide.

LACTOPHENOL COTTON BLUE FOR FUNGI

Phenol crystals	20 g
Lactic acid	20 g
Glycerin	40 g
Distilled water	20 ml

---

*Slides can be held several hours or overnight.

*Slides can be held several hours or overnight.

Dissolve these ingredients by heating gently over a steam bath. Add 0.05 g of cotton blue dye (Poirier's blue). This may be used for yeasts as well as molds and serves as both a mounting fluid and a stain.

1. Place a drop of fluid on a clean slide.
2. Place a small amount of culture in this drop. If the culture is on agar, remove a piece of the medium with the embedded growth.
3. Cover with a coverglass, and press down gently to flatten.
4. Warm gently to remove air bubbles if necessary.
5. Examine under the microscope with high-dry or oil immersion objectives.
6. Ring edges of coverglass with nail polish if a permanent mount is required.

METACHROMATIC GRANULE STAINS FOR *CORYNEBACTERIUM* SPECIES

ALBERT STAIN (CHRISTENSEN MODIFICATION)

(Clark, editor. 1981. Staining procedures, ed. 4. Williams and Wilkins, Baltimore.)

The Albert stain is a differential stain and is recommended for its simplicity in staining *Corynebacterium diphtheriae*.

Toluidine Blue Stain Solution

Toluidine blue O	0.15 g
95% ethanol	2 ml
Glacial acetic acid	5 ml
Distilled water	100 ml

Dissolve the toluidine blue O in the ethanol and then add the distilled water. Add the glacial acetic acid as the final step.

1. Prepare a thin smear of the organism in distilled water, air dry, and heat fix.
2. Flood the slide with acidic toluidine blue and allow to stand for 1 min. Rinse in tap water.
3. Flood the slide with Gram's iodine and allow to stand for 1 min. Rinse in tap water.
4. Counterstain with Gram's safranin counterstain and allow to stand for 1 min. Rinse in tap water and blot dry.
5. Examine under oil immersion (1000 ×).

Granules appear blue-black; the bands appear blue to blue-green; and the cytoplasm appears green. The stain is excellent for demonstrating volutin granules in other bacteria as well.

METHYLENE BLUE STAIN (LOEFFLER'S)

Methylene blue	0.3 g
Ethyl alcohol (95%)	30 ml

When dissolved add:
Distilled water	100 ml

Loeffler methylene blue stain, as formerly used, was prepared by adding alkali to the foregoing solution. Current commercial preparations of methylene blue do not require the addition of alkali. The older preparations contained acid impurities.

This is a simple stain. Prepare a smear of the organism, and fix with heat. Flood smear with Loeffler methylene blue, and allow to react for 1 min. Wash and blot dry. The granules readily absorb the dye and appear deep blue. Overstaining lessens the contrast.

PERIODIC ACID–SCHIFF STAIN FOR OBSERVATION OF FUNGI IN DIRECT SMEARS

(Hendrickson. 1985. Reagents and stains. In Lennette et al., editors: Manual of clinical microbiology, ed. 4. American Society for Microbiology, Washington, D.C. p. 1105.)

The periodic acid step in this stain method hydrolyzes cell wall aldehydes, which are then able to combine with the modified Schiff reagent (the carbolfuchsin and the hydrosulfite solutions), coloring the cell wall carbohydrates red. Either zinc or sodium hydrosulfite may be used, and either picric acid or light green counterstain may be used in this method with good results. A control slide (a suspension of hyphal forms of yeast is adequate) should be run concurrently with each patient specimen.

1. Prepare basic fuchsin solution as follows:
Basic fuchsin	0.1 g
95% ethanol	5 ml
Distilled water	95 ml

   Mix together and store at room temperature in tightly capped Coplin jars.
2. Prepare zinc (or sodium) hydrosulfite solution as follows:
Zinc (or sodium) hydrosulfite	1.0 g
Tartaric acid	0.5 g
Distilled water	100 ml

   Mix together and store at room temperature in tightly capped Coplin jars.
3. Prepare saturated aqueous picric acid as follows: Place 100 ml of distilled water into a flask and stir continuously on a slightly warm hotplate stirrer. Add crystals of picric acid slowly until the

crystals no longer go into solution. Store tightly stoppered at room temperature.

4. Prepare light green counterstain as follows:

Light green	1 g
Glacial acetic acid	0.25 ml
80% ethanol	100 ml

   Mix together and store at room temperature.

5. Prepare the slides by spreading material thinly (respiratory secretions, body fluids, and other viscous specimens), air dry, and heat gently to fix. For skin scrapings and dry material, fix the material to the slide with a small amount of 10% albumin.

6. Flood the slide with 95% alcohol (or immerse in the alcohol in a Coplin jar) for 1 min.

7. Immerse the slide in a Coplin jar containing 5% periodic acid.

8. Immerse the slide in basic fuchsin for 2 min and rinse gently in tap water.

9. Counterstain with either the aqueous picric acid for 2 min or light green for 5 s. Rinse thoroughly in tap water.

10. Dehydrate in 95% ethanol for 10 s, followed by 100% ethanol for 1 min.

11. Clear through two quick changes in xylene and mount with Permount or other mounting medium while the slide is still wet with xylene.

12. Examine for the presence of fungal elements, which stain bright red or purplish against an orange (picric acid) or green (light green) background.

POTASSIUM HYDROXIDE (10% KOH) WET PREPARATION FOR DIRECT OBSERVATION OF FUNGI IN CLINICAL MATERIAL

See also Chapters 7 and 43.

1. Prepare 10% KOH as follows:

Potassium hydroxide	10 g
Glycerin	10 ml
Distilled water	80 ml

   Mix together and store at room temperature. Dispense into small dropper bottles for use.

2. Place the material to be stained on the slide and add a drop of 10% KOH. Equal amounts of 10% KOH and viscous material (sputum, etc.) should be mixed on the slide. A drop of lactophenol cotton blue or diluted India ink will enhance contrast.

3. Cover the material with a coverslip, and allow to remain at room temperature for approximately 10 min. Gentle heating may hasten the breakdown of protein and allow better visualization of fungal elements.

4. Examine under all objectives for hyphal elements, budding cells, spherules, and other fungal morphologies. Reducing the light passing through the condensor or using phase microscopy may be helpful.

PPLO (MYCOPLASMA) STAIN

(Dienes and Weinberger. 1951. Bacteriol. Rev. 15:245.)

Methylene blue	2.5 g
Azure II	1.25 g
Maltose	10 g
Sodium carbonate	0.25 g
Distilled water	100 ml

Dissolve the ingredients in the water.

1. Spread a drop of stain on a grease-free coverglass, and allow it to dry.

2. With a sterile scalpel, cut out a small block of agar medium containing a few *Mycoplasma* colonies and place, with colonies up, on a clean glass slide.

3. Lay coverglass, stain side down, carefully on the agar block, without rubbing.

4. Seal the preparation with a mixture of 3 parts petrolatum and 1 part paraffin to prevent drying.

5. Examine under low-power objective.

   Mycoplasma colonies are quite distinct with dense blue centers and light blue peripheries.

RHODAMINE-AURAMINE FLUOROCHROME STAIN FOR ACID-FAST CELLS

See also Chapter 41.

RHODAMINE-AURAMINE FLUOROCHROME STAIN (TRUANT METHOD)

(Truant, Brett, and Thomas. 1962. Henry Ford Hosp. Med. Bull. 10:287.)

By staining a smear with fluorescent dyes, such as auramine and rhodamine, and examining by fluorescence microscopy using an ultraviolet light source, acid-fast bacilli, when present, appear to glow with a yellow-orange color. They are visible under lower magnifications of the microscope; thus, a stained smear can be examined in much less time than is required by conventional methods. Numerous modifications of the procedure have been introduced; that reported by Truant and co-workers is recommended.

Auramine O*	1.5 g
Rhodamine B†	0.75 g
Glycerol	75 ml
Phenol	10 ml
Distilled water	50 ml

Combine the solutions, mix well (using a magnetic stirring device for 24 h or heating until warm and stirring vigorously for 5 min), filter through glass-wool, and store in a glass-stoppered bottle at 4° C. The stain is stable for several months under refrigeration.

1. Heat fix on a slide warmer‡ at 65° C for 2 h or overnight.
2. Cover the smear with the rhodamine-auramine solution.
3. Stain for 15 min at room temperature or at 35° C.
4. Rinse off with distilled water.
5. Decolorize with 0.5% hydrochloric acid in 70% ethanol for 2 to 3 min; then rinse thoroughly with distilled water.
6. Flood the smear with counterstain, a 0.5% solution of potassium permanganate (filter and store in amber bottle), for 2 to 4 min (no longer—excessive exposure results in loss of brilliance).
7. Rinse with distilled water, dry, and examine.

Ultraviolet light source. The smears are examined under a binocular microscope using an ultraviolet light source. The Leitz, Zeiss, and Reichert fluorescent microscopy units are highly recommended and are equipped with Osram HBO 200 maximum pressure mercury vapor lamps as light sources, BG 12 (3 or 4 mm) or C 5113 (2 mm) violet exciter filters, and OG 1 deep yellow barrier filters in the eyepieces. This recommended filter combination results in *bright yellow-orange* staining bacilli against a dark background; nonspecific background debris fluoresces a pale yellow, quite distinct from the yellow-orange bacilli.

It is suggested that a drop of immersion oil be placed on the darkfield condenser, the slide inserted, and the microscope first focused under bright light until a clear central area is seen on the slide. The microscope should then be switched over to the ul-traviolet source. Smears may be rapidly examined under low- or high-power objective (25 or 40 ×) with a 10 × eyepiece; after a little practice, all smears may be examined at these magnifications or lower in a matter of seconds. Occasionally, it may be necessary to switch to the oil immersion objective to confirm typical morphologic characteristics, such as beading and cording. It is recommended that microscopic examination be carried out in a darkened room for maximum efficiency.

Quartz-halogen illuminator

(Runyon et al. 1980. In Lennette et al., editors: Manual of clinical microbiology, ed. 3. American Society for Microbiology, Washington, D.C.)

Excellent demonstration of fluorochrome-stained mycobacteria is obtained by use of a microscope equipped with a quartz-halogen illuminator and the proper combinations of primary (exciter) and secondary (barrier) filters. This system provides the same benefits as an ultraviolet apparatus with the added advantages that the *blue light apparatus* does not require a special dark room (though subdued lighting is recommended), does not require oil on the condenser or slide, is simpler and more economical, and does not present radiation hazards. The following recommendations based on use of the Zeiss RA 38 microscope and attachments are applicable to other equipment having comparable features.

The equipment needed is a standard binocular microscope with an illuminator containing a collector lens and a 12 V, 100 W quartz-halogen lamp or high-intensity tungsten bulb, front-surface reflecting mirrors, brightfield condenser, low-power objectives (10 or 25 ×) for scanning, and high-dry (63 ×) plan-achromat (flat field; if the high-dry objective is corrected for coverslip, then a coverslip must be placed, not mounted, over the smear), a 100 × oil immersion objective for more critical examination of acid-fast (fluorescent) bodies, and 10 × compensating eyepieces. A turret or intermediate tube with holders for secondary filters located in the tube body between the objectives and the eyepieces facilitates filter changing. The optics and light path must be precisely aligned to avoid loss of light intensity. The light source is adjusted for Köhler illumination by centering and focusing the lamp filament on the closed iris diaphragm of the condenser. Maximal intensity is obtained by making small adjustments of

---

*Chroma 1B339, Chroma Gesellschaft, Schmid GmbH, available from Roboz Surgical Instrument Co., Washington, D.C.
†Matheson, Coleman, and Bell. CI 45170. Norwood, Ohio.
‡Microslide staining and drying bath are available from Baxter/Scientific Products, Division of American Hospital Supply Corp., McGaw Park, Ill.

the condenser while viewing an auramine-stained mycobacterial smear.

Combinations of primary and secondary filters are selected to provide good contrast between a dark background and the fluorescing yellow bacillus. However, the background must be sufficiently light that nonfluorescing debris can be seen for maintaining focus while scanning the slide. A BG 12 primary filter transmitting only wavelengths less than about 500 nm (peak 404 nm) in combination with secondary filters that transmit only wavelengths above 500 or 530 nm, as Zeiss No. 50 or 53, respectively, provides satisfactory demonstration of fluorescing mycobacteria. The particular combination of complementary exciter and barrier filters determines the color of the background. The greater the overlap of transmission curves, the lighter the background, and vice versa. Therefore, the user should have on hand BG 12 filters of various thicknesses (1, 1.5, 2, and 3 mm; Fish-Schurman Corp.) for neutral density purposes and secondary filters having transmission cutoffs at 500, 515, and 530 nm to determine which combinations provide optimal background-contrast qualities. The following exciter and barrier filter combinations have been found to be excellent for demonstrating fluorochrome-stained mycobacteria: 3-mm BG 12 and No. 50, light green background; 4-mm BG 12 and No. 50, dark green; 3-mm BG 12 and No. 53, light brown; 3.5-mm BG 12 and No. 53, dark brown. Another primary filter, the fluorescein isothiocyanate (FITC) interference filter, used in combination with a 3-mm BG 12 and a No. 50 or 53 barrier filter, results in excellent dark green and dark red-brown backgrounds, respectively. The FITC laminated to a BG 38 (to reduce red transmission) and in combination with a 1.5-mm BG 12 produces a reddish-tinged gray background with the No. 50 and a red field with the No. 53.

RICKETTSIAL STAINS

CASTAÑEDA STAIN

Stain Solution A

Potassium phosphate (KH_2PO_4) (1% aqueous)	100 ml
Sodium phosphate ($Na_2HPO_4 \cdot 12H_2O$) (25% aqueous)	100 ml

Mix and add 1 ml of formalin.

Stain Solution B

Methyl alcohol	100 ml
Methylene blue	1 g

Working Stain Solution

Mix 20 ml of solution A with 0.15 ml of solution B and add 1 ml of formalin.

Solution C (Counterstain)

Safranin O (0.2% aqueous)	25 ml
Acetic acid (0.1%)	75 ml

1. Prepare a homogeneous film, and dry in air.
2. Cover film with stain (mixture of solutions A and B).
3. Drain off stain. Do not wash.
4. Counterstain with safranin O (solution C) for 1 to 4 s.
5. Wash with tap water. Blot dry.
6. Examine under oil immersion lens.

The rickettsiae stain blue, whereas the cellular elements stain red.

GIEMSA METHOD*

1. Prepare a homogeneous film on a clean glass slide. Air dry.
2. Flood with methyl alcohol for 1 min.
3. Drain off alcohol, and allow to dry.
4. Cover film with Giemsa stain (15 drops; see Giemsa Stain for Chlamydia), and allow to react for 1 min.
5. Add distilled water (30 drops), and continue staining for 5 min.
   Drain off.
6. Wash with distilled water.
7. Place slide on end, and allow to dry in air.
8. Examine under oil immersion lens. The rickettsiae stain a bluish-purple.

SILVER STAINS

See also Grocott's Gomori methenamine–silver nitrate stain for visualization of *Pneumocystis carinii* in respiratory specimens. These GMS stains also stain fungal elements very well. Fungal elements appear black or gray-to-black against a turquoise and gray background.

80° C METHENAMINE–SILVER NITRATE STAIN

(Modified by Lynne Garcia and the UCLA Parasitology Laboratory from Pintozzi, R. 1978. J. Clin. Pathol. 31:803.)

1. Prepare reagents as follows:

Chromic acid (10% solution)	
Chromic acid (Fisher Scientific)	100 g

---

*This stain may also be used for spirochetes, which stain blue.

Distilled deionized water   1,000 ml

Weigh out 100 g chromic acid and dissolve in 1 L distilled water. Solution usable for up to 1 year.

Methenamine (3% solution)

| Hexamethylenetetramine (Fisher Scientific) | 12 g |
| Distilled deionized water | 400 ml |

Weigh out 12 g hexamethylenetetramine and dissolve in 400 ml distilled water. Solution usable for up to 6 months.

Silver nitrate (5% solution)

| Silver nitrate (Fisher Scientific) | 5 g |
| Distilled deionized water | 100 ml |

Weigh out 5 g silver nitrate and dissolve in 100 ml distilled water. Solution is usable for up to 6 months.

Stock methenamine–silver nitrate

| Methenamine (3% solution) | 400 ml |
| Silver nitrate (5% solution) | 20 ml |

A white precipitate forms when reagents are added together but immediately clears with mixing. Store at 4° C. The solution is usable for up to 1 month.

Borax (5% solution)

| Borax (sodium borate; Fisher Scientific) | 5 g |
| Distilled deionized water | 100 ml |

Dissolve sodium borate in distilled water. Solution usable for up to 1 year.

Sodium bisulfite (1% solution)

| Sodium bisulfite (Fisher Scientific) | 5 g |
| Distilled deionized water | 500 ml |

Weigh out sodium bisulfite and add to distilled water. Solution usable for up to 1 year.

Gold chloride (0.2% solution)

| Gold chloride (chloroauric acid; Sigma Chemical Co.) | 0.5 g |
| Distilled deionized water | 250 ml |

Weigh out gold chloride and add to distilled water. Solution usable for up to 1 year.

Sodium thiosulfate (2% solution)

| Sodium thiosulfate (Fisher Scientific) | 10 g |
| Distilled deionized water | 500 ml |

Solution usable for up to 1 year.

Stock light green solution

Light green SF-Yellowish (Harleco)	0.2 g
Distilled deionized water	100 ml
Glacial acetic acid	0.2 ml

Solution usable for up to 1 year.

Working light green solution

| Stock light green solution | 10 ml |
| Distilled deionized water | 40 ml |

Solution usable for up to 1 month.

2. Fill two Coplin jars each with absolute ethanol and 95% ethanol. These jars may be sealed with screw caps, and the reagents can be reused until they become cloudy.
3. Fill two Coplin jars with xylene. These jars may be sealed, and the xylene can be reused.
4. Immediately before each staining procedure, prepare working methenamine–silver nitrate as follows:

Stock methenamine–silver nitrate	37.5 ml
Distilled deionized water	37.5 ml
Borax (5% solution)	3 ml

This solution must be prepared fresh in a Coplin jar for each set of slides stained. It is not reusable, even for a second staining procedure performed immediately afterward.

5. Staining procedure
   a. Turn on water bath, allowing 45 to 60 min to reach 80° C.
   b. Prepare smears and air dry. Heat fix all smears at 70°C for 10 min on a heating block.
   c. Fix smears in absolute methanol for a minimum of 3 min.
   d. Place two Coplin jars, one containing 5% chromic acid (approximately 50 ml) and the other containing working methenamine solution into 80° C water bath for 5 min.
   e. Place smears into heated 5% chromic acid. Incubate in water bath at 80° C for 2 min.
   f. Remove slides from chromic acid and place in Coplin jar with distilled water. Rinse slides in three changes of distilled water.
   g. Place slides in 1% sodium bisulfite for 30 s.
   h. Rinse in three changes of distilled water.
   i. Place slides in heated methenamine working solution. Incubate in water bath at 80° C for 4½ min.
   j. Place slides in Coplin jar with distilled water. Rinse in three changes of distilled water.
   k. Wipe the back of slides with a paper towel to remove excess methenamine.

l. Tone in 0.2% gold chloride for 30 s; background lightens in this step.
m. Rinse in three changes distilled water.
n. Place slides in 2% sodium thiosulfate for 30 s to remove unreduced silver.
o. Rinse in three changes of distilled water.
p. Counterstain in light green working solution for 30 s.
q. Rinse in three changes of distilled water.
r. Dehydrate and clear for 30-s intervals in two changes each of 95% ethanol, 100% ethanol, and xylene, respectively.
s. Place coverslips on slides with Permount while the slides are still wet with xylene. Slides are ready to be read.
6. Interpretation: Background will be green, and *Pneumocystis* cysts will appear gray to black. They are spherical, may be punched in and cup shaped, and may show black parentheses-like structures in the center (See Figure 44.10). The cysts tend to occur in groups, often surrounded by foamy-looking green exudative background material.

WARTHIN-STARRY SILVER STAIN

The Warthin-Starry silver stain for visualization of the agent of cat-scratch disease is described in Chapter 40.

SPORE STAINS

DORNER METHOD

1. Make a heavy suspension of organisms in distilled water in a test tube, and add an equal volume of freshly filtered carbolfuchsin (Kinyoun; see Acid-fast Stains).
2. Place tube in boiling water bath for 5 to 10 min.
3. Mix a loopful of the aforementioned combination with a loopful of boiled and filtered 10% aqueous solution of nigrosin on a clean slide.
4. Spread out and dry film quickly with gentle heat.
5. Examine under oil. The spores stain red, and the bacterial cells are almost colorless against a dark gray background.

A modification of the Dorner method may be employed whereby a smear of the culture is prepared and fixed. The smear is then covered with a strip of filter paper to which carbolfuchsin is added. The dye is heated to steaming for 5 to 7 min with a Bunsen burner, and the filter paper is removed. Wash with water, blot dry, and cover with a thin film of nigrosin using a second slide or a needle. The appearance of the cells is as previously described.

WIRTZ-CONKLIN METHOD

(Paik. 1980. In Lennette et al., editors: Manual of clinical microbiology, ed. 3. American Society for Microbiology, Washington, D.C.)

Flood the entire slide with 5% aqueous malachite green. Steam for 3 to 6 min, and rinse under running tap water. Counterstain with 0.5% aqueous safranin for 30 s. Spores are seen as green spherules in red-stained rods or with red-stained debris.

SUDAN BLACK B FAT STAIN FOR *BACILLUS* SP. AND OTHER BACTERIA

(Burdon. 1946. J. Bacteriol. 52:665.)

Sudan black B	0.3 g
Ethanol, 70%	100 ml

Mix together and shake the solution thoroughly at intervals during the day, and allow it to stand overnight before use. Dry and fix the smear with heat. Stain the slide with Sudan black for 10 min, drain, and blot dry. Wash and clear the smear with xylene. Counterstain with a 0.5% aqueous solution of safranin for 10 to 15 s. Wash in tap water; blot dry. The cells stain red; the highly refractile poly-β-hydroxybutyrate granules are blue-black. For *Legionella pneumophila*, counterstain for 1 min.

TOLUIDINE BLUE-O STAIN FOR DETECTION OF *PNEUMOCYSTIS* IN RESPIRATORY SECRETIONS

See Chapter 44.

TRICHROME STAIN FOR INTESTINAL PROTOZOA

See Chapter 44.

WARTHIN-STARRY STAIN

See Chapter 40.

WAYSON STAIN

Dissolve 0.2 g of basic fuchsin and 0.75 g of methylene blue in 20 ml of absolute ethanol. Add the dye solution to 200 ml of a 5% solution of phenol in distilled water. Filter. Stain smears for a few seconds. Wash, blot, and dry. This stain is useful in detecting polar staining morphology.

WRIGHT STAINS

These stains are used for demonstrating parasites in blood and occasionally in tissue. Because of its superior staining characteristics, the Giemsa stain is used more frequently. The following stain yields sharper results than the classic Wright formula does. Because of differences in lots of Wright stain, control slides should be stained with the reagents to ensure suitable results.

Wright Stain (Lille's Modification)

(Clark, editor. 1981. Staining procedures, ed. 4. Williams and Wilkins, Baltimore.)

1. Prepare stock Wright stain as follows:

Wright stain powder*	1 g
(available commercially)	
Glycerol	50 ml
Methanol (100%)	50 ml

   Mix the alcohol and glycerol together before adding the stain powder. Store at room temperature.

2. Prepare working solution immediately before use as follows:

Stock stain solution	4 ml
Acetone	3 ml
Phosphate buffer (1/15 M, pH 6.5)	2 ml
Distilled water	31 ml

   Mix together in a Coplin jar. The solution may be used for two staining procedures if they are performed one after the other.

3. Prepare blood or tissue films by spreading ma-

---

*Biological Stain Commission certified.

terial thinly over slide using a second slide. Fix immediately in absolute methanol for 2 to 3 min.

4. Allow the fixed slides to air dry.
5. Immerse the slides in a Coplin jar containing the working solution for 5 min.
6. Wash gently in distilled water and air dry.
7. Examine for parasitic forms under several different magnifications. Structures appear blue, purplish, and red.

Wright-Giemsa Method for Staining Conjunctival Scrapings

The Wright-Giemsa stain, along with a Gram stain of the scrapings, gives immediate information to the ophthalmologist regarding conjunctivitis of bacterial origin, inclusion body conjunctivitis and trachoma, or eosinophilia of allergic conjunctivitis.

1. Two slide preparations of scrapings are made; one is stained by the Gram method and one by the Wright-Giemsa technique.
2. To carry out staining by the Wright-Giemsa technique, apply Wright stain to the slide for 1 min. Add an equal volume of neutral distilled water (pH 7.0), and stain for 4 min.
3. Shake off stain; then apply dilute Giemsa stain (1 drop to 1 ml of neutral distilled water), and allow to stain for 15 min.
4. Shake off, decolorize lightly with ethanol, and air dry (do not blot).

Appendix C Selected Product Suppliers for Clinical Microbiology

Although we have attempted to list many major sources of products, not all manufacturers or suppliers are listed here. Regional supply houses and other sources should be considered.

ANAEROBIC BACTERIAL PRODUCTS

Anaerobe Systems, Inc.
2200 Zanker Rd., Suite C
San Jose, CA 95131

Bartels Immunodiagnostics
12729 North East 20th St.
Bellevue, WA 98005

Becton-Dickinson Microbiology Systems
P.O. Box 243
Cockeysville, MD 21030

Bellco Glass, Inc.
340 Edrudo Rd.
Vineland, NJ 08360

Carr-Scarborough Microbiologicals, Inc.
P.O. Box 1328
Stone Mountain, GA 30086

Difco Laboratories, Inc.
P.O. Box 1058
Detroit, MI 48232

H. B. Company (Rosco disks)
4141 Ball Rd., Suite 217
Cypress, CA 90630

Kontes (Kimble div. of Owens-Illinois)
1022 Spruce St.
Vineland, NJ 08360

Oxoid U.S.A., Inc.
9107 Red Branch Rd.
Columbia, MD 21045

Scott Laboratories, Inc.
771 Main St.
Fiskeville, RI 02823

ANTIBIOTICS

See Chapter 13.

ANTIBODY DETECTION SYSTEMS

Abbott Laboratories
Abbott Park 6C4, Dept. 49B
Abbott Park, IL 60064

American Dade
P.O. Box 520672
Miami, FL 33152

Analytab Products
200 Express St.
Plainview, NY 11803

Behring Diagnostics
10933 N. Torrey Pines Rd.
La Jolla, CA 92037

Bio-Diagnostic Systems, Inc.
1 Wall St., Research Park
Princeton, NJ 08540

Calbiochem-Behring Corp.
10933 N. Torrey Pines Rd.
La Jolla, CA 92037

Cetus Corp.
1400 53rd St.
Emeryville, CA 94608

Clinical Sciences Inc.
30 Troy Rd.
Whippany, NJ 07981

Cooper Biomedical, Inc.
One Technology Court
Malvern, PA 19355

Cordis Laboratories, Inc.
2140 North Miami Ave.
Miami, FL 33127

DuPont Co.
Barley Mill Plaza
Wilmington, DE 19898

Electro-Nucleonics, Inc.
7101 Riverwood Dr.
Columbia, MD 21046

Flow Laboratories, Inc.
7655 Old Springhouse Rd.
McLean, VA 22102

Gull Laboratories
890 East 5400 South
Salt Lake City, UT 84107

ICL Scientific (Hybridoma Sciences, Inc.)
18249 Euclid St.
Fountain Valley, CA 92708

Immuno-Mycologics, Inc.
P.O. Box 1151
Norman, OK 73070

International Diagnostic Technology, Inc.
2050 Concourse Dr.
San Jose, CA 95131-1701

Kallestad Laboratories Inc.
2000 InterFirst Tower
Austin, TX 78701

Labsystems
P.O. Box 48723
Chicago, IL 60648

MarDx Diagnostics, Inc.
847 Jerusalem Rd.
Scotch Plains, NJ 07076

MeDiCa
Camino Vida Roble, Suite 1
Carlsbad, CA 92009

Meridian Diagnostics
3471 River Hills Dr., P.O. Box 44216
Cincinnati, OH 45244

Organon Teknika
100 Akzo Ave.
Durham, NC 27704

Ortho Diagnostic Systems
Route 202
Raritan, NJ 08869

Sclavo Inc.
5 Mansard Court
Wayne, NJ 07470

Syva Co.
900 Arastradero Rd.
Palo Alto, CA 94303

Wampole Laboratories
Half Acre Rd., P.O. Box 1001
Cranbury, NJ 08512-0181

Whittaker M.A. Bioproducts
P.O. Box 127, Biggs Ford Rd.
Walkersville, MD 21793

Zeus Scientific, Inc.
St. John and Elizabeth Streets
Raritan, NJ 08869

ANTIBODY SEPARATION SYSTEMS

Gull Laboratories
890 East 5400 South
Salt Lake City, UT 84107

Isolab, Inc.
Drawer 4350
Akron, Ohio 44321

Whittaker M.A. Bioproducts
P.O. Box 127, Biggs Ford Rd.
Walkersville, MD 21793

ANTIGEN DETECTION SYSTEMS

Abbott Laboratories
Abbott Park 6C4, Dept. 49B
Abbott Park, IL 60064

Ames (div. of Miles Laboratories).
P.O. Box 70
Elkhart, IN 46515

Antibodies Incorporated
P.O. Box 1560
Davis, CA 95617

Becton-Dickinson Microbiology Systems
P.O. Box 243
Cockeysville, MD 21030

Binax, Inc.
95 Darling Ave.
South Portland, ME 04106

Burroughs-Wellcome Co.
(see Wellcome Diagnostics Division)

Difco Laboratories, Inc.
P.O. Box 1058
Detroit, MI 48232

Electro-Nucleonics, Inc.
7101 Riverwood Dr.
Columbia, MD 21046

Enzo Biochem, Inc.
325 Hudson St.
New York, NY 10013

E-Y Laboratories, Inc.
127 N. Amphlett Blvd.
San Mateo, CA 94401

Flow Laboratories, Inc.
7655 Old Springhouse Rd.
McLean, VA 22102

Genetic Systems
3005 First Ave.
Seattle, WA 98121

Gen-Probe, Inc.
9880 Campus Point Dr.
San Diego, CA 92121

Gene-Trak Systems
31 New York Ave.
Framingham, MA 01701

Hybritech, Inc.
11095 Torreyana Rd., P.O. Box 269006
San Diego, CA 92126

Immuno-Mycologics, Inc.
P.O. Box 1151
Norman, OK 73070

Meridian Diagnostics
3471 River Hills Dr., P.O. Box 44216
Cincinnati, OH 45244

Microbiological Associates
(see Whittaker M.A. Bioproducts)

Micro-Media Systems
6200 El Camino Real
Carlsbad, CA 92008

Molecular Biosytems, Inc.
10030 Barnes Canyon Rd.
San Diego, CA 92121

Orion Research, Inc.
(Medical Technology Corp.)
71 Veronica Ave.
Somerset, NJ 08873

Ortho Diagnostic Systems
Route 202
Raritan, NJ 08869

Ramco Laboratories, Inc.
3801 Kirby Dr., Suite 170
Houston, TX 77098

Syva Co.
900 Arastradero Rd.
Palo Alto, CA 94303

Ventrex Laboratories, Inc.
217 Read St.
Portland, ME 04103

Wampole Laboratories
Half Acre Rd., P.O. Box 1001
Cranbury, NJ 08512

Wellcome Diagnostics Division
3030 Cornwallis Rd.
Research Triangle Park, NC 27709

Whittaker M.A. Bioproducts
P.O. Box 127, Biggs Ford Rd.
Walkersville, MD 21793

Zeus Scientific, Inc.
St. John and Elizabeth Streets
Raritan, NJ 08869

ANTISERA

Becton-Dickinson Microbiology Systems
P.O. Box 243
Cockeysville, MD 21030

Burroughs-Wellcome Co.
(see Wellcome Diagnostics Division)

Cooper Animal Health, Inc.
P.O. Box 27-406
Kansas City, MO 64180-0001

Dan-Serum Inc. (div. of Statens Seruminstitut)
2920 Wolff St.
Racine, WI 53404

Difco Laboratories, Inc.
P.O. Box 1058
Detroit, MI 48232

Fisher Scientific Co.
711 Forbes Ave.
Pittsburgh, PA 15219

Flow Laboratories, Inc.
7655 Old Springhouse Road
McLean, VA 22102

Hazleton Biologics, Inc.
P.O. Box 14848
Lenexa, KS 66215

Immuno-Mycologics, Inc.
P.O. Box 1151
Norman, OK 73070

Kallestad Laboratories Inc.
2000 InterFirst Tower
Austin, TX 78701

Meridian Diagnostics
3471 River Hills Dr., P.O. Box 44216
Cincinnati, OH 45244

Northeast Biomedical, Inc.
R.R. No. 1, Inland Farm Dr.
South Windham, ME 04082

Ortho Diagnostic Systems
Rte. 202
Raritan, NJ 08869

Roach Laboratories Inc.
Route 5, Donald Dr.
Loganville, GA 30249

Scott-Nolan Laboratories
4958 Hammermill Rd.
Tucker, GA 30084

Statens Seruminstitut (see also Dan-Serum Inc.)
Amager Blvd. 80
DK 2300 Copenhagen S
Denmark

Whittaker M.A. Bioproducts
P.O. Box 127, Biggs Ford Rd.
Walkersville, MD 21793

AUTOMATED MICROBIOLOGY SYSTEMS (DETECTION, IDENTIFICATION, SUSCEPTIBILITY, ETC.)

Abbott Laboratories, Analytical Systems
P.O. Box 152020
Irving, TX 75015

Analytab Products
200 Express St.
Plainview, NY 11803

Analytical Luminescence Laboratory
11760 Sorrento Valley Rd., #E
San Diego, CA 92121

Baxter Healthcare Corp., MicroScan Division
1584 Enterprise Blvd.
W. Sacramento, CA 95691

BBL Microbiology Systems
P.O. Box 243
Cockeysville, MD 21030

Biolog, Inc.
3447 Investment Blvd., Suite 3
Hayward, CA 94545

Difco Laboratories, Inc.
P.O. Box 1058
Detroit, MI 48232

Hewlett-Packard Co.
Route 41
Avondale, PA 19311

Johnston Laboratories
P.O. Box 20086
Towson, MD 21204

MCT Diagnostics
1997 Sloan Pl., Suite 26
St. Paul, MN 55117

Mesa Diagnostics, Inc.
3700 Osuna N.E., Suite 604
Albuquerque, NM 87109

Microbial ID, Inc.
115 Barksdale Professional Center
Newark, DE 19711

Micro-Media Systems
6200 El Camino Real
Carlsbad, CA 92008

Organon Teknika Corp.
100 Akzo Ave.
Durham, NC 27704

Shandon Inc.
171 Industry Dr.
Pittsburgh, PA 15275

Spiral System Instruments, Inc.
4853 Cordell Ave., Suite A-10
Bethesda, MD 20814

Turner Designs
920 West Maude Ave.
Sunnyvale, CA 94046

Vista Laboratories, Ltd.
8432 45th Street
Edmonton, Alberta, T6B 2N6 Canada

Vitek Systems, Inc.
595 Anglum Dr.
Hazelwood, MO 63042

BACTERIAL AND FUNGAL IDENTIFICATION REAGENTS

Abbott Laboratories Diagnostics Division
One Abbott Park Rd.
Abbott Park, IL 60064-3500

American MicroScan Div. of Baxter Healthcare, Inc.
1584 Enterprise Blvd.
W. Sacramento, CA 95691

Analytab Products
200 Express St.
Plainview, NY 11803

Austin Biological Laboratories, Inc.
6620 Manor Rd.
Austin, TX 78723

Becton-Dickinson Microbiology Systems
P.O. Box 243
Cockeysville, MD 21030

Binax
95 Darling Ave.
S. Portland, ME 04106

Bio-Spec, Inc.
179A Mason Circle
Concord, CA 94520-1213

California Integrated Diagnostics, Inc.
433 Industrial Way
Benicia, CA 94510

Cambridge BioScience Corp.
365 Plantation St.
Worcester, MA 001605

Carr-Scarborough Microbiologicals, Inc.
P.O. Box 1328
Stone Mountain, GA 30086

Diagnostic Technology, Inc.
240 Vanderbilt Motor Parkway
Hauppauge, NY 11788

Difco Laboratories, Inc.
P.O. Box 1058
Detroit, MI 48232

DuPont Co.
Barley Mill Plaza
Wilmington, DE 19898

E-Y Laboratories, Inc.
127 N. Amphlett Blvd.
San Mateo, CA 94401

H. B. Company (Rosco disks)
4141 Ball Rd., Suite 217
Cypress, CA 90630

ICL Scientific
11040 Condor Ave.
Fountain Valley, CA 92708

Integrated Diagnostics, Inc.
P.O. Box 24124
Baltimore, MD 21227

Immuno-Mycologics, Inc.
P.O. Box 1151
Norman, OK 73070

Key Scientific Co.
P.O. Box 66307
Los Angeles, CA 90066

Meridian Diagnostics
3471 River Hills Dr., P.O. Box 44216
Cincinnati, OH 45244

Micro-Bio-Logics
217 Osseo Ave. North
St. Cloud, MN 56301

Oxoid USA, Inc.
9017 Red Branch Rd.
Columbia, MD 24015

Pharmacia LKB Biotechnology, Inc.
800 Centennial Ave.
Piscataway, NJ 08854-9932

Remel
12076 Santa Fe Dr.
Lenexa, KS 66215

Roche Products, Ltd.
Welwyn Garden City
Hertfordshire, England

Scott Laboratories, Inc.
771 Main St.
Fiskeville, RI 02823

Serono-Baker Diagnostics
100 Cascade Dr.
Allentown, PA 18103

Stanbio Laboratories Inc.
2930 E. Houston St.
San Antonio, TX 78202

University Micro Reference Laboratory, Inc.
611(P) Hammonds Fery Rd.
Linthicum, MD 21090

Vitek Systems, Inc.
595 Anglum Dr.
Hazelwood, MO 63042

Wampole Laboratories
Half Acre Rd.
Cranbury, NJ 08512

Wellcome Diagnostics Division
3030 Cornwallis Rd.
Research Triangle Park, NC 27709

BACTERIAL AND FUNGAL IDENTIFICATION SYSTEMS, MULTICOMPONENT AND NONAUTOMATED

Analytab Products
200 Express St.
Plainview, NY 11803

Austin Biological Laboratories, Inc.
6620 Manor Rd.
Austin, TX 78723

Bartels Immunodiagnostics
12729 North East 20th St.
Bellevue, WA 98005

Baxter Healthcare, MicroScan Division
1584 Enterprise Blvd.
W. Sacramento, CA 95691

Becton-Dickinson Microbiology Systems
P.O. Box 243
Cockeysville, MD 21030

Biolog, Inc.
3447 Investment Blvd., Suite 3
Hayward, CA 94545

DuPont Co.
Barley Mill Plaza
Wilmington, DE 19898

Flow Laboratories, Inc.
7655 Old Springhouse Rd.
McLean, VA 22102

Innovative Diagnostic Systems, Inc.
3404 Oakcliff Rd., Suite C-1
Atlanta, GA 30340

Organon Teknika Corp.
100 Akzo Ave.
Durham, NC 27704

Roche Diagnostic Systems
340 Kingsland St.
Nutley, NJ 07110

Winfield Laboratories, Inc.
670 International Parkway
Suite 150, P.O. Box 2616
Richardson, TX 75080

BLOOD CULTURE SYSTEMS

BBL Microbiology Systems
P.O. Box 243
Cockeysville, MD 21030

Difco Laboratories, Inc.
P.O. Box 1058
Detroit, MI 48232

DuPont Co.
Barley Mill Plaza
Wilmington, DE 19898

Johnston Laboratories
P.O. Box 20086
Towson, MD 21204

Organon Teknika Corp.
100 Akzzo Ave.
Durham, NC 27704

Roche Diagnostic Systems
340 Kingsland St.
Nutley, NJ 07110

CHEMICALS

Aldrich Chemical Co.
P.O. Box 355
Milwaukee, WI 53201

Allied Chemical and Dye Co.
1411 Broadway
New York, NY 10018

American Can Co. (Parafilm Products)
American Lane 2A3
Greenwich, CT 06830

Baker Chemical Co.
(see J.T. Baker)

Behring Diagnostics Division,
American Hoechst Corp.
10933 N. Torrey Pines Rd.
La Jolla, CA 92037

Bio Spec, Inc.
6499 Sierra Ln.
Dublin, CA 94566

Boehringer Mannheim
9115 Hague Rd.
Indianapolis, IN 46250

Colab Laboratories, Inc.
3 Science Rd.
Glenwood, IL 60425

E. Merck Darmstadt
480 Democrat Rd.
Gibbstown, NJ 08027

Eastman Chemical Co.
343 State St.
Rochester, NY 14650

Fisher Scientific Co.
711 Forbes Ave.
Pittsburgh, PA 15219

Hazelton Research Products, Inc.
Box 7200
Denver, PA 17517

ICN Pharmaceuticals, Inc.
222 N. Vincent Ave.
Covina, CA 91722

J.T. Baker Chemical Co.
600 N. Broad St.
Phillipsburg, NJ 08825

Mallinckrodt, Inc.
675 McDonnell Blvd.
St. Louis, MO 63134

Marion Scientific Corp.
9233 Ward Parkway, Suite 350
Kansas City, MO 64114

Medical Chemical Corp.
P.O. Box 445
Santa Monica, CA 90404

Merck Chemical Co.
P.O. Box 2000
Rahway, NJ 07065

Meridian Diagnostics
P.O. Box 44216
3471 River Hills Dr.
Cincinnati, OH 45244

Polysciences, Inc.
400 Valley Rd.
Warrington, PA 18976

Sargent-Welch Scientific Co.
7300 N. Linder Ave., P.O. Box 1026
Skokie, IL 60077

Sigma Chemical Co.
3050 Spruce St.
St. Louis, MO 63103

Trend Scientific, Inc.
13895 Industrial Park Blvd., Suite 175
Minneapolis, MN 55441

Winthrop Laboratories
90 Park Ave.
New York, NY 10018

DISINFECTANTS

Alcide Corporation
125 Main St.
Westport, CT 06880

National Laboratories
225 Summit Ave.
Montvale, NJ 07645

Sporicidin Co.
4000 Massachusetts Ave. N.W.
Washington, D.C. 20016

Stanbio Laboratory, Inc.
2930 E. Houston St.
San Antonio, TX 78202

FILTERS

See Membrane Filters.

INOCULATING LOOPS

Elkay Products, Inc.
800 Boston Turnpike
Box 5247, Turnpike Station
Shrewsbury, MA 01545

Medical Wire & Equipment Co. (USA)
Hamilton Business Park Unit 9B, Franklin Rd.
Dover, NJ 07801

Micro-Bio-Logics
217 Osseo Ave. North
St. Cloud, MN 56303

Microdiagnostics
601 Stones Levee
Cleveland, OH 44113

Science Center Inc.
P.O. Box 994
Santa Fe, NM 87504-0994

INSTRUMENTS

ELISA INSTRUMENTS AND SUPPLIES

Abbott Laboratories, Diagnostics Division
One Abbott Park Rd.
Abbott Park, IL 60064-3500

Bio-Tek Instruments
Highland Park, Box 998
Winooski, VT 05404-0998

Cambridge Biotechnology, Inc.
23 Elm St.
Watertown, MA 02172

DiaMedix
2140 N. Miami Ave.
Miami, FL 33127

Dynatech Laboratories, Inc.
14340 Sullyfield Circle
Chantilly, VA 22021

Flow Laboratories
7655 Old Springhouse Rd.
McLean, VA 22102

Labsystems, Inc.
6200 West Oakton St.
Morton Grove, IL 60053

Skatron, Inc.
P.O. Box 530
Sterling, VA 22170

SLT Labinstruments Inc., USA
2110 Smithtown Ave., #3
Ronkonkoma, NY 11779

VWR Scientific, Inc.
P.O. Box 7900
San Francisco, CA 94120

Whittaker M.A. Bioproducts
P.O. Box 127
Biggs Ford Rd.
Walkersville, MD 21793

INSTRUMENTS (OTHER)

Bellco Glass, Inc.
340 Edrudo Rd.
Vineland, NJ 08360

Biotek Instruments
Highland Industrial Park
Winooski, VT 05404

Cetus Corp.
1400 53rd St.
Emeryville, CA 94608

Dynatech Laboratories, Inc.
900 Slaters Lane
Alexandria, VA 22314

New Brunswick Scientific Co., Inc.
44 Talmadge Rd., P.O. Box 986
Edison, NJ 08817

Spiral System Instruments, Inc.
4853 Cordell Ave., Suite A10
Bethesda, MD 20814

Tekmar Co.
P.O. Box 37202
Cincinnati, OH 45222

TOMTEC, Inc.
607 Harborview Rd.
Orange, CT 06477

Ultra-Violet Products, Inc.
5100 Walnut Grove
San Gabriel, CA 91778

Wescor, Inc.
459 South Main St.
Logan, UT 84321

MEDIA (PREPARED AND DRY)

BACTERIOLOGIC MEDIA

Anaerobe Systems
2200 Zanker Rd., Suite C
San Jose, CA 95131

BBL/Becton-Dickinson Microbiology Systems
P.O. Box 243
Cockeysville, MD 21030

Carr-Scarborough Microbiologicals, Inc.
P.O. Box 1328
Stone Mountain, GA 30086

Difco Laboratories, Inc.
P.O. Box 1058
Detroit, MI 48232

Edge Diagnostics
P.O. Box 1198
Memphis, TN 38111

Flow Laboratories, Inc.
7655 Old Springhouse Rd.
McLean, VA 22102

Gibco Laboratories
(Life Technologies, Inc.)
421 Merrimack St.
Lawrence, MA 01843

Hana Biologicals, Inc.
626 Bancroft Way
Berkeley, CA 94710

Hardy Media
205 W. Montecito St.
Santa Barbara, CA 93101

Micro-Bio-Logics
217 Osseo Ave. North
St. Cloud, MN 56301

Oxoid U.S.A., Inc.
9107 Red Branch Rd.
Columbia, MD 21045

Remel
12076 Santa Fe Dr.
Lenexa, KS 66215

Scott Laboratories, Inc.
771 Main St.
Fiskeville, RI 02823

VIRAL CULTURE MEDIA

Bartels Immunodiagnostics
12729 North East 20th St.
Bellevue, WA 98005

Difco Laboratories
P.O. Box 1058
Detroit, MI 48232

Earl-Clay Laboratories, Inc.
7075 Redwood Blvd.
Novato, CA 94947

Flow Laboratories, Inc.
7655 Old Springhouse Rd.
McLean, VA 22102

Genus Diagnostics
225 Wildwood
Woburn, MA 01801

Northeast Biomedical, Inc.
R.R. No. 1, Inland Farm Dr.
South Windham, ME 04082

Ortho Diagnostic Systems
Route 202
Raritan, NJ 08869

Viromed Laboratories, Inc.
5100 Gamble Dr., Suite 55
Minneapolis, MN 55416

Whittaker M.A. Bioproducts, Inc.
Biggs Ford Rd., Building 100
Walkersville, MD 21793

MEMBRANE FILTERS

Amicon Corporation
17 Cherry Hill Dr.
Danvers, MA 01923

Gelman Sciences, Inc.
600 South Wagner Rd.
Ann Arbor, MI 48106

Millipore Corporation
Ashby Road
Bedford, MA 01730

Nuclepore Corporation
7035 Commerce Circle
Pleasanton, CA 94566-3294

Sartorius Filters Inc.
30940 San Clemente, Bldg. D
Hayward, CA 94544

MICROORGANISMS (FOR QUALITY CONTROL)

American Type Culture Collection
12301 Parklawn Dr.
Rockville, MD 20852

Difco Laboratories, Inc.
P.O. Box 1058
Detroit, MI 48232

Micro-Bio-Logics
217 Osseo Ave. North
St. Cloud, MN 56301

Remel
12076 Santa Fe Dr.
Lenexa, KS 66215

Roche Diagnostic Systems
340 Kingsland St.
Nutley, NJ 07110

Scientific Device Laboratory, Inc.
508 Zenith Dr., P.O. Box 88
Glenview, IL 66025

Scott Laboratories, Inc.
771 Main St.
Fiskeville, RI 02823

Trend Scientific Inc.
P.O. Box 41203
Minneapolis, MN 55441

PARASITE CONCENTRATING DEVICES

Evergreen Scientific
2300 East 49th St.
Los Angeles, CA 90058

Trend Scientific Inc.
P.O. Box 41203
Minneapolis, MN 55441

PLASTICS

American Scientific Products
1430 Waukegan Rd.
McGaw Park, IL 60085

Becton-Dickinson & Co.
299 Webro Rd.
Parsippany, NJ 07054

Corning Glass Works: Science Products
P.O. Box 1150
Elmira, NY 14902-9944

Costar
205 Broadway
Cambridge, MA 02139

Dynalab Corporation
P.O. Box 112
Rochester, NY 14692

Falcon Plastics (Becton-Dickinson)
1950 Williams Dr.
Oxnard, CA 93030

Miles Scientific
2000 N. Aurora Rd.
Naperville, IL 60566

Nunc InterMed
Postbox 280, Kamstrup-DK
4000 Roskilde, Denmark
Distributed by:
Vangard International, Inc.
1111-A Green Grove Rd.
Neptune, NJ 07753

Scientific Device Laboratory, Inc.
508 Zenith Dr., P.O. Box 88
Glenview, IL 60025

SPECIMEN-TRANSPORT SYSTEMS AND SUPPLIES

Anaerobe Systems, Inc.
2200 Zanker Rd., Suite C
San Jose, CA 95131

Bartels Immunodiagnostics
12729 North East 20th St.
Bellevue, WA 98005

BBL/Becton Dickinson Microbiology Systems
P.O. Box 243
Cockeysville, MD 21030

Becton-Dickinson Vacutainer Systems
301 Route 17 North
Rutherford, NJ 07070

BioSpec Products, Inc.
P.O. Box 722
Bartlesville, OK 74005

Difco Laboratories, Inc.
P.O. Box 1058
Detroit, MI 48232

Electro-Nucleonics, Inc.
368 Passaic Ave.
Fairfield, NJ 07006

Evergreen Scientific
2300 East 49th St.
Los Angeles, CA 90058

Flow Laboratories, Inc.
7655 Old Springhouse Rd.
McLean, VA 22102

Hardy Media
205 W. Montecito St.
Santa Barbara, CA 93101

Masterseal Corporation
711 W. 17th St.—G6
Costa Mesa, CA 92627

Medical Chemical Corp., Medi-Chem, Inc.
1909 Centinela Ave., P.O. Box 445
Santa Monica, CA 90404

Medical Wire & Equipment Co. (USA)
Hamilton Business Park Unit 9B
Franklin Rd.
Dover, NJ 07801

Micro-Bio-Logics
217 Osseo Ave. North
St. Cloud, MN 56301

Microdiagnostics
601 Stones Levee
Cleveland, OH 44113

Ortho Diagnostic Systems, Inc.
Route 202
Raritan, NJ 08869

Precision Dynamics Corp.
13880 Del Sur St.
San Fernando, CA 91340-3490

Remel
12076 Santa Fe Dr.
Lenexa, KS 66215

Sage Products, Inc.
680 Industrial Dr.
Carey, IL 60013

Scott Laboratories, Inc.
771 Main St.
Fiskeville, RI 02823

Spectrum Diagnostics, Inc.
3 Science Rd.
Glenwood, IL 60425

Trend Scientific, Inc.
P.O. Box 41203
1848 Berkshire Lane North
Minneapolis, MN 55441

Glossary

A Acid.

abscess Localized collection of pus.

accessioning Receipt and recording of specimens delivered to laboratory.

accolé Early ring form of *Plasmodium falciparum* found at margin of red cell.

acid-fast Characteristic of certain bacteria, such as mycobacteria, that involves resistance to decolorization by acids when stained by an aniline dye, such as carbolfuchsin.

acquired immunodeficiency syndrome (AIDS) Severe immune deficiency disease caused by human immunodeficiency virus (HIV-1) infection of the T cells, characterized by opportunistic infections and other complications.

acute serum Serum collected for antibody determination early in course of an illness when there would have been little or no antibody produced.

acute urethral syndrome Lower urinary tract infection that may be difficult to differentiate from cystitis; seen most commonly in younger, sexually active females and caused by *Escherichia coli* (counts as low as 100 per milliliter may be significant in this situation), *Chlamydia*, and other organisms.

aerobe, obligate Microorganism that lives and grows freely in air and cannot grow anaerobically.

aerogenic Producing gas (in contrast to anaerogenic: non-gas-producing).

aerosol Atomized particles suspended in air; in context of this book, microorganisms suspended in air.

aerotolerant Ability of an anaerobic microorganism to grow in air, usually poorly, especially after initial anaerobic isolation.

AFB Acid-fast bacilli.

affinity Inherent attraction and relationship.

agarose gel electrophoresis Separation of proteins based on molecular weight by electrical-current-stimulated movement through a semisolid gel matrix. (See Figure 10.6.)

agglutination Aggregation or clumping of particles, such as bacteria when exposed to specific antibody.

AIDS Acquired immunodeficiency syndrome.

AIDS-related complex (ARC) Prodromal symptoms in patients infected with HIV virus, including lymphadenopathy, fever, weight loss, and malaise.

Alk (or K) Alkaline.

alopecia Baldness.

AMI Antibody-mediated immune response.

aminoglycosides Group of related antibiotics including streptomycin, kanamycin, neomycin, tobramycin, gentamicin, and amikacin.

amniotic Pertaining to the innermost fetal membrane forming a fluid-filled sac.

anaerobe, obligate Microorganism that grows only in complete or nearly complete absence of air or molecular oxygen.

anaerogenic Non-gas-producing.

analytic reagent (AR) Grade of chemical.

anamnestic response More rapid production of antibodies in response to exposure to an antigen previously encountered.

anergy Absence of reaction to antigens or allergens.

antagonism Diminution of activity of one drug by a second one.

antibiogram Distinctive pattern of susceptibility of an organism to a battery of antimicrobial agents.

antibiotic Substance, produced by a microorganism, that inhibits or kills other microorganisms; a broad-spectrum antibiotic is therapeutically effective against a wide range of bacteria.

antibody Substance (immunoglobulin), formed in blood or tissues, that interacts only with antigen that induced its synthesis (e.g., agglutinin).

antigen Molecular structure that is capable of stimulating production of antibody.

antigenic determinant Antigen.

antimicrobial Chemical substance, either produced by a microorganism or by synthetic means, that is capable of killing or suppressing growth of microorganisms.

antiseptic Compound that stops or inhibits growth of bacteria without necessarily killing them.

arboviruses Arthropod-borne viruses.

ART Automated reagin test for syphilis.

arthritis, septic Infection of synovial tissue and joint fluid of one or more joints; characterized by joint pain, stiffness, swelling, and fever.

arthroconidium Spore formed by septation of a hypha and subsequent separation of septa.

ascitic fluid Serous fluid in peritoneal cavity.

assimilation Utilization of nutrients. Assimilation tests are used to determine whether yeasts are able to grow with only a single carbohydrate or nitrate; these tests are useful for classification of yeasts.

ATCC American Type Culture Collection.

autotroph Organism that can utilize inorganic carbon sources (CO_2).

auxotroph Differing from the wild strain (prototroph) by an additional nutritional requirement.

avid The property of binding strongly, such as an antibody that strongly binds to an antigen.

avidity Firmness of union of two substances; used commonly to describe union of antibody to antigen.

B cells Lymphocytes involved in antibody production.

bacteremia Presence of viable organisms in blood.

bacterial vaginosis Noninflammatory condition in vagina characterized by foul-smelling vaginal discharge and presence of mixed bacteria.

bactericidal Term used to describe a drug that kills microorganisms.

bacteriocins Antibiotic-like substances, produced by bacteria, that exert a lethal effect on other bacteria.

bacteriophage Virus that infects a bacterial cell, sometimes bringing about its lysis.

bacteriostatic Term used to describe a drug that inhibits growth of an organism without killing it.

bacteriuria Presence of bacteria in urine.

BAP Blood agar plate.

BCG Bacille Calmette-Guerin, an attenuated strain of *Mycobacterium tuberculosis* used for immunization.

benign tertian malaria Malaria caused by *Plasmodium vivax*.

Beta-lactamases Enzymes that destroy penicillins and/or cephalosporins and are produced by a variety of bacteria.

BFP Biological false-positive.

bifurcated Divided into two branches.

biological safety cabinet Enclosure in which one can work with relatively dangerous organisms without risk of acquiring or spreading infection due to them. These cabinets, also called biosafety hoods, vary in design according to nature of agents to be worked with. The simpler ones maintain a negative pressure within the work area and a laminar air curtain, both of which operate to prevent escape of organisms from interior of hood. Air that is exhausted may be passed through a high-efficiency bacterial filter that will trap all micro-organisms that are anticipated or may be passed through a furnace that will incinerate any organisms. (See Chapter 2 for more information.)

bioluminescence Light generation by living organisms.

biopsy Removal of tissue from a living body for diagnostic purposes (e.g., lymph node biopsy).

biotin Small vitamin with two binding sites, one of which can bind covalently with nucleic acid leaving the other free to form a strong bond with the protein avidin, which in turn can be bound to enzymes. The system is used as a label for nucleic acid probe detection.

biotype Biological or biochemical type of an organism. Organisms of the same biotype will display identical biological or biochemical characteristics. Certain key markers are used to define and recognize biotypes in tracing the spread of organisms in the environment and in epidemics or outbreaks.

blackwater fever Condition in which the diagnostic symptom is passage of reddish or red-brown urine, which indicates massive intravascular hemolysis *(Plasmodium falciparum)*.

blastoconidium A spore formed by budding, as in yeasts.

blepharitis Inflammation of eyelids.

blind loop A condition in which continuity of the bowel has been interrupted in such a way that a segment of bowel receives material from higher in the bowel in the usual way but cannot empty normally because it ends in a blind sac. This leads to proliferation of microorganisms, especially anaerobes, in the blind loop of bowel and may produce profound pathophysiologic effects. There are other situations in which there may be bacterial overgrowth in a segment of the bowel by other mechanisms.

B-lymphocytes (or B cells) Bursa-derived lymphocytes important in humoral immunity.

breakpoint Level of an antibacterial drug achievable in serum; organisms inhibited by this level of drug are considered susceptible. In certain situations, clinicians strive to achieve serum or body fluid levels several times that of the breakpoint.

brightfield microscopy Conventional microscopy in which the object to be viewed is illuminated from below.

bronchial lavage Similar to bronchial washings but this term implies instillation of a larger volume of fluid before aspiration. Alveolar organisms may be present in the lavage.

bronchial washings Fluid that may be aspirated from bronchial tree during bronchoscopy.

bronchitis Inflammation of mucous membranes of bronchi; often caused by infectious agents, viruses in particular.

bronchoscopy Examination of bronchi through a bronchoscope, a tubular illuminated instrument introduced through the trachea (windpipe).

bubo Inflammatory enlargement of lymph node, usually in the groin or axilla.

buffy coat Layer of white blood cells and platelets above red blood cell mass when blood is sedimented.

bullae Large blebs or blisters, filled with fluid, in or just beneath the epidermal layer of skin.

bursitis Inflammation of a bursa, which is a small sac lined with synovial membrane and filled with fluid interposed between parts that move on each other.

butt Lower portion or medium in a tube that has the medium dispensed in such a way that the lower portion fills the tube entirely while the upper portion is distributed in the form of a slanted surface leaving an air space between the slant and the opposite wall of the tube.

butyrous Butterlike consistency.

C & S Culture and sensitivity.

calibrated loop Bacteriological loop that is carefully calibrated to deliver a specified volume of fluid providing that directions are followed carefully and the loop has not been damaged; used as a simple means of quantitating the number of organisms present, especially for urine culture.

CAMP Lytic factor named after Christie, Atkins, and Munch-Peterson.

candle jar A jar with a lid providing a gas-tight seal in which a small white candle is placed and lit after the culture plates have been placed inside. Candle will burn only until the oxygen concentration has been lowered to the point where it will no longer support the flame. Atmosphere of such a jar has a lower oxygen content than room air and a carbon dioxide content of about 3%.

cannula An artificial tube for insertion into a tube or cavity of the body.

CAP Chocolate agar plate.

CAPD Chronic ambulatory peritoneal dialysis.

capneic incubation Incubation under increased CO_2 tension, as in a candle extinction jar (approximate 3% CO_2).

capnophilic Term used to describe microorganisms that prefer an incubation atmosphere with increased carbon dioxide concentration.

capsule Gelatinous material surrounding bacterial cell wall. Usually of polysaccharide nature.

carrier One who harbors a pathogenic organism but is not affected by it.

caseation necrosis Tissue death with loss of cell outlines and a cheeselike, amorphous appearance.

catalase Bacterial enzyme that breaks down peroxides with liberation of free oxygen.

catheter Flexible tubular (rubber or plastic) instrument used for withdrawing fluids from (or introducing fluids into) a body cavity or vessel (e.g., urinary bladder catheter).

cation A positive ion.

CDC Centers for Disease Control.

cell line, continuous Line of tissue cells that is maintained by serial culture of an established cell line.

cell line, primary Line of tissue cells established by cutting up fresh tissue, often kidney, into tiny pieces, trypsinizing, and putting in a flask with appropriate medium.

cellulitis Inflammation of subcutaneous tissue.

cerebriform With brainlike folds.

cervical Pertaining either to the neck or to the cervix of the uterus.

CF Complement fixation.

CFU Colony-forming unit (i.e., colony count).

Charcot-Leyden crystals Slender crystals shaped like a double pyramid with pointed ends, formed from the breakdown products of eosinophils and found in feces, sputum, and tissues: indicative of an immune response that may have parasitic or nonparasitic causes.

chemotherapeutic Chemical agent used in the treatment of infections (e.g., sulfonamides).

chlamydospore Thick-walled spore formed from a vegetative cell.

chromatography Method of chemical analysis by which a mixture of substances is separated by fractional extraction or adsorption or ion exchange on a porous solid.

chromogen Bacterial species whose colonial growth is pigmented (e.g., *Flavobacterium* species, yellow).

chromogenic Giving rise to color, as chromogenic substrates for colored products of biochemical reactions or chromogenic bacteria that produce pigmented colonies.

CIE Counterimmunoelectrophoresis.

clavate Club-shaped.

clone Group of microorganisms of identical genetic makeup derived from a single common ancestor.

CMI Cell-mediated immunity.

CNS Central nervous system.

coagglutination Agglutination of protein A–containing cells of *Staphylococcus aureus* coated with antibody molecules when exposed to corresponding antigen.

colitis Inflammation of mucosa of colon.

colony Macroscopically visible growth of a microorganism on a solid culture medium.

colorimetry Chemical analysis by color determination.

commensal Microorganism living on or in a host but causing the host no harm.

complement fixation test Antigen-antibody test based on fixation of complement in the presence of both elements and use of an indicator system to determine whether or not complement has been fixed.

congenital Existing before or at birth.

conjugation Passing genetic information between bacteria by transferring chromosomal material, often via pili.

conjunctivitis Inflammation of the conjunctivae or membranes of the eye and eyelid.

convalescent serum Serum collected later in the course of an illness than the acute serum, usually at least 2 weeks after initial collection.

counterimmunoelectrophoresis (CIE) Detection of antibody or antigen by precipitin reaction that occurs in solid-phase (gel or paper) system that uses electric current to carry reactants toward each other.

CPC Clinical pathologic conference.

CPE Cytopathogenic (cytopathic) effect; visual effect of virus infection on cell culture.

Creutzfeld-Jakob disease Debilitating prion-caused disease characterized by dementia, ataxia, delirium, stupor, coma, and death: has been transmitted by organ transplant.

croup Inflammation of upper airways (larynx, trachea) with respiratory obstruction, often due to virus infections in children.

CRP C-reactive protein.

CSF Cerebrospinal fluid.

culdocentesis Aspiration of fluid from the cul-de-sac by puncture of the vaginal vault.

CYE Charcoal yeast extract (agar plate).

cystitis Inflammation of urinary bladder, most often caused by bacterial infection.

cytotoxin Toxin that produces cytopathic effects in vivo or in a tissue culture system.

darkfield microscopy Technique used to visualize very small microorganisms or their characteristics by a system that permits light to be reflected or refracted from surface of objects being viewed.

debridement Surgical or other removal of nonviable tissue.

decontamination Process of rendering an object or area safe for unprotected people by removing or making harmless biological or chemical agents.

decubitus ulcer A craterlike defect in skin and subcutaneous tissue caused by prolonged pressure on the area. This occurs primarily over bony prominences of the lower back and hips in individuals who are unable to care for themselves well and unable to roll or move periodically; also known as pressure sore or bedsore.

definitive host Host in which the sexual reproduction of a parasite occurs.

dermatophyte A fungus parasitic on skin, hair, or nails.

desquamation Shedding or scaling of skin or mucous membrane.

DFA Direct fluorescent antibody test.

DIC Disseminated intravascular coagulation.

dichotomous Branching in two directions.

diluent Fluid used to dilute a substance.

dimorphic fungi Fungi with both a mold phase and a yeast phase.

direct wet mount A preparation from clinical material suspended in sterile saline or other liquid medium on a glass slide and covered with a coverslip; used for microscopic examination to detect microorganisms in clinical material and, in particular, to detect motility directly.

disinfectant Agent that destroys or inhibits microorganisms that cause disease.

DNA Deoxyribonucleic acid, the lipoprotein molecule that contains the genetic code for most living things.

DNase Deoxyribonuclease, an enzyme that depolymerizes DNA.

DRGs Diagnosis related groups; system introduced to control rising medical costs under which hospitals are reimbursed for costs of caring for patients based on the primary diagnoses of the patients and what is considered to be a fair dollar value for treatment of usual patients with those diagnoses.

droplet nucleus A tiny aerosolized particle that, because of its lack of mass, may stay suspended in air for extended periods of time.

Durham tube Small tube placed in an inverted position below the surface of a growth-supportive broth and filled completely with the broth solution. Gas produced by the organism displaces the broth in the Durham tube and the resulting gas bubble is visual evidence of gas production.

Dx Diagnosis.

dysentery Inflammation of the intestinal tract, particularly the colon, with frequent bloody stools (e.g., bacillary dysentery).

dysgonic Growing poorly (bacterial cultures).

ectoparasite Organism that lives on or within skin.

ectothrix Outside of hair shafts.

edema Excessive accumulation of fluid in tissue spaces.

effusion Fluid escaping into a body space or tissue (e.g., pleural effusion).

Eh Oxidation-reduction potential.

elementary body The infectious stage of *Chlamydia* or a cellular inclusion body of a viral disease.

elephantiasis Condition caused by inflammation and obstruction of the lymphatic system, resulting in hypertrophy and thickening of the surrounding tissues, usually involving the extremities and external genitalia (often as a result of filariasis).

ELISA Enzyme-linked immunosorbent assay.

elution Process of extraction by means of a solvent.

EMB Eosin-methylene blue (agar plate).

emetic Inducing vomiting.

empyema Accumulation of pus in a body cavity, particularly empyema of the thorax or chest.

encephalitis Inflammation of the brain.

endocarditis A serious infection of the endothelium of the heart, usually involving leaflets of the heart valves where destruction of valves or distortion of them by formation of vegetations may lead to serious physiologic disturbances and death: also, an inflammation of the endocardial surface (much less common).

endocervix Mucous membrane of the cervical canal.

endogenous Developing from within the body.

endoparasite Parasite that lives within the body.

endophthalmitis Inflammation of internal tissues of eye; may rapidly destroy the eye.

endothelium Squamous epithelium lining blood vessels.

endothrix Within the hair shaft.

endotoxin Substance containing lipopolysaccharide complexes found in the cell wall of bacteria, principally gram-negative bacteria; felt to play an important role in many of the complications of sepsis such as shock, DIC, and thrombocytopenia.

enteric fever Typhoid fever; paratyphoid fever.

enteroinvasive Capable of invading the mucosal surface and sometimes the deeper tissues of the bowel.

enteropathogenic *Escherichia coli* (EPEC) Specific serotypes of *E. coli* isolated from feces of patients with diarrhea, usually associated with nursery epidemics.

enterotoxigenic Producing an enterotoxin (e.g., enterotoxigenic *Escherichia coli*).

enterotoxin Toxin affecting the cells of the intestinal mucosa.

enzyme-linked immunosorbent assay (ELISA) An immunologic assay similar to RIA that uses an enzyme conjugated to antibodies to produce a visible endpoint. (See Figure 10.5.)

EPEC Enteropathogenic *Escherichia coli*.

epidemiology The study of the occurrence and distribution of disease and factors that control presence or absence of disease.

epididymitis Inflammation of the epididymis characterized by fever and pain on one side of the scrotum; seen as a complication of prostatitis and cystitis.

epiglottiditis Inflammation of the epiglottis, a structure that prevents aspirating swallowed food and fluids into the tracheobronchial tree; a serious infection because the swollen epiglottis may block the airway.

epithelium Tissue composed of contiguous cells that forms the epidermis and lines hollow organs and all passages of the respiratory, digestive, and genitourinary systems.

erysipelas An acute cellulitis caused by group A streptococci.

erythema Redness of the skin from various causes.

erythema chronicum migrans Characteristic radial skin lesion of Lyme disease.

erythrasma A minor, superficial skin infection caused by *Corynebacterium minutissimium*.

erythrocytic cycle Developmental cycle of malarial parasites within red blood cells.

eschar A dry scar, particularly one related to a burn.

ETEC Enterotoxigenic *Escherichia coli*. Strains of *E. coli* that produce a choleralike toxin; have been implicated as causes of diarrhea.

etiology Cause or causative agent.

eugonic Growing luxuriantly (bacterial cultures).

eukaryotic Organisms with a true nucleus, in contrast to bacteria and viruses.

exanthem Skin eruption as a symptom of an acute disease, usually viral.

exoerythrocytic cycle Portion of the malarial life cycle occurring in the vertebrate host in which sporozoites, introduced by infected mosquitoes, penetrate the parenchymal liver cells and undergo schizogony, producing merozoites, which then initiate the erythrocytic cycle.

exogenous From outside the body.

exotoxin A toxin produced by a microorganism that is released into the surrounding environment.

exudate Fluid that has passed out of blood vessels into adjacent tissues or spaces; high protein content.

facultative anaerobe Microorganism that grows under either anaerobic or aerobic conditions.

fascia Membranous covering of muscle.

favus Dermatophyte infection of the scalp produced by *Trichophyton schoenleinii*.

fermentation Anaerobic decomposition of carbohydrate.

filamentous Threadlike.

fimbriae Proteinaceous fingerlike surface structures of bacteria that provide for adherence to host surfaces.

fistula Abnormal communication between two surfaces or between a viscus or other hollow structure and the exterior.

Fitz-Hugh-Curtis syndrome Inflammation of the capsule of the liver that may be seen in course of gonococcal or chlamydial infection in the female.

floccose Cottony, in tufts.

flocculation test Antigen-antibody test in which a precipitin end product forms macroscopically or microscopically visible clumps.

fluorescent Emission of light by a substance (or a microscopic preparation) while acted on by radiant energy, such as ultraviolet rays, as in the immunofluorescent procedure.

fluorescent immunoassays (FIAs) Similar to RIA but employ fluorescent molecules as labels.

fluorochrome A dye that becomes fluorescent or self-luminous after exposure to ultraviolet light.

fomite Any inanimate object that may be contaminated with disease-causing microorganisms and thus serve to transmit disease.

FTA Fluorescent treponemal antibody.

FTA-ABS Fluorescent Treponemal Antigen-Antibody absorption test; indirect fluorescent antibody stain used to detect antibodies directed against whole cell antigens of *Treponema pallidum* (syphilis bacillus).

fungemia Presence of viable fungi in blood.

FUO Fever of unknown origin.

fusiform Spindle-shaped, as in the anaerobe *Fusobacterium nucleatum*.

gangrene Death of a part of tissue resulting from disease, injury, or failure of blood supply.

gas-liquid chromatography (GLC) A method for separating substances by allowing their volatile phase to flow through a heated column with a carrier gas and measuring the time required to detect their presence at the distal end of the column.

gastric aspirate Fluid that may be aspirated from the stomach via a tube placed in the stomach by way of the nose or mouth.

gastroenteritis Inflammation of the mucosa of the stomach and intestines.

GC Gonococcus.

germicide An agent that destroys germs; disinfectant.

germ tube Tubelike process, produced by a germinating spore, that develops into mycelium.

glabrous Smooth.

GLC Gas-liquid chromatography.

glove box A device with flexible, semirigid, or rigid plastic walls used for cultivation of anaerobic bacteria. Bacteriologist must work by way of glove ports, and materials are brought into and out of the anaerobic work area by way of an interchange (airlock) that can be evacuated and refilled with an anaerobic atmosphere repeatedly until it itself is anaerobic. The interchange has one door leading into the glove box per se and another door to the outside. Some glove boxes have incubators within them. Also called anaerobic chamber or anaerobic cabinet.

GN Gram-negative (broth).

granulocytopenia Reduced number of granulocytic white blood cells in the blood.

granuloma Aggregation and proliferation of macrophages to form small (usually microscopic) nodules.

HAA Hepatitis-associated antigen.

HAI Hemagglutination inhibition.

halophilic Preferring high halide (salt) content.

HATTS The hemagglutination treponemal test for syphilis.

headspace gas Gas generated during growth of an organism in a closed tube that accumulates between the upper surface of the broth in the tube and the top of the tube.

hemagglutination Agglutination of red blood cells caused by certain antibodies, virus particles, or high molecular weight polysaccharides.

hematogenous Disseminated by the bloodstream.

hemolysis, alpha Partial destruction of, or enzymatic damage to, red blood cells in a blood agar plate, leading to greenish discoloration about the colony of the organism producing the alpha hemolysin.

hemolysis, beta Total lysis of red blood cells about a colony on a blood agar plate, leading to a completely clear zone surrounding the colony.

hemolysis, gamma No hemolysis is seen with organisms classed as gamma hemolytic; nonhemolytic would be a better designation.

HEPA High-efficiency particulate air filter; used in biological safety cabinets to trap pathogenic microorganisms.

herpes Inflammation of the skin characterized by clusters of small vesicles (e.g., caused by herpes simplex); disease caused by herpes simplex virus.

heterotroph Organism that requires an organic carbon source.

hidradenitis suppurativa Inflammation of certain sweat glands leading to formation of abscesses and draining sinuses.

high-pressure liquid chromatography (HPLC) Similar to GLC but capable of higher resolution because of increased pressure of liquid carrier that runs through the column.

hilum of lung Central area where major vessels and bronchi begin to branch.

HPLC High-pressure (or performance) liquid chromatography.

humidophilic Organisms preferring or requiring an increased moisture content; can be achieved by placing cultures in sealed jars or bags. For some organisms that do better in a candle jar than in the ambient atmosphere, it is the increased moisture content rather than the change in the gas content that is important.

humoral immunity Immunity effected by antibody.

hyaline Colorless, transparent.

hybridoma The product of fusion of an antibody-producing cell and an immortal malignant antibody-producing cell.

hydrolysis Breakdown of a substrate by an enzyme that adds the components of water to key bonds within the substrate molecule.

hyperalimentation Process by which nutrition (literally, extra nutrition) is provided; typically done by the intravenous route in subjects who are not able to absorb foods well from the gut because of disease of the bowel, in subjects in whom it is desirable to put the bowel "at rest" to promote healing, and in malnourished individuals to improve the nutritional status (e.g., before surgery), usually done over an extended period of time and requires use of a special access IV catheter such as a Hickman catheter.

hyperemia Increased blood in a part, resulting in distention of blood vessels.

hypertonic Hyperosmotic.

hypertrophy Increased size of an organ resulting from enlargement of individual cells.

hypha Tubular cell making up the vegetative portion of mycelium of fungi.

hypoxia Decreased oxygen content of tissues.

ID Infectious disease; identification; immunodiffusion.

IE Infectious endocarditis.

IFA Indirect fluorescent antibody; test that detects antibody by allowing an antibody to react with its substrate and adding a second fluorescein dye–labelled antibody that will bind to the first.

Ig, IgG, etc. Immunoglobulin, immunoglobulin G, etc.

immunodiffusion Detection of antigen or antibody by observing the precipitin line formed in a semisolid gel matrix when homologous antigens and antibodies are allowed to diffuse toward each other and react.

immunofluorescence Microscopic method of determining the presence or location of an antigen (or antibody) by demonstrating fluorescence when the preparation is exposed to a fluorescein-tagged antibody (or antigen) using ultraviolet radiation.

immunoglobulin Synonymous with antibody; five distinct classes have been isolated: IgG, IgM, IgA, IgE, and IgD.

immunoperoxidase stain Combination of an enzyme that catalyzes production of a colored product with an antibody to facilitate detection of certain antigens, particularly viral antigens.

immunosuppression Depression of the immune response caused by disease, irradiation, or administration of antimetabolites, antilymphocyte serum, or corticosteroids.

impedance Apparent resistance of a circuit to the flow of an alternating electric current.

impetigo Acute inflammatory skin disease, caused by streptococci or staphylococci, characterized by vesicles and bullae that rupture and form yellow crusts.

inclusion bodies Microscopic bodies, usually within body cells; thought to be virus particles in morphogenesis.

indigenous flora Normal or resident flora.

induced malaria Malaria infection acquired by parenteral inoculation (e.g., blood transfusion or sharing of needles by drug addicts).

induration Abnormal hardness of a tissue or part resulting from hyperemia or inflammation, as in a reactive tuberculin skin test.

infection Invasion by and multiplication of microorganisms in body tissue resulting in disease.

inhibitory quotient Ratio of the average peak achievable level of antibiotic in a body fluid from which an organism was isolated to the MIC of that organism.

in situ hybridization Detection of nucleic acid of a pathogenic organism in tissue sections by separating the DNA into single-stranded molecules and allowing a labeled strand of homologous DNA to bind to the target. The target is visualized by developing the label (either enzymatic precipitate, fluorescence, or radiolabel).

inspissation Process of making a liquid or semisolid medium thick by evaporation or absorption of fluid.

intermediate host Required host in the life cycle in which essential larval development must occur before a parasite is infective to its definitive host or to additional intermediate hosts.

intertrigo Erythematous skin eruption of adjacent skin parts.

intramuscular (intraperitoneal, intravenous) Within the muscle (peritoneum, vein), as in intramuscular injection.

in vitro Literally, within glass (i.e., in a test tube, culture plate, or other nonliving material).

in vivo Within the living body.

involution forms Abnormally shaped bacterial cells occurring in an aging culture population.

ion-exchange chromatography Separation of components of a solution by chromatography based on the reversible exchange of ions in the solution with ions present in or on an external matrix.

isotonic Of the same osmolality of body tissues, red blood cells, bacteria, etc.

K Alkaline.

Kawasaki disease Mucocutaneous lymph node syndrome; disease of children that may involve more serious phenomena such as cardiac disease.

keratitis Inflammation of the cornea.

KIA Kligler's iron agar (tube).

KOH Potassium hydroxide.

Köhler illumination Modification of brightfield microscopy in which a substage condenser is used to avoid glare from illuminating source.

lag phase Period of slow microbial growth that occurs following inoculation of the culture medium.

laked blood Hemolyzed blood; hemolysis may be effected in various ways, but alternate freezing and thawing is a simple method.

laminar flow Nonturbulent flow of air in layers (flowing in a vertical direction in the case of a biosafety hood).

latent Not manifest; potential.

latex agglutination Agglutination of latex particles coated with antibody molecules when exposed to the corresponding antigen.

lectin Naturally produced proteins or glycoproteins that can bind with carbohydrates or sugars to form stable complexes.

Leishman-Donovan body Small, round intracellular form (called amastigote or leishmanial stage) of *Leishmania* species and *Trypanosoma cruzi*.

leukocytosis Elevated white blood cell count.

leukopenia Low white blood cell count.

L form Cell wall–deficient form of a bacterium.

***Limulus* amebocyte lysate** Product of white blood cells of the horseshoe crab used in an assay for endotoxin.

lipopolysaccharide Carbohydrate-lipid complex; integral substance in gram-negative cell walls. Also known as "endotoxin".

liposome Small closed vesicle consisting of a single lipid bilayer.

logarithmic phase Period of maximal growth rate of a microorganism in a culture medium.

LPA Latex particle agglutination.

LPS Lipopolysaccharide; see **endotoxin.**

lysis Disintegration or dissolution of bacteria or cells.

lysogeny Process by which a viral genome is integrated into that of its host bacterium.

MAC MacConkey (agar plate).

macroconidia Large, usually multiseptate, club- or spindle-shaped fungal spores.

malignant tertian malaria Malaria caused by *Plasmodium falciparum*.

mass spectrometry Method for determining composition of a substance by observing its volatile products during disintegration and comparing them with known standards.

MBC Minimum bactericidal concentration.

meconium Pasty greenish mass in intestine of fetus; made up of mucus, desquamated cells, bile, and such.

media, differential Media that permit ready recognition of a particular organism or group of organisms by virtue of facilitating recognition of a natural product of the organism being sought or by incorporating an appropriate substrate and indicator system so that organisms possessing certain enzymes will be readily recognized.

media, enrichment Media, usually liquid, that favor the growth of one or more organisms while suppressing most of the competing flora in a specimen with a mixture of organisms.

media, selective Culture media that contain inhibitory substances or unique growth factors such that one particular organism or group of organisms is conferred a real advantage over other organisms that may be found in a mixture. Efficient selective media will select out only the organism or organisms being sought, with little or no growth of other types of organisms.

media, supportive Culture media that provide adequate nutrition for most nonfastidious microorganisms and that permit each organism to grow normally without conferring any special advantage to one organism over another.

mediastinum Space in the middle of the chest between the medial surfaces of the two pleurae.

meningitis Inflammation of the meninges, the membranes that cover the brain and spinal cord (e.g., bacterial meningitis).

merozoite Product of schizogonic cycle in malaria that will invade red blood cells.

mesenteric adenitis Inflammation of mesenteric lymph nodes.

mesentery A fold of the peritoneum that connects the intestine with the posterior abdominal wall.

metastatic Spread of an infectious (or other) process from a primary focus to a distant one via the bloodstream or lymphatic system.

MHA-TP Microhemagglutination test for antibody to *Treponema pallidum*.

MIC Minimum inhibitory concentration.

microaerophile, obligate Microorganism that grows only under reduced oxygen tension and cannot grow aerobically or anaerobically.

microcalorimetry Study of microcalories, a measure of heat production.

microconidia Small, single-celled fungal spores.

microfilaria Embryos produced by filarial worms and found in the blood or tissues of individuals with filariasis.

miliary Of the size of a millet seed (0.5 to 1.0 mm); characterized by the formation of numerous lesions of the above size distributed rather uniformly throughout one or more organs.

minimum bactericidal concentration (MBC) The minimum concentration of antimicrobial agent needed to yield a 99.9% reduction in viable colony forming units of a bacterial or fungal suspension. (See Figure 13.2.)

minimum inhibitory concentration (MIC) The minimum concentration of antimicrobial agent needed to prevent visually discernible growth of a bacterial or fungal suspension. (See Figure 13.2.)

mixed culture (pure culture) More than one organism growing in or on the same culture medium, as opposed to a single organism in pure culture.

monoarticular Occurring in only one joint.

monoclonal antibody Antibody that is derived from a single cell producing one antibody molecule type that reacts with a single epitope.

monolayer A confluent layer of tissue culture cells one cell thick.

MOTT Mycobacteria other than *Mycobacterium tuberculosis*.

mucopurulent Term used to describe material containing both mucus and pus (e.g., mucopurulent sputum).

mucosa A mucous membrane.

multiple myeloma Malignancy involving antibody-producing plasma cells.

mycelium Mass of hyphae making up a colony of a fungus.

mycetoma Chronic infection, usually of feet, caused by various fungi or by *Nocardia* or *Streptomyces*, resulting in swelling and sinus tracts; pulmonary mycetoma is a mass of fungal hyphae ("fungus ball") growing in a cavity formed during previous tuberculosi infection or other pathologic condition.

mycoses Diseases caused by fungi (e.g., dermatomycosis, fungal infection of the superficial skin).

myocarditis Inflammation of the heart muscle.

myositis Inflammation of a muscle, sometimes caused by infection as in pyomyositis, an infection due to *Staphylococcus aureus* that leads to small abscesses within the muscle substance.

nares External openings of nose (i.e., nostrils).

nasopharyngeal Pertaining to the part of the pharynx above the level of the soft palate.

necrosis Pathologic death of a cell or group of cells.

necrotizing fasciitis A very serious, painful infection involving the fascia (membranous covering) of one or more muscles, may spread widely in short periods of time since there is no anatomic barrier to spread in this type of infection.

neonatal First 4 weeks after birth.

nephelometry Determination of the degree of turbidity of a fluid by light scatter.

neuritis Inflammation of a nerve; most often not caused by an infectious agent.

neurotrophic Having a selective affinity for nerve tissue. Rabies is caused by a neurotrophic virus.

NFB Glucose nonfermenting gram-negative bacteria.

NGU Nongonococcal urethritis.

nick translation Use of enzymes to break DNA and re-polymerize small sections of the molecule, usually for purposes of labeling the DNA with a radioactive nucleotide.

nonphotochromogens Slow-growing, nonpigmented mycobacteria.

nonsporulating Does not produce spores.

nosocomial Pertaining to or originating in a hospital, as nosocomial infection.

nucleic acid hybridization Process by which the single-stranded probe unites with complementary DNA in an unknown sample.

nucleic acid probe Piece of labeled single-stranded DNA used to detect complementary DNA in clinical material or a culture and thus to specifically identify the presence in these materials of an organism identical to that used to make the probe.

O & P Ova and parasites.

O-F Oxidation-fermentation medium.

octal numbers Numbers employed in computer data bases to identify biochemical profiles of organisms and thus their identification.

oil immersion microscopy Use of immersion oil to fill the space between the slide being studied and the special objective of the microscope; this keeps the light rays from dispersing and provides good resolution at high magnification (total magnification of $1000\times$).

ONPG *o*-nitrophenol-β-galactopyranoside (β-galactosidase test).

operculated ova Ova possessing a cap or lid.

opsonize To facilitate destruction of pathogens by phagocytic ingestion or lysis by complement through the action of adherent antibodies.

osteomyelitis Inflammation of the bone and the marrow.

otitis Inflammation of the ear from a variety of causes, including bacterial infection; otitis media: inflammation of the middle ear.

oxidation A metabolic pathway of the microorganism that involves use of oxygen as a terminal electron acceptor. This type of reaction occurs in air.

oxidation-reduction potential Electromotive force exerted by a nonreacting electrode in a solution containing the oxidized and reduced forms of a chemical, relative to a standard hydrogen electrode; the more negative the value, the more anaerobic conditions are.

pandemic Epidemic over a wide geographic area, or even worldwide.

paracentesis Surgical transcutaneous puncture of the abdominal cavity to aspirate peritoneal fluid.

parasite Organism that lives on or within and at the expense of another organism.

parenteral Route of administration of a drug other than by mouth; includes intramuscular and intravenous administration.

paronychia Purulent inflammation about margin of a nail.

parotitis Inflammation of the parotid gland, the largest of the salivary glands; mumps is the most common cause of this.

paroxysm Rapid onset (or return) of symptoms; term usually applies to cyclic recurrence of malaria symptoms, which are chills, fever, and sweating.

pathogenic Producing disease.

pathologic Caused by or involving a morbid condition, as a pathologic state.

PCR Polymerase chain reaction.

penicillinase (β-lactamase I) Enzyme produced by some bacterial species that inactivates the antimicrobial activity of certain penicillins (e.g., penicillin G).

percutaneous Performed through the skin (e.g., percutaneous bladder aspiration).

pericarditis Inflammation of the covering of the heart (pericardium).

perineum The portion of the body bounded by the pubic bone anteriorly, the coccyx posteriorly, and the bony prominences (tuberosities) of the ileum on both sides.

peritoneal cavity Space between the visceral and parietal layers of the peritoneum; the serous membrane lining the abdominal cavity and surrounding the contained viscera.

peritonitis Inflammation of the peritoneal cavity, most often caused by bacterial infection.

petechiae Tiny hemorrhagic spots in the skin or mucous membranes.

phase-contrast microscopy Technique for direct observation of unstained material in which light beams pass through the object to be visualized and are partially deflected by the different densities of the object. These light beams are deflected again when they impinge on a special objective lens, increasing in brightness when aligned in phase.

photochromogens Mycobacteria that produce pigment after exposure to light but whose colonies remain buff-colored in the dark.

PID Pelvic inflammatory disease.

pili Structures in bacteria similar to fimbriae that participate in bacterial conjugation and transfer of genetic material.

pilonidal cyst Hair-containing cyst in the skin or subcutaneous tissue, often with a sinus tract, commonly in the sacrococcygeal area.

plasma Fluid portion of blood; obtained by centrifuging anticoagulated blood.

plasmids Extrachromosomal DNA elements of bacteria carrying a variety of determinants that may permit survival in an adverse environment or successful competition with other microorganisms of the same or different species.

pleomorphic Having more than one form, usually widely different forms, as in pleomorphic bacteria.

pleura The serous membrane enveloping the lung and lining the internal surface of the thoracic cavity.

pleuropulmonary Pertaining to the lungs and pleura.

PMC Pseudomembranous colitis.

pneumonia Inflammation of the lungs, primarily caused by infectious agents.

pneumonia, aspiration Pneumonia caused by aspiration of oropharyngeal or gastric contents.

pneumothorax Introduction of air (usually inadvertently) into the pleural space, leading to collapse of the lung on that side.

polyarticular Occurring in more than one joint.

polymerase chain reaction (PCR) A method for expanding small discrete sections of DNA by binding DNA primers to sections at the ends of the DNA to be expanded and using cycles of heat (to create single-stranded DNA) and cooler temperatures (to allow a DNA polymerase enzyme to create new sections of DNA between the primer ends).

PPD Purified protein derivative (skin test antigen for tuberculosis).

PPNG Penicillinase-producing (i.e., penicillin-resistant) *Neisseria gonorrhoeae*.

PRAS Prereduced, anaerobically sterilized.

precipitin test Detection of antigen by allowing specific antibody to diffuse through liquid or gel until an antigen-antibody complex forms, which can be viewed as a line of precipitated material.

prion Proteinaceous infectious agent associated with Creutzfeld-Jakob disease and perhaps other chronic, debilitating central nervous system diseases.

proctitis Inflammation of the rectum.

prodromal Early manifestations of a disease before specific symptoms become evident.

proglottid Segments of the tapeworm containing male and female reproductive systems; may be immature, mature, or gravid.

prognosis Forecast as to the possible outcome of a disease.

progressive bacterial synergistic gangrene Serious polymicrobial infection of skin and soft tissue, often a postoperative complication, involving a mixture of microaerophilic streptococci and *Staphylococcus aureus* classically. At times the streptococci are anaerobic or gram-negative bacilli are seen in lieu of the staphylococci.

prokaryotic Organisms without a true nucleus.

prophylaxis Preventive treatment (e.g., the use of drugs to prevent infection).

prostatitis Inflammation of the prostate gland, usually due to infection, characterized by fever, low back or perineal pain, and at times urinary frequency and urgency; a common background factor for recurrent cystitis in males.

prosthesis An artificial part such as a hip joint or eye.

protein A A protein on the cell wall of strains of *Staphylococcus aurus* (Cowan strain) that binds the Fc portion of antibodies.

prototroph Naturally occurring or wild strain.

pseudomembrane Necrosis of mucosal surface simulating a membrane.

pseudomembranous colitis (PMC) Syndrome in the large bowel characterized by a layer of necrotic tissue and dead inflammatory cells often caused by the toxin of *Clostridium difficile*.

psychrophilic Cold-loving (e.g., microorganisms that grow best at low [4° C] temperatures).

purulent Consisting of pus.

pus Product of inflammation, consisting of fluid and many white blood cells; often bacteria and cellular debris are also present.

pyelonephritis Infection of the kidney and renal pelvis and the late effects of such infection.

pyocin Pigment produced by a bacterium that has antibacterial properties against other strains or species of bacteria.

pyoderma Any of the pus-producing lesions of the skin such as boils or impetigo.

pyogenic Pus-producing

QC Quality control.

QNS Quantity not sufficient.

quartan malaria Malaria caused by *Plasmodium malariae*.

radioimmunoassay (RIA) A very sensitive competitive binding assay that uses radioactively labeled antigen and specific homologous antibody to determine the amount of antigen in a sample. The antigen could also be an antibody.

radioisotope Unstable molecule that emits detectable radiation (gamma rays, X-rays, etc.) for a known period of time (half-life). Can be incorporated into other compounds as a label for later detection by X-ray film exposure or by measurement in a scintillation counting instrument.

radiometric analysis Determination of an element that is not itself radioactive by means of an interaction with a radioactive element.

reagin An antibody that reacts in various serologic tests for syphilis.

reservoir Source from which an infectious agent may be disseminated; for example, humans are the only reservoir for *Mycobacterium tuberculosis*.

resin Plant product composed largely of esters and ethers of organic acids and acid anhydrides.

restriction endonuclease Enzyme that breaks nucleic acid (usually DNA) at only one specific sequence of nucleotides.

reticulate body The metabolically more active form of elementary bodies.

reticuloendothelial system Macrophage system, which includes all the phagocytic cells of the body except for the granulocytic leukocytes.

R factor Plasmid that carries gene coding for resistance to one or more antibacterial agents.

rheumatoid factor IgM antibodies produced by some patients against their own IgG.

rhizoid Rootlike absorbing organ.

RIA Radiometric immunoassay (radioimmunoassay).

RNA Ribonucleic acid.

RPR Rapid plasma reagin, nontreponemal test for antibodies developed in response to syphilis infection.

saccharolytic Capable of breaking down sugars.

saprophytic Nonpathogenic.

SBA Suprapubic bladder aspiration.

SBE Subacute bacterial endocarditis.

schizogony Stage in the asexual cycle of the malaria parasite that takes place in the red blood cells of humans.

Schlichter test Synonym for the serum bactericidal level test.

sclerotic Hard, indurated.

scolex (pl., scolices) Head portion of a tapeworm; may attach to the intestinal wall by suckers or hooklets.

scotochromogens Mycobacteria that are pigmented even in the absence of exposure to light.

sensitivity Ability of a test to detect all true cases of the condition being tested for; absence of false negative results. (Also see "specificity".)

septate Having cross walls.

septic shock Acute circulatory failure caused by toxins of microorganisms, often leads to multiple organ failure and is associated with a relatively high mortality.

septicemia (sepsis) Systemic disease associated with presence of pathogenic microorganisms or their toxins in the blood.

sequestrum A detached or dead piece of bone within a cavity, abscess, wound, or area of osteomyelitis.

Sereny test Test for bacterial invasiveness; involves applying a suspension of the organism to the conjunctiva of a small mammal and observing for development of conjunctivitis.

serosanguineous Like serous but with some blood present grossly.

serous Like serum.

serum Cell- and fibrinogen-free fluid after blood clots.

serum bactericidal level Lowest dilution of a patient's serum that kills a standard inoculum of an organism isolated from that patient; this, of course, is related to antibiotic level achieved in the patient's serum and the bactericidal activity of the drug being employed.

sinus Suppurating tract; paranasal sinus, hollows, or cavities near the nose (e.g., frontal and maxillary sinuses).

slant See definition of "butt." The slant is the upper surface of the medium in the tube described. It is exposed to air in the tube.

solid-phase immunosorbent assay (SPIA) ELISA test in which the capture antigen or antibody is attached to the inside of a plastic tube, microwell, or to the outside of a plastic bead, in a filter matrix, or some other solid support. Allows faster interaction between reactants and more concentrated visual endproducts than ELISA tests performed in liquid.

somatic Pertaining to the body (of a cell) (e.g., the somatic antigens of *Salmonella* species).

Southern blot Identification of specific genetic sequences by separating DNA fragments by gel electrophoresis and transferring them to membrane filters in situ. Labeled complementary DNA applied to the filter will bind to homologous fragments, which can then by identified by detecting the presence of the labeled DNA in association with bands of certain molecular size. Named after its discoverer, E. M. Southern.

specificity Ability of a test to correctly yield a negative result when the condition being detected is absent; absence of false positive results. (Also see "sensitivity".)

SPIA Solid-phase immunosorbent assay.

spore Reproductive cell of bacteria, fungi, or protozoa; in bacteria, may be inactive, resistant forms within the cell.

sporogony Stage in the sexual cycle in the malarial parasite that takes place in the mosquito.

sporozoite Slender, spindle-shaped organism that is the infective stage of the malarial parasite; it is inoculated into humans by an infected mosquito and is the result of the sexual cycle of the malarial parasite in the mosquito.

sputum Material discharged from the surface of the lower respiratory tract air passages and expectorated (or swallowed).

stab culture Culture in which the inoculation of a tube of solid medium is made by stabbing with a needle to encourage anaerobic growth in the bottom.

stat Statim (Latin); immediately.

stationary phase Stage in the growth cycle of a bacterial culture in which the vegetative cell population equals the dying population.

STD Sexually transmitted disease.

sterile (sterility) Free of living microorganisms (the state of being sterile).

strobila Entire chain of tapeworm proglottids, excluding the scolex and neck.

substrate A substance on which an enzyme acts.

sulfur granule Small colony of organisms with surrounding clublike material; yellow-brown; resembles grain of sulfur.

superinfection Strictly speaking, this refers to a new infection superimposed on another being treated with an antimicrobial agent. The new infecting agent is resistant to the therapy initially employed and thus survives and causes persistence of the infection (now resistant to the treatment) or a new infection at a different site. Term is also used to indicate persistence or colonization with a new organism without any evidence of resulting infection.

suppuration Formation of pus.

suprapubic bladder aspiration Obtaining urine by direct needle puncture of the full bladder through the abdominal wall above the pubic bone.

syndrome Set of symptoms occurring together (e.g., nephrotic syndrome).

synergism Combined effect of two or more agents that is greater than the sum of their individual effects.

synovial fluid Viscid fluid secreted by the synovial membrane; formed in joint cavities, bursae, and so forth.

T cells Lymphocytes involved in cellular immunity.

TB Tuberculosis.

TDM Therapeutic drug monitoring, testing serum for levels of antibiotics or other therapeutic agents.

T-M Thayer-Martin (agar plate).

tenesmus Painful, unsuccessful straining in an attempt to empty the bowels.

therapy, antimicrobial Treatment of a patient for the purpose of combating an infectious disease.

thermolabile Adversely affected by heat (as opposed to thermostable, not affected by heat).

thoracentesis Drainage of fluid from the pleural space.

thoracic Pertaining to the chest cavity.

thrush A form of *Candida* infection that typically produces white plaquelike lesions in the oral cavity.

tinea Dermatophyte infection (tinea capitis, tinea of scalp; tinea corporis, tinea of the smooth skin of the body; tinea cruris, tinea of the groin; tinea pedis, tinea of the foot).

titer Level of substance such as antibody or toxin present in material such as serum; reciprocal of the highest dilution at which the substance can still be detected.

T-lymphocytes (or T cells) Thymus-derived lymphocytes important in cell-mediated immunity.

tolerance A form of resistance to antimicrobial drugs; of uncertain clinical importance. *See* tolerant.

tolerant Characteristic of an organism that requires a great deal more antimicrobial agent to kill it than to inhibit its growth.

TORCH Toxoplasmosis, rubella, cytomegalovirus infection, and herpes infection; acronym used for illnesses or tests.

TPI *Treponema pallidum* immobilization test, a test for antibodies against the agent of syphilis that uses live treponemes.

trachoma Serious eye infection caused by *Chlamydia trachomatis;* often leads to blindness.

transduction Moving genetic material from one prokaryote to another via a bacteriophage or viral vector.

transposon Genetic material from a plasmid that can move between plasmids or from a plasmid to a chromosome; so-called "jumping genes."

transtracheal aspiration Passage of needle and plastic catheter into the trachea for obtaining lower respiratory tract secretions free of oral contamination.

transudate Similar to exudate but with low protein content.

trophozoite Feeding, motile stage of protozoa.

TSI Triple sugar iron (agar tube).

TSS Toxic shock syndrome.

TTA Transtracheal aspiration.

typing Methods of grouping organisms, primarily for epidemiologic purposes (e.g., biotyping, serotyping, bacteriophage typing, and the antibiogram).

urethritis Inflammation of urethra, the canal through which urine is discharged (e.g., gonococcal urethritis).

URI Upper respiratory tract infection.

UTI Urinary tract infection.

VD Venereal disease.

VDRL Venereal Disease Research Laboratory; classic nontreponemal serologic test for syphilis antibodies. Uses cardiolipin, lecithin, and cholesterol as cross-reactive antigen that flocculates in the presence of "reaginic" antibodies produced by patients with syphilis. Best test for cerebrospinal fluid in cases of neurosyphilis.

vector An arthropod or other agent that carries microorganisms from one infected individual to another.

vegetation In endocarditis, the aggregates of fibrin and microorganisms on the heart valves or other endocardium.

vesicle A small bulla or blister containing clear fluid.

villi Minute, elongated projections from the surface of intestinal mucosa that are important in absorption.

Vincent's angina An old term, seldom used presently, referring to anaerobic tonsillitis.

viremia Presence of viruses in the bloodstream.

virulence Degree of pathogenicity or disease-producing ability of a microorganism.

viscus (pl., viscera) Any of the organs within one of the four great body cavities (cranium, thorax, abdomen, and pelvis).

V-P Voges-Proskauer.

Weil-Felix test Whole cell agglutination assay that uses Proteus cell surface antigens to detect cross-reactive rickettsial antibodies.

Western blot Similar to Southern blot, except that antigenic proteins of an organism are separated by gel electrophoresis and transferred to membrane filters. Antiserum is allowed to react with the filters, and specific antibody bound to its homologous antigen is detected using labeled anti-antibody detectors.

Whipple's disease A disease thought to be caused by a bacterium and characterized by diarrhea, arthritis, and neurologic manifestations.

xenodiagnosis Procedure involving the feeding of laboratory-reared triatomid bugs on patients suspected of having Chagas' disease; after several weeks, the feces of the bugs are checked for intermediate stages of *Trypanosoma cruzi*.

zoogleal mass Jellylike matrix in which microorganisms may be embedded.

zoonoses Diseases of lower animals transmissible to humans (e.g., tularemia).

Zygomycetes Group of fungi with nonseptate hyphae and spores produced within a sporangium.

Index

A

Abbott Quantum II system, 757
Abortion, 275
Abscess
  autopsy and, 298
  microorganisms in, 279-281
Absidia
  classification of, 705, 706
  diabetic ketoacidosis and, 280
  mucormycosis and, 284
  working schema for, 709
  zygomycosis and, 746, 748
Acanthamoeba
  biopsy specimen for, 802
  body sites of, 777
  cerebrospinal fluid specimen for, 797
  culture techniques for, 805, 806
  keratitis and, 303
  meningitis and, 214, 216
  visual examination of, 307
Acanthamoeba culbertsoni, 779
Acanthocephala, 777
Accessioning of specimen, 18
Accreditation Manual for Hospitals, 17
Acetate agar formula, A1
Acetate buffer solution formula, A2
N-Acetyl-L-cysteine–sodium hydroxide method, 605-607
Acholeplasma laidlawii, 565
Achromobacter
  identification of, 402
  taxonomy of, 386
Achromobacter xylosoxidans
  identification of, 402
  taxonomy of, 386
Acid-fast organisms, 604-610
Acid-fast stains
  formulas for, A35-A36
  fungi and, 687
  lower respiratory tract infections and, 234-235
  method for, 70-73
  Mycobacterium and, 611-615
  parasites and, 790
Acid lability test, 674
Acid-wash, 580
Acidaminococcus
  characteristics of, 549, 550
  identification of, 554-557
Acidaminococcus fermentans, 556
Acinetobacter
  characteristics of, 392-393
  disk diffusion test and, 183
  epidemiology and pathogenesis of, 388
  hospital-acquired, 315
  identification of, 402-403
  keratitis and, 303

Acinetobacter—cont'd
  peritoneal dialysis fluid and, 292
  pneumonia and, 231
  respiratory tract and, 224
  taxonomy of, 386
  treatment of, 406
  urinary tract infection and, 255
  vancomycin and, 103
Acinetobacter baumannii, 402, 403
Acinetobacter calcoaceticus
  in blood, 198
  identification of, 402, 403
  nitrate reduction test for, 114
Acinetobacter haemolyticus, 402, 403
Acinetobacter johnsonii, 402, 403
Acinetobacter junii, 402, 403
Acinetobacter lwoffii, 402, 403
Acquired immunodeficiency syndrome
  cat-scratch disease and, 589
  Cryptococcus neoformans and, 748, 750
  gastrointestinal tract and, 245
  infections in patients with, 317-319
  laboratory-acquired infection and, 12-13
  laboratory safety and, 8
  Mycobacterium and, 604
  Mycobacterium avium and, 597
  Mycobacterium avium-intracellulare and, 600, 635-636
  Pneumocystis carinii and, 798-802
  serologic tests for, 658-659
Acremonium
  classification of, 707
  identification of, 767
  specimen of, 683
  sporulation of, 703
  working schema for, 709
Acremonium falciforme, 690
Acremonium kiliense, 690
Acremonium recifei, 690
Acridine orange stain
  formula for, A37
  use of, 74-75
Actinobacillus
  carbohydrate fermentation reaction and, 31
  characteristics of, 409, 423, 424
  identification of, 422
Actinobacillus actinomycetemcomitans
  characteristics of, 424
  classification of, 415
  differentiating from *Haemophilus aphrophilus* and, 419, 420
  head and neck and, 302
  identification of, 422
Actinobacillus capsulatus, 422
Actinobacillus equuli, 422, 424
Actinobacillus lignieresii, 422, 424
Actinobacillus suis, 422, 424